Intraoperative Monitoring

Silvia Mazzali Verst
Maria Rufina Barros
Marcos Vinicius Calfat Maldaun
Editors

Intraoperative Monitoring

Neurophysiology and Surgical Approaches

Springer

Editors
Silvia Mazzali Verst
Instituto de Ensino e Pesquisa
(Research and Teaching Institute)
Hospital Sírio Libanês
São Paulo, Brazil

Maria Rufina Barros
Neurophisiology Department
Vitoria Apart Hospital
Serra, Espírito Santo, Brazil

Marcos Vinicius Calfat Maldaun
Neurosurgery Department
Hospital Sírio Libanês
São Paulo, São Paulo, Brazil

ISBN 978-3-030-95729-2 ISBN 978-3-030-95730-8 (eBook)
https://doi.org/10.1007/978-3-030-95730-8

This Springer imprint is published by the registered company Springer Nature Switzerland AG
The registered company address is: Gewerbestrasse 11, 6330 Cham, Switzerland

From Silvia:

To my husband Heinz and our children Thomas and Lisa, for enabling me to fly high.

From Rufina:

To Jefferson (in memoriam), my beloved husband, best friend, and supporter, who rose to other dimensions during this project, and to Catarina, our daughter.

"We are what we repeatedly do; excellence, then, is not an act but a habit."

Aristotle

Foreword

This book is the culmination of all the collective shared experiences of the authors. When the idea of writing this book came about, it was because of a desire to share our knowledge and experience that we have gained over the many years in performing intraoperative neurophysiologic monitoring (IONM). Some of us, including my good friend and compadre Dr. Ricardo Ferreira and I, were self-taught and learned how to conduct IONM essentially "on the job." Of course, we had the proper clinical neurophysiology foundation to be able to build on, but we "learned" IONM because we found the field fascinating and understood that we could have a direct and profound impact on patient care during surgery. Not having been previously exposed to IONM, once I did my first case in 1993, I realized that there is another world of clinical neurophysiology where it can be applied in a very dynamic fashion and where our clinical neurophysiologist's decisions can have immediate impact on the patient's surgical outcome. We realized that we could prevent neurologic injury, including stroke, spinal cord, and peripheral nerve injury among others. We could also guide and alter surgical management. All these things were completely new and addictive to those of us who started before there were any formal training programs in IONM. An important point to make is that all the contributors are individuals who actually "do" IONM. By that I mean they know how to setup cases, place electrodes on patients, run the IONM equipment, and troubleshoot technical problems, and they are available throughout the patients' operative procedure. That's the way we train our IONM fellows at Stanford. Many of the authors, especially those in South American countries, take it a step further and run their cases from beginning to end without help from technologists.

Thus, it has been our desire and drive to teach and pass the knowledge and experience that we have gained "the hard way" to those now coming into the field. This book helps to serve that purpose. Here is our collective knowledge and experience gained over many years, from thousands of cases; from research, conferences, collaborative work, and recommendations; and from colleagues' advice. Our intent is to present IONM in a comprehensive but concise and practical manner so that all practitioners in the field will find it useful and can take the information and apply it to their patients.

The inspiration and impetus for creating this book come from many; however, the heart and driving forces behind this come from Rufina Barros and Silvia Verst. Without them, this collective work, which took 2 years to complete, would not have materialized. Recruiting authors, coaxing them to write their chapters, and trying to adhere to a deadline, all of which occurred while they still had to fulfill their IONM clinical duties in the middle of a global pandemic, were truely colossal efforts. I hope that the contents of this book become a practical reference in the comprehensive education of IONM and can form a foundation for those starting in the field.

My ultimate desire is that all who read this book get a chance to monitor a case covered in each chapter and that for every novel case you monitor, you contact the author of the chapter that it corresponds.

Stanford, CA, USA Jaime R. López
August 20, 2021

Preface

The completion of this project has been quite a challenge since it was undertaken during a pandemic that affected most of the authors. Many lost their loved ones and suffered under personal and familiar illnesses. We cannot sufficiently express our thankfulness to those who managed to complete their chapters.

This book started with the desire to share the experience and expertise of neurophysiologists who deal with many difficulties in the operating room during their daily practice and yet manage to hold on to high standards of care. IOM quality relies in technical details that must not be overlooked. As Rufina says, "the frog jumps out due to necessity." The frog in this case is the neurophysiologist overcoming economic and scientific barriers present in underdeveloped countries. It includes travelling abroad to refine technical knowledge and buying intraoperative systems at their own expense. It goes further by not having the possibility of using expensive and specially designed electrodes. Despite that, the neurophysiologist can perform the "proper jump."

Aage Moller told Rufina in Croatia in 2009 that "neurosurgeons started intraoperative neurophysiology monitoring, but it is up to neurophysiologists to bring it a step forward." It has become true in many ways. Innovations are occurring quickly, leading to refinements in many techniques, like in motor-evoked potentials, awake craniotomies, and peripheral nerves approach, to name a few. Innovations start anywhere in the world, and we could successfully add some to the book.

Many of the authors are global pioneers in IOM since they debuted at a time when not even motor-evoked potentials were available in the operating room. Since then, accumulated development has resulted in renowned books on this subject. It was challenging to develop a project that equalized with those. This book does not aim to exhaust the subject of IOM but to contribute to the field.

We have been engaged in educational projects and activities over the years. We simply love teaching because it enables us to translate complex subjects into easily understandable content. Besides that, we are directly engaged in fellowship programs for neurosurgeons in neuro-oncology (Maldaun) and neurophysiologists in intraoperative monitoring (Verst), aiming to fill a gap and share our experience in the field. Training is a difficult task, but it is rewarding if you achieve to inspire others to strive for high quality in healthcare.

We were able to manage this project because of our long trajectory in the search for excellence. It was a life's choice since it held us apart from familiar and social living. Thus, it is paramount to thank the most important people:

- To our families whose selflessness has allowed us to spend a large part of our lives in the pursuit of knowledge. It would not have been possible without their love, understanding, and partnership.
- To our patients who trusted their lives in our hands.
- To the surgeons who see us as a fundamental member of the teamwork.
- To our medical associates, technicians, and fellows, whose daily conviviality gives us support, responsibilities, and focus.

We would like to individually name everyone who supported our project, but that is not feasible. Yet, there are some that we cannot miss because of their great help at critical moments.

Our special thanks to Ricardo Ferreira who encouraged and helped many authors during their writing and took over many chapters on his own, as well as to

- Partha Thirumalla, who believed and jumped into this project since the very beginning
- Kathleen Seidel, whose care and kindness was a refreshment along the way
- Linda Wilson-Pauwells, João Tiago Alves, and Luana Bulgarelli, whose incredible illustrations enrich many chapters
- The Springer staff, who helped us throughout the editorial process

São Paulo, SP, Brazil — Silvia Mazzali Verst
Serra, ES, Brazil — Maria Rufina Barros
São Paulo, SP, Brazil — Marcos Vinicius Calfat Maldaun

Contents

Part I Overview

1 **History of Intraoperative Neurophysiological Monitoring in Brazil: Reports from the Pioneers and a Glance in Latin America** ... 3
Andreya Fonseca Cardoso Cavalcanti and Francisco Soto

2 **Intraoperative Neurophysiological Monitoring in Brazil: Regulatory Aspects, Training, and Evidence Level** ... 39
Carlo Domênico Marrone and Andréa Broisler Sucena Caivano

3 **Muscle Motor Point Atlas and Needling Pitfalls** ... 57
Bruno Nogueira da Silva and Tae Mo Chung

4 **Safety and Troubleshooting** ... 89
Jose Alberto Nunes Sobrinho, Monica Nascimento de Melo, and Silvia Mazzali Verst

5 **Central Nervous System Anesthesia: Asleep Approach** ... 111
Nelson Mizumoto

Part II Neurophysiological Modalities Applied to IOM

6 **Brainstem Auditory Evoked Potentials** ... 129
Jamison Beiriger, Varun Shandal, Josh Sunderlin, and Parthasarathy D. Thirumala

7 **Evoked Potential – Visual Pathways Approach beyond Visual Evoked Potentials** ... 143
Monica Nascimento de Melo and Silvia Mazzali Verst

8 **Somatosensory Evoked Potentials** ... 165
Jamison Beiriger, Varun Shandal, Josh Sunderlin, and Parthasarathy D. Thirumala

9 **Motor Evoked Potential** 181
Carla Ferreira and Silvia Mazzali Verst

10 **Intraoperative Monitoring: Electroencephalogram** 203
Maria Lucia Furtado de Mendonça and Francisco José Carchedi Luccas

11 **Electromyography** 225
Francisco Tellechea Rotta, Carlo Domênico Marrone, and Ana Maria Hoppe

12 **Brainstem Reflexes** 237
Isabel Fernández-Conejero and Sedat Ulkatan

Part III Brain Functions: Eloquent Areas

13 **The Brain Surface** 253
Eduardo Carvalhal Ribas and Guilherme Carvalhal Ribas

14 **Brain Functions: Eloquent Areas – Motor and Somatosensory** 269
Kathleen Seidel and Marcos Vinicius Calfat Maldaun

15 **Anesthesia: Awake Approach** 287
Vinicius Gonçalves Vieira

16 **Anatomy: Language Network and DTI** 301
João Tiago Alves-Belo

17 **Awake Surgery: Performing an Awake Craniotomy** 327
Silvia Mazzali Verst, Juliana Ohy, Cleiton Formentin, and Marcos Vinicius Calfat Maldaun

18 **Language and Cognitive Tests: A Target-Guided Protocol** 357
Silvia Mazzali Verst, Tatiana Vilasboas Alves, and Leonardo Dornas de Oliveira

Part IV Brainstem and Cranial Nerve Function

19 **Cranial Nerve Monitoring III to XII** 387
Silvia Mazzali Verst, Maria Rufina Barros, and Rayssa Addiny Modenesi Lozano

20 **Fourth Ventricle's Floor Mapping** 421
Kathleen Seidel and Andreas Raabe

21 **Microvascular Decompression** 431
Jamison Beiriger, Varun Shandal, Josh Sunderlin, and Parthasarathy D. Thirumala

Part V Spine and Spinal Cord Surgery

22 Spinal Deformity Surgery ... 459
Ricardo José Rodriguez Ferreira, Emília Caram Bordini, André Cleriston J. dos Santos, Roberto Waldesmand Farias Pontes, Paulo Tadeu Maia Cavali, and Tiago Bertacini Gonzaga

23 Lumbar Interbody Fusion Surgeries: LIFS ... 495
Ricardo José Rodriguez Ferreira, Marcus Vinícius Magno Gonçalves, Emília Caram Bordini, and Alexandre Fogaça Cristante

24 Cervical Spinal Surgery ... 513
Ricardo José Rodriguez Ferreira, Patrícia Toscano, Emília Caram Bordini, and Arthur Werner Poetscher

25 Tethered Cord Syndrome ... 539
Vanise Campos Gomes Amaral, Sérgio Cavalheiro, Ricardo José Rodriguez Ferreira, and Maria Lucia Furtado de Mendonça

26 Selective Dorsal Rhizotomy and Intraoperative Neurophysiological Monitoring: Theory to Practice ... 565
Carlo Domênico Marrone, André Bedin, Ana Maria Hoppe, Cristiane Soveral D'Aviz, and Jorge Wladimir Junqueira Bizzi

27 Intramedullary Spinal Cord Tumors ... 587
Andreya Fonseca Cardoso Cavalcanti, Karina Maria Alécio de Oliveira, Monica Nascimento de Melo, and Silvia Mazzali Verst

Part VI Vascular Surgery

28 Intraoperative Neurophysiologic Monitoring of Cerebrovascular Disorders ... 611
Jaime R. López and Felix W. Chang

29 Intraoperative Neurophysiologic Monitoring for Thoracic and Thoracoabdominal Aortic Procedures ... 661
Felix W. Chang and Jaime R. López

Part VII Pheripheral Nerve Surgery

30 Peripheral Nerve: Neurophysiology as a Tool to Optimize Topographic Accuracy and Surgical Planning ... 711
Maria Rufina Barros

Part VIII Head and Neck Surgery

31 Monitoring in Facial, Neck, and Ear Surgeries 745
Karina Maria Alécio de Oliveira, Estela Lladó-Carbó, Ricardo José Rodriguez Ferreira, Marcus Vinícius Magno Gonçalves, and Marina Azzi Quintanilha

Part IX Epilepsy Surgery

32 Intraoperative Monitoring in Epilepsy Surgery 781
Vera Cristina Terra, Marcelo Volpon, and Hélio Rubens Machado

Part X Movement Disorders Surgery

33 Neurophysiological Guidance for Movement Disorder Surgery 817
Denise Spinola Pinheiro and Erich Fonoff

Part XI Special Topics

34 IOM in Pelvic Floor: Gynecological and Urological Surgeries 839
Ricardo José Rodriguez Ferreira, Emília Caram Bordini, Guillermo Martín-Palomeque, Lidia Cabañes-Martinez, and Nucelio Luiz De Barros Moreira Lemos

Index 865

Contributors

Tatiana Vilasboas Alves Neurosurgeon at São Camilo Hospital, Unit Pompéia, São Paulo, Brazil

João Tiago Alves-Belo Neurosurgery Department, Hospital Felício Rocho, Belo Horizonte, MG, Brazil

Vanise Campos Gomes Amaral Universidade do Estado do Amazonas/Escola Superior de Ciências da Saúde-UEA/ESA, Manaus, AM, Brazil

Maria Rufina Barros Department of Intraoperative Monitoring, Neurological Institute of Espirito Santo, Vitória, ES, Brazil

Department of Neurophysiology, Vitoria Apart Hospital (VAH), Vitória, ES, Brazil

André Bedin Brazilian Society of Pediatric Surgery, Porto Alegre, RS, Brazil

Jamison Beiriger School of Medicine, Drexel University, Philadelphia, PA, USA

Jorge Wladimir Junqueira Bizzi Pediatric Neurosurgery Department, Clinical Hospital of the Medical School of the University of Rio Grande do Sul, Porto Alegre, RS, Brazil

Emília Caram Bordini AACD - Disabled Child Care Association, São Paulo, SP, Brazil

Dr Ricardo Ferreira Clinic, São Paulo, SP, Brazil

Spine Surgery Department at Orthopedics and Trauma Institute of Clinical Hospital of the University of São Paulo Medical School, São Paulo, SP, Brazil

Lidia Cabañes-Martinez Clinical Neurophysiology, Hospital Ramón y Cajal, Madrid, Spain

Andréa Broisler Sucena Caivano Biomedical Technologist, Brain Spine Neurofisiologia, São Paulo, São Paulo, SP, Brazil

Andreya Fonseca Cardoso Cavalcanti Department of Neurology and Neurophysiology, Neurocol Neurofisiologia Avançada, São Paulo, SP, Brazil

Sérgio Cavalheiro Department of Neurosurgery, Universidade Federal de São Paulo, São Paulo, SP, Brazil

Paulo Tadeu Maia Cavali Scoliosis Group, AACD - Disabled Child Care, Association, São Paulo, SP, Brazil

Scoliosis Department at Sirio Libanês Hospital, São Paulo, SP, Brazil

Felix W. Chang Department of Neurology and Neurological Sciences, Stanford University, Stanford, CA, USA

Tae Mo Chung Clinical Neurophysiology Coordinator, Physical Medicine and Rehabilitation Department at the Clinical Hospital of University of São Paulo Medical School, São Paulo, SP, Brazil

Alexandre Fogaça Cristante Spine Surgery Department at Orthopedics and Trauma Institute of Clinical Hospital of the University of São Paulo Medical School, São Paulo, SP, Brazil

Cristiane Soveral D'Aviz Department of Neurophysiology – Santa Casa de Misericórdia de Porto Alegre/RS, Porto Alegre, RS, Brazil

Isabel Fernández-Conejero University Hospital of Bellvitge, Barcelona, Spain

Ricardo José Rodriguez Ferreira AACD - Disabled Child Care Association, São Paulo, SP, Brazil

Dr Ricardo Ferreira Clinic, São Paulo, SP, Brazil

Spine Surgery Department at Orthopedics and Trauma Institute of Clinical Hospital of the University of São Paulo Medical School, São Paulo, SP, Brazil

Carla Ferreira Clinical Hospital of the Federal University of Minas Gerais, Belo Horizonte, MG, Brazil

Erich Fonoff Department of Neurology, University of São Paulo, São Paulo, SP, Brazil

Cleiton Formentin Researcher at Instituto de Ensino e Pesquisa (Teaching and Research Institute) of Hospital Sirio Libanês, São Paulo, SP, Brazil

Marcus Vinícius Magno Gonçalves Neurologist and Neurophysiologist, Neurology at the University of the Region of Joinville (UNIVILLE), Joinville, Brazil

Tiago Bertacini Gonzaga Anesthesiology Department, AACD - Child Care Association, São Paulo, SP, Brazil

Ana Maria Hoppe Department of Neurophysiology, Santa Casa de Misericórdia de Porto Alegre, Porto Alegre, RS, Brazil

Nucelio Luiz De Barros Moreira Lemos Gynecology Department, University of Toronto, Toronto, ON, Canada

Estela Lladó-Carbó Clinical Neurophysiology Department, Neurotoc - Intraoperative Neuromonitoring company- (Spain), HM Catalunya Hospital, Barcelona, Spain

Jaime R. López Department of Neurology and Neurological Sciences, Stanford University, Stanford, CA, USA

Department of Neurosurgery (Courtesy), Stanford University, Stanford, CA, USA

Rayssa Addiny Modenesi Lozano Clinical Neurophysiologist at Brain Spine Neurofisiologia, São Paulo, Brazil

Francisco José Carchedi Luccas Clinical Neurophysiology, Hospital São Luiz – Morumbi – Rede D'Or, São Paulo, SP, Brazil

Hélio Rubens Machado Center for Epilepsy Surgery, Department of Surgery and Anatomy, Ribeirao Preto Medical School, University of Sao Paulo, Ribeirao Preto, Sao Paulo, Brazil

Marcos Vinicius Calfat Maldaun Instituto de Ensino e Pesquisa (Teaching and Research Institute) of Hospital Sirio Libanês, São Paulo, SP, Brazil

Neurosurgery Department, Hospital Sirio Libanês, São Paulo, São Paulo, Brazil

Carlo Domênico Marrone Past President of the Brazilian Clinical Neurophysiology Society, Porto Alegre, RS, Brazil

Intraoperative Neurophysiological Monitoring, Department Coordinator of Hospital da Criança Santo Antônio, Porto Alegre, RS, Brazil

Universidade Federal de Ciências da Saúde de Porto Alegre - UFCSPA, Porto Alegre, RS, Brazil

Clínica Marrone, Clinical Neurophysiology, Porto Alegre, RS, Brazil

Guillermo Martín-Palomeque Clinical Neurophysiology, Hospital Ramón y Cajal, Madrid, Spain

Silvia Mazzali Verst Instituto de Ensino e Pesquisa (Research and Educational Institute) of Sírio Libanês Hospital, São Paulo, Brazil

Brain Spine Neurofisiologia, Jundiaí, SP, Brazil

Monica Nascimento de Melo Department of Neurophysiology, Integrated Neuroscience Institute, Goiânia, GO, Brazil

Maria Lucia Furtado de Mendonça Clinical Neurology and Neurophysiology, Intraoperative and Critical Care Clinical Neurophysiology, Neuro Logical Clinica Médica, Rio de Janeiro, RJ, Brazil

Nelson Mizumoto Anesthesiology Coordinator at the Neurosurgery Department, Clinical Hospital of University of Sao Paulo Medical School, Sao Paulo, Brazil

Juliana Ohy Researcher at Instituto de Ensino e Pesquisa (Teaching and Research Institute) of Hospital Sirio Libanês, São Paulo, SP, Brazil

Leonardo Dornas de Oliveira Hospital das Clínicas da Universidade Federal de Minas Gerais, Belo Horizonte, MG, Brazil

Karina Maria Alécio de Oliveira Department of Neurology and Neurophysiology, Clinica Stela de Monitoramento Clínico e Cirúrgico em Neurologia, Brasília, DF, Brazil

Denise Spinola Pinheiro Department of Neurology, Universidade Federal de São Paulo, São Paulo, SP, Brazil

Arthur Werner Poetscher Neurosurgery Department at Hospital Israelita Albert Einstein, São Paulo, SP, Brazil

Roberto Waldesmand Farias Pontes Neurology and Neurophysiology Department, Ribeirão Preto Medical School of the, University of São Paulo, Ribeirão Preto, SP, Brazil

Marina Azzi Quintanilha Cervical and Head Surgery Department, CICAP, Centro Clínico Sudoeste, Brasília, DF, Brazil

Andreas Raabe Department of Neurosurgery, Inselspital, Bern University Hospital, University of Bern, Bern, Switzerland

Eduardo Carvalhal Ribas Hospital Israelita Albert Einstein, São Paulo, SP, Brazil

University of São Paulo Medical School, São Paulo, SP, Brazil

Guilherme Carvalhal Ribas Hospital Israelita Albert Einstein, São Paulo, SP, Brazil

University of São Paulo Medical School, São Paulo, SP, Brazil

Francisco Tellechea Rotta Intercoastal Medical Group, Sarasota, FL, USA

André Cleriston J. dos Santos Neurology and Neurophysiology Department, Ribeirão Preto Medical School of the, University of São Paulo, Ribeirão Preto, SP, Brazil

Kathleen Seidel Department of Neurosurgery, Inselspital, Bern University Hospital, University of Bern, Bern, Switzerland

Varun Shandal Department of Neurological Surgery, Center for Clinical Neurophysiology, University of Pittsburgh, Pittsburgh, PA, USA

Bruno Nogueira da Silva Clinical Neurophysiologist by Brain Spine Neurofisiologia, Jundiai, SP, Brazil

Jose Alberto Nunes Sobrinho Department of Neurophysiology, Stela Clinic, Brasilia, Brazil

Francisco Soto Department of Neurology, Las Condes Clinic, Santiago, Chile

Josh Sunderlin Procirca, Clinical Neurophysiology, University of Pittsburgh Medical Center, Pittsburgh, PA, USA

Vera Cristina Terra Centro de atendimento Integral das Epilepsias, Nossa Senhora das Graças Hospital, Rua Alcides Munhoz, Curitiba – PR, Brazil

Parthasarathy D. Thirumala Department of Neurological Surgery, Center for Clinical Neurophysiology, University of Pittsburgh, Pittsburgh, PA, USA

Department of Neurology, University of Pittsburgh, Pittsburgh, PA, USA

Department of Neurological Surgery and Neurology, University of Pittsburgh, Pittsburgh, PA, USA

Patrícia Toscano Neurology Department, Ribeirão Preto Medical School of the University of São Paulo, Ribeirão Preto, SP, Brazil

Sedat Ulkatan Mount Sinai West Hospital, New York, NY, USA

Vinicius Gonçalves Vieira Anesthesiology Department, Sírio Libanês Hospital, São Paulo, SP, Brazil

Marcelo Volpon Center for Epilepsy Surgery & Department of Surgery and Anatomy, Ribeirão Preto Medical School of the University of São Paulo, Ribeirão Preto, SP, Brazil

Part I
Overview

Chapter 1
History of Intraoperative Neurophysiological Monitoring in Brazil: Reports from the Pioneers and a Glance in Latin America

Andreya Fonseca Cardoso Cavalcanti and Francisco Soto

Introduction

Writing history is complex and has inaccuracies and biases as it can depend on the author's point of view. Therefore, it is understandable that there are different versions of the same period of history. However, there is only one truth and it is essential to recognize that it is often not possible to fully know it.

Over the past 40 years, intraoperative neurophysiological monitoring (IOM) has grown from an investigational procedure into a widely used method, aiming to protect patients from neurologic injury during surgery. However, it was only more recently, in the last 20 years, with the introduction and popularization of the use of motor evoked potential (MEP) in the operating room (OR), that the evaluation of motor pathways boosted the spread of IOM around the world.

Companies invested in equipment and production of supplies to this emerging medical field. IOM clinical papers popped up and departments were structured in Universities Medical Centers.

Despite or due to the great growth of knowledge in IOM, the number of properly trained and qualified professionals is still far below the world demand. And Brazil is no exception.

Latin America had a creative, early, and robust development in this area of clinical neurophysiology, which was recognized worldwide by different international societies that approached the continent to participate and foster this development.

A. F. C. Cavalcanti (✉)
Department of Neurology and Neurophysiology, Neurocol Neurofisiologia Avançada,
São Paulo, SP, Brazil
e-mail: andreya@neurocol.com.br

F. Soto
Department of Neurology, Las Condes Clinic, Santiago, Chile

S. M. Verst et al. (eds.), *Intraoperative Monitoring*,
https://doi.org/10.1007/978-3-030-95730-8_1

This achievement was based on the hard and consistent work of a few Latin American neurophysiologists, initially scarce, but many more were added over time.

To systematize the global, Latin American, and Brazilian context of the IOM, the chapter is subdivided into three large sections:

1. Timeline of IOM Evolution in the World
2. Overview of IOM History in Latin America
   - 2.1 Origins of IOM in Latin America
   - 2.2 Influence of International Mentors and Societies
   - 2.3 Special Interest Group in IOM and Latin American IOM Events
   - 2.4 Congress and Course of the International Society of Intraoperative Neurophysiology (ISIN) Rio 2015
3. History of IOM in Brazil
   - 3.1 Overview of the Late 1980s and Early 1990s
   - 3.2 Experience and Reports of the Brazilian Pioneers
   - 3.3 Academic Training in IOM in Brazil
   - 3.4 Evolution of IOM Equipment and Its Arrival in Brazil
   - 3.5 Brazilian Society of Clinical Neurophysiology (SBNC)
     - 3.5.1 IOM Events by SBNC
     - 3.5.2 Development of IOM Department at SBNC
   - 3.6 Current Status of IOM in Brazil and Latin America

Timeline of IOM Evolution in the World

- 1898: Fedor Krause stimulated the facial nerve to observe its functioning [1].
- 1937: Penfield used direct cortical stimulation to define the homunculus of human motor and sensory cortex [2].
- 1949: Electrocorticography (ECoG) was used to identify regions of epileptic discharges [3, 4].
- 1959: Penfield & Robert: First language mapping during awake craniotomy [5].
- Late 1960s and early 1970s: Electroencephalogram (EEG) was carried out in carotid endarterectomy [6–8].
- Early 1970s: Ojeman proposed a methodology for language mapping during awake craniotomy [9]. Directly recorded spinal potentials from the epidural space after direct spinal stimulation [10–13].
- 1974: Middle- and long-latency somatosensory evoked cortical potentials (SEP) started to be applied in the OR [14].
- 1977: Nash in the USA and Tamaki in Japan started monitoring spinal deformities in young children [15, 16].
- Late 1970s and early 1980s: Technical improvements on SEP, which became a widely adopted method of spinal cord monitoring [17].

- Early 1980s: IOM began to be mentioned in academic meetings [18].
- 1981: Commercial IOM equipment became available [18].
- 1985: Use of auditory evoked potentials and electroneuromyography during surgery around cranial nerves [19, 20].
- Mid-1980s: IOM-specific meetings began to be offered [18].
- 1986: The first IOM textbook (Nuwer) was published [18].
- 1988: The second IOM textbook (Moller) was released [18].
- Late 1980s: IOM became an established technique widely used.
- 1991: Hicks and Burke described the use of transcranial electrical stimulation with epidural recording as a corticospinal evaluation technique for use under anesthesia [21, 22].
- 1993: Taniguchi described the technique of transcranial electrical stimulation with muscle registration for use under anesthesia: Popularization of MEP in the OR [23].
- 1998: Deletis, Kothbauer, and Epstein implemented transcranial electrical single pulse stimulation with D wave spinal cord recording with multipulse transcranial stimulation with myogenic recording in intramedullary spinal cord tumors [24].
- 2002: Food and Drug Administration (FDA) approval of the first commercially available transcranial electrical stimulator (Digitimer D185) [25].

Overview of IOM History in Latin America

Origins of IOM in Latin America

In 1994, the Head of the Department of Neurosurgery at the Las Condes Clinic (Santiago, Chile), the prestigious neurosurgeon Professor Luciano Basauri, MD, contacted the neurologist Francisco Soto, MD, to give him a mission: to develop intraoperative neurophysiological monitoring in complex surgeries of the Central and Peripheral Nervous System.

There was nothing similar in Chile. Basauri recommended Soto to a personal friend at New York University (NYU), Fred Epstein, MD (†). Epstein was a world famous and charismatic neurosurgeon. His skill was to operate inoperable Central Nervous System tumors, especially intramedullary tumors.

In 1996, the NYU Department of Neurosurgery organized a course, not knowing that the first steps were being taken to found intraoperative monitoring in Latin America. In this course, the enthusiastic Professor Epstein stated bluntly: "*Intraoperative neurophysiological monitoring constitutes the greatest revolution in neurosurgery at the end of the 20th century*". The secret that Epstein kept for the resection of inoperable tumors with the least possible neurological deficit was the intraoperative neurophysiology.

Epstein generously shared that he used it in all his surgeries. It was implemented by Vedran Deletis, MD, PhD, a brilliant neurophysiologist, inquisitor, rigorous, and passionate about developing neurophysiological techniques for use in the intraoperative environment and obsessed with the neurophysiology of the motor system.

Together with Professor Vahe Amassian, MD, Deletis taught Soto and others a new world by monitoring the motor system, using transcranial electrical motor evoked potentials.

In Latin America in those early years, at the beginning of the 1990s, Soto and other pioneering Latin American neurophysiologists, including Brazilians, implemented intraoperative monitoring with somatosensory potentials and continuous and stimulated electromyography in their first cases of tethered cord and scoliosis. In some cases, they added auditory evoked potentials, as in cerebellopontine angle tumors.

The need for monitoring the motor pathway has become evident since cases of motor neurological deficits began to be described in which somatosensory potentials remained unaltered.

With the lessons learned at NYU, Soto performed for the first time in Chile, in 1999, the transcranial motor electrical stimulation, with the train stimulation technique, with equipment imported directly from Great Britain (Digitimer®).

Soto focused on implementing these techniques on his patients in Santiago. Without knowing each other, in different countries, other pioneering neurophysiologists in Latin America were following the same path, such as the Brazilians Ricardo Ferreira, Silvia Verst, and Adauri Camargo, from São Paulo, Martín Segura, from Buenos Aires, and many others who will still be mentioned in this chapter.

Those were times when neurosurgeons and orthopedic surgeons did not know about monitoring or had only heard about it in international symposia. Therefore, it was necessary to make them aware of its benefits for patients' safety and present it again and again in the congresses of these specialties.

Influence of International Societies and Mentors

Some international mentors and societies played a crucial role in the development of IOM in Latin America.

The mentors who have always been in Latin America giving lectures at courses and conferences are professors Marc Nuwer (University of California), MD, PhD, Jaime López (Stanford University), MD, PhD, and Aatif Husain (Duke University), MD, PhD.

All of them have contributed a lot to the dissemination of knowledge in IOM in Latin America, including receiving many Latin American neurophysiologists for IOM training in their institutions.

The International Federation of Clinical Neurophysiology (IFCN) and its Latin American Chapter (LAC) have supported every one of the renowned Latin American Intraoperative Neurophysiology Symposia.

IFCN's support has been consistent, not only in allocating funds but and especially in academic support. History must always acknowledge these symposia that have motivated many physicians in Latin America to dedicate themselves to this specialty.

The other scientific society that has been pivotal is the International Society of Intraoperative Neurophysiology (ISIN). It was founded in 2006 by Vedran Deletis and Beatrice Cioni in Rome, and since then has contributed immensely with valuable guidelines in this discipline.

However, it was only in 2009 that an ISIN speaker, Francesco Sala, MD, PhD, a brilliant neurosurgeon from Verona, visited Latin America for the first time, at an event in Porto Alegre, Brazil. Sala motivated many people with one of the first and most robust articles on the evidence that monitoring improves and impacts surgical outcomes: In a historical case-control study, with 50 cases without the use of monitoring and 50 cases with its use, operated by the same team, in strictly matched and comparable patients. Sala has received several neurophysiologists from Latin America at his center and has visited the continent many times after 2009: Chile, Argentina, Brazil (again), and Mexico. ISIN, with its brightest members, began to generously nurture Latin American neurophysiologists with the participation of its members on different occasions and countries. A special section will be devoted later to how ISIN organized one of its Biannual congresses for the first time in Latin America, ISIN Rio 2015.

Special Interest Group (SIG) and IOM Events in Latin America

The Special Interest Group (SIG) on IOM of the Latin American Chapter (LAC) of the IFCN (SIG-IOM-LAC-IFCN) was founded in 2009 by Ricardo Ferreira, Martin Segura, Francisco Soto, Francisco Luccas, and Daniel Cibils.

Throughout its existence, the SIG has been fruitful and has organized the biannual Latin American symposia: in Montevideo organized by Daniel Cibils (Fig. 1.1), Porto Alegre organized by Ricardo Ferreira and Carlo Domenico Marrone, Viña del Mar organized by Francisco Soto, Buenos Aires organized by Martín Segura, Guadalajara organized by Armando Tello, and Bogotá organized by Jorge Gutierrez.

The role of the members of the IOM SIG has been fundamental in organizing and promoting high-level scientific events in Latin America.

The SIG and its five founding members have been modified (Fig. 1.2) after the resignation of Francisco Jose Luccas and then Daniel Cibils, incorporating the Chairman of the Guadalajara Symposium, the prominent Armando Tello, representative of Latin America at the IFCN, and then the Chairman of the Symposium from Bogotá, Jorge Gutierrez, past President of the IFCN LAC and current member of the IFCN Board of Directors.

In 2015, Ferreira created the Latin American Institute of Intraoperative Neurophysiology – ILANI. It is restricted to his ex-fellows and invited friends from Latin America, USA, and Europe. It aims to promote lectures to the 68 members.

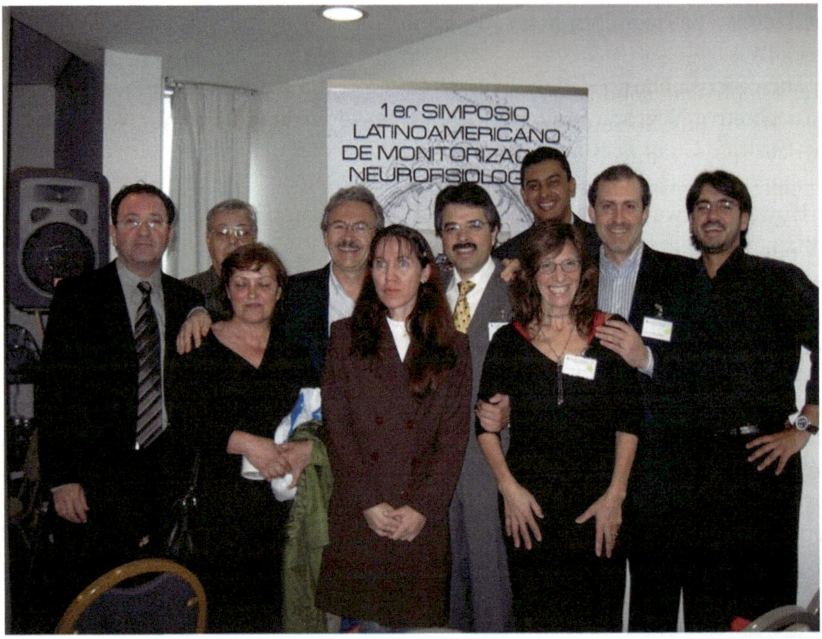

Fig. 1.1 First Latin American Symposium on Intraoperative Neurophysiology (Montevideo, 2007). (Courtesy of Soto's personal file)

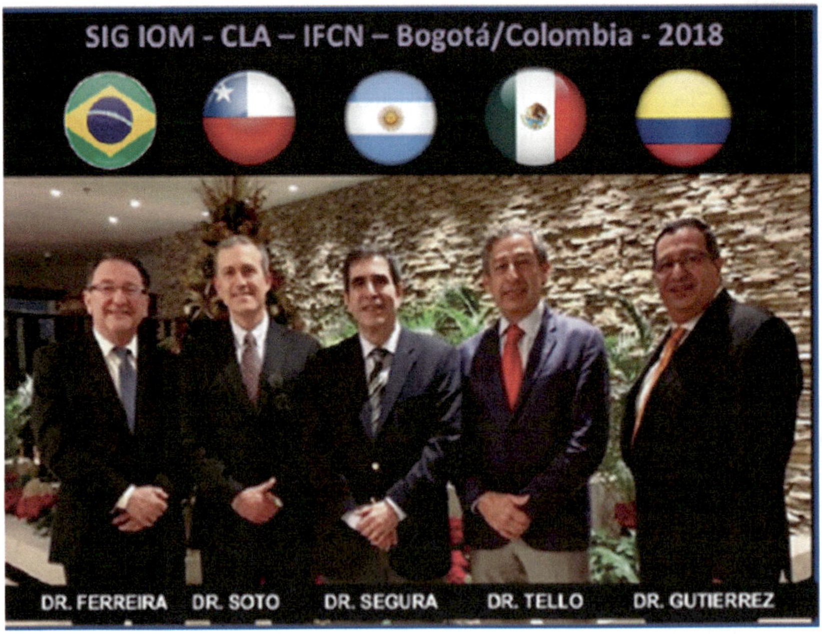

Fig. 1.2 Special Interest Group on Intraoperative Neurophysiology of the Latin American Chapter of the IFCN. (Courtesy of Soto's personal file)

ISIN Rio 2015

After establishing solid academic relationships with the ISIN and becoming active members of this Society, two Latin Americans, Ricardo Ferreira and Francisco Soto, were encouraged to assume a more significant challenge, organize the Biannual Congress and annual Educational Course in Rio de Janeiro.

They had to compete against other venues in the world that presented attractive and powerful proposals. However, the ISIN Board elected them in Cape Town, South Africa. In this Congress in the year 2013, Ferreira proudly presented the next venue of the 5th Congress of the History of the ISIN without knowing that it would become one of the best and most vibrant events in History in the field of Intraoperative Neurophysiology.

It was a titanic effort, which had to be financed from scratch, in one of the most beautiful and expensive cities globally. Latin America's reaction was of joy and jubilation to have this opportunity to attend an event of this level in the continent, which was reflected in 400 attendees.

Finally, it was a beautiful event lasting one whole week, in a beautiful hotel on Copacabana beach, where joy was breathed and an academic and scientific level that is still remembered worldwide.

One of the ISIN Congress lights was born in a breakfast in Istanbul 2014, in one of the Educational Courses of the ISIN. Ferreira, Soto, and the remembered Scientific Committee Chairman of the ISIN at that time, Karl Kothbauer (†), raised the idea of holding a Session on the warning criteria for motor evoked potentials.

This idea became a reality at ISIN Rio 2015, by five brilliant speakers: Martín Segura, brilliant neurologist and neurophysiologist from Hospital Garrahan in Buenos Aires, David Mac Donald, Editor in Chief of the IOM Section of Clinical Neurophysiology, Karl Kothbauer, Austrian-born professor at Lucerne in Switzerland, a world-renowned neurosurgeon and direct disciple of Fred Epstein, Louis Journee, leading Dutch neurologist from the beautiful city of the University of Groningen, one of the world authorities on motor evoked potentials and that with Langeloo published the alarm criterion of a decrease of 80% in motor potentials during scoliosis surgery, and Blair Calancie, the author of the threshold criterion in motor potentials.

It was a vibrant session, full of scientific discussion that reflected an article in the Journal of Clinical Neurophysiology on this topic; with all the participants at this ISIN Rio round table, this article remains as the Gold Standard.

The list of invited professors to ISIN Rio was incredible. It included 34 professors (Fig. 1.3).

It was a great effort, but without a doubt, it was rewarded for the mark it left on Latin America.

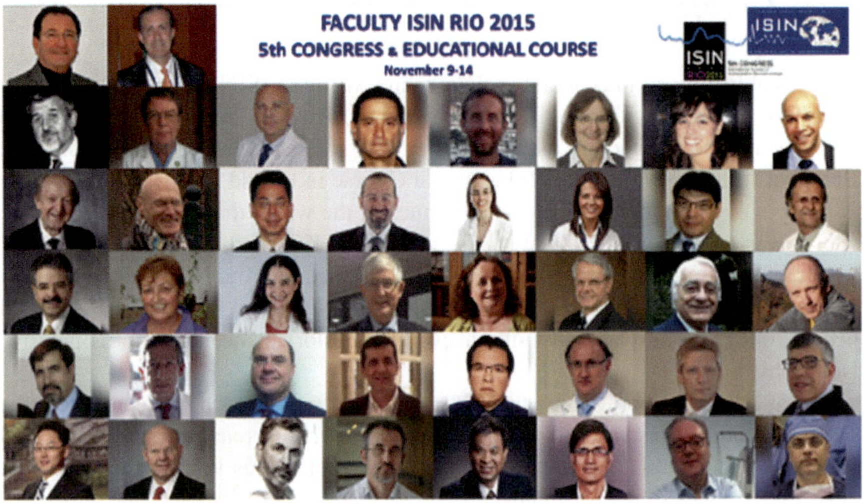

Fig. 1.3 Faculty ISIN Rio 2015. (Courtesy of Soto's personal file)

History of IOM in Brazil

An Overview of Late 1980s and Early 1990s

In the late 1980s and early 1990s, the study and use of evoked potentials (EP) emerged. Brazilian neurophysiologists interested in the area traveled annually to the United States to participate in courses of the American Society of Clinical Evoked Potentials (ASCEP). In these events, the lectures by Donald York, Aage Moller, and Neil Spielholz on the application of EP in the intraoperative environment aroused the interest of Brazilians.

This period coincides with the emergence of magnetic resonance imaging (MRI), a milestone in the advancement of the diagnosis of demyelinating neurological diseases, such as multiple sclerosis (MS). MS represented one of the main outpatient indications for the use of EP. MRI eventually replaced the EP as the first exam for MS diagnosis. Hence, IOM came to renew the use and re-signify the importance of the EP in a new context: the OR.

However, it is worth mentioning that the earliest experiences of IOM in Brazil date back to the 1970s. Electrocorticography (ECoG) and direct cortical stimulation (DCS) in epilepsy surgeries have been carried out by professor Raul Marino Junior (Fig. 1.4), MD, PhD, since 1971, at the Institute of Psychiatry (IPQ) of the University of São Paulo (USP) [26]. He learned the methodology with professors Theodore Rasmussen and Wilder Penfield, during his Fellowship in Functional Neurosurgery at Montreal Neurological Institute (MNI), Canada [27].

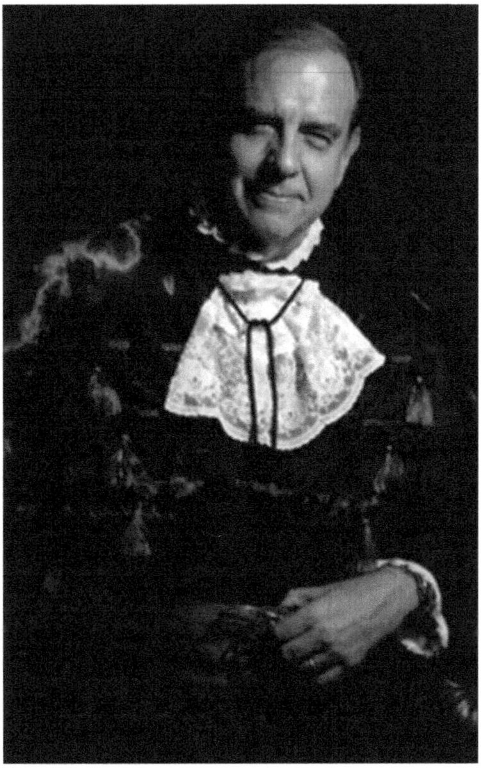

Fig. 1.4 Professor Raul Marino Junior, the first Brazilian neurosurgeon to perform awake craniotomies with motor and language mapping. (*Source*: Marino Jr., Raul. *Um cirurgião sob o olhar de Deus: uma introdução às ciências do cérebro, da mente e do espírito.* Barueri: Manole, 2020, with permission)

Marino was the first Brazilian neurosurgeon to perform awake craniotomies (Fig. 1.5) with motor and language mapping, initially on his own and later with the collaboration of physiatrist and neurophysiologist Gary Gronich (Fig. 1.6).

Meanwhile, the neurologist and neurophysiologist Francisco José Carchedi Luccas (Fig. 1.7) started in 1986 to perform EP in OR for skull base surgeries at Hospital Israelita Albert Einstein (HIAE), in Sao Paulo. He showed some of his cases at the symposia by the Company Berger (1990–1995).

From the mid-1990s came a more favorable moment for the expansion of IOM in Brazil: the country's economic stability, better access to technology, and a greater number of specialists in Neurophysiology besides Epilepsy and EEG. In addition, the use of Neurophysiology in an intraoperative environment in Europe and in the USA was also advancing.

Experience and Reports of Brazilian Pioneers

Most of the pioneering neurophysiologists in IOM in Brazil were self-taught, but all of them had a very solid base in Clinical Neurophysiology.

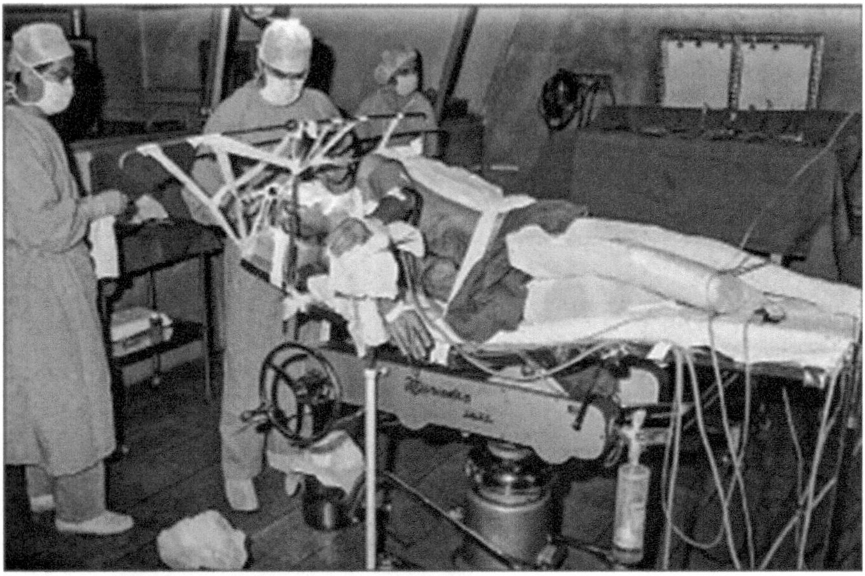

Fig. 1.5 Preparation for epilepsy surgery with patient awake in 1971, by the team of Professor Raul Marino Junior. (*Source*: Marino Jr., Raul. *Um cirurgião sob o olhar de Deus: uma introdução às ciências do cérebro, da mente e do espírito*. Barueri: Manole, 2020, with permission)

Fig. 1.6 Gary Gronich, the first Brazilian neurophysiologist to perform intraoperative neurophysiological monitoring in the 1970s. (*Source*: Marino Jr., Raul. *Um cirurgião sob o olhar de Deus: uma introdução às ciências do cérebro, da mente e do espírito*. Barueri: Manole, 2020, with permission)

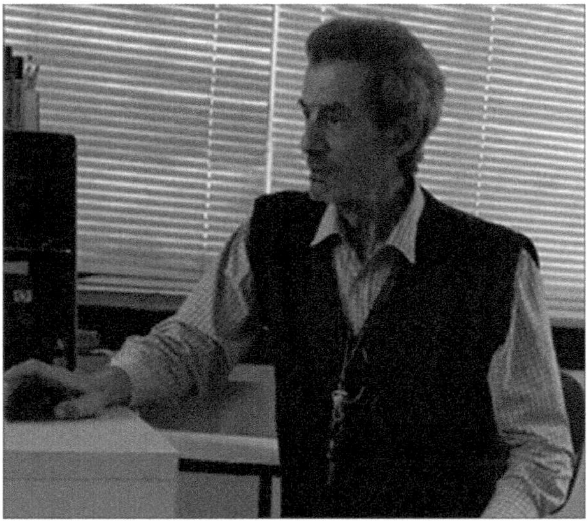

Gary Gronich, MD

Physiatrist and neurophysiologist Gary Gronich's interest in intraoperative neurophysiology dates back to the early 1970s, when he was still a student at USP Medical School (FMUSP). He attended Luccas in intraoperative EEG monitoring in animal models undergoing liver transplantation.

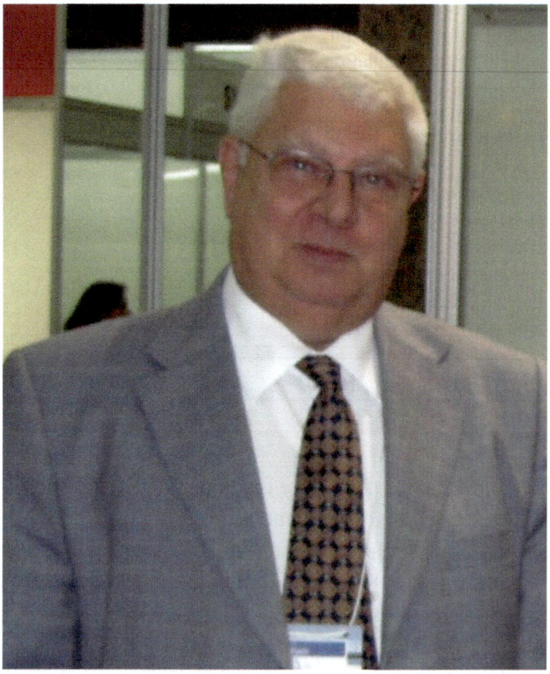

Fig. 1.7 Francisco José Carchedi Luccas, neurophysiologist who started in 1986 to perform evoked potentials in the operating room. (Courtesy of Luccas' personal file)

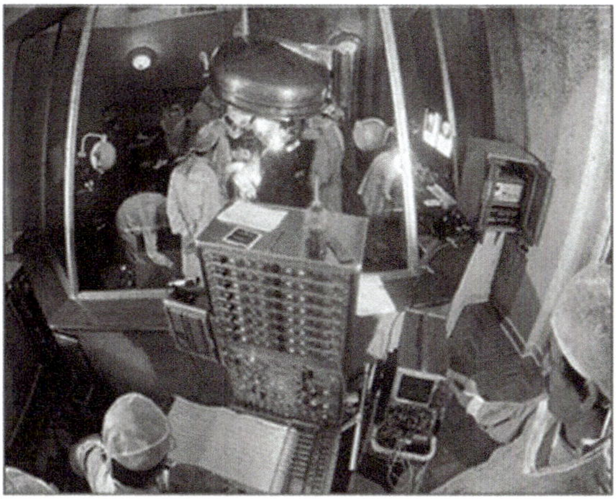

Fig. 1.8 Transoperative electrocorticographic record, performed by Gary Gronich in the 1970s. (*Source*: Marino Jr., Raul. *Um cirurgião sob o olhar de Deus: uma introdução às ciências do cérebro, da mente e do espírito*. Barueri: Manole, 2020, with permission)

From 1972, Gronich began to participate in the activities of the Department of Neurophysiology of USP, performing ECoG records in laboratory animals. Short after that, a damage compromised the DCS device that Professor Marino used in his pioneering surgeries. Aware of Gronich skills as a self-taught electronics technician, Marino called him to repair the device and invited him to join the studies on epilepsy surgeries at IPQ.

Hence, in mid-1974, they founded CENEPSI, Center for Neuropsychosurgery at USP. Gronich was responsible for ECoG and DCS (Figs. 1.8 and 1.9) and also

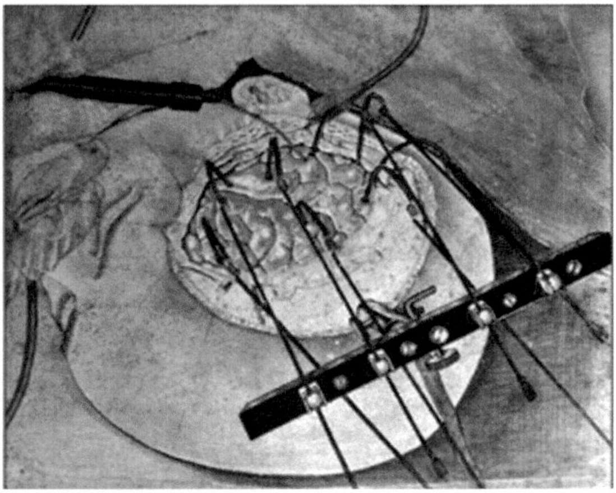

Fig. 1.9 Brain mapping with electrocorticography and electrical stimulation for epilepsy surgery, performed at HCFMUSP. (*Source*: Marino Jr., Raul. *Um cirurgião sob o olhar de Deus: uma introdução às ciências do cérebro, da mente e do espírito.* Barueri: Manole, 2020, with permission)

became head of the newly formed CENEPSI Bioengineering Laboratory. A hundred other specialists joined the team and formed the embryo of what would become USP's Functional Neurosurgery Division (DNF).

In the late 1970s, Gronich became director of the entire IPQ EEG Department and was responsible for restructuring the Service, transforming it into a Clinical Neurophysiology Laboratory.

"In addition to ECoG, we also performed DCS on awake patient in surgeries for epilepsy of the temporal lobe and in surgeries for resection of tumors in eloquent areas, talking to the patient during stimulation. We performed DCS with current intensity from 0.5 to 5 mA, pulse duration of 1 ms and frequency from 5 Hz to 60 Hz.

We developed several electrodes and probes by hand, always aiming to better adapt to the intraoperative circumstances that we would face. All the electrodes and devices created for the group were developed by me in the bioengineering laboratory of CENEPSI.

In 2009, I retired after more than 40 years dedicated to Neurophysiology at IPQ. I made great friendships and also enmities. And I was able to solve part of the immense curiosity that had always motivated me to better understand how the nervous system works", reported Gronich.

Francisco José Carchedi Luccas, MD

Francisco José Carchedi Luccas was responsible for introducing EP in OR during tumors resection at cerebellopontine angle, in 1986, at the Hospital Israelita Albert Einstein (HIAE), in São Paulo.

Luccas has been performing EEG since 1972 and EP since 1982 in outpatients. In 1986, he started to monitor carotid endarterectomies with EEG and several other types of brain surgeries with SEP, visual evoked potential (VEP) and brainstem auditory evoked potential (BAEP).

"The initial difficulties were due to the lack of portability of the equipment at the time and mainly because the surgeons did not know exactly how the

neurophysiologist could help. They did not accept very well the team with biomedical technicians in neurophysiology. Additionally, it was tiring for the neurophysiologist to stay many hours in the OR while there were other hospital calls to see patients in Intensive Care Units (ICUs) and elective exams. I dedicated myself to IOM from 1986 until 1998 and as I grew older, I got tired of the arduous routine of the OR", stated Luccas.

After Luccas, during the 1990s, Ricardo José Rodriguez Ferreira, Adauri Bueno de Camargo, and Silvia Mazzali-Verst began their practice in an almost simultaneous chronology. Since 2000, many others have emerged: Maria Lúcia Furtado de Mendonça (Rio de Janeiro), Carlo Domênico Marrone (Rio Grande do Sul), Alfredo Torres Castellon (São Paulo), Maria Rufina Barros (Espírito Santo), Rachel de Alvarenga Boy Lanna (Minas Gerais), Karina Maria Alécio de Oliveira, and José Alberto Nunes Sobrinho (Distrito Federal).

Ricardo José Rodriguez Ferreira, MD

The history of IOM in Brazil is an integral part of the personal and professional history of the physiatrist and neurophysiologist Ricardo José Rodriguez Ferreira.

In 1990, Ferreira assumed the service of Electroneuromyography (EMG) and EP of the Association for Assistance to Disabled Children (AACD), in São Paulo. In 1994, he received a mission from the chief spine surgeon Ivan Ferraretto: to study and carry out the first IOM during a spine surgery in a year to come at Abreu Sodré Hospital.

Self-taught, initially reading papers and EP books, Ferreira began his research on and soon realized that his main obstacles would be the limitations of equipment and the anesthetic regime. In February 1995, he performed his first IOM: one case of Acoustic Neurinoma resection surgery with the neurosurgeon Jean -Luc Fobe, at Hospital Santa Paula, in São Paulo (Fig. 1.10).

It is worth remembering that Fobé has always been one of the greatest enthusiasts and supporters of the use of IOM and that his name is also often mentioned by three other important Brazilian pioneers in IOM, Adauri Bueno de Camargo, Silvia Mazzali-Verst, and Luiz Henrique Cuzziol who, together with Ferreira, constituted the so-called AACD group.

Ferreira relied on Jorge Florêncio Cardoso, from the company Alfamedic, to optimize several necessary adaptations in his EMG/EP equipment for the spinal surgery to come.

At that time, as MEP did not yet exist, it was mandatory to perform the Wake-up test (Stagnara test). It consisted of an intraoperative clinical motor test created in 1973, which was the gold standard for scoliosis approach.

He asked AACD anesthesiologists to study on how to accomplish a total intravenous anesthetic regimen. It was a challenge at the time, since there were no continuous infusion pumps and no shorter half-life drugs to facilitate this activity. Additional difficulties were lack of evaluation of the anesthetic depth (bispectral index – BIS) and absence of neuromuscular block reversals.

Thus, in 1995 the AACD team was ready to perform SEP and EMG during the first Brazilian IOM of a spine surgery (Fig. 1.11). Since then, they have

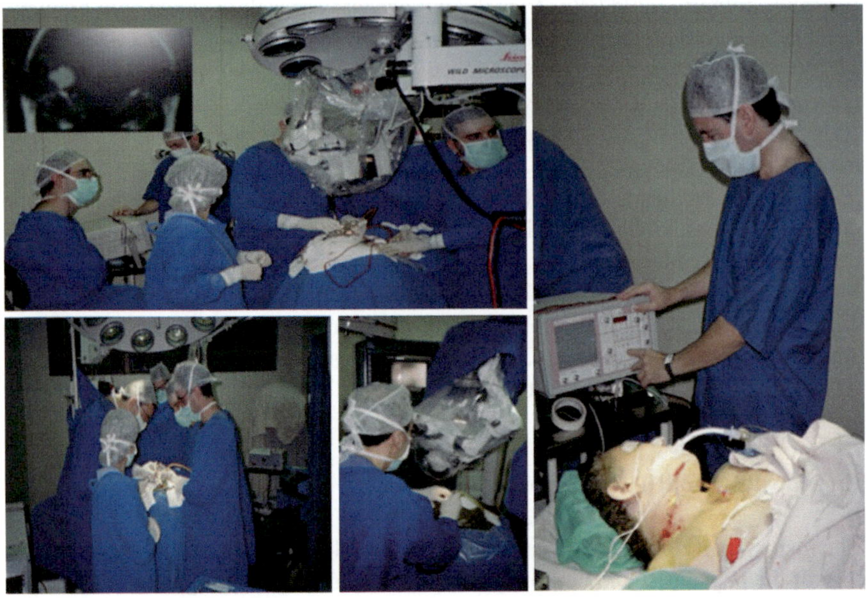

Fig. 1.10 First IOM performed by Ricardo Ferreira (February 1995): Acoustic Neurinoma resection surgery. (Courtesy of Ferreira's personal file)

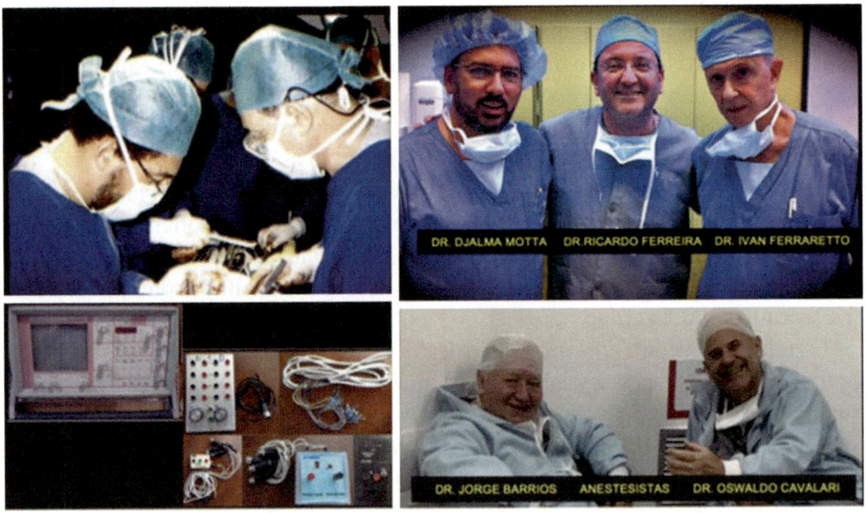

Fig. 1.11 Left: First Brazilian IOM in spine surgery and equipment of the time (at AACD, September 1995). Right: Ricardo Ferreira and the anesthesia and surgery teams. (Courtesy of Ferreira's personal file)

increasingly improved the protocols and equipment, spreading the knowledge about IOM to the surgeons, stimulating and teaching neurophysiologists about this area of expertise.

In 1997, Ferreira went to Chicago (USA) to participate in a Congress of an American society exclusively devoted to IOM – American Society of Neurophysiology Monitoring – ASNM. That year, cork-screw needle electrodes were launched, which would revolutionize both the transcranial electrical stimulation and recordings from the scalp.

Next, Ferreira encouraged Silvia Mazzali-Verst and Adauri Bueno de Camargo to accompany him to the ASNM Congresses in Philadelphia (1998) and in Denver (1999) (Fig. 1.12). These meetings led the AACD team to familiarize with IOM particularities, in a "step by step" way.

Ferreira led many courses and congresses in Brazil and Latin America in the following years (see topics "Special Interest Group (SIG) and IOM Events in Latin America", "ISIN Rio 2015", and "IOM Events by SBNC"). These meetings were in the origin of the spread of the IOM in this side of the world.

Jaime Lopez, Head of Intraoperative Neurophysiology at Stanford University, was a frequent guest by Ferreira's meetings. They first met in 2002, during an

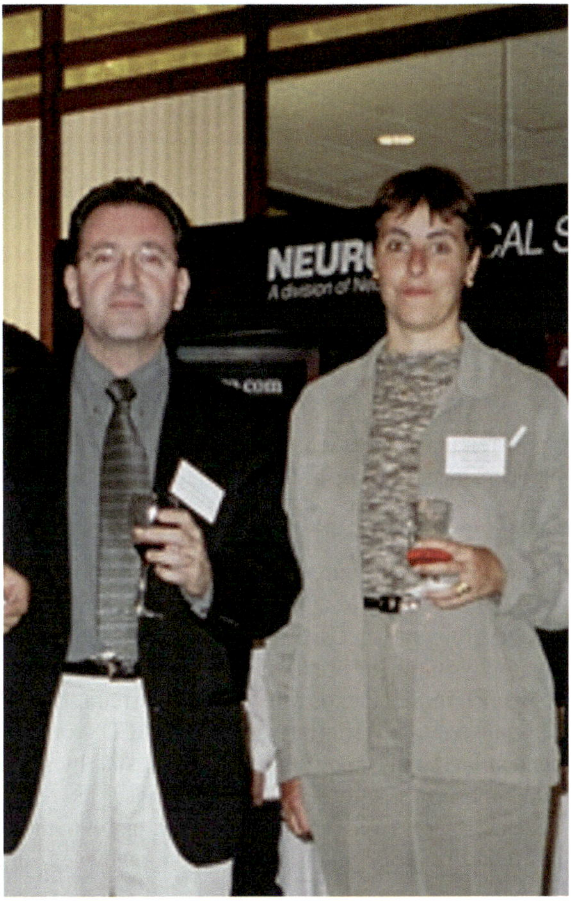

Fig. 1.12 Ricardo Ferreira and Silvia Verst at the opening ceremony of the ASNM Congress in Denver (1999). (Courtesy of Ferreira's personal file)

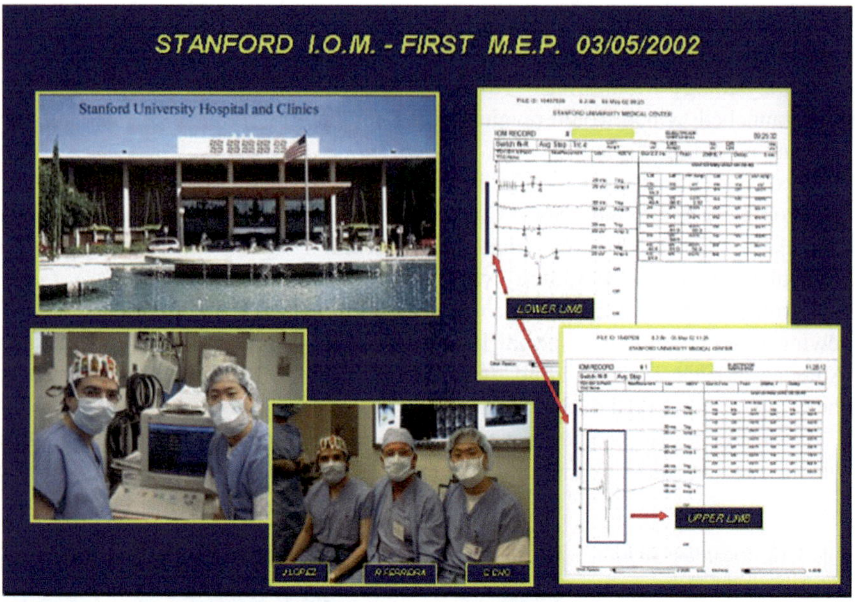

Fig. 1.13 Jaime Lopez, Ricardo Ferreira, and Charlie Cho at Stanford University, in 2002. (Courtesy of Ferreira's personal file)

observational training at Stanford University, in Palo Alto-California (USA). On the occasion, Ferreira helped Lopez's team to carry out their first MEP with transcranial electrical stimulation in an upper thoracic spine surgery (Fig. 1.13). Since then, Lopez has been several times in Brazil to exchange knowledge.

In 2018, Ferreira and Segura presented their "Joint proposal of a Conduct Algorithm in MEP alarm in spine deformities" at the IFCN World Congress in Washington (USA). In 2020, in New Orleans (USA), Ferreira's team has been awarded the prize of "Young Investigator".

Ferreira is a remarkable figure in the history of Brazilian IOM, since almost all pioneers mentioned his influence in their reports.

Adauri Bueno de Camargo, MD

Adauri Bueno de Camargo is one of the most prominent physiatrists in Neurophysiology in Brazil. From 1994 to 1999, he worked as a Neurophysiologist at AACD, in São Paulo, with Ricardo Ferreira, Luiz Henrique Cuzziol, and Silvia Mazzali Verst. This was the so-called "AACD group". They formed a group of independent neurophysiologists who worked side by side in some hospitals and separated most of the time. They exchanged many experiences and collaborated whenever necessary. They reported that, in 1996, the neurosurgeon Jean-Luc Fobe, returning from his Fellowship with the renowned surgeon Marc Sindou, in Lyon,

France, started working at AACD and operating children, especially those with spasticity, submitted to rhizotomy.

"One day Fobe came knocking on our door, in the Neurophysiology Department, asking us to assist him at the surgical center. From there, we started to study, investigate and inform ourselves about Intraoperative Neurophysiology. We started to "venture" into the AACD surgical center, relying on Fobe's goodwill and patience", reported Camargo.

At that time, there was no dedicated or suitable equipment for IOM. EP and EMG devices were used, configuring the protocols for what was believed to be appropriate. Ferreira soon located a congress in the USA, the 1997 Congress of the ASNM, returning very excited and full of plans. His excitement motivated the "AACD group" to start with their trajectories in IOM.

From 1999 to 2001, Camargo specialized in Intraoperative Neurophysiology, at the Institute of Neurology and Neurosurgery, with Vedran Deletis (Department of Neurophysiology), Fred Epstein (Department of Neurosurgery), and Alex Berenstein (Department of Neuroradiology), at Beth Israel Medical Center (Albert Einstein College of Medicine, Yeshiva University, New York). The service offered two fellowship seats annually and Camargo took the seat left by Francesco Sala. At the time, his fellow colleague was Andrea Szelenyi. After 2 years of fellowship, he was invited to remain in the same service, this time training new fellows (Klaus Novak and Sedat Ukatan), supervising and guiding intraoperative monitoring and participating in research activities.

In 2003, Camargo received a proposal to set up the Intraoperative Neurophysiology Hospital Service at HIAE in São Paulo and ended up returning to Brazil. He worked at HIAE establishing the first intra-hospital intraoperative neurophysiological monitoring service (although other colleagues had already been practicing IOM in the country, it was performed independently, privately, and there was not yet an "in-house" hospital service established and entirely dedicated to IOM). Camargo became responsible for the entire Department of Neurophysiology, when Luccas left his position.

In 2005, Camargo went to New York accepting an invitation to work with the same group of Neurosurgery with which he had worked at the time of his Fellowship. They had divided the Neurosurgery group after the death of Fred Epstein. Deletis went to the campus at St. Luke's-Roosevelt Hospital, and Camargo was invited to Montefiore Medical Center, another campus of Albert Einstein College of Medicine.

Meanwhile (2005–2011), Camargo kept ties with Brazil through guidance and consultancy to Brazilian professionals in the area, with special attention to Silvia Verst, who had assumed his position at HIAE after his return to the USA.

Camargo conducted part of the training of countless IOM technicians in the USA from 2005 to the present. In 2010, he went to work at the New York University School of Medicine and, in 2012, returned to São Paulo again, where he lived until 2018. In 2019 he returned to New York to work in the IOM Department at New York University, under the leadership of Aleksander Beric. He is actually co-responsible for the Continuing Education in IOM at the institution.

Silvia Mazzali-Verst, MD, PhD

Silvia Mazzali-Verst is, without a doubt, one of the Brazilian intraoperative neurophysiologists with greater national and international prominence. She has published six papers in international medical journals as author and many others as co-author. In 1995, Verst started to work at the AACD with Ferreira. There, she received training in EP with Adauri Bueno de Camargo and Luiz Henrique Cuzziol and became interested in IOM.

In 1998, Verst, Ferreira, and Camargo participated in the Congress of the ASNM, in Philadelphia, USA. Since then, Verst started a tireless way to acquire knowledge in IOM. Twice, she has visited the IOM service at the Albert Einstein School of Medicine (New York, USA), coordinated by Professor Vedran Deletis, during Camargo's fellowship.

In 2002, when her first child was born, she sold her Digitimer device to Alfredo Torres Castellon and left IOM and São Paulo for 2 years. She came back in 2004, to take over the department of EMG, EP, and IOM at HIAE.

Over the following years, she spent some time learning with Georg Neuloh, at the University Hospital of Bonn (Bonn, Germany), with Andrea Szelenyi, at the University Hospital of Düsseldorf (Düsseldorf, Germany) and with Hughes Duffau, at the University of Montpellier (Montpellier, France). She was also spent precious time with the Brazilian colleague Camargo, at Montefiore Medical Center, in New York, USA (Fig. 1.14). She had participated in the ASNM Congresses and in all the meetings of the ISIN around the world.

In 2011, Verst concluded her Physical Degree by the Neurology Department of FMUSP with the orientation of Professor Paulo Henrique Pires de Aguiar. She proposed the use of C5-Cz and C6-Cz as an option assembly for eliciting corticobulbar-MEP during skull base surgeries.

She is involved with several educational activities: (1) coordination of an IOM Fellowship at Brain Spine Neurofisiologia, (2) invited professor by the Latu Sensu Post-Graduate Program in Neuro-Oncology at the Teaching and Research Institute (IEP) of the Hospital Sírio-Libanês (HSL), and (3) invited professor by Post-Graduate Program in Neuro-Anesthesia of FMUSP. At HSL-IEP in 2019, she coordinated the first dedicated course on Awake Craniotomy with a 360° view on this approach, involving anatomy, imaging, anesthesia, surgery, language evaluation, and rehabilitation.

The difficulties of the first years of practice were overcome with a lot of creativity and persistence: *"In the beginning, we were unaware of the influence of anesthetics, there was still no MEP and the surgeries files were saved on floppy disks. In 2001, I acquired a Digitimer D185 device, but it was difficult to adapt it to my Sapphire four-channels EMG equipment. Besides, there was a shortage of books on the subject. During my visits to the Department of Professor Deletis in New York, I used to stay until late evening, making copies of the papers on the subject. I always came back home with my suitcase crammed with this printed material, many bare needles, cork-screw electrodes and pedicle stimulating probes. After that, I started*

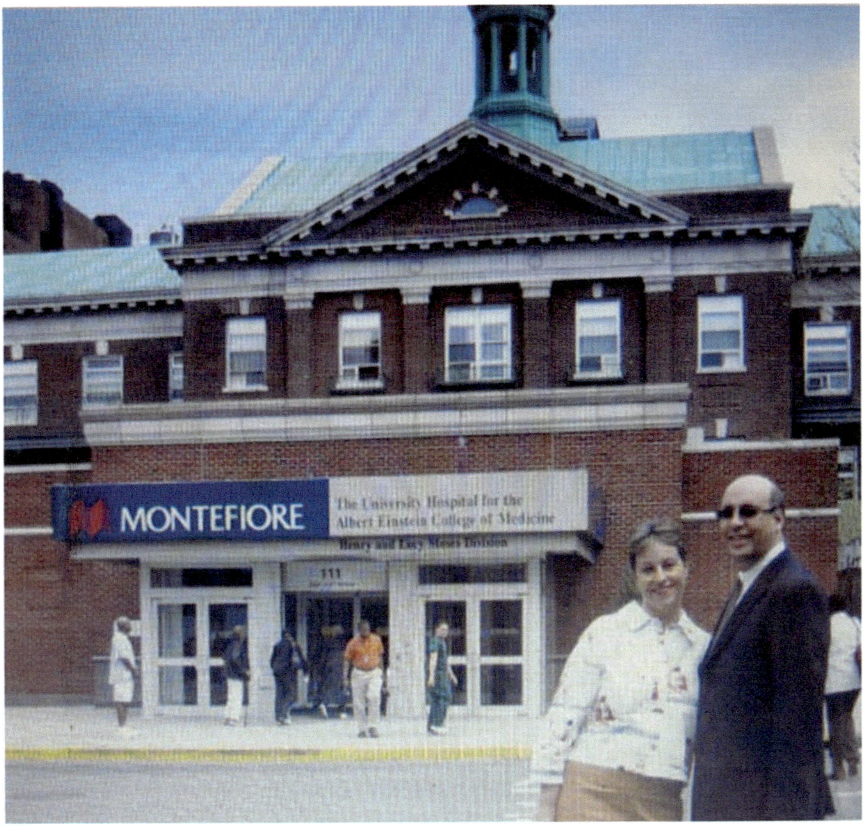

Fig. 1.14 Silvia Verst and Adauri Camargo, at Montefiore Medical Center, in New York, USA. (Courtesy of Verst's personal file)

to bring strips and epidural electrodes. Camargo taught me a lot about setting up, protocols and reasoning in IOM", comments Verst.

At the beginning of her career, Verst dedicated herself to Tethered Cord and Scoliosis surgeries at AACD. In general, most Brazilian neurophysiologists with basic training in IOM tend to be more skillful and focused on spine procedures. Verst is an exception, since she steps herself as passionate for Neurosurgery. "*My soul mate in IOM is Maria Rufina Barros, who shares this passion. We were immediately aware of this neurophysiological compatibility when we first met in Croatia during ISIN meeting in 2009"*.

Her main research interests are in the field of Neurosurgery. Verst's trajectory in awake craniotomy began in 2007, with the return of the Brazilian neurosurgeon Marcos Vinicius Calfat Maldaun, MD, PhD from his Fellowship at the MD Anderson Cancer Center, in Texas (USA). They developed together the monopolar high-frequency technique for awake craniotomies.

"It is very difficult to be a pioneer. We insisted on our language mapping protocol because we obtained good results for the patients. This led us to develop a better intraoperative language test and to perform different tasks, such as drawing, semantics, due task, writing, visual field, syntax, memory and repetition. We perform tasks tailored to the individual and the region of the brain being operated on. Nowadays, we are pleased to use a dynamic approach and receive visitors in the OR to see our work", stated Verst in an interview for the Clinical Neurophysiology Practice Journal, 2020.

Based on the first 20 pictures that Maldaun had brought from Texas, they validated a language test composed of 420 images among native Brazilian Portuguese speakers [28]. Their language task is called Verst-Maldaun Language Assessment for object naming and semantic, which is available under vemotests.com (more details in Chap. 18). This dedication resulted in four papers about awake craniotomy and language assessment [28–31].

She is also involved in a cryoablation research project being held by Ricardo de Freitas, MD, PhD at the Neurology Department of FMUSP, using an animal model [32]. Their experience was presented at the European Congress of Radiology in 2020.

She is proud to be have been part of the team of Evandro de Oliveira, MD, PhD† (until his retirement in 2019). Many other neurosurgeons that directly influenced her career are authors and co-authors in this book.

Alfredo Torres Castellon, MD, PhD

Alfredo Torres Castellon is a physiatrist and neurophysiologist. He has been working with EMG since 1991. His interest in IOM started in 1999 after his fellowship with Ferreira.

"My activity in the IOM area had the fundamental incentive of Ricardo Ferreira. During the 10 years of this partnership, we worked not only in São Paulo, but also explored several regions of Brazil, which did not yet have intraoperative neurophysiologists.", said Castellon.

During 22 years of uninterrupted practice, Castellon contributed to the evolution of IOM in Brazil; held a master's degree in "Intraoperative Neurophysiological Monitoring in spinal fractures" from the Hospital Santa Casa de Misericórdia de São Paulo; and trained other neurophysiologists in the field.

Maria Lúcia Furtado de Mendonça, MD

Maria Lúcia Furtado de Mendonça has always been the greatest Brazilian reference in IOM of cardiovascular procedures. Here is her personal account of the beginnings of her practice:

"I was fortunate enough to meet Francisco Luccas in 1992, when a multidisciplinary team from HIAE came to Rio de Janeiro (RJ) to assess the coma prognosis of the mother of the former president of Brazil, Fernando Collor de Melo, in the midst of a political impeachment. This event resulted in the beginning of a friendship, companionship and admiration for life.

In 1993, under the guidance of Luccas and inspiration from Kenneth Jordan, MD (California, USA), I started EEG monitoring in critical patients at Pró-Cardíaco Hospital, in RJ.

In that same year, we also started the monitoring of carotid endarterectomies and cardiac surgeries, initially unimodal monitoring, with continuous EEG. In 1999, we started multimodal IOM (EEG, transcranial doppler, and SEP) for cardiac, aortic, and carotid surgeries. Between 1993 and 2012, approximately 3.500 cardiovascular procedures were monitored at the Pró-Cardíaco Hospital.

In 2002, I met Ricardo Ferreira at the Congress of Brazilian Society of Clinical Neurophysiology (SBNC), in Arraial da Ajuda (Bahia) (Fig. 1.15). *Ferreira encouraged me to expand the monitoring to neurological and spine surgeries, providing all*

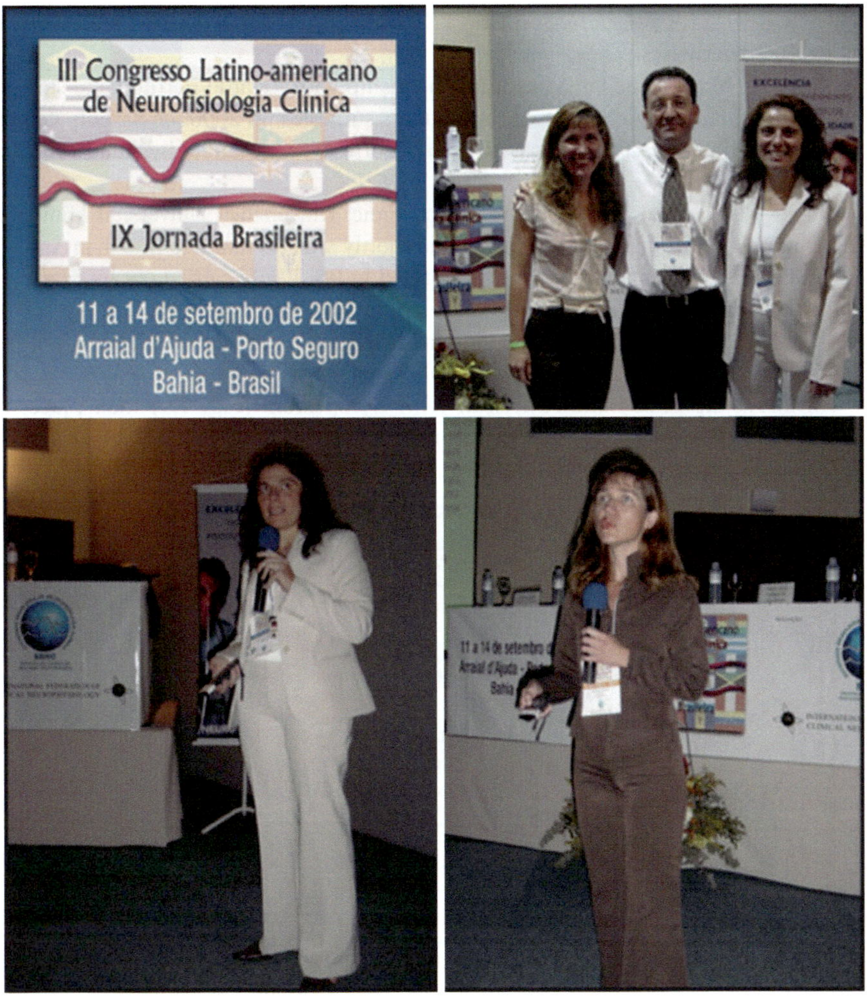

Fig. 1.15 Maria Lucia F. Mendonça (left) and Karina Maria A. Oliveira (right) at the South American Congress of CLA/IFCN, in 2002. (Courtesy of Ferreira's personal file)

the support, from the orientation to purchase the equipment to the assistance in surgeries in which I was not self-confident.

In 2009, I acquired equipment for monitoring neurological surgeries, which represented a new step in my career", reported Mendonça.

Carlo Domênico Marrone, MD

Although root monitoring with EMG in spinal surgeries had been carried out since 1970 in Porto Alegre (Rio Grande do Sul-RS) and EcoG for epilepsy surgeries since 1990, it was only in 1998 that IOM emerged in RS with Carlo Domênico Marrone.

At the time, Marrone performed mapping and monitoring of peripheral nerves at São Lucas Hospital of the Pontifical Catholic University of Rio Grande do Sul (PUCRS) with surgeon Jefferson Braga Silva. He used to make his own electrodes with Kirschner wires.

In 1999, Marrone began a beautiful friendship with Ricardo Ferreira and started making regular trips to São Paulo to watch his surgeries. In 2000, he participated in the first IOM course at São Lucas Hospital (Porto Alegre), taught by Adauri Bueno de Camargo.

In 2001, he held IOM Fellowship at Freie Universität, Universitätsklinikum Benjamin Franklin, in Berlin, Germany. And shortly after his return to Brazil, in August 2001, the first multimodal IOM was performed in RS. It was carried out by Marrone with the neurosurgeon Arlindo D'Ávila, in a lumbosacral spine stenosis surgery.

In 2005, at SBNC Congress, in Gramado (RS), together with Ferreira, Marrone held the first Brazilian Symposium on IOM (Fig. 1.16).

In 2007, the First Latin American IOM Symposium (Fig. 1.1) took place in Montevideo (Uruguay), chaired by Daniel Cibils, MD. In 2009, the Second Latin

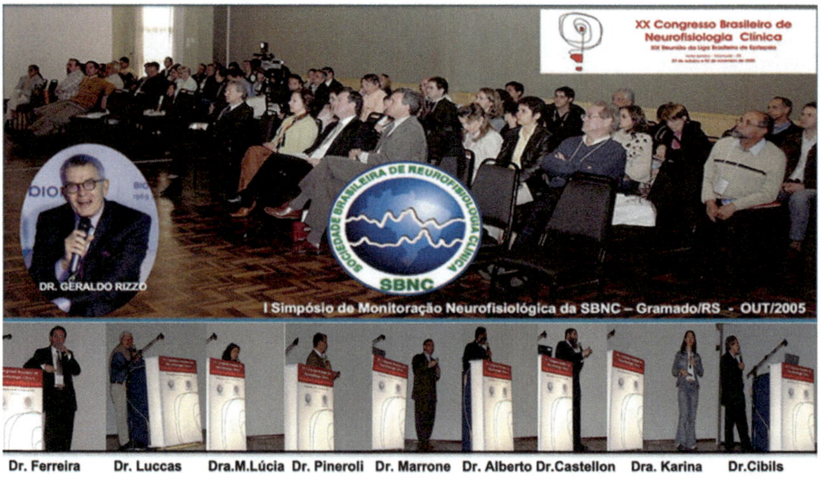

Fig. 1.16 I Brazilian IOM Symposium in the SBNC Brazilian Congress, in Gramado-RS, in 2005. (Courtesy of Ferreira's personal file)

American IOM Symposium was held in Brazil, with Ferreira as Chairman and Marrone as Co-Chairman. From that point, the spread of IOM throughout Latin America was gradually increasing.

In the teaching field, Marrone has already participated and still actively participates in IOM training of neurophysiologists, having trained so far 11 professionals.

Marrone is the current president (2019–2021) of the SBNC. During his tenure, the Continuing Education Project in Neurophysiology was implemented. It consists of weekly online academic meetings, comprising all procedures in neurophysiology. Once a month, the subject is IOM.

Karina Maria Alécio de Oliveira, MD

Karina Maria Alécio de Oliveira had as a mentor in her training in Clinical Neurophysiology Roberto Low, MD. Like Luccas, Low and Oliveira are Brazilian references in EP.

Oliveira concluded IOM Fellowship in 1999 at the Toronto Western Hospital, Canada. Upon her returning to Brazil, she started her practice with difficulties and a lot of self-teaching. Below is her testimony:

"My experience and learning are mainly due to the setting up of the IOM Department for brain tumors resection involving eloquent areas at the Hospital de Base do Distrito Federal (HBDF, Brasília-DF). There, I monitored the cases of neurosurgeon Luiz Cláudio Modesto Pereira, MD, PhD. His Awake Craniotomies between 1998 and 2008 were part of this project: "Efficacy of craniotomy with fully awake patient for resection of primary supratentorial tumors in eloquent area" (Fig. 1.17).

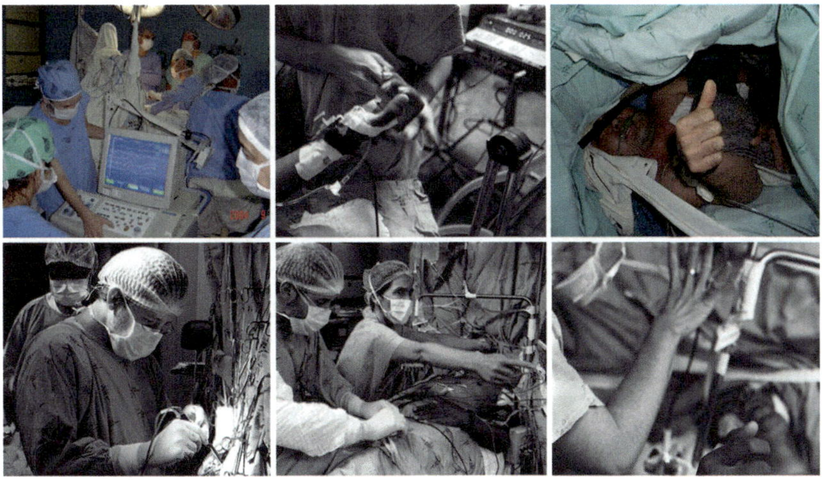

Fig. 1.17 IOMs performed by Karina Oliveira in 1998 in craniotomies with fully awake patient for resection of primary supratentorial tumors in eloquent area at the Hospital de Base do Distrito Federal. (Courtesy of Oliveira's personal file)

In 2009, I met José Alberto Nunes Sobrinho, MD, who became my partner and great companion in IOM. We founded Stela Clinic and, in 2012, we created an IOM Fellowship in partnership with HBDF and the Foundation for Teaching and Research in Health Sciences of the Federal District (FEPECS). It was a 1 year long, full-time, remunerated fellowship. It was indeed the first Brazilian Fellowship in IOM officially linked to the Ministry of Education (MEC). We trained Andreya Fonseca Cardoso Cavalcanti, MD.

And a story that saddens me a lot is that I have never been able to leverage IOM in Functional Neurosurgery as there are companies with commercial interests that take non-medical technicians and software engineers to perform this activity. However, I never stopped studying and I feel ready for the opportunity whenever it comes."

José Alberto Nunes Sobrinho, MD

Until 2009, before forming a team with Oliveira, José Alberto Nunes Sobrinho was little known for his experience in IOM. He had been practicing high standard IOM by Sarah Network of Hospitals.

"I first learned about IOM at Sarah Hospital in the year 2000, when we performed tibial nerves SEP during scoliosis approaches. We used a Nihon Kohden device and complemented the assessment with a wake-up test.

At that time, I read about the Digitimer D185 equipment and soon after, in 2002, Sarah Hospital Brasília acquired one. Yet, we still had a limited number of recording channels. We solved some technical difficulties thanks to Ricardo Ferreira who told us how to obtain boxes with selector keys and extension cables. From that, I was able to perform all other possible neurophysiological modalities.

Over time, I looked for better devices that could be used exclusively for IOM. In 2004, in my opinion, the German company Inomed's equipment was the most modern.

At that time, the first Latin American IOM symposium took place. There I met other renowned neurophysiologists who had been dedicating themselves to IOM for years. They also were dealing with national limitations, but with utmost creativity: Karina Alécio, Maria Lúcia Mendonça, Carlo Marrone, Rachel Boy, Alfredo Castellon, Daniel Cibils and Francisco Soto. This group was the embryo for the next Latin American symposia and congresses, when there was an exponential increase in the number of people in the area.", stated Sobrinho.

Maria Rufina Barros, MD

It was 1998 when Maria Rufina Barros asked her chief of the EMG Residency at the Clinic Hospital of the Ribeirão Preto Medical School (FMUSP-RP), Wilson Marques Júnior, MD, PhD to contact Ricardo Ferreira. She was willing to do an IOM internship at AACD, in São Paulo. However, at that time, only SEP was performed with a Wake-up Test for scoliosis surgeries.

After Barros ended her first internship in IOM at AACD, she set with Ferreira that she would return to learn MEP as soon as it would come up.

She began her IOM department in Vitória-ES in 1999. Back then, she used a four-channel electromyographer to monitor facial nerve discharges in surgeries for cerebellopontine angle tumor resection.

It took her 10 years to return to learn MEP with Ferreira, at AACD. After that, she immediately bought her first IOM equipment with a transcranial motor stimulator.

In 2010, due to a request made by Ferreira, Barros was received by Jaime Lopez at the Clinic Hospital of Stanford University (USA). Her third internship in IOM enabled her to improve her practice and protocols, especially in posterior fossa and vascular surgeries.

Barros is perhaps the Brazilian Neurophysiologist with greater expertise in IOM for traumatic injuries of the brachial plexus and peripheral nerves in general. She has a peculiar experience in the area as she performs a preoperative EMG planning as part of the IOM in cases of spine, spinal cord, and peripheral nerves IOM.

"For about 10 years, our team, composed by surgeons and neurophysiologist, has been doing IOM planning together based on patient preoperative exams. According to the surgeons' report, the improvement of the result with the use of IOM is unquestionable. Neurolysis and Anastomosis are techniques that have been used for 25 years; the difference highlighted by the surgeons is that now neurophysiology tells them what to do and where to do it", explains Barros.

Just like the rocky road endured by several other pioneers in IOM, Barros' search for knowledge could not be left out:

"Yes, we had to travel a lot, not only searching for symposia, congresses and courses, but also looking for our IOM stuff. We had no option but to buy more delicate manufacture stimulating probes and even the common electrodes outside the country. It was already part of our travel itinerary; we usually placed the order in advance and had it delivered to the hotel.

Even after over two decades of IOM in Brazil, we still suffer a lot with the extremely limited supply and variety of material. Nowadays we are no longer allowed to buy the latest products abroad and return back with them, even if we declare them to custom. This bureaucracy to register new material and equipment is something that needs to change urgently. It enormously delays progress and the acquisition of new technologies."

In 2009, Barros attended her first ISIN meeting, in Dubrovinik (Croacia). At this event, she had the opportunity to approach and talk in private with Aage Moller, questioning critically the details of the IOM protocols of the posterior fossa surgeries and showing him her records. After a pleasant and productive conversation on the topic, Moller ended up encouraging the reasoning of Barros and said to her: *"we are neurosurgeons, we started this. But you are neurophysiologists and you will do much more and better than us"*.

Another event that deserves to be mentioned on this trip is highlighted by Barros: *"It was when I met Silvia Verst, who challenged me with a series of questions in a conversation about IOM during the flight. I believe that I did well because since then we have cultivated a friendship, affection and admiration that I cherish immensely."*

Barros owes to Ricardo Ferreira all her training, guidance, and motivation in the area of IOM. She has been participating in almost all the Symposia and Conferences organized by him since the end of the 1990s. It gave her the opportunity to meet with several international personalities of IOM.

Finally, Barros could never dissociate her trajectory in IOM from the figure of the renowned neurosurgeon Paulo Melo Jacques, MD, PhD. He has always allowed her to take innovative ideas, techniques, and concepts to the surgical protocols, under the justification of his professional motto: *"What matters is the final result, even if it costs us more dedication".*

Technicians in Neurophysiology

As for the role of non-medical health professionals in the IOM area in Brazil, we emphasize that SBNC recognizes the activity of technicians in Neurophysiology (biomedical, nurses, among others), provided they are directly supervised by a neurophysiologist [33, 34].

The technician is not allowed to indicate, plan, analyze, or interpret the data acquired during IOM. The technician may be trained to assist the neurophysiologist but never to replace him [33, 34].

In Brazil, the training of technicians in Neurophysiology has always been more focused on outpatient procedures (EEG, Polysomnography, and EP). There is a shortage of well-trained and qualified IOM technicians to work in the area.

Andrea Broisler Sucena Caivano represents one of the pioneering neurophysiological technical professionals in the IOM field. She is biomedical and has been working as a Clinical Neurophysiology General Technician since 1988 and as IOM technician since 2004.

"I did my specialization in Clinical Neurophysiology in 1988 with Francisco Luccas, working for many years with EEG and EP at HIAE, in São Paulo.

I first learned about IOM in 2002, when I participated in the IV International Symposium on Intraoperative Neurophysiological Monitoring at Beth Israel Medical Center, in New York. During this period, at HIAE, we used to perform EEG in endarterectomies and BAEP and SEP in brain tumors. In 2004, I did a specialization at St. Luke's Hospital (New York) with Vedran Deletis and at John Hopkins Hospital (Baltimore) with Adauri Camargo.

In 2007, I started working exclusively with IOM with the team of Silvia Verst. As a technical assistant I acquired skills to understand all the neurophysiological tests that are performed during the procedure, assisting the physician responsible for IOM with the setting up and acquisition of the records. ", stated Caivano.

Academic Training in IOM in Brazil

Denise Spinola Pinheiro, MD

The neurologist and neurophysiologist Denise Spinola Pinheiro has been coordinating the IOM Fellowship program at the Federal University of São Paulo (Unifesp-SP) for many years now. It is the only current IOM Fellowship offered by a Brazilian public university.

"*I was a little self-taught. As I was extremely interested in the area, I joined a co-worker, Carmelinda Campos, MD and together we started to study IOM. We published a paper on neurological endovascular procedures. Afterwards, the university bought an IOM equipment, sponsored by funds from the São Paulo State Research Support Foundation (Fapesp). That enabled us to implement the IOM service. In 2015, I started the Fellowship program, which today has become an official specialization course at Unifesp. Since 2015, we have trained 24 neurophysiologists in IOM.*", reported Pinheiro.

Pinheiro, Oliveira, and Jessie Navarro, MD stand as the few Brazilian neurophysiologists with experience in IOM for Functional Neurosurgery, especially in Deep Brain Stimulation (DBS) procedures.

Training Challenges

Regarding academic training in IOM, there are practically no formal institutional training centers. Over the years, Ferreira, Verst, Marrone, and Pinheiro were responsible for IOM training of many neurophysiologists and technical assistants. Many of their fellows were pioneers in IOM in their states, allowing the spread of the technique throughout Brazil. Paulo Kimaid, MD, PhD (who will be mentioned in a topic ahead) structured an informative course, with intensive and short duration theoretical and practical steps. Recently, training criteria created by SBNC are detailed in Chap. 2.

Yet, many neurophysiologists interested in IOM still need to spend some time training outside Brazil. Many IOM departments throughout the USA and in shorter terms in Europe, welcome and tutor colleagues in short (a month) and long term (1–2 years). There is still no consensus on the ideal period of training.

Carla Juliana Araújo Ferreira, MD (Belo Horizonte-Minas Gerais) is a young neurophysiologist who can give a testimony on this matter. Her training was based on a mixed educational model, partly done in Brazil and partly abroad. Her training in IOM in Brazil was mentored by Silvia Verst, Andreya Cardoso, and Wilson Scapini, MD. Afterward, Araújo Ferreira went to the United States, where she did a Research Fellow in IOM at the University of Pittsburgh Medical Center with a scholarship from the International Federation of Clinical Neurophysiology (IFCN). Here is her clarifying testimony drawing a comparative parallel between Brazilian education and training abroad.

"Little by little, I learned that IOM's pioneers in Brazil took the responsibility of developing programs in order to teach new professionals to work in the area.

I started training in IOM in 2016 with the team of Silvia Verst, Andreya Cardoso and Wilson Scapini, who all work in different hospitals in and around São Paulo, hospitals with different quality and complexity. I participated in almost 100 procedures between 2016 and 2017 and at the end of 2017, I went to Pittsburgh for a Fellow with an IFCN scholarship for young neurophysiologists. Along the six-month period, I experienced an immersion in a different reality, but not necessarily more enriching.

The level of professionalism of the American medical system is contrasting. Each hospital has its own team, which takes the relationship between surgeons and neurophysiologists to a different level of interaction and quality of communication. The teams are structured with professionals of different levels of training: technicians, non-medical neurophysiologists and neurophysiologists neurologists. Each has a very well-defined role and surgeries of different complexities demand more or less participation of each member. Telemedicine is very well structured. Teamwork is highly organized to allow regular rest for professionals, thus avoiding overload. Practice and research go hand in hand. All in all, the systemic organization is admirable.

However, I still think that despite everything, the service provided by the good Brazilian neurophysiologist to the patient manages to be somehow superior. Perhaps because there is no or less intermediation by a technician, perhaps because we are almost exclusively focused on assistance.

The person who manages the equipment (press the buttons) is the same person who has full medical knowledge and thus manages to have a broader view, greater interpretative capacity and greater "neuroplasticity" in the protocols.

I realized that multimodality was limited under the justification that too much information would end up being difficult to manage, what they call "cognitive noise", which does not apply to the good Brazilian neurophysiologist.

At the end of the day, I see that my training in IOM in different services was complementary and not at all redundant, with different aspects being addressed in each stage of the training. And despite the frequently unfavorable system, or because of it, the good doctor is especially good".

Evolution of IOM Equipment and Its Arrival in Brazil

The evolution of the IOM equipment followed the development of our pioneers. They always brought to Brazil each of the latest models of equipment.

"When I started IOM, I used a device that allowed me to perform SEP and, with some adaptations, also a few EMG channels. In 1998, I acquired a 4-channel Dantec device (Fig. 1.18). *Afterwards, I ordered a 12-channel device from an Argentinian company to carry out EMG",* stated Ferreira.

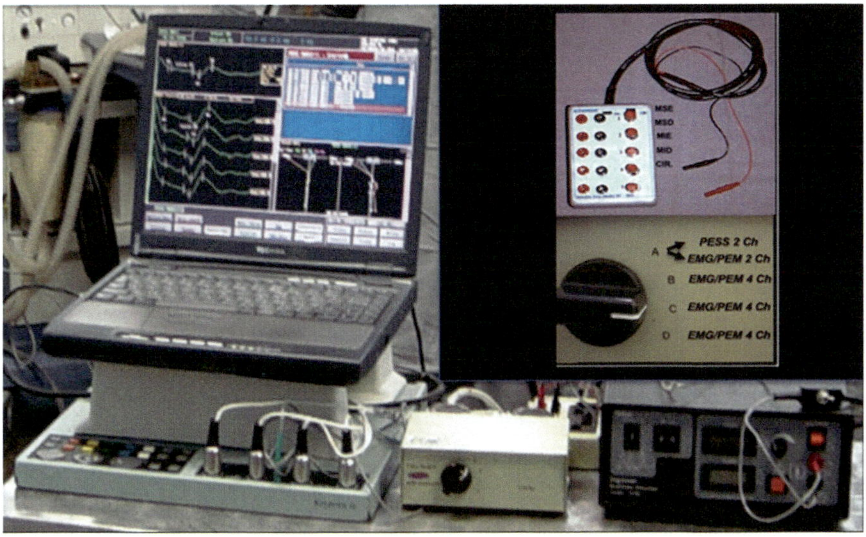

Fig. 1.18 4-Channel Dantec device – Digitimer D185 – switch boxes from Alfamedic. (Courtesy of Ferreira's personal file)

"In order to enhance recording channels, my husband, a German engineer called Heinrich Verst, built us a shielded cable with 64 twisted and shielded numbered wires. I remember that it was very difficult to find a dealer of touch-proof connectors. The 4 meters-cable allowed us to connect the muscle recording needles at one end and the other end to equipment. It became possible to switch between muscle channels, as required by scoliosis surgery. We enhanced our recordings capability. The cable was very heavy though. Later on, we introduced a switch stimulation box (Fig. 1.19), *first created by Vedran Deletis, that had given to me"* stated Silvia Verst.

Regarding the use of the MEP in Brazil, Ferreira and Silvia Verst brought the first transcranial electric stimulators (Digitimer D-185) in 2001 (Fig. 1.18). *"Step by step, we demonstrated to surgeons that there was no longer need to perform the Wake-Up test in scoliosis*", stated Ferreira.

"In 2004, a 16-channel IOM device had been brought to HIAE, however, the hospital gave up buying it. I acquired the first 16-channel device in Brazil. And in 2008, Marrone and I acquired the first two 32-channel devices in the country.

Today, young intraoperative neurophysiologists cannot even imagine how difficult our daily lives at the OR were at that time. Since then, the equipment has improved a lot. They developed into a dedicated IOM software and greater number of recording and stimulating channels. Currently, there are several companies in Brazil that have electrodes and equipment ready for delivery, with online support and repair services, a real luxury.

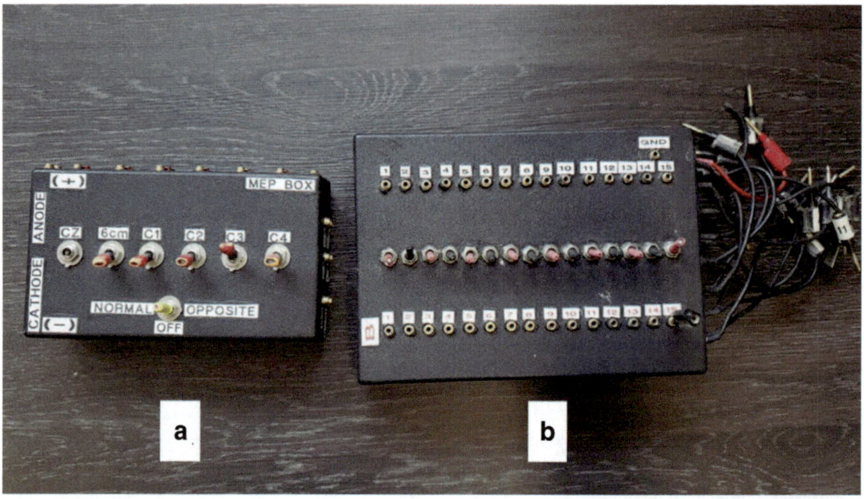

Fig. 1.19 Stimulation and recording boxes developed by Vedran Deletis and given as a gift to Silvia Verst in 1999, during her first visit. (**a**) MEP stimulation box connected to Cz, Cz+6 cm, C1, C2, C3, and C4. At that time, six stimulating corkscrew electrodes were placed for every surgery. It was unclear which combination would work better. It was possible to set the pin direction to anode or cathode and then invert them to "normal or opposite". Only one combination could be used per turn. (**b**) Recording box with 15 channels and ground electrode. This box was connected to the four-channel EMG machine and it was possible to enable 4 channels for analysis as needed. Thus, all recording cables were "in reach", and it was easily possible to switch between channels. (Courtesy of Verst's personal file)

I emphasize that despite this truly simple arsenal and full of adaptations, we carried out procedures within the established protocols and with enormous ethical and technical commitment. We still have these records today", reported Ferreira.

Brazilian Society of Clinical Neurophysiology (SBNC)

IOM Events by SBNC

The first IOM courses, symposia, and congresses in Brazil were of paramount importance for the spread of this field among Brazilian neurophysiologists. They were led by Ferreira with the contribution of many others, like Luccas, Mendonça, Barros, Oliveira, and Marrone.

- 2000: IOM lecture in the VIII Brazilian Conference on Clinical Neurophysiology (Belo Horizonte-MG), including an IOM Workshop at Hospital Arapiara (Fig. 1.20).
- 2002: Session about IOM in the South American Congress of the Latin American Chapter of the International Federation of Clinical Neurophysiology (LAC/IFCN), in Porto Seguro-BA (Fig. 1.15).

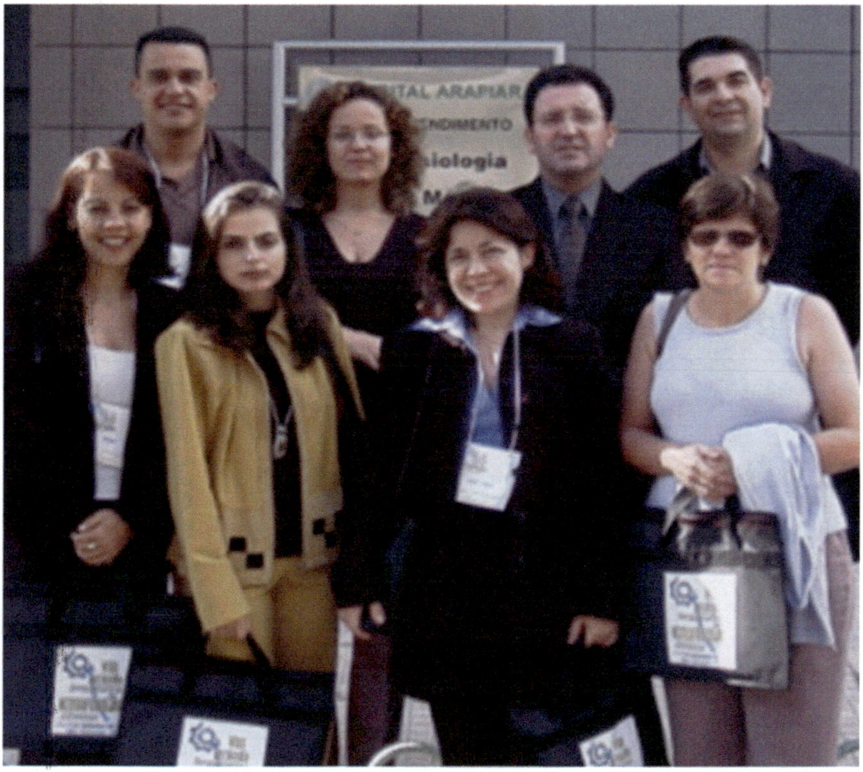

Fig. 1.20 IOM Workshop at Hospital Arapiara (MG)/VIII Brazilian Conference on Clinical Neurophysiology (2000). (Courtesy of Ferreira's personal file)

- 2005: I Brazilian IOM Symposium in the SBNC Brazilian Congress, in Gramado-RS (Fig. 1.16). During this meeting, Luccas, Marrone, and Ferreira achieved to create IOM as an area of interest inside SBNC.
- 2007: II Brazilian IOM Symposium in the SBNC Brazilian Congress, in São Paulo-SP (Fig. 1.21).
- 2009: XXII SBNC Brazilian Congress (Florianópolis-SC): SBNC IOM Department was created by Andréa Julião de Oliveira, MD, current SBNC president.
- Since then, every SBNC Congress has IOM sessions in its scientific program.
- 2011: XXIII SBNC Brazilian Congress/VI LAC/IFCN's Congress, in Punta Del Este (Uruguai): the first SBNC examining board for IOM certification exam was composed.
- 2013–2015-2017: Relevant IOM sessions in the SBNC congresses in Rio de Janeiro (2013), Natal (2015), and Goiânia (2017).
- In 2019, in São Paulo, was held the XXVII SBNC Brazilian Congress/VII LAC/IFCN's Congress. Several international renowned specialists were there. All

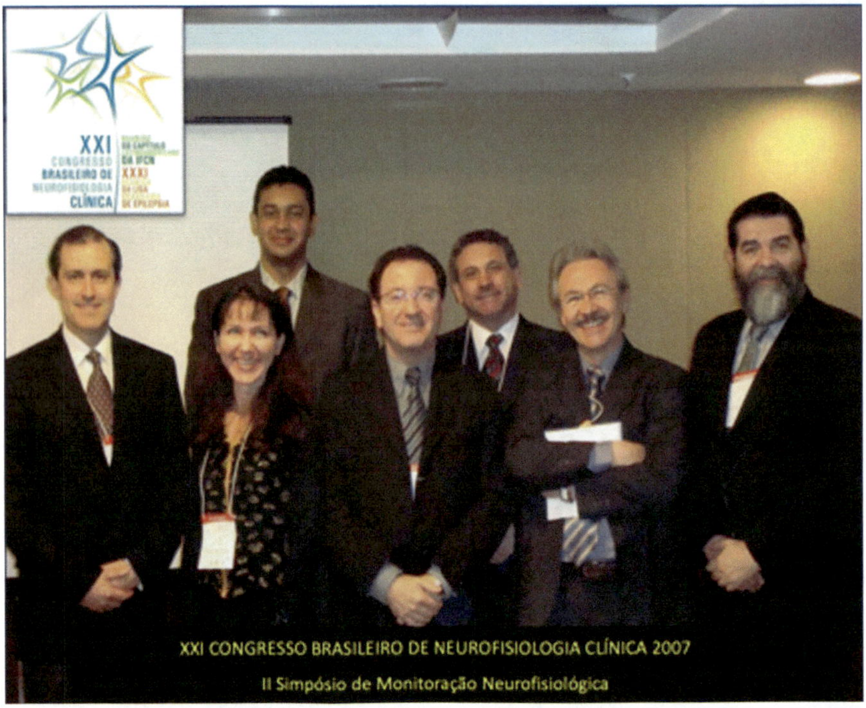

Fig. 1.21 II Brazilian IOM Symposium in the SBNC Brazilian Congress, in São Paulo, in 2007. From left to right: Soto, Oliveira, Sobrinho, Ferreira, Marrone, Cibils and Castellon. (Courtesy of Sobrinho's personal file)

IOM lectures were full. It took place exactly 14 years after the first Symposium, which had gathered few Brazilians interested in IOM. Nowadays, there are over a hundred neurophysiologists performing IOM in Brazil.

Development of IOM Department at SBNC

Paulo André Teixeira Kimaid, MD, PhD first became interested in IOM in 2004. He declares himself as self-taught.

In 2011, Kimaid assumed the presidency of SBNC. During his tenure, the first SBNC examining board for IOM certification exam was composed. It approved the first candidates ever: Ricardo Ferreira and Rafael de Castro, who had recently arrived from his Fellowship with Aaatif Hussein at Duke University, North Carolina (USA). The first examining board was comprised by Maria Lúcia Furtado de Mendonça (RJ), Karina Maria Alécio de Oliveira (DF), Carlo Domenico Marrone (RS), and Rinaldo Claudino (SC).

Kimaid participated in the examining boards of SBNC from 2012 to 2019. He could count on Castro for heading the IOM scientific department of SBNC during this period. As an interesting note, Castro and José Alberto Campos da Silva Júnior, MD were the first neurophysiologists to perform IOM in Northeastern Brazil.

In 2015, Kimaid assisted the Neurology Technical Chamber of the Federal Council of Medicine (CFM) to write and publish a resolution that regulates IOM practice in Brazil [33, 35]. At this same year, he started teaching IOM. His course has the peculiarity of compressing the classes in short-days period with observational surgeries. Since 2018, Kimaid has been part of the IFCN Educational Committee.

As part of his interest in teaching, Kimaid managed to publish the first Brazilian book in IOM in 2019.

Current Status of IOM in Brazil and Latin America

Every neurophysiologist who joined this world had a mentor who encouraged them to follow this path. This path is still under construction as it is the last frontier of clinical neurophysiology.

There are areas of darkness that are not yet understood, complete areas of the nervous system that cannot yet be monitored; a person has to have a unique spirit to persevere in a discipline like this, with a grueling operating room and no schedule.

All Latin American countries have already joined this discipline. There are several working groups; without a doubt, tens of thousands of cases of the most varied pathologies are carried out per year. But it is important to emphasize that there are threats to the healthy development of the IOM.

Intraoperative neurophysiology is a medical act that benefits a patient facing a complex surgery: Reason why the physician should carry out the monitoring. A person with in-depth knowledge of neurophysiology, neuroanatomy, and systemic factors can speak correctly with an anesthesiologist and surgeon. When the situation justifies the temporary or permanent suspension of surgery, it is an enormous responsibility; the neurophysiologist cannot abandon the patient.

Intraoperative neurophysiologists should try give their best to teach new generations in this discipline, developing gentle, rigorous, patient-centered professionals.

Conclusion

IOM's arrival in developing countries faced many more difficulties than its introduction in Europe and in the United States. In Brazil, its practice has become more expressive in the last fifteen years, after the registration of equipment and materials to carry it out.

The availability of the new technology has been accompanied by disorderly growth, resulting in concern about the indications, the training of those who carry it out and also how it should be carried out.

Knowledge in intraoperative neurophysiology in Brazil continues to flourish, thanks not only to the dedicated and persistent pioneers, but also to the young neurophysiologists who have emerged in the area.

Multimodality is a term that refers not only to the diversity and complementarity of neurophysiological techniques used in IOM, but also characterizes the versatility and creativity of its practitioners.

We hope that this chapter will inspire surgeons, neurophysiologists, anesthesiologists, and technologists to work together and in a "multimodal way", using a lot of creativity, versatility, and scientific knowledge to reduce postoperative neurological deficits.

References

1. Bacigaluppi S, Bragazzi NL, Martini M. Fedor Krause (1857–1937): the father of neurosurgery. Neurosurg Rev. 2020;43:1443–9.
2. Penfield W, Boldrey E. Somatic motor and sensory representation in the cerebral cortex of man as studied by electrical stimulation. Brain. 1937;37:389–443.
3. Jasper HH. Electrocorticograms in man. Electroencephalogr Clin Neurophysiol. 1949;2:16–29.
4. Marshall C, Walker AE. Electrocorticography. Bull Johns Hopkins Hosp. 1949;85:344–59.
5. Penfield W, Roberts L. Speech and brain mechanisms. Princeton: Princeton University Press; 2014.
6. Thompson JE. Surgery for cerebrovascular insufficiency (stroke) with special emphasis on carotid endarterectomy. Springfield: Charles C Thomas; 1968. p. 96.
7. Wylie EJ, Ehrenfeld WK. Extracranial occlusive cerebrovascular disease: diagnosis and management. Philadelphia: W.B. Saunders Company; 1970. p. 231.
8. Sharbrough FW, Messick JM Jr, Sundt TM Jr. Correlation of continuous electroencephalograms with cerebral blood flow measurements during carotid endarterectomy. Stroke. 1973;4:674–83.
9. Ojeman's testimony at International Video Symposium on Brain Mapping (IamBrain.org) 20–21 Mar 2021.
10. Shimoji K, Higashi H, Kano T. Epidural recording of spinal electrogram in man. Electroencephalogr Clin Neurophysiol. 1971;30:236–9.
11. Imai T. Human electrospinogram evoked by direct stimulation on the spinal cord through epidural space. J Jpn Orthop Assoc. 1976;50:1037–56.
12. Tamaki T, Yamashita T, Kobayashi H, Hirayama H. Spinal cord monitoring. J Jpn Electroencephalogr Electromyogr. 1972;1:196.
13. Tamaki T, Tsuji H, Inoue S, Kobayashi H. The prevention of iatrogenic spinal cord injury utilizing the evoked spinal cord potential. Int Orthop. 1981;4:313–7.
14. Nash CL Jr, Schatzinger L, Lorig R. Intraopertive monitoring of spinal cord function during scoliosis spine surgery. J Bone Joint Surg Am. 1974;56:1765.
15. Nash CL Jr, Lorig RA, Schatzinger LA, Brown RH. Spinal cord monitoring during operative treatment of the spine. Clin Orthop Relat Res. 1977;126:100–5.
16. Tamaki T, Kobayashi H, Yamane T, Egashira T, Tsuji H, Inoue S. Clinical application of evoked spinal cord evoked potential. Seikeigeka (Orthop Surg). 1977;28:681–9.
17. Nuwer MR, Dawson EC. Intraoperative evoked potential monitoring of the spinal cord: enhanced stability of cortical recordings. Electroencephalogr Clin Neurophysiol. 1984;59:318–27.
18. Nuwer MR. Intraoperative monitoring of neural function. Amsterdam: Elsevier; 2008.
19. Møller MB, Møller AR. Loss of auditory function in microvascular decompression for hemifacial spasm. Results in 143 consecutive cases. J Neurosurg. 1985;63:17–20.
20. Moller AR. Evoked potentials in intraoperative monitoring. Baltimore: Williams & Wilkins; 1988. p. 224.

21. Hicks RG, Burke DJ, Stephen JP. Monitoring spinal cord function during scoliosis surgery with Cotrel- Dubousset instrumentation. Med J Aust. 1991;154:82–6.
22. Burke D, Hicks R, Stephen J, Woodforth I, Crawford M. Assessment of corticospinal and somatosensory conduction simultaneously during scoliosis surgery. Electroencephalogr Clin Neurophysiol. 1992;85:388–96.
23. Taniguchi M, Cedzich C, Schramm J. Modification of cortical stimulation for motor evoked potentials under general anesthesia: technical description. Neurosurgery. 1993;32(2):219–26. https://doi.org/10.1227/00006123-199302000-00011. PMID: 8437660.
24. Kothbauer KF, Deletis V, Epstein FJ. Motor-evoked potential monitoring for intramedullary spinal cord tumor surgery: correlation of clinical and neurophysiological data in a series of 100 consecutive procedures. Neurosurg Focus. 1998;4(5):e1.
25. Calancie B, Harris W, Brindle GF, Green BA, Landy HJ. Threshold-level repetitive transcranial electrical stimulation for intraoperative monitoring of central motor conduction. J Neurosurg. 2001;95(Suppl. 2):161–8.
26. Amaro JWF. A história do Instituto de Psiquiatria do Hospital das Clínicas e do Departamento de Psiquiatria da Faculdade de Medicina da Universidade de São Paulo. Arch Clin Psychiatry (São Paulo). 2003;30(2):44–71.
27. Marino JR. Um cirurgião sob o olhar de Deus: uma introdução às ciências do cérebro, da mente e do espírito. 1st ed. Barueri-São Paulo: Manole; 2020.
28. Verst SM, de Castro I, Scappini-Junior W, de Melo MN, de Oliveira JR, de Almeida SS, Alvarez NRC, Sucena ACB, Barros MR, Marrone CD, Maldaun MVC. Methodology for creating and validating object naming and semantic tests used by Verst-Maldaun Language Assessment during awake craniotomies. Clin Neurol Neurosurg. 2021;202:106485. https://doi.org/10.1016/j.clineuro.2021.106485. PMID: 33476885.
29. Verst SM, de Aguiar PHP, Joaquim MAS, Vieira VG, Sucena ABC, Maldaun MVC. Monopolar 250-500 Hz language mapping: results of 41 patients. Clin Neurophysiol Pract. 2018;10(4):1–8. https://doi.org/10.1016/j.cnp.2018.11.002. PMID: 30619979; PMCID: PMC6312792.
30. Mathias RN, de Aguiar PH, da Luz Oliveira EP, Verst SM, Vieira V, Docema MF, Calfat Maldaun MV. “Next Door” intraoperative magnetic resonance imaging for awake craniotomy: preliminary experience and technical note. Surg Neurol Int. 2016;7(Suppl 40):S1021–7. https://doi.org/10.4103/2152-7806.195587. PMID: 28144477; PMCID: PMC5234280.
31. Verst SM, Melo MND, Caivano AS, Fonseca US, Mathias LR, Alves TV. Awake surgery versus VEP in tumors of visual pathway: case report. Interdiscip Neurosurg. 2020;20:100675.
32. de Freitas RMC, Caldas JGMP, Verst SM, Hoff AO, Bezerra Neto JE, Fragoso MCBV. Crossed-probes cryoablation for the treatment of a sclerotic vertebral metastasis abutting the spinal canal. J Vasc Interv Radiol. 2020;31(2):284–5. https://doi.org/10.1016/j.jvir.2019.11.006. PMID: 31997752.
33. Diário Oficial da União de 01 de março de 2016,seção 1, p.71. Resolução CFM 2136-2015 de 11 de dezembro de 2015.
34. Kimaid PAT. Monitorização Neurofisiológica Intraoperatória: Conceitos Básicos e Técnicas. 1st ed. Brazil: Thieme Revinter; 2019. p. 4.
35. Recommendation document for the exercise of Clinical Neurophysiology in Brazil. Executive Committee – Brazilian Society of Clinical Neurophysiology – Affiliated to the Brazilian Medical Association. https://sbnc.org.br/legislacao/

Chapter 2
Intraoperative Neurophysiological Monitoring in Brazil: Regulatory Aspects, Training, and Evidence Level

Carlo Domênico Marrone and Andréa Broisler Sucena Caivano

Abbreviations

AMB	Brazilian Medical Association
CDC	Código de Defesa do Consumidor
CFBM	Conselho Federal de Biomedicina
CFBM	Federal Council of Biomedicine
CFM	Conselho Federal de Medicina
CME	Comissão Mista de Especialidades – Joint Specialties' Commission
CRM	Conselho Regional de Medicina
EBM	Evidence-Based Medicine
EBP	Evidence-Based Practice
EEG	Electroencephalography
EMG	Electromyography
GRADE	Grading of Recommendations Assessment, Development and Evaluation
IONM	Intraoperative neurophysiological monitoring
IT	Information technology
MEP	Motor potentials
NP	Clinical Neurophysiology

C. D. Marrone (✉)
Brazilian Clinical Neurophysiology Society, Porto Alegre, RS, Brazil

Intraoperative Neurophysiological Monitoring, Department Coordinator of Hospital da Criança Santo Antônio, Porto Alegre, RS, Brazil

Universidade Federal de Ciências da Saúde de Porto Alegre - UFCSPA, Porto Alegre, RS, Brazil

Clínica Marrone, Clinical Neurophysiology, Porto Alegre, RS, Brazil
e-mail: Drmarrone@clinicamarrone.com.br

A. B. S. Caivano
Biomedical Technologist, Brain Spine Neurofisiologia, São Paulo, São Paulo, SP, Brazil

S. M. Verst et al. (eds.), *Intraoperative Monitoring*,
https://doi.org/10.1007/978-3-030-95730-8_2

NPh	Neurophysiologist
OR	Operating room
RCT	Randomized controlled trials
SBNC	Brazilian Society of Clinical Neurophysiology
SSEP	Somatosensory evoked potentials
TA	Technical assistant

Introduction

Clinical neurophysiology (NP) analyzes the generated or provoked signals present in tests such as electromyography (EMG), electroencephalography (EEG), polysomnography, EEG video, visual, auditory, somatosensory evoked potentials (SSEP) of upper and lower limbs, and motor potentials (MEP). It aims to assist in the diagnosis of several pathologies by assessing the central and peripheral nervous systems.

IONM combines in real time several tests according to the profile of each surgery and is individualized to patient needs. Tests are performed in a continuous and interspersed manner for an accurate and updated evaluation, meaning in multimodality. Frequently there is a short time opportunity for multifactorial data review before the reaction of the surgeon. It means that it is of cornerstone importance that the neurophysiologist (NPh) provides the best accurate analysis possible.

IONM fundamental goals are to avoid and reduce the risk of postoperative neurological deficits, to help the surgeon identify ambiguous neurological structures (e.g., tumor or normal brain? tumor or normal spinal cord?) and reversible neurophysiological changes. Hence, surgery has become safer since damage can be defined early on and the surgeons´ reaction can prevent deficits. It has a pedagogical role for the team involved in the surgery, especially for surgeons, who can master their skills, by identifying functional/physiological abnormalities related to their acts. This process will ultimately benefit the patient.

There are essential requirements for a safe IONM. First, *IONM is a medical procedure* performed by a NPh. Initial steps include clinical evaluation, analysis of preoperative tests, planning with the surgeon and the anesthesiologist the best strategy for the approach. NPh is responsible for the correct neurophysiological protocol planning and set-up, placement of needles and special electrodes (which demands knowledge of anatomy and physiology), connecting and checking wires, cables, and system, and ensuring that electrical safety and grounding steps were properly carried out. Planning steps include the correct allocation of the system in the crowded OR, where many people are circulating, and other electrical equipments are functioning. The NPh should properly communicate with the other members of the surgical and anesthesia team. Interpretation of IONM alterations should start an immediate interventional cascade. It is fully dependent on the ability of the NPh to *promptly* exclude technical errors, anesthesia influence, clinical lability (like decreased mean blood pressure or SO_2, hypercapnia), limb ischemia, and positional nerve compression, among others.

Medical Legal and Ethics Aspects

IONM is well established in Brazil according to the Federal Board of Medicine (Conselho Federal de Medicina – CFM) by resolution No. 2136, from 11th of December, 2015 [1]. We point out some of its important issues:

- Art. 1. "Intraoperative neurophysiological monitoring is a medical act".
- Art. 2. "The doctor is not authorized to perform surgical procedures with intraoperative neurophysiological monitoring conducted by a non-physician".
- Art. 6. "The surgeon is not authorized to perform intraoperative neurophysiological monitoring concomitantly with the surgical procedure".

The above-mentioned resolution also states that "Acts that support the performance of IONM may be shared with other professionals. These professionals might promote equipment setup, placement and removal of electrodes under on-site supervision by the physician in charge".

The role of technicians in the scope of INOM is discussed in item 4.

Yet, there is a civil law that states that any physician can perform any medical procedure [2]. Ethically it is clear that only skilled professionals should perform complex procedures like IONM, which directly affects patient's health. The most used example of this contradiction is if a non-specialized physician submitted a patient to a cardiac surgery. This physician is legally allowed to do that, according to law 3.268/1957, but it would be ethically reprehensible. Hence, the physician would be submitted to a lawsuit for malpractice, because of any impairment caused to the patient.

Last but not least, qualification control should start with hospitals, clinics, health insurance operators, and healthy managers [2]. Therefore, although this is a technical and highly specialized book, one cannot fail to contextualize the responsibilities of all those involved in patient care.

In Brazil, from the legal standpoint, civil liability in the medical field is generally governed by the Consumer Protection Code (Código de Defesa do Consumidor – CDC) [3]. Special attention should be paid to Article 14 and paragraph 4:

"Art. 14. The service provider is liable, regardless of guilt, for the compensation of the damage caused to customers for defects in the provision of the services, as well as for insufficient or inadequate information about their fruition and risks. [...]. [...] § 4 – Personal accountability of self-employed professionals shall be determined through the verification of guilt".

According to CDC, in cases of medical error, physicians shall be responsible for the damage caused if proved guilty because of malpractice, recklessness, or negligence. Hospitals, for example, are accountable for the damage caused regardless of proof of guilt, objectively in joint liability [3]. Just as there is joint civil liability of health insurance operators due to malpractice, i.e., "The health insurance operator and the benefits' administrator are jointly liable for the damage caused to beneficiaries, since both are part of the service supply chain in the consumption relationship" [4].

Additionally, hospitals and operating room (OR) managers (nurses/physicians) and healthcare personnel fail to inhibit medical material dealers to provide technicians to operate a system, as if it were IONM. This situation violates articles 1, 2, and 6 of the CFM resolution 2136/15 above-mentioned [1]. Besides, it is an illegal practice of medicine as described in the Brazilian penal code, Article 282. It identifies a criminal action as being the act of practicing a profession without authorization from the competent board or outside the limits imposed by the legislation [5].

The Brazilian Society of Clinical Neurophysiology (SBNC), aiming to assist the health assistance chain, i.e., physicians, hospital clinical and technical directors, and health insurance operators and administrators, issued Alert Statement 001/2020 [11]. It recalls normative resolution 2136/15 on the action of IONM and its legal malpractice consequences [1].

Which Medical Professional Is Qualified to Perform IONM?

The law 3.268/1957 states in its article 17 that "physicians may only legally practice medicine in any of its branches or specialties, after prior registration of their titles, diplomas or certificates under the Ministry of Education and Culture and under the Regional Board of Medicine (Conselho Regional de Medicina – CRM), in their due jurisdictions" [2].

It is required for the medical professionals to have proper training while dealing with a highly specialized area. To perform IONM they should master the knowledge of neuroanatomy, neuropathology, neurophysiological tests (instrumentation, electrical safety, application, and interpretation, etc.), anesthesia, and surgical approaches. Therefore, the most skilled and legally certified medical professional to perform IONM in Brazil is the clinical neurophysiologist.

Certification by competent boards ensures that proper qualification has been achieved. The Brazilian Medical Association (AMB) has granted the Brazilian Society of Clinical Neurophysiology (SBNC) the duty to apply a proficiency test in this area of activity for decades [6].

The resolution by the Federal Board of Medicine 2148/2016 decrees CME (Comissão Mista de Especialidades – Joint Specialties' Commission) from January 2016 in Article 5 states that "The CME will only recognize a medical specialty with a minimum of two-year training time and area of activity with a minimum of one-year training time, with a mandatory minimum annual workload of 2880 h". Moreover, in paragraph 2, it *clearly states* that "The competence matrix from which the time of medical specialty training or area of activity in AMB training programs accredited by a medical specialty society, shall be approved by the CME...". These requirements are contemplated by the SBNC, which provides a proof of knowledge based on the matrix of competence as determined by the CFM, granting the necessary expertise to the clinical NPh to perform IONM [7, 8].

Regarding medical colleagues who are not clinical NPh and are performing IONM, in Brazil, their performance is a medical act. There is no contention among physicians of different specialties, but we must conceptualize terms, so that we practice what we are empowered to perform, especially, but not only, in Head and Neck Surgery and Otorhinolaryngology. They perform laryngeal recurrent and facial nerves mapping, for which they have received proper training during medical residency. Yet, it should be considered totally different from the complex and multimodal tests performed by a NPh, which are included in the term IONM.

Mapping Versus Monitoring

There should be a comprehensive understanding of the terms "*Monitoring*" and "*Mapping*". In Portuguese, the words "*monitorizar*" or "*monitorar*" can be used without any distinction. They mean to do surveillance, to monitor, control, supervise, assess, and inspect. "Mapping", on the other hand, refers to making the map of, representing an area defined in a map, and in biology to locate and determine the relative distribution of the different parts of a whole [9]. From a neurophysiological point of view, these terms have different but complementary meanings [10, 11].

Monitoring refers to the multimodality and simultaneous neurophysiological techniques aiming to evaluate several neurological functions, i.e., somatosensory evoked potential, motor evoked potential, brain stem auditory evoked potential, electroencephalogram, electrocorticography, free running electromyography, triggered electromyography, bulbocavernosus reflex, etc. Among these techniques, several mappings of peripheral and central nervous system structures are included, such as mapping of the spinal cord dorsal column, medullary and brainstem nucleus, fourth ventricle floor, direct cortical and subcortical mapping for motor, language and cognitive eloquent areas, nerve roots, peripheral and cranial nerves, etc. Hence, *Mapping* is only a single part of a "world" represented by the act of monitoring.

In Brazil, a clinical neurophysiologist spends 2880 h of training in "*monitoring*". It is remarkable the difference with a training course of a *particular mapping technique*, like for laryngeal recurrent nerve, which duration reaches at most 270–280 h.

How to Teach IONM?

Proper training in IONM is a current concern worldwide. IONM is growing faster than the capability of training enough physicians. As a complex procedure that involves several types of neurophysiological tests, it takes time for the physician to build skills. Regarding how a physician should be trained in IONM some concepts are fundamental:

(a) The trainer (institution and/or individual) should have one or more personnel in-charge, with unquestionable experience, proficiency, and with certification from the legal Board (SBNC) [1, 6].

(b) Provide the appropriate means to conduct the training, with dedicated equipment and proper supplies, surgical approaches in different fields of Medicine (neurosurgery, orthopedics, vascular, head neck and otorhinolaryngology, and peripheral nerves).
(c) Respect the workload and the competency matrix determined by the certifier (SBNC) [7, 8].
(d) Theoretical classes on basics and advanced IONM clinical discussions.
(e) Provide a face-to-face and ongoing teaching/learning program. That is, the student should be in the OR time enough to fill the necessary number of supervised procedures and to discuss the multifactorial events happening during the approaches. The learning curve in IONM requires the student's presence in OR, handling the device, performing, and interpreting the neurophysiological tests. These requirements make online training impossible and inadmissible. Hence, IONM visualization through a virtual way, even if the surgery is taking place "in the room next door", is only *demonstration, never training*. Finally, training is an almost individual task, requiring a maximum of two students per monitoring. It is necessary for better learning purposes, and mainly for patient's safety not to have a crowdy OR. The above-mentioned criteria are not feasible during a "weekend" model of training, in which a group of 5–10 people huddle together to watch, not to participate in the neurophysiological procedure. "Weekend" training is not suitable for any neurophysiological modalities, like EMG, EEG, and EP. Most frequently it suits only the course-giver pocket.

What Is the Role of Medical Assistants/Technicians in IONM?

The Federal Board of Biomedicine (Conselho Federal de Biomedicina – CFBM) edited the Resolution 245/2014 on this subject [12]. Hence, the medical and the biomedical federal boards clearly stated in their resolutions that IONM is a medical procedure, and that the technical assistant (TA) can assist on IOM performance under on-site medical supervision.

TA may assist in terms of equipment, tests performing and electrodes placing and removal. They are not allowed to carry out the planning, decision making, analysis, and interpretation of tests according to the resolutions of regulatory agencies [1, 12]. The TA must be in the OR throughout the entire procedure [13, 14].

TA needs to have proper IOM skills and training. It is ideal to have a degree in any Health area like Biomedicine, Nursing or Physiotherapy, which provides knowledge and experience in patients care. Besides, knowledge of the anatomy and functions of the nervous system (Table 2.3) and knowledge of the electrophysiological parameters (Table 2.4) are required for optimal performance. In addition to the degree, TA's specific certification in IONM is recommended according to the standards of practice of each country. The sole Brazilian professional representation board that regulates the scope of TAs in IONM is the Federal Council of Biomedicine (CFBM).

They edited the Resolution 245/2014 [12], which states:

- "Art. 1: It is a duty of the Biomedical Professional to act *under medical supervision* in Transoperative Neurophysiological Monitoring, *operating specific equipment* for the activity and using electrophysiological methods such as EEG, EMG and SSEP to monitor the integrity of specific nerve structures during surgery."
- "Art. 2: The practice of the professional activity for Transoperative Neurophysiological Monitoring requires a specialization course, duly registered and approved by the Ministry of Education. The minimum disciplines should include Neuroanatomy, Neurophysiology, Basic and Advanced Neuropathology, Theory of Surgical Techniques, Applied Technologies and practical internship in Transoperative Neurophysiological Monitoring services duly registered and under professional supervision and Sanitary Surveillance."

Thus, the legally qualified biomedical is absorbed by specific segments of the labor market, naturally those related to diagnosis, research, and education, with the operation/handling of biomedical equipment and systems, and their participation in IONM is regulated by resolution 245/14 [13, 14].

In daily practice, TA arrives in the OR in advance to prepare the equipment and listed supplies. They set up the equipment, placing it in the room in the best spot not to interfere with other systems, adjusting boxes and cables. Under supervision of the NPh, he/she separates the electrodes that will be used and sets all the material organized and ready for placement. He/she assists in the placement of electrodes as planned by the NPh, allocating wires and cables in the best way so as not to harm patients and not to *run* the risk of being removed during patients positioning and along the procedure. He/she ensures all connections are properly set in the boxes according to the selected protocol and measures impedance. After baseline recordings, he/she follows the surgery, adjusting the system boxes, and assists with recordings when necessary. When the surgery is finished, the TA turns off the equipment, disassembles and puts everything away in the case, removes the electrodes, assisting until the end of the surgery.

The IONM system might be operated by TA under NPh supervision. For this task, it is required that the TA is trained in the software and hardware and masters knowledge about signals, waveforms, stimulation, filters, artifacts, electrode impedance and positioning, and troubleshooting. As Skinner and Holdefer say, the teamwork enhances results [15].

Is There Evidence and Level of Recommendation for IONM?

The experience of each physician or group of physicians in a given situation undoubtedly has its value in the handling decision-making. However, it is necessary to refine medical reasoning, to reduce the biases which may occur and, at the same time, produce more comprehensive knowledge. Thus, evidence-based medicine (EBM), a term coined by Guyatt in 1991, using epidemiological principles from Cochran and Feinstein, aims to improve medical reasoning. In 1992, the Evidence-Based Working Group proposed a systematic process of discovering, assessing, and using research to support clinical decision-making [16].

Jenicek (1997) organized the principles for this systematic process, that is, (a) formulation of a clear clinical question based on the patient's problem which needs to be responded to, (b) searching the literature for other relevant articles/sources of information, (c) critical assessment of the evidence, (d) selection of the best piece of evidence, (e) linking evidence with clinical experience, knowledge, and practice, (f) implementation of useful findings in clinical practice, (g) assessment of the overall performance and implementation by the MBE professional, and (h) teaching other physicians how to practice EBM [17, 18].

In the hierarchical pyramid of the evidence quality classification (Chart 2.1) and strength of recommendation (Table 2.1), controlled and randomized clinical trials have been at the top for many years, especially in the comparative assessment of

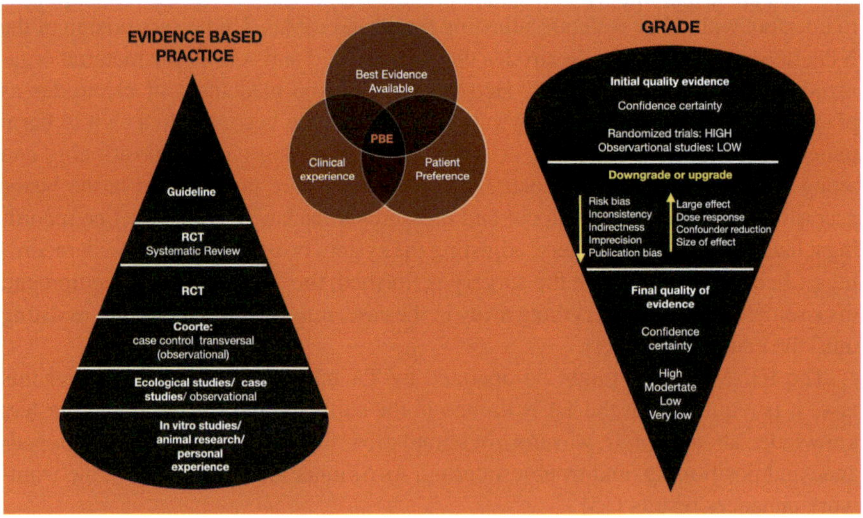

Chart 2.1 Evidence-based practice (EBP) and how we can relate it to GRADE (Grading of Recommendations Assessment, Development and Evaluation)

Table 2.1 Quality of evidence [25]

Class I	One or more prospective, blind and well-designed controlled studies
Class II	One or more well-designed clinical studies (case-control, cohort, etc.)
Class III	Expert opinion, non-randomized historical control and case reports

Table 2.2 Strength of recommendation [25]

Type A	Strongly positive based on Class I or very strong Class II
Type B	Positive in Class II
Type C	Positive based on strong Class III consensus
Type D	Negative based on conflictive or inconclusive Class II
Type E	Negative based on ineffective evidence
Type U	No recommendation based on insufficient data or divided expert opinion

randomized and non-randomized (observational) studies. In recent years, a great movement has been taking strength to consider how the study is conducted, identifying the specific sources of bias and the confidence limitations regarding the treatment effects [19, 20]. Although very relevant, randomized controlled trials (RCT) that assess treatment/outcomes may have serious limitations resulting from biases that have not been duly identified. On the other hand, observational studies for treatment and outcomes, which would normally have lower weight in the hierarchy of evidence quality classification, if well adjusted for confounding situations, may play an important role in supporting the evidence [21].

The evidence quality assessment by the GRADE (Grading of Recommendations Assessment, Development and Evaluation) method is used by several agencies (WHO, BMJ, NIH, etc.) and is a key element for better understanding in systematic reviews, randomized controlled trials, and non-randomized controlled (observational) trials [22]. *GRADE* aims to provide a high, moderate, low, or very low Evidence Certainty rating through domain assessments that serve as a grading tool. The domains are divided into risk of bias, inconsistency, indirect evidence, inaccuracy, and publication bias, among others. RCTs enter the GRADE method with a high level of evidence quality but depending on how they behave in the domains (risk of bias, inconsistency, indirect evidence, inaccuracy, publication bias, etc.), they may be downgraded, whereas the opposite may occur with observational studies [21].

Most studies on IONM are conducted as observational (they are not randomized controlled trials) and class I evidence is not found, being classified as class II and III – Tables 2.1 and 2.2 [19, 23]. However, as Sala (a neurosurgeon by the way) argues, much of the evidence used in neurosurgical treatment cases are also classified as class II and III (acute spinal cord injuries, aneurysms, traumatic head and brain injury, benign tumors, etc.). Thus, the level of evidence-based medicine in IONM is no worse than what is found in neurosurgery in general [23].

There is little research with comparative designs on the effects of treatment [21]. An explanation has been attributed to ethical and legal restrictions to perform randomized studies on IONM in surgeries with high risk of neurological injury [24]. Therefore, as an example, it would not be ethical/legal to conduct a research in scoliosis approach to: (a) assess the outcome of absence or presence of spinal cord injury having one group making use of IONM and not the other, (b) making surgeons and neurophysiologists blind to IOM alterations.

Therefore, as Holdefer and Skinner stated, comparative studies on the effectiveness of IONM on outcomes are both necessary and urgent. One cannot accept new technologies such as IONM as a "fad"/"hype cycle" (all that is new is good!), nor should we think that it will never be possible to design new studies based on the knowledge gathered by IONM [21, 23].

Concerning RCTs and IONM, there may be ethical/legal restrictions for surgeries with greater potential of causing harm to the nervous system. For those with less potential of harm there might be the possibility of RCT designs, despite the difficulties regarding trial costs and number of patients. If RCT is not possible, observational comparative studies can be conducted with all scientific rigor (e.g., using GRADE) to improve methods and, mainly, to adjust confounding factors (Chart 2.1). As Howick et al. stated, data records with perspectives of monitored and unmonitored controls offer the possibility of enough statistical power to detect small reductions in the already very low incidence of iatrogenic injuries [25]. A multi-centric collaboration in an attempt to constitute an observational cohort study might represent an excellent alternative to the difficulties of conducting a controlled trial in IONM [25]. As a matter of fact, given the expertise of countless colleagues among us, why not do this in Brazil and Latin America? (Table 2.3).

The 2021–2022 SBNC directory's recommendations for the several types of IONM were under construction by the time of release of this book. The process includes the systematic review phase according to the GRADE method with the elaborated questions under discussion using the PICO method – Patients,

Table 2.3 Description of basic knowledge for TA

Decubitus
Median, sagittal, frontal, transversal planes
Central and peripheral nervous system – which are the structures
Anatomy of the brain – frontal, parietal, temporal, and occipital lobes – spatial vision and main functions
Sympathetic and parasympathetic autonomous system – basic function
Peripheral nervous system – basic function
Anatomy of cranial pairs, muscles to be needled

Interventions, Comparison and Outcomes [26]. Recommendations and degrees of evidence of the American Society of Clinical Monitoring dated 2013 are available elsewhere [17].

Remote or On-Site Neurophysiologist? From Dream to Reality in Brazil

Nowadays, the possibility of assisting the patient with the most diverse and modern technologies is a fact, even if one does not have them all in one place. Telemedicine is a practice of distance medicine, whose interventions, diagnoses, treatment decisions, and recommendations are based on data, documents, and other information transmitted through telecommunications systems. It can contribute in an important way to patients' well-being as Tel Aviv Declaration [27].

In Neurology there are areas supported by adequate technological and care-related infrastructures, which can be safely applied via teleneurology, such as the Neurovascular area (with its Stroke units) and Neurointensive care. According to Maldonado et al. (2016) telemedicine has an interdisciplinary nature, requiring integration from different fields of knowledge, like information technology (IT), telecommunications, equipment development, security protocols of data transmission, etc. [28].

INOM is inserted in the context of modern technologies which greatly assist patients and the anesthesia-surgical teams and, in many countries, is remotely performed [29]. However, technical conditions (the dream) are not readily available for remote IONM via telemedicine in Brazil and many other countries, at least nowadays (reality) (Table 2.4).

The topic has already led to heated discussions. Even though remote INOM is carried in some places around the world, one must respect the particularities of each country. After a careful review and peers´ discussion, SBNC decided to strongly recommend in-site NPh (in the OR) – IONM. This complex topic was analyzed in different perspectives to improve the SBNC level of recommendation, as shown below.

Table 2.4 Basic understanding requirements of electrophysiological parameters

What is electrical activity?
What is amplitude?
What is an electrode?
What is potential?
What is an amplifier?

Remote IONM

IONM, similarly to anesthesia, is traditionally performed by an in-site physician. Most important, classical proof of the efficacy of IONM in surgeries according to class I and II evidence was established in this traditional model, i.e., NPh in the OR [30].

Which Would Be the Best Way to Convey IONM in a Remote Technique (Dream)?

In the USA, there is a rule guide for remote IOM detailing physician supervision. It describes each participant's role, including which media might be used for external communication among them [29]. Yet, there is no consensus on the most suitable way to collect, transmit, supervise, etc., data in IONM. Some even suggest that supervision could be done via mobile phone (call, text message, chat, WhatsApp, etc.), whereas others criticize this situation fervently [29, 31].

For EMG outpatient examination, an attempt has been made to establish a protocol via telemedicine. It required installation of real-time capture cameras with accurate focus on needle placement, sound registration, and data image/charts of the system screen, among other requirements. It proved to be an ineffective tool for a correct diagnosis decision [32].

Comparisons between remote IONM with the "telestroke initiative" were held by Skinner and Sala [31, 33–36]. They pointed out that the main concern in a stroke situation is deciding whether to use a thrombolytic agent, whereas in IONM there is "an ongoing flow of neurophysiological data integrated to the surgical context that is in constant change".

Regarding remote IONM, difficulties like data confidentiality, exposure of medical data in communication systems, and adoption of the in-site-remote-physician real-time connection should be overcome [31]. For ethical reasons, the patient should be offered the same technical conditions (including personnel and others), either at in-site or in-remote physician assessment [37]. Hence, IONM should be interpreted in both endings of the chain by skilled physicians specialized in neurophysiology, allowing real-time full access to images and sounds from the OR, and encompassing at least the following [38]:

1. Operating table with patient positioning.
2. Wiring and cabling of IONM equipment and IONM screen in real time.
3. Verbal communication between the physicians involved in IONM and the anesthesiologist, without disturbing the ongoing surgery.
4. Straightforward view of the anesthetist screen for immediate access to data on mean arterial pressure, oximetry, capnography, heart rate, etc.
5. Straightforward communication, that is, sound and image from surgical team.
6. Visualization of surgical field through cameras placed on light spots and/or on microscopes.

What Is the Ideal Distance from the OR? Should the Physician In-Charge Be Inside or Outside the Same Hospital Where IONM Is Taking Place? Could He/She Be Out of Town, Outside the State or Abroad? How Many IONMs Could be Supervised Simultaneously by the NPh In-Charge?

The acceptable distance which the PHh could keep from the OR (we must never forget that IONM should be patient-centered) and the number of simultaneous IONM one physician could carry out are very controversial. The American Academy of Neurology conducted an e-mail survey asking neurologists about the volume, types of cases, duration, number of simultaneous cases, and location of the monitoring physician [39]. Among those who responded to the survey, 86% did it locally, 37% of which did it only inside the OR, 65% were close-by, entering the room if necessary, and it was observed that some did both (sum greater than 100%). Out of the 23% who did it "online", 15% did it only remotely. Most neurologists who conducted the remote cases did 2.2 cases at a time. People who monitored locally, performed many more intracranial cases whereas those who did remote monitoring had typically more spinal cases.

Dormans, 2010, in reference to remote IONM, did the following questions [40]:

(a) "How well can an individual outside the OR interpret fluctuating IONM data and develop a plausible explanation for this?
(b) How is it possible for a remote professional to deliver an appropriate level of surveillance if multiple cases are being monitored?
(c) How can an individual who has never done IONM and who is at a distance from the OR have or develop the necessary skills and expertise to make accurate and reliable decisions?
(d) What happens if remote connectivity is lost?
(e) What forensic accountability will be taken by the remote professional in case of misinterpretation, negligence, etc.?"

What Is the Reliability of IONM Performed by Telemedicine?

If communication interruption via connection means even in the best centers happens, more so would it in developing countries [36]. Thus, there may be a serious breach in the neurophysiological procedure safety, especially if it happens at a crucial moment of the surgery.

Even if the above-mentioned situations do not occur (dream), some crucial issues about communication and reliability between the anesthesia-surgery-neurophysiology teams should be considered. According to the Joint Commission on Accreditation of Healthcare Organization, communication dysfunction has caused medical errors, though in sentinel events, 65% of the time between 1995 and 2004 [41]. Yet, neither the usage of any sophisticated technology in order to enable a remote IONM, nor any telemedicine support and devices, even if well applied, could replace personal interaction. Easy communication between specialists is what ultimately reduces and avoids errors [36, 42].

An IONM intervention cascade can be summarized by the following sequence: performance of test, interpretation of findings, communication between the team, intervention, and outcome [42]. For this cascade to really work, an essential element is trust between peers during surgery. It may sound simple, but it is of vital importance and must be established long before a possible moment of crisis (e.g., signal loss in the MEP [36, 42]. The clear dialogue between doctors follows the same line, both "spoken" and visual/gestural, especially in urgent situations, because straightforward communication between physicians through posture, gestures, expressions, visual contact, etc., helps in the interpretation and adds meaning to the information being shared [43].

Therefore, familiarity between teams in the OR is also a factor that has influence on good performance, significantly reducing interruption in the surgical flow and leading to fewer errors per case [44]. There is evidence, according to Neilly [45] that communication between teams in the OR and awareness of what is happening goes along with better patient outcomes.

Skinner et al. [42] believe that despite good intentions, professionals outside the OR can be frustrated by hindrances that block essential medical information, inadequate ability to deal with a given situation, burden of multiple supervised cases, and insufficient technology. They may have difficulty in collaborating with teams during surgery and reduced awareness of the severity of the threatening situation. These conditions may affect IONM reliability, even when the NPh is present in the room. So, how can one expect reliability with the NPh at a distance or when IONM is done by an unskilled person?

Although technological barriers exist, especially in a country of the size and diversity such as Brazil (low-speed and unstable internet, instability of electricity; electrical interference of the OR in IONM equipment, etc.) it is expected that in the future such difficulties could be overcome. Yet, it is not only a matter of better communication infrastructure, enabling better data transmission (the dream), but also of what can be effectively accomplished to ensure the total safety of the patient (reality). Additionally, there is the lack of skilled personnel to be overcome worldwide (reality).

Conflict of Interest

It is important that institutions ensure good medical practice for their patients, supervising to prevent malpractice and surgical approaches from being performed by non-experts and not properly trained personnel.

A tough issue is the relation between medicine, business, and profit. Any relationship involving people (physicians and their patients), institutions (hospitals), dealers, and healthcare companies should practice the four principles of bioethics: (a) beneficence, (b) non-maleficence, (c) autonomy, and (d) justice. Withdrawing from this way might result in losing the focus on the patient and on the relief from his/her ailments. Hence, the doctor-patient relationship should always be based on trust, honesty, and best possible evidence for handling the illness. It should exclude external interferences which may lead to improper care.

There has been a growing interest from system manufacturers and medical suppliers in IONM worldwide. It has resulted in better devices, stimulators, probes, and electrodes. Yet, in Brazil, some companies, aiming to increase their profits, sell supplies and provide "monitoring operators" included in the price. Most frequently those operators are non-medical personnel or physicians without proper skills. In this situation a relevant question arises: If there is a bad outcome, whose responsibility, is it? Usually, the surgeon, hospital, and healthcare insurance are issued to pay for the damage. It is strongly recommended that the service supplier be included in this equation.

Conclusion

By now we cannot take the risk to perform remote IONM in Brazil and in many other countries. We shall be careful not to mistake "IONM expansion", meaning more skilled physicians, with increasing business profits at the expense of patient safety.

Finally, this chapter aimed to bring up tough issues that are usually left behind in textbooks, but strongly interferes with daily work. Bringing them to real life context, where the main actors of the play are (patients, surgeons, NPh, hospital managers, professional councils, health care insurance, and regulatory agencies), may contribute to the reflection on how to improve patient care.

References

1. Medicina CF. RESOLUÇÃO N° 2.136, DE 11 DE DEZEMBRO DE 2015 – Disciplina o procedimento de monitorização neurofisiológica intraoperatória como ato médico exclusivo. Diário Oficial da União. 2016, 01 março;Ed. 40:70.
2. Brasil. Lei 3.268/1957 artigo 17.
3. BRASIL. Lei n°.8.078 de 11 de Setembro de 1990: Código de Defesa do Consumidor. Disponível em: http://www.planalto.gov.br/ccivil_03/leis/l8078.htm. Acesso em: Mar. de 2017b.
4. Código de Defesa do Consumidor Arts. 7°, parágrafo único; 25, § 1°; e 34, todos do CDC. Entendimento do TJDFT de 15/01/2020.
5. Código Penal – Decreto-Lei n° 2.848, de 7 de dezembro de 1940, artigo 282.
6. www.sbnc.org.br/titulos (edital de concurso para obtenção do certificado de área de atuação em neurofisiologia clínica).
7. Resolução do Conselho Federal de Medicina 2148/2016,portaria CME 01/2016 (www.sbnc.org.br/informativos/22-02-19).
8. www.sbnc.org.br/titulos (matriz de competência).
9. https://www.infopedia.pt/dicionarios/lingua-portuguesa/mapear
10. www.sbnc.org.br (newsletter sbnc n° 20 – 10 de abril de 2020 – Alerta 001/2020).
11. https://www.infopedia.pt/dicionarios/lingua-portuguesa/monitorar

12. Resolução do CFBM 2457/2014. http://crbm1.gov.br/novosite/wp-content/uploads/2013/12/RESOLU%C3%87%C3%83OCFBM-n%C2%BA-245.2014.Monitoramento.pdf
13. https://crbm1.gov.br/site2019/wpontent/uploads/2021/03/Manual_do_Biomedo_2021_V4.pdf
14. Nuwer MR. Regulatory and medical-legal aspects of intraoperative monitoring. J Clin Neurophysiol. 2002;19(5):387–95.
15. Skinner AS, Holdefer RN. The intraoperative neurophysiological monitoring team. Neurophysiol Neurosurg. 2020;44:607–21.
16. Evidence-Based Working Group. Evidence-based medicine. A new approach to teaching the practice of medicine. JAMA. 1992;268:2420–5.
17. Jenicek M. Epidemiology, evidenced-based medicine, and evidence-based public health. J Epidemiol. 1997;7(4):187–97.
18. Cartiel LD, Póvoa ED. Medicina Baseado em Evidência: Novo Paradigma assistencial e pedagógico? Interface-Comunicação, Saúde, Educação. 2002;11:113–32.
19. MacDonald DB, Skinner S, Shils J, Yingling C. Intraoperative motor evoked potential monitoring – a position statement by the American Society of Clinical Monitoring. Clin Neurophysiol. 2013;124:2291–316.
20. Djulbegovic B, Guyatt GH. Progress in evidence-based medicine: a quarter century on. Lancet. 2017;390(10092):415–23.
21. Holdefer RN, Skinner AS. Evidence-based medicine and intraoperative neurophysiology. Neurophysiol Neurosurg. 2020;43:607–21.
22. Guyatt GH, Oxman AD, Vist GE, Kunz R, Falck-Ytter Y, Alonso-Coello P, Schünemann HJ, GRADE Working Group. GRADE: an emerging consensus on rating quality of evidence and strength of recommendations. BMJ. 2008;336(7650):924–6.
23. Sala F. Intraoperative neurophysiology is here to stay. Childs Nerv Syst. 2010;26(4):413–7.
24. Nuwer MR, Emerson RG, Galloway G, Legatt AD, Lopez J, Minahan R, et al. Evidence-based guideline update: intraoperative spinal monitoring with somatosensory and transcranial electrical motor evoked potentials: report of the Therapeutics and Technology Assessment Subcommittee of the American Academy of Neurology and the American Clinical Neurophysiology Society. Neurology. 2012;78(8):585–9.
25. Howick J, Cohen BA, McCulloch P, Thompson M, Skinner SA. Foundations for evidence-based intraoperative neurophysiological monitoring. Clin Neurophysiol. 2016;127(1):81–90.
26. Guyatt G, Rennie D, Meade M, Cook D, editors. Users' guides to the medical literature: a manual for evidence-based clinical practice. American Medical Association; 2015.
27. Declaração de Tel Aviv sobre responsabilidades e normas éticas na utilização da telemedicina [Internet] 1999.
28. Maldonado JM, Marques AB, Cruz A. Telemedicine: challenges to dissemination in Brazil. Cad Saude Publica. 2016;32(Suppl 2):e00155615.
29. Gertsch JH, Moreira JJ, Lee GR, Hastings JD, Ritzl E, Eccher MA, et al. Practice guidelines for the supervising professional: intraoperative neurophysiological monitoring. J Clin Monit Comput. 2019;33(2):175–83.
30. Emerson RG, Husain AM. Blurring of local and remote practice models threatens IOM's future. Neurology. 2013;80(12):1076–7.
31. Skinner SA, Aydinlar EI, Borges LF, Carter BS, Currier BL, Deletis V, et al. Is the new ASNM intraoperative neuromonitoring supervision "guideline" a trustworthy guideline? A commentary. J Clin Monit Comput. 2019;33(2):185–90.
32. Simmons SC, Moore DP, Wells J. Evaluation of technical approaches to tele-electromyography via internet protocol networks. Telemed e-Health. 2007;13(1):33–9.
33. Wechsler LR, Tsao JW, Levine SR, Swain-Eng RJ, Adams RJ, Demaerschalk BM, et al. Teleneurology applications: report of the telemedicine work Group of the American Academy of Neurology. Neurology. 2013;80(7):670–6.
34. Sarfo FS, Adamu S, Awuah D, Ovbiagele B. Tele-neurology in sub-Saharan Africa: a systematic review of the literature. J Neurol Sci. 2017;380:196–9.

35. Martins SC, Pontes-Neto OM, Alves CV, de Freitas GR, Filho JO, Tosta ED, et al. Past, present, and future of stroke in middle-income countries: the Brazilian experience. Int J Stroke. 2013;8(Suppl A100):106–11.
36. Skinner S, Sala F. Communication and collaboration in spine neuromonitoring: time to expect more, a lot more, from the neurophysiologists. J Neurosurg Spine. 2017;27(1):1–6.
37. Skinner S. Patient-centered care model in IONM: a review and commentary. J Clin Neurophysiol. 2013;30(2):204–9.
38. Stoecklein VM, Faber F, Koch M, Mattmuller R, Schaper A, Rudolph F, et al. Optional real-time display of intraoperative neurophysiological monitoring in the microscopic field of view: avoiding communication failures in the operating room. Acta Neurochir. 2015;157(11):1843–7.
39. Nuwer MR, Cohen BH, Shepard KM. Practice patterns for intraoperative neurophysiologic monitoring. Neurology. 2013;80:1156–60.
40. Dormans JP. Establishing a standard of care for neuromonitoring during spinal deformity surgery. Spine. 2010;35(25):2180–5.
41. Joint Commission on Accreditation of Healthcare Organizations. National patient safety goals for 2005 and 2004, 2006. Available at: https://www.jointcommission.org/assets/1/6/2006_Annual_Report. Accessed 3 Aug 2016.
42. Skinner S, Holdefer R, McAuliffe J, Sala F. Medical error avoidance in intraoperative neurophysiological monitoring: the communication imperative. J Clin Neurophysiol. 2017;7:1–7.
43. Solet DJ, Norvell JM, Rutan GH, Frankel RM. Lost in translation: challenges and opportunities in physician-to-physician communication during patient handoffs. Acad Med. 2005;80:1094–9.
44. ElBardissi AW, Wiegmann DA, Henrickson S, Wadhera R, Sundt TM III. Identifying methods to improve heart surgery: an operative approach and strategy for implementation on an organizational level. Eur J Cardiothorac Surg. 2008;34:1027–33.
45. Neily J, Mills PD, Young-Xu Y, et al. Association between implemen- tation of a medical team training program and surgical mortality. JAMA. 2010;304:1693–700.

Chapter 3
Muscle Motor Point Atlas and Needling Pitfalls

Bruno Nogueira da Silva and Tae Mo Chung

Abbreviations

CMAP	compound muscle action potential
EMG	electromyography
IOM	intraoperative monitoring
M	muscle
mMEP	muscle motor evoked potential
MU	motor unit
TES	transcranial electrical stimulation

Motor Point Concept

The motor point concept as we will apply in this section will have a practical purpose and will be referred to the intramuscular region with the highest density of motor plates (motor plate zone). This region rich in motor plate terminals is the preferred neurophysiologic target for measuring the electrical phenomena of motor units. Its privileged position near the region of onset of depolarization of the muscle fiber produces less phase cancellation effect and higher recording amplitudes translating finally to a better signal-to-noise ratio.

Extramuscular motor point, a term applied to the region of entry of the motor branch in the muscle belly, does not correspond anatomically to the region of the

B. N. da Silva (✉)
Clinical Neurophysiologist by Brain Spine Neurofisiologia, Jundiai, SP, Brazil

T. M. Chung
Clinical Neurophysiology Coordinator, Physical Medicine and Rehabilitation Department at the Clinical Hospital of University of São Paulo Medical School, São Paulo, SP, Brazil

S. M. Verst et al. (eds.), *Intraoperative Monitoring*,
https://doi.org/10.1007/978-3-030-95730-8_3

motor plate zone and has other practical purposes (e.g., phenolic chemo denervation and application of functional electrical currents for rehabilitation). Despite the availability of practical manuals on the subject, the conceptual confusion between these different muscle sub-regions and the absence of specific anatomical and histological research of the regions of concentration of plaques per muscle in the body make attempts to formulate these so-called motor point maps inaccurate [1, 8, 9]. Considering these limitations, we have drawn up a small suggested topographical guide for positioning muscle needle recording electrodes targeting the motor plate zone.

Production of Muscle Potentials

This subject has already been covered in other chapters. We will go through some basic concepts that will help you understand how the recording of muscle potentials can be optimized.

The nomenclature of intraoperative monitoring (IOM) sometimes uses the term compound muscle action potentials (CMAP) for both muscle action potentials generated by transcranial electrical stimulation (TES) discharged in the central nervous system and potentials originating from direct stimulation of peripheral nerves (peripheral CMAP). Yet, a distinction is reasonable and already stablished [13] since the methodology applied for generating the peripheral CMAP and muscle motor evoked potentials (mMEP) are different. Peripheral CMAP are obtained by a single pulse while mMEP generally requires a synchronized "bombardment" of excitatory potentials in the lower motor neuron.

As the stimulus intensity increases, a progressive number of motor units (MU) are recruited in an almost linear fashion until the total number of MUs is reached (supramaximal stimulation). By TES, the sequence of stimuli causes recruitment of fractions of the MUs at the motor point and is triggered from the first to the nth pulse (usually 3–7 pulses). The amount of MUs recruited per pulse is variable and theoretically the same unit can be recruited at different moments within the train of stimuli provided the absolute refractory time of the neuron involved in impulse generation has passed.

Additionally, spontaneous electromyography (EMG) activity recordings are also dependent on proper needling.

Muscle-Potentials Generators (the Motor UNIT)

The depolarization of the MU is the elementary phenomenon that will produce the muscle potentials (CMAP and mMEP). MU is the peripheral motor functional unit composed of the body of the second motor neuron (located at the anterior horn of the spinal cord), its axon, neuromuscular junction (motor plate), and all the muscle fibers it innervates.

The amplitude of a CMAP, mMEP and spontaneous EMG activity recording is influenced by the amount of muscle fibers per MU of the muscle in question, the average diameter of the muscle fibers, and the spatial distribution of the MU within the muscle belly. Each muscle in the body has a quantitative pattern of muscle fibers per MU and the greater this number, the larger the size of the MU. Thus, one MU can supply 6–10 muscle fibers in the orbicular eye muscle to hundreds of fibers as in the bicipital muscle [7]. The area of motor fibers influenced by a particular motor neuron is called the MU territory and varies depending on the muscle [17], with an estimated diameter of 5–10 mm in the biceps brachii [16]. As for muscle fiber size, we know that appendicular muscles of the upper and lower limbs have an average fiber diameter of 40–50 and 50–60 μm, and a smaller number in facial muscles (20–30 μm diameter/fiber) [2, 14]. Thus, reduced recording amplitudes are expected in smaller muscles.

These concepts can help to understand the extreme variation in morphology between the different stimulus trains according to the muscle studied, reinforcing the importance of bringing the recording electrode as close as possible to the motor point region for the best electrical representation of the muscle in question. In this way, the sum of the MU potentials recorded after a stimulation will determine the amplitude of the final CMAP or mMEP. The deflagration of the action potential of each MU is of the all-or-nothing type. Thus, an isolated MU of great amplitude that is close to the recording electrode and that has its excitability varying between stimuli (or eventually becoming difficult to obtain as the anesthetic fading phenomenon evolves) can become a source of concern during surgery and eventually triggers a false-positive alarm.

Recording Electrodes

The proximity of the recording electrode to the generator source according to the generator electric dipole and conduction volume theory influences the amplitudes and morphology of the recorded responses in different ways. The types of electrodes available for muscle recording have been covered in the EMG Chap. 11. Here we will reinforce the electrical generators recording theory according to the electrodes available and how their proximity to the muscle and motor point can influence the amplitudes and morphology of the potentials.

Available for motor recordings are surface electrodes, insulated and non-insulated needle electrodes. In surface recording a larger amount of distant MU fibers contribute to the potential [15].

Each type of needle electrode has different recording characteristics as in Table 3.1.

Although not well studied, the area of recording of non-insulated needles occurs throughout the whole needle surface. The region of recording is along the entire

Table 3.1 Characteristics of recordings according to electrode type

Electrode	Recording surface	Recording area
Monopolar insulated needle	640 μm	0.12–0.34 mm^2 (10–20 fibers)
Concentric needle	150 and 580 μm	0.07 mm^2 (10–20 fibers)
Single fiber needle	25 μm	0.0005 mm^2 (2 muscle fibers)
MacroEMG	Un-insulated distal 15 mm of needle	Large 300–2000 fibers

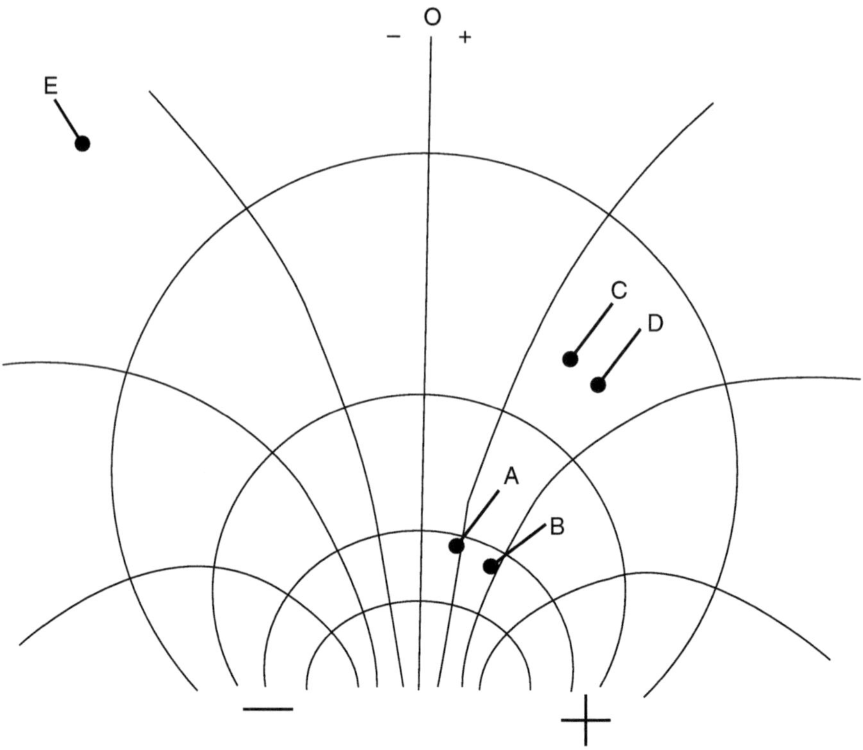

Fig. 3.1 Potential generators in relation to source generators. (A, B): near-field bipolar recording, (C, D): far-field bipolar recording, (A, E): near-field monopolar recording. (D, E): far-field monopolar recording. (This figure was published in Daniel Dumitru, Machiel J Zwarts, Anthony A. Amato (Editors), Electrodiagnostic medicine, 2nd ed. Chapter 2 Electrical sources and volume conduction, Page 28, Copyright Elsevier (2002). Reprinted with permission)

needle and the resulting potential is an average of the electrical fields in proximity to the entire needle denudated surface.

According to the theory of conduction volume and electric dipole recording, assemblies embracing more isopotential lines and closer to the electrical generators record higher values of electric dipole voltage (Fig. 3.1). Thus, the monopolar or near-field reference assembly (A-E and B-E) will exhibit potentials of higher amplitudes, followed by the bipolar near-field assembly (A-B). The lowest amplitudes would be registered in the bipolar far-field (C-D) and monopolar far-field (C-E or D-E) assemblies. These last two assemblies would be representative of the recording method with short (non-insulated) subdermal needles.

Beyond the concept of isopotential lines, the closer the point chosen for the study of the motor point (the main generator of the muscle electric dipole, due to containing the highest concentration of motor plates), the greater the chance of recording more robust CMAP/mMEP. The distance between the generating unit (MU motor plate zone) and the capture electrode is a very important component for higher CMAP/mMEP amplitudes (Fig. 3.2). It relies on Faraday's electric field law

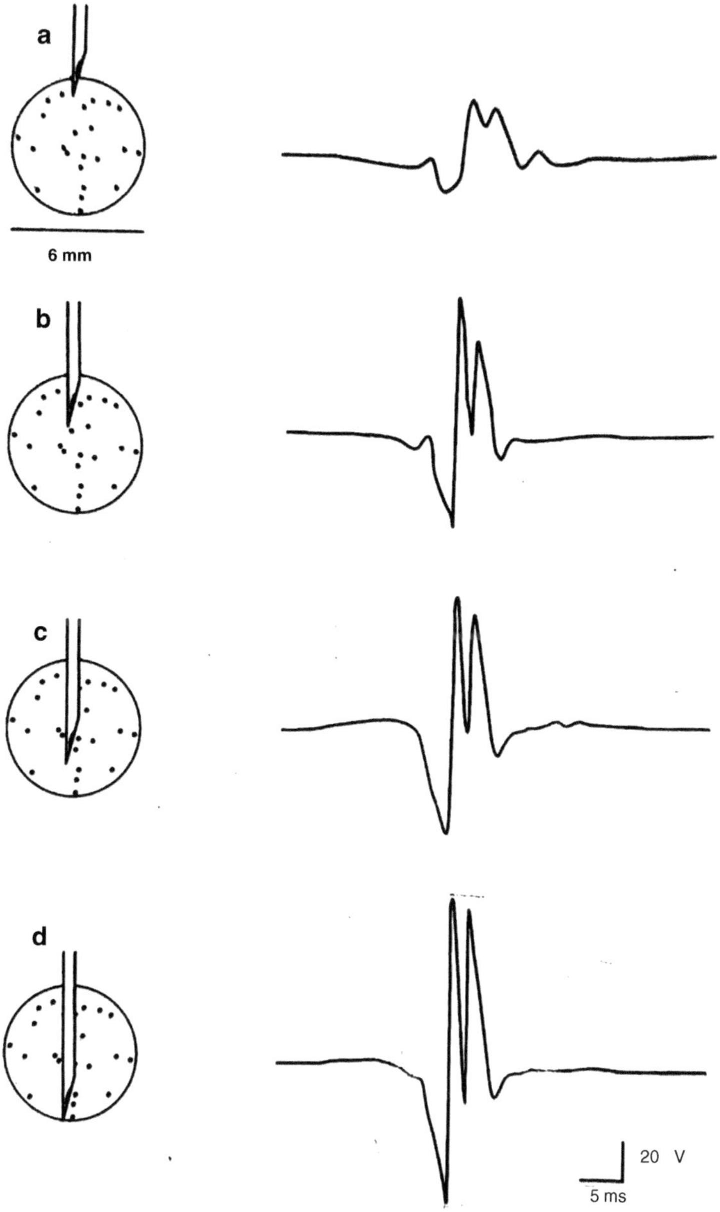

Fig. 3.2 Muscle Fiber Motor Unit Territory. Position of the recording needle in relation to the muscle motor point directly relates to CMAP/mMEP amplitude and EMG activity recording. Muscle fibers belonging to one MU are randomly distributed within a 6 mm-oval territory. Four separate CMAP waveforms (all representing the same MU) are recorded from four different locations: close to (A) or within the MU (B-D). The more the recording tip is located within the MU territory (B-D), the greater the resulting potential. (This figure was published in Daniel Dumitru, Machiel J Zwarts, Anthony A. Amato (Editors), Electrodiagnostic medicine, 2nd ed. Chapter 2 Electrical sources and volume conduction, Page 72, Copyright Elsevier (2002). Reprinted with permission)

($F = kQq/d^2$), which states that the magnitude of the circulating electrical field is directly related to the area enclosed in the loop. Hence, the amplitude of the recorded potential is directly related to the current density, which decreases with an increase in distance from the generator [6]. The greater the distance between the needle and the muscle motor point, the smaller the amplitude of the recorded potential. This principle substantiates the optimized positioning of needles near the electrical generator during any IOM recording.

An important and under-discussed aspect is the effect that bare and insulated needles have on recorded muscle activity and CMAP/mMEP. In general, larger recording surfaces result in slighter smaller potentials. Although larger electrodes will obviously record from a larger area of volume conductor, they will "average out" different contributions from individual MUs [6]. Yet, insulated needles or hook-wire electrodes selectively record over the distal tip area. There is an absence of specific studies on needles differences in IOM. Hence, a parallel can be established with the concepts gained from the electromyography (EMG) laboratory. Monopolar needles and macro-EMG needles have similar recording areas as 13–15 mm-bare needles [10]. Experiments with progressive Teflon denudation (thus enlarging recording surface) of reusable EMG monopolar needles points to impairment of spontaneous muscle activity and recruitment pattern analysis [3].

Obese Patients

The muscle electric dipole field in response to stimulation attenuates exponentially as the distance between the record electrode and the generating muscle fibers increases (Faraday's 2nd law). Signal attenuation will be higher in the presence of thicker adipose tissue, which will enlarge this distance.

Jahangiri [11] studied 13 patients comparing the use of paired 13 mm and paired 18 mm, 25 mm, 37 mm, and 50 mm insulated needles for recording mMEPs from the rectus femoris muscle. Records were obtained in 12 patients (92.3% of cases) with 37 and 50 mm insulated needles and in only one patient with 13 mm needle. Recordings through the 37 and 50 mm needles increased the chances of acquiring MEPs even with lower TES thresholds.

Kim et al. [12] showed a relationship between obesity and the risk of false positives, possibly related to small mMEPs.

Morphology and Amplitude of Motor Potentials as a Function of the Position of the Needles in the Muscle Belly

The central positioning of the motor plate in muscles is strategic and provides a better dispersion of the action potential bidirectionally along the muscle fiber membrane. Although there are anatomic scattered motor plates throughout the muscle body, the zone of greatest concentration is generally located near the midpoint of the muscle belly.

The motor plate location within a muscle is directly influenced by the muscle morphology [18]. Histological studies with acetylcholinesterase staining are gold-standard for analysis but are scarce. The presumed location of the motor point in a given muscle is in the middle of the muscle belly, especially in fusiform muscles [4]. In longitudinal muscles such as sartorius and gracilis the motor plate zones tend to be more distributed in a scattered manner along the entire long muscle belly. In unipennate muscles, a transverse band rich in motor plates has been found in the middle of the muscle, whereas in bipennate muscles the motor plate band would tend to be concave [2]. A more comprehensive understanding of muscle anatomy and motor plate distribution is not the scope of this chapter.

Relationship Between CMAP and mMEP

Peripheral nerve stimulation can be used to measure pharmacological neuromuscular junction blockage. A four-stimulus repeatedly applied results in equal number of CMAPs if there is no blockage. Degree of blockage will be inferred by the number of acquired CMPAs. For example, 2 CMAPs in 4 stimulus represents 50% blockage.

Establishing the comparison between CMAP and mMEP improves IOM quality in many aspects, for example, during peripheral nerve approach (Chap. 31). If there is no proper previous EMG study, identifying atrophied muscles by peripheral nerve stimulation in operating room allows to consider better strategies for recording, such as adding muscles to the protocol or changing the insertion point of the needles.

Another way to correlate CMAP and mMEP is to perform supramaximal peripheral nerve and TES stimulation. The comparison between them would predict the quantity of MUs elicited. For example, by corticonuclear MEP it is supposed that only one-fifth of the motor pathway is activated by TES [5]. Moreover, if only low amplitude CMAP can be recorded, most probably there will be equally low amplitude mMEP. It is the expected situation for small or atrophied muscles, or for inadequate needles placement. Last but not least, there is an unpredictable pattern of atrophy within a MU and among MUs.

Conclusion

As sophisticated and complex as IOM might be, it does not preclude from very basic concepts of neurophysiology. IOM comprises several steps that must be observed individually. The technique of electrode placement is a fundamental one since repositioning is frequently impossible once the procedure has begun. The goal is to elicit the best, the greatest, and more well-defined mMEP, CMAP, and EMG activity as possible. It optimizes the recording using basic concepts regarding electrical generators and conduction volume theories.

Needle placement should be the closest to the region of greatest concentration of motor plates as possible. Thus, understanding the different muscle morphologies provides ballast for the needling technique.

The accumulation of knowledge will point to the most effective types of needles for intraoperative muscle recordings. Costs versus benefits should not be overlooked. At present, there is a lack of uniformity of opinions and practice regarding IOM needle selection.

Muscle Motor Points

M. frontalis (Picture 3.3)

<table>
<tr><td>Origin: Skin of the eyebrow.</td><td rowspan="5">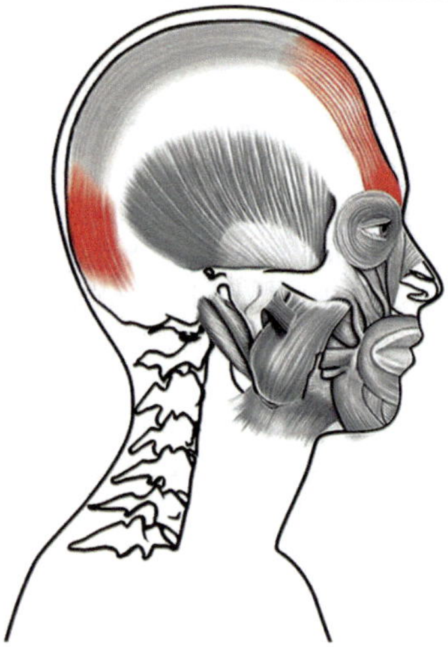</td></tr>
<tr><td>Insertion: Joins the occipital muscle in the aponeurotic galea.</td></tr>
<tr><td>Innervation: Facial nerve</td></tr>
<tr><td>Action: Pulls the forehead skin upward, wrinkling the forehead.
Active electrode: Pupillary line in the middle of forehead</td></tr>
<tr><td>Morphology: Wide muscle with parallel fibers.</td></tr>
<tr><td>Depth 0.5 cm</td><td></td></tr>
</table>

M. Occipitalis (Picture 3.4)

<table>
<tr><td>Origin: Occipital bone.
Insertion: The two venters come together, inserting into the aponeurotic galea.
Innervation: Facial nerve (VII cranial pair)
Action: Pulls the forehead skin upward, wrinkling the forehead.
Active electrode: Three centimeters above the superior nuchal line.
Morphology: Wide muscle with parallel fibers.
Depth: 0.5 cm</td><td>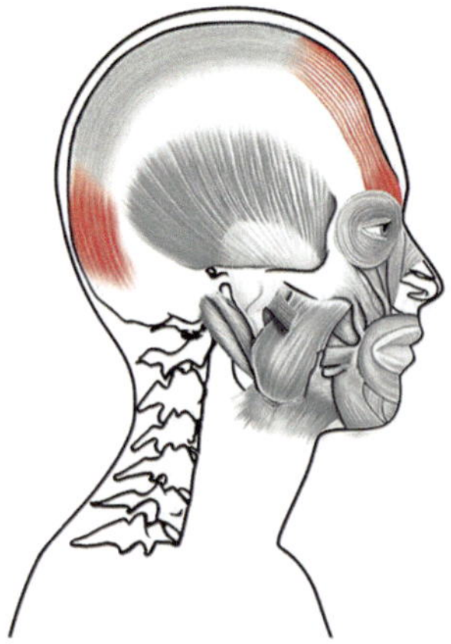</td></tr>
</table>

M. Orbicularis oculi (Picture 3.5)

Origin
Orbital portion: medial palpebral ligament, frontal, and maxillary bones.
Pre-septal portion: medial palpebral ligament and lacrimal ridge.
Pre-tarsal portion: medial palpebral ligament (lateral border).
Insertion
Orbital portion: orbital cutis on maxillary, frontal, and zygomatic bones.
Pre-septal portion: middle layer of the lateral palpebral raphe.
Pre-tarsal portion: innermost layer of the lateral palpebral fold.
Innervation: Facial nerve (VII cranial pair).
Action: Closes the eyelids and wrinkles the skin around the eyes.
Active electrode: Directs the needle externally to the eyeball.
Morphology: Wide muscle with circular fibers.
Subcutaneous depth

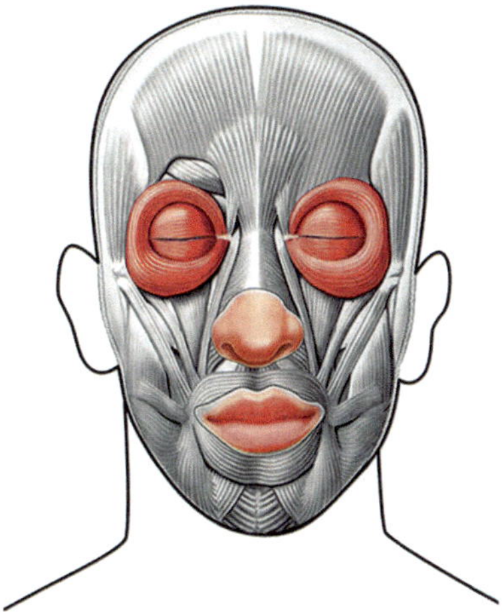

M. Levator labii superioris alaeque nasi (Picture 3.6)

Origin: Frontal process of the maxilla.
Insertion: Nose wing and medial portion of the orbicular muscle of the mouth.
Innervation: Facial nerve (VII cranial pair).
Action: Discrete elevation of the upper lip and the nose wing (dilates the nostril).
Active electrode: At the midpoint of the lateral sulcus formed by the nose wing.
Morphology: Long muscle with parallel fibers.
Depth: 0.3–0.5 cm

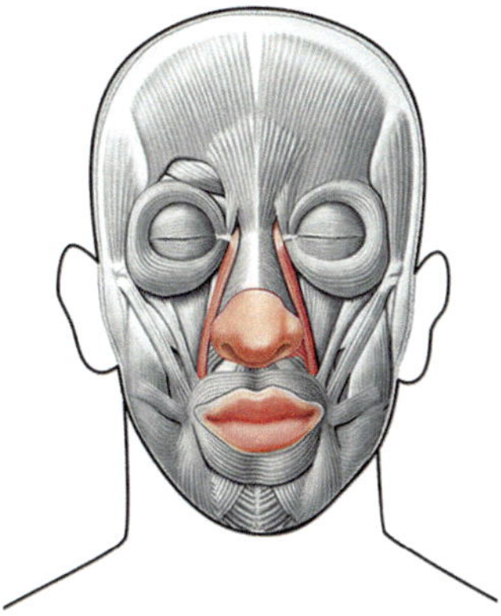

M. orbicularis oris (Picture 3.7)

Origin: Most originate from the perioral skin and from the incisive fovea of the jaw and mandible.
Insertion: Skin and mucosa of the lips.
Innervation: Facial nerve (VII cranial pair).
Action: Closes the mouth and protracts the lips.
Active electrode: Approximately one centimeter from the labial border.
Morphology: Wide muscle with parallel fibers.
Depth: 0.5 cm

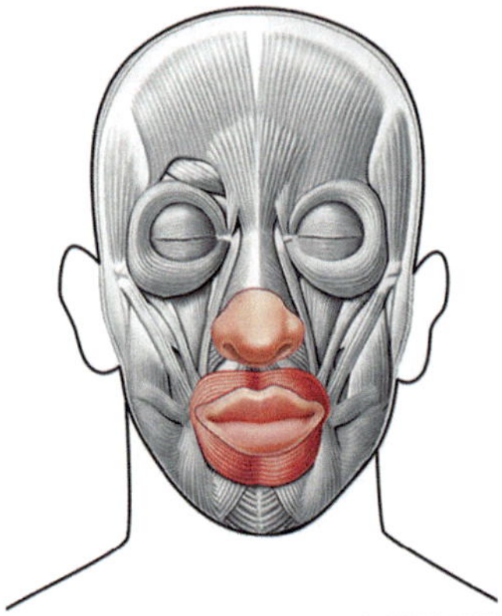

M. Mentalis (Picture 3.8)

Origin: Mentonian fossae above the mentonian tubercle
Insertion: Skin of the chin.
Innervation: Facial nerve (VII cranial pair).
Action: It wrinkles the skin of the chin and folds the lower lip.
Active electrode: One centimeter lateral to the midline of the face, between the labial line and the lower border of the mandible.
Morphology: Short muscle with parallel fibers.
Depth: 0,5–1 cm

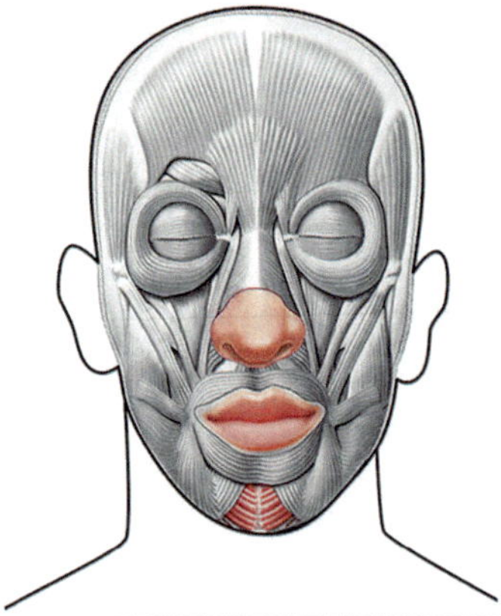

M. Platysma (Picture 3.9)

Origin: Lower edge of the mandible.
Insertion: Skin of the neck, clavicle, and anterior face of the first rib.
Innervation: Facial nerve (VII cranial pair).
Action: wrinkles the skin of the neck, slightly lowers the jaw, and lowers the angle of the mouth.
Active electrode: Multiple possible points arranged between the inferior border of the mandible and the superior border of the clavicle (from its sternal end to the acromial end).
Morphology: Wide muscle with parallel fibers.
Subcutaneous depth

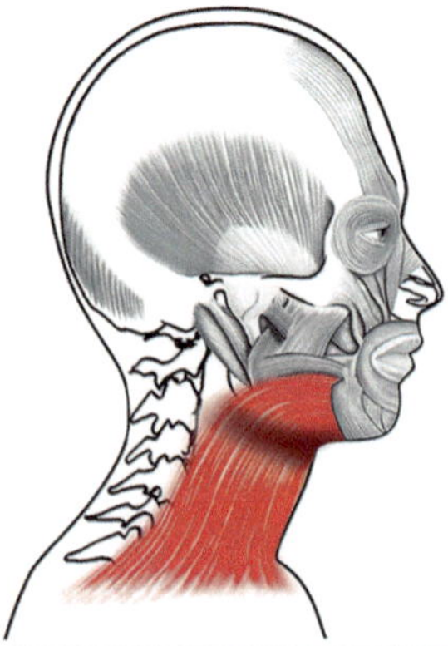

M. Genioglossus (Picture 3.10)

Origin: Internal surface of the mandible, in the upper genian spine, just above the geniohyoid muscle.
Insertion: Tongue body and lingual aponeurosis.
Innervation: Hypoglossal nerve (XII cranial pair)
Action: Mainly protrudes the tongue, but also acts as a depressor.
Needle position: One centimeter lateral to the midpoint between the inferior surface of the symphysis of the mandible and the body of the hyoid bone. Introduce the needle 45° obliquely over the transverse plane in the anteroposterior direction.
Morphology: Wide muscle with parallel fibers.
Depth: 2.5–3 cm

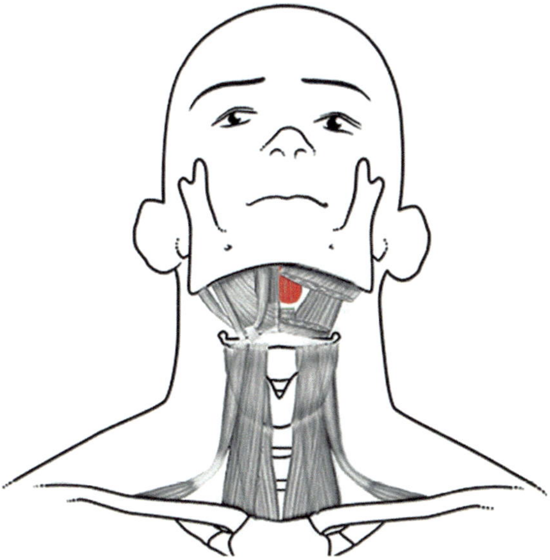

M. Crycothyroid (Picture 3.11)

Origin: Anterolateral portion of the cricoid cartilage
Insertion: inferior margin of the thyroid cartilage
Innervation: superior laryngeal nerve
Action: pulls the thyroid cartilage anteriorly and inferiorly, tensioning the vocal folds (high-pitched sounds).
Active electrode: palpate the space between the lower margin of the thyroid cartilage and the upper margin of the cricoid. Insert 2 cm from the midline between the two margins directing the needle 45° externally.
Morphology: Short with oblique fibers.
Depth: 1.5 cm.

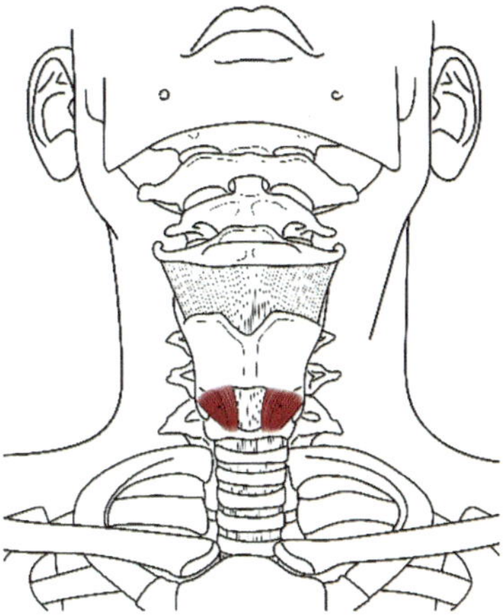

M. Temporalis (Picture 3.12)

Origin: External face of the temporal bone and fascia. Insertion: Anterior border and medial face of the mandibular coronoid process. Innervation: Trigeminal nerve (V cranial pair). Action: Elevation (occlusion) and retraction of the mandible. Active electrode: Midpoint of the temporal fossa. Morphology: Wide muscle with parallel fibers. Depth: 1.5 cm	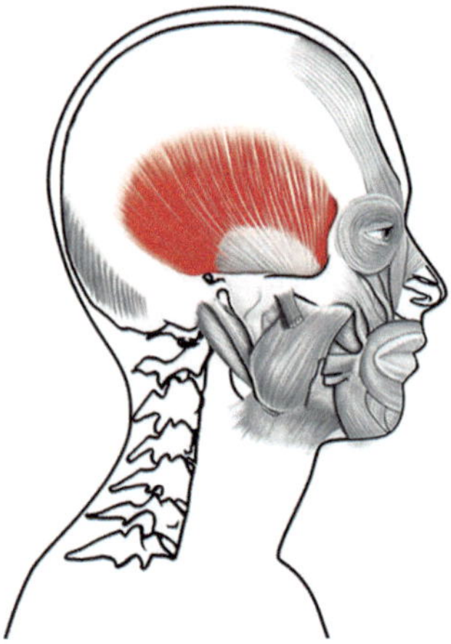

M. masseter (Picture 3.13)

Origin: Inferior margin of the zygomatic bone and zygomatic arch. Insertion: Lateral face of the mandibular angle. Innervation: Trigeminal nerve (V cranial pair). Action: Elevation (occlusion) of the mandible. Active electrode: Two to three centimeters anterior to the mandibular angle. Morphology: Wide muscle with parallel fibers. Depth: 1.0–1.5 cm	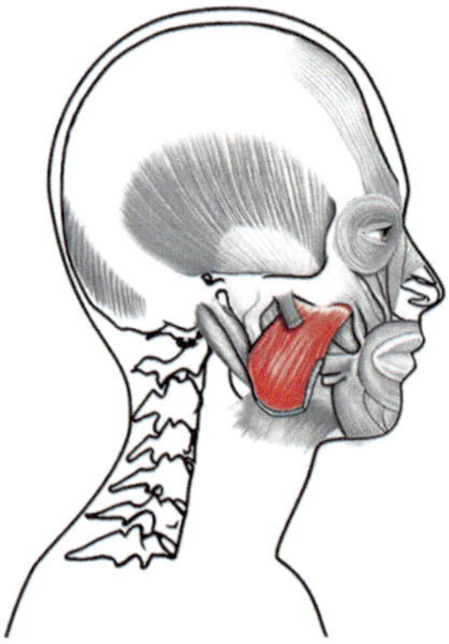

M. Sternocleidomastoid (Picture 3.14)

Origin
Clavicular head: medial third of the superior surface of the clavicle.
Sternal head: anterior face of the sternal notch and sternoclavicular joint.
Insertion: Lateral third of the superior nuchal line and mastoid process of the temporal bone.
Innervation: Accessory nerve (XI cranial pair) and cervical plexus (C1-C2-C3).
Action: On unilateral contraction it rotates the head to the opposite side and can also, at the same time, flex it to the same side. On contraction of both muscles, the head is stretched and pulled anteriorly.
Active electrode: midpoint between mastoid process and the jugular notch of the sternal bone.
Morphology: Long muscle, with two main heads and parallel fibers.
Depth: 0,5–1 cm

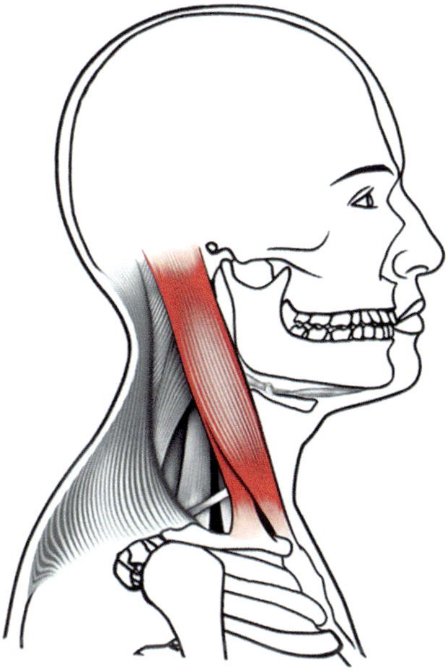

M. trapezius (Picture 3.15)

Origin: External occipital protuberance and
spinous processes of C1 to C7
Insertion: Lateral third of clavicle
Innervation:: Accessory nerve and motor branches of C2, C3, and C4
Action: Mainly shoulder elevation
Active electrode: Midpoint between the acromion and the occipital region
Morphology: Wide
Depth: 1.5–2.5 cm

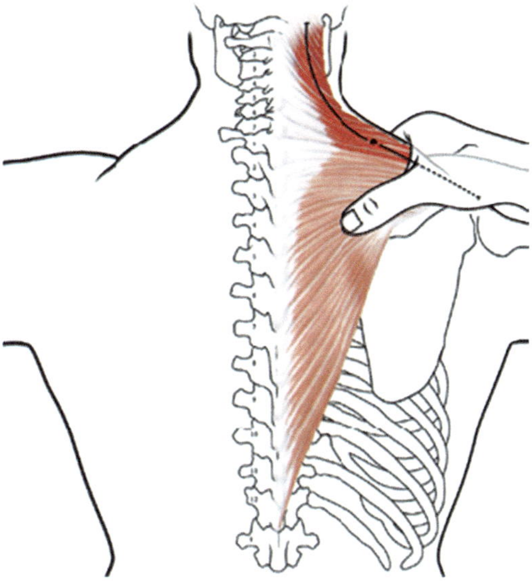

M. supraespinatus (Picture 3.16)

Origin: Supraspinatus fossa of scapula
Insertion: Greater tubercle of humerus
Innervation: Suprascapular nerve (C5, C6)
Action: Arm abduction
Active electrode: Midpoint of its belly. For most appropriate recording recommended insulated and long needles to isolate from more superficial trapezius muscle.
Morphology: Fusiforme
Depth: 3–4 cm

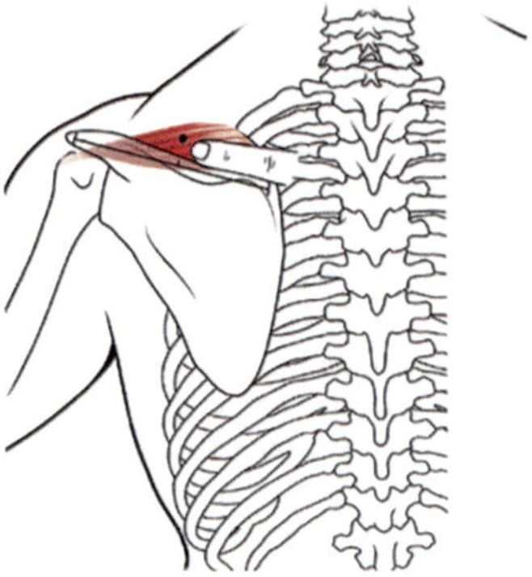

M. infraspinatus (Picture 3.17)

Origin: Supraspinatus fossa of scapula
Insertion: Greater tubercle of humerus
Innervation: suprascapular nerve (C5, C6)
Action: External rotation
Active electrode: Half of an imaginary line between the midpoint of the scapular spine and its inferior angle. For the same reason as the supraspinalis, insulated long needles are recommended.
Morphology: Oblique and multipenate
Depth: 2 cm

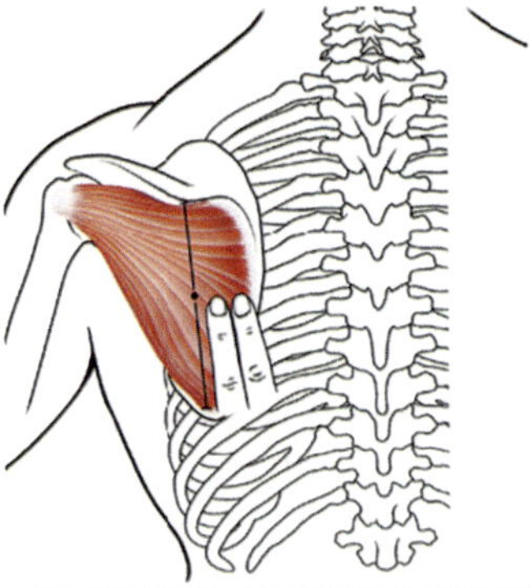

M. Deltoid (Picture 3.18)

Origin: Acromion
Insertion: Humerus
Innervation: Axillary nerve (C5, C6)
Action: Abduction
Active electrode: Midpoint of its medial segment
Morphology: Oblique and multipenate
Depth: 1–2 cm

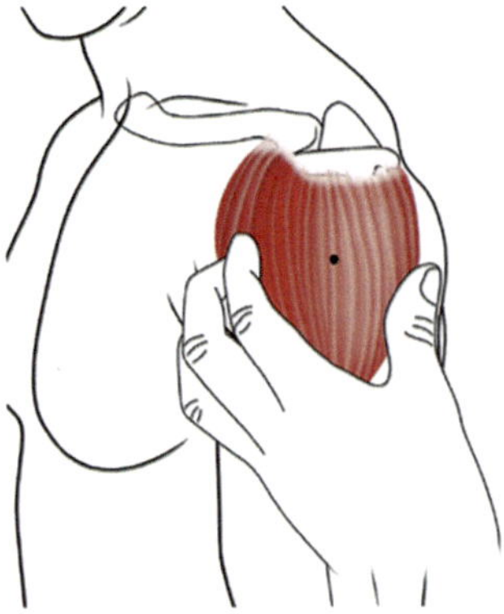

M. Biceps brachii (Picture 3.19)

Origin Short head: coracoid process of the scapula Long head: supraglenoid supraglenoidal tubercle of the scapula Insertion: radius tuberosity Innervation: Musculocutaneous nerve (C5, C6) Action: Supination of the forearm and flexion of the upper arm. Active electrode: Midpoint of the anterior segment of the arm Morphology: Parallel and fusiform Depth: 2 cm	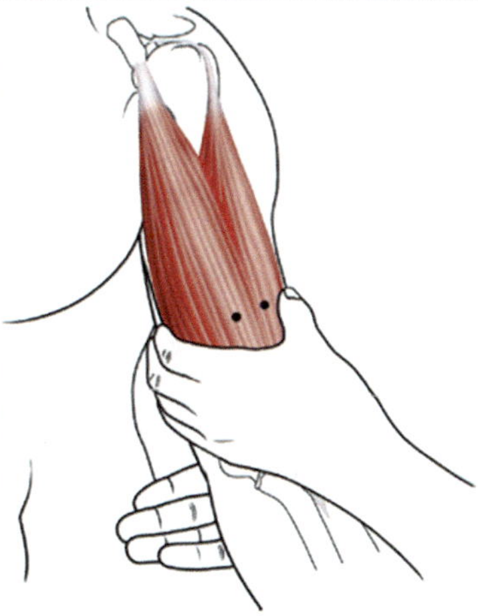

M. triceps brachii (long head) (Picture 3.20)

Origin: Infraglenoid tubercle of the scapula Insertion: Olecranon Innervation: Radial nerve (C6, C7, C8) Action: Extension of the forearm Active electrode: Distal third of the posterior portion of the humerus Morphology: Parallel Depth: 1.5 cm	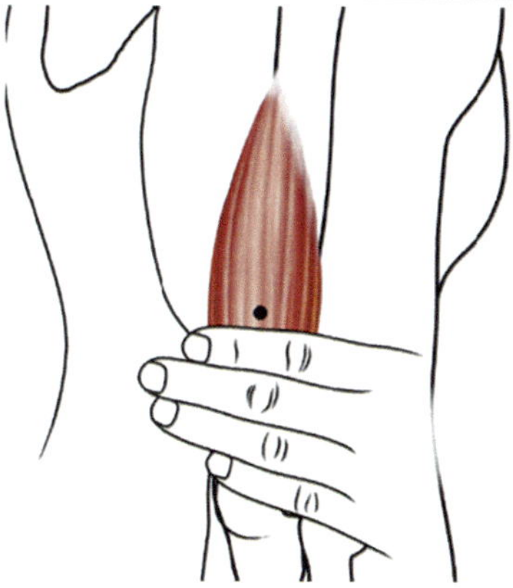

M. extensor carpi radialis (Picture 3.21)

Origin: Lateral supraepichondylar crest of the humerus Insertion: Base of the 2nd metacarpal Innervation: Radial nerve (C6, C7) Action: Extension and radial deviation of the hand Active electrode: 2 cm distal to the lateral epicondyle. Morphology: Long Depth: 1–2 cm	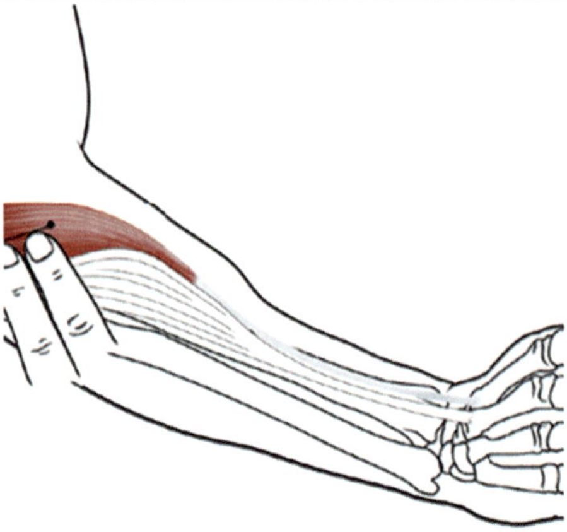

M. extensor digitorum (Picture 3.22)

Origin: Lateral epicondyle of the humerus Insertion: Extensor expansions of the four fingers Innervation: Radial nerve (C7, C8) Action: Extension of the fingers Active electrode: the extensor digitorum is the second muscle belly laterally to the brachioradialis in the proximal third of the forearm. Morphology: Long Depth: 1 cm	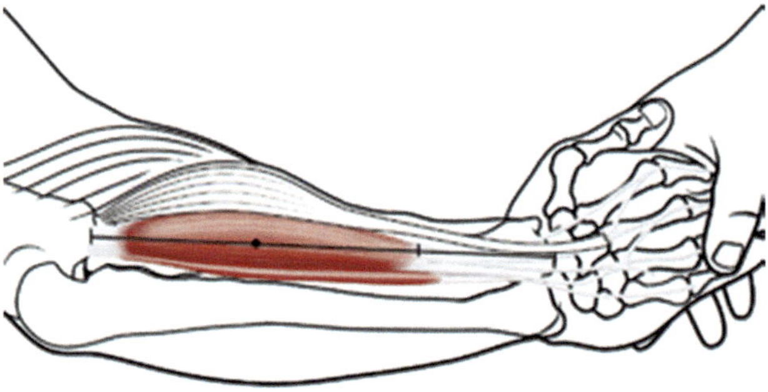

M. brachiorradialis (Picture 3.23)

Origin: Supracondylar process of humerus Insertion: Distal extremity of the radius Innervation: Radial nerve (C5, C6) Action: Flexion of the forearm in neutral position Active electrode: With the forearm flexed and in neutral position, the muscle is in its proximal third. Morphology: Parallel Depth: 2 cm	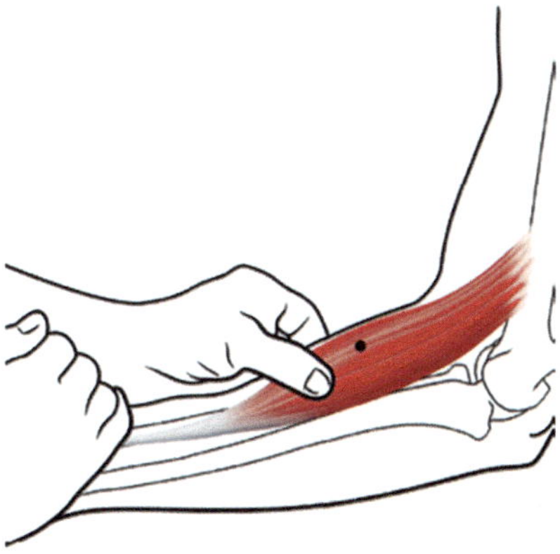

M. pronator teres (Picture 3.24)

Origin: Coronoid process and medial epicondyle of humerus Insertion: Proximal lateral face of the radius Innervation: Median nerve (C6, C7) Action: Pronation of the forearm Active electrode: Palpate the medial border of the biceps tendon and draw a line from this point to the medial epicondyle. At the midpoint of this imaginary line, descend three fingers distally. Morphology: Short and longitudinal Depth: 1–1.5 cm	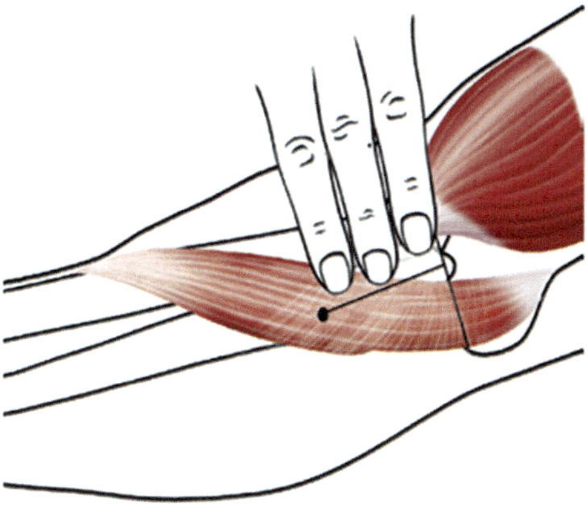

M. flexor carpi radialis (Picture 3.25)

Origin: Medial epicondyle of the humerus Insertion: Base of the 2nd metacarpal Innervation: Median nerve (C6, C7) Action: Flexion and radial deviation of the hand Active electrode: Identify the tendon of the flexor carpi radialis at the wrist and follow proximally to the myotendinous transition (point where it is more difficult to palpate the tendon). At this point, draw an imaginary line to the medial epicondyle. The muscle is at the midpoint of this line. Morphology: Long and bipenate Depth: 1 cm	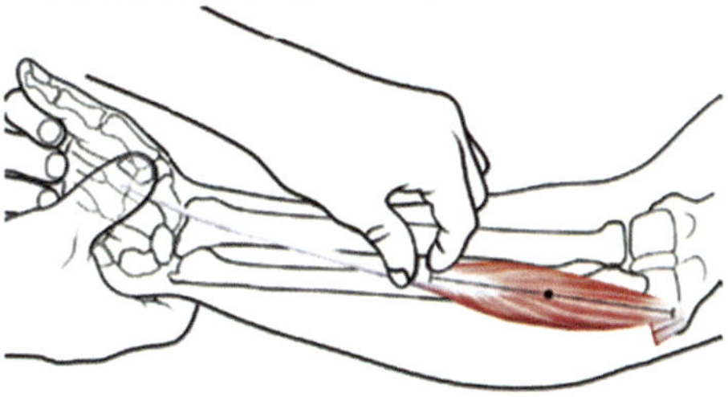

M. flexor carpi ulnaris (Picture 3.26)

Origin: Medial epicondyle of the humerus
Insertion: Pisiform, hamate, and 5th metacarpal
Innervation: Ulnar nerve (C8, T1)
Action: Flexion and ulnar deviation of the hand
Active electrode: Identify the tendon of the flexor carpi ulnaris at the wrist
the wrist and follow proximally to the myotendinous transition (point where it becomes more difficult to palpate
of the tendon). At this point, draw an imaginary line to the medial epicondyle. The muscle is located at the midpoint of this line.
Morphology: Long and fusiform
Depth: 1–2 cm

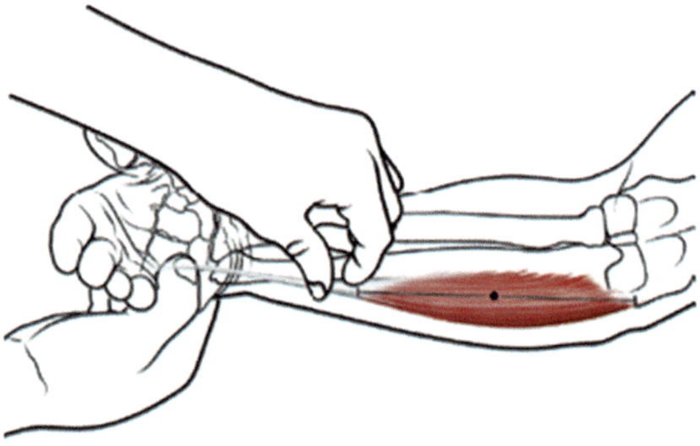

M. extensor indicis (Picture 3.27)

Origin: Distal third of the ulna
Insertion: Expansion of the extensor muscle of the 2nd finger
Innervation: Radial nerve (C7, C8)
Action: Extension of the index finger
Active electrode: With the hand in pronation, the muscle is three fingerbreadths above the styloid process of the ulna.
Morphology: Long
Depth: 0.5

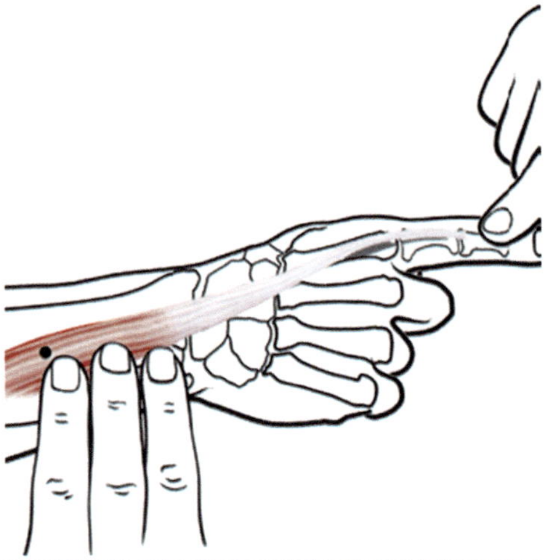

M. Abductor pollicis brevis (Picture 3.28)

Origin: Retinaculum of flexors
Insertion: Lateral face of the 1st metacarpal
Innervation: Median nerve
Action: Abduction of the thumb (C8, T1)
Active electrode: Midpoint of the 1st metacarpal bone, close to the medial edge of the bone.
Morphology: Short
Depth: 0.5 cm

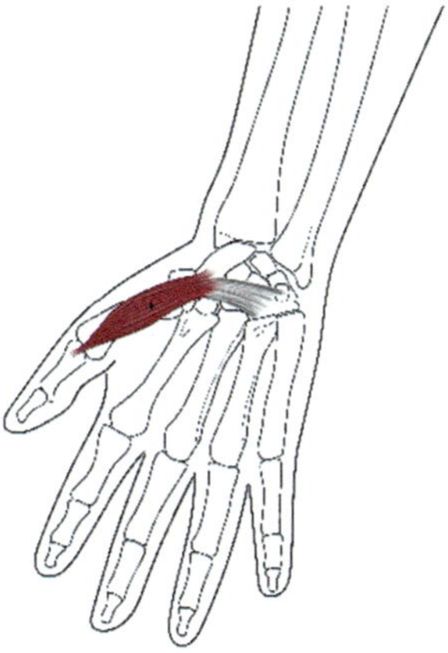

M. abdutor digiti minimi (Picture 3.29)

Origin: Pisiform
Insertion: Base of the proximal phalanx of the minimum finger
Innervation: Ulnar nerve
Action: Little finger abduction (C8, T1)
Active electrode: On the medial border, midpoint of the 5th metacarpal
Morphology: Short and fusiform
Depth: 0.5 cm

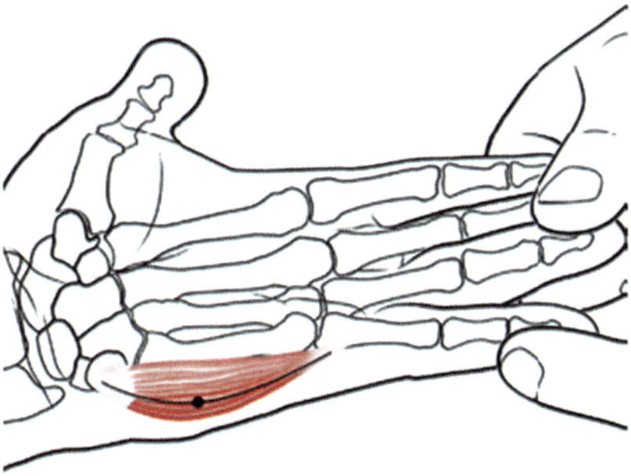

M. diaphragm (Picture 3.30)

Origin: Internal surfaces of lower costal cartilages na ribs 7–12
Insertion: Central tendon of diaphragm
Innervation: Nervo frênico (C3, C4, C5)
Action: Primary muscle of breathing (inspiration)
Active electrode: At the anterior axillary line superior to the 9th or 10th rib. Ultrasound Image Guidance Is recommended.
Morphology: Large muscle with radial fibers
Depth:

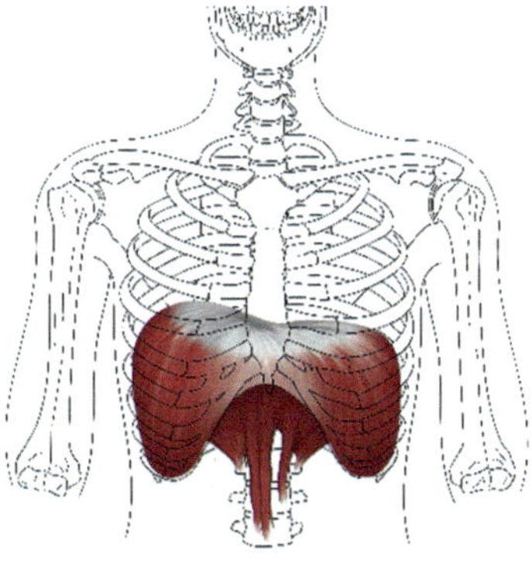

M. obliquus abdominis (Picture 3.31)

Origin: External surfaces of ribs 5–12 Insertion: Linha Alba, pubic tubercle and anterior half of iliac crest Innervation: Intercostal nerves (T7-T11) and subcostal nerve (T12) Action: ipsilateral trunk lateral flection, contralateral trunk rotation, and trunk flection (bilateral contraction) Active electrode: Halfway between linea alba and midaxillary line. Morphology: Large with oblique fibers Depth: 1,5–2 cm 1, cm	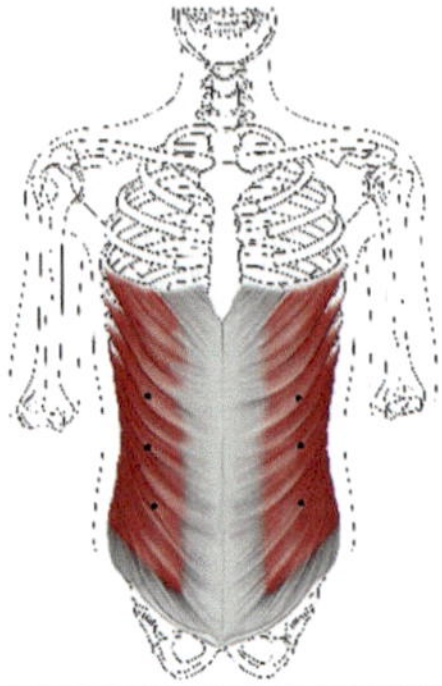

M. intercostalis (Picture 3.32)

Origin: Costal groove of ribs Insertion: Superior border Innervation: Intercostal nerve Action: Depress ribs during forced expiration Active electrode: Half way between costocondral articulations and axilary line. Morphology: Short with oblique fibers Depth:	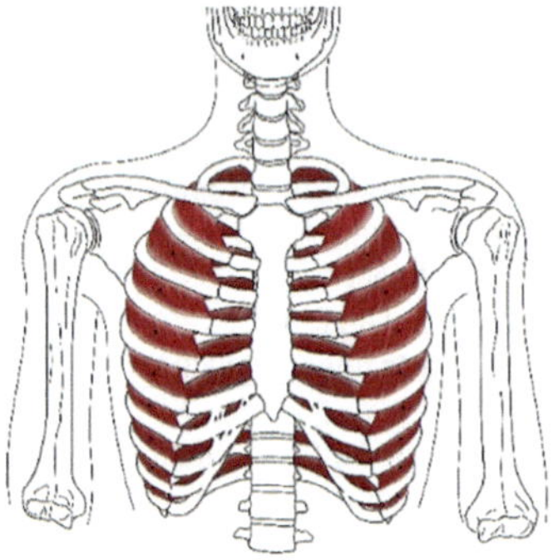

M. Rectus abdominais (Picture 3.33)

Origin: Pubic Symphysis Insertion: Xiphoid process and costal cartilages of ribs 5–7 Innervation: Ictecostal nerves (T7-T11) and subcostal nerve (T12) Active electrode: 10 points disposed 5 cm from the midline. Depth: 2–3 cm	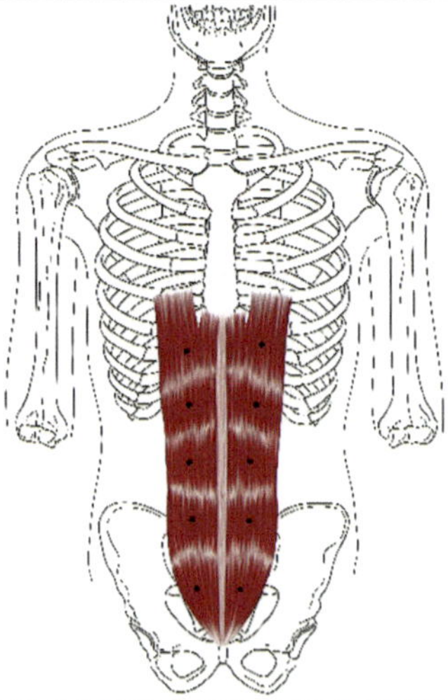

M. iliacus (Picture 3.34)

Origin: Iliac crest, iliac fossa, and sacral wing
Insertion: Psoas major and lesser trochanter
Innervation: Femoral nerve (L2, L3)
Action: Flexion of the thigh
Active electrode: Midpoint between the anterosuperior iliac spine and the femoral artery, directly below the inguinal ligament (tilt the needle 45° toward the internal face of the iliac bone).
Morphology: Wide
Depth: 5–9 cm

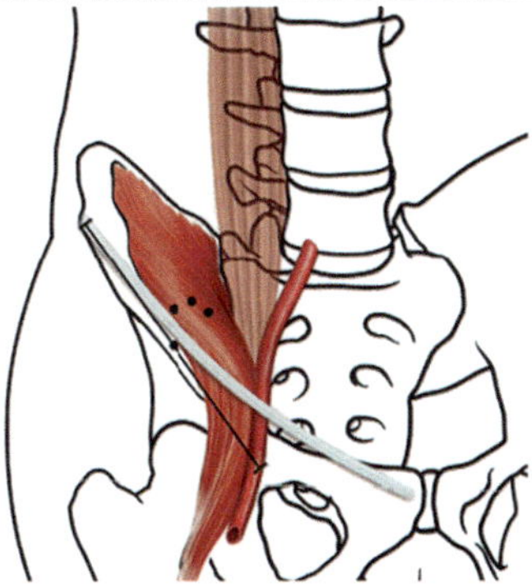

M. adductor longus (Picture 3.35)

Origin: Body of pubis
Insertion: Middle third of femur
Innervation: Obturator nerve (L2, L3, L4)
Action: Adduction of the thigh
Active electrode: Proximal third of the medial aspect of the thigh
Morphology: Wide
Depth: 2–4 cm

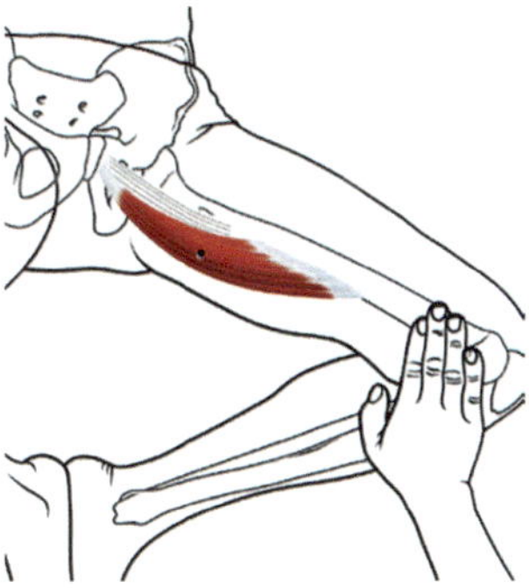

M. Addcutor brevis (Picture 3.36)

Origin: Body of pubis
Insertion: Pectineal line
Innervation: Obturator nerve (L2, L3)
Action: Adduction of the thigh
Active electrode: Proximal third of the medial aspect of the thigh
Morphology: Wide and longitudinal
Depth: 2–4 cm

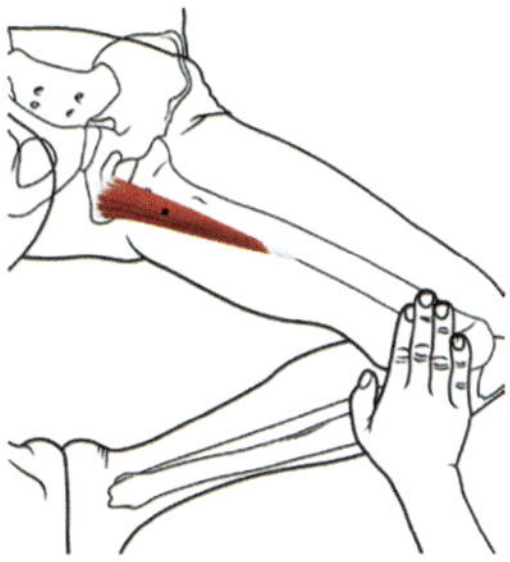

M. rectus femoris (Picture 3.37)

Origin: Anteroinferior iliac spine
Insertion: Tibial tuberosity
Innervation: Femoral nerve (L2, L3, L4)
Action: Knee extension, flexion of the thigh
Active electrode: Midpoint between anterosuperior iliac spine and the superior border of the patella.
Morphology: unipenate
Depth: 1–2 cm (from 3 cm depth on, the vastus muscle the vastus intermedius)

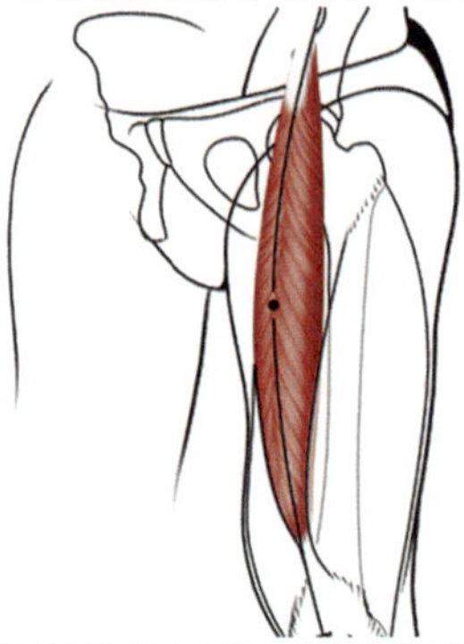

M. tibialis anterior (Picture 3.38)

Origin: Lateral condyle of the tibia
Insertion: Medial cuneiform and base of 1st metatarsal
Innervation: Deep peroneal nerve (L4, L5)
Action: Dorsiflexion and inversion of the foot
Active electrode: Proximal third of the tibia, 1 cm lateral to its anterior margin.
Morphology: long and with parallel fibers
Depth: 1 cm

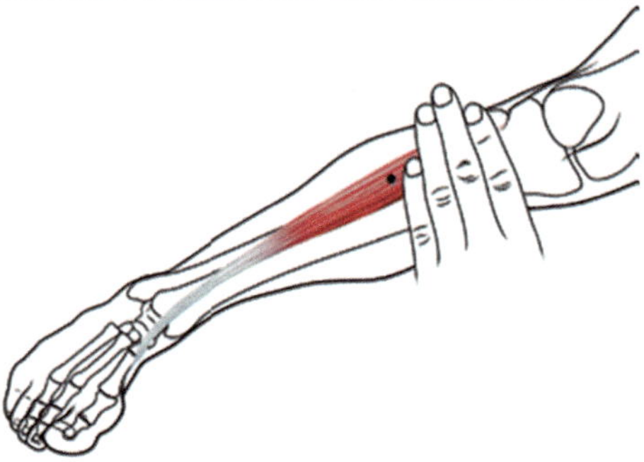

M. extensor hallucis longus (Picture 3.39)

Origin: Anterior face of the fibula and interosseous membrane
Insertion: Base of the distal phalanx of the hallux
Innervation: Deep peroneal nerve (L5, S1)
Action: Hallux extension
Active electrode: Four to five toes and 1 cm lateral to the midpoint of the bimalleolar line.
Morphology: Oblique and bipennate
Depth: 1–2 cm

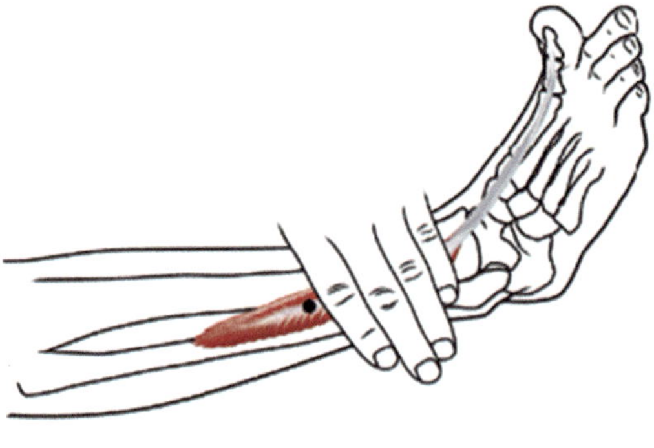

M. gastrocnemius (Picture 3.40)

Origin
Lateral head: Lateral condyle of the femur
Medial head: Medial condyle of the femur
Insertion: Posterior surface of the calcaneus
Innervation: Tibial nerve (S1-S2)
Action: Mainly plantar flexion
Active electrode: Upper third of the posterior aspect of the leg (lateral head in the lateral portion and medial head in the medial portion).
Obs: By performing digit pressure on the lower part of the popliteal fossa fossa, two protrusions (medial and lateral gastrocnemius) are observed that correspond to the motor points of the portions of this muscle.
Morphology: Oblique and bipennate
Depth: 2–3 cm

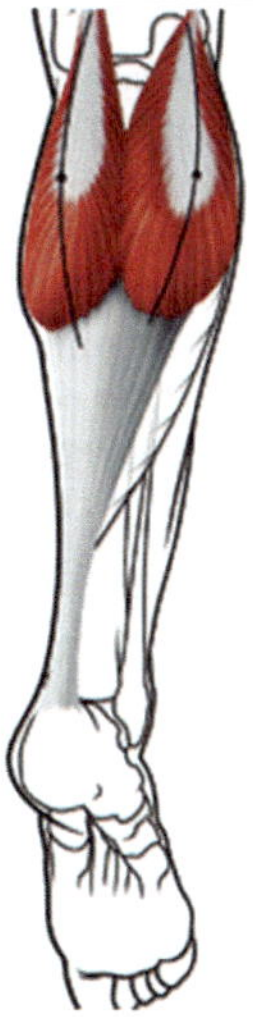

M. Abductor hallucis (Picture 3.41)

Origin: Medial process of calcaneal tuberosity and plantar aponeurosis
Insertion: Proximal phalanx of great toe
Innervation: Medial plantar nerve (S1-S2)
Action: Toe abduction and flexion
Active electrode: 2 points are possible. In the proximal third of metatarsus and 2 fingerbreadths below and anterior to talus bone.
Morphology: Long with oblique fibers
Depth: 1–1.5 cm.

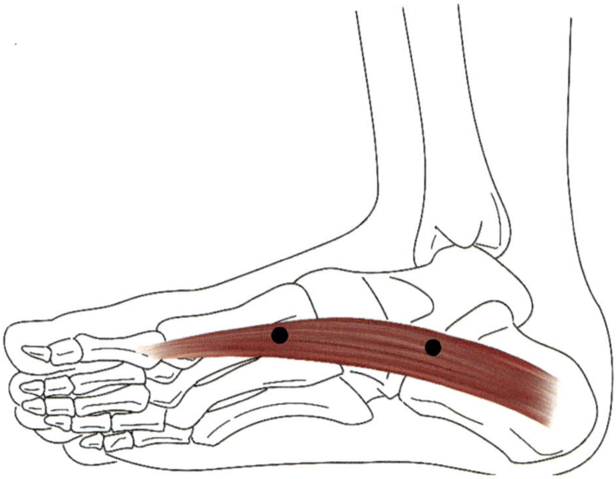

M. gluteus maximus (Picture 3.42)

Origin: Ilium posterior to the posterior gluteal line, dorsal aspect of the sacrum and coccyx
Insertion iliotibial tract
Innervation: Inferior gluteal nerve (L5, S1, S2)
Action: Extension of the thigh
Active electrode: Four fingerbreadths inferiorly to the posterior most prominent posterior portion of iliac crest, insert the needle obliquely toward the greater trochanter
Morphology: Large and oblique
Depth: 3 cm

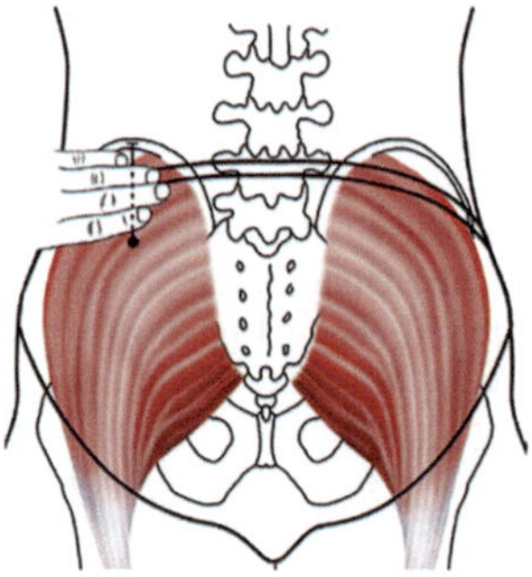

M. gluteus medius (Picture 3.43)

Origin: External face of the ilium
Insertion: Femoral greater trochanter
Innervation: Upper gluteal nerve (L5, S1)
Action: Abduction and medial rotation of the thigh
Active electrode: Two centimeters inferior to the anterior third of the iliac crest
Morphology: Oblique
Depth: 3 cm

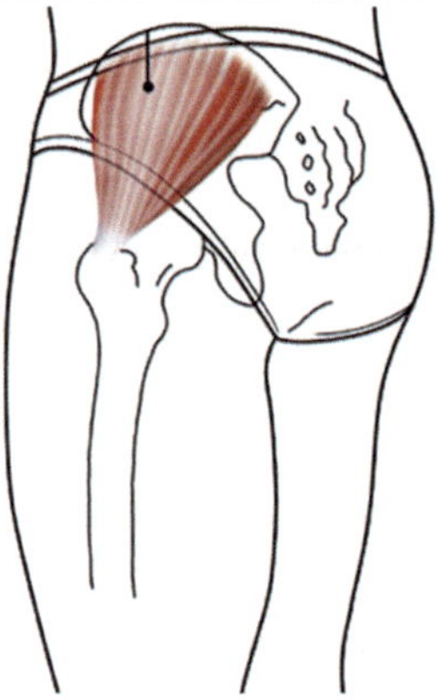

Gluteus minimus (Picture 3.44)

Origin: External face of the ilium
Insertion: Femoral greater trochanter
Innervation: Upper gluteal nerve (L5, S1)
Action: Medial rotation of the thigh
Active electrode: Midpoint between greater trochanter femoris and the midline posterior border of the iliac crest.
Morphology: Oblique
Depth: 3–4 cm

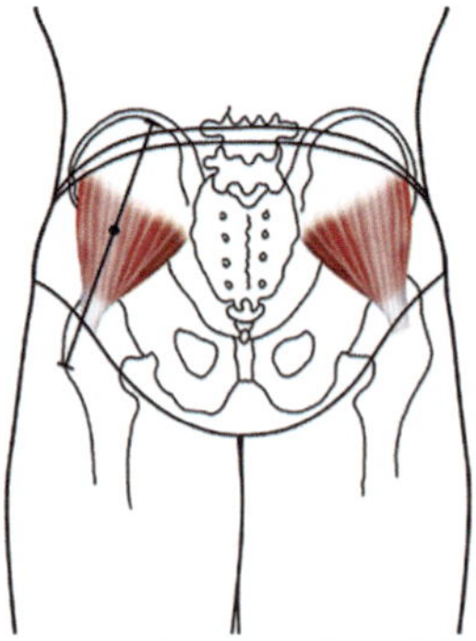

M. semitendinosus (Picture 3.45)

Origin: ischial tubercle
Insertion: Upper part of the medial aspect of the tibia (tibial plateau)
Innervation: Tibial division of the sciatic nerve (L5, S1, S2)
Action: Hip extension, flexion, and internal rotation of the leg
Active electrode: Midpoint between tuber ischium and medial tibial plateau. Displace 2 cm lateral.
Morphology: Parallel
Depth: 2.5–4 cm

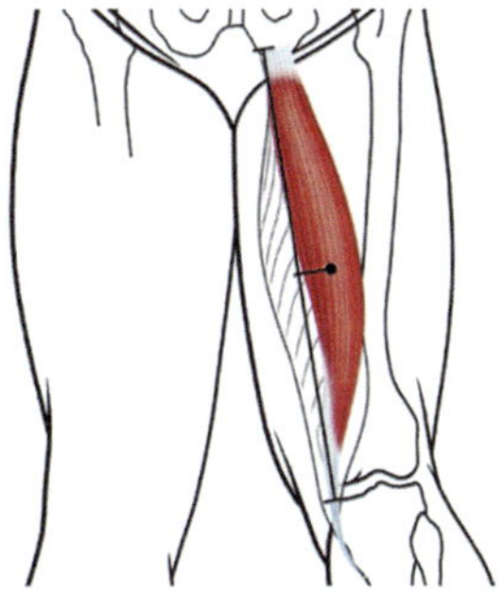

M. Semimembranosus (Picture 3.46)

Origin: ischial tubercle
Insertion: Upper part of the medial aspect of the tibia (tibial plateau)
Innervation: Tibial division of the sciatic nerve (L5, S1, S2)
Action: Hip extension, flexion, and internal rotation of the leg
Active electrode: Midpoint between ischial tubercle and medial tibial plateau.
Morphology: Parallel
Depth: 2.5–4 cm

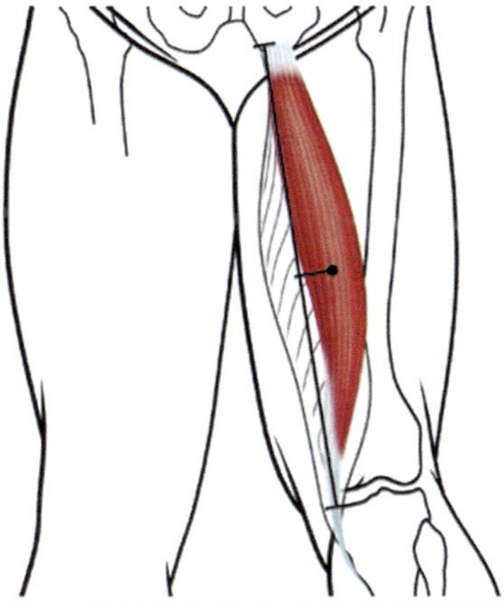

M. bíceps femoris – long head (Picture 3.47)

Origin: ischial tuber
Insertion: Fibula head
Innervation: Tibial portion of the sciatic nerve (L5, S1, S2)
Action: Hip extension, flexion, and external rotation of the leg
Active electrode: Midpoint between the ischial tubercle and fibular head.
Morphology: Oblique
Depth: 2.5–4 cm

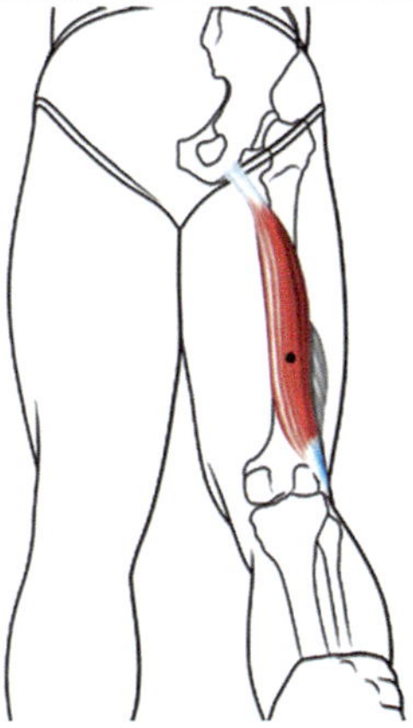

M. biceps femoris- short head (Picture 3.48)

Origin: Lateral supracondylar line of the femur
Insertion: Fibula head (L5, S1, S2)
Innervation: Common fibular division of the sciatic nerve
Action: Hip extension, flexion, and external rotation of the leg
Active electrode: Distal third between the ischial tubercle and fibular head.
Morphology: Oblique
Depth: 2.5–4 cm

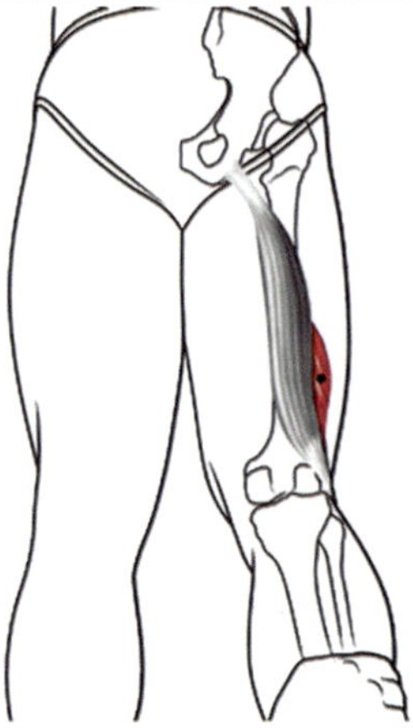

M. tensor fasciae latae (Picture 3.49)

Origin: Anterosuperior iliac spine
Insertion: Lateral condyle of the tibia
Innervation: Upper gluteal nerve (L4, L5, S1)
Action: Abduction and medial rotation of the thigh
Active electrode: Two fingers medially to the greater trochanter
Morphology: Parallel
Depth: 2 cm

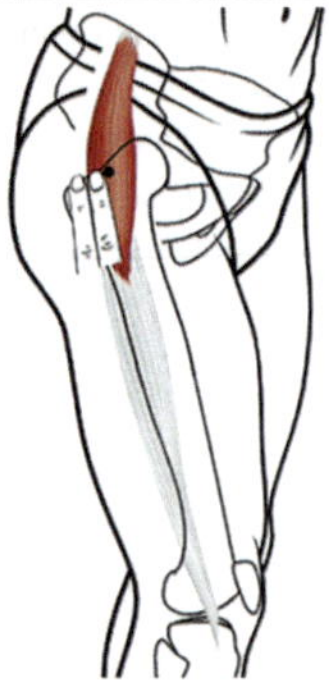

M. perineal transversus (deep and superficial portions) (Picture 3.50)

Origin: Inferior rami of the ischium Insertion: Deep transverse perineal muscle of the opposite side Innervation: Pudendal nerve Action: Constricts urethra and vagina Active electrode in women: 2 ponts 3 cm away from midline lateral to vaginal introitus, just between midline and ischium. Active electrode in men: Halfway between ischial tuberosity and pênis crus just between middle line and ischium. Morphology: Large with parallel fibers Depth: 3 cm	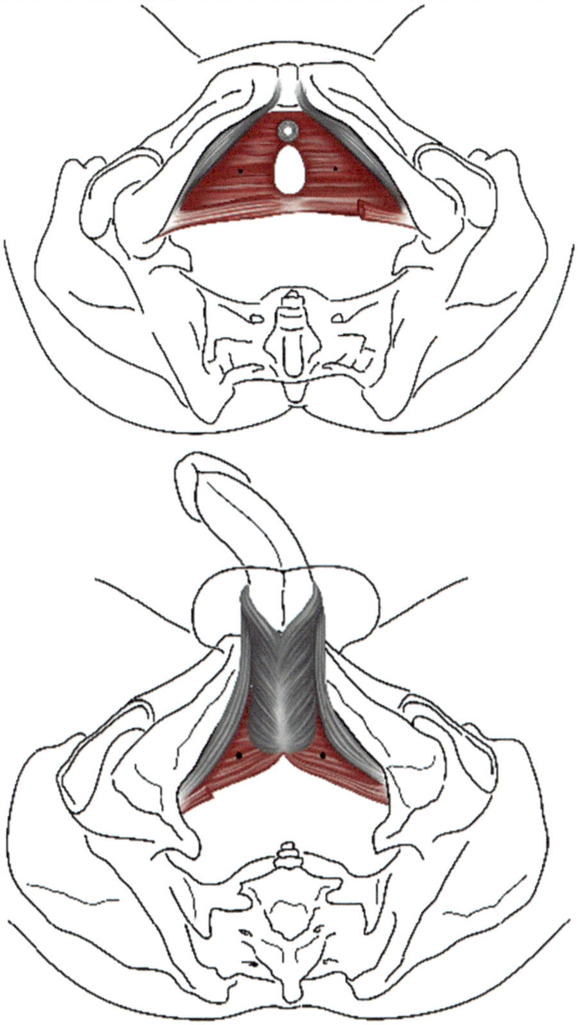

M. Ischiocavernosus (Picture 3.51)

Origin: Ischial tuberosity and ramus Insertion: crus of clitoris or penis Innervation: Deep branch of pudendal nerve (S2-S4) Action: Maintains erection of penis/clitóris, pushes blood from root to body of clitóris/penis Active electrode: Halfway between the ischial tuberosity and penis/clitoris crus just medial to ischium. Morphology: long with parallel fibers Depth: 2 cm	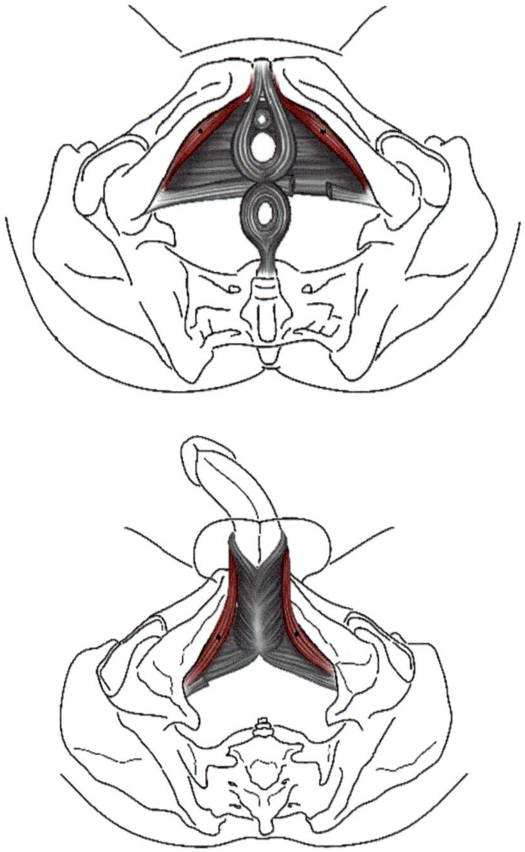

M. Bulboespongiosus (Picture 3.52)

Origin: Perineal body, median penile raphe
Insertion: Pubic arch, fascia of corpora cavernosa and clitoris (female).
Perineal membrane, fascia of vulv of penis, and dorsal aspect of corpus spongiosum.
Innervation: Deep branch of pudendal nerve
Action: Assists in erection of clitóris/pênis, supports perineal body
Active electrode in men: 4 points 2 cm away from the midline between testicle and anal sphincter. Active electrode in women: Halfway between external urethral sphincter and vaginal introitus, 2 cm from the midline.
Morphology: n/s
Depth: 2 cm

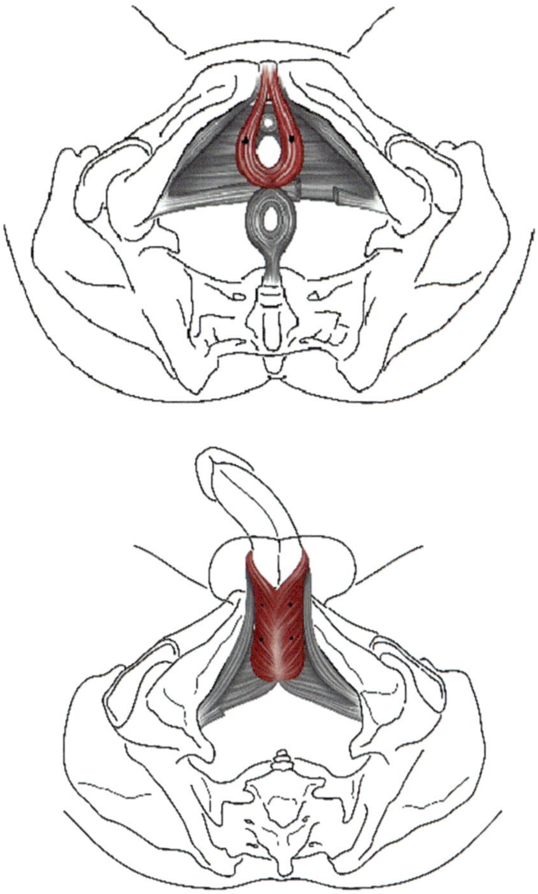

M. external urethral sphincter (Picture 3.53)

Origin and insertion: encircles membranous urethra Innervation: Deep branch of pudendal nerve Action: Maintains urinary continence and prevents retrograde ejaculation Active electrode: 2 points 1 cm away from the external urethral orifice (just in women). Morphology: sphincter Depth: 2 cm	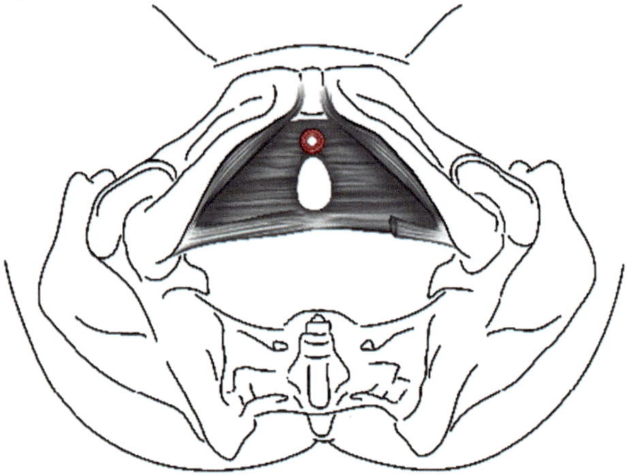

M. internal anal sphincter (Picture 3.54)

Origin and insertion: surrounds the upper 2/3 of the anal canal. Innervation: Inferior anal/rectal branch of pudendal nerve (S2-S4) Action: Fecal continence Active electrode: 2 points 1 cm away from the anal orifice. Morphology: sphincter Depth: 2, 5 cm	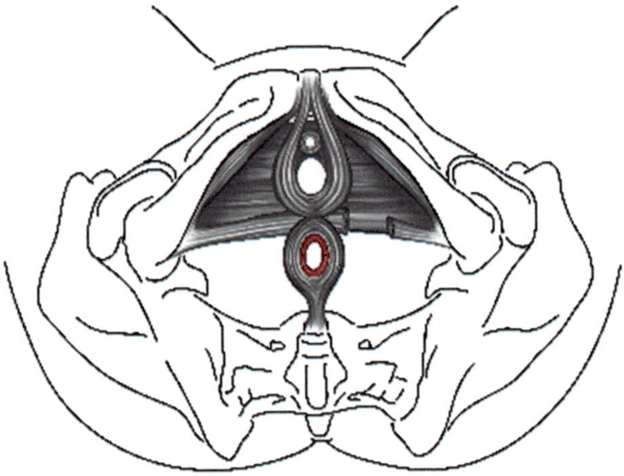

M. external anal sphincter (Picture 3.55)

Origin: Skin and fascia around anus Insertion: Perineal body and anococcygeal ligament Innervation: Inferior anal/ rectal branch of pudendal nerve (S2–S4) Action: Constricts anal canal and supports pelvic floor Active electrode: 4 points in a radial fashion 3 cm away from the anal orifice in each of 4 quadrants. Insert neele in a 45° direction towards the anal orifice. Morphology: sphincter Depth: 1 cm	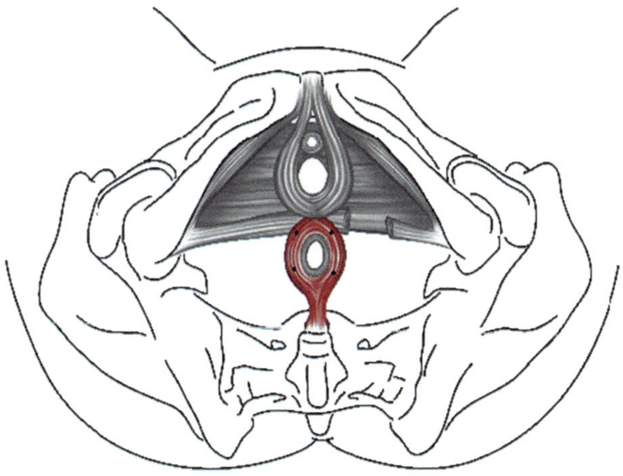

References

1. Botter A, Oprandi G, Lanfranco F, Allasia S, Maffiuletti NA, Minetto MA. Atlas of the muscle motor points for the lower limb: implications for electrical stimulation procedures and electrode positioning. Eur J Appl Physiol. 2011;111(10):2461–71. https://doi.org/10.1007/s00421-011-2093-y. PMID: 21796408.
2. Christensen E. Topography of terminal motor innervation in striated muscles from stillborn infants. Am J Phys Med. 1959;38(2):65–78. PMID: 13637190.
3. Chu J, Chan RC, Bruyninckx F. Progressive teflon denudation of the monopolar needle: effects on motor unit potential parameters. Arch Phys Med Rehabil. 1987;68(1):36–40. PMID: 3800622.
4. Coers C, Durand J. La répartition des appareils cholinestérasiques en cupule dans divers muscles striés [Distribution of cup-shaped cholinesterase apparatus in various striated muscles]. Arch Biol (Liege). 1957;68(2):209–15. French. PMID: 13445292.
5. Dong CCJ, MacDonald DB, Akagami R, Westerberg B, AlKhani A, Kanaan I, Hassounah M. Intraoperative facial motor evoked potential monitoring with transcranial electrical stimulation during skull base surgery. Clin Neurophysiol. 2005;116(3):588–96.
6. Dumitru D, Zwarts MJ, Amato AA, editors. Elctrodiagnostic medicine. 2nd ed. Elsevier; 2002.
7. Feinstein B, Lindegard B, Nyman E, Wohlfart G. Morphologic studies of motor units in normal human muscles. Acta Anat (Basel). 1955;23(2):127–42. https://doi.org/10.1159/000140989. PMID: 14349537.

8. Gobbo M, Gaffurini P, Bissolotti L, Esposito F, Orizio C. Transcutaneous neuromuscular electrical stimulation: influence of electrode positioning and stimulus amplitude settings on muscle response. Eur J Appl Physiol. 2011;111(10):2451–9. https://doi.org/10.1007/s00421-011-2047-4. PMID: 21717122.
9. Gobbo M, Maffiuletti NA, Orizio C, Minetto MA. Muscle motor point identification is essential for optimizing neuromuscular electrical stimulation use. J Neuroeng Rehabil. 2014;25(11):17. https://doi.org/10.1186/1743-0003-11-17. PMID: 24568180; PMCID: PMC3938308.
10. Jabre JF. Concentric macro electromyography. Muscle Nerve. 1991;14(9):820–5. https://doi.org/10.1002/mus.880140904. PMID: 1922175.
11. Jahangiri FR, Trausch C. Utilizing longer intramuscular needle pair electrodes: what are we missing in our intraoperative muscle recordings? EC Neurol. 2019;11(4):288–94.
12. Kim DH, Zaremski J, Kwon B, Jenis L, Woodard E, Bode R, Banco RJ. Risk factors for false positive transcranial motor evoked potential monitoring alerts during surgical treatment of cervical myelopathy. Spine (Phila Pa 1976). 2007;32(26):3041–6. https://doi.org/10.1097/BRS.0b013e31815d0072. PMID: 18091499.
13. AAEE glossary of terms in clinical electromyography. Muscle Nerve. 1987;10(8 Suppl):G1–60. PMID: 3657851.
14. Polgar J, Johnson MA, Weightman D, Appleton D. Data on fibre size in thirty-six human muscles. An autopsy study. J Neurol Sci. 1973;19(3):307–18. https://doi.org/10.1016/0022-510x(73)90094-4. PMID: 4716847.
15. Skinner SA, Transfeldt EE, Savik K. Surface electrodes are not sufficient to detect neurotonic discharges: observations in a porcine model and clinical review of deltoid electromyographic monitoring using multiple electrodes. J Clin Monit Comput. 2008;22(2):131–9. https://doi.org/10.1007/s10877-008-9114-3. PMID: 18335318.
16. Stålberg E. Macro EMG, a new recording technique. J Neurol Neurosurg Psychiatry. 1980;43(6):475–82. https://doi.org/10.1136/jnnp.43.6.475. PMID: 7205288; PMCID: PMC490586.
17. Stålberg E, Antoni L. Electrophysiological cross section of the motor unit. J Neurol Neurosurg Psychiatry. 1980;43(6):469–74. https://doi.org/10.1136/jnnp.43.6.469. PMID: 7205287; PMCID: PMC490585.
18. Van Campenhout A, Molenaers G. Localization of the motor endplate zone in human skeletal muscles of the lower limb: anatomical guidelines for injection with botulinum toxin. Dev Med Child Neurol. 2011;53(2):108–19. https://doi.org/10.1111/j.1469-8749.2010.03816.x. PMID: 20964675.

Chapter 4
Safety and Troubleshooting

Jose Alberto Nunes Sobrinho, Monica Nascimento de Melo, and Silvia Mazzali Verst

Abbreviations

DCS	direct cortical stimulation
DBS	deep brain stimulator
EEG	electroencephalography
EMG	electroneuromyography
EP	evoked potentials
IOM	intraoperative monitoring
OR	operating room
MEP	motor evoked potential
TES	transcranial electrical stimulation
SSEP	somatosensory evoked potential

Supplementary Information The online version contains supplementary material available at [https://doi.org/10.1007/978-3-030-95730-8_4].

J. A. Nunes Sobrinho (✉)
Department of Neurophysiology, Stela Clinic, Brasilia, Brazil

M. N. de Melo
Department of Neurophysiology, Integrated Neuroscience Institute, Goiânia, GO, Brazil

S. M. Verst
Instituto de Ensino e Pesquisa (Research and Educational Institute) of Sírio Libanês Hospital, São Paulo, Brazil

Brain Spine Neurofisiologia, Jundiaí, SP, Brazil

S. M. Verst et al. (eds.), *Intraoperative Monitoring*,
https://doi.org/10.1007/978-3-030-95730-8_4

Introduction

IOM advances as a medical specialty that combines neurological signals analysis in real-time with surgical approaches. Integration of multimodal analysis offers a better understanding of neurological reactions, enhancing surgeon's maneuvers to avoid neural damage. The modalities of evoked potentials (EP), electroneuromyography (EMG), and electroencephalography (EEG) are interspersed as frequently as possible since simultaneity is neither desired nor possible.

As the sophistication of neurophysiological signal modalities ensues, it is paramount to hasten the development of systems that safely stimulate and record, without posing a hazard to the patient's integrity. Neurophysiological practice involves the interaction of two large electrical systems: the human body and a recording machine. Both are sources of electric current generation, energy dissipation, resistance to transmission, charge storage, and production of electric and magnetic vectors, and, as such, are subject to the same physical laws. The dynamics of electrical interaction and induction of magnetic fields created by electron displacement establish the basic notions for obtaining the most appropriate recordings [1–3]. It reduces interference as well as enhances the electrical safety of the patient and examiner, thus preventing injuries.

The direct effect of the electric current on the corticospinal tract produces physical effects on the body such as movements with possible biting of the tongue and lips, seizures, and arrhythmia. The use of invasive electrodes such as needles, cortical grids, and spinal electrodes increases the risk of infection and bleeding. It is paramount for good practice that the neurophysiologist predicts these risks and minimizes them whenever possible.

In the OR numerous electrical devices are simultaneously and competitively connected to or close to the patient, like mechanical ventilators, catheters, infusers, body warmers, electrosurgical devices, cardioverters, neuronavigators, aspirators, lamps, and cleaning devices. All these connections increase both the presence of artifacts and electrical noise in the IOM recordings, and the electrical risk to which the patient is exposed. The catastrophic event occurs when an amount of current, over the estimated, enters the body, and/or follows the flow to exit via an unexpected route. Therefore, for better prevention and minimization of risks, the knowledge of the basic elements of physics and its application becomes primordial.

Physics Applied to Neurophysiology

The displacement of the electrons follows the principle of energy saving, starting from the largest orbit to the least energy orbit, and is titled *electric current* (i) to its flow during the time, whose vector representation has opposite direction to the movement. As a result, we have as fundamental concept that the electric current is directly proportional to the amounts of charges *(Q)* that moves during a unit of time in which the movement *(t)* occurs, deducting the formula below:

$$i = Q / t$$

where current is measured in *Amp (A)* and represents the charge of 1 Coulomb *(C)* in 1 second.

The ease of losing or gaining electrons determines the conductivity of the material (conductive and non-conductive), and the more uniform its composition, the more predictable its behavior will be. For example, consider the differences in pedicle screw composition and the impact it results in determining threshold values (see Chap. 23 for details). To generate the current, it is necessary to establish a difference in charges between two points (in neurophysiology, two electrodes), since equilibrium is assumed as the natural state. Without this maintenance of the differential, the tendency of electrons is to occupy their orbits of stable movements tending to neutrality.

Concepts Applied to IOM

Electrical Current and Charges

The favorable property of materials for displacement of loads depends on their structure, giving their nature to be conductive or non-conductive. The easier the electrons pass through the material, the lower its resistivity or electrical resistance, and the greater its conductivity. Conversely, the more difficult the displacement, the greater resistivity, less conductivity, and more suitable for charges storage is the material in question. It can be anticipated that non-conductive materials are used in the production of capacitors for charge storage (see below), and mixed compounds that use different materials can function both as conductor and as storage according to the predominant characteristic in a particular situation, as in the case of the human body.

Important concepts reflected in electrical safety are established:

(a) The higher the voltage of the electrical source *(V)*, the greater the amount of current *(i)* generated by the greater amount of charge *(Q)* in motion
(b) Joules' Law (James P. Joules, 1849): the heat/energy raised by the passage of the electric current is proportional to the conductor's resistance, to the square of the voltage intensity, and to the time during which it passes in the conductor. If only the relationship among voltage and current is considered, regardless of time, we arrive at the definition of work (*T*, in watt). The kinetic energy of the electron movement correlates the work directly proportional to the amount of charge (*Q*) and the voltage that prints this displacement (*V*) over time (in joules).

Thus,

$$\mathrm{T} = V \times i$$

$$E = V \times Q \therefore E = V \times i \times t$$

what enables us to accurately predict that higher the voltage or current, and longer the time involved, more energy or heat will be produced. Consequently, it is greater the risk of burns. Classic consequences of electric current flow through the body include direct effects on cell membranes (e.g., cellular depolarization or electroporation), at nerve and muscle cells, burns and deep necrosis (in alternating current accidents) [4]. *However, brain damage and kindling are highly unlikely* [5].

Electric currents can be either alternated or pulsed, in consonance to the variation over time, defining the shape of the wave (square, triangular, sinusoidal, exponential, etc.), and according to the direction that the charges move (single-phase or two-phase). According to international conventions and safety parameters, IOM equipment uses low voltage direct current (4).

Regarding biphasic waves, they can have equal (symmetrical) or different (asymmetric) amplitudes. **The duration or width of the pulse (*D*) determines the duration of time that the charges will pass on each pulse. Altogether, taking a square wave as an example, the total charge dispensed will depend on the current intensity, the pulse duration, the number of pulses, and the wave morphology**

$$\mathrm{Qt} = i \times D \times N\mathrm{pulse}\left(\times 2, \mathrm{if\ biphasic}\right)$$

If the wave is sinusoidal, it is corrected with a factor of 0.637; if the current has an exponential decay (charge generated by a capacitor), it is multiplied by the time constant related to the discharge [6].

Caution with electrical safety is an important step in IOM protocols and the stimulus parameters cannot be set randomly. The amount of charge delivered is a product of ***Intensity x Pulse Duration x Stimulator Electrode Diameter*** (Coulomb's Law). Electrode diameter is directly responsible for charge density.

Resistance, Impedance, and Reactance

One must ponder the resistance *(R,* measured in Ω), whose usefulness is to disperse the kinetic energy of electron movement in heat. If there was no interposition of this element, the amount of energy that would reach the poles of the source would quickly destroy them. At this point it is worth remembering two significant laws, namely:

I. **Ohm's Law (Georg S. Ohm, 1826): voltage results from the product of resistance versus current. If we have a constant resistance, the electric current will be proportional to the system voltage.** On the other hand, the greater the resistance of the material, the lower the current.

$$V = R \times i \therefore i = V / R$$

In a circuit where the resistors are arranged in a series system, the total resistance will be the direct sum of the resistances.

According to Ohm's law, in a constant voltage stimulator the delivered charge will not overcome tissue resistance variation and can be lower of the established. Conversely, by a constant current stimulator, the final charge will be established since it will adapt to tissue resistance. This directly impacts many tests in IOM. Taking as an example TES for corticobulbar tract, if there is a variation due to scalp edema or air inside the skull, the final delivered current may be not enough for supramaximal activation of the motor pathway (more details in Chap. 21).

II. Kirchhoff's Laws (Gustav Kirchhoff, 1845): the energy in one system can be transformed into another, but its total will be the sum of the values (general law of energy conservation). The same is true about the current: the total current entering a node in the closed system will be equal to the sum of the leaving currents. Likewise, the voltage in a mesh system of that node will be the same for all devices. Therefore, in a parallel system, the sum of the resistances will be represented by its inverse, according to the formula below

$$it = i1 + i2 \ldots \therefore V / R\mathrm{t} = V / R1 + V / R2 \ldots$$

$$\text{or, simplifying } V,$$

$$1 / Rt = 1 / R1 + 1 / R2 \ldots$$

Energy can also be defined as the function among voltage, electric current, charge, and resistance, established by Joules' law combined with Ohms' law. Thus, we will have the formulas:

$$E = i \wedge 2 \times t \times R \therefore E = V \wedge 2 / R \times t \therefore E = i \wedge 2 \times D \times R,$$

where time is replaced by the duration of the stimulus to determine the total charge.

However, we must consider the equivalent resistance applied to the neurophysiological routine. There will be both resistances from different equipment in parallel connected to the patient and the human body also acting as another equivalent total resistance in parallel (resulting from the sum of several "resistances" in series of the different tissues). The calculation is not an easy task since body resistance is not stable. It depends on many factors that are neither accessible nor controllable, such as the dynamic variation of the body reacting to the variation in volume of the instilled fluids, organic composition, stature, size, and thickness of the organs, to mention some examples.

Being this the case, in an equipment composed of several electrical elements constituted of different materials, it is not appropriate to call it resistivity and resistance, which is the peculiar property of each of them, but impedance (*Z*), measured in Ω), the same relationship remaining in accordance with Ohms' law. Example: a copper resistor has its resistivity and resistance checked by the material of the alloy that composes it, and it is perfectly calculated. However, equipment resistance is not spoken when several compound electronic components are integrated and made of different materials, but, instead, impedance.

Although the impedance translation is mistaken for the "resistance" to the electrical passage, it goes beyond the characteristic heat dissipation nature and includes the storage of electrical charges and energy (capacitance), and the reason for the associated magnetic flux that passes through the circuit (inductance). The combination of these properties determines reactance (*X*) of the system. *The same situation is applied to the human body, which offers a variable reactance according to its individual composition, able to accumulate charges, dissipate, transfer, and induce currents according to its variable composition, its physical-chemical state, and according to its content.*

$$Z = R + X$$

The risks arising from elements of low resistance arranged on the surface or inside the human body, such as catheters, metal electrodes, or wires, appear to be more understandable, making it easier to drain incoming or accumulated charges. The human body itself has areas of greater or lesser conductivity, and depending on the physiological state, presenting greater or lesser reactance.

The arrangement of tissues makes the human body a semiconductor system with heterogeneous charge storage capacity, making its reactance fluctuate constantly. As the dry skin, dermis, tendons, and bones offer greater impedance, damp skin, muscles, nerves, and the bloodstream behave in the exact opposite manner. Following the same line of reasoning, the conditions surrounding the body favor the reduction of impedance, such as wet surfaces or even their immersion in water or contact with conductive or non-conductive materials. *Considering IOM practice, the insertion of catheters, subdermal or intramuscular electrodes, plates, surface electrodes with conductive gel, among several others, are favorable means for the transmission of charges, and are sometimes more relevant due to the decrease in reactance* [7].

Recalling, electric displacement obeys the rule of energy saving: where there is less impedance, less resistivity, less difficulty to flow, and greater conductivity, this will be the path of choice for the stream of electron flow [2].

Capacitor and Filters

The charge rate of the capacitor depends on the variation of the voltage of the source for the accumulation of charges, and the current generated by its discharge depends on the frequency of variation of the voltage of the source, both following an exponential relationship with the time constant. *A practical importance regarding the study of the system's capacitance is found in the generation of electrical artifacts: the lower this property of the device, the greater the chance that the current generated by the system source reaches electrodes and causes electrical artifacts* [8, 9].

The neurophysiology device combines resistance and capacitor connected to the same source, that is, one element that disperses and another that accumulates energy. This alliance between antagonistic elements allows modulation in

obtaining signals, where the restriction of high frequencies and the passage of low frequencies correspond to the capacitive property of the system, while the inverse takes place when it comes to the resistance. The time constant, which is directly proportional to capacitance and resistance, and represents the time for the current to charge the capacitor could be compared to the width of a narrow gap: the wider, the greater the composition of slow frequencies, and the narrower, the greater the composition of fast frequencies.

The high- and low-frequency filters consist of the parallel association of the resistor or the capacitor, whose determination of which of the two is connected in series with the source will define which type of frequency will have its passage restricted. To provide a better understanding of the process, we return to the capacitor reactance concept (X_C) to establish the relationship with the frequency of the waves (f) using the formula below:

$$Xc = 1 / 2\pi fC$$

C is the capacitance (invariant constant) of the capacitor. We can predict that higher frequencies will produce lower reactance X and this will make it harder for low-frequency waves to pass, and consequently lower frequencies will determine higher reactance X, which will offer a barrier to the passage of higher frequencies. If the capacitor is connected in series with the power source, it will prevent low frequencies from passing and will favor the passage of high frequencies (low-frequency filter). If the capacitor is connected in parallel with the source, the low frequencies will not be restricted to the passage, but the resistance connected in series will hinder the passage of the high frequencies. Defining the resistance value, we will restrict the cut of the high frequency that we want (high-frequency filter).

This cutoff frequency is defined as the value that will produce the attenuation of 30% of the input value, which corresponds to equal values of the reactance and the capacitance ($R = XC$). In high-frequency filters, values above the stipulated cutoff frequency are attenuated by 70%, while in low-frequency filters the reverse occurs (frequencies below the cutoff value will be reduced by 70%).

Filtering is an important issue regarding IOM success. Since there is a direct influence between the filter band and the potential amplitude, the narrower the band, the smaller the amounts of axons visualized within the potential.

For practical purposes, the arrangement of the capacitor in series with the source defines the low-frequency filter, and the capacitor in parallel with the source specifies the high-frequency filter, whose cut will be determined by the resistance.

Grounding in IOM

It is fundamental to ensure that unwanted or unforeseen currents do not circulate through patient's body, since it can trigger catastrophic or unpleasant events. To avoid risks, it is imperative to eliminate these charges out of the circuit by draining through grounding. Its primary function is to offer a safe path to eliminate this energy, protecting the system from damage (both the equipment and the individual connected to it). The ideal ground is one that offers low resistance, high conductivity, and dispersion of charges (guarantee of low density of charges), while remaining neutral. Although this ideal element does not exist in the practical reality, the Earth represents the closest thing that can be reached due to its characteristics (mass dimension and distribution of charges over its surface, resulting in low density, added to the equipotential distance given by the radius of the planet).

By extension, any electrical element that favors the dispersion of charges is called ground, although this nomination might produce confusion in certain circumstances. **The ground of the electrical network to which the ground of the device box (chassis) is connected (for the dispersion of charges to the Earth) is not the same for "patient ground" (for dispersion of charge from the recording electrodes). Patient's ground is related to impedances measurement to reduce artifacts at the registration site** [10, 11]. **It represents the establishment of a point of comparison between differential amplifiers to reject signals in common mode and are arranged electronically isolated from all other grounds. Meanwhile, the electrical network ground (true ground) consists of the electrical component for draining the current, even that produced by the magnetic induction generated by the circulation of electrons in the electrical components (leakage currents).** Exceptionally, in anomalous conditions of true ground operation, flow of electrical charges through this route offers a high risk of an overload to the patient and the system.

Hence pronounced attention ought to be paid to the conditions of the ground. The protection recommendations require the existence of effective grounding of the devices, and this must not be the neutral pole of the power line. It is recommended not adding more than one ground to the patient to avoid loop current formation between both points (Fig. 4.1). *All electrical equipment connected to the patient must be connected to the same set of sockets to ensure the same equipotential ground* (Fig. 4.2). *It is recommended never to use devices other than medical/hospital devices in the same network system to which the patient is connected. The reason is that non-electronic biomedical devices can have leakage current greater than the determined safety limit* [10, 11].

In conditions of malfunction of the device, the generation of leakage current can have its draining flow interrupted in the presence of a ground break. It could be any of the system's ground: the internal ground cable of the device connected to the chassis, the ground of the cable of the voltage cable, or the ground system of the electrical network. Under these conditions, the generated charge may use another route of less reactance to escape, passing through the electrodes and going to the patient. For safety reasons, the exhaust current is set below 100μV or 100μA for medical and electronic medical devices in normal conditions (and 500μA for the patient when not connected to devices). Intensity of 20μV or 10μA, if applied directly to the endocardium or to smaller individuals, can generate ventricular fibrillation [6, 10].

Bearing in mind the risks of electrical current passing through the myocardium and subsequent severe and symptomatic arrhythmia, the International

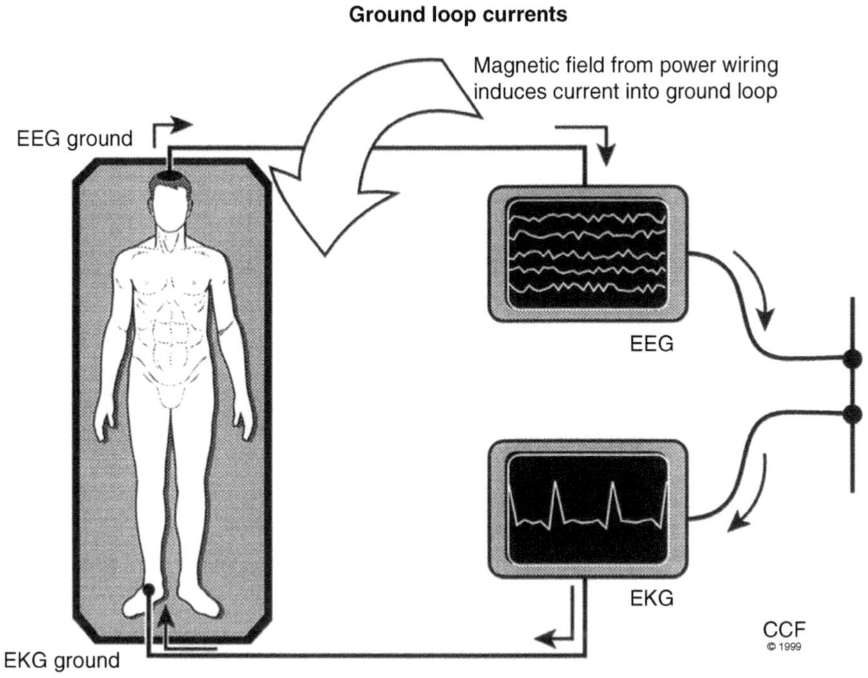

Fig. 4.1 Non-equipotential grounds. The magnetic field generated by the power wiring induces current into ground loop. If, due to the positioning of the cables of the different equipment, the patient becomes a conducting part of this loop and conducts the current, an injury can occur. (From Levin KH, Luders HO (2000). Comprehensive Clinical Neurophysiology, WB Saunders)

Electrotechnical Commission establishes the heart current factor as the ratio of the risk of rhythm disturbance and cardiac conduction (the most deleterious being ventricular fibrillation) compared to the passage of current through the left hand and foot ($F = 1$) according to possible pathways (Table 4.1) [6]. The awareness of this notion enables the proposal of the strategy of placing the grounding plates on the patient's body according to the lowest values of F, minimizing the severity in unwanted events. Besides to foot (F), other body regions can be considered as current input and output ports, having their values estimated for the impedance calculation comparatively [10]. For example, the impedance between the neck and the left hand is 60% less than between the left hand and the left foot, resulting in the passage of a greater amount of current (Ohm's law). By IOM there is the usage of multiple materials simultaneously. Thus, it is recommended to adopt the lowest impedance value aiming to prevent harm. It must be kept in mind that such calculations are considered as a reference possibility, and do not include intravascular and intracardiac devices, which reduce the general reactance.

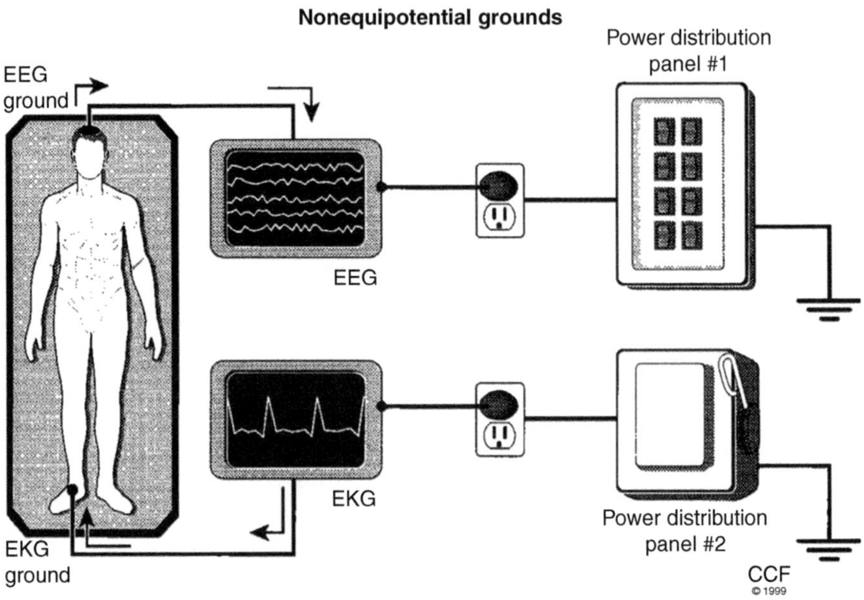

Fig. 4.2 Ground loop currents. When the equipment connected to the patient is powered by circuits derived from circuit breakers on different panels, the grounding between them may not be equipotential and the patient may carry current between them. (From Levin KH, Luders HO (2000). Comprehensive Clinical Neurophysiology, WB Saunders)

Table 4.1 Correction factor for current path

Path of the electric current passing through the human body	F
From the left hand to the left foot, to the right foot or to both feet	1,0
From both hands to both feet	1,0
From the left hand to the right hand	0,4
From the right hand to the left foot, the right foot or both feet	0,8
From the back to the right hand	0,3
From the back to the left hand	0,7
From the chest to the right hand	1,3
From the chest to the left hand	1,5
Left hand, right hand or both hands and buttocks	0,7

Adapted from: IEC-479-1, Effects of Current on human beings and livestock. Accessed on July 20th, 2021. https://www.abntcatalogo.com.br/norma.aspx?ID=410528

Safety Paradigms

In a systematic review (including 26,750 publications), Dechent et al. (2002) found four reports of mild adverse effects (burns and skin lesions) associated with TES.

As safe as a modern IOM system might be, every precaution must be taken to prevent unwanted events. Perhaps the worst of all causes is to ignore or minimize the risks of accidents, thus providing the cascade of errors and their dire consequences. Indeed, all body tissues and organs can be affected by the current flow.

Electric Stimulation

The threats of injury by shock or stimulation are due to the intensity and displacement of the electric current, and the energy. The consequences of the shock are also proportional to the physical variables that act in the propagation of the current through the body, like the frequency of the event, to the body region involved, and to the path through the body. It is considered more relevant if (a) proximal to the heart, (b) involves a large area of the body, and (c) if there is a system integrity disruption (dependent on component impedance and skin characteristic), (d) duration of the flow, and (e) humidity of the environment [4]. These factors affect the intensity of current and energy generated.

The intensity of the current will depend on the potential difference, amounts of displaced charges, duration and number of pulses, area of the electrodes, resistance/impedance of the system, and discharge duration.

Other factors should be added, such as the propagation path, the reactance of the body and materials, and the dispersion of energy. The same current intensity over a tissue or body area differs according to its characteristics. For instance, differences in the integrity and physiological conditions of the skin (temperature and skin type) contribute to fluctuating impedance values [12].

The intensity of the stimulus needed to generate a neural action potential and consequent muscle response varies with the duration of the pulse, rheobase, and chronaxie. Using a rectangular pulse, rheobase is related to the smallest value of current applied when considering an infinite pulse width (250 to 1000 μs), while chronaxie is the smallest pulse width to generate muscle contraction, considering twice the rheobase [13]. Parameters that limit the strength of the stimulus make IOM safer. Accordingly, current, charge, and energy are interrelated and if in imbalance, are potentially harmful. Reducing the duration of the stimulus leads to increase in the current threshold and, if too high, it favors electrochemical damage. Increasing the duration of the pulse, on the other hand, can increase the offered charge and consequently the risk of excitotoxic damage.

Leakage Current or Equipment Malfunction

The main concern about current leakage or excessive load output is their potential of finding a pathway through the heart, causing severe arrhythmias like ventricular fibrillation. The presence of central venous access of lower resistance can facilitate this situation. The risk is higher by alternating current and is directly related to its final strength and frequency. The connection of several devices in the OR increases voltage sources and the possibility of grounding paths between the equipment and the patient. However, some simple precautions can minimize these risks [13]:

A. Periodic electrical safety testing – identifies possible leakage currents outside the safety limits and possible malfunction of cables and equipment connections that can generate a difference between the current set on the screen and the current offered to the patient.
B. Pay attention to the device's notifications during IOM – modern equipment has its own protection systems that inform the neurophysiologist when there is an inadequate connection. It automatically interrupts stimulation when there is an overload and limits the intensity of stimulation according to the other parameters used (duration, frequency, inter-stimulus interval). For safety reasons, the modern IOM system performs auto-checking when turned on.
C. Avoid extension cables, and tin soldered plugs and cables. Preferably, choose touch proof connectors – these measures help maintain the protective grounding.
D. Use stimulus parameters established in the literature.
E. Never place the IOM boxes under intravenous drip holders, bladder tubes, or where fluids may enter. Direct contact of liquid with the boxes can reduce impedance to a value lower than that of the plate, turning into an alternative and unwanted area for current flow. Listed situations would be a) incidental leakage of serum, or urine, b) excessive sweating due to thermal blanket. Additionally, avoid locating the grounding plate arranged in a region with a high concentration of hair, which could lead in low contact and greater impedance than desired. The dynamic nature of the skin must be controlled and anticipated, particularly in prolonged surgical procedures, to prevent accidents.

Excitotoxicity and Electrochemical Damage

Load, charge density, and current intensity can create a peri-cellular electric field due to the movement of ions. During direct stimulation on the nervous tissue, as occurs in subcortical cathodal stimulation, the higher intracellular concentration of negative charges can result in a reduction in proteins. Conversely, anodic cortical stimulation generates a higher concentration of positive ions, facilitating oxidation. Although both processes are correlated to a plethora of neurodegenerative diseases [14, 15], experimental evidence of injury was found only in the animal model after prolonged monophasic stimulation [16]. Yuen et al. in 1981 identified that biphasic pulse trains at 50 Hz caused neuronal damage within 15 h of the experiment [17]. It is far more prolonged than that performed in surgical procedures.

Specifically, during TES there is an important dissipation of charge in the ratio of 20:1 through the skin and skull [8]. Thus, due to the absence of reports of excitotoxicity in humans, the technique is apparently quite safe, since the intracranial charge and charge density are probably below the lesion threshold. Nevertheless, some cautions deserve attention. Very small electrodes increase the charge density, and the use of 1cm^2 electrodes is indicated in DCS [13]. Pulses of 0.2 ms limit the charge when compared to longer pulses and are also preferable. Always use stimuli with parameters well established in the literature and only with the intensity necessary to obtain the responses.

Thermal Injury and Burns

Considering the energy measured in joules by the relationships between voltage, electric current, and resistance, stimuli from constant electric current vary the intensity of the voltage (Ohm's law). In extreme cases of intense resistance, the current would be limited by the capacity to increase the voltage inherent in the device, whose intrinsic limit could even prevent its generation. On the other hand, stimuli produced by constant voltage, in the face of changing resistance, tend to produce variable electric current. Thus, energy is also estimated to be unstable.

The energy released by the electric current is translated into heat. The best perception of the action of energy on tissues comes from devices used in electrosurgery or diathermy, and their consequent denaturing effect on cellular proteins and tissues: coagulation and vaporization. During fever of 40 degrees, some enzymes can have their tertiary and quaternary conformation reversibly modified, partially altering their function. Above 50 degrees, denaturation for more than 6 minutes leads to cell death.

Thermal injuries occur due to inadequate heat dissipation, and their incidence in IOM is estimated at 0.01%. As previously described, energy is related to current intensity, pulse duration, and resistance, and its empirical safety limit in TES is 50 mJ at 1 k resistance [6, 18]. Very short pulses increase energy and can facilitate thermal injury. Durations of 0.01 ms should be avoided in DCS. Ideally, the pulse duration should be adjusted to tissue chronaxie, but this parameter is not always known or the adjustment feasible. Evidence suggests that the average chronaxie in DCS MEP is 0.2 ms [19], which is why stimuli of this duration are preferable and considered safer.

Another way to minimize the risk of thermal injury is to avoid intensities above what is needed for optimal responses and to avoid high intensities in TES using a pulse duration of 0.05 ms. The effects of the controlled current expended during the somatosensory evoked potential (SSEP) or TES are easy to quantify [17], even though the heat generated can affect structures unevenly. *The calculated current densities in direct cortical MEP application range between 0.029 mA/cm^2 and 0.057 mA/cm^2, thus far below the safety limit of 14.29 mA/cm^2* [4].

Electrocautery represents a direct transmission of heat to the tissue, with no current flowing through it, since the pathways are contained at a single end. It employs high frequencies that do not depolarize nerves and muscles but interfere with neurophysiological screen recordings. Yet, the current transits between the tip and the plate positioned in contact with the patient's skin. Generally, the plate has a large surface area, which reduces the local charge density and generates less heat. But if the plate comes loose, or in presence of malfunctions or breaks in the cable, current can leak through lower impedance points and nearby electrodes. In these cases, IOM's needle electrodes are potentially harmful because their small surface area causes high energy density and heat, with possible burns. Whenever possible, IOM equipment, cables, and connections should be kept away, and needle electrodes should not be placed close to the plate.

Preventive Measures

There is the risk posed by a device without adequate preventive maintenance to cause the passage of electrical current beyond what is recommended. It could cause tissue damage near the entrance, or at a distance depending on the intensity. Yearly system check-up hinders the risk of accidents.

Reuse of electrodes poses a higher risk of injury since in this case the electrodes have a far higher resistivity up to a factor of 10,000 [4]. It is strictly not recommended.

Adverse Effects

Biting and Movement

In TES, some degree of movement is always expected, and the proximity of the stimulus point to the temporal muscles and trigeminal nerve promotes strong activation of the masseter muscle and risk of tongue biting. The incidence of such an event is approximately 0.2%, and the use of soft protectors between the teeth (silicone protectors or gauze roll) is indicated whenever the technique is used [17, 20]. Rigid guards should be avoided as they offer the additional risk of tooth breakage. Injuries are usually restricted to bruising or minor lacerations of lips and/or tongue, and the need for surgical repair is rare (Fig. 4.3).

Body movement in TES can be reduced by using more selective montages such as C3-CZ, C4-CZ, C1-C2, and midline instead of C3-C4 and avoiding the use of high stimulus intensities (more details of topographic-guided MEP refer to Chap. 9). Not least, good communication between neurophysiologist and surgeon is essential so that the stimulations are performed at a timely moment within the times of the surgery. Thus, the surgeon can quickly stop manipulation near a neural structure so that TES can be performed.

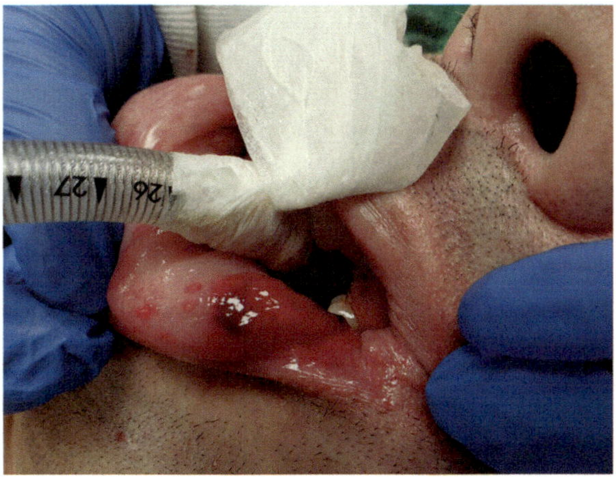

Fig. 4.3 Bite injury due to TES

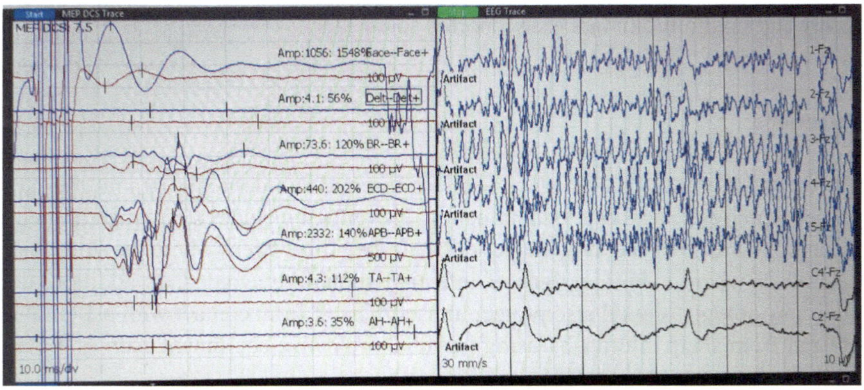

Fig. 4.4 Seizure triggered by DCS

Seizures and Afterdischarges

Particularly, patients with a history of epilepsy, diffuse brain lesions, and during the use of the Penfield technique are more likely to have ictic or epileptiform discharge events after direct electric stimulation [5, 17, 18].

Seizures and afterdischarges are rare with high-frequency TES (0.03%) [18], but may occur in DCS or direct subcortical stimulation, especially when the 50-60 Hz technique is used. During direct brain stimulation, there is an estimated incidence of seizures in 5 to 20% of patients using low frequency, while with high-frequency technique the incidence is about 1% [18] (Fig. 4.4). The use of cold serum irrigation is recommended to control the event (the use of anticonvulsant drugs may prevent language mapping, although its use in refractory cases is strongly advised). For more a comprehensive understanding read Chap. 17.

Arrhythmias

Cardiac arrhythmias are rarely reported in the literature. Besides the excessive current output and its intracardiac passage, arrhythmias can occur by electric stimulation at brainstem autonomic centers, especially during the mapping of lesions in IV-ventricle floor [18]. The lack of reports might be related to low morbidity rate.

Risk Due to the Use of Invasive Electrodes

Bleeding and Bruising

The placement of cortical grids or D-wave electrodes in the epidural/subdural space can potentially cause traction and rupture of vessels leading to bleeding or hematoma formation. However, usually, the surgeon performs the maneuver quite delicately and no morbidity has been reported so far [13].

Infections

To record responses, needle electrodes are inserted sub-dermally or into muscles bellies which pose a risk of local infection. Prevention includes skin preparation by cleaning it with 70% alcohol or alcoholic chlorhexidine. Areas where the skin is not healthy or where there are signs of infection should be avoided. In addition, the neurophysiologist should also protect himself/herself from contact with patient fluids and from sharp injuries by using personal protective equipment such as gloves and goggles.

Needle electrodes, cortical grids, D-wave electrodes, and stimulators should be sterile and discarded after use.

Contraindications to IOM

The risk-benefit of IOM must be considered and weighted in face of relative contraindications, like pacemakers and/or implantable bioelectric devices, DBS, epilepsy, vascular clips or shunts, and skull deformities. Adaptations of the technique can enable testing targeted to patients' needs.

Electronic Implants

Modern electronic devices are built with amplification of electrical and motion signals to detect and trigger responses or set for continuous or alternate stimulation. It allows for increased sensitivity to those who are interested in correcting dysfunction but leaves them more subject to interference, either electrical or mechanical, originating from the organism itself or external, as well as exogenous magnetic and radioactive. The list includes pacemakers of fixed or variable demand (cardiac or *vagus* nerve), deep stimulators of the nervous or substance release system, cochlear implants, etc. In general, they have filters that select the frequency of deflagration, or mechanisms that prevent the passage of currents, setting the activation of safety modes. However, the possibility of interference is common to all, with greater or lesser risk of deregulation of the device [21, 22]. Yellin et al. (2015) described the successful use of TES in two pediatric patients with cochlear implants [23]. Thus, risks and benefits should be analyzed according to patient's needs.

Pacemakers

Specially about pacemakers, their circuits amplify, filter, and identify the cardiac potentials, correcting bradycardia and tachycardia. External electrical interferences can provoke dysfunction, leading to inhibition, asynchronous reversion, or inappropriate defibrillation [24]. A strong electrical charge could damage its components or overheat the electrode-myocardia junction without possible repair. So electrical bistoury, thermocautery, MRI, radiotherapy, radiofrequency, diathermia, and TES are normally avoided. Several protection mechanisms have been created to avoid continuous current to enter the pacemaker or to short cut high-intensity currents before they damage it. Such mechanisms are bipolar electrodes, electronic filtering, and spectral detection. Under a skilled specialist, the pacemaker program can be modified during a specific procedure to stand a hostile situation. The recommendation is that during the IOM to rely on the presence of a technician in the OR for adjusting the specific configuration and tracking of the device. If necessary, set to asynchronous mode [22] (Fig. 4.5). A practical alternative is also to modify the stimulation frequency to produce desynchronization between the electronic device artifact and the wave to be studied, or the application of cardiac stimulus with bipolar electrodes, reducing the extension of the artifact.

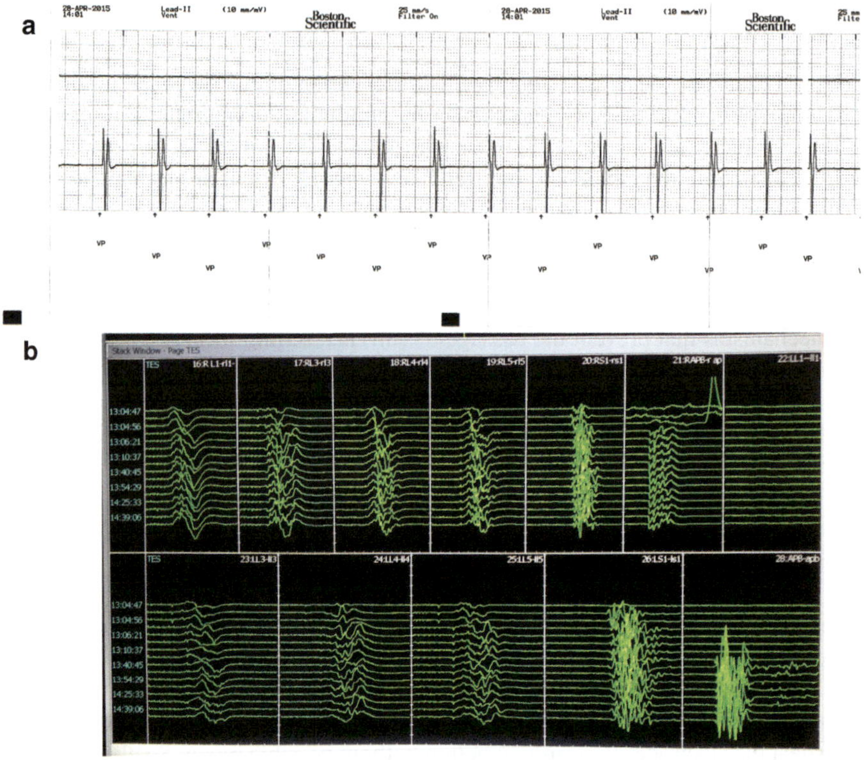

Fig. 4.5 MAS, female, 75y.o., going through a L3-L5 lumbar stenosis decompression. TES was performed with C3-C4 stimulation, train of 6 pulses, 0,5 ms duration, 4 ms interpulse interval, 300 V. The patient had a bicameral pacemaker due to total AV blockage. Immediate after the positioning of the patient, the cardiologist turned the pacemaker to an assincronic function, which stimulated the ventricle with 6,5 V, 1 ms duration, and 80 bpm. In an assincronic function the pacemaker was not influenced for an external electrical source and TES was registered several times during the decompression maneuver. (**a**) Pacemaker registration during TES. (**b**) TES

Troubleshooting

Electrical Artifacts

Artifacts or noise are broadly defined as any signal captured that is not of interest to the purpose of the study. Usually, biological signals of interest are made up of a set of frequencies. Thus, in the examination of SSEP, muscle contractions studied on EMG, electrocardiogram, or respiratory movement captured during the EEG, environmental noise during language testing would be characterized as noise. On the other hand, eye movement recorded during sleep is a useful activity for staging the REM phase, or even drowsiness, aiding in the diagnostic interpretation. Noises/artifacts are, therefore, signals from multiple sources (biological and non-biological) registered within the chosen spectrum of the frequencies to be analyzed, or which impair their interpretation.

The first action to minimize the effects of the artifacts is knowing the frequency range of the biological signals under study and applying a bandwidth filtering to improve their recording but not causing distortion to the point of misinterpretation [25]. Additionally, limiting the time window with an appropriate sweep time for detecting the studied potentials mitigate irrelevant signals.

Some simple measures can help, like (a) keeping the IOM system (including recording boxes) distant from the potential sources of electromagnetic fields (electrocautery, microscopes, radioscopy), (b) not sharing electrical sockets, (c) joining or braiding the electrodes cables.

There is no single protocol to be followed to minimize or eliminate noise, although recognizing the most common ones surely helps in dealing with its source. A helpful sequence could be (a) correctly distinguish between an artifact and an electrode leakage, break or disconnection, (b) guide following actions according to the most likely suspicions. Unfortunately, it is not uncommon to be unable to identify where the major cause is coming from in environments with numerous competitors.

Troubleshooting in Non-biological Electrical Artefacts

(a) Check if the sockets are grounded and preferably on a mutual ground, i.e., exclusively for the flow of charges from medical equipment used to care of that patient (do not connect the patient directly to this electrical ground). Connecting to outlets with different grounds can generate uneven ground loops.
(b) All equipment connected to the patient must have its own isolation system, producing no leakage currents greater than 10–20 μA (optimal). It is assumed that the insulation tests and prophylactic maintenance of the equipment are carried out routinely to ensure good and proper electrical operation, with leakage currents through the chassis up to 100 μA. The devices must be previously connected to their connection with the patient, and turned off only after proceeding with their disconnection, ensuring that leakage currents do not move.
(c) 50 Hz or 60 Hz artifacts can come from the socket itself, whose grounding is not adequate, network overload due to the amount of equipment connected, proximity between devices (Video 4.1) and/or crossing of capture and stimulation wires and cables, power cables, etc. (Video 4.2). Stimulation outside harmonic frequencies helps to reduce this type of artifact (Video 4.3). Expandable equipment for patient care should be turned off and disconnected from the network.

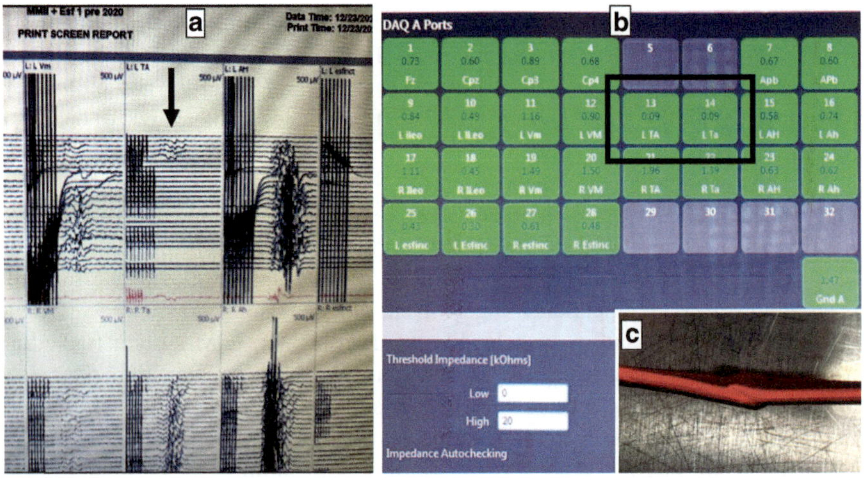

Fig. 4.6 (**a**) Loss of motor potentials in left tibialis anterior muscle. (**b**) Impedance test showing same impedance value. (**c**) Checking of electrodes revealed bending and electrode breakage

(d) The electrodes and stimulators must be in proper conditions of use, and have their impedances correctly assessed. Higher than expected impedances can indicate wire breakage, increased resistivity, or adhesion, and zero impedances can indicate the formation of electrical bridges (Fig. 4.6). Additionally, unbalanced impedance values between a pair of electrodes (>1kOhms) should be promptly corrected.

(e) The use of high- and/or low-frequency filters should be done with discretion, considering the changes they generate on biological signals. Over-filtration may lead to the error of generating waves that do not correspond to physiological signals.

Troubleshooting in Biological Electrical Artifacts

(a) Use of differentiated parameters (scan time, stimulation frequency, mediation, disposition of capture electrodes) can minimize the recording of artifacts.

(b) Environmental and patient control: (a) temperature stability prevents prolongation of latency due to temperature drop and alteration of signal amplitude; (b) control of level of consciousness during anesthesia using EEG and spectral edge frequencies avoid administration of drugs *bolus* or that modify the generation or capture of signals (Video 4.4).

Conclusion

Understanding basic concepts of bioelectricity and its effects on the human body greatly improves the recognition of possible risks to which a patient is exposed during IOM. When strictly performed within the recommended parameters, IOM does not cause irreversible cellular damage and is not related to high morbidity. Mostly, events are related to patient movements (which may disturb the surgeon), seizures, and bite injuries. However, under inappropriate conditions, like excessive electrical current output or passage of current through the heart, the risk of excitotoxicity, electrochemical and thermal injury, or arrhythmias increases.

The rich electromagnetic environment in OR can generate artifacts or noise that impair the interpretation of the recorded responses. It is part of a good practice of the neurophysiologist to understand these situations to correctly deal with them.

References

1. Halliday D, Resnick R, Walker J. Fundamentals of physics. 10th ed. Wiley Publisher; 2013.
2. Chaves A. Basic physics: electromagnetism. 1st ed. LTC Publisher; 2007.
3. Bauer W, Westfall GD, Dias H. Physics for university students: electricity and magnetism. 1st ed. AMGH Publisher; 2013.
4. Dechent D, Emonds T, Stunder D, Schmiedchen K, Kraus T, Driessen S. Direct current electrical injuries: a systematic review of case reports and case series. Burns. 2020;46(2):267–78. https://doi.org/10.1016/j.burns.2018.11.020.
5. Dineen J, Maus DC, Muzyka I, See RB, Cahill DP, Carter BS, Curry WT, Jones PS, Nahed BV, Peterfreund RA, Simon MV. Factors that modify the risk of intraoperative seizures triggered by electrical stimulation during supratentorial functional mapping. Clin Neurophysiol. 2019;130:1058–65.
6. IEC-479-1. Effects of current on human beings and livestock - part 1: general aspects. Publication 479–1 International Electrotechnical Commission; 1994.
7. Brazilian Standard of ABNT NBR IEC (2012) 60601–1 addendum 1, subsection 3, page 36 and subsection 4.8; 2016.
8. Brazilian Standard of ABNT NBR IEC 60601-1. 2nd edition. 2010:p.180. https://www.abntcatalogo.com.br/norma.aspx?ID=410528. Accessed on 20 July 2021.
9. Misulis KE. Basic electronics for clinical neurophysiology. J Clin Neurophysiol. 1989;6(1):41–74.
10. Kindermann G. Electric Shock. 4th edition of the author. Santa Catarina: LabPlan; 2013.
11. Burgess RC. Electrical safety. In: Levin KH, Chauvel P, editors. Handbook of clinical neurology, vol. 160. Elsevier; 2019. p. 67–81.
12. Brazilian Technical Standards Association (ABNT) NBR 5410. Low voltage electrical installations. 2004 (revised version 2008). pp. 30–31.
13. Macdonald DB, Seidel K, Shils JL. Safety. In: Deletis V, Shils JL, Sala F, Seidel K, editors. Neurophysiology in neurosurgery – a modern approach. Elsevier; 2020. p. 581–96.
14. Gandhi S, Abramov AY. Mechanism of oxidative stress in neurodegeneration (review). OxiMed and Cellular Longevity. 2012:1–11.

15. Matthew D, Matthew R, Namakkal SR, Victor DU, Jianhua Z. KEAP1 – NRF2 Signalling and autophagy in protection against oxidative and reductive proteotoxicity. Biochem J. 2015;469(3):347–55.
16. Merril DR, Bikson M, Jeffreys JGR. Electrical stimulation of excitable tissue: design of efficacious and safe protocols. J Neurosci Methods. 2005;141:171–98.
17. Macdonald DB. Safety of intraoperative transcranial electrical stimulation motor evoked potential monitoring. J Clin Neurophysiol. 2002;19(5):416–29.
18. Macdonald DB, Skinner S, Shills J, Yingling C. Intraoperative motor evoked potential monitoring – a position statement by the American Society of Neuropysiological Monitoring. Clin Neurophysiol. 2013;124:2291–316.
19. Abalkhail TM, Macdonald DB, AlThubaiti I, AlOtaibi FA, Stigsby B, Mokeem AA, AlHamoud IA, Hassounah MI, Baz SM, AlSemari A, AlDhalaan HM, Khan S. Intraoperative direct cortical stimulation motor evoked potentials: stimulus parameter recommendations based on rheobase and chronaxie. Clin Neurophysiol. 2017;128(11):2300–8. https://doi.org/10.1016/j.clinph.2017.09.005. Epub 2017 Sep 28
20. MacDonald DB, Deletis V. Safety issues during surgical monitoring. In: Nuwer MR, editor. Intraoperative monitoring of neural function, Handbook of clinical neurophysiology, vol. 8. Amsterdam: Elsevier; 2008. p. 88298.
21. Merrit WT, Brinker JA, Beattie C. Pacemaker-mediated tachycardia induced by intraoperative somatosensory evoked potential stimuli. Anesthesiology. 1988;69:766–8.
22. Schneider R, Machens Q, Bucher M, Raspé C, Heinroth K, Dralle H. Continuous intraoperative monitoring of vagus and recurrent laryngeal nerve function in patients with advanced atrioventricular block (rapid communications). Langenbeck's Arch Surg. 2016;401(4):551–6. https://doi.org/10.1007/s00423-016-1433-0. Epub 2016 Apr 30
23. Yellin JL, Wiggins CR, Franco AJ, Sankar WN. Safe transcranial electric stimulation motor evoked potential monitoring during spinal fusion in two patients with cochlear implants. J Clin Monit Comput. 2016;30:503–6.
24. Elmqvist R, Senning Ä. Implantable pacemaker for the heart. Proceedings of the second international conference on medical electronics, Paris. Jun 24–27, 1959.
25. Burgess RC. Filtering of neurophysiologic signals. In: Levin KH, Chauvel P, editors. Handbook of clinical neurology, vol. 160. Elsevier; 2019. p. 51–65.

Chapter 5
Central Nervous System Anesthesia: Asleep Approach

Nelson Mizumoto

Abbreviations

BBB	blood-brain barrier
BIS	Bispectral Index
CBF	cerebral blood flow
CBV	cerebral blood volume
$CMRO_2$	cerebral metabolic rates
CNS	central nervous system
CPP	cerebral perfusion pressure
ECoG	electrocorticographic
EEG	electroencephalography
Hb	hemoglobin
ICP	intracranial pressure
IOM	neurophysiological monitoring
MAP	median arterial pressure
MEP	motor-evoked potential
SSEP	somatosensory evoked potential
TIVA	total intravenous anesthesia

N. Mizumoto (✉)
Anesthesiology Coordinator at the Neurosurgery Department, Clinical Hospital of University of Sao Paulo Medical School, Sao Paulo, Brazil

S. M. Verst et al. (eds.), *Intraoperative Monitoring*,
https://doi.org/10.1007/978-3-030-95730-8_5

Intracranial Pressure (ICP) and Cerebral Blood Flow (CBF)

ICP normal range values are 10–15 mmHg and result from the interaction of liquor volume with the intracranial pressure, the cellular interstitial fluid, and the water volume inside neurons and astrocytes. Excessive water in the brain results in cerebral edema thus affecting its plasticity. Brain swelling leads to loss of vascular reactivity and causes increase in the cerebral blood volume. The intracranial compensation mechanism relieves the ICP increase when small volumes are added inside the skull [1, 2]

When the volume of one of the ICP constituents increases, this compensation mechanism decreases the volume of the other players in order to keep a constant ICP and to prevent the reduction of the CPP.

Cerebral Blood Volume and Cerebral Blood Flow

The intracranial blood volume may increase due to the augment of arterial dilation caused by increased cerebral metabolism, hypercapnia, hypoxia, or by the action of encephalic vasodilator drugs. The loss of arterial constriction (e.g., loss of cerebral autoregulation) elevates cerebral blood volume, which may worsen in the presence of systemic hypertension. Moreover, increased intracranial venous blood can occur with the obstruction of the brain's venous drainage system, either by expansive intracranial processes or by increased extracranial venous resistance such as high intrathoracic pressure, or yet, due to excessive neck rotation or patient's head positioned below the heart.

Factors which alter cerebral blood flow According to Ohm's law, the flux of fluids inside a rigid tube depends: (a) on the difference between the entrance pressure and the exit pressure in this tube, (b) as well as the fluid resistance in the tube. The flux equation is obtained by considering the fluid resistance degree as the tube's radius increase, and the fluid resistance increase as long is the tube; or more viscous is the fluid (Hagen-Poiseuille relation):

$$\boldsymbol{F} = \frac{(\boldsymbol{P1} - \boldsymbol{P2}).\boldsymbol{r}^4}{\mathbf{8}.\boldsymbol{l}.\eta}$$

[wherein *F* is the flux, *P*1 the entrance pressure, *P2 the* exit pressure, *r* is the tube radius, *l* the tube's length, and η is the fluid viscosity].

That equation is applied to the Newtonian fluids which yield flux without turbulence inside rigid tubes. As a rational exercise, we may apply the equation to the blood flux in the cerebral artery and the arterioles, despite the arterial variation in diameter. Therefore, we consider ***F*** as the encephalic blood flux, ***P1*** as the median arterial pressure (MAP), ***P2*** as the intracranial pressure (ICP), ***r*** as the encephalic artery radius, ***l*** as the length of encephalic circulation, and η as the blood viscosity. This equation does not apply to brain capillaries due to the size of the red cells in relation to the capillary lumen. The mean global blood flow to the brain is approximately 53.5 ml/100 g/min.

Cerebral blood flow and cerebral blood volume may vary during anesthesia, as the diameter of cerebral arteries and arterioles changes with cerebral metabolic activity, arterial carbon dioxide ($PaCO_2$), and/or arterial oxygen (PaO_2) concentrations as well as the systemic arterial pressure.

Cerebral Blood Flow (CBF) and Cerebral Metabolic Rate ($CRMO_2$)

Under normal conditions the brain controls its blood flux to maintain the supply of energy substrate according to its needs [3–5]. In other words, the brain coordinates the cerebral metabolic requirements and the brain vascular reactivity by keeping constant the relationship between cerebral blood flow (CBF) and cerebral oxygen metabolic rate ($CMRO_2$). Therefore, when the metabolic rate is reduced, the cerebral blood flow is reduced as well, as it occurs during barbituric-induced coma. Conversely, in the convulsive crises the metabolic rate and the blood flux are both increased [6]. Conversely, anesthetics which relax the smooth muscle fibers of cerebral arteries disrupt that relationship and despite the metabolic rate reduction, the halogenates increase cerebral blood flow due to the arterial dilation. Barbiturates which induce vasoconstriction keep constant the relationship between decreased cerebral metabolic rate and reduced cerebral blood flow.

Therefore, in the normal brain, the relationship between cerebral blood flow and cerebral metabolic rate is constant (CBF/CMRO2 = 15), with the blood flow being modified by the metabolic activity. The factors that modify that relationship are (a) halogenate anesthetics (despite reducing metabolic rates they increase blood flow, thus changing the relation $CBF/CMRO_2$); and (b) the relationship between metabolic rate and blood flow is modified in the brain as a result of traumatic injury and in the swollen peritumoral areas as vascular reactivity is compromised.

Cerebral Blood Flow and $PaCO_2$

Carbon gas concentrations in the blood modify both the diameter and flow in the arteries and arterioles [7, 8]. Hyperventilation causes hypocapnia, also known as hypocarbia, which leads to liquor alkalinization, cerebral vasoconstriction, and reduced CBF. Respiratory acidosis or alkalosis change CBF whereas blood metabolic acidosis or alkalosis have almost no effect on the CBF because there is no immediate passage of bicarbonate or hydrogen ions through the (healthy/intact)?

blood-brain barrier (BBB). CBF is altered in 2–3% with 1 mmHg change in $PaCO_2$ [8].

The normal global CBF is 52 ml/100 g/min. When $PaCO_2$ is at 20 mmHg the intense vasoconstriction excessively reduces the blood flow (20 to 25 ml/100 g/min) and may cause cerebral ischemia by reducing neuron activity and flattening the electroencephalographic (EEG) tracing. Cerebral vasodilator drugs such as halogenate barbiturates displace the CO_2 curve to the left. Cerebral vasoconstrictor drugs (e.g., barbiturates, benzodiazepines, and etomidate) shift the curve to the right. The vascular reactivity to CO_2 is ineffective in the arteries present in the peritumoral area. In that area the blood flow is augmented, providing an increased supply of oxygen which is known as *luxury perfusion* because such excess of blood and extra oxygen supply is not needed by the peritumoral nervous tissue [9] .

Cerebral Blood Flow and Arterial Pressure

CPP is the gradient difference between median arterial pressure (MAP) and ICP, **CPP = MAP-ICP**. The brain has autoregulation mechanisms which keep constant the blood flow when the arterial variation occurs within certain limits. Therefore, cerebral arterial dilation occurs during a systemic arterial hypotension whereas cerebral arterial constriction occurs during a systemic arterial hypertension. CBF may be understood as fluid flow in conduction vessels. In other words, because of the existing variation in the encephalic perfusion pressure, the radius of arteries and arterioles change to keep CBF constant. Such autoregulation is effective with arterial median pressures within the lowest limit of 50 mmHg and the upper threshold of 150 mmHg [10, 11].

When the MAP is higher than 150 mmHg, the contraction of the muscle fibers in arterioles becomes ineffective, which increases brain blood flow and volume. Situations that modify vascular reactivity to MAP variation are as follows: (a) the self-regulation curve threshold where the flow is constant is shifted to higher values with hypercapnia or to lower values with hypocapnia; (b) drugs that cause brain vasodilation, such as halogenated anesthetics, shift the autoregulation from the upper limit to lower blood pressure values; and (c) CBF self-regulation capacity is reduced in damaged areas of the brain, such as those presenting peritumoral edema.

Effects of Anesthetics on the Cerebral Blood Flow and the Metabolic Rate

Inhaled halogenated anesthetics of major or lesser intensity (halothane, isoflurane, sevoflurane, and desflurane) reduce brain metabolism [12, 13], depending on the administered dose concentration. Nevertheless, they act on the smooth muscle fibers of encephalic arteries and arterioles inducing vasodilation and increased blood flow. The higher the dose concentration of halogenated anesthetic, the greater the shift from the autoregulation upper limit curve (150 mmHg) to lower values. Besides considering the effect of halogenated anesthetics on CBV, the effect on systemic peripheral resistance should also be considered, as it may cause a certain degree of systemic arterial hypotension. Sevoflurane shows a lesser impact on the encephalic vascular reactivity and causes a minor effect on encephalic vasodilation than the other halogenated anesthetics [14].

Enflurane, when associated with deep hypocapnia, can generate EEG readings alike the state of epilepsy [15]. Nitrous oxide is associated with increased CBF and the cerebral metabolic rate [16, 17], but these effects can be minimized with intravenous anesthetics that reduce metabolic rates and cause vasoconstriction. Except for ketamine, intravenous anesthetics cause cerebral vasoconstriction which increases brain activity [18, 19]. The vasoconstriction reduces cerebral blood volume and intracranial pressure. As the reduction in blood flow is due to a depressant action on the neuron's metabolic rate, at adequate levels it does not cause brain damage since it also reduces the oxygen demand. Although anesthetics reduce the metabolic rate, they do not fully protect nerve cells from the induced blood flow reduction resulting from deep hypocapnia.

Intravenous barbiturates decrease the functional activity of neurons. In other words, they reduce the neurotransmission-induced activity [20, 21] in those brain areas that still respond to vascular reactivity mechanisms [22] .

Barbiturate-induced coma aiming at metabolic reduction should be monitored through continuous EEG activity, as it has not an additional effect in reducing the intrinsic activity of neurons and the excess of barbiturates causes significant depression on the cardiovascular system plus arterial hypotension. Methohexital may cause EEG activity and induce seizures in epileptic patients [23]. It was used in the past to evoke epileptic activity for mapping brain activity in patients who had no brain activity due to depression caused by deep general anesthesia during craniotomy.

Like barbiturates, etomidate reduces the metabolic rate and CBF [24, 25], but not in a linear fashion. The maximum reduction of CBF occurs with a smaller dose than that necessary to reduce the maximum possible metabolic rate, which suggests that etomidate acts in two distinct pathways: direct action on cerebrovascular constriction and on suppression of metabolic activity [26].

As previously mentioned, etomidate can trigger tonic-clonic muscle activity and EEG spams like seizures [27, 28], which enabled its use for brain stimulation in patients undergoing general anesthesia with EEG activity suppression, in replacement of methohexital. However, dose increases of etomidate cause depression of brain activity [29] .

Hypothermia reduces neuron intrinsic activity because it decreases the total metabolic activity by 7% per each reduced degree of temperature in the brain [30, 31].

Benzodiazepines reduce in approximately 25% the metabolic rate and CBF. The flow reduction seems to be related to the metabolism [32, 33]· and to the reduction in intracranial pressure. Flumazenil reverses the effects of benzodiazepines on CBF,

$CMRO_2$, and ICP, so it may have unintended effects when used to reverse anesthesia [32].

Propofol reduces the metabolic rate, cerebral blood flow, and intracranial pressure [34–36]. However, since it also reduces the systemic blood pressure [37], a red flag should be raised to the risk of reducing cerebral perfusion if systemic arterial hypotension occurs [38, 39] in neurosurgical patients.

Opioid anesthetics have the least direct effect on cerebral blood flow, metabolic rate, and intracranial pressure [40]. Ketamine is a potent cerebral vasodilator capable of significantly increasing CBF [41] which may worsen the patient's condition with pre-existent intracranial hypertension or seizures [42].

Succinylcholine may increase ICP, likely due to ICP increases caused by the nociceptive stimuli reaching the brain [43–45]. Therefore, before the administration of succinylcholine, deep anesthesia must be instituted with anesthetics that reduce ICP in patients with intracranial hypertension. Competitive muscle relaxants should not be used when monitoring with motor evoked potential (MEP). If the use of competitive muscle relaxants is necessary, they must have their action reversed before starting motor stimulation [46].

General Anesthesia and the CNS Monitoring

When deep enough anesthesia is administered to reduce the CNS metabolic rate, a relaxed brain with a reduced volume occurs that does come out of the cranial space. This facilitates the surgical handling by the neurosurgeon because the deeper the anesthesia the lower the metabolic rate and smaller the brain volume. Such brain-volume reduction is due to cerebral arterial vasoconstriction, which depends on the arterial regulation, induced by the changes in neuronal metabolic rates.

However, too deep anesthesia may cause unintended adverse effects on the neurosurgical procedure when intraoperative monitoring of the CNS is performed. Anesthetic drugs may depress evoked sensitive and motor responses in a major or minor intensity, depending on the chosen anesthetic and the administered concentrations. Therefore, it is crucial the understanding of CNS physiology and of its interactions with the effects of systemic changes and/or the effects of the administered drugs.

The goal of intraoperative monitoring is the prompt detection of ischemic aggression in the brain or in the spinal medulla, to stop or decrease the intensity of surgical handling, thus avoiding harmful and irreversible events. Moreover, one should keep in mind other factors that hinder the CNS monitoring such as: (a) hyperventilation that induces hypocapnia, followed by vasoconstriction and ischemia; (b) hypothermia that decreases neuronal metabolism; (c) arterial hypotension that causes ischemia; and (d) mechanical compression of peripheral nerves which affects the conduction of nerve stimuli.

Intravenous and inhaled anesthetics affect the neural synaptic and axonal functional activities, and the response depends on the affected pathway and on the mechanism of action of the anesthetic agent. In other words, the inhibition effect may be direct or indirect, depending on changes between inhibitory or excitatory inputs [47]. The synaptic effects of inhalation anesthetic agents are more highly dependent responses on the synaptic function that will have marked reductions in amplitude and increases in latency. The use of intravenous anesthetics will require much higher doses to achieve the same effect. Intravenous anesthetics like etomidate, ketamine, and fentanyl allow better registry of the evoked motor potential than halothane.

For intraoperative CNS monitoring and brain mapping, general anesthesia cannot be too deep otherwise the interpretation of the electrocorticographic (ECoG) readings will be difficult. Conversely, two shallow anesthesia may induce awakening, so it is important to previously orient the patient for the possibility of awakening during ECoG. Sudden and agitated awakening may lead to excitation, heart frequency, and arterial pressure increase, causing elevation of cerebral blood volume and augmentation of brain volume. In cases of too much excitation, convulsive crises may occur with the disorderly activity of brain neurons, brain-volume increase, and risk of cortical hemorrhage. In such extreme situation the cerebral cortex must be perfused with a very cold physiologic solution to reduce neuronal metabolism and to stop the convulsive crisis. If such procedure is not enough to cease the epileptic activity, anticonvulsant anesthetic drugs such as propofol (10–30 mg) in bolus should be administered. If still necessary, midazolam (1–2 mg) in bolus can be administered as well. In the latter case, consider that the subsequent recording of ECoG activity may be impaired if high doses of benzodiazepines were administered [48]. The use of a muscle relaxant impedes the MEP registry and when its administration is necessary, the use of an antagonist should be administered before the next motor-evoked potential reading [46].

Under some circumstances, too deep anesthesia affects the interpretation of the EcoG reading, even after superficializing the anesthetic dose. If cortical mapping is not possible, anesthetic drugs that increase activity in brain foci should be administered. Methohexital was the most used anesthetic to evoke this excitement [49, 50], but due to the irregular response regarding the required dose and the intensity of the epileptic crises, it was replaced by other drugs. Low-dose etomidate may activate epileptic foci whereas in high doses it may depress the entire brain [27, 51].

Patients who develop intraoperative convulsive crises may be kept under anticonvulsant drugs of long duration, such as phenytoin, during the post-surgery period [48].

The choice of short half-life intravenous hypnotics (propofol, dexmedetomidine) with remifentanil and/or fentanyl has been frequently adopted as it permits rapid anesthesia superficializing and brain volume reduction. When halogenated inhalation anesthetics are used, they should be administered in low concentrations and in association with other intravenous anesthetics. When choosing the anesthetic drug, it should be considered its effects on ECoG and on the evoked sensitive and motor potentials. An exchange of ideas with the neurophysiologist who will perform the monitoring could be very productive.

Electroencephalogram (EEG), Bispectral Index (BIS), and Evoked Potential

The anesthetized state is comprised by two factors: (a) sedation/hypnosis (mental blocking); and (b) analgesia (sensitive suppression). Deep hypnosis without analgesia does not prevent hemodynamic changes in response to nociceptive stimuli. Conversely, deep analgesia does not guarantee an unconscious state. Therefore, deep anesthesia is obtained with a combination of anesthetics or by an anesthetic drug which yields both anesthesia and unconsciousness, simultaneously [52].

Those two components are intimately associated since the unconscious state impedes pain perception, which could be magnified if the patient were awake during the procedure whereas the lack or insufficient analgesia could induce patient's awakening due to the pain caused by the nociceptive stimulus [53].

EEGs to study the action of anesthetic drugs in the CNS have been used for years, and an extensive EEG data bank of patients submitted to diverse types of anesthetics is currently available [54]. In anesthetized patients the EEG readings show a shift from high-frequency and low-amplitude waves – which are present in the awake state – to lower frequencies and higher amplitude waves, characteristic of deep anesthesia.

High-frequency low-amplitude occurs predominantly in light anesthetic levels. Alpha-waves (8–12 Hz) appear with the increase of anesthetic depth and replace the higher frequency β-activity (13–30 Hz). As the anesthesia progresses, low-frequency high-amplitude θ-waves (5–7 Hz) and δ-waves (1–4 Hz) occur [55].

The bispectral analysis (BIS) of the EEG by a mathematical process has obtained a bispectral index which is dependent on the coherence measure of the EEG quantitative components [56]. The BIS obtained by processing of EEG parameters is used to measure the anesthesia depth, thus helping to schedule faster awakening from anesthesia and reduced recovery time, which are associated with keeping the BIS between 50 and 65 [57, 58].

Monitoring with BIS helps in the anesthetic drug titration to obtain the desired depth and reduces the consumption of anesthetics, whether inhaled or intravenous [59], which contributes to the reduction of adverse side effects, such as arterial hypertension or hypotension as well as post-operative cognitive dysfunctions during recovery [60, 61].

During neurosurgery with CNS monitoring, a too deep anesthesia can make it difficult to obtain adequate readings for possible mechanic aggression to certain CNS areas. The use of certain anesthetic agents that further depress the CNS can also make monitoring difficult. Therefore, the combined use of EEG, BIS, and evoked potentials will allow more accuracy in the anesthetic dose adjustment and the adequate level of analgesia and hypnosis for each patient, while avoiding too deep anesthesia which would hinder the CNS monitoring.

Total intravenous anesthesia (TIVA) facilitates the evoked monitoring interpretation when compared to balanced anesthesia [46, 62, 63] being preferred by neurophysiologists during intraoperative monitoring.

Drugs with neurophysiologic and pharmacokinetic properties, such as propofol, remifentanil, ketamine, and midazolam, favor the better intraoperative quality of the MEPs and reduce surgical morbidity [64] because they facilitate the CNS mapping and interpretation.

Propofol is the most used anesthetic to perform ECoG recording during surgeries requiring the cerebral cortex mapping, although there are some case reports in the literature correlating propofol with the induction of tonic-clonic seizures, as above mentioned [63].

Dexmedetomidine is a short-acting α-2 agonist with no respiratory-depressive effects and properties of anxiolysis, analgesia, sedation, and sympatholysis. As it does not interfere with the motor-stimulatory effect and ECoG activity, it has a good indication for awake craniotomy in epileptic patients [63]. Further details on awake-approach anesthesia are addressed in Chap. 15.

Synthetic opioids (alfentanil, fentanyl, sufentanil, and remifentanil) can be used in awake craniotomy as they do not have a significant risk of causing perioperative seizures or changes in ECoG activity. However, high doses of synthetic opioids can increase interictal spike activity [65–68].

Note that myoclonus, which occurs as a side effect of etomidate, coincides with an increase in the components of the somatosensory evoked potential (SSEP), which could indicate a disinhibitory or excitatory cortical effect, although in spike-wave complexes it is seen at the EEG after etomidate [69].

The pharmacokinetics and pharmacodynamics of anesthetic drugs are modified in senior patients and may lead to deep and lasting effects or even unintended side effects. BIS is a useful monitoring tool to help adequate titration of anesthetics in elderly patients [61, 70].

BIS has a good correlation to assess the anesthesia depth regardless of age, even though age-related differences in the EEG may exist in the normal population. However, BIS values can be much lower during anesthesia when there is senile dementia [71], probably due to extensive atrophy of the cerebral cortex. Besides monitoring anesthesia depth with BIS, evoked potentials also help in this assessment. BIS gradually increases during the superficializing of anesthesia, helping to monitor awareness and end of anesthesia. However, the auditory evoked potential better identifies the transition state between awake and sleeping than BIS [72]. Similarly, to BIS, auditory evoked potential helps titrate the anesthetic dose, improving post-anesthetic recovery [73].

Intraoperative neurophysiological monitoring (IOM) using SSEPs and MEPs contributes to the intraoperative decision with the patient under general anesthesia, thus reducing surgical risk. However, the IOM is under the influence of the anesthetic agent administered since both inhaled and intravenous anesthetics have their effects on neural synaptic and axonal activities. Hence the effect of the anesthetic on the evoked responses depends on which pathway is affected by the anesthetic and its mechanism of action, e.g., as a result from direct inhibition or indirect effects on the scale between inhibitory or excitatory inputs. The greatest decrease in amplitude and increase in latency occur in responses that are highly dependent on synaptic function, such as with inhalation anesthetics or high doses of intravenous anesthetics [74].

At certain concentrations, inhaled anesthetics can make IOM difficult. For instance, during the recording of the MEP, the amplitude reduces in a dose-dependent manner with sevoflurane at the concentration for clinical use [75].

Inhaled anesthetics can cause α-wave activity in the frontal region, which can resemble sleep spindles [76]. Inhaled anesthetics affect ECoG by suppressing the spontaneous interictal spikes. Nitrous oxide (N_2O) alone or in combination with sevoflurane depresses the interictal spike activity [77, 78]. Isoflurane inhibits more than propofol the IOM in spinal surgery [79].

The Voss LJ and colls' review on seizures and general anesthetic drugs [47] followed the definitions proposed by the International League Against Epilepsy and the International Bureau for Epilepsy [80, 81].

A seizure is characterized by episodes of abnormal enhanced synchrony in neuronal activity. Therefore, the term *seizure* is used when the event is recorded by EEG whereas *Epileptiform activity* refers to small areas (<1 cm^2) of neuronal hypersynchrony. Based on these definitions, it can be said that anesthetic drugs usually induce epileptiform activity but rarely seizures. Epileptiform activity is more likely to occur in patients with epilepsy [81–83].

Some anesthetics such as sevoflurane, enflurane, and etomidate may induce epileptiform EEG activity. Enflurane, etomidate, methohexital, and potent opioids have been used to facilitate the identification of the epileptic focus for surgical resection [84–86].

Most anesthetic drugs alter neural transmission, with excitatory or inhibitory effects on the cerebral cortex activities, which can make difficult the interpretation of ECoG and the mapping of the cerebral cortex. Apparently, this mechanism depends on the ratio between excitatory and inhibitory neurons affected in the cortical and subcortical structures of the brain, as anesthesia deepens [47].

IOM of MEPs has been useful in cerebral aneurysm surgeries which require temporary clipping of the artery with aneurysm or when the aneurysm may burst, being therefore necessary to induce deep arterial hypotension [87].

Factors that May Interfere with CNS Monitoring

- *Neuromuscular blockers can interfere with the amplitude of the MEPs* [46].
- *Hypothermia increases the cortical SSEPs amplitude* [88].
- *Acute anemia with hemoglobin (Hb) concentrations of 7–8 g/dL may be associated with cerebral injury in perioperative patients* [89]. If anemia becomes deeper (Hb up to 5–6 g/dL), deficits of cognitive function may occur [90].
- *Abnormally slow BIS values decrease, or abrupt drop may indicate hypoperfusion and cerebral ischemia* [91, 92].
- *Interference from electrical equipment used during surgery* [93, 94].

In addition to being aware of these factors which cause misreading in CNS monitoring, the anesthesiologist must avoid possible complications derived from inadequate anesthesia that may lead to an overdose or underdose of the anesthetics.

Final Thoughts

The requirements for a good anesthesia performance in patients under neurosurgery with CNS monitoring are many and there is not a hierarchical degree of importance among them, since they are all necessary and interactive on their effect upon the CNS. When used in combination, they provide a better reading and interpretation of possible aggressions to be avoided.

Before the beginning of anesthesia it is crucial the following procedures (a) a dialogue with the neurosurgeon to understand which encephalic conditions he requires to approach the lesion to be surgically resected, and which should be the positioning of the patient on the surgical table as well as the position and level of the head in relation to the body, which is important for the CNS reflux of venous blood, considering that if the patient needs to be awake during surgery for conscious assessment, such positioning should be comfortable; (b) to discuss with the neurophysiologist the choice of anesthetic technique which may offer the best condition for the CNS monitoring, and which level of anesthesia should be necessary.

We must be constantly alert to the non-anesthetic interference factors as mentioned before, which interfere with CNS monitoring as they can cause diagnostic errors and misreading. Monitoring with BIS, EEG, and motor and/or sensory evoked potentials is an important procedure to determine the appropriate level and depth of anesthesia, because when it is too deep the CNS monitoring becomes difficult whereas too superficial anesthesia may lead to the patient abrupt awake.

When brain mapping must be performed with the awake patient, before the resection of the pathologic area, his awakening must be planned to be gradual and smooth, without the risk of arterial hypertension or psychomotor agitation, or pain, or cough.

References

1. Shapiro HM. Intracranial hypertension: therapeutics and anesthetics. Anesthesiology. 1975;43:445–71.
2. Marmarou A, et al. Contribution of CSF on vascular factors to the elevation of ICP in severely head-injured patients. J Neurosurg. 1987;66:883–90.
3. Frackowiak RS, et al. Regional cerebral oxygen utilization and blood flow in normal man using oxygen-15 and positron emission tomography. Acta Neurol Scand. 1980;62:336–44.
4. Siesjo BK. Cerebral circulation and metabolism. J Neurosurg. 1984;60:883–908.
5. Sokoloff L. Circulation and energy metabolism of the brain. In: Siegel G, et. Al., editors. Basic neurochemistry: molecular, cellular and medical aspects. New York: Raven Press; 1989. p. 565–91.
6. Plum F, et al. Cerebral metabolic and circulatory responses to induced convulsions in animals. Arch Neurol. 1968;18:1–13.
7. Reivich M, et al. Reactivity of cerebral vessel to CO2 in the newborn rhesus monkey. Eur Neurol. 1971;6:132–6.
8. Reivich M. Arterial PCO2 and cerebral hemodynamics. Am J Phys. 1964;1:25–35.

9. Lassen N. The luxury perfusion syndrome and its possible relation to acute metabolic acidosis localized within the brain. Lancet. 1967;2:1113–5.
10. Harper AM. Autoregulation of cerebral blood flow: influence of arterial blood pressure on the blood flow through the cerebral cortex. J Neurol Neurosurg Psychiatry. 1966;29:398–403.
11. McHenry JLC, et al. Cerebral autoregulation in man. Stroke. 1974;5:695–705.
12. Cucchiara RF, et al. The effects of isofluran on canine cerebral metabolism and cerebral flow. Anesthesiology. 1974;40:571–4.
13. Theye RA, Michenfelder JD. The effect of halothane on canine cerebral metabolism. Anesthesiology. 1968;29:113–8.
14. Takahashi H. Sevoflurane does not increase intracranial pressure in hyperventilated dogs. Br J Anaesth. 1993;71:551–5.
15. Lebowitz MH, et al. Enflurane-induced central nervous system excitation and its relation to carbon dioxide tension. Anesth Analg. 1972;51:355–63.
16. Baughman VL, et al. Cerebrovascular metabolic effects of N2O in unrestrained rats. Anesthesiology. 1990;73:269–72.
17. Pelligrino DA, et al. Nitrous oxide markedly increases cerebral cortical metabolic rate and blood flow in the goat. Anesthesiology. 1984;60:405–12.
18. Ferrer-Allado, et al. Ketamine induced electro-convulsive phenomena in the human limbic and thalamic regions. Anesthesiology. 1973;38:333–44.
19. Rosen I, Hagerdale M. Electroencephalographic study of children during ketamine anesthesia. Acta Anesthesiol Scand. 1976;20:32–9.
20. Kassell NF, et al. Influence of changes in arterial pCO2 on cerebral blood flow and metabolism during high-dose barbiturate therapy in dogs. J Neurosurg. 1981;54:615–9.
21. Michenfelder JR. The interdependency of cerebral functional and metabolic effects following massive doses of thiopental in dogs. Anesthesiology. 1974;41:231–6.
22. Shapiro HM, et al. Rapid intraoperative reduction of intracranial pressure with tiopentone. Br J Anaesth. 1998;5:798–803.
23. Wyler AR, et al. Methoexital activation of the epileptogenic foci during acute electrocorticography. Epilepsia. 1987;28:490–4.
24. Milde L, et al. Cerebral functional metabolic, and haemodinamic effects of etomidate in dogs. Anesthesiology. 1985;63:371–17.
25. Davis DW, et al. Regional brain glucose utilization in rats during etomidate anesthesia. Anesthesiology. 1986;64:751–7.
26. Newberg Milde L, et al. Cerebral functional metabolic, and haemodinamic effects of etomidate in dogs. Anesthesiology. 1985;63:371–17.
27. Ebrahim KY, et al. Effect of etomidate on electroencefalogram of patients with epilepsy. Anesth Analg. 1986;65:1004–6.
28. Gancher S, et al. Activation of epileptogenic activity by etomidate. Anesthesiology. 1984;61:616–8.
29. Yeoman P, et al. Etomidate infusion for the control of refractory status epilepticus. Intens Care Med. 1989;15:255–9.
30. Zanatta P, Bosco E, Comin A, Mazzarolo AP, Di Pasquale P, Forti A, Longatti P, Polesel E, Stecker M, Sorbara C. Effect of mild hypothermic cardiopulmonary bypass on the amplitude of somatosensory evoked potentials. J Neurosurg Anesthesiol. 2014;26(2):161–6. https://doi.org/10.1097/ANA.0000000000000016.
31. Madhok J, Wu D, Xiong W, Geocadin RG, Jia X. Hypothermia amplifies somatosensory evoked potentials in uninjured rats. J Neurosurg Anesthesiol. 2012;24(3):197–202. https://doi.org/10.1097/ANA.0b013e31824ac36c.
32. Fleischer JE, et al. Cerebral effects of high-dose midazolam and subsequent reversal with Ro 15-1788 in dogs. Anesthesiology. 1988;69:145–7.
33. Nugent M, et al. Cerebral metabolic, vascular and protective effects of midazolam maleate: comparison of diazepam. Anesthesiology. 1982;56:172–6.
34. Van Hemelrijck J, et al. Effect of propofol on cerebral circulation and autoregulation in the baboon. Anesth Analg. 1990;71:49–54.

35. Artru AA, Shapira Y, e Bowdle. Electroencephalogram, cerebral metabolic, and vascular responses to propofol anesthesia in dogs. J Neurosurg Anesthesiol. 1992;4:99–109.
36. Karsli C, et al. Propofol decreases cerebral blood flow velocity in anesthetized children. Can J Anaesth. 2002;49:830–4.
37. Pinaud M, et al. Effects of propofol on cerebral hemodynamics and metabolism in patients with brain trauma. Anesthesiology. 1990;73:404–9.
38. Cuebras X, et al. Propofol incresead cerebral perfusion as compared with isoflurane during a cerebral angiography in a child with moyamoya disease. J Neurosurg Anesthesiol. 2003;1:50–4.
39. Smith JH, et al. Cerebral blood flow velocity increases when propofol is changed to desflurane, but not when isoflurane is changed to desflurane in children. Acta Anaest Scan. 2005;49:23.
40. Jobes DR, et al. Cerebral blood flow and metabolism during morphine-nitrous oxide anesthesia in man. Anesthesiology. 1977;47:16–8.
41. Takeshita K, et al. The effects of ketamine on cerebral circulation and metabolism in man. Anesthesiology. 1972;1:69–75.
42. Shapiro H, et al. Ketamine anaesthesia in patients with intracranial pathology. Br J Anaesth. 1972;44:1200–4.
43. Cottrell JE, et al. Intracranial and hemodynamics changes after succinilcholine administration in cats. Anaest Analg. 1983;62:1006–9.
44. Lanier WL, et al. Cerebral stimulation succinilcholine in dogs. Anesthesiology. 1986;64:551–9.
45. Lanier WL, et al. Cerebral blood flow and afferent muscle activity following the succinilcholine in dogs. Anesthesiol Rev. 1987;14:60–1.
46. Yamamoto Y, Kawaguchi M, Hayashi H, Horiuchi T, Inoue S, Nakase H, Sakaki T, Furuya H. The effects of the neuromuscular blockade levels on amplitudes of post tetanic motor-evoked potentials and movement in response to transcranial stimulation in patients receiving propofol and fentanyl anesthesia. Anesth Analg. 2008;106(3):930–4, table of contents. https://doi.org/10.1213/ane.0b013e3181617508.
47. Voss LJ, Sleigh JW, Barnard JP, Kirsch HE. The howling cortex: seizures and general anesthetic drugs. Anesth Analg. 2008;107:1689–703.
48. Chui J, Manninen P, Valiante T, Venkatraghavan L. The anesthetic considerations of intraoperative electrocorticography during epilepsy surgery. Anesth Analg(Review). 2013;117:479–86.
49. Musella L, Wilder BJ, Schmidt RP. Electroencephalographic activation with intravenous methohexital in psychomotor epilepsy. Neurology. 1971;21:594–602.
50. Hufnagel A, Burr W, Elger CE, Nadstawek J, Hefner G. Localization of the epileptic focus during methohexital-induced anesthesia. Epilepsia. 1992;33:271–84.
51. Gancher S, et al. Activation of epileptogenic activity by etomidate. Anesthesiology. 1984;61:616–8.
52. Shafer SL, Stanski DR. Defining depth of anesthesia. Handb Exp Pharmacol. 2008;182:409–23. https://doi.org/10.1007/978-3-540-74806-9_19. Review. PMID: 18175102
53. Bischoff P, Schneider G, Kochs E. Anesthetics drug pharmacodynamics. Handb Exp Pharmacol. 2008;182:379–408. https://doi.org/10.1007/978-3-540-74806-9_18.
54. Rampill IJ. A primer for EEG signal processing in anesthesia. Anesthesiology. 1998;89:980–1002.
55. Kiersey DK, Bickford RG, Faulconer A Jr. Electro-encephalographic patterns produced by thiopental sodium during surgical operations; description and classification. Br J Anaesth. 1951;23:141–52.
56. Nunes RP, Chaves IMM, Alencar JCG, Franco SB, Oliveira YGBR, Menezes DGA. Bispectral index and other processed parameters of electroencephalogram: an update. Rev Bras Anestesiol. 2012;62(1):105–17.
57. Rosow C, Manberg PJ. Bispectral index monitoring. Anesthesiol Clin North Am. 2001;19(4):947–66, xi. https://doi.org/10.1016/s0889-8537(01)80018-3.
58. Johansen JW, Sebel PS, Sigl JC. Clinical impact of hypnotic-titration guidelines based on EEG bispectral index (BIS) monitoring during routine anesthetic care. J Clin Anesth. 2000;12(6):433–43. https://doi.org/10.1016/s0952-8180(00)00187-2. PMID: 11090728

59. Paventi S, Santevecchi A, Metta E, Annetta MG, Perilli V, Sollazzi L, Ranieri R. Bispectral index monitoring in sevoflurane and remifentanil anesthesia: analysis of drugs management and immediate recovery. Minerva Anestesiol. 2001;67(6):435–9.
60. Wang D, Song Z, Zhang C, Chen P. Bispectral index monitoring of the clinical effects of propofol closed-loop target-controlled infusion: systematic review and meta-analysis of randomized controlled trials. Medicine (Baltimore). 2021;100(4):e23930. https://doi.org/10.1097/MD.0000000000023930. Meta-Analysis
61. Lewis SR, Pritchard MW, Fawcett LJ, Punjasawadwong Y. Bispectral index for improving intraoperative awareness and early postoperative recovery in adults. Cochrane Anaesthesia Group, Cochrane Database Syst Rev. 2019;2019(9):CD003843. Published online 2019 Sep 26. https://doi.org/10.1002/14651858.CD003843.pub4.
62. Taniguchi M, Nadstawek J, Pechstein U, Schramm J. Total intravenous anesthesia for improvement of intraoperative monitoring of somatosensory evoked potentials during aneurysm surgery. Neurosurgery. 1992;31(5):891–7.
63. Struys MMRF, Vereecke H, Moerman A, Erik W, Verhaeghen D, De Neve N, Dumortier FJE, Mortier EP. Ability of the bispectral index, autoregressive modelling with exogenous input-derived auditory evoked potentials and predicted propofol concentrations to measure patient responsiveness during anesthesia with propofol and remifentanil. Anesthesiology. 2003;99(4):802–12.
64. Scheufler KM, Zentner J. Total intravenous anesthesia for intraoperative monitoring of the motor pathways: an integral view combining clinical and experimental data. J Neurosurg. 2002;96(3):571–9.
65. Elbakry AE, Ibrahim E. Propofol-dexmedetomidine versus propofol-remifentanil conscious sedation for awake craniotomy during epilepsy surgery. Minerva Anestesiol. 2017;83(12):1248–54. https://doi.org/10.23736/S0375-9393.17.11873-0. Epub 2017 Jun 14. PMID: 28631453
66. Manninen PH, Balki M, Lukitto K, Bernstein M. Patient satisfaction with awake craniotomy for tumor surgery: a comparison of remifentanil and fentanyl in conjunction with propofol. Anesth Analg. 2006;102(1):237–42. https://doi.org/10.1213/01.ANE.0000181287.86811.5C.
67. Berkenstadt H, Perel A, Hadani M, Unofrievich I, Ram Z. Monitored anesthesia care using remifentanil and propofol for awake craniotomy. J Neurosurg Anesthesiol. 2001;13(3):246–9. https://doi.org/10.1097/00008506-200107000-00013. PMID: 11426102
68. Sridharan K, Sivaramakrishnan G. Comparison of fentanyl, remifentanil, Sufentanil and Alfentanil in combination with propofol for general anesthesia: a systematic review and meta-analysis of randomized controlled trials. Curr Clin Pharmacol. 2019;14(2):116–24. https://doi.org/10.2174/1567201816666190313160438.
69. Kochs E, Treede RD, Schulteam Esch J. Increase in somatosensory evoked potentials during anesthesia induction with etomidate. Anaesthesist. 1986;35(6):359–64. PMID:3752481
70. Renna M, Venturi R. Bispectral index and anaesthesia in the elderly. Minerva Anestesiol. 2000;66(5):398–402. PMID: 10965724.
71. Gajraj RJ, Doi M, Mantzaridis H, Kenny GN. Comparison of bispectral EEG analysis and auditory evoked potentials for monitoring depth of anaesthesia during propofol anaesthesia. Br J Anaesth. 1999;82(5):672–8. https://doi.org/10.1093/bja/82.5.672.
72. Litvan H, Jensen EW, Maestre ML, Galán J, Campos JM, Fernández JA, Caminal P, Landeira JM. Comparison of an auditory evoked potentials index and a bispectral index versus clinical signs for determining the depth of anesthesia produced by propofol or sevoflurane. Rev Esp Anestesiol Reanim. 2000;47(10):447–57.
73. White PF, Ma H, Tang J, Wender RH, Sloninsky A, Kariger RM. Does the use of electroencephalographic bispectral index or auditory evoked potential index monitoring facilitate recovery after Desflurane anesthesia in the ambulatory setting? Anesthesiology. 2004;100(4):811–7.
74. Links Sloan TB, Heyer EJ. Anesthesia for intraoperative neurophysiologic monitoring of the spinal cord. J Clin Neurophysiol. 2002;19(5):430–43.
75. Kawaguchi M, Inoue S, Kakimoto M, Kitaguchi K, Furuya H, Morimoto T, Sakaki T. The effect of sevoflurane on myogenic motor-evoked potentials induced by single and paired

transcranial electrical stimulation of the motor cortex during nitrous oxide/ketamine/fentanyl anesthesia. J Neurosurg Anesthesiol. 1998;10(3):131–6.
76. Modica PA, Tempelhoff R, White PF. Pro- and anticonvulsant effects of anesthetics (part I). Anesth Analg. 1990;70:303–15.
77. Sato Y, Sato K, Shamoto H, Kato M, Yoshimoto T. Effect of nitrous oxide on spike activity during epilepsy surgery. Acta Neurochir. 2001;143:1213–5.
78. Kurita N, Kawaguchi M, Hoshida T, Nakase H, Sakaki T, Furuya H. Effects of nitrous oxide on spike activity on electro-corticogram under sevoflurane anesthesia in epileptic patients. J Neurosurg Anesthesiol. 2005;17:199–202.
79. Chen Z. The effects of isoflurane and propofol on intraoperative neurophysiological monitoring during spinal surgery. J Clin Monit Comput. 2004;18(4):303–8. https://doi.org/10.1007/s10877-005-5097-5.
80. Fisher RS, van Emde BW, Blume W, Elger C, Genton P, Lee P, Engel J. Epileptic seizures and epilepsy: definitions proposed by the International League Against Epilepsy (ILAE) and the International Bureau for Epilepsy (IBE). Epilepsia. 2005;46:470–2.
81. Zhao X, Wang X. Anesthesia-induced epilepsy causes and treatment. Expert Rev Neurother. 2014;14(9):1099–113. https://doi.org/10.1586/14737175.2014.948851. Epub 2014 Aug 13. PMID: 25115173
82. Kumar A, Sharma S. Complex Partial Seizure. In: StatPearls [Internet]. Treasure Island: StatPearls Publishing; 2021. 2021 Jan–. PMID: 30085572. REF REF.
83. Kumar A, Maini K, Arya K, Sharma S. Simple Partial Seizure. In: StatPearls [Internet]. Treasure Island: StatPearls Publishing; 2021. 2021 Jan–. PMID: 29763181.
84. Flemming DC, Fitzpatrick J, Fariello RG, Duff T, Hellman D, Hoff BH. Diagnostic activation of epileptogenic foci by enflurane. Anesthesiology. 1980;52:431–3.
85. Musella L, Wilder BJ, Schmidt RP. Electroencephalographic activation with intravenous methohexital in psychomotor epilepsy. Neurology. 1971;21:594–602.
86. Hufnagel A, Burr W, Elger CE, Nadstawek J, Hefner G. Localization of the epileptic focus during methohexital-induced anesthesia. Epilepsia. 1992;33:271–84.
87. Takebayashi S, Kamiyam AH, Takizawa K, Kobayashi T, Saitoh N. The significance of intraoperative monitoring of muscle motor evoked potentials during unruptured large and giant cerebral aneurysm surgery. Neurol Med Chir (Tokyo). 2014;54:180.
88. Zanatta P, Bosco E, Comin A, Mazzarolo AP, Di Pasquale P, Forti A, Longatti P, Polesel E, Stecker M, Sorbara C. Effect of mild hypothermic cardiopulmonary bypass on the amplitude of somatosensory evoked potentials. J Neurosurg Anesthesiol. 2014;26(2):161–6. https://doi.org/10.1097/ANA.0000000000000016.
89. Hare GM, Tsui AK, McLaren AT, Ragoonanan TE, Yu J, Mazer CD. Anemia and cerebral outcomes: many questions, fewer answers. Anesth Analg. 2008;107(4):1356–70. https://doi.org/10.1213/ane.0b013e318184cfe9. PMID: 18806052
90. Floyd TF, McGarvey M, Ochroch EA, Cheung AT, Augoustides JA, Bavaria JE, Acker MA, Pochettino A, Detre JA. Perioperative changes in cerebral blood flow after cardiac surgery: influence of anemia and aging. Ann Thorac Surg. 2003;76(6):2037–42. https://doi.org/10.1016/s0003-4975(03)01074-9.
91. Myles PS. Bispectral index monitoring in ischemic–hypoxic brain injury. J Extra Corpor Technol. 2009;41(1):P15–9.
92. Villacorta J, Kerbaul F, Collart F, Guidon C, Bonnet M, Guillen JC, Gouin F. Perioperative cerebral ischaemia in cardiac surgery and BIS. Anaesth Intensive Care. 2005;33(4):514–7. https://doi.org/10.1177/0310057X0503300415.
93. Myles PS. Bispectral index monitoring in ischemic–hypoxic brain injury. J Extra Corpor Technol. 2009;41(1):P15–9.
94. Villacorta J, Kerbaul F, Collart F, Guidon C, Bonnet M, Guillen JC, Gouin F. Perioperative cerebral ischaemia in cardiac surgery and BIS. Anaesth Intensive Care. 2005;33(4):514–7. https://doi.org/10.1177/0310057X0503300415.

Part II
Neurophysiological Modalities Applied to IOM

Chapter 6
Brainstem Auditory Evoked Potentials

Jamison Beiriger, Varun Shandal, Josh Sunderlin, and Parthasarathy D. Thirumala

Brainstem Auditory Evoked Potentials

Overview

Evoked potentials are electrical responses of the sensory pathways in the nervous system to sensory or electrical stimuli. Stimulation and subsequent recording of these potentials allows for evaluation of both peripheral sensory function and integrity of the central nervous system (CNS) sensory pathways. Evoked potentials are used to assess three main stimuli – visual, somatosensory, and auditory via pattern visual evoked potentials (PVEP), somatosensory evoked potentials (SSEP) and brainstem auditory evoked potentials (BAEP), respectively. This chapter focuses on brainstem auditory evoked potentials.

Brainstem auditory evoked potentials (BAEPs) are electrical responses of the nervous system to acoustic stimulation. Despite the name, the first component of the

J. Beiriger
School of Medicine, Drexel University, Philadelphia, PA, USA

V. Shandal
Department of Neurological Surgery, Center for Clinical Neurophysiology, University of Pittsburgh, Pittsburgh, PA, USA

J. Sunderlin
Procirca, Clinical Neurophysiology, University of Pittsburgh Medical Center, Pittsburgh, PA, USA

P. D. Thirumala (✉)
Department of Neurological Surgery, Center for Clinical Neurophysiology, University of Pittsburgh, Pittsburgh, PA, USA

Department of Neurology, University of Pittsburgh, Pittsburgh, PA, USA
e-mail: thirumalapd@upmc.edu

S. M. Verst et al. (eds.), *Intraoperative Monitoring*,
https://doi.org/10.1007/978-3-030-95730-8_6

response arises outside the brainstem in the auditory nerve. While somewhat of a misnomer, BAEP remains the accepted terminology as it is widely used and understood [1]. The remainder of the response is from the brainstem and possibly higher subcortical structures, although this remains controversial. Responses are measured using electrodes placed on the skin. Measuring potentials with low electrical activity of <1 μV on a background spontaneous brain electrical activity of ~100 μV presents a challenge. Repetitive auditory stimulation allows electrical activity recorded from the scalp to be averaged in order to single out time-locked electrical activity, which is a response to the auditory stimulus [2]. Although distinct waves are recorded, each measured wave is a summation of responses from multiple sources rather than a single wave for each portion of the pathway. BAEPs are useful for detecting and localizing auditory dysfunction. This includes intraoperative monitoring during procedures with potential for hearing loss. It is important to note that performing auditory evoked potentials is a tool to predict hearing, not a definitive hearing test.

Purpose

Intraoperative monitoring of BAEPs is a rapid, effective technique for assessing the integrity of auditory pathway. Real-time monitoring of auditory pathway during surgical procedures allows for correction or elimination of techniques and maneuvers that could cause auditory pathway dysfunction resulting in hearing loss [3–8]. BAEPs can accurately and reliably predict postoperative hearing loss [5, 9]. In some procedures, BAEPs have drastically reduced the rate of hearing loss [8, 10–14]. In particular, BAEPs have nearly eliminated hearing loss in microvascular decompression for both hemifacial spasm and glossopharyngeal neuralgia [3–7, 15].

Qualifications

Training for interpretation of clinical evoked potential studies is accomplished through at least a year-long post-residency fellowship in clinical neurophysiology. A part of the American Board of Clinical Neurophysiology two-part examination is devoted to clinical evoked potentials. Passing this exam and subsequently becoming credentialed demonstrates competency in interpretation of clinical evoked potential studies. Along with interpreters, technologists are necessary to conduct these studies. Becoming an evoked potential technologist requires a formal training program in neurophysiology. Additionally, technologists need training and experience of at least 1 year with proficiency in the following areas: explaining the purpose of the study to the patient, addressing patient fears, obtaining necessary medical history, getting high-quality data, recording all pertinent information, and maintaining equipment. These constitute the qualifications required to become an entry-level technologist. More prerequisites are necessary for complicated studies including more training, more experience, initiative, and ability for independent assessment [16].

Equipment

To obtain reliable evoked potentials, equipment must comply with certain guidelines. Often, newer commercially available equipment will exceed these requirements, but any equipment that meets the guidelines is satisfactory.

Amplifier

An amplifier is necessary to transform the low voltage electrical responses into signal waveforms. The goal of the amplifier is to amplify stimulus response while filtering out noise. Different specifications are needed based on the context of monitoring (i.e., intraoperative), but there are minimal acceptable criteria. In order to keep background noise to a minimum, the amplifier must have a great common-mode rejection ratio of at least 80 dB with recommendations of above 120 dB for use in the operating room. Likewise, the input impedance should be high, at least 100 MΩ. Lastly, gain should be finely adjustable in steps of no more than 2.5 to 1. Gain should be set to the maximum possible without generating excessive artifact production. Meeting these specifications will allow for enhanced signal recording while reducing noise [16].

Averager

The average allows for compiling the electrical responses of many trials into one output while simultaneously eliminating artifact-contaminated trials. Amplitude resolution of 12 bits at the analog-to-digital converter (A–D) is preferred, but an 8 bit A–D is sufficient. The averager must be capable of averaging at least 4000 trials. BAEP studies require a minimum of two channels and a time resolution of $\leq$20 μs per data point [16].

Display and Writeout

An easily readable cathode ray tube or similar display shows the average waveforms and the unaveraged EEG. In addition to the display output, there needs to be a permanent printout of the evoked potentials. Any data manipulations should be clearly and obviously presented on the display as well as the printout because these modifications can affect the study's reliability [16].

Indications

Intraoperative monitoring of auditory function with BAEPs is useful in several surgeries. Removal of acoustic neuromas as well as a number of posterior fossa procedures requires monitoring as hearing loss is a potential complication. Intraoperative monitoring allows for real-time warning and subsequent correction (if possible) of auditory pathway impairment acquired during surgery. BAEPs can also be used to monitor for hearing restoration, albeit much less frequently. Lastly, BAEPs are useful in assessing and monitoring the brainstem function intraoperatively. Specifically, changes in wave V during tumor resection or procedures involving the posterior circulation can signify alter brainstem function [17].

Generation of Potentials

Anatomy

Each wave generated in the BAEP corresponds to synapses in various locations along the auditory pathway. The knowledge of auditory pathway anatomy is critical for understanding the generated potentials, and their significance in lesion localization when abnormal findings are present. The auditory pathway begins in the modiolus of the cochlea. Dendritic processes of the auditory nerve travel from the cochlea through the spiral ganglia to the internal auditory canal. In the temporal bone, the acoustic and vestibular portions merge to form the auditory nerve. The auditory nerve exits the skull, terminating in either the posterior ventral cochlear nucleus or anterior ventral cochlear nucleus situated on the lateral surface of the inferior cerebellar peduncle in rostral medulla. The auditory pathway fibers synapsing at the posterior ventral cochlear nucleus also connects to the dorsal cochlear nucleus. Once fibers reach the dorsal cochlear nucleus, there are a number of available pathways, but most fibers cross to the contralateral brainstem via the trapezoid body. Both the medial and lateral superior olivary nuclei in caudal pons receive some fibers, while others travel through the lateral lemniscus to the inferior colliculus. Of note, the superior olivary nucleus on each side receives input from bilateral cochlear nuclei, more so from contralateral cochlear nucleus, and acoustic information is bilaterally represented from this point onwards in the auditory pathway. The ascending pathway includes synapses at the inferior colliculus, the mediate geniculate body of the thalamus, and finally, the primary auditory cortex [17].

BAEP Waveforms

BAEPs are measured as a series of seven vertex positive waves within 10 msec of the stimulus. Wave amplitude, wave latencies, and interpeak latencies are all useful for assessing hearing function. In the standard recording between the vertex and mastoid or earlobe electrodes, the seven waves are sequentially numbered I-VII. Between the waves, vertex negative components are labeled I-VI. Waves IV and V are often observed as a single complex or barely discernable from one another. Convention states that this can be regarded as wave V [1]. Most studies place the most importance on waves I, III, and V as they serve as the best measurement parameters [1, 18]. Wave I primarily correspond to the synchronous firing of CN VIII fibers in the distal part of the nerve. Thus, Wave I measurement allows for interpretation of nerve integrity. Wave II represents activity in the proximal CN VIII adjacent to the brainstem and/or synaptic activity in the cochlear nucleus. Wave III represents signal transmission to the superior olivary nucleus located in the inferior pons. This is the first potential from the brainstem. Waves IV and V are from the lateral lemniscus and inferior colliculus, respectively. Waves VI and VII are not always measured clinically but indicate transmission to the medial geniculate body and the thalamocortical pathways. These are generalizations as each wave can correspond at least in part to synapses in multiple places. Assessment of the waves includes their presence, reproducibility, amplitude, absolute latencies, and interpeak latencies [18]. The American Clinical Neurophysiology Society Guidelines require several measurements for intraoperative monitoring including: peak latencies for waves I, III, and V; amplitude of waves I and V; interval latencies for I-III, III-V, and I-V; and amplitude ratio of wave IV-V/I [1].

Stimulation and Recording Technique

Stimuli used to generate evoked potentials can vary; however, for the purpose of intraoperative monitoring certain stimuli are preferred. Click stimuli are most commonly used because of their broad spectrum. Broadband 2 ms long clicks are produced by a 100 μs square wave pulse to the diaphragm of the speaker membrane. Generally, these clicks are at 100 μs intervals, allowing response synchronization resulting in well-defined peaks in the recorded evoked potentials [17]. More than 10 stimuli per second result in decreased amplitude of waves I, II, VI, and VII, so stimuli at rates of 8–10 per second are generally preferred. However, high stimulus rates (50–70/s) may aid in identification of wave V [1]. Stimuli can be at variable frequencies usually between 10 and 40 Hz. One technique is to begin at a fast rate for a timelier response to the surgeon then to progressively decrease the rate if the low amplitude becomes an issue. Generally, the responses from 1000 to 4000 stimuli are averaged to produce BAEPs. Click intensity is determined based upon hearing threshold using decibel sensation level (dBSL), decibel hearing level (dBHL), or decibel peak equivalent sound pressure level (dBpeSPL). dBSL and dBHL are subjective measures assessing the patient's ability to hear a pure tone stimulus at a given intensity, while dBpeSPL is a more objective measure determined by the amplitude of the headphone speaker's membrane response to a click stimulus. An optimal stimulus intensity is 65–70 dB above dBSL or dBHL or 100 to 110 dBpeSPL. Polarity can also affect the recorded potentials. Rarefaction, or the movement of the speaker membrane away from the ear drum, is typically used due to easier wave I identification along with separation of waves IV and V. Alternatively, condensation, or moving the speaker membrane toward the eardrum, can prolong the latency of wave I and help identify wave V. Alternating polarity can also be used and this is especially helpful in delineating wave I when it is obscured by the stimulus artifact. Stimuli to the ipsilateral ear also affect the contralateral ear through bony conduction, resulting in undesired responses. To avoid this, white noise consisting of an equal mix of frequencies that encompasses the entire human auditory range is applied to the contralateral ear at an intensity of 40 dB less than the click stimulus. Clicks and other broadband stimuli tend to underestimate hearing loss [19]. Responses to clicks may be more precise for interpreting sensorineural hearing loss rather than conductive hearing loss [20]. This makes clicks more useful in intraoperative monitoring in conditions where sensorineural hearing loss is more likely. Frequency-specific stimuli present an alternative. The most commonly used specific frequencies are administered as tone bursts and tone pips [19]. Frequency-specific stimuli are more accurate for pure tone audiometry [21]; however, more research is needed to make a definitive determination in the intraoperative environment [19, 22]. Stimuli should be delivered to one ear at a time [23].

Recording the BAEP waveforms generated by these stimuli involves electrode recording from the scalp. Standard electrode placement involves placing the noninverting (+) electrode on the high forehead or at the vertex (C_z) and the inverting electrode (−) is preferred on the mastoid (M1 or M2) or earlobe (A1 or A2) but may be placed on the skin just anterior to the earlobe or the tragus of the ear if the operating space impedes the desired areas. The ground can be placed anywhere on the body. Other recording channels may prove useful. For instance, hearing can be monitored bilaterally with an additional inverting electrode (−) on the contralateral side [17]. This montage is recommended for intraoperative monitoring to help with identification of waves IV and V by simultaneously recording the ipsilateral and contralateral pathways [1, 23, 24]. The preoperative baseline BAEP data can be obtained in the outpatient clinic (Fig. 6.1) and dBSL/dBHL can be determined. Also, having the outpatient baseline BAEP data is helpful in the case of inability to obtain the BAEP waveforms just prior to the start of the surgical procedure. This signifies a technical error, and all efforts are then made by the neurophysiology team to troubleshoot the technical issue to obtain the BAEP waveforms for intraoperative monitoring.

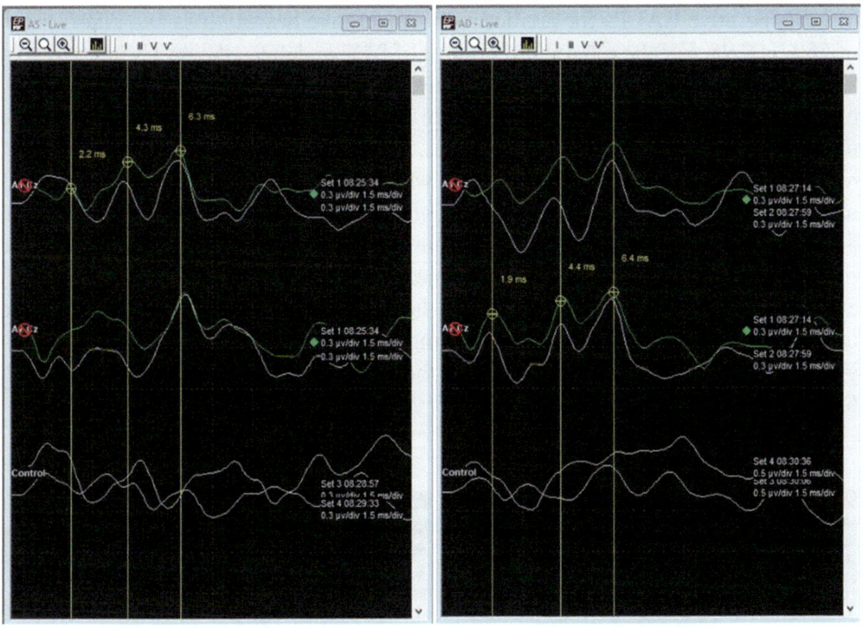

Fig. 6.1 A single set of BAEPs (white) compared to baseline (green) captured in clinic for a patient in preoperative testing before microvascular decompression for trigeminal neuralgia. These are the BAEP waveforms from the left ear (left window) and right ear (right window) at baseline obtained preoperatively in the clinic. This BAEP study shows normal wave I, III, and V peak latencies and their interpeak latencies bilaterally

Warning Criteria

A widely debated question in intraoperative monitoring of BAEPs is when to signal the surgeon. Standard warning criteria according to the American Clinical Neurophysiology Society include: absence of all waves; absence of all waves after wave I, II, or III; prolongation of any of the three aforementioned interpeak intervals; decreased IV-V/I amplitude ratio; and increased difference of interpeak intervals between the two ears [1]. Sensitivity and specificity vary between the measurements. Interpeak intervals are more informative than peak latencies since peak latency is influenced more by age and other external factors [25]. Loss of wave V and prolonged latency of ≥1 ms coupled with a wave V amplitude decrease of >50% have been identified as the most predictive of postoperative hearing loss [7]. Reduction in the amplitude of wave V is the best predictor for abnormal BAEPs. It can be used as a sliding scale warning. A 34% reduction should be monitored, a 46% reduction should be reported to the surgeon, and a 55% reduction should serve as warning of potential postoperative hearing loss. The area under the curve (AUC) of intraoperative BAEPs for predicting postoperative hearing loss at a cutoff value of 55% is 0.98. For the other cutoff values of 34% and 46%, the AUCs are 0.92 and 0.84 respectively [26]. While these values are accurate for microvascular decompression in hemifacial spasm (HFS), there is evidence that different cutoffs may be more appropriate for different procedures. Cerebellopontine angle tumor resection requires a higher suspicion for warning, while hearing loss in nontumor surgery is usually only at risk with permanent loss of wave V [27]. Some early studies found delay in wave V latency as most important, but this is disputed by larger and more recent studies demonstrating the preeminence of wave V amplitude [3, 7]. In fact, even interpeak latency may be more predictive than wave V latency [26]. Despite these variabilities, the incidence of hearing loss due to posterior cranial fossa surgeries has declined substantially through the use of BAEPs. Please refer to Figs. 6.2, 6.3, and 6.4 for illustrations.

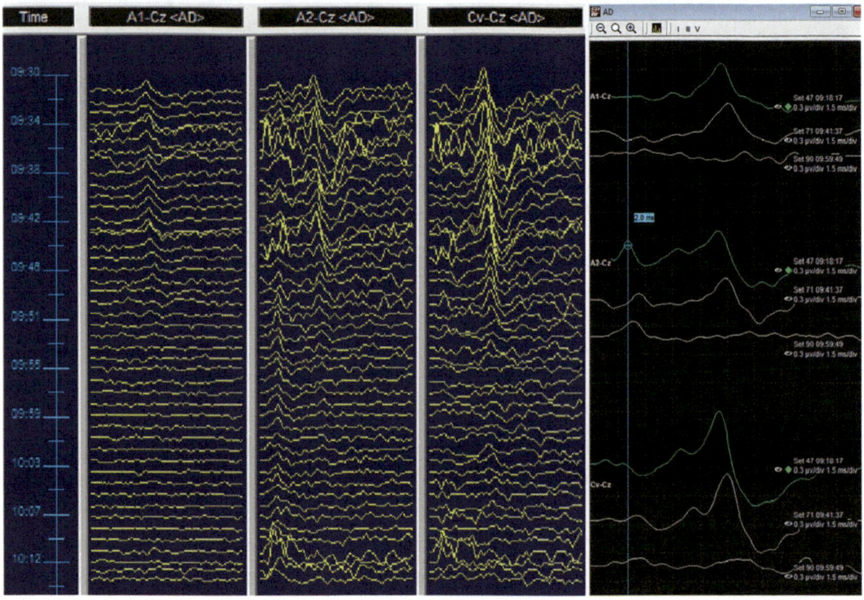

Fig. 6.2 (LEFT) "Waterfall" view of BAEP data during right-sided microvascular decompression showing significant changes. BAEP wave V latency delay from baseline is noted around 9:41, followed by complete loss of amplitude in waves II-V after around 09:59. Wave I was maintained. (RIGHT) displays two sets of BAEPs from the same procedure at 9:41 (set 71) and 9:59 (set 90) (white) compared to baseline (green) for more clarity. This patient suffered immediate postoperative hearing loss in the right ear

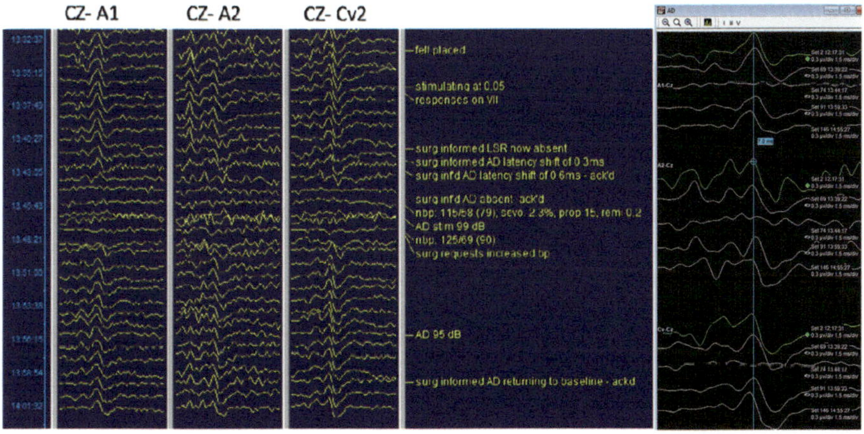

Fig. 6.3 (LEFT) "Waterfall" view of BAEP data during right-sided microvascular decompression. Latency shift of 0.3 ms and 0.6 ms were successively communicated to the surgeon at around 13:43. Subsequent loss of wave I-V amplitude can be observed between 13:43 and 13:45 and was communicated to the surgeon. The surgeon requested increased blood pressure. BAEP returned to baseline after this intervention. (RIGHT) displays multiple sets of data taken at various times during the procedure (white) compared to baseline (green) from the same case. Loss of amplitude in all waves can be observed in the recording from 13:44 with return to baseline by 13:59. The patient suffered no discernable hearing loss after the procedure

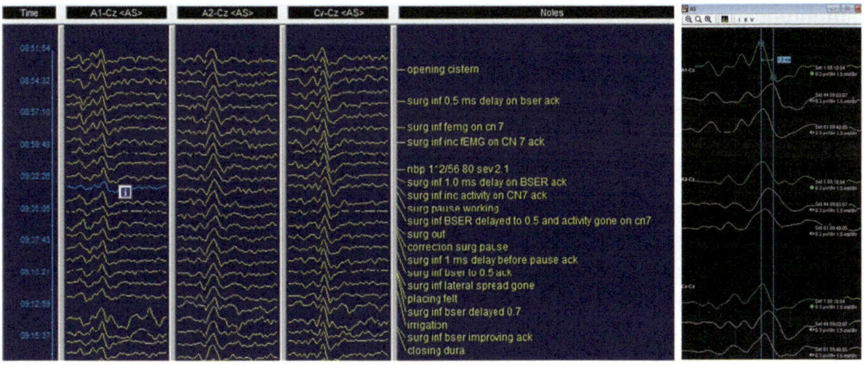

Fig. 6.4 (LEFT) "Waterfall" view of BAEP data during left-sided microvascular decompression. A maximal latency shift of 1 ms without loss of amplitude was observed during this procedure. At this point of time, the surgeon released the retraction on the cerebellum for some time. After the latency delay decreased to 0.5 ms, the procedure was resumed with eventual latency recovery to baseline by closure. (RIGHT) displays two sets of data from different times during the procedure (white) compared to baseline (green) showing the maximal latency shift of 1 ms at 09:03 from baseline which later returned to near baseline by 09:40. This patient did not report postoperative hearing loss

Considerations

BAEPs are useful in sleep or awake states and in infancy through adulthood [1]. Sedation is not problematic and may be preferred in some cases to restrict tension or movement from affecting results. One necessary consideration, however, is that hypothermia may result in BAEP changes similar to those observed in pathological hearing impairment [28]. Anesthesia, drilling, and cerebellar retraction may also affect the recording accuracy, elaborated below. For measurement in children less than 3 years old, special considerations are necessary [29].

Anesthesia

Anesthesia and core body temperature are major considerations for any intraoperative monitoring procedure. BAEPs are mildly affected by inhaled halogenated anesthetic agents in a dose-dependent manner [30, 31]. Both amplitude and latency are affected. However, non-halogenated anesthetic agents minimally affect BAEPs and therefore are preferred for use where intraoperative monitoring is required [32]. A technique to trivialize this effect is to record the baseline measurement while the patient is under anesthesia. This helps mitigate any changes that are a result of the anesthesia. Body temperature may also affect the responses, with temperatures below 35 °C resulting in prolonged interpeak intervals and latency with decreased amplitude [28, 33].

Drilling and Cerebellar Retraction

Monitoring BAEPs while drilling should be avoided to avoid false warnings. Drilling creates bone conducted noise masking the desired acoustic stimulation. It is important the surgeons understand that BAEPs are ineffective while drilling to avoid any expectations. Likewise, retraction of the cerebellum, indicated in many posterior fossa procedures, can increase the I-V interpeak interval. Typically this increase is transient, although it may sometimes be related to hearing loss [3, 34].

Children

BAEPs are generally higher amplitude in children and neonates because of electrode proximity to waveform generators due to thinner skulls and smaller heads. However, these factors do not reduce interpeak variability in normalized data. In children, BAEPs are significantly altered by age, with the effect decreasing as age increases. In neonates, wave I is particularly variable. Wave V and interpeak latency are less variable and should be preferred indicators for this age group. The higher variability of wave I is due to the presence of amniotic fluid in the middle ear cavity causing a transient conductive hearing loss in some children [35]. A multicenter database for BAEPs in children has established normative values at different age groups, allowing for BAEPs to effectively assess hearing function in children [36]. Premature infants may lack BAEPs, however by 3 to 6 months of age the values should be approximately normal. Abnormal BAEPs at 6 months of age in a premature infant may indicate developmental delay [37].

Efficacy

There are five potential outcomes for BAEPs measurement: 1 – No change; 2 – reversible significant change; 3 – irreversible significant change; 4 – reversible loss of response; and 5 – irreversible loss of response. It is widely debated whether significant change has an effect, or if loss of response should be the sole measurement for predicting postoperative hearing loss [38–40]. In a recent meta-analysis of microvascular decompression surgeries, an overall incidence of hearing loss was 4.88% [9]. Hearing loss occurred in 1.81% of patients without any change in BAEPs. Change in BAEPs was demonstrated to be correlated with hearing loss as 8.97% of patients with significant change and 31.14% of patients with loss of response suffered hearing loss. Overall, hearing loss occurred in 15.01% of patients with some significant change or loss of BAEPs. Specificity and sensitivity of hearing loss with loss of response of BAEP are 98% and 74% respectively. The high specificity shows that loss of response should be avoided and reversed if possible. Low sensitivity indicates that hearing loss is still a risk without BAEP loss. Adjusting the alarm criteria to include significant change increases the sensitivity to 88%. Positive likelihood ratio is higher when measuring loss of response alone, while negative likelihood ratio is higher when including significant change and loss of response. Based on this analysis, both criteria have merit for predicting postoperative hearing loss in microvascular decompression surgery. Intraoperative monitoring of BAEPs is currently classified by the American Society of Neurophysiological Monitoring as a Guideline, Type C, Class III recommendation for assessing brainstem function in procedures involving the brainstem, assessing brainstem function in procedures involving risk of injury to the posterior circulation, and assessing function of CN VIII in surgeries involving the cerebellopontine angle [17]. This classification indicates there is consensus expert opinion in favor of monitoring.

Limitations

The effectiveness of monitoring BAEPs is limited by certain factors. Monitoring of BAEPs is unable to completely eliminate hearing loss as an adverse outcome. Certain surgical manipulations, such as injury to a perforator, may result in immediate and irreversible loss of BAEPs. This limits the usefulness of monitoring as damage can occur without the opportunity for correction. Hearing loss may also occur without loss of BAEPs through unknown mechanisms.

References

1. American Clinical Neurophysiology Society. Guideline 9C: guidelines on short-latency auditory evoked potentials. J Clin Neurophysiol. 2006;23:157.
2. Sampath N, Subramaniam S, Sankaran V, Kumar R, Bapu KR. Brainstem auditory evoked potentials for intraoperative neurophysiological monitoring. J Neuroanaesth Crit Care. 2016;3:1.
3. Polo G, Fischer C, Sindou MP, Marneffe V, Bricolo A, Sala F, et al. Brainstem Auditory Evoked Potential monitoring during microvascular decompression for Hemifacial spasm: intraoperative brainstem auditory evoked potential changes and warning values to prevent hearing loss - prospective study in a consecutive series of 84. Neurosurgery. 2004;54:97.
4. Polo G, Fischer C. Intraoperative monitoring of brainstem auditory evoked potentials during microvascular decompression of cranial nerves in cerebellopontine angle. Neurochirurgie. 2009;55:152.
5. Huang BR, Chang CN, Hsu JC. Intraoperative electrophysiological monitoring in microvascular decompression for hemifacial spasm. J Clin Neurosci. 2009;16:209.
6. Sindou MP. Microvascular decompression for primary hemifacial spasm. Importance of intraoperative neurophysiological monitoring. Acta Neurochir. 2005;147:1019.
7. Park SK, Joo BE, Lee S, Lee JA, Hwang JH, Kong DS, et al. The critical warning sign of real-time brainstem auditory evoked potentials during microvascular decompression for hemifacial spasm. Clin Neurophysiol. 2018;129:1097.
8. Brock S, Scaioli V, Ferroli P, Broggi G. Neurovascular decompression in trigeminal neuralgia: role of intraoperative neurophysiological monitoring in the learning period. Stereotact Funct Neurosurg. 2004;82:199.
9. Thirumala PD, Carnovale G, Loke Y, Habeych ME, Crammond DJ, Balzer JR, et al. Brainstem Auditory Evoked Potentials' diagnostic accuracy for hearing loss: systematic review and meta-analysis. J Neurol Surg Part B Skull Base. 2017;78:43.
10. Barker FG, Jannetta PJ, Bissonette DJ, Larkins MV, Jho HD. The long-term outcome of microvascular decompression for trigeminal neuralgia. N Engl J Med. 1996;334:1077.
11. Radtke RA, Erwin CW, Wilkins RH. Intraoperative brainstem auditory evoked potentials: significant decrease in postoperative morbidity. Neurology. 1989;39:187.
12. Simon MV. Neurophysiologic intraoperative monitoring of the vestibulocochlear nerve. J Clin Neurophysiol. 2011;28:566.
13. Moller AR, Moller MB. Does intraoperative monitoring of auditory evoked potentials reduce incidence of hearing loss as a complication of microvascular decompression of cranial nerves? Neurosurgery. 1989;24:257.
14. Joo BE, Park SK, Cho KR, Kong DS, Seo DW, Park K. Real-time intraoperative monitoring of brainstem auditory evoked potentials during microvascular decompression for hemifacial spasm. J Neurosurg. 2016;125:1061.
15. Habeych ME, Crammond DJ, Gardner P, Thirumala PD, Horowitz MB, Balzer JR. Intraoperative neurophysiological monitoring of microvascular decompression for glossopharyngeal neuralgia. J Clin Neurophysiol. 2014;31:337.
16. American Clinical Neurophysiology Society. Guideline 9A: Guidelines on evoked potentials. J Clin Neurophysiol. 2006;23:125.
17. Martin WH, Stecker MM. ASNM position statement: intraoperative monitoring of auditory evoked potentials. J Clin Monit Comput. 2008;22:75.

18. Gathe BM, Gandhe MB, Gandhe SM, Puttewar AN, Saraf C, Singh R. Brainstem auditory evoked potentials (BAEP)- a pilot study conducted on young healthy adults from Central India. J Clin Diagn Res. 2014;8:BC16.
19. Ren W, Ji F, Zeng J, Zhao H. Intra-operative hearing monitoring methods in middle ear surgeries. J Otol. 2016;11:178.
20. Abdala C, Folsom RC. The development of frequency resolution in humans as revealed by the auditory brain-stem response recorded with notched-noise masking. J Acoust Soc Am. 1995;98:921.
21. Stapells DR, Oates P. Estimation of the pure-tone audiogram by the auditory brainstem response: a review. Audiol Neuro-Otol. 1997;2:257.
22. Ren W, Ji F, Zeng J, Hao Q, Liu R, Xu G, et al. Preliminary application of intra-operative hearing monitoring by tone pip ABR via loudspeakers. Acta Otolaryngol. 2017;137:167.
23. Stockard JJ, Stockard JE, Sharbrough FW. Nonpathologic factors influencing brainstem auditory evoked potentials. Am J EEG Technol. 1978;18:177.
24. Chiappa KH, Gladstone KJ, Young RR. Brain Stem Auditory Evoked Responses: studies of waveform variations in 50 normal human subjects. Arch Neurol. 1979;36:81.
25. Markand ON. Brainstem auditory evoked potentials. J Clin Neurophysiol. 1994;11:319.
26. Zhang Y, Ren H, Jia G, Zhang L, Fan G, Bi Q, et al. Predictive values of maximum changes of brainstem auditory evoked potentials during microvascular decompression for hemifacial spasm. Acta Neurochir. 2020;162:2823.
27. James ML, Husain AM. Brainstem auditory evoked potential monitoring: when is change in wave V significant? Neurology. 2005;65:1551.
28. Markand ON, Lee BI, Warren C, Stoelting RK, King RD, Brown JW, et al. Effects of hypothermia on brainstem auditory evoked potentials in humans. Ann Neurol. 1987;22:507.
29. Stapells DR. Auditory brainstem response assessment of infants and children. Semin Hear. 1989;10:229.
30. Grundy BL, Jannetta PJ, Procopio PT, Lina A, Boston JR, Doyle E. Intraoperative monitoring of brain-stem auditory evoked potentials. J Neurosurg. 1982;57:341.
31. Kim SM, Kim SH, Seo DW, Lee KW. Intraoperative neurophysiologic monitoring: basic principles and recent update. J Korean Med Sci. 2013;28:1261.
32. Saito T, Yamamoto I, Huang XL, Yukawa N, Osawa M, Takeichi S. Effects of muscle relaxants on EEG, ABR and EMG in rabbits. Hum Exp Toxicol. 1999;18:718.
33. Markand ON, Warren C, Mallik GS, Williams CJ. Temperature-dependent hysteresis in somatosensory and auditory evoked potentials. Electroencephalogr Clin Neurophysiol Evoked Potentials. 1990;77(6):425.
34. Rizvi SS, Goyal RN, Calder HB. Hearing preservation in microvascular decompression for trigeminal neuralgia. Laryngoscope. 1999;109(4):591.
35. Priner R, Freeman S, Perez R, Sohmer H. The neonate has a temporary conductive hearing loss due to fluid in the middle ear. Audiol Neuro-Otol. 2003;8(2):100.
36. Scaioli V, Brinciotti M, Di CM, Lori S, Janes A, Pastorino G, et al. A multicentre database for normative Brainstem Auditory Evoked Potentials (BAEPs) in children: methodology for data collection and evaluation. Open Neurol J. 2009;3(1):72.
37. Wang X, Carroll X, Wang H, Zhang P, Selvaraj JN, Leeper-Woodford S. Prediction of delayed neurodevelopment in infants using brainstem auditory evoked potentials and the Bayley II scales. Front Pediatr. 2020;8:485.
38. Ojemann RG, Levine RA, Montgomery WM, McGaffigan P. Use of intraoperative auditory evoked potentials to preserve hearing in unilateral acoustic neuroma removal. J Neurosurg. 1984;61(5):938.
39. Colletti V, Fiorino FG, Mocella S, Policante Z. ECochG, CNAP and ABR monitoring during vestibular schwannoma surgery. Int J Audiol. 1998;37(1):27.
40. Oh T, Nagasawa DT, Fong BM, Trang A, Gopen Q, Parsa AT, et al. Intraoperative neuromonitoring techniques in the surgical management of acoustic neuromas. Neurosurg Focus. 2012;33(3):E6.

Chapter 7
Evoked Potential – Visual Pathways Approach beyond Visual Evoked Potentials

Monica Nascimento de Melo and Silvia Mazzali Verst

Abbreviations

AH	Abductor hallucis
APB	Abductor pollicis brevis
Bsl	Baseline
BR	Brachioradialis
DELT	Deltoid
DES	Direct electrical stimulation
DBS	Deep brain stimulation
EDC	Extensor digitorum communis
ERG	Electroretinogram
IFOF	Inferior occipito-frontal fascicle
ILF	Inferior longitudinal fascicle
IOM	Intraoperative neurophysiological monitoring
MEP	Motor evoked potential
OO	Orbicular oris
OP	Optic nerve(s)
PKAN	Pantothenate kinase-associated neurodegeneration
SEF	Spectral EEG frequency

Supplementary Information The online version contains supplementary material available at [https://doi.org/10.1007/978-3-030-95730-8_7].

M. N. de Melo (✉)
Department of Neurophysiology, Integrated Neuroscience Institute, Goiânia, GO, Brazil

S. M. Verst
Instituto de Ensino e Pesquisa (Research and Educational Institute) of Sírio Libanês Hospital, São Paulo, Brazil

Brain Spine Neurofisiologia, Jundiaí, SP, Brazil

S. M. Verst et al. (eds.), *Intraoperative Monitoring*,
https://doi.org/10.1007/978-3-030-95730-8_7

SSEP	Somatosensory evoked potential
SS	*Sagittal Striatum*
TA	Tibialis anterior
TES	Transcranial electrical stimulation
TIVA	Total intravenous anesthesia
VEP	Visual evoked potential(s)
VM	Vastus medialis
VP	Visual pathways

Introduction

The light stimulus upon reaching the retina is converted into an electrical input that travels through the VP to the visual processing cortex in the occipital lobes. Optic nerves (ON), optic chiasm, optic tracts, and lateral geniculate bodies make up the anterior part of this pathway, while optic radiation and visual cortex make up its posterior part. The responses evoked by these stimuli are called VEP. Its landmark is a three-phase wave, whose main component is P100.

Tumor resection along the VP can cause lesions, resulting in partial or complete visual deficit. Hence, VEP is indicated in any procedure with risk to the visual structures, like orbital, transsphenoidal, parasellar, temporal, occipital, and parieto-occipital transition surgeries. Additionally, VP monitoring is useful in functional surgeries, including microelectrode placement in the globus pallidus for deep brain stimulation (DBS) and in stereotactic pallidotomies.

Classically, during intraoperative neurophysiology monitoring (IOM), visual function is studied through VEP with flash-light stimulation. First described in 1973 by Wright et al. [16], the technique was not promising, since under general anesthesia, the resulting potential was unstable and with low reproducibility. The spread of total intravenous anesthesia and the development of devices with higher luminescence improved the technique. Consequently, better correlation between VEP potential and postoperative visual function became more reliable.

Yet, intraoperative usage of VEP is still very challenging. VEP reflects the activation of fibers from the macular region of the retina. Peripheral retina is not fully activated with the technique. Changes in amplitude and latency have limited value in focal lesions in the optic radiation and associative cortex. As dependent on a polysynaptic pathway, VEP is susceptible to anesthetic agents and systemic factors. Hypotension, hypothermia, hypoxemia, hypovolemia, and hematocrit below 15% should be discharged when interpreting the amplitude drop of the N75-P100 complex [16, 20].

Mapping the VP in awake craniotomies aims to highlight the topography of the anatomical pathways and their functional connectivity with other eloquent areas, such as language [5–7, 11, 26, 44, 45, 48].

This chapter deals with the anatomy of the VP, intraoperative mapping, and monitoring techniques under general anesthesia and in the awake craniotomies. Technical limitations are also discussed.

Anatomy of the Visual Pathways

The light stimulus penetrating the pupil is captured by specialized cells in the retina (photoreceptors – cones and rods), converted into an electrical input, and transmitted via bipolar cells to the retinal ganglion cells, whose axons form the ON. After leaving the orbit through the optic canal in the lesser sphenoid wing the ON proceeds through the middle fossa. In the optic chiasm, the nasal fibers of each nerve cross the midline and join the temporal fibers of the other eye, constituting the optic tract. Each optic tract proceeds posteriorly to the lateral geniculate nucleus of the thalamus, where it synapses and initiates optic radiation, the final pathway to the primary cortical areas of visual processing (Fig. 7.1). Anatomy and physiology of the circadian reflex and the pupillary reflex are beyond the scope of this chapter.

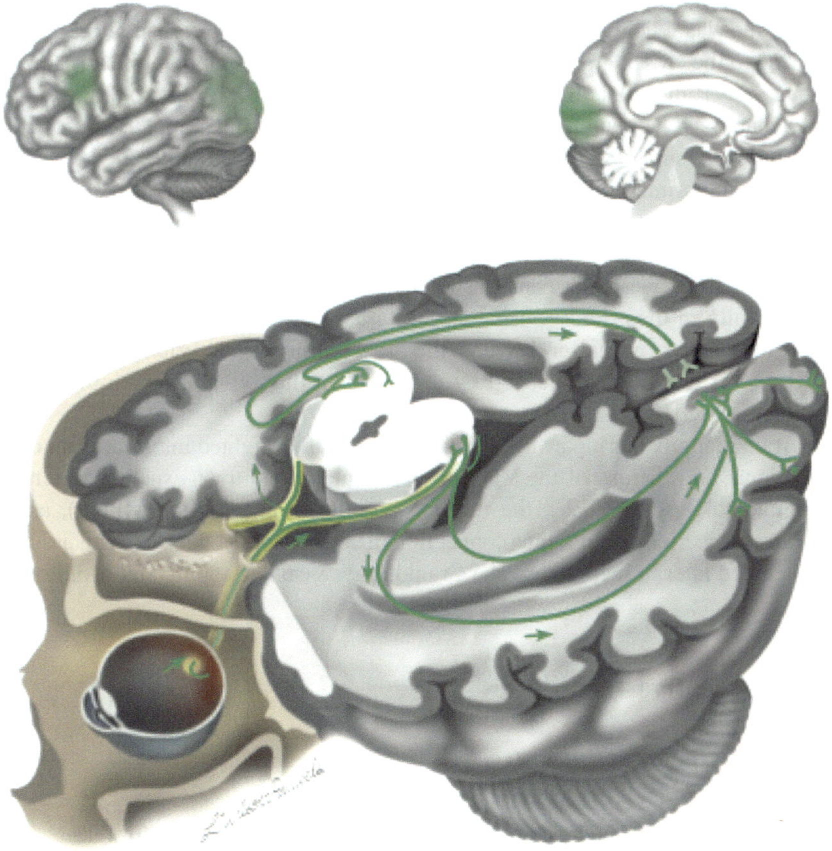

Fig. 7.1 Anatomy of the visual pathways

The optical radiation is divided: one loop courses above and laterally to the inferior horn of the lateral ventricle. The other is Meyer's loop, which courses anteriorly toward the pole of the temporal lobe before heading posteriorly to the cortex. Hence, surgeries in the temporo-occipital transition and in areas immediately anterior to the inferior horn of the lateral ventricle may damage the optic radiation. There is an incidence of an upper quadrantanopia ranging from 68 to 100% in anterior temporal lobectomies [52].

From the retina to the visual cortex there is a wide convergence of signals. In the peripheral retina, the signal from thousands of photoreceptors converges to one ganglion cell, while in the fovea this ratio is almost one to one [51]. This explains the high resolution of central vision and why the cortical representation of the fovea around the calcarine fissure is larger. Another important particularity is how information from the visual fields reaches the visual cortex. The light stimuli are refracted in the lens and when they reach the retina, the image is inverted both vertically and horizontally. Thus, the upper visual field is mapped below the calcarine fissure and the lower visual field above the calcarine fissure, besides the right-left inversion.

Due to the crossing of fibers in the optic chiasm and its topographic organization along the VP, different clinical presentations result from an injury to the VP, including amaurosis, hemianopia, and quadrantanopia. Their anatomical-functional correlation is illustrated in Figs. 7.2 and 7.3.

From the primary visual cortex (area 17), the signals are sent to the association visual cortex for interpretation (areas 18 and 19) and to the frontal ocular cortex, an area related to visual fixation. There may be differences in terms of cortical generator between reverse-pattern and flash-activated VEP. The former seems to be generated mainly in the primary visual cortex (area 17) while the latter is mediated by both the primary visual cortex and the association visual cortex. Flash-activated VEP seems not to be influenced by the point on the retina at which the stimulus occurs [30, 33].

Brain mapping during awake craniotomies has highlighted important anatomical functional correlations of the VP with other subcortical tracts, such as the inferior longitudinal fascicle (ILF), the inferior occipito-frontal fascicle (IFOF), and the U-fiber projection system, interconnecting different eloquent cortex. This issue will be detailed later in section "Awake Craniotomy: Visual Mapping and Monitoring".

Intraoperative Techniques

VEP – Asleep Techniques

The flash visual stimulus is the most commonly used mechanism for retinal activation during VP monitoring. Flash-VEP indicates VP integrity when present, rather than giving details of the visual system. Flash stimulation does not depend on patient compliance and activates luminescence-sensitive channels (cones and rods).

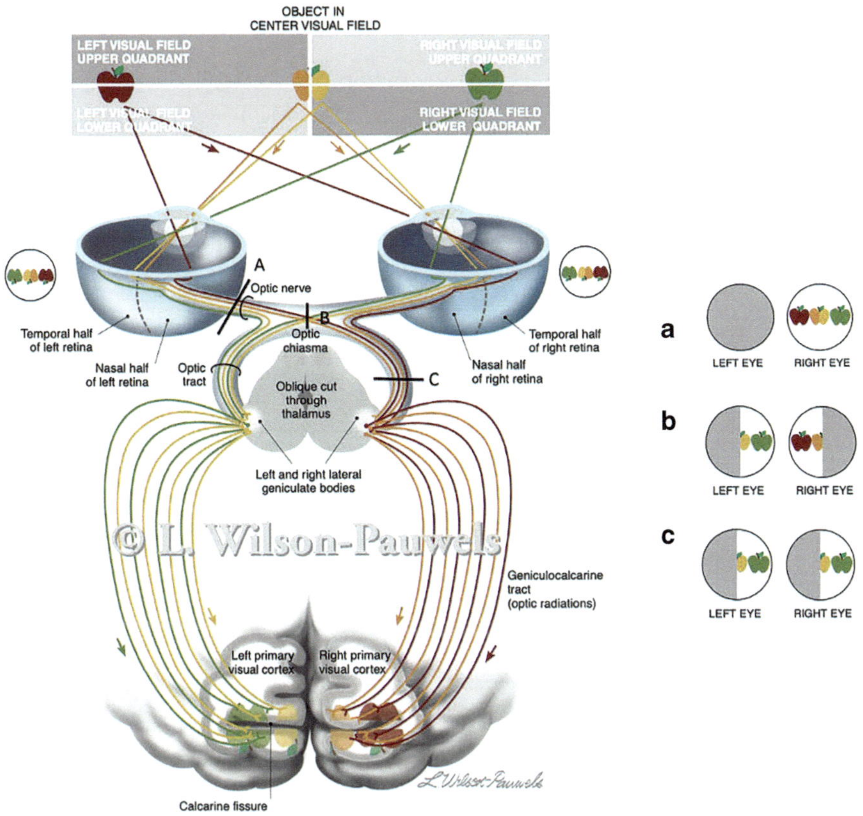

Fig. 7.2 Correlation between injuries at different levels of the VP and visual deficits. (**a**) Injury to the ON causes disruption of nasal and temporal fibers of the same eye. This results in amaurosis ipsilateral to the injury. (**b**) Lesion of the optic chiasma interrupts the crossing of the nasal fibers in each eye, resulting in the loss of peripheral vision, called bi-temporal hemianopia. (**c**) Injury to the optic tract interrupts the ipsilateral and nasal temporal fibers contralateral to the injury. This results in homonymous hemianopia. (Adapted from Wilson-Pauwels, et al. [51] (with permission))

Outpatient reverse-pattern stimulus activates more contrast-sensitive channels (rods) [30, 51]. In people with normal vision, the VEP is recorded eminently as a three-phase potential with a first negative component at 75 ms (N75), a positive component at 100 ms (P100), and a third negative component at 145 ms (N145).

After induction of anesthesia, eyes are taped with a transparent film dressing to avoid exposure and cornea abrasion. Subdermal needle electrodes are inserted in the lower and lateral or medial orbit for electroretinogram (ERG) recordings. ERG continuously evaluates the efficacy of the light stimulation of the retina. Needling of III, IV, and VI is done if indicated in IOM protocol (more details in Chap. 20). Afterward, a goggle-shaped stimulator (Fig. 7.4a) is placed over the closed eyes. Even further care must be taken not to displace the inserted needles. We kindly cover the region

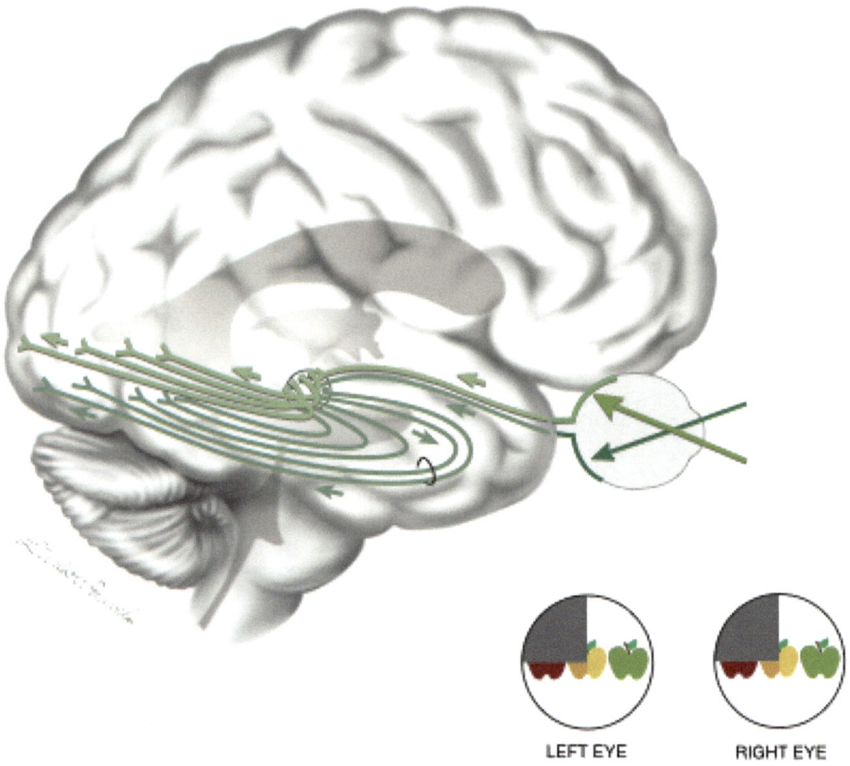

From "Cranial Nerves in Health and Disease" 2002, © Wilson-Pauwels, Akesson, Stewart, Spacey, B C Decker Inc.

Fig. 7.3 Optical radiation injury. A lesion of right Meyer's loop axons results in a loss of vision in the upper contralateral visual quadrants—homonymous quadrantanopia

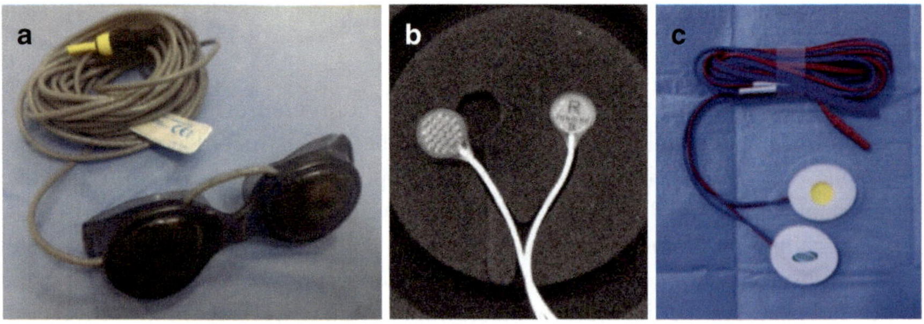

Fig. 7.4 Devices used for monitoring VEP: (**a**) Goggle-shaped stimulator. (**b**) Disk-type stimulator from Inomed GmbH, Germany. (**c**) Adhesive VEP electrodes for single-use and flash stimulation. Compatible with all IOM machines since they have touch-proof connections. Each eye stimulator should be connected to an electrical output for alternating stimulation. Manufactured by Spes Medica, Italy

with gauze and use large adhesive tapes. There is a risk of goggle displacement by frontal skin flap during frontal and frontotemporal craniotomies or during patient's positioning. Disk-type stimulators (Fig. 7.4b) are lighter, more flexible, and easily positioned, and tend to shift less [16, 19]. Yet, they are not available for all IOM machines. Newly released, adhesive low weight VEP electrodes are suitable for all IOM machines (Fig. 7.4c). They connect to a touch-proof electrical output and their luminescence relates to stimulus intensity. These VEP electrodes are available for white or red color flash.

Regardless of the device used, it is important that it is well fitted to the face not to press the eyeballs and to block the entrance of any light beam (Fig. 7.5). Total darkness is essential for the retina to be adequately stimulated only by the deflated flash, and in the operating room several light sources can disrupt the stimulation [14]. Displacement of stimulators is diagnosed by ERG loss.

LEDs with white light are preferable to LEDs with red light for the following reasons: (1) white contains all color spectra, being able to activate even cone-photoreceptors, whose maximum spectral sensitivity is for the colors red, green, and blue [51]; (2), all types of rods, consequently a larger area of the retina [14]; (3) white color keeps the retina adapted to light during long-lasting surgeries [34].

Paradoxically, although flash-VEP activates a wide retina area [14], the activation seems to predominate in fovea. The fovea is richer in cones and saturates less when exposed to bright light. This phenomenon might explain why quadrantanopia is poorly predicted by flash-VEP [20].

Stimulus and recording parameters vary widely among normative studies [53]. Most frequencies used to flash deflagration are inferior to 4 Hz. Most commonly, being around 1.1 Hz. Higher frequencies imply a reduction in the amplitude of the responses and, if done continuously, a greater risk of heat injury to the eyelids [16, 19]. Wiedemayer et al. [50] reported stable VEPs at a frequency of 8.5 Hz using goggles with red light-emitting diodes, but the signal-to-noise ratio was higher than

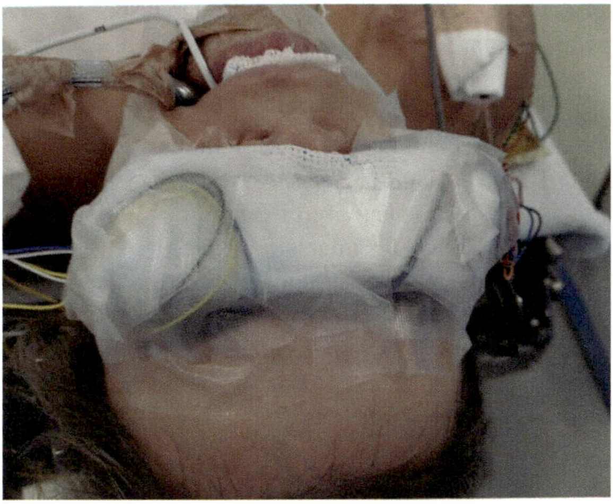

Fig. 7.5 Positioning of goggles: They are placed gently in order not to displace III, IV, and VI muscle needles. The needles should remain straight, leaning against the goggles. By doing so, needles do not damage the eyeballs. Needle cables bend on themselves and are covered by tape so they can't be accidentally pulled off. Special care is taken to avoid goggle displacement with gauze and large adhesive tapes

that often obtained in skull surgery. There is an alternation of the stimulus between eyes.

The brightness of the flash is measured in illuminance, ranging between 10,000 and 20,000 lux (Lx). The intensity of the stimulus is measured in Candela (Cd) and ranges between 0 and 175 mCd, depending on the other parameter sets and differences between IOM machines. Since the retina has the ability to adapt to light, there can be a variation in the amplitude of the responses obtained after the initial stimuli.

For a stable activation of the retina, 1 minute of flash stimulus is recommended before VEP recording [34]. Stable and reproducible VEPs are obtained with stimuli of 10 to 20 ms duration. Kodama and Goto [19] have successfully described the use of stimuli with 40 ms duration. They were able to successfully identify P100 after 40 to 100 sweeps. Moreover, they could perform continuous stimulation for over 30 minutes, without skin burn events. Despite their good results, it is important to keep in mind that longer durations generate more heat, especially if done continuously for a long period of time. The balance between stimulus intensity, duration, frequency, and time is essential to ensure the safety of the technique.

Registration

ERG ensures that the retina is being adequately stimulated. A subdermal needle electrode is placed in the lower corner of the orbit of each eye and referenced to Fz or to ipsilateral medial/lateral orbit corner. Two main components can be identified in the ERG waveform, a negative component (N30 or A) related to photoreceptor activation and a positive component (P50 or B) related to retinal and ON activation [24].

Corkscrew electrodes are positioned at points Oz, O1, and O2 and referenced to Cz and Fz for registration of VEP on the scalp. Some authors suggest the placement of more recording electrodes, such as L10 and R10 (10 cm lateral to Oz), as a safety measure in case of displacement of any of the other electrodes during the approach [19, 34]. Usually, the highest amplitude responses are obtained in Oz-Fz or Oz-Cz, with inter-individual variability of the highest electronegativity.

The number of measured responses varies between 40 and 200, depending on the signal-to-noise ratio. The most important is to obtain stable and reliable VEPs promptly. Recommended filtering ranges from 1-30 Hz (low-frequency filter) and 300–1000 Hz (high-frequency filter) [16, 19, 34, 53]. We generally use 1-100 Hz bandpass filter, sensitivity of 20 μV/division, and 200–300 ms analysis time for adults and 500 ms for infants.

During occipital craniotomies, VEP potentials might be recorded with a strip electrode positioned directly over the visual cortex (cortical VEP) (Fig. 7.6). Ota et al. [33] were able to register P100 with good detectability and stability using a strip. They demonstrated consistency between postoperative clinical changes and findings during surgery. Shahar et al. [39] recorded P100 with subdural recording during awake craniotomies. They stated that P100 presented greater amplitude and spatial resolution than scalp recording.

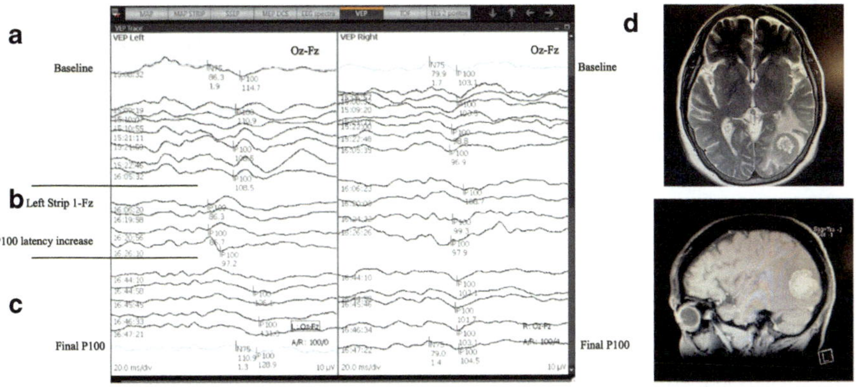

Fig. 7.6 Female, 65 y.o., breast cancer metastasis in the left occipital region. No previous visual deficit. Flash-VEP recording electrodes at Oz-Fz'. Filters: 5-100 Hz Complete IOM protocol included: TES-MEP: C3-Cz and C4-Cz with recordings at APB and AH/SSEP for ulnar and tibial nerves bilaterally/subcortical motor mapping (monopolar & cathodal) and EEG. (**a**) Baselines (bsl) with normal P100 (110.9 ms). (**b**) After dura mater opening, a strip electrode was placed directly over the left occipital cortex: cortical P100 showed 10 ms shorter latency compared to bsl. During tumor resection: cortical P100 latency increased 10 ms. (**c**) After resection and back to corkscrew recordings: P100 latency was delayed (128.9 ms). Total delay = 14 ms in relation to previous corkscrew recordings. P100 amplitude variation <50%. Patient had no new deficit. (**d**) MRI at presentation

Kikuchi et al. [18] studied the correlation between P100 amplitude and the cross-sectional area of the ON. They stimulated ON in the vicinity of the orbit and registered a potential near the chiasma, about 8 mm distance. In this experimental study, the amplitude of the potential is related directly to the cross-sectional area of the nerve, i.e., a reduction of its amplitude with the gradual narrowing of the nerve. The study did not assess the correlation between visual function and changes in the ON potential. Møller et al. [28] recorded ON potential after flash stimulation. The response showed low amplitude and reproducibility, with intraoperative fluctuations. In both techniques, only the exposed ON was evaluated, restricting its use to very specific approaches.

Interpretation and Warning Signs

ERG translates that retina is properly being stimulated and serves as a control technique. A drop in amplitude of the VEP associated with the loss of ERG waves indicates a failure in the visual stimulus, either by inadequate deflagration of the flash, or by stimulator displacement (Fig. 7.7).

VEP is indicated in all surgery in which the VP is at risk, either due to proximity, direct invasion, or compression of its fibers (Fig. 7.8). In this context, the P100 is the most robust, stable, and reliable parameter for VEP analysis during IOM. Each VEP wave relates to a specific generator. Most probably, P40 reflects activation of the ON

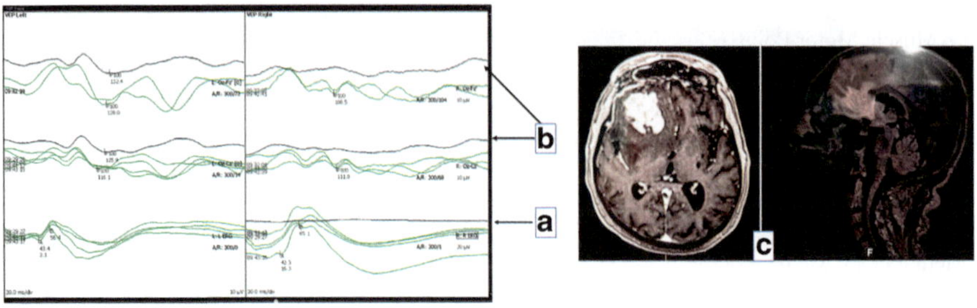

Fig. 7.7 Male, 83 y.o., lung cancer metastasis in the right supraorbital region. Flash-VEP with recording electrodes at Oz-Fz and Oz-Cz'. ERG: inferior orbit-Fz. Filters: LFF - 1 Hz, HFF - 800 Hz. Sweeps: 100. Baselines showed replicable N30(A)/P50(B) and P100 with normal latencies. Right N30/P50 disappeared, as did P100 at the same eye. Due to the wide frontal craniotomy, skin flap displaced the goggles. The diagnose of the situation was fully dependent on ERG recordings. (**a**) Displacement of goggle after frontal skin repair with loss of ERG (black line). Baselines in green. (**b**) Loss of P100 on the right. (**c**) MRI – right supraorbital lesion

[28], and P50 and N80 are generated in central structures distally to the optic chiasm. The origin of N75 has not yet been completely clarified, but it is likely that N75 and P100 have their functional and anatomical origin in different neuronal structures [30, 42]. Although some indications suggest that P100 is generated in the primary visual cortex, studies with magnetoencephalography and depth electrodes have suggested an important contribution from the dorsal extrastriate cortex of the middle occipital gyrus, lingual gyrus, and ventral portion of the fusiform gyrus [33]. Hayashi et al. [16] showed N75-P100-N145 to have more reproducibility under anesthesia than other VEP components.

The use of VEP as a predictor of postoperative visual deficit is still controversial. Some studies have described specific findings to have positive relation to the postoperative outcome. Yet, others showed opposite results and technical difficulties interfering with its reliability and reproducibility. Cedzich et al. [3] reported inconsistent results in their report with great fluctuation of latencies, amplitudes, and even loss of potentials that did not correlate with a significant clinical change. The development of new anesthetic protocols and devices with higher luminescence led to a greater correlation between intraoperative findings and postoperative visual outcomes.

Yet, previous visual impairment or large visual field defects directly affect intraoperative VEP recording feasibility. If obtained, P100 shows low amplitude and reproducibility and is unstable [1, 25, 33]. Hence, a corrected visual acuity greater than 0.4 is an important factor for the acquisition of reliable potentials [16, 20].

To overcome interindividual variability, P100 is compared with patient's intraoperative baseline. P100 amplitude deterioration >50% has been shown to be the most reliable parameter [38]. Transient P100 loss with recovery does not seem to indicate irreversible VP damage. Harding et al. [15] showed that P100 loss for more than 4 minutes related to an increased risk of postoperative deficit. This temporal analysis still has to be confirmed by other studies.

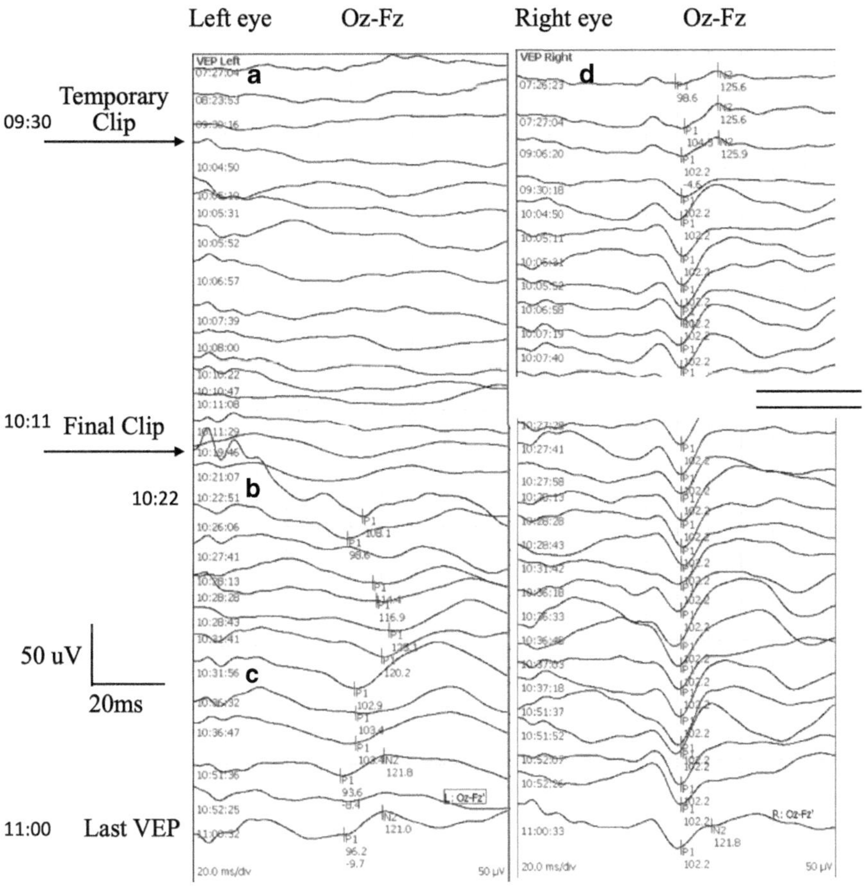

Fig. 7.8 Male, 39 y.o, left ophthalmic artery aneurysm. Flash-VEP: recording electrodes at Oz-Fz and Oz-Cz'. ERG: inferior orbit-Fz. Filters: 1-100 Hz. Sweeps: 35. (**a**) Baseline: absent left P100 (7:27 a.m.). No change with temporary clip. (**b**) Left P100 showing up about 10 minutes after definitive clamping. (**c**) Final left P100. (**d**) Right VEP with normal P100 from baseline to final recordings

Pattern-reversal P100 latency shows great variability between healthy and affected eyes. Yet, flash-VEP P100 latency varies little, resulting in less importance as a diagnostic value [16]. Latency was shown to have an intraoperative spontaneous variation. Therefore, it is ineffective for this purpose (Harding et al., 2015).

Ota et al. [33] stated that direct cortical recordings improve spatial resolution. They were able to register the best cortical P100 in the vicinity of the calcarine fissure. Noachtar et al. [30] showed a variability of lateral extent of area 17 ranging from 4 mm to 24 mm. Hence, it would result in considerable topographic variability of the primary visual cortex.

Type of stimulus, electrodes, and recording parameters directly affect the quality of intraoperative P100. The diversity of reported techniques hinders the direct comparison of efficacy. Hence, it is understandable that controversy about intraoperative VEP still exists.

Special Techniques

Stimulation of the optic tract might be performed in functional surgeries for Parkinson's disease and primary dystonia refractory to drug treatment. The internal globus pallidus is the therapeutic target in some cases of pallidotomies and deep brain stimulation (DBS), and its posterior-inferior-medial part lies a few millimeters above the optic tract. Hence, stimulation of the VP at this point is important for recognition and prevention of injury of the anatomical therapeutic target previously identified by stereotaxis.

For this purpose, Landi et al. [21] described the use of a monopolar electrode for stimulation of the optic tract under general anesthesia. Stimulus parameters were single-phase square pulse with 50 μs duration, 3 Hz frequency, 1 to 4 mA intensity, and 60 sweeps. Recording electrodes were positioned at Oz, O1, and O2 with a non-cephalic reference. They obtained biphasic potentials N40-P70 in scalp. Manohar et al. [27] could successfully reproduce Landi's protocol. In both studies, no patient had visual changes postoperatively.

Regarding parasellar tumor resection, Benedicic and Bosnjak [1] reported a cohort of 11 cases, in which they performed a dual stimulation technique. VEP was elicited by epidural stimulation of the optic nerves (using one needle electrode with a ball tip at each side of the optic nerve) and by flash with scalp recording (Oz-Fz as a control). Direct optic nerve stimulation used 0.2 to 5 mA, pulse duration of 0.1–0.3 ms at a rate of 2 Hz. The responses obtained with direct nerve stimulation consisted of three-phase potentials characterized by a first positive deflection at 20 ms (P20), a negative at 30 ms (N30), and a third small positive deflection at 40 ms (P40). They used as warning signal an amplitude deterioration greater than 30% for P20 and N30. Reversible reduction in responses during manipulation of the anterior VP had statistical significance in preventing postoperative visual deterioration. No deterioration of P100 was registered during the procedure.

We present a case of three-phase wave P20-N30-P40 complex recorded at scalp after subcortical stimulation using a DBS probe (Fig. 7.9). This case covers both methodologies described above and points to possible new frontiers of VP evaluation.

Interestingly, Böex et al. [2] used subcortical-cortical evoked potentials in twelve patients under general anesthesia. They recorded bilateral cortical responses at central, parietal, parieto-occipital, occipital regions. Bipolar stimulation parameters were biphasic pulse of 0.2 ms/phase, 1.3 Hz, 30 sweeps, 5-4000 Hz, and up to 10 mA for optic radiation and Meyer's loop and 5 mA for ON. They aimed to set a correlation between stimulation point and distance to VP. Biphasic P1(2.4–5.4 ms)-P2(15–21.6 ms) complex was successfully evoked at a distance up to 4.5 mm. P1-P2 were registered at ipsilateral occipital cortex after temporal and parietal stimulations and bilateral occipital responses after ON stimulation.

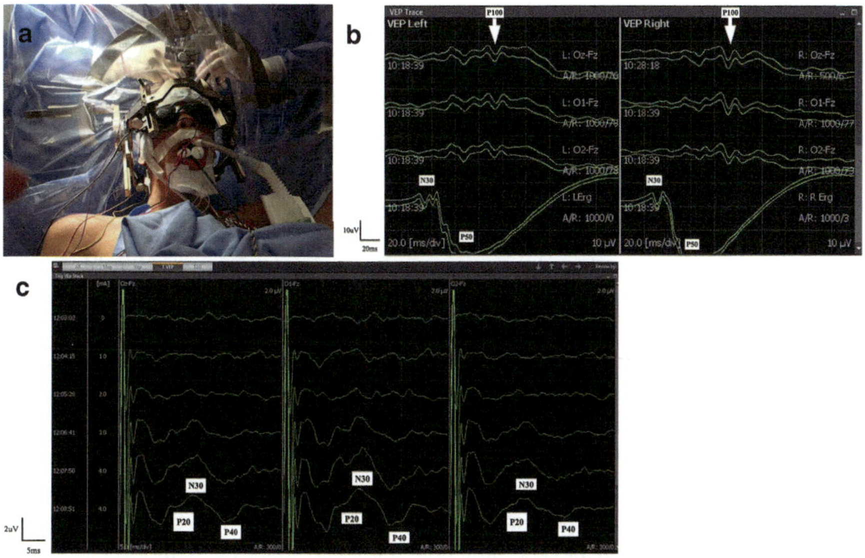

Fig. 7.9 Male, 14 y.o., with dystonia due to pantothenate kinase-associated neurodegeneration (PKAN). DBS approach. IOM protocol: 1. Flash-VEP / 2. MEP (due to proximity to internal capsule: bilateral muscles recordings: *Orbicularis oris*, Deltoid, *Extensor digitorum communis*, *Abductor pollicis brevis*, *Vastus medialis*, *Tibialis anterior* and *Abductor hallucis*) / 3. Optic tract mapping using DBS electrode. (**a**) Googles and patient positioning. (**b**) Baseline. Flash-VEP recording electrodes at Oz-Fz, O1-Fz and O2-Fz. Filters: 30-100 Hz. Sweeps: up to 1000. (**c**) After positioning the DBS electrode, electrical stimulation was performed through the most distal contact to assess the proximity of the optic tract. Parameters: intensity 0.2 to 4 mA, frequency 2 Hz, duration 0.2 ms, sweeps: 50, recordings at Oz-Fz / O1-Fz / O2-Fz. A three-phase wave P20-N30-P40 complex showed up with 3 mA and is greater with 4 mA (last line). (Source: Denise Spinola Pinheiro, MD, PhD and Murilo Martinez Marinho, MD. Unpublished personal data (with permission))

Stimulation along the VP with scalp recordings seems to be a promising technique. The methodology needs to be correlated with outcome in larger cohorts to validate and standardize its application.

Awake Craniotomy: Visual Mapping and Monitoring

Real-time identification of functional networks during brain tumor resection has improved the functional and oncological outcomes. The role of awake craniotomy and eloquent-areas mapping is already well known [4, 9, 32, 47]. New frontiers in cortical and subcortical direct electrical stimulation (DES) of non-motor and non-verbal connections are being searched [6, 8, 11, 48]. VP and DES is the next big thing.

Of utmost interest for DES is optic radiation and visual cortex. The fibers of the optical radiation take a three-dimensional path involving the temporal and occipital horns of the lateral ventricle and terminate in a retinotopic organization in the visual cortex. The central beam of optic radiation contains the macular fibers (central vision) and terminates at the lips of the calcarine fissure, while the anterior (Meyer's loop) and posterior beams represent the upper and lower quadrants of the retina [12, 35] (Figs. 7.2 and 7.3). Optic radiation mapping is important when operating the posterior half of temporal lobe, inferior parietal lobe, and occipital lobe. There is a somatotopic organization of the primary and associative visual cortex regarding shape, color, and motion.

Lee et al. [23] demonstrated that there are specific areas for one type of function, while others relate to more than one image feature. Certainly, there is an inter-individual anatomical and functional variability. They stimulated the lateral temporo-occipital region or temporo-parieto-occipital junction and elicited scotomas or large visual field defects on the contralateral side. The basal temporo-occipital cortical region produced micropsia (shrunken image), macropsia (enlarged image), and metamorphopsia (image distortion). Stimulation of the fusiform gyrus and lingual gyrus produced colorful shapes, and stimulation of areas such as the basal temporo-occipital junction, mesial parieto-occipital junction, or temporo-parieto-occipital junction and occipital pole produced shapes with motion. Complex shapes associated with auditory responses were produced upon stimulation of the superior temporal cortex.

The subcortical DES exposes the interneural connections that associate the captured images with memories, language, and other cognitive aspects. This network is fundamental for perceiving and understanding the surrounding environment.

The processing of the written word, as well as recognition of images and people, and the access to the meaning of this information depends on the connections of the visual system to the other eloquent areas.

The optic radiation is located medially and above the ILF, just below the IFOF. This region of high connectivity between the optic radiation, IFOF, and ILF is called the *Sagittal Striatum* (SS) and should be considered as a functional boundary in occipito-temporal tumor resections [5]. The posterior dorsal portion of ILF is part of the ventral indirect semantic language pathway and connects the occipital lobe with the basal posterior-temporal cortex. This is the area for visual word and visual object formation, visual recognition, and reading [10]. The IFOF is part of the direct ventral semantic language pathway, and relates to written word comprehension, color, and letter recognition [40]. In the right hemisphere, IFOF also seems to be involved in the recognition of facial emotions, especially for feelings of sadness, anger, and fear [48]. The function of the right hemisphere should not be overlooked, as referenced in Chap. 19.

The depth of the temporo-occipito-parietal junction also deserves special attention, since the optic radiation bundles are emerging from the lateral geniculate body at this point.

We use several tasks to evaluate visual network, such as the visual field, Verst-Maldaun-Language-Assessment (VMLA)-Semantic [44, 46], stroop test, line bisection, drawing, description of acts, and reading (Table 7.1). Some of these tests are available for free use at vemotests.com. More details are in Chap. 18.

Table 7.1 Tests used during awake craniotomies for posterior temporal/ inferior parietal and occipital approaches. Tests are available on vemotests.com

Test	Task	Goal
Stroop test	Read the written color or identify the color or the letter	It is an interferential test used as a visual semantic and reading task
VMLA-semantic	Combination of verbal and non-verbal images	Testing visual semantic interconnectivities
Reading	Words and sentences	ILF testing
Visual memory	Non-verbal: The patient is asked to memorize an image from VMLA-ON[a]. After naming 2 other images, he is asked to tell which figure he/she has seen before Verbal: The same task, but using a sequence of written words	Memory
Visual interpretation	The patient is asked to describe a scene from VMLA-ON	Posterior temporal testing
Visual field	Verbal and non-verbal. The patient is asked to fix a red point in the middle of the screen and describe the images present on middle and lateral quadrants (either inferior or superior, alternating positions)	Optic radiation
Movement cadency	Dual task: Tapping of finger-to-finger while performing one of the above tasks	Inferior posterior parietal region

[a]Verst-Maldaun Language Assessment-Object Naming (at vemotests.com)

There is a large inter-individual variability in the shape of the optical radiation. Its surgical manipulation without causing any visual deficits can be challenging [12, 13, 35]. Usually, DES of optical radiation is referred to by the patient as visual blurring, phosphenes, shadows, and less frequently, visual hallucinations. We usually add visuospatial assessment for optic radiation. This task is compounded by objects placed in different quadrants on the screen. Thus, one image should be positioned in the quadrant under interest and another in the opposite quadrant [13]. It is important to ask the patient to fix his gaze on the center of the screen.

Reading and verbal and non-verbal semantic tasks associated with cadence of hand movement complement the evaluation of optical radiation interconnected to Geschwind area.

Despite advances in optical radiation mapping, intraoperative recognition of quadrantanopia is still a frequent limitation. Conti Nibali et al. [29] proposed a new approach for visual field assessment. The numbers 0, 3, or 7 are presented randomly, one at a time and at different points of the extreme peripheral portion of the screen (upper, middle, or lower) for 0.3–0.5 seconds during subcortical mapping. Like by Double Picture Naming Task (DPNT), the patient is encouraged to keep his/her gaze fixed to the center of the screen. Errors of detection and visual discrimination could be separated according to the stimulus of optic radiation and ILF respectively. Naming of a number is a strongly acquired automatism, which decreases the occurrence of errors due to language alteration. Hence, the technique showed great specificity for optic radiation mapping and was able to reduce visual deficits when compared to the control group, submitted to DPNT.

The visual cortex also has important connections with the thalamus, which acts as a gateway to the frontal eye field, supplementary ocular cortex, and lateral prefrontal cortex. Déjerine in 1901 has showed the relationships of pulvinar nucleus with posterior temporal and parietal adjacent regions (cited by [31]). And later on, Walker in 1938 reported pulvinar relation to temporo-parietal occipital association cortex [31]. The dorsomedial, ventrolateral, ventroanterior, and dorsolateral thalamus nuclei act in the control of self-generated eye movements, saccades, and visuospatial attention [22, 41]. Such functional aspects were explored by the author in a recent case (Fig. 7.10, Video 7.1). Awake craniotomy and DES might be useful tools in identifying these connections.

Both bipolar stimulation at 50-60 Hz and monopolar stimulation at 250–500 Hz might be used for VP mapping. The choice of mapping technique should be based on team experience (neurophysiologist and neurosurgeon). Additionally, the patient's clinical presentation, such as presence or absence of seizures, degree of tumor infiltration, edema, and delineation of the tumor borders should also be taken into consideration. More details are in Chap. 18.

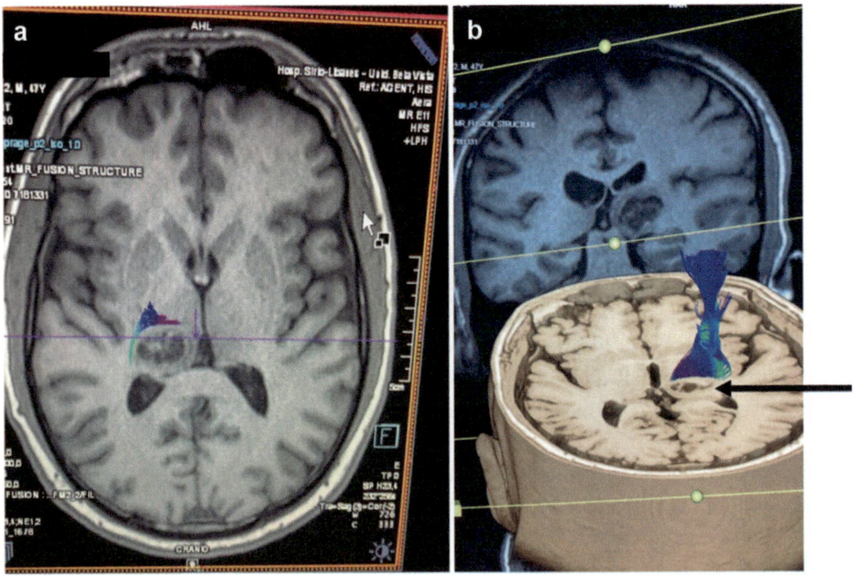

Fig. 7.10 Male, 47 y.o. Left thalamic cavernoma. The patient underwent awake craniotomy for intraoperative visual field and semantic testing. [tests available at vemotests.com]. (**a**) Tractography demonstrating the corticospinal tract in blue. (**b**) Video: During cavernoma manipulation, the patient referred diplopia in the left quadrants. He was instructed to gaze to the center of the screen and name the objects in the quadrants. This case illustrates the role of the thalamus and its connections to eye movement and visuospatial attention

The patient should be comfortably positioned and with wide face exposure. If patient uses glasses, they should be prepared for intraoperative use by removing one or both straps as necessary. A previous clinical evaluation and tractography images analysis are important to set IOM protocol. Switching between appropriate tests directed to the functions of the anatomical resection area optimizes the results. Continuous communication between the tester and the surgeon is of paramount importance.

Mapping of VP during awake craniotomies is a good technique to recognize interindividual anatomical heterogeneity and anatomical-functional relationships [10, 12, 35, 52]. The functional connectivity cannot be assessed with flash-PEV. Tractography has limitations in identifying fiber crossing, underestimating the anterior extent of Meyer's loop, for example. We reported a case, in which we performed awake craniotomy and flash-VEP during two different approaches for left and right occipital lesions [44, 45]. We had the unique opportunity of analyzing the outcome of the same patient after either technique. Awake craniotomy was performed for resection of the left lesion, without new deficits. Asleep approach using flash-VEP was used for the right lesion. The patient evolved with left inferior temporal quadrantanopia.

Awake craniotomy plays an important role in VP mapping and monitoring.

Anesthesia and Systemic Factors

Like other polysynaptic evoked potentials, VEP suffers wide interference from anesthetic drugs. Under total intravenous anesthesia (TIVA), VEP shows less amplitude and latency variability, compared to other anesthetic regimens [16, 43, 49]. Kodama and Goto [19] reported a 97% successful rate for flash-VEP recordings under TIVA in twelve years' experience.

Inhaled anesthetics such as nitric oxide, sevoflurane, and isoflurane markedly depress the amplitude of P100, even at low doses [3]. Conflictingly, Ota et al. [33] reported stable P100 in 14 of 17 patients using sevoflurane and propofol. Kamada et al. [17] used only sevoflurane, and P100 was successfully recorded over the cortex. However, in most surgeries where VEP monitoring is indicated, motor evoked potential is also required, and in this context, inhalational anesthesia should be avoided.

Other venous agents such as Thiopental increase the latency and decrease the amplitude of the VEP in a dose-dependent manner. Its suppressive effect is already considerable at low doses. Ketamine only slightly increases latency, but markedly attenuates amplitude [16].

The brain is an organ of high metabolism, with high and constant demand for oxygen and nutrients. Therefore, alterations in systemic homeostasis compromise the detection and stability of VEP, since they hinder synaptic transmission and/or axonal conduction. Hypoxemia, hypotension, and hemodilution, especially hematocrit below 15%, decrease oxygen transport to the central nervous system, with probable effect on VEP latency increase and amplitude deterioration. In somatosensory evoked potentials (SSEPs), hypocapnia generates changes in pH and ions' balance, with impaired conduction velocity [16]. As a polysynaptic pathway, we could infer that the same changes occur in obtaining P100. Hypothermia, in turn, interferes in synaptic transmission. Russ et al. [37] evidenced that a drop in body temperature by 1° reduces the central conduction of SSEPs by 15%. The increase in the latency of VEPs with hypothermia has already been shown [36].

Conclusion

Different visual stimulus and recording parameters have been described for VEP IOM in the past decade. It led to improvement of the technique, more stable recordings, and improved correlation to postoperative visual outcome. However, differences in reported techniques and interpretation parameters hinder reliability and consensus about intraoperative VEP.

Regarding awake craniotomies for VP cortical and subcortical mapping, reports point to its usefulness for identifying functional interconnections beyond the limitations of flash-VEP technique.

Flash-VEP presents low sensibility for detecting small optical radiation lesions and resulting quadrant impairment.

As with other neurophysiological techniques, VEP is sensitive to the effects of inhaled anesthetic agents and changes in systemic homeostasis. Hence, TIVA is recommended.

Team communication is an essential factor in mitigating existing technical and environmental biases.

References

1. Benedicic M, Bosnjak R. Intraoperative monitoring of the visual function using cortical potentials after electrical epidural stimulation of the optic nerve. Acta Neurochir. 2011;153:1919–27. https://doi.org/10.1007/s00701-011-1098-y.
2. Boëx C, Goga C, Bérard N, Al Awadhi A, Bartoli A, Meling T, Bijlenga P, Schaller K. Intraoperative subcortical-cortical evoked potentials of the visual pathway under general anesthesia. Clin Neurophysiol. 2021; https://doi.org/10.1016/j.clinph.2021.02.399.
3. Cedzich C, Schramm J, Mengedoht CF, Fahlbusch R. Factors that limit the use of flash visual evoked potentials for surgical monitoring. Electroencephalogr Clin Neurophysiol. 1988;71:142–5.
4. Chang EF, Raygor KP, Berger MS. Contemporary model of language organization: an overview for neurosurgeons. J Neurosurg. 2015;122:250–61. https://doi.org/10.3171/2014.10.JNS132647. Epub 2014 Nov 28.
5. Chang-Seng E, Moritz-Gasser S, Duffau H. Awake mapping for low-grade gliomas involving the left saggital stratum: anatomofunctional and surgical considerations. J Neurosurg. 2014;120:1069–77.

6. Coello AF, Moritz-Gasser S, Martino J, Martinoni M, Matsuda R, Duffau H. Selection of intraoperative tasks for awake mapping based on relationships between tumor location and functional networks. J Neurosurg. 2013;119:1380–94.
7. Duffau H. New concepts in surgery of WHO grade gliomas: functional brain mapping, connectionism and plasticity – a review. J Neuro-Oncol. 2006;79:77–115. https://doi.org/10.1007/s11060-005-9109-6.
8. Duffau H. Awake Surgery for Nonlanguage Mapping Neurosurgery. 2010;66:523–9. https://doi.org/10.1227/01.NEU.0000364996.97762.73.
9. Duffau H, Moritz-Gasser S, Mandonnet E. A re-examination of neural basis of language processing: proposal of a dynamic hodotopical model from data provided by brain stimulation mapping during picture naming. Brain & Language. 2014;131:1–10.
10. Duffau H, Schotten MT, Mandonnet E. White matter functional connectivity as an additional landmark for dominant temporal lobectomy. J Neurol Neurosurg Psychiatry. 2008;79:492–5. https://doi.org/10.1136/jnnp.2007.121004.
11. Duffau H, Velut S, Mitchell MC, Gatignol P, Capelle L. Intra-operative mapping of the subcortical visual pathways using direct electrical stimulations. Acta Neurochir. 2004;000:1–6. https://doi.org/10.1007/s(0701-003-0199-7.
12. Ebeling U, Reulen HJ. Neurosurgical topography of the optic radiation in the temporal lobe. Acta Neurochir. 1988;92:29–36.
13. Gras-Combe G, Moritz-Gasser S, Herbet G, Duffau H. Intraoperative subcortical electrical mapping of optic radiations in awake surgery for glioma involving visual pathways. J Neurosurg. 2012;117:466–73.
14. Gutzwiller EM, Cabrilo I, Radovanovic I, Schaller K, Boëx C. Intraoperative monitoring with visual evoked potentials for brain surgeries J Neurosurg. 2018; https://doi.org/10.3171/2017.8.JNS171168. Epub 2018 March 30.
15. Harding GFA, Bland JDP, Smith VH. Visual evoked potential monitoring of optic nerve function during surgery. J Neurol Neurosurg Psychiatry. 1990;53:890–5.
16. Hayashi H, Kawaguchi M. Intraoperative monitoring of flash visual evoked potential under general anesthesia. Korean J Anesthesiol. 2017;70(2):127–35.
17. Kamada K, Todo T, Morita A, Masutani Y, Aoki S, Ino K, Kawai K, Kirino T. Functional monitoring for visual pathway using real-time visual evoked potentials and optic-radiation tractography. Neurosurgery. 2005;57(ONS Suppl 1):ONS-121–7.
18. Kikuchi Y, Sasaki T, Matsumoto M, Oikawa T, Itakura T, Kodama N. Optic nerve evoked potentials elicited by electrical stimulation – experimental and clinical studies. Neurol Med Chir. 2005;45:349–55.
19. Kodama K, Goto T. Neurophysiology of the visual system: basics and intraoperative neurophysiology techniques. Deletis V, Shils JL, Sala F, Seidel K, Neurophysiology in Neurosurgery – A modern approach. Elsevier; 2020.53–64.
20. Kodama K, Goto T, Sato A, Sakai K, Tanaka Y, Hongo K. Standard and limitation of intraoperative monitoring of the visual evoked potential. Acta Neurochir. 2010;152:643–8.
21. Landi A, Pirillo D, Cilia R, Antonini A, Sganzerla EP. Cortical visual evoked potentials recorded after optic tract near field stimulation during GPi-DBS in non-cooperative patients. Clin Neurol Neurosur. 2011;113:119–22.
22. Lappi O. Eye movements in the wild: oculomotor control, gaze behavior & frames of reference. Neurosci Biobehav Rev. 2016;69:49–68.
23. Lee HW, Hong SB, Seo DW, Tae WS, Hong SC. Mapping of functional organization in human visual cortex: electrical cortical stimulation. Neurology. 2000;54:849–54. https://doi.org/10.1212/WNL.54.4.849.
24. Lowitsch K, Hopf HC, Buchner H, Claus D, Jörg J, Rappelsberger P, Tackmann W. Visuell evozierte Potentiale (VEP). In: EP-Buch D, editor. . 1st ed. Stuttgart: Georg Thieme Verlag; 2000.

25. Luo Y, Regli L, Bozinov O, Sarnthein J. Clinical utility and limitations of intraoperative monitoring of visual evoked potentials. PLoS One. 2015;10(3):e0120525. https://doi.org/10.1371/journal.pone.0120525.
26. Mandonnet E, Gatignol P, Duffau H. Evidence for an occipito-temporal tract underlying visual recognition in picture naming. Clin Neurol Neurosur. 2009;111:601–5.
27. Manohar N, Thakkar K, Balasubramaniam A, Palan A. Globus pallidus internum targeted deep brain stimulation placement using optic tract stimulated visual evoked potentials and corticospinal tract stimulation in a case of severe dystonia. Neurol India. 2019;67:600–1.
28. Møller AR, Burgess JE, Sekhar LN. Recording compound action potentials from the optic nerve in man and monkeys. Electroencephalogr Clin Neurophysiol. 1987;67:549–55.
29. Conti Nibali M, Leonetti A, Puglisi G, Rossi M, Sciortino T, Gay LG, Arcidiacono UA, Howells H, Viganò L, Zito PC, Riva M, Bello L. Preserving visual functions during gliomas resection: feasibility and efficacy of a novel intraoperative task for awake brain surgery. Front Oncol. 2020;10:1485. https://doi.org/10.3389/fonc.2020.01485.
30. Noachtar S, Hashimoto T, Lüders H. Pattern visual evoked potentials recorded from human occipital cortex with chronic subdural electrodes. Electroencephalogr Clin Neurophysiol. 1993;88:435–46.
31. Ojemann GA, Fedio P, van Buren JM. Anomia from pulvinar and subcortical parietal stimulation. Brain. 1968;91:99–116. https://doi.org/10.1093/brain/91.1.99.
32. Ojemann GA. The neurobiology of language and verbal memory: observations from awake neurosurgery. Int J Psychophysiol. 2003;48:141–6. https://doi.org/10.1016/S0167-8760(03)00051-5.
33. Ota T, Kawai K, Kamada K, Kin T, Saito N. Intraoperative monitoring of cortically recorded visual response for posterior visual pathway. J Neurosurg. 2010;112:285–94. https://doi.org/10.3171/2009.6.JNS081272.
34. Rajan S, Simon MV. Intraoperative neurophysiologic monitoring and mapping of the visual pathways. In: Simon MV, editor. Intraoperative Neurophysiology – a comprehensive guide to monitoring and mapping. Demos Medical Publishing; 2019. p. 303–11.
35. Rubino PA, Rhoton AL, Tong X, Oliveira E. Three-dimensional relationships of the optic radiation. Neurosurgery. 2005;57(ONS Suppl 3):ONS-219–27. https://doi.org/10.1227/01.NEU.0000176415.83417.16.
36. Russ W, Kling D, Loesevitz A, Hempelmann G. Effect of hypothermia on visual evoked potentials (VEP) in humans. Anesthesiol. 1984;61:207–10.
37. Russ W, Sticher J, Scheld H, Hempelmann G. Effects of hypothermia on somatosensory evoked responses in man. Br J Anaesth. 1987;59:1484–91.
38. Sasaki T, Itakura T, Susuki K, Kasuya H, Munakata R, Muramatsu H, Ichikawa T, Sato T, Endo Y, Sakuma J, Matsumoto M. Intraoperative monitoring of visual evoked potential: introduction of a clinically useful method. J Neurosurg. 2010;112:273–84.
39. Shahar T, Korn A, Barkay G, Biron T, Hadanny A, Gazit T, Nossek E, Ekstein M, Kesler A, Ram Z. Elaborate mapping of the posterior visual pathway in awake craniotomy. J Neurosurg. 2017; https://doi.org/10.3171/2017.2.JNS162757. Epub 2017 August 25.
40. Surbeck W, Hildebrandt G, Duffau H. The evolution of brain surgery on awake patients. Acta Neurochir. 2015;157:77–84. https://doi.org/10.1007/s00701-014-2249-8.
41. Tanaka M, Kunimatsu J. Thalamic roles in eye movements. In: The Oxford Handbook of Eye Movements; 2012. https://doi.org/10.1093/oxfordhb/9780199539789.013.0013.
42. Tobimatsu S, Shima F, Ishido K, Kato M. Visual evoked potentials in the vicinity of the optic tract during stereotactic pallidotomy. Electroencephalogr Clin Neurophysiol. 1997;104:274–9.
43. Uribe AA, Mendel E, Peters ZA, Shneker BF, Abdel-Rasoul M, Bergese SD. Comparison of visual evoked potential monitoring during spine surgeries under total intravenous anesthesia versus balanced general anesthesia. Clin Neurophysiol. 2017;128:2006–13.
44. Verst SM, Castro I, Junior WS, Melo MN, Oliveira JR, Almeida SS, Alvarez NRC, Sucena ABC, Barros MR, Marrone CD, Battistella LR, Vasconcellos MAK, Alves AS, Maldaun

MVC. Verst-Maldaun language assessment (VMLA) validation process database. Mendeley Data. 2020;V2 https://doi.org/10.17632/zjhfk7mm7v.2.
45. Verst SM, Melo MN, Caivano AS, Fonseca US, Mathias LR Jr, Vilasboas T. Awake surgery versus VEP in tumors of visual pathway: case report. Interdiscip Neurosurg. 2020;20:100675.
46. Verst SM, Castro I, Scappini-Junior W, Melo MN, Oliveira JR, Almeida SS, Alvarez NRC, Sucena ACB, Barros MR, Marrone CD, Maldaun MVC. Methodology for creating and validating object naming and semantic tests used by Verst-Maldaun language assessment during awake craniotomies. Clin Neurol Neurosurg. 2021;202:106485.
47. Vigneau M, Beaucousin V, Hervé PY, Duffau H, Crivello F, Houdé O, Mazoyer B, Tzourio-Mazoyer N. Meta-analyzing left hemisphere language areas: phonology, semantics and sentence processing. NeuroImage. 2006;30:1414–32.
48. Vilasboas T, Herbet G, Duffau H. Challenging the myth of right nondominant hemisphere: lessons from corticosubcortical stimulation mapping in awake surgery and surgical implications. World Neurosurg. 2017;103:449–56.
49. Watson KR, Shah MV. Clinical comparison of 'single agent' anaesthesia with sevoflurane versus target-controlled infusion of propofol. Br J Anaesth. 2000;85:541–6.
50. Wiedemayer H, Fauser B, Sandalcioglu IE, Armbruster W, Stolke D. Observations on intraoperative monitoring of visual pathways using steady-state visual evoked potentials. Eur J Anaesthesiol. 2004;21:429–33.
51. Wilson-Pauwels L, Akesson EJ, Stewart PA, Spacey SD. Optic Nerve. In: Decker BC, editor. Cranial Nerves in health and disease. 2nd ed; 2002.
52. Yogarajah M, Focke NK, Bonelli S, Cercignani M, Acheson J, Parker GJM, Alexander DC, McEvoy AW, Symms MR, Koepp MJ, Duncan JS. Defining Meyer's loop-temporal lobe resections, visual field deficits and diffusion tensor tractography. Brain. 2009;132:1656–68.
53. York D. Visual evoked potentials during surgery. In: Nuwer MR, editor. Intraoperative monitoring of neural function. Handb Clin Neurophysiol. Elsevier; 2008. p. 172–7.

Generation of Potentials

Anatomy

Monitoring of SSEPs evaluates the functionality of the somatosensory pathway. Stimulation involves the peripheral nerves in the extremities and propagation of the signal is monitored throughout the pathway. First-order neurons in the somatosensory pathway have cell bodies in the dorsal root ganglion and axons that extend to the periphery. In addition to branching toward the periphery, these pseudo-unipolar neurons extend axons into the dorsal root entry zone and branch up and down through the ipsilateral dorsal column of the spinal cord. Some dorsal root ganglion fibers, instead of ascending the spinal cord, descend or synapse in the spinal cord gray matter. These branches are involved in reflexes, sensory modulation, and proprioception. Ascending fibers from the leg form the gracile fasciculus and fibers from the arm form the cuneate fasciculus. After ascending the spinal cord, these axons synapse with second-order neurons in the gracile and cuneate nuclei, respectively. From there, the axons of the second-order neurons decussate in the medulla as the internal arcuate fibers known as the sensory decussation. It is important to keep in mind that certain rare conditions can predispose patients to lack of decussation resulting in signals remaining ipsilateral, which should be screened for before monitoring [9, 14, 15]. After decussating, the second-order neuron fibers climb the brainstem in the medial lemniscus before synapsing with third-order neurons in the ventral posterolateral thalamic nuclei. Axons from the third-order neurons ascend in the posterior limb of the internal capsule before dispersing in the thalamocortical radiation to their respective areas of the primary sensory gyrus. Upper extremity fibers travel to the lateral convexity and lower extremity fibers go to the mesial parasagittal region. It is important to note that the stimulation technique is particular to the axons in the dorsal system and does not include anterolateral system axons due to differences in threshold and conduction [9].

Blood Supply of Somatosensory Pathway

Disruption in blood flow to various parts of the pathway can alter stimulus propagation. This allows for localization of lesions by observing which SSEPs are diminished. The somatosensory cortex is supplied by the anterior cerebral artery medially and by the middle cerebral artery laterally. This can help with localization of cerebral ischemia, since the tibial nerve pathway would be affected by anterior cerebral artery ischemia and the median nerve pathway by middle cerebral artery ischemia. Thalamocortical sensory axons are supplied by lenticulostriate branches of the middle cerebral and anterior choroidal arteries. Branches of the posterior cerebral artery supply the thalamic sensory nuclei, while branches of the basilar and vertebral arteries supply the medial lemniscus. In the spine, the two posterior spinal arteries supply the dorsal column. The anterior spinal artery supplies the white matter and the remaining grey matter. It has anastomoses with the cervical, aortic, and iliac radicular arteries.

SSEP Waveforms

Recorded SSEPs are summated into waveforms that have a series of peaks and valleys. Nomenclature of the waveforms includes Ns and Ps which represent peaks and valleys respectively. N and P indicate the polarity of the waveform with N being negative (up) and P being positive (down). Different waves are of interest for different recording sites. When monitoring the sensorimotor cortex, the waveform peaks primarily analyzed are N20 and P20 (also referred to as P22). These waveforms originate from median nerve stimulation and are thought to be of thalamic and cortical origin. N20/P30 is recorded over the somatosensory cortex, while P20/N30 are of opposite polarity and recorded over the primary motor cortex. For the cervical spinal cord, Erb's potential (N9), P14, N18, and N20 are assessed. Erb's potential is a peripheral response recorded from Erb's point 2 cm above the mid-clavicle. P14 and N18 potentials are recorded from the centroparietal scalp ipsilateral to the stimulus and are most likely generated by subcortical structures including the caudal medulla, areas of the brainstem, and thalamus. Lastly, for thoracolumbar spinal cord monitoring, the popliteal fossa, P31, N34, and P37 are generally monitored. Recording in the popliteal fossa monitors peripheral responses, while P31, N34, and P37 are recorded from the forehead midline to monitor brainstem response. In each procedure the most readily apparent and robust waveforms should be used to analyze amplitude, morphology, and latency (Figs. 8.1, 8.2, and 8.3).

Stimulation and Recording Technique

SSEPs are used to check the functionality of the somatosensory pathway at various levels from the periphery to the cortex. The stimulation is applied to the distal portion of a peripheral nerve, most commonly the median or ulnar nerve at the wrist for upper extremity SSEPs and the posterior tibial nerve at the ankle or the peroneal nerve at the fibular head for the lower extremity. To monitor the sensorimotor cortex, the median nerve should be stimulated; however, the stimulated nerve should be contralateral to the portion of the cortex at risk. Alternatively, dermatomal SSEPs are elicited by stimulation to the skin of the dermatome at risk. Stimulation points

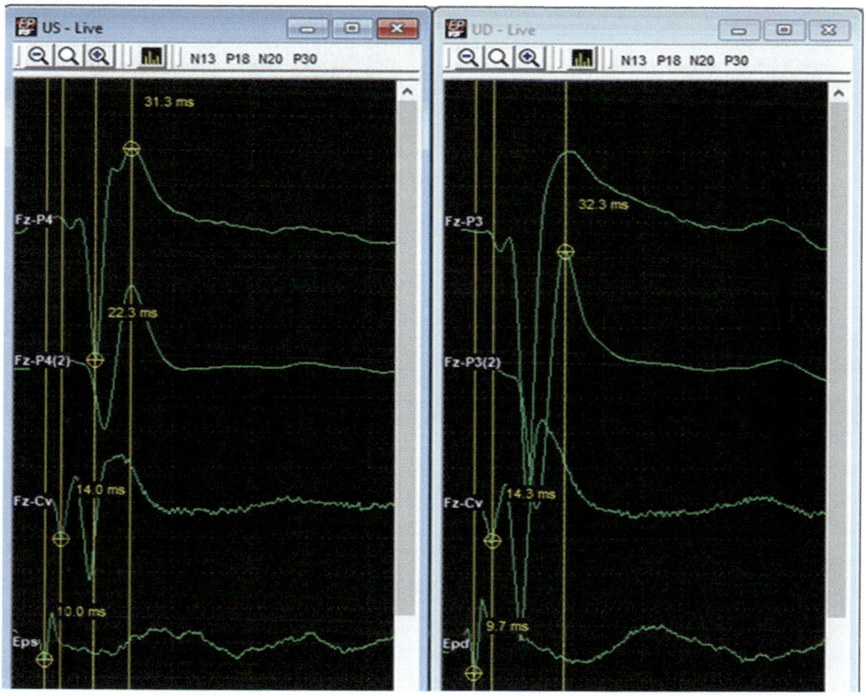

Fig. 8.1 Upper extremity SSEP data from ulnar nerve stimulation. In this dataset, the N9, N13, N20, and P30 waveforms are marked. Note that the active and reference electrodes are reversed to display N's as negative deflection waveforms, and P's as positive inflection waveforms. The Fz-P4 channel in the "US" waveform window shows an N20 with a latency of 22.3 ms and a P30 with a latency of 31.3 ms using a bandwidth of 10-250 Hz. The channel below uses the same two electrodes but has more aggressive filtering (30–100 Hz) which makes the N20 appear to have a longer latency and reduces some of the complexity in the P30. This channel is used primarily to allow for continuous monitoring during high-frequency noise. The Fz-Cv channel utilizes an electrode placed near the inion to record the N13 and P18 (if the inion isn't accessible the mastoid region can be used). Erb's point responses are collected from electrodes placed above the clavicle

are flexible and should be chosen based on ease of access to the site, easily identifiable landmarks, and ability to insert an electrode at the location. Typically for the upper extremities the default location is near the wrist, unless this site is unavailable. To stimulate the median nerve, the cathode of the pair of electrodes should be positioned between the palmaris longus and flexor carpi radialis tendons 2–4 centimeters proximal to the wrist [5, 11, 12]. The anode of the electrode pair should be placed 2–3 centimeters distal to the cathode to prevent an issue with action potential transmission known as anodal block. Anodal block is due to hyperpolarization of the axon under the anode leading to improper action potential initiation by the cathode if the two are in close proximity or the anode is proximal to the cathode. This placement guideline should be followed despite some evidence that anodal block

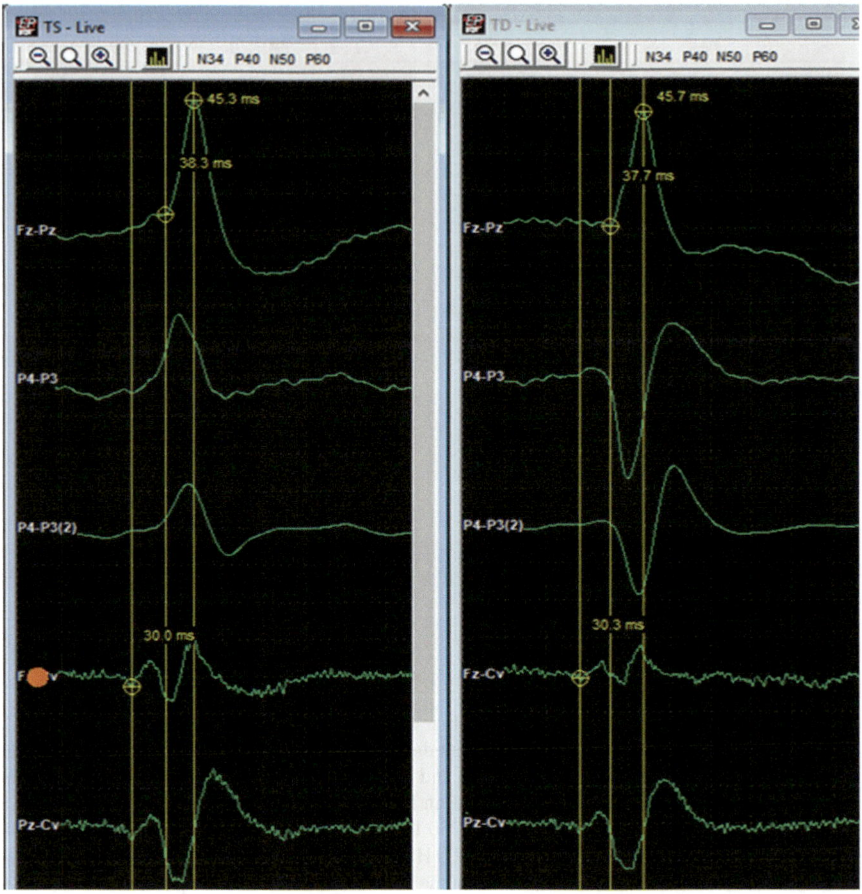

Fig. 8.2 Lower extremity SSEP data from posterior tibial nerve stimulation. In this dataset, the N30, N37, and P40 are marked. As with the upper extremity data, the active and reference electrodes are reversed to make N's negative and P's positive. The Fz-Pz channels show a downward pointing N37 followed by an upward pointing P40. The P4-P3 channel also shows the cortical P40 response but note that the left posterior tibial nerve P40 is upward pointing but the same channel in the right posterior tibial nerve waveform window shows a downward pointing waveform. This is by design and helps to identify left-right mix-up errors that can occur when plugging in the stimulating electrodes. The brainstem-generated responses are clearly present from the Fz-Cv and Pz-CV channels

will not play a significant role in stimulated action potentials [16]. The same setup with the cathode 2-4 cm proximal to the wrist and the anode distal to the cathode can be used for ulnar nerve stimulation, but on the medial side of the forearm next to the flexor carpi ulnaris muscle. The median nerve SSEP amplitude is usually larger than the ulnar nerve SSEP amplitude and is better for monitoring, but in some cases ulnar nerve SSEP monitoring can be more useful, especially cervical spine

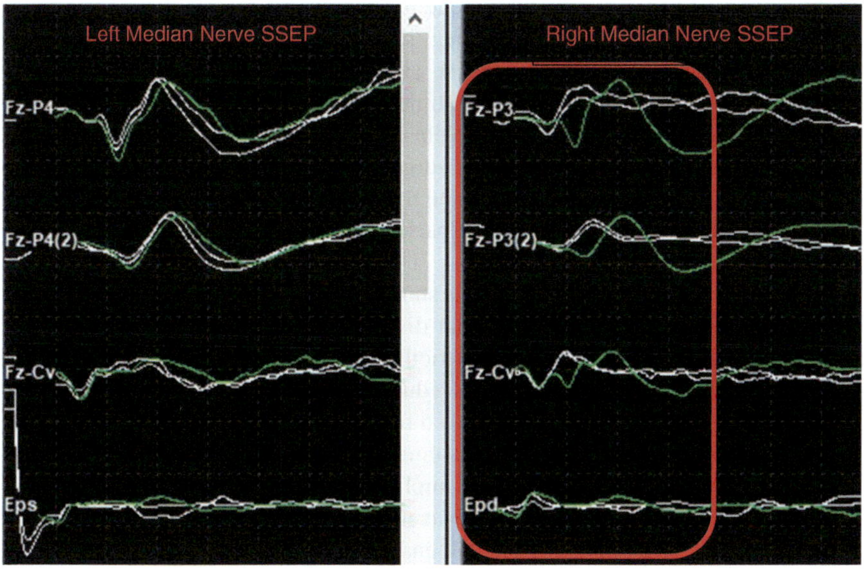

Fig. 8.3 Upper extremity SSEP data from a cardiac procedure showing the effects of a Left MCA occlusion (M1) on the cortically generated N20/P30 responses from the right median nerve. The baseline (green) shows data from the beginning of the procedure, and the two white traces show the data during the large vessel occlusion stroke. Note that the N9 (Erb's point) data remains unchanged, as does the brainstem generated N13. After the complete loss of the N20/P30, a far-field N13 can be seen from the Fz-P3 channels. This brainstem-generated response can mimic a cortical waveform in morphology, but marking the latency reveals that it is too early, and an ominous indicator of severe cortical dysfunction

surgeries depending on what cervical spine level is being operated on. Also, ulnar nerve SSEP monitoring is more sensitive in identifying position-related SSEP changes that can occur either from ulnar nerve compression around the elbow and/or stretch injury to the brachial plexus lower trunk from abnormal positioning. Placement of the cathode for posterior tibial nerve stimulation should be between the medial malleolus and the Achilles tendon with the anode 3 cm distal to the cathode. Alternatively, the peroneal nerve can be stimulated at the fibular head or the tibial nerve can be stimulated in the popliteal fossa. After stimulation, SSEPs are recorded from multiple locations along the sensory pathway. These locations can vary with both subcortical and cortical recording sites.

Certain stimulus parameters allow for accurate and consistent measurement. The stimuli should be constant-current rectangular pulses of 0.2–0.3 ms. [9] Supramaximal signal intensity is different for each patient and is estimated as 2 times motor or 3 times sensory threshold. Supramaximal intensity level is recommended for peripheral nerves, with the exception of proximal nerves at the knee, to avoid fluctuating stimulus to potential propagation and to avoid false alarms due to amplitude changes. In the unparalyzed patient, supramaximal intensity stimulation at the knee may become problematic due to vigorous muscle contractions causing compartment syndrome in the lower leg, although more evidence is necessary to definitively identify SSEP as the cause [15, 17]. However, with neuromuscular blockade, the proximal supramaximal stimulation at knee does not pose any problem. Some evidence suggests this problem can be avoided by waiting to inflate the lower leg pressure cuffs until after the surgery has been completed [17]. Stimulus frequency also depends on the patient and the requirements of the procedure. Faster frequencies allow for more timely feedback but diminish cortical recording amplitude, potentially reducing effectiveness. The recommended optimal frequency is between 4.7 and 5.1 Hz, but ideally this should be adjusted to the individual procedure [13]. Importantly, frequencies that divide evenly into 50 or 60 can produce time-locked artifacts and should be strictly avoided. Interleaving, or alternating stimuli, between all four limbs can reduce the time for monitoring by 50%. Unfortunately, this time cannot be reduced further since there needs to be a decrease in frequency to accommodate all the stimuli; however, a benefit of the lower frequency is improved cortical recording amplitude.

Output of SSEP monitoring is in waveforms that represent the summation of multiple evoked potentials. The recommended number of trials to be averaged varies widely from 300 to 2000 trials, with most systems using 300–500 trials. As the number of trials increases, the time it takes to record increases much more than background noise is reduced. For instance, going from 300 to 1500 samples takes 5 times as long and only reduces the noise by a factor of 2.24. Noise reduction is equal to the square root of the factor of increased number of trials (in this case 5) [5]. Signal to noise ratio and the importance of a rapid alert to the surgeon for a particular surgery ultimately decide the number of trials that should be averaged.

Like stimulation, recording is also done with electrodes. Recording locations are variable, with options for both the upper and lower limb. For the upper limb, the peripheral recording electrode should be at the cubital fossa. The cortical recording is most commonly at the contralateral centroparietal with reference to the midline centroparietal (CPc-CPz) area. Other options include contralateral centroparietal with reference to ipsilateral centroparietal (CPc-CPi) or contralateral centroparietal with reference to the midline frontal area (CPc-Fz). For the lower limb, the peripheral recording electrode should be at the popliteal fossa. The primary cortical recording is midline centroparietal with reference to contralateral centroparietal (CPz-CPc). Other options include midline central with reference to contralateral centroparietal (Cz-CPc), midline parietal with reference to midline centroparietal (Pz-CPz), ipsilateral intermediate centroparietal with reference to contralateral centroparietal (iCPi-CPc), ipsilateral centroparietal with reference to contralateral centroparietal (Cpi-CPc), or midline central with reference to midline parietal (Cz-Pz). Patients with non-decussation should have the same peripheral recording sites and flipped ipsilateral and contralateral recording sites. For instance, the best cortical recording site from upper limb stimulation for a patient with non-decussation is ipsilateral centroparietal with reference to midline centroparietal (Cpi-CPz) [9]. Combining multiple pertinent recording sites into a montage in different channels may allow for more accurate and precise interpretation of the evoked potentials.

Warning Criteria

Classical warning criteria for SSEP monitoring is 50% reduction in peak amplitude and > 10% increase in latency from baseline [18, 19]. These criteria, developed in the 1970s, emphasized the impact of change in latency; however, we now consider amplitude change more diagnostic. Intraoperative pathologic processes mostly result in amplitude reduction while more chronic conditions such as demyelination have a greater effect on latency. Multiple studies corroborate the validity of these criteria [20, 21]. It is important to consider confounding factors when the warning threshold is reached. To account for other causes of amplitude or latency changes, peripheral recording sites or contralateral SSEPs should be used as controls. Factors such as anesthesia, hypothermia, edema, or changes in systemic blood flow may alter SSEPs without indicating the need for surgical intervention. Focal amplitude reductions can also result from nonsurgical causes like limb positioning. Despite not directly resulting from the surgery, the surgeon should still be informed in some cases so underlying issues may be addressed. Aside from confounding factors, other considerations need to be made for the warning criteria. Drift is the progressive change in amplitude over time and may affect the efficacy of the warning criteria. Downward drift to more than 50% of baseline amplitude can be noted without any obvious insult or pathology in up to 20% of scoliosis surgeries [22, 23]. Also, upward drift can reduce the sensitivity of the warning criteria because the amplitude fails to fall below 50% of baseline despite a noticeable decrease from the previous recording. In practice, drift should be accounted for and a less stringent reliance on the traditional warning criteria may allow for more accurate interpretation of the recording [9]. One recommendation for adaptive criterion is obvious reduction in amplitude from the previous values exceeding variability especially when sudden and focal. This recommendation has been demonstrated to reduce the likelihood of incorrect results compared to the traditional criteria. Additionally, the changes must be reproducible for an alarm to be given. This accounts for transient response variability and reduces unnecessary surgical interruptions.

Considerations

Anesthesia

Anesthetic agents and muscle relaxants are important to consider since SSEPs are being recorded intraoperatively. Anesthetic agents have the greatest effect on cortically generated responses and only minor effects on subcortical or peripheral responses. These effects are dose-related, vary by individual, and vary by type of anesthetic. Anesthetic lipid solubility and therefore potency correlate with the effect on SSEPs. These effects most commonly involve decreased amplitude and increased latency. Halogenated agents are particularly potent in the cortex, have some effect on the subcortical responses, and little effect on the peripheral responses. Of the halogenated inhaled anesthetics, enflurane and halothane are least potent, while isoflurane is most potent. In procedures where cortical SSEP monitoring is critical, these agents should be restricted or avoided entirely. For subcortical and peripheral monitoring, low doses (< 0.5 MAC) could be viable as anesthetics. Propofol and opioid total intravenous anesthesia (TIVA) are the recommended anesthetics because of minimal SSEP depression and higher signal to noise ratio. Benzodiazepines, ketamine, or etomidate also may be acceptable alternatives. Unlike anesthetics, muscle relaxants can be beneficial for SSEP monitoring by reducing the interference from muscle groups near the recording electrodes. Additional relaxant can be useful in cases with excessive myogenic artifact [5].

Blood Pressure and Temperature

Blood pressure determines neural tissue perfusion. Decreased perfusion can result in decreased tissue functioning, affecting SSEPs. Cortical SSEPs begin to change when cerebral blood flow drops below 18 ml/100 g/min, resulting in amplitude decrease and latency increase. At cortical blood flow of less than 15 ml/100 g/min, ischemia results in a complete loss of cortical SSEPs [24–26]. This threshold is for tissue function and just above the perfusion threshold for permanent neurologic damage, serving as a warning sign for dangerously low blood pressure. The effect of blood pressure on SSEPs varies by individual; however, systolic pressure above 80 mm is generally sufficient for stable SSEPs [27]. Much of the variability is determined by the patient's normal blood pressure in the outpatient setting. Peripheral and subcortical SSEPs are less affected by changes in blood pressure. Body temperature can also affect SSEPs. Hypothermia tends to prolong latency and can even reduce scalp SSEP amplitude if severe [28].

Efficacy

The American Society of Neurophysiological monitoring positional statement on intraoperative monitoring of SSEPs to prevent postoperative neurologic deficits is strongly in favor, supported by Class II and III, strong Type A recommendation. SSEP works most effectively as a continuously run modality that captures data during nearly every minute of time spent in between surgical incision and closure. This intraoperative neuromonitoring modality (IONM) allows for timely therapeutic interventions to impending iatrogenic injury related to surgical maneuvers that cause time-dependent damage such as compression, traction, and ischemia. Some injuries, however, are irreversible and others may need more rapid identification and intervention than available. In these cases, SSEP still offers utility by helping the surgeon gauge the severity of the situation and take appropriate recourse. Additionally, preservation of SSEPs can serve as a surrogate for overall spinal cord integrity, but damage can occur in other regions without impacting the somatosensory pathway. Damage to the ventral portion of the spinal cord may impact motor function without SSEP deterioration, so MEPs should be monitored simultaneously [3, 29, 30].

Limitations

As is true with any IONM modality, SSEP monitoring has limitations, the most notable of which is that it is a poor measure of nerve root integrity. This is due to the fact that multiple sensory nerve roots contribute to each of the peripheral nerves being stimulated to generate an SSEP. As mentioned, injury to the spinal cord may not impact the dorsal column, resulting in injury without changes in SSEPs. Alternatively, SSEP changes can occur after an irreversible injury resulting in post-operative neurologic deficits. Sometimes this occurs due to the nature of the injury and other times is due to a delay before the intervention. Also, SSEPs are less sensitive than MEPs at detecting spinal cord ischemia since white matter requires less blood flow than gray matter [31]. This can be useful for determining injury mechanism as abrupt SSEP deterioration is more likely a result of compression or another pathologic process rather than ischemia. Other monitoring techniques should be used in conjunction with SSEP monitoring when indicated to fully minimize the risk of an adverse event.

References

1. Larson SJ, Sances A, Christenson PC. Evoked somatosensory potentials in man. Arch Neurol. 1966;15(1):88–93. https://doi.org/10.1001/archneur.1966.00470130092010.
2. MacEwen GD, Bunnell WP, Sriram K. Acute neurological complications in the treatment of scoliosis. A report of the Scoliosis Research Society. J Bone Jt Surg - Ser A. 1975;57(3):404–8. https://doi.org/10.2106/00004623-197557030-00020.
3. Nuwer MR, Dawson EG, Carlson LG, Kanim LEA, Sherman JE. Somatosensory evoked potential spinal cord monitoring reduces neurologic deficits after scoliosis surgery: results of a large multicenter survey. Electroencephalogr Clin Neurophysiol Evoked Potentials. 1995. https://doi.org/10.1016/0013-4694(94)00235-D.
4. Coe JD, Arlet V, Donaldson W, et al. Complications in spinal fusion for adolescent idiopathic scoliosis in the new millennium. A report of the Scoliosis Research Society Morbidity and Mortality Committee. *Spine (Phila Pa 1976)*. 2006;31(3):345–9. https://doi.org/10.1097/01.brs.0000197188.76369.13.
5. ACNS. Guidline 11B: Recommended standards for intraoperative monitoring of somatosensory evoked potentials. Am Clin Neuophysiol Soc Guidel. 2009.
6. Guideline eleven: guidelines for intraoperative monitoring of sensory evoked potentials. J Clin Neurophysiol. 1994;11(1):77–87. https://doi.org/10.1097/00004691-199401000-00012.
7. Stecker MM, Patterson T, Netherton BL. Mechanisms of electrode induced injury. Part 1: theory. Neurodiagn J. 2006;46(4):315–42. https://doi.org/10.1080/1086508x.2006.11079592.
8. Netherton BL, Stecker MM, Patterson T. Mechanisms of electrode induced injury. Part 3: practical concepts and avoidance. Neurodiagnostic J. 2007;47

9. MacDonald DB, Dong C, Quatrale R, et al. Recommendations of the International Society of Intraoperative Neurophysiology for intraoperative somatosensory evoked potentials. Clin Neurophysiol. 2019;130(1):161–79. https://doi.org/10.1016/j.clinph.2018.10.008.
10. Patterson T, Stecker MM, Netherton BL. Mechanisms of electrode induced injury. Part 2: clinical experience. Neurodiagn J. 2007;47(2):93–113. https://doi.org/10.1080/1086508x.2007.11079617.
11. International organisation of societies for electrophysiological technology (OSET): guidelines for performing Eeg and evoked potential monitoring during surgery. Am J Electroneurodiagnostic Technol. 1999;39(4):257–77. https://doi.org/10.1080/1086508x.1999.11079270.
12. Celesia GG, Allison T, Bodis-Wollner I, et al. American electroencephalographic society guidelines for intraoperative monitoring of sensory evoked potentials. J Clin Neurophysiol. 1987;4(4):397–416. https://doi.org/10.1097/00004691-198710000-00005.
13. Nuwer MR, Packwood JW. Somatosensory evoked potential monitoring with scalp and cervical recording. Handb Clin Neurophysiol. 2008;8(C):180–9. https://doi.org/10.1016/S1567-4231(07)08011-2.
14. Vulliemoz S, Raineteau O, Jabaudon D. Reaching beyond the midline: why are human brains cross wired? Lancet Neurol. 2005;4(2):87–99. https://doi.org/10.1016/S1474-4422(05)00990-7.
15. MacDonald DB, Streletz LJ, Al-Zayed Z, Abdool S, Stigsby B. Intraoperative neurophysiologic discovery of uncrossed sensory and motor pathways in a patient with horizontal gaze palsy and scoliosis. Clin Neurophysiol. 2004;115(3):576–82. https://doi.org/10.1016/j.clinph.2003.10.029.
16. Wee AS, Leis AA, Kuhn AR, Gilbert RW. Anodal block: Can this occur during routine nerve conduction studies? Electromyogr Clin Neurophysiol. 2000;40(7):387–91.
17. Divani KG, O'Brien A, Molloy S, Trivedi J, Cowan J, Gibson A. A multicentre retrospective review of muscle necrosis of the leg following spinal surgery with motor evoked potential monitoring: a cause for concern? Eur Spine J. 2016;25(3):801–6. https://doi.org/10.1007/s00586-015-4063-2.
18. York DH, Chabot RJ, Gaines RW. Response variability of somatosensory evoked potentials during scoliosis surgery. Spine (Phila Pa 1976). 1987;12(9):864–76. https://doi.org/10.1097/00007632-198711000-00007.
19. Brown RH, Nash CL, Berilla JA, Amaddio MD. Cortical evoked potential monitoring: a system for intraoperative monitoring of spinal cord function. Spine (Phila Pa 1976). 1984;9(3):256–61. https://doi.org/10.1097/00007632-198404000-00006.
20. Wiedemayer H, Fauser B, Sandalcioglu IE, Schäfer H, Stolke D. The impact of neurophysiological intraoperative monitoring on surgical decisions: a critical analysis of 423 cases. J Neurosurg. 2002;96(2):255–62. https://doi.org/10.3171/jns.2002.96.2.0255.
21. More RC, Nuwer MR, Dawson EG. Cortical Evoked Potential Monitoring During Spinal Surgery. J Spinal Disord. 1988;1(1):75–80. https://doi.org/10.1097/00002517-198801000-00010.
22. MacDonald DB, Al Zayed Z, Al Saddigi A. Four-limb muscle motor evoked potential and optimized somatosensory evoked potential monitoring with decussation assessment: Results in 206 thoracolumbar spine surgeries. In: European Spine Journal. Vol 16. ; 2007. https://doi.org/10.1007/s00586-007-0426-7.
23. MacDonald DB, Al Zayed Z, Khoudeir I, Stigsby B. Monitoring scoliosis surgery with combined multiple pulse transcranial electric motor and cortical somatosensory-evoked potentials from the lower and upper extremities. Spine (Phila Pa 1976). 2003;28(2):194–203. https://doi.org/10.1097/00007632-200301150-00018.
24. Branston NM, Symon L. Cortical EP, blood flow and potassium changes in experimental ischaemia. In: Evoked Potentials. ; 1980:527–30. https://doi.org/10.1007/978-94-011-6645-4_61.
25. Nuwer MR. Intraoperative electroencephalography. J Clin Neurophysiol. 1993;10(4):437–444. https://doi.org/10.1097/00004691-199310000-00005.
26. Prior PF. Eeg monitoring and evoked potentials in brain ischaemia. Br J Anaesth. 1985;57(1):63–81. https://doi.org/10.1093/bja/57.1.63.

27. Cui H, Luk KDK, Hu Y. Effects of physiological parameters on intraoperative somatosensory-evoked potential monitoring: Results of a multifactor analysis. Med Sci Monit. 2009;15(5).
28. Markand ON, Warren C, Mallik GS, King RD, Brown JW, Mahomed Y. Effects of hypothermia on short latency somatosensory evoked potentials in humans. Electroencephalogr Clin Neurophysiol Evoked Potentials. 1990;77(6):416–24. https://doi.org/10.1016/0168-5597(90)90002-U.
29. Ben-David B, Haller G, Taylor P. Anterior spinal fusion complicated by paraplegia: A case report of a false-negative somatosensory-evoked potential. Spine (Phila Pa 1976). 1987;12(6). https://doi.org/10.1097/00007632-198707000-00005.
30. Minahan RE, Sepkuty JP, Lesser RP, Sponseller PD, Kostuik JP. Anterior spinal cord injury with preserved neurogenic "motor" evoked potentials. Clin Neurophysiol. 2001;112(8):1442–50. https://doi.org/10.1016/S1388-2457(01)00567-3.
31. Marcus ML, Heistad DD, Ehrhardt JC, Abboud FM. Regulation of total and regional spinal cord blood flow. Circ Res. 1977;41(1):128–34. https://doi.org/10.1161/01.RES.41.1.128.

Chapter 9
Motor Evoked Potential

Carla Ferreira and Silvia Mazzali Verst

Abbreviations

BAEP	Brainstem auditory evoked potential
CBT	Corticobulbar tract
COR	Class of recommendation
CR	Corona radiata
CST	Corticospinal tract
CMAP	Compound motor unit action potential
DCS	Direct cortical stimulation
EEG	Electroencephalogram
EPSP	Excitatory postsynaptic potential
IOM	Intraoperative neurophysiologic monitoring
ISI	Interstimulus interval
LMN	Lower motor neurons
LOE	Level of evidence
MEP	Motor evoked potentials
MU	Motor unit
mMEP	Muscle motor evoked potentials
TES	Transcranial electrical stimulation
UMN	Upper motor neurons
SSEP	Somatosensory evoked potential

C. Ferreira (✉)
Clinical Hospital of the Federal University of Minas Gerais, Belo Horizonte, MG, Brazil
e-mail: carla.jferreira@ebserh.gov.br

S. M. Verst
Instituto de Ensino e Pesquisa (Research and Educational Institute) of Sírio Libanês Hospital, São Paulo, Brazil

Brain Spine Neurofisiologia, Jundiaí, SP, Brazil

S. M. Verst et al. (eds.), *Intraoperative Monitoring*,
https://doi.org/10.1007/978-3-030-95730-8_9

Anatomic Review

Good knowledge about the anatomy and physiology of the motor system is crucial in the proper execution of the MEP. Its central components begin in the primary motor cortex (Brodmann area 4), usually located in the precentral gyrus, which works in association with other motor areas, including the premotor cortex, the supplementary motor area, posterior parietal cortex, somatosensory cortex, and several subcortical brain regions, to plan and execute movements. Damage to the primary motor cortex will result in permanent weakness. While lesions of the associated areas may also cause a motor disturbance, they tend to be transient as the remaining cortices can take over the lost function [1].

The connection between the motor cortex and motor neurons in the spine/brainstem is made by the pyramidal tract that is composed of the descending axons of the Betz cells, also known as upper motor neurons (UNM), which are part of the corticospinal tract (CST) and part of the corticobulbar tract (CBT) [2]. These descending axons in the corona radiata (CR) progressively converge at the posterior limb and genu of the internal capsule (IC) and continue their path inferiorly through the cerebral peduncle, the base of the pons, and medulla pyramids. Here, most of the CST fibers (80 to 90%) cross the midline constituting the pyramidal decussation and follow as lateral corticospinal tract or, in a smaller proportion, keep uncrossed as the anterior or lateral corticospinal tract. There are significant individual variations. The CST fibers descend along the spinal cord reaching the lower motor neurons (LMNs), whose cell body is located in the ventral gray matter of the spinal cord. A small percentage connects mono synaptically, whereas the majority terminate in propriospinal interneurons [3, 4]. In its turns, the CBT axons diverge from the pyramidal tract at the brainstem by synapse with the contralateral and ipsilateral motor nucleus of the cranial nerves via interneurons or directly (more details in Chap. 21).

Each of these levels is somatotopically organized. At the precentral gyrus, the foot and leg areas are located in the medial surface of the hemisphere, within the interhemispheric fissure. Towards the middle convexity, the thigh, trunk, arm, and forearm are represented, respectively. Further down, there are areas of the hand, face, and mouth; and lastly, next to the Sylvian fissure, it is the area of the tongue and pharynx (Fig. 9.1) [3]. The size of the representation is proportional to its functional importance, being much larger for distal limbs and face. A similar sequence can be seen at caudal levels where the pharyngeal, tongue, and facial muscles are at the genu and medial portion of the cerebral peduncle, distal/ proximal superior limb, trunk, and proximal/ distal inferior limb are represented in the anteroposterior direction of the posterior limb of the IC and mediolateral direction of the cerebral peduncle (Figs. 9.2 and 9.3).

Besides the corticospinal fibers, other indirect motor pathways travel to synapses with the LMNs mostly indirectly by interneurons, including the rubrospinal, reticulospinal, vestibulospinal, and tectospinal tracts. In addition, there are intrinsic spinal cord motor control systems like inputs from inhibitory interneurons and sensory Ia

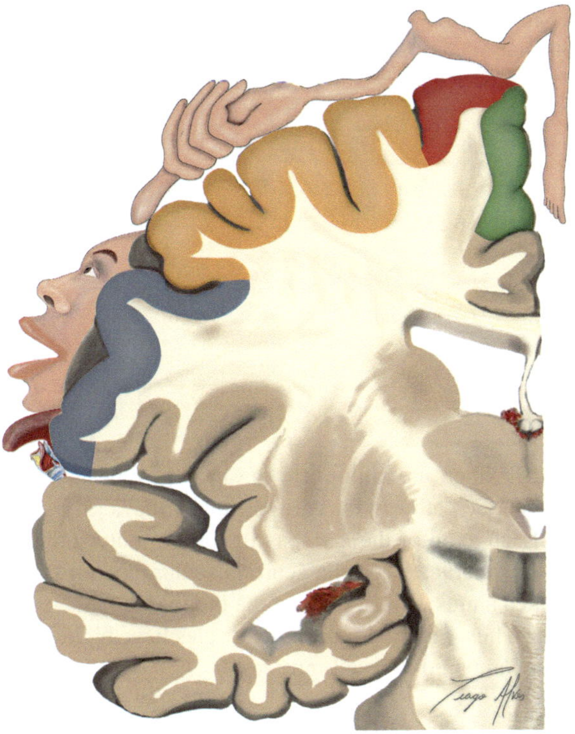

Fig. 9.1 Cortical somatotopic representation of the Penfield motor homunculus

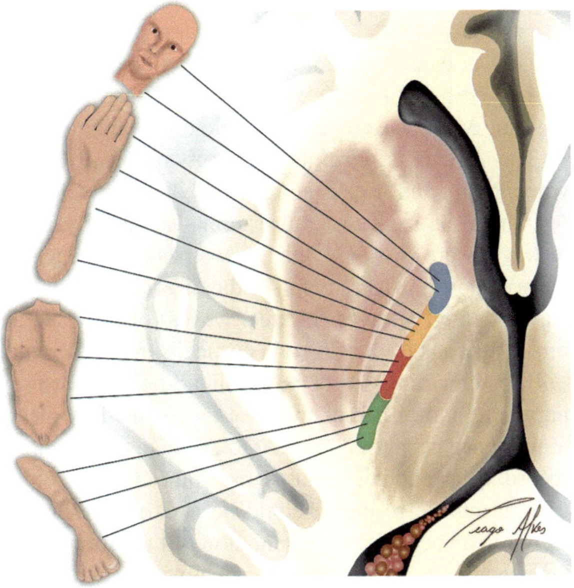

Fig. 9.2 Motor somatotopic representation at the level of the internal capsule

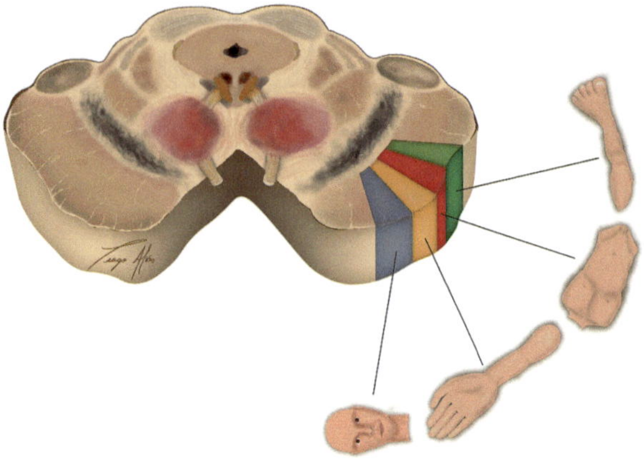

Fig. 9.3 Motor somatotopic representation at the level of the cerebral peduncle

and Ib fibers in addition to the propriospinal neurons, which provide an indirect disynaptic pathway for corticospinal volleys [5, 6].

Each axon of the LMNs will form a motor unit (MU) that includes the muscle fibers innervated and the neuromuscular junctions interposed. The more finely controlled a muscle is, the lesser the number of muscle fibers innervated by each motor unit. Thus, the proximal limb muscles have higher muscle fibers number per motor unit compared to distal muscles.

Brief Historical Review and Physiological Basis

The use of electrical stimulation by Penfield founded intraoperative brain mapping in the first half of the twenty century. However, more than fifty years would pass until the MEPs have become viable to be reliably used for IOM [4, 7–11].

The first neurophysiological registration of an MEP dates back to the 1950s when Patton and Amassian recorded direct traveling waves from the CST stimulating with a single electric pulse applied at the monkey's motor cortex [12]. Two types of waves were observed: the first was a short-latency response called D-wave (direct wave), interpreted as a result of the direct activation of the CST, followed by a set of waves termed I-waves (indirect waves), interpreted as trans-synaptic activation of motor neurons of the CST via cortical synaptic circuits.

The remaining motor path, including the lower spinal cord, nerve roots, and peripheral motor nerves, was not represented by these waves. Thus, different techniques have been tried in order to evaluate them. Stimulation of the spinal cord with recording at another level of the spine, nerves, or muscles was attempted. Even though muscle response could be evoked by spine stimulation, these recordings were not an accurate representation of the motor path since spinal cord stimulation activates other tracts in a non-selectively way, including antidromic volleys in the dorsal column ending at collateral synapses on LMNs [13–15].

Since the 1980s, we can elicit muscle response after transcranial stimulation both electrically and magnetically in conscious humans [11, 16]. However, due to the multi-synaptic nature of these evoked responses, these potentials did not persist under general anesthesia. Then, in 1993, Taniguchi broke this barrier by using a high-frequency train of 3–5 electric pulses with an inter-pulse interval of 2–4 ms applied directly to the human motor cortex, which evoked a muscle MEP (mMEP) intraoperatively in anesthetized patients. This sequence of stimulus in such a short interval seems to allow the summation of excitatory postsynaptic potential (EPSP) of the descendent volleys, mostly D-waves but probably also some I-waves, thus enabling the LMNs to fire [10].

Nowadays, MEP is widely used in the intraoperative practice at different types of surgeries threatening the motor system, either by transcranial electrical stimulation (TES) or by direct cortical stimulation (DCS). The muscle MEP is more versatile and most broadly employed, although the D-waves also have a specific but crucial role in some situations.

D-Waves

As a result of direct and selective activation of the axons of the CST, D-waves are a pure representation of the lateral system at the spinal cord. It comprises axons from the CST, responsible for sophisticated motor control of fine movements of the distal limbs and rubrospinal tract [3]. A single-pulse stimulus is applied over the motor cortex, while the descending volley of the CST is recorded over the spinal cord. I-waves are occasionally obtained in anesthetized patients; however, they are not stable enough to be followable. As the intensity of the stimulus increases, the greater the number of axons is recruited, increasing the amplitude of the registered potential until the maximum amount of CST is activated and the response reaches a point of stability without variation inter trials at the suprathreshold stimulation. An inverse relationship is also observed between the latency and the intensity of the stimulus. The greater the stimulus applied, the shorter the response latency, which can also bifurcate or even trifurcate into earlier components. Thus, it seems that higher intensities activate the CST deeper, and these shorter latencies and earlier components are nothing more than representations of activation at the level of the IC or brainstem [17–19].

The D-wave amplitude is also dependent on the pool of CST axons at the record level. Thus, the D-wave is bigger at cervical levels, and it gets smaller and smaller as the recording electrode goes down in the craniocaudal direction until it is no longer obtained generally around the T10 level [5, 20, 21].

Muscle MEP

Unlike the D-wave, the mMEP results from the activation of a multi-synaptic path mainly mediated by the propriospinal interneurons. This characteristic is of cornerstone importance in understanding the role of mMEP during intramedullary spinal cord tumor resection (more details in Chap. 28). The excitability of the interneurons and alpha motor neurons results from inhibitory and facilitatory impulses from supraspinal sources, such as rubrospinal, reticulospinal, and vestibulospinal tracts. Intraspinal propriospinal tracts are involved in reflexes, posture, and locomotor activity. They interconnect up to six spinal segments (short) and cervical and lumbar enlargements (long) [22]. Stimulation of the somatosensory cortex can also elicit mMEP, but it requires higher intensity.

Under anesthesia, mMEP only will be obtained efficiently if a short train at high frequency is used, thus allowing a temporal and spatial summation of LMN EPSPs [10]. The number of MU firing at intensities near the threshold is unknown and widely variable. Higher intensities of stimulation result in increased amplitude, polyphasia, duration, and short latencies by recruiting more MU and deeper until supramaximal intensity. Nevertheless, even in supramaximal levels, considerable trial to trial variation in amplitude and morphology occurs [5, 21, 23].

Methodology

Of paramount importance, while choosing a methodology, we point out that activated CST must be rostral to the lesion. This principle is going to rule all other variables: (1) DCS or TES, (2) electrode placement, (3) stimulus parameters, and (4) recording protocol. The goal is to match the highest amplitude of compound motor unit action potential (CMUAP) with the lowest intensity, leaving room for further intensity increase during the long-lasting surgery [24].

Electrode Placement

Cortical stimulation, either by DCS or by TES, works better utilizing anodal stimuli, whereas cathodal stimuli are more efficient for subcortical stimulation. Thus the montages are designed as anode-cathode for TES and DCS and vice versa for subcortical stimulation [21, 25]. For direct cortical stimulation, a subdural strip electrode is positioned over the primary motor cortex, and one or more contact can be used as an anode and other channels on the same strip or a subdermal needle, placed in the or near the surgical field, as a cathode [21, 24].

For TES, electroencephalogram (EEG) cups, needles, and corkscrew electrodes can be used. However, the last one provides better fixation and lower impedance and

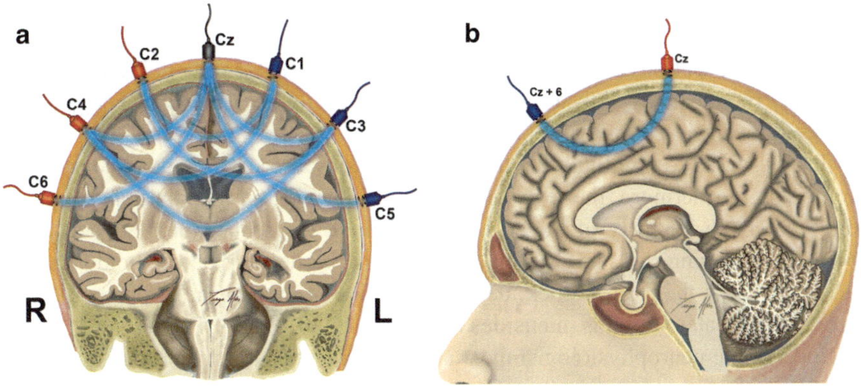

Fig. 9.4 The most used position for TES electrodes: C3, C4, C1, C2, Cz, and 6 cm anterior to Cz as well as C5 and C6, enabling multiple montages, such as C1-C2, C1-C4, C2-C3, C3-C4, C3/C4-Cz, C5/C6-Cz (**a**), and Cz-Cz + 6 cm (**b**). Right (R) and Left (L)

used to be preferred. Stimulation electrodes may be placed at the scalp in various positions, based on the 10–10 system (expanded 10–20) with the arrangement depending on the interest [26, 27]. The electrodes are most commonly placed at C3, C4, C1, C2, Cz, and 6 cm anterior to Cz, enabling multiple montages, such as C1-C2, C1-C4, C2-C3, C3-C4, C3/C4-Cz, and Cz-Cz + 6 cm (Fig. 9.4). Some have proposed a slight anterior positioning as M1, M2, M3, M4 (1cm in front of the traditional C position) [28], although there is no proven efficacy difference between the two sites (C versus M). Based on the motor homunculus distribution, the C3 and C4 positions tend to be more efficient to activate the motor path correspondent to the superior limbs at the same time that the electrodes placed at or near the middle line, namely, C1, C2, Cz, and Cz + 6 cm, preferably activate the lower limbs [20, 21, 29]. We have also suggested C5 and C6 as an interesting position to CBT due to the somatotopic organization of the cortical areas of the face and neck, allowing the use of lower stimulus intensities [30].

The montages are categorized according to their disposition on the scalp as hemispheric, interhemispheric, and midline. The hemispheric montages (C3/5-Cz, C4/6-Cz) activate the corresponding hemisphere, generating a predominantly contralateral response. These montages limit, at least in part, the depth of current penetration and allow the selective activation of upper limbs and face with low-intensity stimuli and minimal patient movement [21, 23, 29, 31]. The interhemispheric montages (C3-C4 and C1-C2) promote deeper current penetration evoking bilateral responses that include upper and lower limbs and often also sphincter and face, with lower threshold and higher amplitude contralateral to the anode [21, 23, 29, 31]. However, the interhemispheric montages are not advisable for CBT evaluation due to their potential to activate the facial nerve peripherally or supratentorial surgeries because of the high risk of bypassing the level of interest [5, 32]. The current shutting through the scalp makes C1-C2 a less efficient assembly than C3-C4, although, on the other hand, it induces less movement and may allow selective activation of the lower limbs [21, 29, 31]. Lastly, the midline montage (Cz-Cz + 6 cm) evokes symmetric leg mMEPs but is much less effective to hand and face [21, 29]. Even to selective leg responses, high intensities are often necessary because the electrical current induced occurs in an anterior-posterior direction, and this may preferentially activate neurons transynaptically since it might not evoke D waves as readily as coronal TES [33].

It is essential to highlight that activation happens already in the axon, not at the cell body. Furthermore, the level of activations depends on the stimulus intensity: the greater the intensity of the stimulus delivered, the deeper the CST activation point. So, keeping the same stimulator position, the depolarization would happen juxtacortical at the axon hillock, deeper at the IC, or even at the brainstem if progressively greater stimulus intensities are used [18–20] (Fig. 9.5).

Indeed, the neurophysiologist must always pay attention to the premise of *staying above the target* (see Fig. 9.6). For example, if the level at risk is the spinal cord, a C1-C2 or C3-C4 interhemispheric transcranial stimulation will activate the four limbs efficiently without major anatomic concerns. On the other side, if this same stimulation is used to evaluate a resection of a juxtacortical tumor, the activation will probably bypass the point of interest. Thus, it will only obtain an intraoperative mMEP registration without any predictive value, which cannot be called monitoring.

In order to avoid such pitfalls, we recommend a *topographic-physiological-guided MEP*. It is a more appropriate way to stimulate each level at risk, and the recorded response works as feedback of adequacy. Hence, we usually prefer

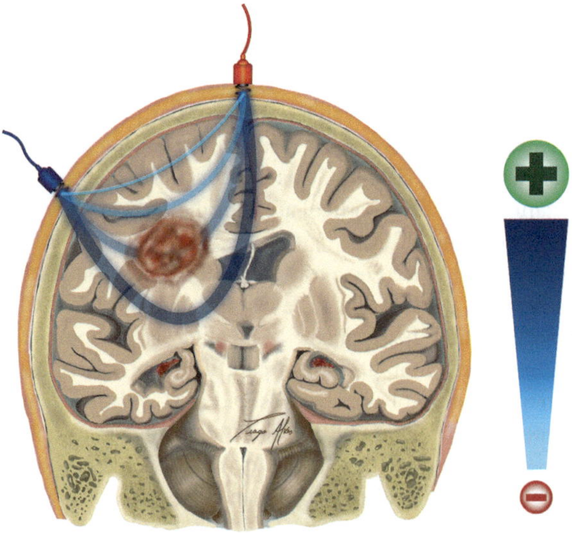

Fig. 9.5 The hemispheric montages activate the corresponding hemisphere, generating a predominantly contralateral response. These montages limit, at least in part, the depth of current penetration and allow the selective activation of upper limbs and face with low-intensity stimuli. Nevertheless, as long as the stimulus intensity increases, the stimulus loop tends to depolarize deeper levels being able to reach the IC or even the brainstem. Thus, is it crucial to stay careful in order to not allow the stimulus bypass the level of interest

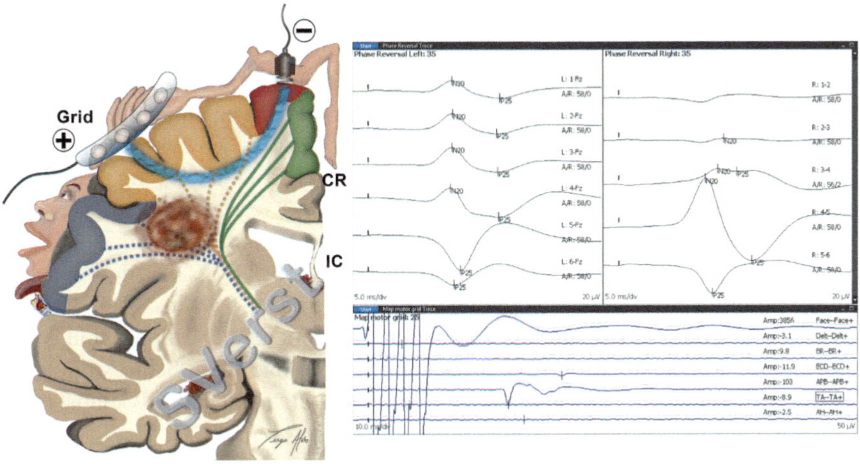

Fig. 9.6 Grid for upper limb: strip selective DCS MEP for upper extremity for lesions sitting at the level of CR. Strip position guided by phase reversal (see details about brain motor mapping technique at Chap. 14). MEP recording at contralateral *Mentalis (Face), Deltoide (Delt), Braquiorradialis (BR), Extensor digiti comunis (ECD), Abdutor pollicis brevis (APB), Tibialis anterior (TA),* and *Abductor hallucis (AH)*

Table 9.1 Reasoning between target and stimulation assembly

Target	Electrodes´ montage	Recording muscles	Notes
Corona radiata (CR)	DCS: Grid electrode Reference: Cz/ Fz or mc. If the tumor is large and separate upper and lower limb stimulation is needed, try to place the grid along the precentral gyrus and stimulate 2 different points of the grid or use 2 grids	A	Lesions in the vicinity of the convexity should always be monitored using DCS. Separate upper and lower limb mMEP should be achieved to infer stimulus is at CR
Internal capsula (CI)/ Insular tumor/ aneurysms/ anterior and media fossa approach	DCS or hemispheric TES: First option: C3 or C4-Cz for upper limbs and Cz-Cz + 6 for lower limbs. If Cz-Cz + 6 fails, try Cz-C4 Second option: C4-C1 and C3-C2	A and B	It is acceptable to get mMEP in all contralateral muscles, provided that ipsilateral mMEPs are absent. In this situation, only one-side IC is being activated
Infratentorial	Interhemispheric C1-C2 or C3-C4	C	

Recording muscles: (A) contralateral: Face, Deltoide, forearm flexor and extensor, *Abductor digiti minimi, Tibialis anterior and abductor hallucis. (AH)*; (B) ipsilateral: *Abductor digiti minimi, and Abductor halluces*; (C) bilateral *Abductor digiti minimi, Tibialis anterior, and abductor hallucis*

hemispheric stimulus for separate upper and lower limb mMEP for supratentorial approaches and interhemispheric assembly for infratentorial and spinal surgeries (Table 9.1). The supratentorial protocol is divided into cortical and CR versus IC. The former is always performed using DCS. So, lower intensities are necessary, and the activation usually happens juxtacortical, generating response in the muscle group represented in the cortex below the active grid (Fig. 9.6). If the IC is treated as surgeries for approaching an insular tumor or clipping an internal carotid or middle cerebral arteries aneurysm, the DCS is still recommended, although not always feasible, because often the primary motor cortex is not exposed by the craniotomy. In such situations, it is also possible to resort to TES stimulation as long as it stimulates upper or lower limbs selectively.

To ensure selective stimulation during the IC-target protocol, it is mandatory to record bilaterally (four limbs). The reasoning is based on the presence or absence of mMEP at the extremities. Since the first CST convergence happens at IC, we suppose that activation of IC results in simultaneous contralateral upper and lower mMEP but no ipsilateral mMEP. It means that only one IC is being stimulated. Eliciting simultaneous ipsilateral mMEP represents activation below IC, most probably by activating bilateral CST at the brainstem (Fig. 9.7).

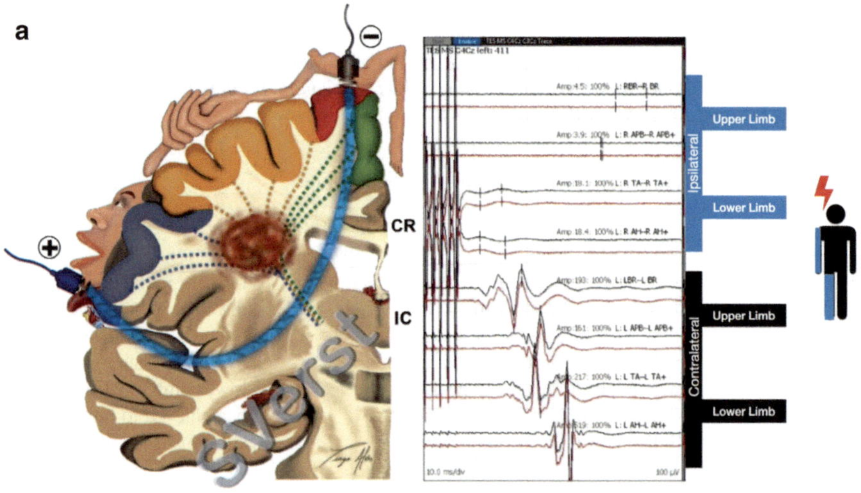

Fig. 9.7 Topographic-guided MEP protocol: bilateral muscle recordings and hemispheric stimulation in order to reach the level above the target. Recording at contralateral *Mentalis (Face), Deltoide (Delt), Braquiorradialis (BR), Extensor digiti comunis (ECD), Abdutor pollicis brevis (APB), Tibialis anterior (TA),* and *Abductor hallucis (AH)* in addition to *ipsilateral to stimulation Abdutor digiti minimi (ADMc)* and *Abductor hallucis (AHc)* or *BR, APB, TA, and AH bilateral.* (**a**) At lower intensity, mMEPs only from contralateral upper limb and face are recorded: probable stimulation site: CR, above the IC. Partial CR activation represented by dashed lines. (**b**) At median intensity, only mMEPs from contralateral upper and lower limb are recorded. There is mMEP response at the ipsilateral body. Probable stimulation site: IC. (**c**) At higher C3-Cz intensity stimulation, recordings of mMEP from contralateral upper and lower limbs + ipsilateral upper limb are present. Probable stimulation site: at the level of bilateral IC, or at the brainstem or below, where bilateral CSTs are being activated. ADM: *adductor digiti minimi*

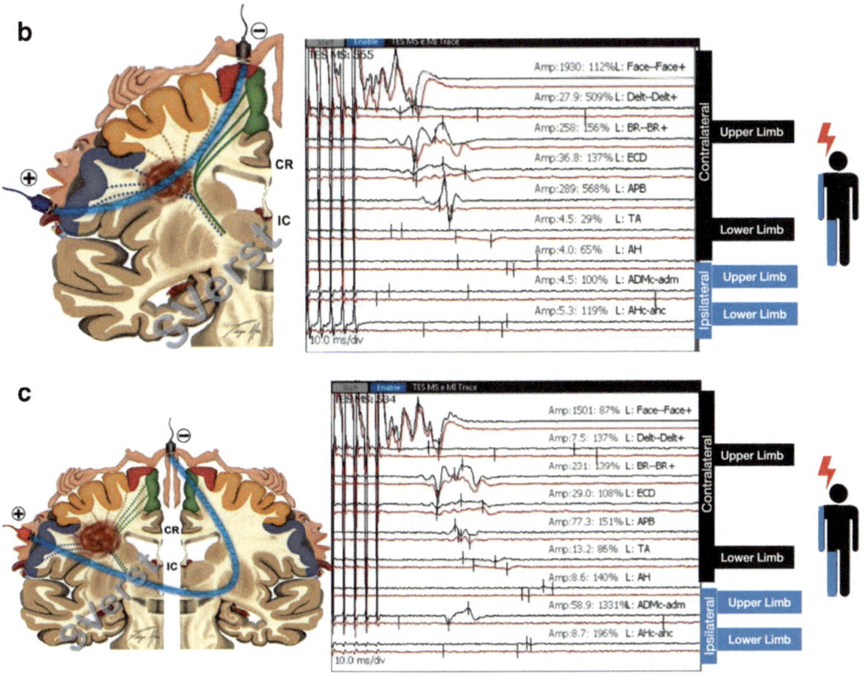

Fig. 9.7 (continued)

The biggest challenge is to achieve separate recordings for lower limbs. It relies on the sparse UMN population and depth of the interhemispheric sulcus. If the lesion is at CR, the grid electrode should be placed in the vicinity of the interhemispheric sulcus or slid inside the sulcus (Fig. 9.8). For lower limb mMEP activation nearby IC, Cz-Cz + 6 cm is effective in 68% [29]. Alternatively, Cz-C4 or C3, using Cz as the anode in the vertex and the cathode in the convexity, is sometimes effective to obtain a selective response of the lower limbs, although it often promotes deeper and less selective activation [5]. Most often, both lower limb mMEPs are recorded simultaneously due to the proximity of bilateral cortices. Yet, it does not compromise topographic-guided MEP (Fig. 9.9).

A combination of two electrodes in each hemisphere in parallel, called quadripolar (C1/M3 - C2/M4 or C3-M1/C4-M2), has recently been proposed by Schwartz and Husain [34]. The concept is expanding the current network to the same applied stimulation since the active electrodes are simultaneously positioned over the arm and leg area. The linked quadripolar method showed the most robust mMEP response in the foot, and the stimulation intensity was lower on average than any of the standard bipolar montages [34]. Some authors have also reported the same advantages to external anal sphincter MEPs with this electrode configuration [24].

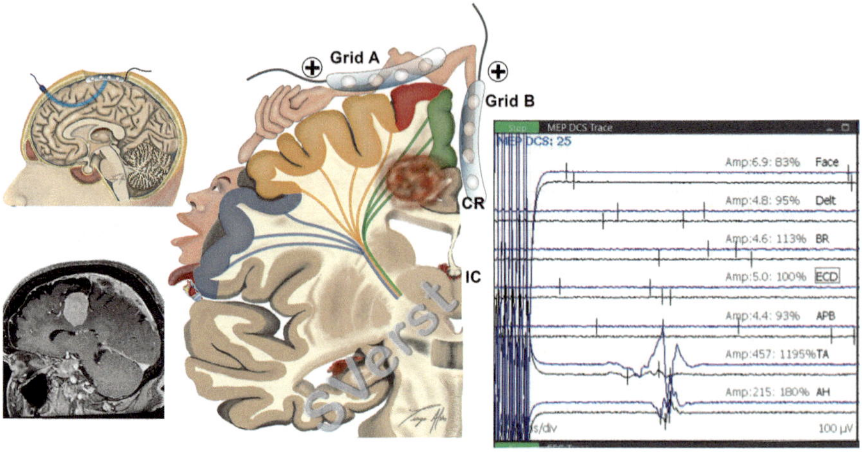

Fig. 9.8 Grid for lower limb: selective DCS MEP for lower extremity for lesions sitting at the level of CR: suggested positions for grid electrode: (A) or (B). Recording at contralateral *Mentalis (Face), Deltoide (Delt), Braquiorradialis (BR), Extensor digiti comunis (ECD), Abdutor pollicis brevis(APB), Tibialis anterior (TA),* and *Abductor hallucis (AH)*

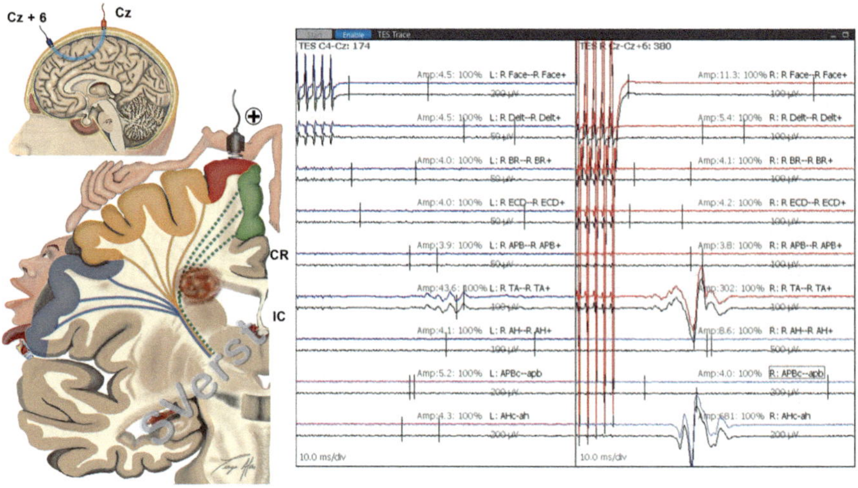

Fig. 9.9 Cz-Cz + 6: woman, 62 y.o., re-operation of glioma at right caudate nucleus. MEP protocol: C4-Cz for upper mMEP and Cz-Cz + 6 for lower limb mMEP. Recording at contralateral *Mentalis (Face), Deltoide (Delt), Braquiorradialis (BR), Extensor digiti comunis (ECD), Abdutor pollicis brevis (APB), Tibialis anterior (TA),* and *Abductor hallucis (AH)* in addition to *ipsilateral Abdutor digiti minimi (ADMc)* and *Abductor hallucis (AHc)* or *BR, APB, TA, and AH bilateral.* Stimulation Cz-Cz + 6 cm at lower intensity results in unilateral response; stimulation at higher intensity results in bilateral lower limb mMEP, without any response at upper limb, which is considered effective for topographic-guided MEP

Stimulus Parameters

When it comes to cortical stimulation, either by TES or ECD, anodal stimulation is more effective than cathodic because the dendrites on the surface of the cortex hyperpolarize under the anode, which depolarizes the descending axons of the CST, thus preferentially activating the D-waves. On the other hand, cathodic stimulation is more favorable to the depolarization of cortical interneurons, preferentially activating the I-waves. As it involves a greater number of synapses, the latter is more susceptible to anesthetic effects. Due to direct contact with the axon at the subcortical level, cathodal stimulation becomes the most effective [12, 35–38].

As pointed above, a high-frequency multipulse technique is necessary to elicit mMEP: multipulse stimulation (3 to 9 stimuli) delivered with a short interstimulus interval (ISI) 1–4 msec, duration of 0.05 to 0.5 msec, preferably at an inter-train frequency of 1 to 2 Hz. A minimum of 3 pulses is usually required to evoke mMEP. However, many patients may require a larger number of pulses, so 4 to 5 pulses seem to be a good starting point; thenceforth, this number can be adjusted as needed, with some practitioners using up to 9 pulses [5, 21, 24, 39]. The ISI is calculated by dividing 1000 by the stimulus frequency (Hz). Shorter ISI, such as 1 or 2 ms, increases the chance of subsequent pulses finding the pathway still in the relative refractory period, whereas ISI longer than 4 ms may not be favorable to the summation of the EPSPs. Therefore, ISI of 3, and especially 4 ms, generally provides the lowest motor thresholds at least for limb mMEP in patients with normal motor status under total intravenous anesthesia [20, 23, 29, 40]. For short-latency facial MEP, a 1-2 ms ISI can be helpful in separating the stimulation artefact at the same time that it brings responses with the highest amplitudes although with the simplest morphology [32]. We prefer to try the 2, 3, and 4 ms ISIs in each patient and choose the one that has worked better.

The stimulus can be delivered both as constant voltage or constant current. In the former, the stimulating current depends on the resistance, which, in its turns, can vary along with the procedure. At the constant current, the voltage fits according to the resistance to deliver the current chosen. The required intensity ranges a lot depending on age, electrode position, previous deficits, and anesthetic depth. It also depends on the other stimulus parameters. The use of a longer pulse duration has the strongest effect on the lowering of the motor threshold.

Nevertheless, the delivered charge increases proportionally by increasing the pulse duration [21, 29, 41]. Comparing slower (0.50 ms) and faster (0.05 ms) charges, there was no significant difference concerning MEP parameters (amplitude or latencies), MEP elicitability, and intraoperative MEP variability [41]. Rheobase is the smallest current value of a rectangular stimulus with pulse width considered infinite (from 250 to 1000 μs) that causes muscle contraction. Chronaxie is the smallest pulse width, also of a rectangular stimulus, but with twice the value of the rheobase, which causes muscle contraction. Short pulses save charge at the expense of a higher current whereas long pulses constrain current at the expense of a higher charge. The balance between current and charge, considered optimal, is in the pulse duration equal to the chronaxie. A pulse width of 0.2 ms has already been demonstrated to be most consistently optimal or near-optimal [21, 29, 40].

Sometimes, even the proper use of the pulse train technique is not enough to evoke robust muscle responses, especially in patients with previous motor pathway dysfunction or unavoidable unfavorable anesthetic regimens. In such situations, facilitation techniques may be saving. Recurrent pulse train stimulus at 1 or 2 Hz is often effective at enhancing mMEP. It has even been proposed using protocols with higher frequencies up to 5 Hz, which augmented the amplitude of the responses by about 2–3 times compared with 1 Hz. It is essential to point out that, in this same study, the facilitation effects tended to peak in the last half of the series of 10 TESs [42].

Another strategy uses the double train, which consists of applying a preconditioning stimulus before the test stimulus. The former would facilitate the action of the main stimulus by depolarizing the LMNs, thus maximizing its excitability. It is called homonymous stimulation because both conditioning and test stimuli are applied at the same site. From a practical point of view, this is done by applying a 3 to 4 pulse train as a conditioning stimulus followed by the 4–6 pulse test stimulus at specific inter-train intervals (ITI). The facilitation is optimal at short ITIs of 10 to 30 ms and longer ITIs of over 100 ms. It seems that short ITIs facilitate depolarization at the level of the LMNs, whereas the facilitation of longer ITIs is likely to be of cortical origin. It is important to be aware that there is a relatively inhibitory effect with an ITI between 30 and 100 ms [43, 44].

It is also possible to enhance the mMEP by employing a preconditioning stimulus delivered at the peripheral level, known as the heteronymous stimulus since the facilitating stimulus is performed in a different site than the test stimulus. Through it, it is possible to amplify the mMEP of a restricted muscle group corresponding to the conditioned nerve by producing a focal sensory afferent LMN facilitation. The advantage of this high spatial selectivity is that it makes possible the reduction of the TES threshold, consequently reducing a disturbing global movement of the patient in a context in which a segment is of particular interest [44, 45].

The stimulus to obtain the epidural motor evoked potential (wave D) is technically more straightforward because there is no synapse involved, and therefore it is little susceptible to anesthesia effects. A single pulse delivered through a C3-C4 montage is suitable. However, it is quite important to ensure that the stimulus intensity is sufficient to activate the CST bilaterally; otherwise, the fibers to the lower limbs or one CST side may be underrepresented. A practical manner to check which fibers are being activated is to record mMEP concomitantly, so it is possible to ensure that a given stimulus intensity is sufficient to elicit the entire path of interest. Another approach is to record separately left and right D-waves corresponding to right and left anodal TES, respectively, although it cannot be admitted that these are purely lateralized [20, 46].

Recording

The mMEP is recorded from muscles in the form of a CMUAP potential from limbs, sphincters, face, and bulbar muscles with surface, subdermal or intramuscular needle. The CMUAP tends to be more polyphasic and show a bigger amplitude when recorded with needle electrodes compared with surface recordings, although both can be considered effective [5]. Proper needling enhances the amplitude of the CMUAP and is discussed in Chap. 3. An atlas of muscle motor points is also available there.

Muscle recordings should be tailored to the procedure, taking into consideration the myotomes at risk. It is strategic to include in the protocol at least one muscle that is not at risk related to surgical manipulation. This channel works as a control, helping to differentiate between signal loss related to systemic/anesthetic changes and those related to direct neurological damage. When it comes to long paths, the distal muscle limbs would be preferred since they have optimal cortical representation in addition to subcutaneous tissue [47]. Therefore, in the upper limb, mMEPs are optimally recorded from hand muscles, as thenar eminence or abductor digiti minimi, and forearm muscles. In the lower limb, the tibialis anterior and abductor hallucis are the muscles most commonly used. Recording parameters include a sweep length of 50 to 200 msec, bandpass filter from 10–100 to 3KHz, and a sensitivity of 15 to 5.000[V/div according to the amplitude of the obtained responses. Averaging is not necessary due to the high signal-to-noise ratio [21, 23, 24, 29].

In comparison to SSEPs, brainstem auditory evoked potential (BAEP), and EEG, which are usually continually monitored throughout the procedure, TES muscle MEPs are usually acquired at certain periodic intervals due to patient movement induced by excessive muscle contraction, and thus, they are generally monitored intermittently. The use of selective montage as well as facilitation techniques are often effective in reducing the patient's movement, sometimes even allowing continuous or near-continuous stimulation without disturbing the surgeon [21, 24, 29–31].

For D-wave registration, a special bipolar recording electrode should be positioned near the spinal cord into the epidural or subdural space by the surgeon after spine exposure or percutaneously into the subarachnoid space through lumbar puncture followed by radiological confirmation of positioning in the last case. Long distances between the recording electrodes reduce in-phase cancellation, which could increase the D-wave amplitude; however, this favors the capture of more noise. Thus a 2 to 3 cm inter-electrode distance is considered appropriate. Recording parameters include a sweep length of 10 to 50 msec, bandpass filter from 0.2 to 3KHz, and a sensitivity of about 2 to 50 [V/div. Few (5 to 20) if no sweep averaging is necessary [5, 20, 21, 48].

A proximal and a distal electrode should be positioned in relation to a medullary lesion so the former can be used as a reference. In some cases, as when there are tumors or the patient has undergone to radiation, there may be a desynchronization in the conduction of CST axons at a segmental level, and the distal D-wave may not be recordable from the beginning of surgery despite large mMEP and preserved cranial D-wave [20].

Interpretation and Alarm Criteria

When a multipulse technique is applied to anesthetized patients' brains, a limited subset of the largest axons of the CST is fired. Even though only a small part of the motor path is tested, the data obtained generally is enough to predict evolution accurately. The sensitivity of mMEP for the deficit is very high in such a way that preservation of MEPs is almost never associated with motor deficits. The rare false-negative results are better explained by technical and interpretive errors of professionals poorly trained in the use of semi-automated IONM devices [21, 49, 50].

Different alarm criteria have been proposed based on changes in amplitude, latency, duration, and complexity of the potential as well as the threshold stimulus intensity. The amplitude peak-to-peak measurement is the most widely used to assess both D-waves and mMEP [51–54].

There is an intrinsic variability of the mMEP trial to trial in the absence of any neurological damage. Therefore, changes until a 50% amplitude decrease are generally meaningless for all different kinds of surgeries. An amplitude decrement greater than 50% is considered critical to cranial procedures (class of recommendation (COR) III and level of evidence (LOE) C). However, it is usually not an appropriate alarm criterion for spinal cord monitoring because it could produce many false alarms. An "all or nothing" approach, i.e., notification only when the mMEP has completely disappeared, certainly is the most specific predictor of postoperative motor deficit (COR II and III and LOE B). However, a better alarm criterion also needs to be sensitive enough to allow that the surgical team is communicated before an irreversible injury is established when immediate and accurate corrective maneuvers can effectively be performed. Thereby, it seems preferable to notify the rest of the team before the disappearance of mMEP when the decrease reaches a limit percentage higher than 50% (e.g., 70%, 80%, or 90%) (COR II and III and LOE C). The criteria are still evolving, and currently, there is no consensus about the best alarm criterion for mMEP monitoring of the spinal cord [23].

An elevation of the stimulus threshold (100 V or greater) or simplification of the morphology (decrease of response duration or waveform complexity) may also be an indicator for impending neurological deficits. Although the correlation with the postoperative deficit is weaker than the amplitude criterion, it is rational to interpret these changes in the excitability, provided that they are focal as a subclinical or preclinical injury indicator. Therefore, changes in surgical strategy should be considered. It is essential to keep in mind that, from a predictive point of view, if the threshold shift does not progress to a significant drop in amplitude (not reversing with increasing stimulus intensity), then the patient will most likely have no clinical motor deficit postoperatively. These changes may be classified as a minor warning criterion in the intraoperative decision-making process (COR II and III and LOE B) [52, 55]. Changes in latency are generally useless in MEP monitoring [23].

The reliability of any of the warning criteria strongly depends on trial-to-trial variations of the responses. The range of these variations, in its turns, is determined by different factors, and anesthesia is one of the main variables, being a critical confounding factor in the interpretation of mMEP [56]. Therefore, it is essential to create steady-state conditions, preferably using total intravenous anesthesia (TIVA) and maintaining adequate blood pressure and hemoglobin levels as well as temperature and good ventilation parameters to minimize mMEP variations (COR II and III and LOE B). When steady-state conditions are maintained, the coefficient of variance of muscle MEPs tends to be minimal. Even with stable anesthetic conditions, it is also important to remember that it could tend to gradual amplitude fade and threshold elevation, a phenomenon called fading effect, particularly in long procedures or in muscle groups with previous dysfunction [20, 21, 46].

The TES parameters are also an important factor in the variation of the mMEP and are under the direct control of the neuromonitorist. Higher TES intensity reduces the trial-to-trial variability. At submaximal intensities levels, the mMEPs will be most sensitive to the contribution of any input giving space to a large variance of the response that is prone to false-positive findings. In such cases, only a lost of 100% of the response can be helpful as an alarm criterion. On the other hand, in the supramaximal voltage range, the sensitivity to the variations becomes reduced at most because the maximum number of LMNs that can be recruited has been reached. Thereby, supramaximal intensity levels allow proper use of more sensitive alarm criteria instead of only the mMEP disappearance [56].

The fact is that the surgical time, the anesthetic context, and the concomitant evolution of other neurophysiological modalities are much more relevant for interpreting the findings than a magic cut-off number itself. The greater the experience of the neurophysiologist, the greater the accuracy of the interpretation of the findings, whatever the threshold percentage the neuromonitorist has chosen as a reference point [21, 46].

Regarding the D-wave, its stability enables a more objective and reliable alarm criterion: a 50% drop in potential amplitude is widely accepted as such for spinal cord surgeries (COR II and III and LOE B). As mentioned above, the D-wave is the purest representation of the CST, and thus, it is considered the "gold standard" to the CST monitoring over mMEP, which receives a contribution from a supportive system. mMEP can disappear without significant changes in the D-wave during surgery for an intramedullary spinal cord tumor. In such cases, the patients wake up with paralysis, which invariably evolved with recovery within hours to days. This is because the support system can have its function assumed by the remaining tracts, while the CST is functionally irreplaceable. If, in addition to the loss of the mMEP, there was a significant drop in the amplitude D-wave, it means that the postoperative deficit will be permanent [20, 48]. In brain surgery, reduction of 30 to 40% in the cervical D-wave amplitude by DCS is a major alarm criterion (COR III and LOE C) [21, 23, 57].

For more details about interpretation in specific kinds of surgeries, see the corresponding chapter in this book.

Applications (Indications and Contraindications) and Safety

The use of MEP monitoring should be considered for any surgery where there is a risk of damage to the motor path at any level. The most common indications include neurosurgical, orthopedic, and vascular procedures: tumor or vascular malformations at or near the motor cortex and corticospinal tract, posterior fossa surgeries, craniocervical junction operations, aneurysm clipping, descending aortic procedures, carotid endarterectomy, spinal cord or cauda equina surgeries, spinal deformity, fracture or tumor vertebral surgeries and spine instrumentations among other procedures. There may be other procedures not cited in this list where potential damage to the motor system may demand MEP monitoring [21].

In some situations, MEP monitoring may not be required as when the patient already has chronic paralysis without any useful function or when the goal of the procedure is complete removal of certain types of pathologies regardless of postoperative paralysis. Therefore, the indication must be individualized for each case.

Intraoperative MEP monitoring is sufficiently safe for clinical use once taking the necessary precautions. Even so, it is not without complications. The most common complication is bite injuries, such as lip and tongue lacerations, with an estimated incidence rate of 0.2%. Most, with not all, of these injuries involve C3-C4 montage certainly because it tends to generate strong muscular contractions even due to its proximity to the temporal muscle and the trigeminal nerve [31, 58]. Most of these lesions are self-healing, although they may eventually require surgical repair. There are also reports of jaw fracture and endotracheal tube rupture. The use of bite blocks (rolled-up gazes or dental blocks) placed between the molars on both sides of the mouth is recommended to minimize this complication, but unfortunately, it does not eliminate these injuries [2, 21, 59].

Seizures are another possible complication that is rare (incidence of 0,03%), self-limited, and free of morbidity for TES but has a significant highest incidence during DCS. It is known that the Penfield technique is more epileptogenic than brief high-frequency pulse trains with incidences ranging from 5 to 20% and 1 to 4%, respectively. Epileptic patients are at higher risk, mainly if the seizure control is poor. Seizures are preferably treated with ice-cold irrigation if the cortex is exposed, which usually halts the seizure within a few seconds. In case of persistence, propofol bolus or benzodiazepines may be necessary, leading to the suppression of MEPs during a significant period for the procedure [39, 46, 58, 60, 61].

Other complications reported include burns under the stimulating electrodes possibly due to stray electrode current, hemorrhagic or infectious complications related to invasive electrodes, and transient cardiac arrhythmia. The movement induced by the stimulation can cause traumatic injuries to neurovascular structures, mainly during microscopic manipulation, so, in these cases, efforts must be made to minimize movements by optimizing the stimulus parameters and using more selective montages. When the movements are unavoidable, careful communication and surgical field video will be crucial to coordinate the time of the stimulus with the surgical manipulation [21, 58, 60].

Relative contraindications include epilepsy, skull defects, pacemakers or other implanted bioelectric devices, intracranial vascular clips, or electrodes but the real risks are uncertain. Moreover, patients with these conditions have had uneventful TES-MEP monitoring. Therefore, the benefits of MEP monitoring must be weighed against the potential risks in each patient [21, 23].

Conclusion

Despite the limitations regarding the quality of evidence and strength of the recommendations, MEP monitoring is strongly recommended by the main experts and medical societies. Proving a positive impact on outcome faces many challenges related to practical and ethical barriers to randomized and blind clinical trials. Furthermore, in most surgeries where the motor tract is threatened, it is much safer than risky to use intraoperative MEP monitoring techniques, provided it is conducted by qualified hands using the appropriate precautions. Therefore, it seems much more reasonable to use MEP monitoring than stay waiting for more robust evidence.

Bibliography

1. MacDonald BK. The incidence and lifetime prevalence of neurological disorders in a prospective community-based study in the UK. Brain. 2000;123:665–76.
2. Davis SF, Kaye AD, editors. Principles of Neurophysiological Assessment, Mapping, and Monitoring [Internet]. Cham: Springer International Publishing; 2020 [cited 2021 Apr 6]. Available from: https://doi.org/10.1007/978-3-030-22400-4.
3. Moller AR. Intraoperative neurophysiological monitoring. 2nd ed. Totowa: NJ: Humana Press; 2006.
4. Penfield W, Boldrey E. Somatic motor and sensory representation in the cerebral cortex of man as studied by electrical stimulation. Brain. 1937;60:389–443.
5. MacDonald DB. Intraoperative motor evoked potential monitoring: overview and update. J Clin Monit Comput. 2006;20:347–77.
6. Dimitrijevic MR, Persy I, Forstner C, Kern H, Dimitrijevic MM. Motor control in the human spinal cord. Artif Organs. 2005;29:216–9.
7. Rodi Z, Deletis V, Morota N, Vodušek DB. Motor evoked potentials during brain surgery. Pflugers Arch. 1996;431:R291–2.
8. Pechstein U, Ceclzich C, Nadstawek J, Schramm J. Transcranial high-frequency repetitive electrical stimulation for recording myogenic motor evoked potentials with the patient under general anesthesia. Neurosurgery. 1996;39:335–44.
9. Jones SJ, Harrison R, Koh KF, Mendoza N, Crockard HA. Motor evoked potential monitoring during spinal surgery: responses of distal limb muscles to transcranial cortical stimulation with pulse trains. Electroencephalogr Clin Neurophysiol. 1996;9
10. Taniguchi M, Cedzich C, Schramm J. Modification of cortical stimulation for motor evoked potentials under general anesthesia: technical description. Neurosurgery. 1993;32:219–26.
11. Merton PA, Morton HB. Stimulation of the cerebral cortex in the intact human subject. Nature Nature Publishing Group. 1980;285:227.

12. Patton HD, Amassian VE. Single and multiple-unit analysis of cortical stage of pyramidal tract activation. J Neurophysiol. 1954;17:345–63.
13. Minahan RE, Sepkuty JP, Lesser RP, Sponseller PD, Kostuik JP. Anterior spinal cord injury with preserved neurogenic "motor" evoked potentials. Clin Neurophysiol. 2001;112:1442–50.
14. Toleikis JR, Skelly JP, Carlvin AO, Burkus JK. Spinally elicited peripheral nerve responses are sensory rather than motor. Clin Neurophysiol. 2000;111:736–42.
15. Deletis V. The "motor" inaccuracy in neurogenic motor evoked potentials. Clin Neurophysiol. 2001;112:1365–6.
16. Barker AT, Freeston IL, Jalinous R, Jarratt JA. Magnetic stimulation of the human brain and peripheral nervous system: an introduction and the results of an initial clinical evaluation. Neurosurgery. 1987;20:100–9.
17. Burke D, Hicks RG, Stephen JP. Corticospinal volleys evoked by anodal and cathodal stimulation of the human motor cortex. J Physiol. 1990;425:283–99.
18. Rothwell J, Burke D, Hicks R, Stephen J, Woodforth I, Crawford M. Transcranial electrical stimulation of the motor cortex in man: further evidence for the site of activation. J Physiol. 1994;481(Pt 1):243–50.
19. Rattay F. Analysis of models for external stimulation of axons. IEEE Trans Biomed Eng. 1986;BME-33:974–7.
20. Deletis V, Shils JL, Sala F, Seidel K, editors. Neurophysiology in neurosurgery: a modern approach. 2nd ed. San Diego: Elsevier; 2020.
21. MacDonald DB, Skinner S, Shils J, Yingling C. Intraoperative motor evoked potential monitoring – a position statement by the American Society of Neurophysiological Monitoring. Clin Neurophysiol. 2013;124:2291–316.
22. Deng L-X, Walker C, Xu X-M. Schwann cell transplantation and descending propriospinal regeneration after spinal cord injury. Brain Res. 1619;2015:104–14.
23. Legatt AD, Emerson RG, Epstein CM, MacDonald DB, Deletis V, Bravo RJ, et al. ACNS guideline: transcranial electrical stimulation motor evoked potential monitoring. J Clin Neurophysiol. 2016;33:42–50.
24. Simon MV. Neurophysiologic test used in the operating room. In: Simon MV, editor. Intraoperative neurophysiology. New York: Demos medical; 2010. p. 1–46.
25. Szelényi A, Senft C, Jardan M, Forster MT, Franz K, Seifert V, et al. Intra-operative subcortical electrical stimulation: a comparison of two methods. Clin Neurophysiol. 2011;122:1470–5.
26. Klem GH, LuÈders HO, Jasper HH, Elger C. The ten±twenty electrode system of the International Federation. In: Recommendations for the Practice of Clinical Neurophysiology: Guidelines of the International Federation of Clinical Physiology (EEG Suppl 52). Elsevier Science B.V.; 1999. p. 3–6.
27. American electroencephalographic society guidelines for standard electrode position nomenclature. J Clin Neurophysiol. 1991;8:200–2.
28. Macdonald DB, Al Zayed Z, Al SA. Four-limb muscle motor evoked potential and optimized somatosensory evoked potential monitoring with decussation assessment: results in 206 thoracolumbar spine surgeries. Eur Spine J. 2007;16(Suppl 2):S171–87.
29. Szelényi A, Kothbauer KF, Deletis V. Transcranial electric stimulation for intraoperative motor evoked potential monitoring: stimulation parameters and electrode montages. Clin Neurophysiol. 2007;118:1586–95.
30. Verst SM, Chung TM, Sucena AC, Maldaun MVC, Aguiar PHP. Comparison between the C5 or C6-Cz electrode assembly and C3 or C4-Cz assembly for transcranial electric motor activation of muscular response of the contralateral facial nerve. Acta Neurochir. 2012;154:2229–35.
31. Hoebink EA, Journée HL, de Kleuver M, Berends H, Racz I, van Hal C. Movement along the spine induced by transcranial electrical stimulation related electrode positioning. Spine. 2016;41:1128–32.
32. Dong CCJ, Macdonald DB, Akagami R, Westerberg B, Alkhani A, Kanaan I, et al. Intraoperative facial motor evoked potential monitoring with transcranial electrical stimulation during skull base surgery. Clin Neurophysiol. 2005;116:588–96.

33. Brocke J, Irlbacher K, Hauptmann B, Voss M, Brandt SA. Transcranial magnetic and electrical stimulation compared: does TES activate intracortical neuronal circuits? Clin Neurophysiol. 2005;116:2748–56.
34. Schwartz SL, Kale EB, Husain AM. T140. Identifying the best stimulation configuration to use for linked-quadripolar motor evoked potentials. Clin Neurophysiol. 2018;129:e56–7.
35. Hern JE, Landgren S, Phillips CG, Porter R. Selective excitation of corticofugal neurones by surface-anodal stimulation of the baboon's motor cortex. J Physiol. 1962;161:73–90.
36. Raabe A, Beck J, Schucht P, Seidel K. Continuous dynamic mapping of the corticospinal tract during surgery of motor eloquent brain tumors: evaluation of a new method: clinical article. JNS. 2014;120:1015–24.
37. Nathan SS, Sinha SR, Gordon B, Lesser RP, Thakor NV. Determination of current density distributions generated by electrical stimulation of the human cerebral cortex. Electroencephalogr Clin Neurophysiol. 1993;86:183–92.
38. Sala F, Lanteri P. Brain surgery in motor areas: the invaluable assistance of intraoperative neurophysiological monitoring. J Neurosurg Sci. 2003;47:79–88.
39. Rossi M, Conti Nibali M, Viganò L, Puglisi G, Howells H, Gay L, et al. Resection of tumors within the primary motor cortex using high-frequency stimulation: oncological and functional efficiency of this versatile approach based on clinical conditions. J Neurosurg. 2020;133:642–54.
40. Abalkhail TM, MacDonald DB, AlThubaiti I, AlOtaibi FA, Stigsby B, Mokeem AA, et al. Intraoperative direct cortical stimulation motor evoked potentials: stimulus parameter recommendations based on rheobase and chronaxie. Clin Neurophysiol. 2017;128:2300–8.
41. Hausmann O. Transcranial electrical stimulation: significance of fast versus slow charge delivery for intra-operative monitoring. Clin Neurophysiol. 2002;113:1532–5.
42. Ushio S, Kawabata S, Sumiya S, Kato T, Yoshii T, Yamada T, et al. A multi-train electrical stimulation protocol facilitates transcranial electrical motor evoked potentials and increases induction rate and reproducibility even in patients with preoperative neurological deficits. J Clin Monit Comput. 2018;32:549–58.
43. Journée HL, Polak HE, de Kleuver M, Langeloo DD, Postma AA. Improved neuromonitoring during spinal surgery using double-train transcranial electrical stimulation. Med Biol Eng Comput. 2004;42:110–3.
44. Journée H-L, Polak HE, De Kleuver M. Conditioning stimulation techniques for enhancement of transcranially elicited evoked motor responses. Neurophysiologie Clinique/Clinical Neurophysiology. 2007;37:423–30.
45. Andersson G, Ohlin A. Spatial facilitation of motor evoked responses in monitoring during spinal surgery. Clin Neurophysiol. 1999;110:720–4.
46. Dineen J, Simon MV. Neurophysiologic tests in the operating room. In: Intraoperative neurophysiology. 2nd ed. Demos Medical Publishing; 2019. p. 21–39.
47. Parikh P, Cheongsiatmoy J, Shilian P, Gonzalez AA. Differences in the Transcranial Motor Evoked Potentials Between Proximal and Distal Lower Extremity Muscles: Journal of Clinical Neurophysiology. 2018;35:155–8.
48. Deletis V, Sala F. Intraoperative neurophysiological monitoring of the spinal cord during spinal cord and spine surgery: a review focus on the corticospinal tracts. Clin Neurophysiol. 2008;119:248–64.
49. Modi HN, Suh S-W, Yang J-H, Yoon J-Y. False-negative transcranial motor-evoked potentials during scoliosis surgery causing paralysis: a case report with literature review. Spine (Phila Pa 1976). 2009;34:E896–900.
50. Nuwer MR, Emerson RG, Galloway G, Legatt AD, Lopez J, Minahan R, et al. Evidence-based guideline update: intraoperative spinal monitoring with somatosensory and transcranial electrical motor evoked potentials*. J Clin Neurophysiol. 2012;29:101–8.
51. Langeloo DD, Lelivelt A, Louis Journée H, Slappendel R, de Kleuver M. Transcranial electrical motor-evoked potential monitoring during surgery for spinal deformity: a study of 145 patients. Spine (Phila Pa 1976). 2003;28:1043–50.

52. Calancie B, Harris W, Broton JG, Alexeeva N, Green BA. "Threshold-level" multipulse transcranial electrical stimulation of motor cortex for intraoperative monitoring of spinal motor tracts: description of method and comparison to somatosensory evoked potential monitoring. J Neurosurg. 1998;88:457–70.
53. Quiñones-Hinojosa A, Lyon R, Zada G, Lamborn KR, Gupta N, Parsa AT, et al. Changes in transcranial motor evoked potentials during intramedullary spinal cord tumor resection correlate with postoperative motor function. Neurosurgery. 2005;56:982–93; discussion 982-993.
54. Langeloo D-D, Journée H-L, de Kleuver M, Grotenhuis JA. Criteria for transcranial electrical motor evoked potential monitoring during spinal deformity surgery a review and discussion of the literature. Neurophysiol Clin. 2007;37:431–9.
55. Kothbauer KF. The interpretation of muscle motor evoked potentials for spinal cord monitoring. J Clin Neurophysiol. 2017;34:32–7.
56. Journée HL, Berends HI, Kruyt MC. The percentage of amplitude decrease warning criteria for transcranial MEP monitoring. J Clin Neurophysiol. 2017;34:22–31.
57. Fujiki M, Furukawa Y, Kamida T, Anan M, Inoue R, Abe T, et al. Intraoperative corticomuscular motor evoked potentials for evaluation of motor function: a comparison with corticospinal D and I waves. J Neurosurg. 2006;104:85–92.
58. MacDonald DB. Safety of intraoperative transcranial electrical stimulation motor evoked potential monitoring. J Clin Neurophysiol. 2002;19:416–29.
59. Shils J. Deletis, Vedran. Moto evoked potentials. Principles of neurophysiological assessment, mapping, and monitoring. Second. Switzerland: Springer; 2020.
60. Szelényi A, Kothbauer K, de Camargo AB, Langer D, Flamm ES. Deletis V. Motor Evoked Potential Monitoring during Cerebral Aneurysm Surgery: Technical Aspects and Comparison of Transcranial and Direct Cortical Stimulation: Operative Neurosurgery. 2005;57:331–8.
61. Riva M, Fava E, Gallucci M, Comi A, Casarotti A, Alfiero T, et al. Monopolar high-frequency language mapping: can it help in the surgical management of gliomas? A comparative clinical study. J Neurosurg. 2016;124:1479–89.

Chapter 10
Intraoperative Monitoring: Electroencephalogram

Maria Lucia Furtado de Mendonça and Francisco José Carchedi Luccas

Introduction

This chapter aims to highlight electroencephalogram (EEG) monitoring value in the acute care settings, especially during surgical procedures with increased cerebral ischemia risks. Intraoperative neurophysiology monitoring (IOM) primary objective constitutes the real-time early detection of reversible neuronal injury, allowing precise and timely intervention. EEG alterations may alert the surgeon for impeding risks. Secondarily, but no less important, there is the opportunity for better injury mechanism comprehension, envisaging future technical improvement, and documenting relevant neurophysiology events.

Our objective: delivering of practical and basic guidelines envisaging intraoperative scalp EEG, not including electrocorticography (ECoG).

Rational Bases of Intraoperative Electroencephalography (EEG) Monitoring

EEG classically represents dynamic and neurophysiological electrocerebral activity evaluation, constituting a high sensitivity test for early detection of the most common causes of brain injury, ischemia and hypoxia. EEG is believed to be generated mainly by sources in neocortex, large pyramidal neurons forming a macrocolumn whose cell

M. L. F. de Mendonça (✉)
Clinical Neurology and Neurophysiology, Intraoperative and Critical Care Clinical Neurophysiology, Neuro Logical Clinica Médica, Rio de Janeiro, RJ, Brazil

F. J. C. Luccas
Clinical Neurophysiology, Hospital São Luiz – Morumbi – Rede D'Or, São Paulo, SP, Brazil

S. M. Verst et al. (eds.), *Intraoperative Monitoring*,
https://doi.org/10.1007/978-3-030-95730-8_10

bodies occupy layers 3 and 5, dependent on postsynaptic excitatory and inhibitory potentials, occurring as a tangential dipole layer situated mostly in gyri surface, with less contribution from sulci activity. Communication among these sources is intense, involving short and long corticocortical fibers, and also between both cerebral hemispheres through commissural fibers, resulting in transcortical and subcortical influences [1].

Pathology involving these cortical layers may cause severe brain impairment, generating the well-known histological pattern of laminar necrosis. This relatively selective vulnerability of pyramidal cells to hypoxia and/or ischemia makes the EEG particularly sensitive to these types of aggression. EEG correlates with brain topography, detects neuronal dysfunctions in reversible stages, deteriorating before cell membrane failure and reduction of tissue ATP levels [2].

EEG Recording – Technical Aspects

Every EEG channel is recorded among three electrodes, according to Fig. 10.1. Signal goes through grids 1 and 2 of the differential amplifier, when reference (Ref) is subtracted and cancelled, leaving potential difference between the two active electrodes. Amplifiers with high common mode rejection rate help to minimize several types of electrical noise in the surgical theater.

EEG electrodes are scalp oriented according to 10–20 international system, as shown in Fig. 10.2. It is important to define how many electrodes will be used, and also their position, considering the surgery type that will be monitored.

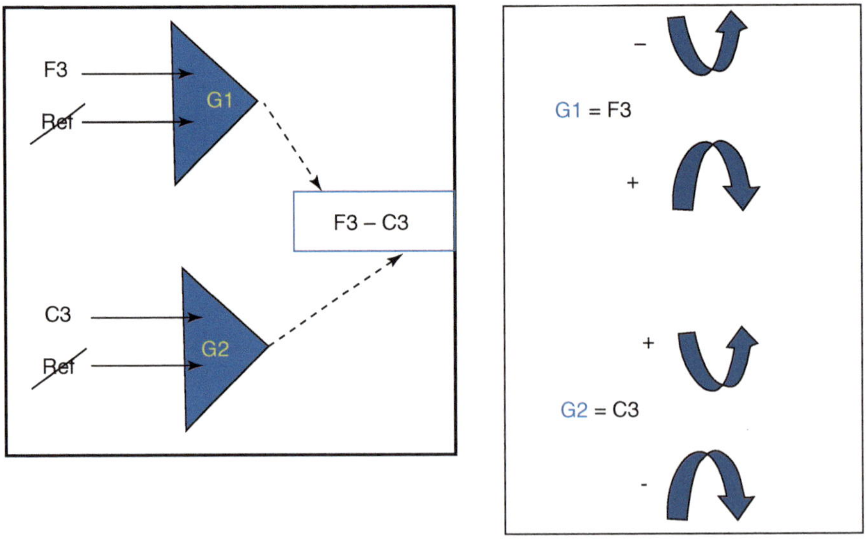

Fig. 10.1 EEG channel schematic representation of a differential amplifier. Left: grids G1 and G2 with connected electrodes, subtracted and cancelled Ref (Reference, not ground), resulting [F3 – C3]. Right minus – and plus + signals indicate wave deflections (relative polarity) in G1 and G2

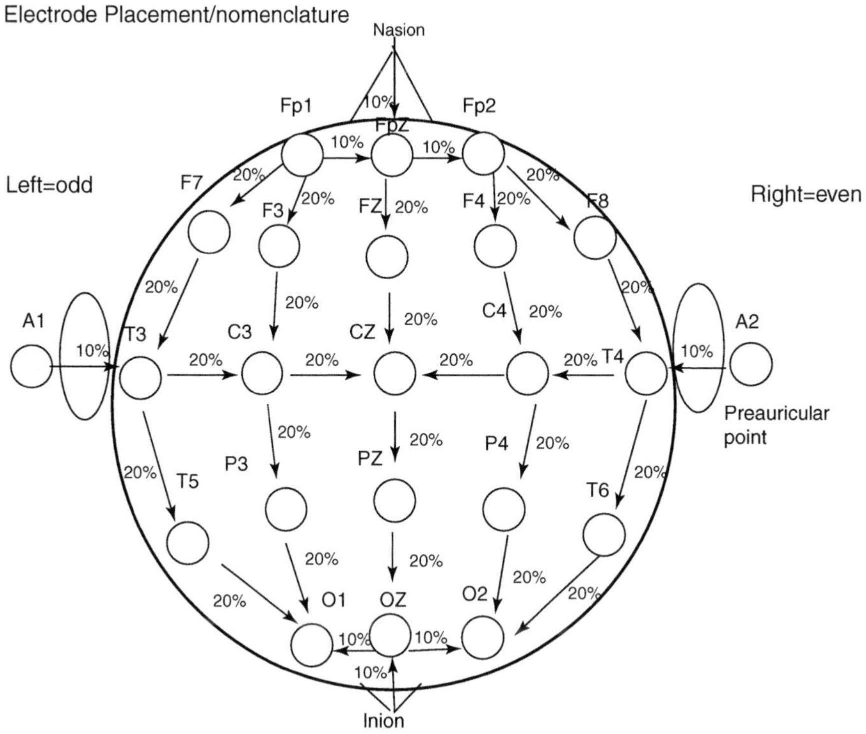

Fig. 10.2 Ten-twenty system electrode placement/nomenclature, and each electrode name follows a logical alphabetical abbreviation that identifies the brain area which it refers to. *F* stands for frontal, *Fp* for frontopolar, *T* for temporal, *C* for central, *P* for parietal, *O* for occipital, and *A* for auricular (ear electrode). The following subscripts in the electrode annotation refer to the specific location of the electrode site within one brain hemisphere. All even numbers identify electrode positions on the right side of the head, whereas all the odd numbers refer to the left hemisphere. The subscript "z" points to electrode sites in the midline of the skull

Electrode Types

Electrode disks are fixed with conductive paste or collodion and conductive gel after proper skin abrasion; collodion application requires little extra time. Impedance electrodes measurement is very important to guarantee good-quality recording. Subdermal electrode needles may also be used, and care must be taken they are not easily removed under surgery dressings. Corkscrew electrodes could be used, but care must be taken with patients receiving anticoagulant therapy. The type and number of electrodes used vary according to the surgical strategy individually.

Montages Selection

EEG montages selection represent channels logical combination displayed in an EEG page. Their selection is dependent on the clear objective of the particular surgery, trying to focus on the expected benefits. There are some usual montage rules: symmetry, left to right and anterior to posterior channels, and most important, avoiding broken lines, such as exemplified by [F3-C3, C3-T3, T3-P3, P3-O1] because different distances are introduced, with a voltage compromise. Most commonly montages used are longitudinal bipolar (temporal, parasagital, and midline), transverse, and common reference such as vertex and common average; laplacean averaged reference may also be used as a more focal montage.

Multimodal intraoperative monitoring includes the association of EEG with other neurophysiologic methods simultaneously, such as somatosensory, auditory, visual, or motor evoked potentials, and transcranial Doppler, causing some degree of channel and screen limitations. In these circumstances, we are directed to apply limited montages, for instance, only eight channels consisting of: [Fp1-C3, C3-O1, Fp1-T3, T3-O1, Fp2-C4, C4-O2, Fp2-T4, T4-O2]. Those patients at risk for ischemic events in the middle cerebral arteries should not have the temporal electrodes disconnected.

Clarifying in a more practical and fast way, in the surgical environment, the brain can be visualized in four quadrants, two anterior and two posteriors, two to the left and two to the right. It has the advantage of covering both cerebral hemispheres, but the disadvantage of distant spatial sampling.

Filter Settings

Filters represent the assumed frequency range limits, since our electrodes "do not know" which type of activity we are looking for. Frequency range is limited by low-frequency filters (high pass) and high-frequency filters (low pass). EEG recording range goes from 0.5 Hz to 70 Hz, with some small variations accepted. Lastly, a 60 Hz (or 50 Hz) notch filter is often necessary to eliminate extraneous, irreducible line artifact noise in the operating room arena.

Display Velocity

EEG can be recorded at the traditional 30 mm/s "paper-speed," having the advantage to be fitted into electroencephalographer brains. Nevertheless, it is a commonplace to use 7.5 mm/s or 15 mm/s "paper-speed." The slower displays allow considerable data compression, turning easier the visual analysis of eventual asymmetry (Fig. 10.3).

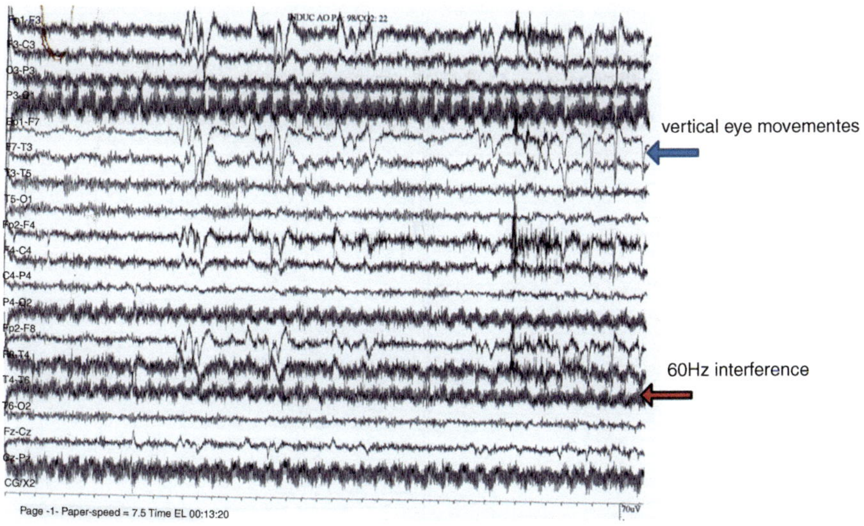

Fig. 10.3 Compressed EEG page during anesthetic induction for cardiac surgery using slower display of 7.5 mm/sec velocity – see the inferior part of the figure, and also showing several artifacts: vertical eye movements at frontopolar derivation (blue arrow) and 60 Hz interference pattern compromising all the record (red arrow)

Sensitivity

The amplifier's sensitivity control output voltage reduces or enhances amplitude screen display. Sensitivity is expressed in microvolts per millimeter (μV/mm) [3]. During EEG recording, the sensitivity is adjusted to optimize the visual analysis (Fig. 10.4).

Artifacts

Artifacts are extracerebral potentials that may interfere with the EEG and is very important to be aware of their existence to avoid wrong interpretation. There are four possible artifact sources, namely installations (proper grounding), equipment, electrodes (representing an especial and important group), and biological.

Line frequency: It occurs in the range of 60 Hz (or 50 Hz) as an interference generated from improper or faulty installations or equipment grounding and is also facilitated by inadequate patient reference electrode (improperly called "ground") application; this situation may be avoided when we connect two reference electrodes. Faulty reference electrodes may record nearby interference from equipment such as ventilators (Fig. 10.3). The 60 or 50 Hz artifact occurring in only one EEG

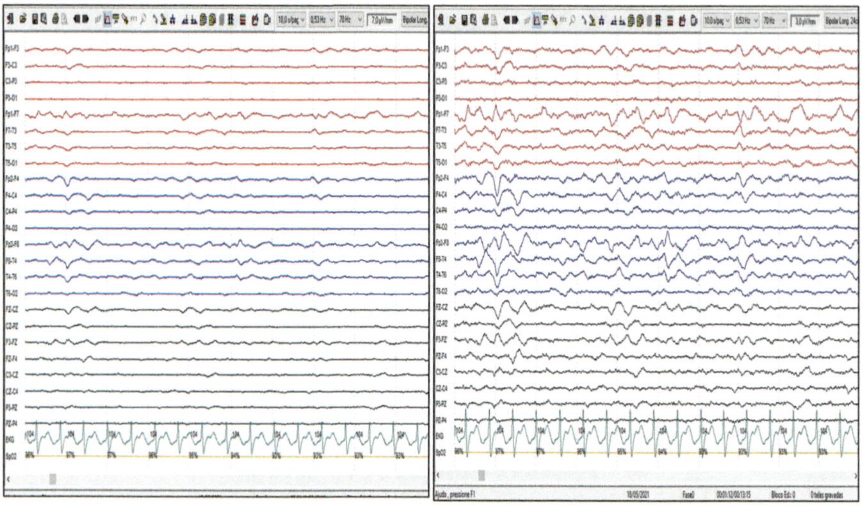

Fig. 10.4 Comparison: same post anoxic EEG page of a 69 yo patient showing different sensitivities, demonstrating the importance of its management. Left: regular SNS = 7 μV/mm with huge generalized attenuation, and few frontal slow waves, besides suggested posterior area depression. Right SNS = 3 μV/mm (more than two times increased) showing continuous frontal slow waves and persistent posterior depression; injury was more severe and probably irreversible in posterior region. The more adequate SNS may help a timely intervention. Small EKG artifacts may be propagated to a depressed EEG

channel is most probably due to unequal, unbalanced, or high impedance electrodes, whose correction should eliminate this artifact.

Care must be taken to avoid saline bridges, caused by paste continuity between a pair of electrodes. Despite impedance measurement assessment, there is no guarantee that electrodes will fulfill their expected function till surgery ends.

Muscle activity may present especially when the anesthetic plan is superficializing and usually involves the frontotemporal region. It may be advisable to inform both the surgeon and the anesthetist before the patient starts to move.

Electrocardiogram (EKG): QRS complex may propagate to the EEG electrodes, mostly to those closer to the heart, such as A1, A2, occipital and temporal, being facilitated by low amplitude EEG signals, for instance, in deep hypothermia. EKG signals may determine interpretation problems when superposing on the brain signals, but its recording in one channel will certainly help (Fig. 10.4).

Artifacts such as eye and eyelid movements, recorded from frontal leads, are rarely seen in anesthetized patients; exception is represented by a waking recording. Eyeball carries an electrical positive potential in the front, also positive at the cornea and an electrical negative potential in the back (at the retina), thus creating a high voltage source of approximately 50–100 mV [1, 4]. Horizontal eye movements are usually recorded at F7 and F8, while vertical eye movements occur at Fp1 and Fp2 (Fig. 10.3).

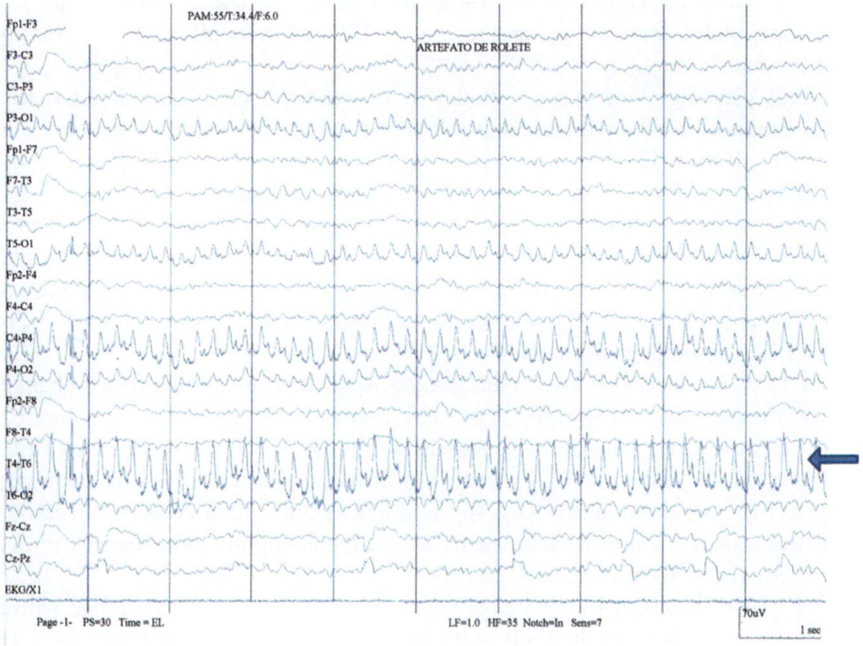

Fig. 10.5 Roller pump artifact, induced during extracorporeal cardiopulmonary bypass surgery, evident in channels involving right and left posterior electrodes

The electrocautery unit in the operating room may represent major monitoring problem, generating high amplitude fast waves in other equipment, also rendering impossible the EEG interpretation. This artifact is easily recognizable, since it correlates with the sound made by electrocautery. Fortunately, it is not used during all surgery phases.

Other artifacts: Roller pump artifact during cardiopulmonary bypass occurs within the frequency range of interest for EEG and may be recognized by their regularity (Fig. 10.5). Train-of-four twitch stimulator and somatosensory evoked potential stimulator may also create a patterned artifact in the EEG [5].

EEG Interpretation – Graphics and Their Importance

EEG is usually presented as an *XY* Cartesian coordinates graphic, depicting *X* time dominion in the abscissa, usually in 10 second pages and the ordinates *Y* showing amplitude in μV/mm. Four main activity types are identified by the frequency (Hertz – Hz) and are known by Greek letters: delta [0.5–3.5 Hz], theta [4–7.5 Hz], alpha [8–13 Hz], and beta [over 13 Hz].

Some of the activities may constitute rhythms that includes, besides frequency, also topography, morphology, and reactivity; EEG analysis also includes polarity and symmetry.

Many years ago, one of the authors (FJCL) was involved in carotid endarterectomy monitoring of three patients, utilizing an EEG eight channel analog paper recording Kaiser TR60. After carotid exposition, the surgeon proceeded to the clamping test, whose protocol demanded waiting 1–2 minutes to see if the EEG changed into any abnormal pattern; surgeon patience was limited, and the neurophysiologist was repeatedly instigated to report if any abnormality was present, when a shunt could be inserted. The problem: paper ran at 10 seconds per page and after 60 seconds (1 minute) it was kind of cumbersome to go back and forth six or more EEG pages to reach a conclusion.

In 1986, we started to overcome turning pages difficulty using a two-channel fronto-mastoid derivation equipment – Neurotrac I (USA). It was very limited, paper recording, no data transfer or saving, but presented some formats: raw EEG, compressed spectral array (CSA) frequency histogram and frequency bands; it was easy to turn into different formats. We used this machine in more than 120 carotid endarterectomies, and it became easier to see the clamping consequences in one page only (Figs. 10.6, 10.7, 10.8, and 10.9).

CSA also presented spectral edge frequency (SEF), marking every line with a small square pointing to the limit of 95–97% of global spectral energy (Figs. 10.8 and 10.9). SEF is very useful to show in a page the monitoring trend and helps to detect ischemic changes at a short sight. SEF trends may receive the influence of

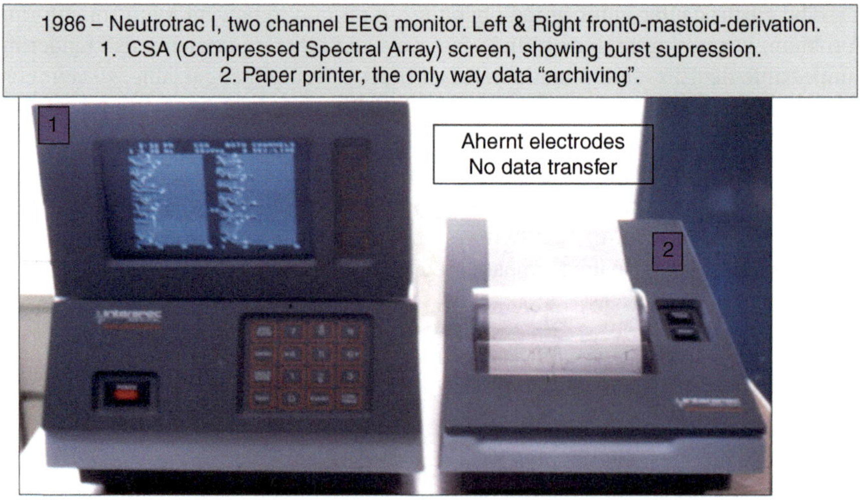

Fig. 10.6 Two channel fronto-mastoid derivation old EEG equipment (Neurotrac I, 1986, USA), used for ICU and OR monitoring through adherent electrodes. Part 1: two channel Left & Right fronto-mastoid derivation; in the screen CSA (compressed spectral array) is depicted, and a burst suppression pattern is identifiable. Part 2: paper printer, the only way for data "archiving"; no data transfer was possible

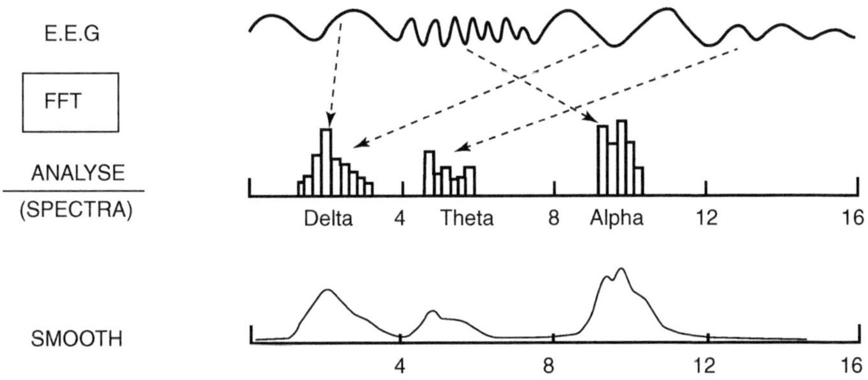

Fig. 10.7 Two channel spectral frequency analysis: the first line shows an EEG signal that is submitted to Fast Fourier Transform (Cooley & Tukey, 1965) generating EEG spectra (second line) in a histogram format. The third line shows spectral energy "hills and valleys" after smoothing, turning analysis visually easier

many aspects, such as: a shift to the left may be induced by anesthetic deepening level with more slow waves, cerebral hypoperfusion (ischemia), and defective electrodes. Right shift may be induced by anesthetic superficializing, muscle artifacts that have higher frequencies, 60 Hz interference such as caused by electrodes bad contact. It is fundamental to understand that isolated trends use may determine interpretation errors, causing monitoring risks that can be detrimental for the patient; trends must be accompanied by raw EEG curves and its correct reading. Other suggested variables are the median power frequency (MPF), under which 50% of the global power is contained, and main dominant frequency (MDF), the mean frequency in the 8–15 Hz frequency band [6].

Fortunately, digital EEG was fully introduced, with many advantages: more channels, reformatting parameter changes, sensitivity, and filters manipulation. EEG acquisition starts with analog-to-digital conversion (ADC), bringing lots of numbers, and ends with digital-to-analog conversion (CDA), generating the classical curves we are used to interpret. An important criticism appeared after some years: neurophysiologists analysis took few advantages of digital EEG, continuing to interpret only in the same way of classical "paper" analog EEG.

Remembering our old CSA experience, an innovation was suggested: the possibility of SIMULTANEOUSLY viewing classical 24 EEG channels together (in the same screen) with 4 CSA channels, two for left and two for right, allowing time dominion analysis, and at the same time, spectral analysis, based in digital EEG numbers and developing Fast Fourier Transform (FFT) to create the power spectral squaring the amplitudes of the individual frequency components [5] (Figs. 10.10 and 10.11).

Our preference was centered on a program named Monitor (Neurotec, Pesquisa & Desenvolvimento, Brazil) that simultaneously showed the classical EEG together with four-channel compressed spectral array (CSA), depicting "mountains and

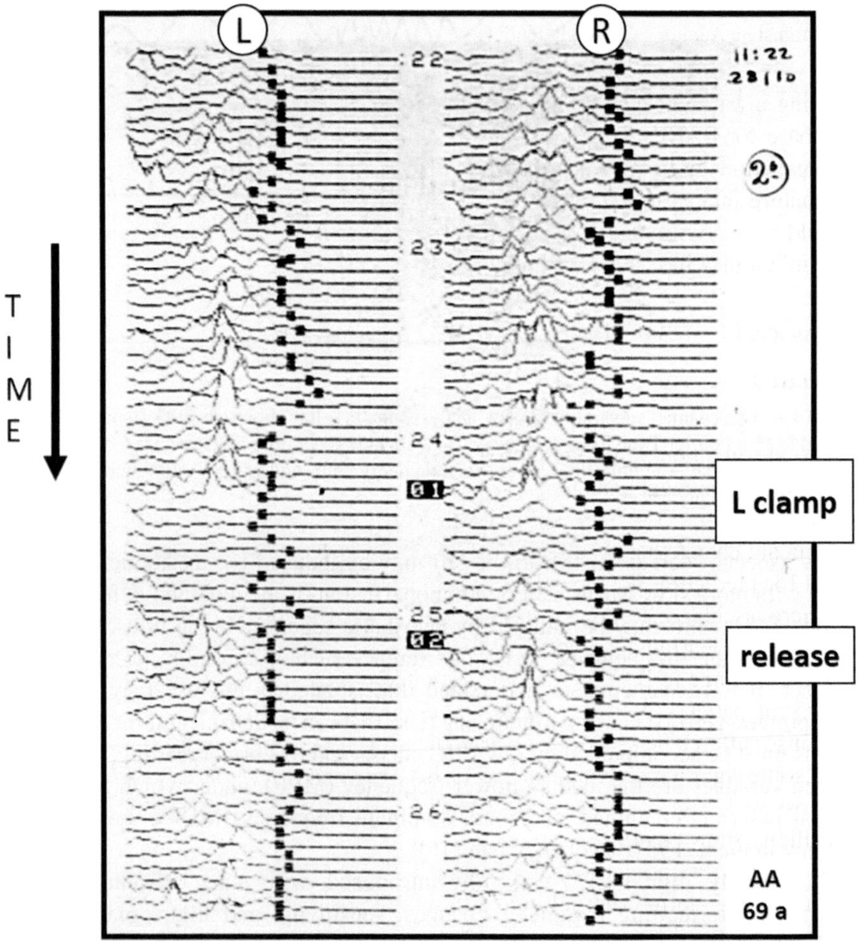

Fig. 10.8 Left carotid artery clamping during carotid endarterectomy using old Neurotrac I. The arrow shows time going down. Symmetrical left and right basal recording (above the mark 01); at this mark the left artery clamping test occurs; SEF (spectral edge frequency) black squares show minimal changes, signaling uneventful recording. Mark 02 shows clamp release to allow better reposition and surgery continuation

valleys" in different colors: black (delta), red (theta), blue (alfa), and violet (beta). SEF was included, with 95% marking superior limit of the spectral energy. Lastly, an amplitude asymmetry index (AAI) was included [7] (Figs. 10.10 and 10.11). CSA may be substituted for the format density spectral array (DSA). Monitor seemed very useful and fully entered our routine. It is well known that spectral analysis does not allow wave morphology definition, but the classical EEG waves are always available, so the clinical neurophysiologist may be very comfortable.

Electroencephalogram has a high sensitivity, complexity, and variability requiring a complex and dynamic visual analysis on the surgical setting using the classical

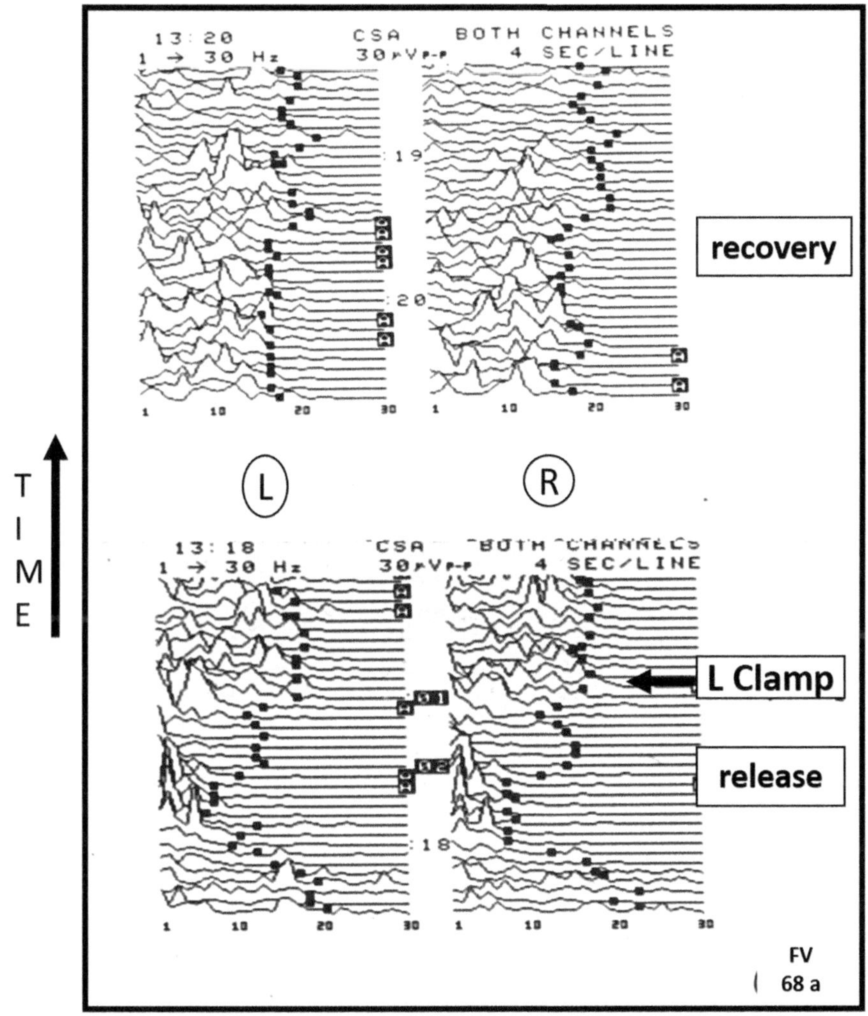

Fig. 10.9 Left and right CSA EEG recording; time goes up in these graphs. Inferior graph mark 01 signals left carotid artery clamping: after a few seconds bilateral intense amplitude reduction is noted, soon followed by huge slow delta waves. CSA EEG shows bilateral and intense ischemic changes, demonstrating left carotid importance for both hemispheres. Mark 02 indicates quick release after 28 seconds, determined by the intensity of the alteration. Left artery was important for both hemispheres! Even after the clamp release, during many seconds there is a clear bilateral attenuation. Upper graph shows amplitude recovery with predominant slow wave activity and progressive installation of a normal EEG under anesthesia. Shunt installation was of fundamental importance to continue the surgery

XY graphic. This information can be *complemented* by signal processing, and the goal of these methods is to make the intraoperative EEG monitoring a more objective and reliable technique.

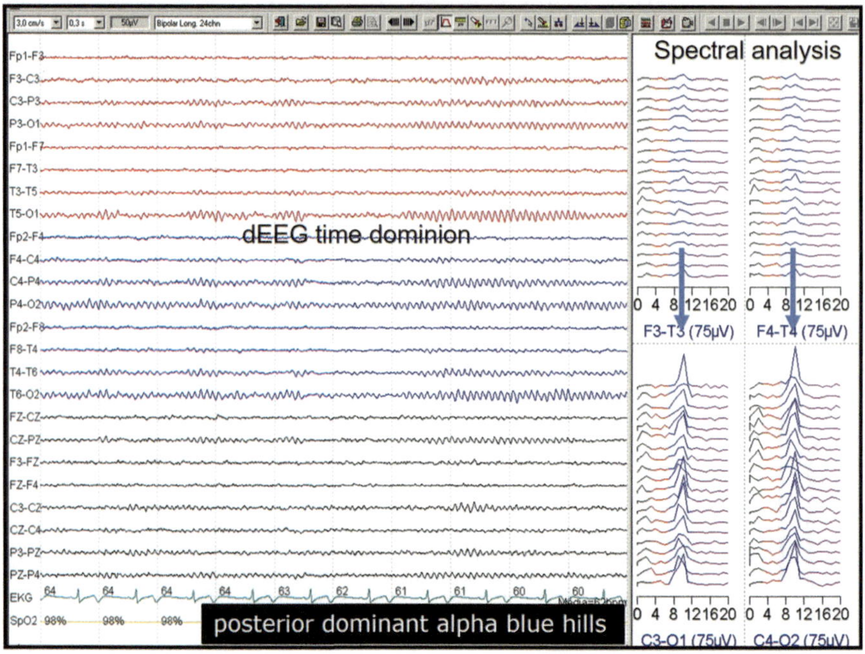

Fig. 10.10 EEG page demonstrating simultaneous acquisition of raw EEG (time dominion) and CSA spectral analysis; the patient is awake showing alpha blue hills posterior dominant (blue arrows). This is not a surgery example and was inserted to reinforce the interpretation advantages of seeing classical EEG curves. It is not recommended to use only processed EEG signals; Wave morphology is preserved in raw EEG

With the numbers generated by the ADC, many different quantitative formats can be developed, but its discussion is beyond the purpose of this chapter. Nevertheless, classical EEG is the golden standard for monitoring some surgeries, and the presence of automated trends can be useful in supplementing raw EEG analysis, even in providing some relevant numerical data, capable of detecting subtle interhemispheric asymmetries [8, 9]. In summary, these formats may aggregate to the analysis, but they don't substitute the raw EEG.

It is important to discuss the BIS (bispectral index) that utilizes a processed parameter to help surgery monitoring and substituting classical EEG. It depends on "coherency" measurement and numerically states different degrees of clinical correlation; the proposed indexes are: 90–100 awaken, 70–90 light-to-moderate sedation, 60–70 superficial anesthesia, 45–60 adequate anesthesia, and 0–45 deep anesthesia. We agree that BIS may be helpful to indicate anesthesia level in non-neurologic patients, prompting shorter surgery times and awakenings, also reducing patient hospital permanence. Nevertheless, there is no discussion if it is successful in children and younger patients, when the EEG has not acquired its mature patterns. Additionally, its application to old age patients whose distinctions to adult

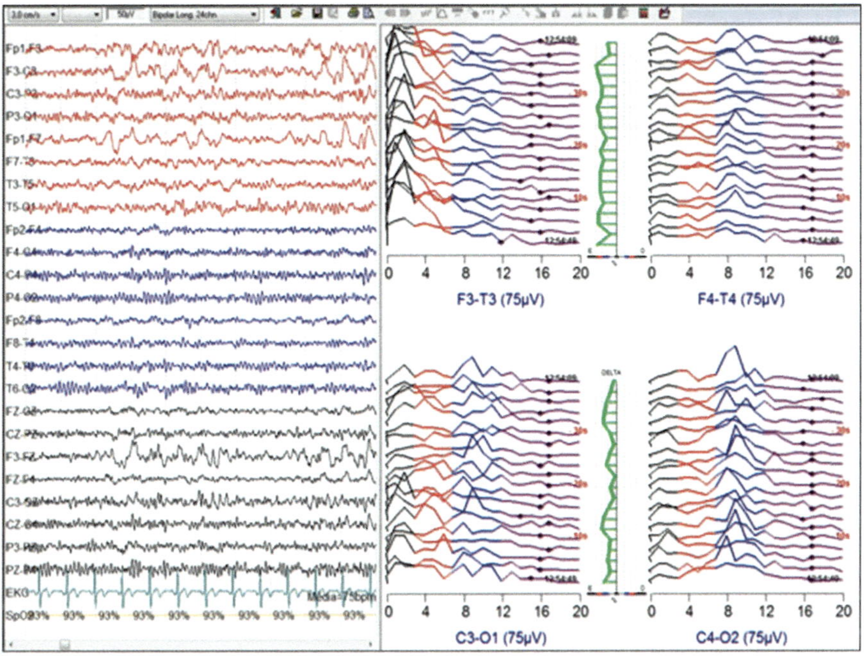

Fig. 10.11 Left graph: compressed raw EEG showing asymmetry, normal in the right hemisphere channels (blue lines), and abnormal, with many slow waves delta and theta range, in the left hemisphere (red lines); the EEG black lines represent z line electrodes recording. Right graph: compressed spectral array (CSA) depicting four channel quadrant spectral analysis, comparing left and right anterior and posterior region; montage [F3-T3, C3-O1, F4-T4, C4-O2]. Frequencies are colors separated: more delta and theta activity on the left (black and red) easily compared to the right side; SEFs (black dots in every line) indicate 90% of the spectral energy to its left. The asymmetry is easier to note with the vertical green line (Amplitude Asymmetry Index), showing clear shift to the left, more important for the anterior channels

population are not accompanied by any modification of the proposed indexes is not detailed. In our opinion, the major BIS drawback is the employment of only one frontal channel; even if new BIS systems are able to show a raw frontal EEG view, it is impossible to even imagine EEG curves over both hemispheres, either considering 16 or 8 channels [10].

EEG Analysis in the Operating Room

Ideally, whenever possible, a routine EEG should be performed before the surgery day. Reasons: a normal EEG will give us the sensation that even light alterations could be valorized; on the contrary, abnormalities, when present, will help to delineate the monitoring protocol, even participating the information to the surgeon. The

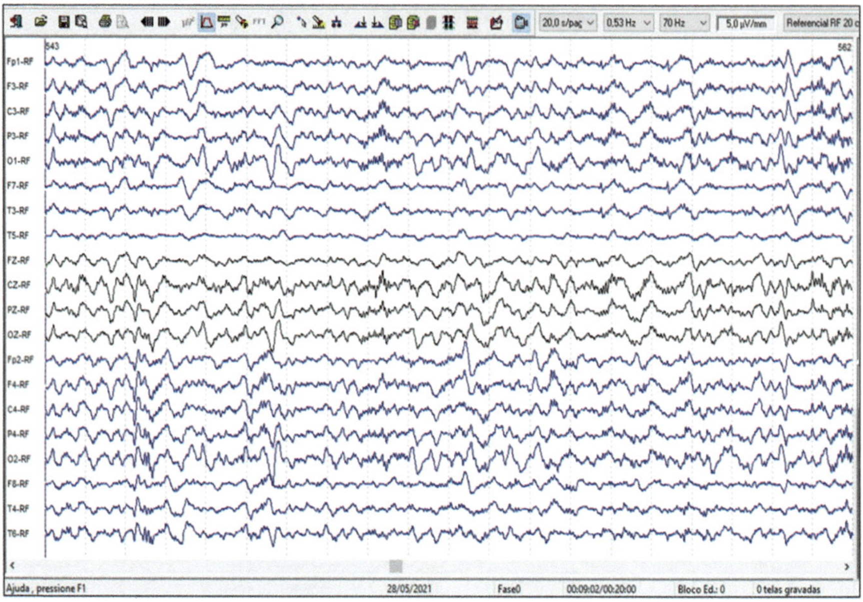

Fig. 10.12 EEG page of an anesthetized stabilized adult patient, showing slow waves and fast rhythms, using dexmedetomidina 5 ml/hour

complexities of EEG signals, with variations either normal (patient age) or abnormal (previous pathology), must be considered in the operation theater.

Secondly, the EEG will be submitted to the action of drugs (anesthesia) and will be interpreted as a basal recording, acting like a model to observe future and eventual alterations. Different agents may produce variable EEG patterns. EEG changes, including burst suppression and even generalized depression, may occur, notably with halogenated agents. It is also important to state that drugs influence the cortical EEG more than subcortical evoked potentials (Fig. 10.12).

Anesthesia complexity evolved with sub-specialization in neuro-anesthesia through expertise in clinical neurology and cerebral physiology, orienting anesthetic technique choices. Since anesthetic agents affect both EEG and evoked potentials, the neurophysiologist should understand the principles that dictate their choices and concentration. Some requests aiming to facilitate neurophysiological monitoring may drastically alter the anesthetic plan, so it is important that the neurophysiologist understands the role of the anesthetist. The goals of the anesthesia are: (1) amnesia; (2) analgesia; (3) unconsciousness, and (4) obtundation of noxious reflexes. These goals are met by a combination of intravenous agents, inhalational anesthetic gases, and somatic muscle relaxants. Since the level of surgical stimulation varies throughout the operation, the anesthetic level and the administered drugs may vary constantly [11]. Anesthetic strategy must be in consonance with the surgical proceedings, and in good harmony with intraoperative neurophysiologic monitoring methods. Inhalational agents, depending on their concentration, the patient's age, and surgical strategy may even be impeditive of the monitoring, particularly focusing on composed muscle action potentials (CMAP). The same difficulties apply to neuromuscular blocking agents, preventing muscle activity recording during electromyography or CMAP monitoring. The importance of good communication and adequate teamwork must be reemphasized at the surgical theater, all working in the best interest of the patient.

We remember arriving to the surgical room, with the patient already anesthetized, and the installed EEG showed burst suppression, a condition most unfavorable to monitor; a drug change was recommended to continue the monitoring. During the surgery, it is also challenging to deal with the complex variability of different surgical times and processes. EEG analysis requires proper training and expertise to be correctly performed. This may include the definition of how many electrodes, which montage will be preferred, always considering the surgical-proposed strategy.

Intraoperative EEG: Interesting Patterns Deserving Discussion

Normal background activity usually appears during stabilized general anesthesia, showing a composition of slow waves (mainly theta) with fast frequencies in the beta range. The EEG may change after anesthetic induction, discovering light asymmetries (Fig. 10.12).

Unexpected awakening: This EEG looks desynchronized, with lower amplitude, and higher frequency patterns such as beta, together with muscle activity and eye movements as artifacts.

Epileptiform activity/seizures: Interictal paroxysmal spikes or sharp waves may sometimes be detected during the surgical monitoring, but don't imply the necessity to change the process. Differently, the occurrence of epileptic seizures imposes immediate treatment and interferes with the surgery. The electroencephalographer is entitled to advert the anesthetist of an impending seizure risk, which may be characterized by an increasing number of rhythmic sharp waves. However, epileptic seizure incidence is low, even in patients submitted to electrical transcranial or direct cortical and subcortical electrical stimulation [12, 13].

There are some patterns that may occur during the surgery and deserve further discussion:

- Experimental evidence suggests that when cerebral blood flow (CBF) falls under 25–30 ml/100 g/min, the EEG starts to demonstrate frontally localized fast frequency reduction. When hypoperfusion goes under 18–25 ml/100 g/min, there is an increase of slow wave activity, beginning with theta, and moving to slower delta in the 12–18 ml/100 g/min range. EEG depression and electrocerebral silence occur with CBF under 10–12 ml/100 g/min, accompanied by cell membrane disruption [14] (Figs. 10.9 and 10.11).

- EEG and CBF correlation allows for a therapeutic intervention window comprising initial CBF reduction and EEG first alteration, always taking great care to avoid cell death. Its importance is highlighted whenever patient clinical observation is limited, such as the case for anesthetized surgical situations. Anesthesia depth can, when profound, make the recognition of focal or generalized ischemic abnormalities much more difficult. Other neuromonitoring modalities, like somatosensory evoked potentials, motor evoked potentials, and transcranial Doppler, may collaborate with cerebral perfusion and cerebrovascular hemodynamic status evaluation, each within its own limitation.

Generalized slowing: Diffuse hemisphere involvement, both cortical and subcortical, either structural or metabolic, shows delta polymorphic activity, probably caused by subcortical association fibers lesion [15], together with fast frequency attenuation. This pattern may be observed at the end of cardiac surgeries with extracorporeal circulation, correlating to diffuse encephalopathy and postoperative systemic inflammatory response [16] (Fig. 10.13).

Burst suppression: EEG pattern showing periods of relative flattening or inactivity intermixed with bursts of higher-amplitude slow and sharp waves, which may represent complete thalamocortical disconnection [17]. During surgery monitoring burst suppression may be caused by anesthetic drug overdose, mainly after bolus, and can be correlated to systemic arterial hypotension or deep hypothermia (Figs. 10.6 and 10.14). The association of EEG intraoperative suppression and systemic arterial hypotension may be correlated to postoperative increased mortality [18, 19].

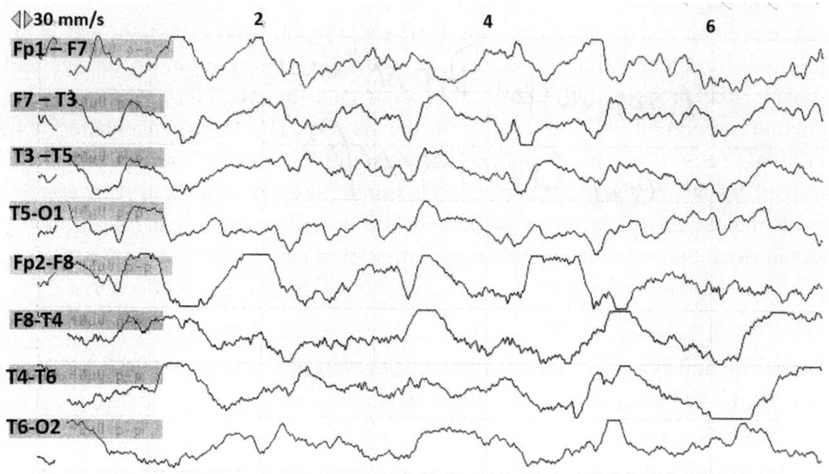

Fig. 10.13 Abnormal generalized EEG pattern showing polymorphic slow waves at the end of cardiac surgery

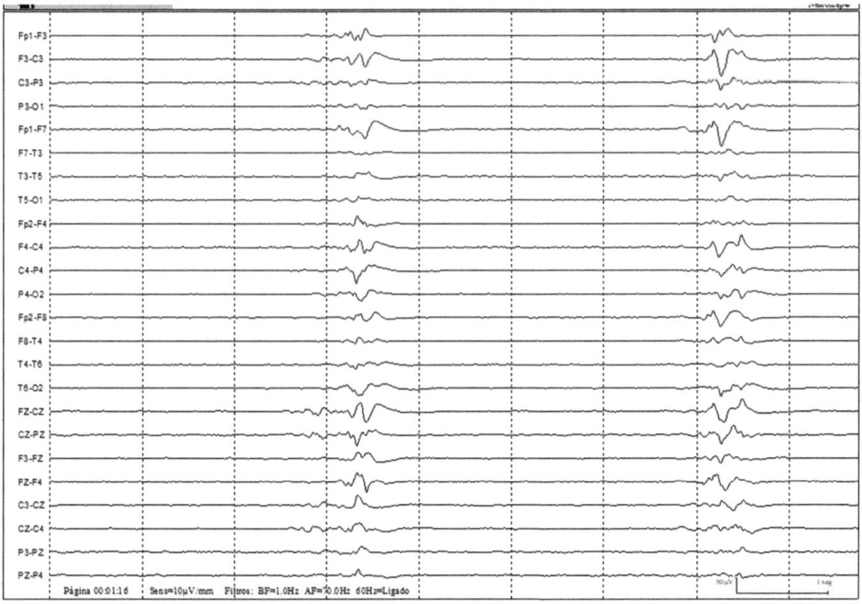

Fig. 10.14 Bilateral, synchronous, and symmetric burst suppression pattern, observed during deep anesthetic level caused by thiopental

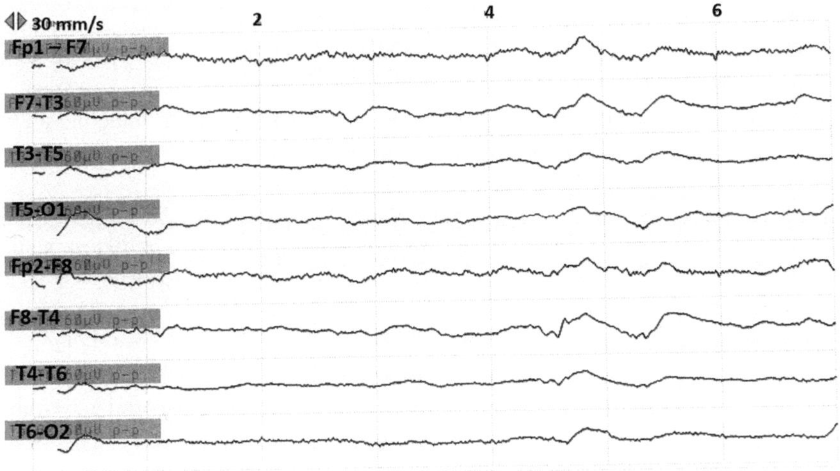

Fig. 10.15 EEG abnormal generalized of bilateral attenuation and slowing

Bilateral and generalized attenuation: It may be characterized as a more severe burst suppression pattern with continuous or very prolonged depression, which may correlate to cerebral vascular collapse, anesthetic overdose, or electrocerebral inactivity induced by deep hypothermia, such as during aorta surgery with circulatory arrest (Figs. 10.9 and 10.15).

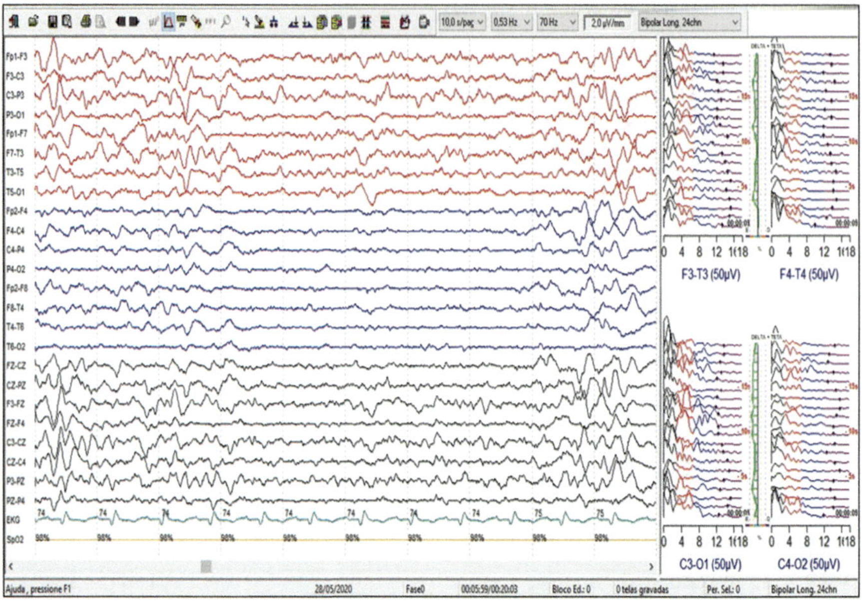

Fig. 10.16 A 78-year-old patient immediate postoperative day of large right temporo-parietal hematoma with uncus herniation; fentanil 5 ml/h + propofol 20 ml/h. EEG asymmetrical burst suppression, more intense in the right hemisphere. ICP 11 mmHg

Interhemispheric asymmetry: Significative when showing a reduction of more than 50% of the fast frequencies in one of the cerebral hemispheres [15]. In some procedures in which the perfusion defcit worsens, we can obseve an increment of slow waves is seen, and with further increasing a depression installs affecting all the frequencies, evolving with irreversible neuronal lesion [1] (Figs. 10.11 and 10.16).

Carotid endarterectomy: It is very important to ascertain with the surgeon which is the involved side; besides, every information regarding preop circulatory status, mainly the collateral circulation, must be considered. In the surgery, EEG is considered a good monitor, noninvasive and continuous, presenting no risks. The asymmetrical interhemisphere pattern observed after shunt placement (carotid clamping test) may represent a fundamental indication for vascular shunt installation. With stabilized anesthesia and paCO2 levels, EEG showed accuracy to correlate intraoperative CBF measuring with postoperative neurological function and impose shunt colocation [20] (Figs. 10.8 and 10.9).

Discussion on monitoring methods for carotid endarterectomy: Many years ago, a vascular surgeon insisted that EEG was not necessary – distal stump pressure had all the necessary information. After some EEGs were made, he admitted EEG's importance.

Years later transcranial Doppler (TCD) was associated with EEG in carotid surgies, to study clamping effects, but not many association cases were available to allow a definite conclusion; our opinion: the association was useful, mostly after surgery flow restoration, when TCD could demonstrate some "blips" embolus (micro embolic signals), not apparent on the EEG. These emboli were attributed to small surgery debris that did not interfere with patient evolution.

There are also possible contributions of somatosensory median nerve evoked potentials (SSEP) to carotid surgery monitoring, on the basis that SSEP is better than EEG for subcortical monitoring, since EEG represents mainly cortical activity. In our experience, the most important surgery risk is the carotid clamping, for which a waiting time of 1–2 minutes is determined. EEG has the advantage of bringing continuous information. On the contrary, a classical SSEP protocol suggests 500 stimuli averaging at a frequency of 4.7 Hz; each evoked response has an implicit time delay of 106.38 seconds, almost 2 minutes! Even reducing the averaging stimuli number, this information is discontinuous. SSEP advantage is to be associated with EEG, then representing cortico-subcortical monitoring.

Cardiac surgery: It may determine brain lesion basically through three different mechanisms, hypoperfusion, embolization, and systemic inflammatory response whose magnitude is dependent on and secondary to the ischemic aggression. Cerebral hemorrhagic complications are rare during cardiac surgery.

Hypoperfusion may be regional or generalized, pending on collateral circulation both intra- and extracranial of patients that usually have previous vascular disease and compromised vascular autoregulation, defining the necessity to individually optimize the cerebral perfusion pressure, which can be attained with the help of continuous EEG. Vascular transition areas are more prone to ischemic hypoperfusion, and these areas are represented by the transition between anterior and media cerebral arteries, and by the transition among superficial and deep media cerebral artery rami.

A major source of micro-emboli is debris originating in aorta canulation [21], and particles coming from extracorporeal circulation equipment, easily detected by continous transcranial Doppler (TCD).

Electroencephalographic alterations at the end of the surgery correlates well with generalized slowing and attenuation pattern, postoperative encephalopathy [22], and the intensity of systemic inflammatory response. The load of microembolization signals TCD detected may also correlate to systemic inflammatory response observed 24 hours after extracorporeal circulation ending [23].

IOM Documentation

An intraoperative neuromonitoring log is made after every surgery, and one of the IOM main goals is represented by medicolegal recording of neurophysiological events during surgery.

This report must contemplate patient demographic data, hospital information, time of the day, proceeding's duration, clinical diagnosis, surgery type, neurophysiological techniques used, as well as eventual surgery problems together with corrective strategy used, and the corresponding results. Events recording graphics should be available, and the final document printed to be sent to the surgeon and medical records.

Conclusion

EEG's objective is to reduce or avoid neurological injury, thus contributing to safety. EEG conveys valuable advantages in intraoperative monitoring: it is noninvasive and continuous and shows a good correlation with changes in CBF and metabolic activity, allowing fast intervention; it represents a method coherent with the dynamic of eventual variables during a surgical intervention.

It is important to correlate the EEG observed patterns with surgical processes and anesthetic conduct, being able, as neurophysiologists, to deliver sound and precise real-time alert information, letting the surgeon change or maintain his strategy. We have always to remember that an isolated EEG alteration, without the clinical correlate, will not identify the cause, the same way that hypotension may be derived from bleeding or vasodilation.

EEG monitoring belongs to multimodal monitoring context, and information gathered from other neurophysiological methods, together with hemodynamical variation, body temperature, hemoglobin level, ventilation parameters, anesthetic report, and systemic dysfunctions; and all these variables need to be focused by the neurophysiologist, who must be team integrated. We believe that only by utilizing this full cooperation, the IOM may have a positive impact in the prognosis.

References

1. Ebersole J. Cortical generators and EEG voltage fields. In: Ebersole JS, Pedley TM, editors. Current practice of clinical electroencephalography. 3rd ed. New York: Lippincott Williams and Wilkins; 2003. p. 12–31.
2. Heuser D, Guggenberger H. Ionic changes in brain ischaemia and alterations produced by drugs. Br J Anaesth. 1985;57:23–33. https://doi.org/10.1093/bja/57.1.23.
3. Connolly MB, Sharbrough FW, Wong PK. Electrical fields and recording techniques. In: Ebersole JS, Pedley TA, editors. Current practice of clinical electroencephalography. 3rd ed. Lippincott Williams &Wilkins; 2003. p. 72–99.
4. Klem GH. Artifacts. In: Ebersole JS, Pedley TA, editors. Current practice of clinical electroencephalography. 3rd ed. Lippincott Williams &Wilkins; 2003. p. 271–87.
5. Rampil IJ. A primer for EEG signal processing in anesthesia. Anesthesiology. 1998;89:980–1002.
6. Archibald JE. Changes in EEG/CSA seen during carotid endarterectomy intraoperative monitoring: EEG, vol. 2. American Society of Electroneurodiagnostic Technologist, Inc; 1996. p. 20–42.

7. Luccas FJC, Bártolo T, Silva NL, Cavenaghi B. Clinical electroencephalogram (EEG) evaluation is improved by the amplitude asymmetry index. Arq Neuropsiquiatr. 2016;74(7):536–43.
8. Vespa PM, Nuwer MR, Juhász C, Alexander M, Nenov V, Martin N, Becker DP. Early detection of vasospasm after acute subarachnoid hemorrhage using continuous EEG ICU monitoring. Electroencephalogr Clin Neurophysiol. 1997;103:607–15. https://doi.org/10.1016/S0013-4694(97)00071-0.
9. Heyer E, Adams D, Moses C, et al. Erroneous conclusion from processed electroencephalogram with changing anesthetic depth. Anesthesiology. 2000;92:603e7.
10. Nunes RR, Chaves IMM, de Alencar JCG, Franco SB, de Oliveira YGBR, de Menezes DGA. Bispectral index and other processed parameters of electroencephalogram: an update. Braz J Anesthesiol. 2012;62(1):105–17. https://doi.org/10.1016/S0034-7094(12)70109-5.
11. McPherson RW. Neuroanesthesia and intraoperative neurological monitoring. In: Niedermeyer E, da Silva FL, editors. Electroencephalography. Basic principles, clinical applications, and related fields. 4th ed. Lippincott Williams & Wilkins; 1999. p. 1092–106.
12. Ulkatan S, Jaramillo AM, Téllez MJ, Kim J, Deletis V, Seidel K. Incidence of intraoperative seizures during motor evoked potential monitoring in a large cohort of patients undergoing different surgical procedures. JNS. 2017;126:1296–302. https://doi.org/10.3171/2016.4.JNS151264.
13. MacDonald DB. Safety of intraoperative transcranial electrical stimulation motor evoked potential monitoring. J Clin Neurophysiol. 2002;19:416–29. https://doi.org/10.1097/00004691-200210000-00005.
14. Schneider AL, Jordan KG. Regional Attenuation WithOut Delta (RAWOD): a distinctive EEG pattern that can aid in the diagnosis and management of severe acute ischemic stroke. Am J Electroneurodiagnostic Technol. 2005;45:102–17. https://doi.org/10.1080/1086508X.2005.11079517.
15. Gloor P, Ball G, Schaul N. Brain lesions that produce delta waves in the EEG. Neurology. 1977:326–33.
16. Luccas FJC, Cibils D, Zanovello JF. III Latin-American Chapter Congress of IFCN and IX Brazilian Symposium of Clinical Neurophysiology, Porto Seguro, Bahia, Brazil, 11–14 September 2002. Clin Neurophysiol. 2003;114:154–65. https://doi.org/10.1016/S1388-2457(02)00341-3.
17. Steriade M, Amzica F, Contreras D. Cortical and thalamic cellular correlates of electroencephalographic burst-suppression. Electroencephalogr Clin Neurophysiol. 1994;90:1–16.
18. Willingham M, Ben Abdallah A, Gradwohl S, Helsten D, Lin N, Villafranca A, Jacobsohn E, Avidan M, Kaiser H. Association between intraoperative electroencephalographic suppression and postoperative mortality ‡. Br J Anaesth. 2014;113:1001–8. https://doi.org/10.1093/bja/aeu105.
19. Watson PL, Shintani AK, Tyson R, Pandharipande PP, Pun BT, Ely EW. Presence of electroencephalogram burst suppression in sedated, critically ill patients is associated with increased mortality. Crit Care Med. 2008;36:3171–7.
20. Sundt TM, Sharbrough FW, Anderson RE, Michenfelder JD. Cerebral blood flow measurements and electroencephalograms during carotid endarterectomy. JNS. 2007;107:887–97. https://doi.org/10.3171/JNS-07/10/0887.
21. Hogue CW, Sundt TM, Goldberg M, Barner H, Dàvila-Román VG. Neurological complications of cardiac surgery: the need for new paradigms in prevention and treatment. Semin Thorac Cardiovasc Surg. 1999;11:105–15. https://doi.org/10.1016/S1043-0679(99)70003-1.
22. MLAF M, HTFM M-F, FJC L, Fagundes FE. Predictive Value of Continuous Intraoperative Electroencephalographic Monitoring (CEEGM) in Neurological Complication During Open Heart Surgery (OHS). In: American Academy of Neurology Annual Meeting, vol. 54. San Diego: Neurology; 2000. p. A131.
23. Mendonca MLAF, Bezerra DC, Gomes RV, Rouge A, Fagundes FE, Prado IC, Mattos AC, Mendonça-Filho HTFM. High loads of microembolic signals and electroencephalographic attenuation are associated with increased inflammatory markers following heart surgery. In: American Academy of Neurology Annual Meeting. San Diego; 2006.

Chapter 11
Electromyography

Francisco Tellechea Rotta, Carlo Domênico Marrone, and Ana Maria Hoppe

Abbreviations

EMG	Electromyography
IOM	Intraoperative neurophysiologic monitoring
SED	Suprasegmentally induced EMG discharge

Introduction

Electromyography (EMG) was incorporated into intraoperative neurophysiologic monitoring (IOM) initially in cerebellopontine angle tumor surgeries as a tool to identify the facial nerve and prevent its injury [1]. Currently both free-run and stimulus triggered EMG are used, as part of multimodal neurophysiological monitoring, in procedures in which cranial nerves, peripheral nerves, or nerve roots are at risk

F. T. Rotta (✉)
Intercoastal Medical Group, Sarasota, FL, USA
e-mail: rotta.francisco@intercoastalmedical.com, frotta@intercoastalmedical.com

C. D. Marrone
Brazilian Clinical Neurophysiology Society, Porto Alegre, RS, Brazil

Intraoperative Neurophysiological Monitoring, Department Coordinator of Hospital da Criança Santo Antônio, Porto Alegre, RS, Brazil

Universidade Federal de Ciências da Saúde de Porto Alegre - UFCSPA, Porto Alegre, RS, Brazil

Clínica Marrone, Clinical Neurophysiology, Porto Alegre, RS, Brazil

A. M. Hoppe
Department of Neurophysiology, Santa Casa de Misericórdia de Porto Alegre, Porto Alegre, RS, Brazil

S. M. Verst et al. (eds.), *Intraoperative Monitoring*,
https://doi.org/10.1007/978-3-030-95730-8_11

of being injured [2]. More recently, the role of continuous EMG in central nervous system surgeries has also been studied, which we will discuss later in this chapter.

Concepts of EMG in IOM

EMG refers to the graphic representation of muscle fiber electric activity identified as difference of electrical potential between a pair of electrodes, one considered the active and the other the reference. Muscle fiber depolarization is captured by the active electrode as a negative charge in relation to the reference and causes an upward graphic deflection. Subsequent hyperpolarization turns the active electrode positive in relation to the reference and causes a downward deflection of the tracing. Diagnostic EMG performed outside the operating room uses intramuscular needle electrodes (either concentric bipolar or monopolar plus a separate reference electrode). It aims to record the single fiber muscle activity such as fibrillation potentials and positive sharp waves, or depolarization of a whole motor units such as fasciculation potentials and motor unit action potentials [3]. In IOM, electrodes record the activity of individual or groups of motor units during the procedure either continuously (free run – fEMG) or by triggered stimulus (tEMG).

fEMG detects spontaneously evoked muscle activities throughout the surgery, with graphic and, if necessary, audible representation. Discharges may result from several surgical maneuvers (such as traction, thermal, mechanical, or metabolic injury), incomplete muscle relaxation (as in cases of superficial sedation), or chronic denervation, as in cases of previous radiculopathies. Its great advantages include not interfering with the surgical field (by not inducing patient movement) and allowing real-time feedback, correlating with operative stages and maneuvers [4].

tEMG consists of applying a stimulus directly to the nerves or roots to generate a muscle action potential in the muscles of corresponding myotome. It can also be used for stimulation of fibrous or tumoral structures adjacent to a nerve at risk, identifying its proximity when direct visualization is impaired [4].

Since intraoperative EMG monitoring is not dependent on central nervous system activity, it is not affected by general anesthesia. On the other hand, the use of neuromuscular blocking agents is a limiting factor. A short acting or reversible agent may be used during intubation or in noncritical moments of the surgery, when monitoring is not necessary. In this case, obtaining a train-of-four response is useful to confirm that neuromuscular blocking has been reversed before monitoring data can be accurately interpreted. Despite that, as EMG is part of a multimodal monitoring system, anesthesia requirements for the other neurophysiological modalities used should be respected [5].

EMG Electrodes

Different types of electrodes may be used for EMG recording. The choice is based on the region and type of recording being monitored [6]. They are placed in (or in close proximity to) muscles innervated by the nerves/roots of interest. Subdermal and intramuscular monopolar needles are most used, with the ideal needle length varying with muscle depth and size.

Surface Electrodes

Surface electrodes are placed on the skin, with the active electrode ideally over the muscle motor point, the area where neuromuscular junctions are concentrated and where the smallest electric current can induce muscle contraction [7]. Localization of motor points of frequently recorded muscles during IOM is identified in Chap. 3. The reference electrode is placed over the tendon or an electric neutral area. Surface electrodes have a large recording area, which improves sampling, so depolarization of a small number of motor units may be detected. Unfortunately, as contamination from nearby muscle activity may occur, there is a decreased specificity especially when dealing with small muscles. This is of particular importance when monitoring cranial nerves, as overlap of muscles innervated by different nerves makes it difficult to properly identify the nerve at risk.

Surface electrodes have a higher impedance and skin and subcutaneous tissue act as a low-pass filter, distorting the muscle signals recorded and impairing the ability to evaluate the morphology of motor unit action potentials. In IOM, surface electrodes may be useful for recording compound muscle action potentials from limb muscles, either from transcranial or motor root/nerve stimulation. Another specific use of surface electrodes is monitoring thyroarytenoid muscle activity recording from electrodes placed in the external surface of an endotracheal tube [8].

Subdermal and Intramuscular Electrodes: Bare/Insulated Needles and Hook Wires

Subdermal needle electrodes (Fig. 11.1) are widely used and have a variable exposed recording tip of 10–50 mm in length. Unlike surface electrodes, the recorded signal

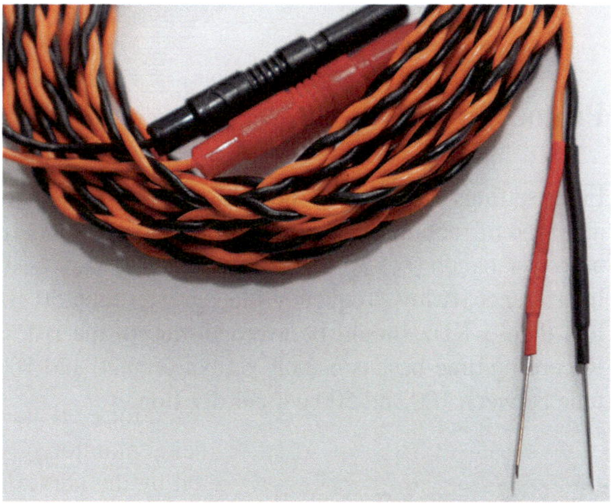

Fig. 11.1 Pair of subdermal needle electrodes

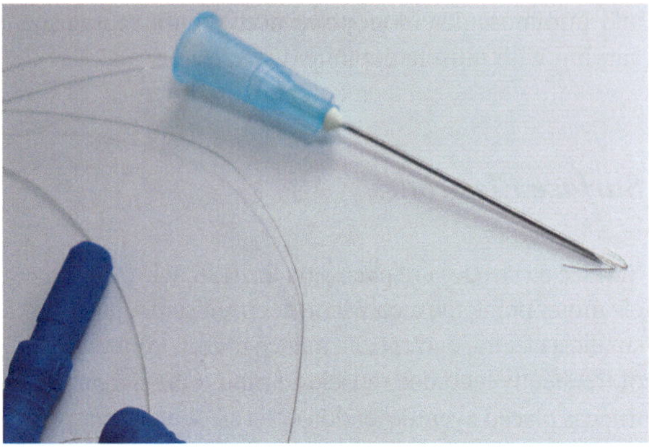

Fig. 11.2 Hook wire electrodes

is little affected by tissue filtering effect. Their exposed surfaces capture electric signals from the sampling area. Both motor unit action potentials and compound muscle action potentials can be recorded, and it is used to register "free run" or evoked activity from most muscles monitored intraoperatively. Subcutaneous needle recordings are less specific when dealing with deep muscles or patients with abundant subcutaneous tissue. In these cases, a longer needle length can be used.

Because of their size and proximity to each other, cranial nerve innervated muscle activity should be registered with needle electrodes that have a smaller recording area, decreasing the risk of capturing activity from adjacent muscles. In this case, subdermal needle electrodes or hook wires are useful. For more details on this subject, refer to Chap. 21.

Hook wires consist of a pair of insulated wires, with an exposed tip of 0.5–2 mm, that are placed intramuscularly using a hypodermic needle (Fig. 11.2). The small recording area limits their usefulness in larger muscles, where activation of distant motor units may go undetected.

Muscle recording is commonly done with both active and reference electrodes in the same muscle for selective root identification. The placement of electrodes in different muscles (gastrocnemius and tibialis anterior, for example) does not allow the precise location of the abnormal activity and should not be used in surgeries that require greater recording specificity [9].

Protocol

Filter settings are variable, depending on the characteristics of the recorded wave and type of recording electrode. A wide band of 2 Hz–5000 Hz may be used, but narrower bands (i.e. 30–50 Hz to 3000 Hz) may be necessary to reduce baseline interference. A low-frequency filter greater than 50 Hz and a high-frequency filter less than 3 KHz should be avoided, due to the risk of distorting potentials [10]. Recording time-base is usually set between 20 and 100 ms per division and amplitude between 100 and 500 μV per division.

EMG parameters vary according to the technique in use: for fEMG time-base is commonly kept between 100 and 200 ms, so that the duration of a continuous discharge is readily detected. Thus, the duration of a continuous discharge is readily detected (sustained responses can last for seconds), as well as an abrupt or gradual onset, the interval between bursts and spikes and the persistence after interruption of surgical maneuvers. The time-base can be reduced (20 ms) after the detection of discharges (with image freezing) for better visualization of the morphology and firing frequency of each motor potential [2, 4, 9, 10].

In tEMG, potentials are triggered and appear on screen with the same latency after each stimulus. The latency of potentials after stimulation of cranial nerves may be less than 10 ms and may reach 20–30 ms for lower limbs distal muscles. Therefore, the time-base cannot be the same used in fEMG and varies from around 3 ms/div for face to 7–10 ms/div for limbs.

When recording peripheral nerve potentials (NAP), bot stimulation and recording are performed in the nerve itself and not in the muscle, with a smaller distance between stimulating and recording electrodes and no synaptic delay. For those reasons, a sweep of 0.5 ms/div may be needed for potentials to be detected on screen. More details about this technique will be described in Chap. 31.

Role in IOM

Free-Run EMG

The use of fEMG is well established in peripheral nerve, spine, cauda equina, and skull base surgeries. Any procedure that requires manipulation or dissection of a nerve (nucleus or axon) or root will be more safely performed with EMG.

Recording can be done in any somatic muscle, including extraocular, intercostal, abdominal wall, anal sphincter – the choice of muscles depending on surgery type and location. In addition to the specific role of protecting nervous structures, it also helps with general information about the surgical environment and the patient's clinical status by demonstrating possible ambient noise, artifacts, impedance changes, electrode displacement, anesthetic depth assessment, and neuromuscular blockage.

Mechanical stimulation or injury to a motor nerve may elicit an EMG discharge in its innervated muscles. This is observed in the free-run recording as either transient or sustained discharges. Transient discharges are referred to as spikes (depolarization of only one motor unit) or bursts (depolarization of multiple motor units) [11]. They are caused by increased ionic channel conductance induced by membrane stretching that do not indicate nerve injury but are useful to alert the surgeon that an area near the motor nerve is being manipulated [12]. Chronically compressed or partially injured nerves have a decreased threshold for mechanical stimulation and may depolarize with distant tissue manipulation and even spontaneously. The

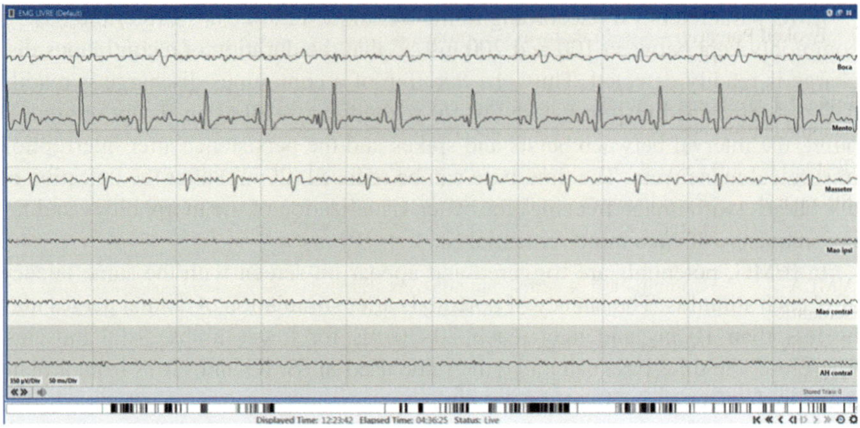

Fig. 11.3 Train of EMG discharges in facial muscles during posterior fossa surgery

neurophysiologist needs to know how to identify these discharges, using this information in conjunction with the knowledge of surgical technique and critical moments, to avoid alarming the surgeon unnecessarily.

Repetitive discharges of one or multiple motor units that are sustained after stimulus cessation are called trains or neurotonic discharges and may last from seconds to several minutes (Fig. 11.3). Trains of discharges are signs of a stronger mechanical stimulus that is causing some degree of nerve fiber injury. The duration of the repetitive discharges may correlate with the degree of nerve irritation and risk of nerve injury [13]. On the other hand, not all neurotonic discharges indicate nerve damage. In spinal surgery, Gunnarsson et al. found neurotonic EMG signals to be 100% sensitive but only 23.7% specific in predicting postoperative paralysis [14].

Free-run EMG monitoring is most useful to record facial nerve innervated muscle activity during posterior fossa surgery. In this setting, different types of sustained discharges have been identified and referred to as A, B, and C trains. A trains, consisting of sinusoidal waves of variable frequency and amplitude with abrupt onset and ending, correlate best with facial nerve injury. Romstock et al. found a sensitivity of 86% and a specificity of 89% for the A train to predict facial nerve injury [11]. This will be further discussed in Chap. 21.

It is noteworthy that this high sensitivity is only achieved with recording in several channels simultaneously, increasing the chance of recording neurotonic responses in time to prevent postoperative injuries, since they can occur in only one muscle or channel. Romstock et al. recommend at least 3 muscles for facial monitoring [11]. Most muscles in the upper and lower limbs receive innervation from more than one root (adjacent roots), so a precise location of the level in case of neurotonic discharges is only possible with the recording of multiple muscles simultaneously [2].

The firing frequency of motor units correlates with the degree of irritation and risk of postoperative injury. Continuous discharges (firing of one or more motor unit with interferential pattern) of high frequency (30 Hz for up to 200 Hz) and prolonged duration (milliseconds to several seconds), when associated with risky maneuvers (traction, cauterization, dissection), indicate intense irritation with greater risk of injury. This risk increases if the activity persists after stopping the maneuver [15]. Bursts are less than 200 ms in duration and consist of single or multiple MUPs firing at 30–100 Hz. They appear as single or multiple repetitive bursts and are typically elicited by touching, rubbing, traction, or other mechanical manipulations of the nerve [4, 11].

Recently, sparse and continuous muscle discharges in fEMG have been described in spinal cord and central nervous system surgeries. These activities are considered possible signs of mechanical irritation of the corticospinal tract, with consequent depolarization of the anterior horn and generation of motor unit potentials in the limbs. As they do not represent direct nerve or root irritation, they are called suprasegmentally induced EMG discharge (SED) and defined as potentials recorded in the contralateral limb during the manipulation of motor pathways in the brain or at least two levels below surgical spinal manipulation. Skinner et al. graded these discharges into mild and severe and demonstrated that the appearance of severe SEDs may precede the drop in transcranial motor potential, being potentially useful as a warning criterion for the interruption or modification of spinal decompression [16].

Triggered EMG

Electric stimulation triggered EMG (Fig. 11.4) is helpful in identifying proximity to motor nerves or roots, either during surgical dissection or the placement of pedicle screws in spinal surgery. With monopolar or bipolar stimulators, the cathode depolarizes the nerve axons, and a compound muscle action potential (CMAP) is captured in the correspondent muscle. Direct stimulation of intact cranial or peripheral nerves may be achieved with as little as 0.05 mA to 2 mA currents, with a constant pulse duration between 100 and 200 ms. Most important is the charge delivered in milicoulomb (mC) since it correlates with neurological damage and is affected by current spread. Delivered charge is calculated by multiplying current (I, in mA) by the duration of the pulse (D, in msec): $Q = I \times D$ [17]. In contrast to their increased susceptibility for spontaneous discharge, partially injured nerves may require higher

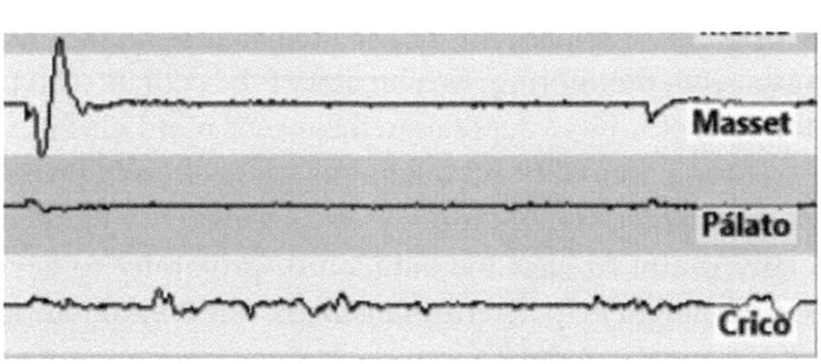

Fig. 11.4 Stimulated EMG of masseter muscle with stimulation of the trigeminal nerve

currents to be stimulated [18]. Based on this, an increase in stimulation threshold during the procedure can be an indication of nerve injury [19].

Situations such as chronic radiculopathies or neuropathies can result in higher stimulation thresholds and false-negative results. Children under the age of two, in whom peripheral myelination is not complete, may also require increased stimulation for depolarization. It is nonetheless important not to increase stimulus intensity too much since current could be conducted across a focal injury and depolarize a distal nerve segment.

To reduce false negatives in the presence or suspicion of previous lesions with axonal degeneration (due to clinical symptoms or preoperative electroneuromyography), or in young children, it is recommended that the threshold intensity of the motor response in direct stimulation or screw placement be tested individually on that segment and compared, if possible, to the threshold of healthy structures from the same patient [2, 18, 20]. More details in Chap. 23.

tEMG is used in surgeries with the risk of injury to peripheral or cranial nerves, nerve roots, and structures such as plexus and cauda equina. In tethered cord surgery, it is essential to differentiate – through direct stimulation – the fibrous tissue to be sectioned (filum) from functional lumbosacral roots [2]. More details in Chap. 26.

In spine surgery, recording electrodes are placed according to the levels that will be decompressed, and pedicles and screws are stimulated. The generation of a CMAP usually indicates a breach in cortical bone with the depolarization of adjacent root fibers [20].

Following the same reasoning, in peripheral nerves or plexus surgeries the choice of muscles to be recorded is not standard but varies according to the involved structures. In posterior fossa surgeries, stimulation also contributes to finding safe entry zones in or nearby the tumor, mapping the brainstem and correctly identifying cranial nerves. More details about stimulation parameters and techniques in each type of surgery will be covered in the corresponding chapters.

Monopolar Stimulation

In monopolar stimulation, the anode is placed at a distance from the cathode. Current is distributed radially from the tip of the stimulator, making a loop with the distant cathode. This setting allows for regional current spread that may depolarize nerve fibers far from the stimulator, reaching deep into tissues and providing greater sensitivity (depolarizing larger areas). It is mainly used for spinal pedicle screws placement monitoring, as a breach of the pedicle wall provides a low resistance path for current flow to depolarize the motor root [21, 22].

During cranial or peripheral nerve dissection procedures, the wide electric field of monopolar stimulation increases sensitivity but decreases specificity. It is especially useful to alert the surgeon of proximity to nerve fibers that are not readily visible and to help determining areas where stimulation does not depolarize a nerve, as safe entry zones [23].

Depending on the type of structure to be stimulated, the polarity of monopolar stimulation changes: in peripheral nerve, roots, brainstem, or subcortical motor tract stimulation the stimulus is cathodal, while in cortical, mapping the polarity must be anodal (reversed). This is due to the different polarities of the axon and the neuronal body. For more details on this subject, refer to Chap. 17.

The presence of blood or cerebrospinal fluid (CSF) in the surgical field, below the tip of the probe, can create a deviation (shunting) of the current and difficulties in stimulation because of low fluid resistance [24].

Bipolar Stimulation

Bipolar probes, with cathode and anode located in proximity from each other, have a narrow field of stimulation and are useful to precisely locate neural structures, albeit with lower sensitivity [25]. Cathode and anode are positioned side by side or concentrically. Current spreads focally between the two components and not radially. This allows for more precise localization, especially of structures very close to the stimulator [2].

Normally, a 5 mm-distance tips probe is selected, which results in 5 mm spread of the current. In nerve surgeries, the distance between the tips can be smaller (3 mm), although the distance is dictated by the size of the nerve. Larges nerves (such as the sciatic nerve) demand a larger interelectrode distance, such as 7 mm. Care must be taken, because short inter-tip distances with high current can create electrical bridging and reduction of potentials [9, 22].

In peripheral nerve surgeries, proper orientation of the stimulating electrodes is important and current should enter the axon perpendicularly. The stimulator must be oriented longitudinally along the nerve with the cathode closer to the recording electrodes. Visual confirmation of the correct orientation should be obtained. Generation of a current immediately under the stimulator prevents propagation (spread) to nearby tissues. However, it is also subject to current deviation (shunting) if there is liquid or blood in the surgical field [2, 25, 26].

While radial spreading of the electric field of a monopolar probe decreases the importance of optimal orientation between probe and target in subcortical stimulation, the more elliptic electric field of a bipolar probe and its larger dimension might alter the activation according to the electrode position and angulation [26, 27].

In cases where the stimulus is very close to the recording electrodes, as in the recording of nerve action potentials (NAP), the stimulator can be tripolar (anode-cathode-anode) to reduce stimulation artifacts.

Bipolar stimulation is the most widely used method for awake craniotomies with 60 Hz technique. Further details on cortical and subcortical monopolar and bipolar stimulation are detailed in Chaps. 17 and 19. For cranial nerves, refer to Chap. 21 and for peripheral nerves to Chap. 31.

Pitfalls: The Importance of Filtering and Sources of Error

Technical parameters of equipment setup and screen display are fundamental for an adequate wave visualization and interpretation. Filters are electronic components with variable resistive and capacitive properties capable of excluding certain determined frequencies from the analyses. The high-frequency (low-pass) filter limits higher frequencies and allows lower-frequency signals to pass unaffected. The opposite occurs with the low-frequency filter (high-pass), which restricts the passage of lower frequencies. Analog filters can eliminate about 70% of the bands below or above the set frequency, so the values of the high- and low-frequency filters should be about two times the frequency of interest [28].

Raising the low-frequency filter above the frequencies contained in the desired potential reduces amplitude, decreases peak latency and duration, and increases the number of phases of the potentials. On the other hand, reducing the high-frequency filter below the frequencies contained in the response under analysis reduces the amplitude (less markedly), prolongs the onset and peak latency, and increases the potential duration [28].

It is essential to be aware of the frequency ranges of each method used in IOM, which is be discussed in the specific chapters. Use of improper scanning, sensitivity, or filtering may produce distortion or decrease the ability to register potentials.

When interpreting fEMG, it is important to correlate any type of discharge with the surgical moment. Muscle activity (motor unit potentials – MUPs) may occur since the beginning of the procedure, due to more superficial anesthesia, absence of neuromuscular blockage (some muscles may maintain tone continuously, such as sphincter, frontalis, ileopsoas), and reversal of neuromuscular block (isoelectric line that changes to noisy lines and episodic discharges). These situations must be identified and not confused with the result of surgical manipulation. Knowing anesthetic techniques, maintaining a dialogue with the anesthesiologist, understanding the mechanism of each medication, and controlling the level of neuromuscular blockade are necessary for proper monitoring and avoiding unnecessary alarms [15]. Artifacts from different sources in the room that can interfere with EMG (60 Hz current cycles, respirators, aspirators, cautery, etc.) are usually easily distinguished by an experienced professional.

In cases of superficial anesthesia, there is a random muscle activity, similar to voluntary MUP, which does not correlate with maneuvers or surgical step, usually with single or small muscle groups activation, at a frequency of ~10–30 Hz, without generating a continuous interferential pattern (trains) [4]. Fibrillations, positive sharp waves, and complex repetitive discharges can be seen in previously denervated muscles. It is essential to distinguish among all these muscle activities the neurotonic discharges, which are sensitive to predict or reflect nerve damage. Another situation that requires attention is at the time of field irrigation, when neurotonic discharges can occur if saline solution is placed directly over the nerve [4].

During peripheral nerve surgeries, at the beginning of lesion manipulation, frequent discharges (trains or bursts) may occur. Damage to myelin, epineurium, and perineurium increases the degree of depolarization in response to irritative maneuvers. In these cases, the reduction of discharges (continuous activity that reduces to bursts or MUPs) must be interpreted with caution, as it may indicate a reduction in mechanical irritation or a damage increase with progressive axonal lesion since the rupture of the axonal structure reduces excitability and modifies thresholds discharges, which may indicate the continuation of a nerve injury [15]. More details in Chap. 31.

Free EMG may not show discharges after nerve section, ischemia, and electrocautery injury. Especially in cases of ischemic injury, the damage can produce axonal blockage, leading to injury without the presence of concomitant EMG activity (false negative). In these cases, stimulation distal to the peripheral nerve injury can generate normal muscle responses (false positive), while the response is absent in proximal stimulation, indicating conduction block or axonal section at the level of surgical manipulation [2, 15]. In addition, previous (chronic) axonal injuries can modify the threshold and reduce motor unit discharges. These difficulties must be known by the neurophysiologist, and the patient's medical history and physical examination must be evaluated before surgery. The use of multimodal IOM, with different techniques for the same surgery (motor potentials by transcranial stimulation, fEMG, tEMG, cranial nerve motor potentials, sensory potentials), analyzes different information at the same time, complementing each other and reducing the chance of error.

Conclusion

This chapter is just an introduction to the use of EMG, either spontaneous or stimulated, in IOM. More information about this technic in specific procedures can be found in specific chapters.

References

1. Rand RW, Kurze TL. Facial nerve preservation by posterior fossa transmeatal microdissection in total removal of acoustic tumours. J Neurol Neurosurg Psychiatry. 1965;28(4):311–6.
2. Holland NR. Intraoperative electromyography. J Clin Neurophysiol. 2002;19(5):444–53.
3. Rubin DI. Needle electromyography: basic concepts. Handb Clin Neurol. 2019;160(3rd series):243–56.
4. Harper CM. Intraoperative cranial nerve monitoring. Muscle Nerve. 2004;29(3):339–51.
5. Nunes RR, Bersot CDA, Garritano JG. Intraoperative neurophysiological monitoring in neuroanesthesia. Curr Opin Anaesthesiol. 2018;31(5):532–8.
6. Mishler ET, Smith PG. Technical aspects of intraoperative monitoring of lower cranial nerve function. Skull Base Surg. 1995;5(4):245–50.
7. Franz A, Klaas J, Schumann M, Frankewitsch T, Filler TJ, Behringer M. Anatomical versus functional motor points of selected upper body muscles. Muscle Nerve. 2017;57(3):460–5.
8. Pearlman RC, Isley MR, Ruben GD, Sandler SC, Wiesbaum B, Ali Khan M, Greene BS, Charles V, Shah A. Intraoperative monitoring of the recurrent laryngeal nerve using acoustic, free-run, and evoked electromyography. J Clin Neurophysiol. 2005;22(2):148–52.

9. Crum BA, Strommen JA. Peripheral nerve stimulation and monitoring during operative procedures. Muscle Nerve. 2007;35(2):159–70.
10. Leppanen RE. Intraoperative monitoring of segmental spinal nerve root function with free-run and electrically-triggered electromyography and spinal cord function with reflexes and F-responses. A position statement by the American Society of Neurophysiological Monitoring. J Clin Monit Comput. 2005;19(6):437–61.
11. Romstock J, Strauss C, Fahlbusch. Continuous electromyography monitoring of motor cranial nerves during cerebellopontine angle surgery. J Neurosurg. 2000;93(4):586–93.
12. Julian FJ, Goldman DE. The effects of mechanical stimulation on some electrical properties of axons. J Gen Physiol. 1962;46(2):297–313.
13. Prell J, Ramp S, Romstock J, Fahlbush R, Strauss C. Train time as a quantitative electromyographic parameter for facial nerve function in patients undergoing surgery for vestibular schwannoma. J Neurosurg. 2007;106(5):826–32.
14. Gunnarsson T, Krassioukov AV, Sarjeant R, Fehlings MG. Real-time continuous intraopera tive electromyographic and somatosensory evoked potential recordings in spinal surgery: correlation of clinical and electrophysiologic findings in a prospective, consecutive series of 213 cases. Spine (Phila Pa 1976). 2004;29:677–84.
15. Minahan RE, et al. Basic neurophysiologic intraoperative monitoring techniques. In: Husain AM, editor. A practical approach to neurophysiologic intraoperative monitoring. New York, NY: Demos Medical Publishing; 2008. p. 21–30.
16. Skinner SA, Transfeldt EE, Mehbod AA, Mullan JC, Perra JH. Electromyography detects mechanically-induced suprasegmental spinal motor tract injury: review of decompression at spinal cord level. Clin Neurophysiol. 2009;120(4):754–64.
17. Clinical practice guidelines for intraoperative neurophysiological monitoring: 2020 update. Ann Clin Neurophysiol. 2021;23(1):35–45.
18. Holland NR, Lukaczyk TA, Riley LH 3rd, Kostuik JP. Higher electrical stimulus intensities are required to activate chronically compressed nerve roots. Implications for intraoperative electromyographic pedicle screw testing. Spine. 1998;23(2):224–7.
19. Mandpe AH, Mikulec A, Jackler RK, Pitts LH, Yingling CD. Comparison of response amplitude versus stimulation threshold in predicting early postoperative facial nerve function after acoustic neuroma resection. Am J Otol. 1998;19(1):112–7.
20. Lall RR, Lall RR, Hauptman JS, Munoz C, Cybulski GR, Koski T, Ganju A, Fessler RG, Smith ZA. Intraoperative neurophysiological monitoring in spine surgery: indications, efficacy, and role of the preoperative checklist. Neurosurg Focus. 2012;33(5):E10.
21. Calancie B, Madsen P, Lebwohl N. Stimulus-evoked EMG monitoring during transpedicular lumbosacral spine instrumentation. Initial clinical results. Spine. 1994;19(24):2780–6.
22. Kartush JM, Niparko JK, Bledsoe SC, Graham MD, Kemink JL. Intraoperative facial nerve monitoring: a comparison of stimulating electrodes. Laryngoscope. 1985;95(12):1536–40.
23. Moller AR, Jannetta PJ. Preservation of facial function during removal of acoustic neuromas: use of monopoly constant voltage stimulation and EMG. J Neurosurg. 1984;61(4):757–60.
24. Schucht P, Seidel K, Jilch A, Beck J, Raabe A. A review of monopolar motor mapping and a comprehensive guide to continuous dynamic motor mapping for resection of motor eloquent brain tumors. Neurochirurgie. 2017;63(3):175–80.
25. Schekutiev G, Schmid U. Coaxial insulated bipolar electrode for monopolar and bipolar mapping of neural tissue: technical note with emphasis on the principles of intra-operative stimulation. Acta Neurochir. 1996;138(4):470–4.
26. Szelényi A, Senft C, Jardan M, Forster MT, Franz K, Seifert V, Vatter H. Intra-operative subcortical electrical stimulation: a comparison of two methods. Clin Neurophysiol. 2011;122(7):1470–5.
27. Wongsarnpigoon A, Grill WM. Computational modeling of epidural cortical stimulation. J Neural Eng. 2008;5(4):443–54.
28. Dumitru, et al. Instrumentation. In: Dumitru D, Amato AA, Zwarts MJ, editors. Electrodiagnostic medicine. 2nd ed. Philadelphia: Hanley & Belfus; 2002. p. 79–85.

Chapter 12
Brainstem Reflexes

Isabel Fernández-Conejero and Sedat Ulkatan

Introduction

Brainstem and posterior fossa surgery represent a challenge for neurosurgeons due to the high risk of iatrogenic injury of vital neurological structures. Therefore, important efforts in improving the surgical and imaging techniques together with intraoperative neurophysiology have been made. In this sense, the last decade has been marked by the development of methods to evaluate the functional integrity of cranial motor nerves. Dong et al. [16] described a consistent method to elicit facial nerve motor evoked potentials by transcranial electrical stimulation. Deletis et al. defined an intraoperative neurophysiological technique to evaluate the functional integrity of the vagal nerve by recording corticobulbar motor evoked potentials (CoMEPs) from vocal [13] and cricothyroid [14] muscles. The same methodology is feasible and reliable to continuously assess the normal function of the motor part of trigeminal, glossopharyngeal, accessory spinal, and hypoglossal nerves [15]. All together represent a significant advance in preserving the motor function of cranial nerves, but they do not avoid deficits related to lesions to the nuclei of sensory fibers. As an example, it has been documented that swallowing problems may develop in the site of intraoperatively preserved CoMEPs. Therefore, it is evident that besides the descending cortical control of the motor nuclei of cranial nerves, preserving the afferent arch is necessary for preserving normal function [6].

I. Fernández-Conejero (✉)
University Hospital of Bellvitge, Barcelona, Spain
e-mail: isabelfernandez@bellvitgehospital.cat

S. Ulkatan
Mount Sinai West Hospital, New York, NY, USA
e-mail: sedat.ulkatan@mountsinai.org

S. M. Verst et al. (eds.), *Intraoperative Monitoring*,
https://doi.org/10.1007/978-3-030-95730-8_12

It has been an outstanding achievement to develop methods to elicit some complex brainstem reflexes intraoperatively from this perspective. They provide valuable information on the brainstem's functional integrity and allow the afferent and efferent pathways and the nuclei and nuclei interconnections of these reflexes to be assessed.

We present in this chapter a description and review of the available methodologies to elicit blink reflex, masseteric reflex, and laryngeal adductor reflex.

Blink Reflex

In 1952 Kugelberg was the first to report the presence of two components of the electrically elicited blink reflex (BR): R1 and R2 [25]. The R1 response corresponds to the oligosynaptic reflex arc, which includes trigeminal afferents, brainstem connections between the sensory part of the trigeminal nucleus, the motor nucleus of the facial nerve, the facial nerve proper, and the orbicularis oculi muscle. The R2 component is more complex in its central, polysynaptic connections within the brainstem, but it has the same afferent and efferent pathways as the R1. Clinically, the blink reflex is elicited after a gentle brush to the cornea or the eyelashes or after a glabellar percussion [17].

This reflex has become an important tool in neurophysiology [40]. It has also found a place as an additional diagnostic tool in investigating pathology involving the reflex arc.

Attempts were made to evoke this reflex in anesthetized patients but with limited results [30].

Mourisse et al. demonstrated the effect of hypnotic drugs on the elicitability of the blink reflex and concluded that it is a good marker of the depth of anesthesia due to its sensitivity, especially to sevoflurane and to propofol [32].

Previous studies have reported the inability to elicit the BR in unconscious patients who had received doses of anesthetics compatible with those used for surgery [28, 30, 31]. The exception was in patients with hemifacial spasm in whom the R1 component could be elicited [29].

In this chapter, we describe the method for eliciting the R1 component of the BR in patients under general anesthesia using a short train of electrical stimuli applied over the supraorbital nerve [12, 13].

The methodology for eliciting MEPs in awake patients or healthy subjects by applying a single stimulus transcranially was not successful in the patient under general anesthesia. Once a short train of stimuli was used, it became the standard for eliciting MEPs under general anesthesia [35]. Furthermore, the ability of a short train of stimuli to overcome the inhibitory effects of anesthetics has been shown in other intraoperative neurophysiological methods such as bulbocavernosus reflex monitoring [10, 36] or for mapping Broca's area in patients under general anesthesia [11]. The same concept was applied to elicit blink reflexes by delivering a short train of stimuli on the supraorbital nerve, which overcomes the inhibitory action of anesthetics due to temporal summation and building-up of excitatory postsynaptic potentials in the interneuronal chain involved in the blink reflex in the brainstem.

The possibility of recording blink reflex intraoperatively opens a new door at the intraoperative neuromonitoring field since it eventually allows assessing the functional integrity of all anatomical structures involved in the reflex arc.

Methodology

Stimulation Parameters

Stimulation of the supraorbital nerve of either side of the face is performed using a pair of electroencephalographic needle electrodes inserted subcutaneously over the supraorbital nerve. The cathode should be inserted in the supraorbital notch and the anode 2.5 cm superior and lateral to the cathode. One to seven rectangular constant-current stimuli with an interstimulus interval (ISI) of 2 ms, intensity of 20–40 mA, and train repetition rate of 0.4 Hz are used. In case no response is obtainable, a method of facilitation could be useful, such as a double train of stimuli, with the intertrain interval ranging from 20 to 40 ms [12, 13].

Recording Parameters

The recording is done with needle electrodes identical to those used for stimulation. The electrodes are inserted in the low lateral part of the orbicularis oculi muscle ipsilateral to the stimulating side after identifying muscle twitches evoked by stimulating facial nerve branches. The recording is performed after averaging two single sweeps. After the first sweep, the stimulating electrode's polarity might be reversed to avoid a large stimulus artifact. Recordings are made by using a 50-ms epoch and bandpass digital filters of 70 and 1219 Hz. Recording of the BR is attempted after intubation, during surgery, and after starting skin closure. Recording can be done very frequently since it does not produce any twitching in the surgical field, providing real-time information about the functional integrity of the structures involved in the reflex during the riskiest moments of the tumor resection.

Anesthetic Considerations

In 2007, Mourisse et al. stated that BR is elicitable in patients under halogenated agents and propofol regime [32]. However, they demonstrated that BR is more sensitive to gases than to propofol. We had a similar experience in our work a few years ago [12, 13]. In practical settings, BR is usually monitored together with other neurophysiological tests, which are not reproducible under halogenated agents. Therefore, the anesthesia regime that allows intraoperative BR monitoring and other neurophysiological responses consist of a constant infusion of propofol and remifentanyl. A short-acting muscle relaxant is administered for intubation purposes only. The anesthesia regime, blood pressure, and temperature are kept constant throughout the surgery. Recovery from muscle relaxation is monitored by the train-of-four technique and is recorded from the abductor pollicis brevis muscle after the stimulation of the median nerve at the wrist.

Previous studies reported the inability to elicit the BR with a single stimulus in anesthetized patients who had received doses of anesthetics compatible with those used for surgery [28, 30, 32]. The exception was in patients with hemifacial spasm in whom the R1 component could be elicited [19, 29].

Clinical Assessment

According to our article, the recordability of BR is up to 86.2%.

The R1 component of BR in anesthetized patients has a latency ranged between 8.9 and 16.5 ms. The amplitude range of the R1 response varies between 7 and 798 μV. Latency should be calculated from the beginning of the train's stimuli that produce the response (Fig. 12.1).

The R2 component of BR in the patients under general anesthesia is not commonly elicitable. Most likely, this is due to the influence of anesthetics on the polysynaptic pathways of the R2 component of the BR.

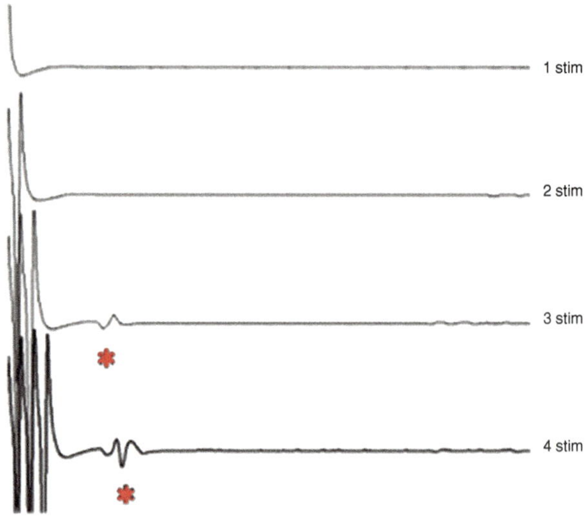

Fig. 12.1 Blink reflex elicitability: Elicitability of the first component of blink reflex after a short train of stimuli applied on the supraorbital nerve. Note that one single stimulus does not produce any response, but a train of three stimuli produces BR. The last trace shows optimal BR after a train of four stimuli

At least three stimuli with an ISI of 2 ms are necessary to elicit a consistent response in most patients. Exceptions can occur under the following circumstances: (a) patients under light anesthesia and (b) patients with hemifacial spasms.

The R1 component of BR is highly reproducible and shows a very similar configuration, amplitude, and latency in each recording (Fig. 12.2).

In some patients, BR is absent, but when a double train of stimuli is applied, the BR is recordable after the second train (Fig. 12.3). If the BR is still not recordable

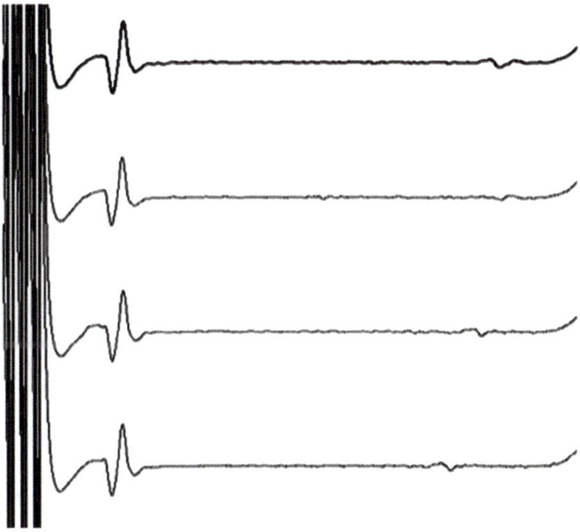

Fig. 12.2 Blink reflex reliability: Recording of the R1 of BR showing the high reproducibility of responses

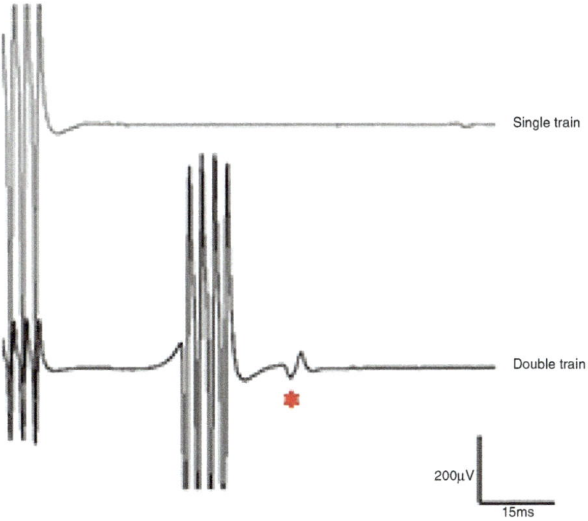

Fig. 12.3 Blink reflex, single train vs. double train: Recording of BR after a double train of identical electrical characteristics with an intertrain interval of 30 ms while a single train cannot elicit BR. Asterisc: blink reflex

after delivering a double train, some other factors should be considered, such as administration of one bolus of propofol or lesion in any anatomical structure involved in the reflex arc before surgery.

Practical Application

The BR can be monitored practically in all patients without severe preoperative deficits involving the anatomical structures related to the reflex. Recording can be done very frequently since stimulation does not produce any twitching in the surgical field, providing real-time information about the functional integrity of the reflex structures during the entire surgical procedure. The presence of BR represents the preservation of functional integrity of trigeminal nerve afferents, trigeminal and facial nerve nuclei, connections between them, and branch of facial nerve innervating oculi muscle. The disappearance of BR during surgery may have different reasons. First, it must be considered a lesion to any structure involved in the reflex. It will be easy to understand which structure has been damaged if we put the moment of disappearance and the surgical maneuver in context. In addition, it will be helpful to observe the behavior of other neurophysiological responses such as corticobulbar motor evoked potentials (CoMEPs) for facial and trigeminal nerve and then correlate changes with BR disappearance if possible. The second cause of BR disappearance could be an increment in the depth of anesthesia. In this case, probably the other neurophysiological tests will still be present since they are less sensitive to propofol than BR.

An essential pitfall of interpretation of facial CoMEPs concerning BR deserves a detailed explanation [18]. The response in the upper facial muscle (orbicularis oculi) after transcranial electrical stimulation (TES) can result from not only the stimulation of corticobulbar pathways for the upper facial muscle but also the stimulation of branches of the supraorbital nerve (trigeminal afferents activation). This effect very often occurs after high-intensity TES due to the spreading of current over the anterior scalp, which activates the branches of the supraorbital nerve. When a strong TES with a short train of stimuli is used, the same stimulation parameters are appropriate for eliciting the first component (R1) of the BR in the orbicularis oculi muscle [12, 13].

Furthermore, transcranial magnetic stimulation studies did reveal that the R1 component of the BR has about the same latency as CoMEPs; therefore, this latter response may be influenced by the BR [9]. Since the upper facial nucleus has bicortical (bihemispheric) innervation, the patient still will not have "central" facial nerve palsy on the upper face in the surgically induced lesion at the cortical/subcortical level. Facial paresis/palsy will be evident only if the lesion is close to the facial nucleus.

Furthermore, in infratentorial surgery, if CoMEPs are the BR, any lesion of trigeminal afferents from the upper face will result in the intraoperative changes or disappearance of the response, while the postoperatively volitional movement of the upper face will be preserved.

One strategy to distinguish these two responses may be to simultaneously monitor CoMEPs, elicited by TES and BR, by stimulating the supraorbital nerve using a short train of stimuli.

In summary, the recording of CoMEPs from the orbicularis oculi muscle cannot be qualified solely as a cortical/subcortical origin since it may also be a BR. So far, no established methodology exists to distinguish these two responses (BR and CoMEPs for upper face) in the setting of intraoperative monitoring, especially since they have similar latencies and behaviors.

As the importance of using a multimodal protocol during surgical procedures has been demonstrated, the observed correlation between the behavior of blink reflex and the trigeminal and facial corticobulbar motor evoked potentials during surgery is remarkable. They complement each other and may help understand if injury to the structures involved occurs and, therefore, change the surgeon's strategy to avoid a permanent new neurological deficit.

Masseteric Reflex

The masseter reflex is a monosynaptic proprioceptive reflex that provides feedback information about masticatory actions. Afferent sensory information from the trigeminal nerve is transmitted to the mesencephalic nucleus of the trigeminal nerve. From the trigeminal mesencephalic nucleus, fibers descend to the mid-pons to the trigeminal motor nucleus monosynaptically and activating the jaw-closing motoneurons of the ipsilateral masseter muscle [20, 24, 46].

The masseter reflex can be elicited by electrical stimulation of the masseter nerve, then termed H of the masseter, or can be elicited by a tap-stretch of the masseter muscle, then termed the jaw jerk reflex. The masseter reflex has an anatomical localization value. Abnormal masseter reflex has been reported ipsilateral to midbrain lesions [8, 34, 50] as the masseter reflex is strictly unilateral.

Methodology

For intraoperative neuromonitoring purposes of masseter H reflex, total intravenous anesthesia (TIVA) is required. Once Intubation was completed, a bite block was placed. However, it is not certain; bite block placement gave mandible specific position such as the semi-open mouth, and masseter muscle would be stretched. Therefore bite block is an integral part of the Masseter H reflex setup.

A pair of monopolar EMG needle electrodes or hook-wire electrodes were introduced at a specific location to stimulate the masseteric nerve electrically. This specific location for percutaneous access to the masseteric nerve was located under the zygomatic arch, 0.5 cm anterior to the temporomandibular joint, as previously described by Godaux and Desmedt. Muscle responses were recorded by a pair of subdermal needle electrodes inserted in the belly of the ipsilateral masseter and temporalis muscles. Temporalis muscle may not be available in all craniotomies.

A single-stimulus of 0.2 ms duration at a repetition rate of 0.7 Hz was steadily increased from zero intensity until the H reflex was elicited. The intensity was further increased after eliciting the H reflex until a direct motor response (M) was elicited. A response was accepted as a reflex when meeting the criteria of an H reflex [24]. Additionally, to prove the reflex origin of the H masseter response, one should be able to elicit the H reflex in the temporalis muscle (if available) [27]. The activation of the Ia proprioceptive fibers from the masseter muscle elicited the pure reflex excitation of the temporalis motoneurons with no antidromic influences on their excitability [7].

The H reflexes in the masseter muscles; mean onset latencies of the masseter H reflex and M response were 5.4 ± 1.3 ms and 2.6 ± 0.6 ms (mean ± SD), respectively. The maximum amplitude of the H reflex was approximately 21% of the maximum M response in the same subject [49].

Practical Application

Publications using Masseter H reflex as a monitoring method are extremely few. This reflex might be more helpful than the blink reflex whenever trigeminal nerve integrity is in question due to surgery. Masseter H reflex is a monosynaptic reflex, and in theoretical perspective, it should be more resistant to anesthesia-related influences than the blink reflex. Using Masseter H reflex and Blink reflex together as a monitoring method gives unique advantages for trigeminal and facial nerve monitoring.

Laryngeal Adductor Reflex

Laryngeal adductor reflex (LAR) is the most critical vital brainstem reflex, followed by cough reflex from the physiological function perspective. The evolution of the human voice box created a disadvantageous laryngeal anatomical position, which moved caudally compared to all mammals and increased significantly to choking and aspiration risk during swallowing in human physiology. Therefore LAR is robust, resistant to general anesthetic agents, and overrides other motor behaviors such as swallowing, respiration, and speech [3, 21]. The LAR is triggered by afferent sensations from the supraglottic mucosa, allowing the protective function of the larynx to be entirely reflexive and involuntary [26, 37].

Physiological reflex organization of the LAR in animals and humans has been described [1, 5]. The sensation from supraglottic mucosa, which makes an afferent loop, travels through the ipsilateral internal branch of the superior laryngeal nerve (iSLN) and vagus nerve to the nucleus of the solitary tract [2, 41]. These afferents run rostral or caudally along the length of the nucleus. From the solitary tract nucleus, fibers project to the –ipsi and contralateral nucleus ambiguus, which runs the length of the ventrolateral part of the medulla within the reticular formation [45]. The caudal reticular formation of the pons and medulla comprises nuclei and local circuit interneurons that generate motor patterns and coordinate reflexes. The laryngeal motor neurons are located in the nucleus ambiguus [4]. These efferent neurons travel to the larynx via the vagus nerve and its recurrent laryngeal branch (RLN) to the laryngeal musculature. All laryngeal muscles are innervated by the RLN, except the cricothyroid muscle, which is innervated by the external branch of the superior laryngeal nerve. Vocal fold adduction happens by the contraction of thyroarytenoid and lateral cricoarytenoid muscles (main adductor forces) and inter-arytenoid muscles [33]. To block foreign body aspiration to the airway, LAR must activate bilateral vocal fold closure [22].

Recent studies contradict prior research in some aspects and give evidence that the early R1 component of the LAR is always bilateral in awake humans and patients under general anesthesia, comprising an ipsi- (iR1) and contralateral (cR1) components relative to the stimulating side [42, 47].

Methodology

There are commercially available endotracheal tubes from different manufacturers. However, these tubes are only available for adult or early teenage groups of patients. In general, the tube contains surface electrodes on the right and left sides that directly contact the right and left vocal folds, respectively. The reader should acknowledge that every manufacturer has a different design, but for simplicity and methodology explanation, we refer to the electromyographic endotracheal tube (EET) with a paired electrode on both sides.

Patients are intubated with an EET that monitors vocal fold contraction by surface electrodes on the endotracheal tube surface. After the patient is positioned for the surgical procedure, intubation should be performed preferably by direct visualization with GlideScope Video Laryngoscope (Verathon, ULC, Burnaby, Canada) [23]. Video laryngoscope is reported as an optimal method for placing this type of ETT [23]. Most of the available tubes have a colored band that can be used for correct positioning, which can be visualized best with a video laryngoscope. Various fastening methods and devices can be used; the standard way of taping the ETT around the mouth is usually suboptimal and causes significant monitoring reliability issues.

A critical key to success rests on choosing the correct endotracheal tube size. This choice is partly dictated by the gender of the patient and partly by the patient's laryngeal anatomy. In adults, the glottic diameter is 4 mm larger in men than in women [39]. Weight should not be a criterion for selecting the tube size.

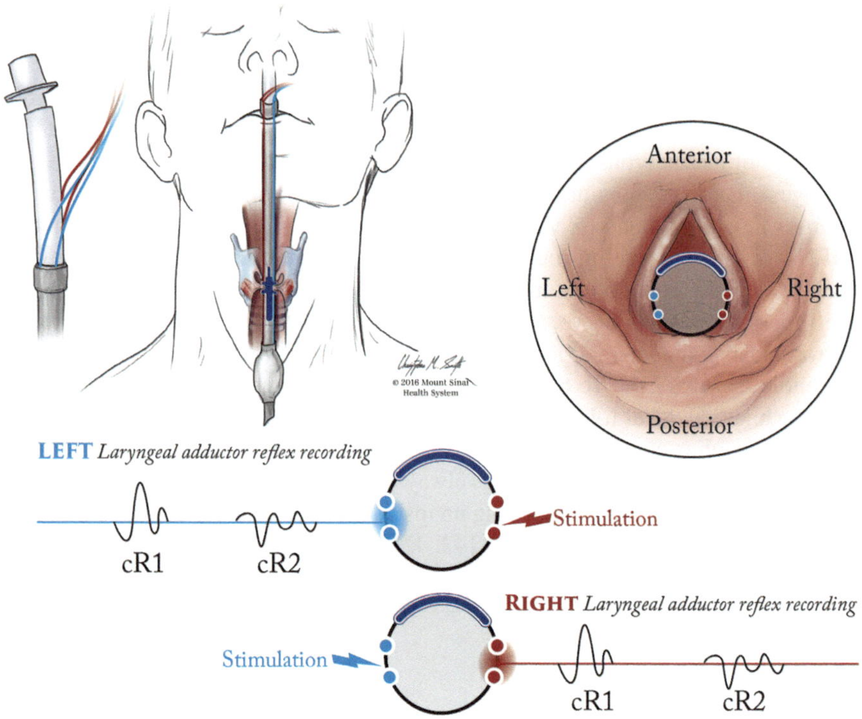

Fig. 12.4 Schematic illustration of the methodology for eliciting the laryngeal adductor reflex by using an endotracheal tube containing bilaterally embedded surface electrodes for stimulating and recording. These electrodes, right (red) and left (blue), come into direct contact with the right and left vocal folds, respectively. The monitoring interest side of LAR is elicited by electrical stimulation of the laryngeal mucosa on the contralateral side. Laryngeal adductor reflex: R1 and R2 components

For LAR elicitation, the two electrodes of one side of the tube electrically stimulate the laryngeal mucosa. A single stimulus between 3 and 20 mA (0.1–1 ms duration) or a short train of 3–4 pulses (Interstimulus Interval 2–4 ms) is applied. Stimuli are delivered at 0.4 Hz to 0.7 Hz repetition rate. Two responses elicited by stimuli of reverse polarity can be averaged to minimize stimulus artifact, if necessary.

For LAR recording, the two electrodes of the tube contralateral to the stimulating side are used to record vocal fold adduction. Thus, the recorded vocal fold responses are the cR1 and cR2 components of the LAR (Fig. 12.4). Signals are filtered at a bandwidth of 30–1000 Hz. Sweep time 100 ms is usually adequate to analyze both components of LAR response.

The amplitude of the LAR is critically dependent on adequate contact between laryngeal mucosa and endotracheal electrodes. Mean LAR amplitudes for patients with normal laryngeal function are 313.5 ± 167.4 μV [14]. We use three different derivations to optimize our recordings and minimize phase cancellation with the available commercialized endotracheal tubes: V+/V−, V+/reference, and V−/reference. The V+/V− array refers to the two electrodes in contact with one vocal fold (either right or left), and the reference is a subcutaneous needle placed at the sternum (along with a subdermal needle acting as a ground electrode). We track changes in all three derivations during monitoring, but we rely on the most stable LAR elicited for monitoring purposes, regardless of the derivation. On the contrary, onset latency of the LAR by electrical mucosa stimulation is highly variable (22.4 ± 2.5 ms) and is not a suitable parameter to predict nerve injury.

Warning criteria for impending nerve injury change during different types of surgery. If RLN or the peripheral part of vagal nerve is monitored, the LAR response amplitude decrement >50% compared to baseline amplitude value, impending nerve injury is possible, the surgeon should be warned and tissue released. If the amplitude decreases >60% of baseline and does not recover with tissue relaxation, postoperative nerve and vocal fold dysfunction are likely [42]. LAR amplitude decrement for warning criteria should be 50% in the brainstem and posterior fossa surgeries [48]. The difference in warning criteria between peripheral and central nervous surgery stems from sensitivity and specificity values compared in Brainstem surgery [48].

LAR interpretation during brainstem surgery is more complicated than peripheral surgery. The reader must consider the location of the brainstem and posterior fossa surgery. Particularly intraaxial brainstem surgery monitoring-related changes interpreted cautiously in case of false-positive results [38]. LAR reflex motor and sensory parts can be affected separately during intraaxial brainstem surgery; the reflex loss due to sensory central lesion may not reflect complete neurological deficit. It is advised that all functional laryngeal assessments should be done objectively, such as video laryngoscopy, not a bedside patient voice assessment.

Anesthesia and LAR

R1 component can be elicited bilaterally at all depths of anesthesia in 100% of patients provided total intravenous anesthesia (TIVA) is used [42].

Previous reports investigating the LAR in humans under general anesthesia using inhalational anesthetic agents reported no discernable R2 (oligo-polysynaptic component) responses at any level of anesthesia. Although R2 components in some patients under TIVA may be present, these responses are less reliable than the R1 component and prone to fade [43].

Sometimes it is used topical lidocaine (4%) during intubation. This drug may abolish LAR and recovery could be slow, even hours. Therefore LAR monitoring necessitates avoiding Lidocaine usage altogether [44].

Practical Application

LAR is a recently developed methodology in IOM and is promising to fill a significant gap for surgeries involving lower medulla and lower cranial nerves. However, the reader should understand that technical aspects of LAR methodology requires further refinement. Young children's technical limitations and electrode placement have severe practical difficulties.

LAR represents one of the most critical functions of the larynx, which cannot be monitored by any other methods for preventing aspiration risk.

Conclusions

The brainstem reflexes are elicitable under general anesthesia, therefore opening a new door for intraoperative neuromonitoring. The evaluation of brainstem reflexes during surgery offers the opportunity to assess continuously, and in real-time, the functional integrity of all anatomical structures involved in the reflex arc since it does not produce any movement of the patient and the surgical field is not disturbed.

From the IOM perspective, brainstem reflexes give us a substantial advantage to continuously monitor the integrity of the cranial nerves involved, but we should also consider the reflex function and consequences, not only general nerve functions.

To conclude, the methodology to elicit brainstem reflexes is feasible and reliable, and it might be implemented in the routine of intraoperative neuromonitoring protocols.

References

1. Ambalavanar R, et al. Neuronal activation in the medulla oblongata during selective elicitation of the laryngeal adductor response. J Neurophysiol. 2004;92(5):2920–32.
2. Andreatta RD, et al. Mucosal afferents mediate laryngeal adductor responses in the cat. J Appl Physiol (1985). 2002;93(5):1622–9.
3. Barkmeier JM, et al. Modulation of laryngeal responses to superior laryngeal nerve stimulation by volitional swallowing in awake humans. J Neurophysiol. 2000;83(3):1264–72.
4. Bieger D, Hopkins DA. Viscerotopic representation of the upper alimentary tract in the medulla oblongata in the rat: the nucleus ambiguus. J Comp Neurol. 1987;262(4):546–62.
5. Bolser DC, et al. Role of the dorsal medulla in the neurogenesis of airway protection. Pulm Pharmacol Ther. 2015;35:105–10.
6. Bricolo A, Sala F. Surgery of Brainstem lesions. Neurophysiology in Neurosurgery. A modern intraoperative approach. Academic Press; 2002. Ed Ch 12. p. 267–89.
7. Cruccu G, Truini A, Priori A. Excitability of the human trigeminal motoneuronal pool and interactions with other brainstem reflex pathways. J Physiol. 2001;531:559–71.
8. Cruccu G, Iannetti GD, Marx JJ, Thoemke F, Truini A, Fitzek S, et al. Brainstem reflex circuits revisited. Brain. 2005;128:386–94.
9. Cruccu G, Hallet M. Brainstem function and dysfunction. Clin Neurophysiol. (Suppl.). 2006;58:4.
10. Deletis V, Vodušek DB. Intraoperative recording of bulbocavernosus reflex. Neurosurgery. 1997;40:88–93.
11. Deletis V, Ulkatan S, Cioni B, Meglio M, Colicchio G, Amassian V, Shrivastava R. Responses elicited in the vocalis muscles after electrical stimulation of motor speech areas. Rivista Med. 2008;14(2):159–65.

12. Deletis V, Urriza J, Ulkatan S, Fernandez-Conejero I, Lesser J, Misita D. The feasibility of recording blink reflexes under general anesthesia. Muscle Nerve. 2009a;39(5):642–6.
13. Deletis V, Fernandez-Conejero I, Ulkatan S, Costantino P. Methodology for intraoperatively eliciting motor evoked potentials in the vocal muscles by electrical stimulation of the corticobulbar tract. Clin Neurophysiol. 2009b;120(2):336–41.
14. Deletis V, Fernández-Conejero I, Ulkatan S, Rogić M, Carbó EL, Hiltzik D. Methodology for intra-operative recording of the corticobulbar motor evoked potentials from cricothyroid muscles. Clin Neurophysiol. 2011;122(9):1883–9.
15. Deletis V, Fernández-Conejero I. Intraoperative monitoring of the functional integrity of the brainstem. J Clin Neurol. 2016;12(3):262–73.
16. Dong CC, Macdonald DB, Akagami R, Westerberg B, Alkhani A, Kanaan I, Hassounah M. Intraoperative facial motor evoked potential monitoring with transcranial electrical stimulation during skull base surgery. Clin Neurophysiol. 2005;116(3):588–96.
17. Esteban A. A neurophysiological approach to brainstem re- flexes. Blink Reflex Neurophysiol Clin. 1999;29:7–38.
18. Fernández-Conejero I, Ulkatan S, Deletis V. Upper facial nerve motor evoked potentials can be a misinterpretation of the blink reflex. J Neurol Neurosurg Psychiatry. 2008. Letter to Editor.
19. Fernández-Conejero I, Ulkatan S, Sen C, Deletis V. Intra-operative neurophysiology during microvascular decompression for hemifacial spasm. Clin Neurophysiol. 2012;123(1):78–83.
20. Godaux E, Desmedt JE. Human masseter muscle: H- and tendon reflexes. Their paradoxical potentiation by muscle vibration. Arch Neurol. 1975;32(4):229–34.
21. Henriquez VM. Laryngeal reflex responses are not modulated during human voice and respiratory tasks. J Physiol. 2007;585(Pt.3):779–89.
22. Heitmiller RF, Tseng E, Jones B. Prevalence of aspiration and laryngeal penetration in patients with unilateral vocal fold motion impairment. Dysphagia. 2000;15(4):184–7.
23. Kanotra SP. GlideScope-assited nerve integrity monitoring tube placement for intraoperative recurrent laryngeal nerve monitoring. J Laryngol Otol. 2012;126(12):1271–3.
24. Kimura J. Electrodiagnosis in diseases of nerve and muscle: principles and practice. F.A. Davis Company; 1989. p. 361–2.
25. Kugelberg E. Facial reflexes. Brain. 1952;75:385–96.
26. Ludlow CL. Central nervous system control of the laryngeal muscles in humans. Respir Physiol Neurobiol. 2005;147(2–3):205–22.
27. Macaluso GM, De Laat A. H-reflexes in masseter and temporalis muscles in man. Exp Brain Res. 1995;107(2):315–20.
28. Marelli RA, Hillel AD. Effects of general anesthesia on the human blink reflex. Head Neck. 1989;11:137–49.
29. Moller AR, Jannetta PJ. Hemifacial spasm: results of electro- physiologic recording during microvascular decompression operations. Neurology. 1985;35:969–74.
30. Mourisse J, Gerrits W, Lerou J, van Egmond J, Zwarts MJ, Booij L. Assessment of blink and corneal reflexes during midazolam administration: useful methods for assessing depth of anesthesia? Acta Anaesthesiol Scand. 2003;47:593–600.
31. Mourisse J, Lerou J, Zwarts M, Booij L. Electromyographic assessment of blink reflexes correlates with a clinical scale of depth of sedation/anaesthesia and BIS during propofol ad- ministration. Acta Anaesthesiol Scand. 2004;48:1174–9.
32. Mourisse J, Lerou J, Struys M, Zwarts M, Booij L. Multi-level approach to anaesthetic effects produced by sevoflurane or propofol in humans: 1. BIS and blink reflex. Br J Anaesth. 2007;98:737–45.
33. Murakami Y, Kirchner JA. Mechanical and physiological properties of reflex laryngeal closure. Ann Otol Rhinol Laryngol. 1972;81(1):59–71.
34. Ongerboer de Visser BW. Afferent limb of the human jaw reflex: electrophysiologic and anatomic study. Neurology. 1982 May;32(5):563–6.
35. Pechstein U, Cedzich C, Nadstawek J, Schramm J. Transcranial high-frequency repetitive electrical stimulation of recording myogenic motor evoked potential with the patient under general anesthesia. Neurosurgery. 1996;39:335–44.

36. Rodi Z, Vodušek DB. Intraoperative monitoring of bulbocavernous reflexthe method and its problems. Clin Neurophysiol. 2001;112:879–83.
37. Sasaki CT. Laryngeal physiology for the surgeon and clinician. San Diego, CA: Plural Publishing, Inc; 2017. p. 1. online resource (xii, 115 pages).
38. Satomaa AL, Vanttinen S, Mattila H. The intraoperative laryngeal adductor reflex (LAR) in brainstem tumor removal: a case of unilateral loss of LAR signal. Clin Neurophysiol. 2019;130:1253–5.
39. Seymour AH, Prakash N. A cadaver study to measure the adult glottis and subglottis: defining a problem associated with the use of double-lumen tubes. J Cardiothorac Vasc Anesth. 2002;16(2):196–8.
40. Shahani B. The human blink reflex. J Neurol Neurosurg Psychiatry. 1970;33:792–800.
41. Sinclair CF, Tellez MJ, Ulkatan S. Human laryngeal sensory receptor mappingilluminates the mechanisms of laryngeal adductor reflex control. Laryngoscope. 2018a;128(11):E365–70.
42. Sinclair CF, Tellez MJ, Ulkatan S. Noninvasive, tube-based, continuous vagal nerve monitoring using the laryngeal adductor reflex: Feasibility study of 134 nerves at risk. Head Neck. 2018b;40(11):2498–506.
43. Sinclair CF, Tellez MJ, Tapia OR, Ulkatan S. Contralateral R1 and R2 components of the laryngeal adductor reflex in humans under general anestehsia. Laryngoscope. 2017a;127(12):443–8.
44. Sinclair CF, Tellez MJ, Ulkatan S. A novel methodology for assessing laryngeal and vagus nerve integrity in patients under general anesthesia. Clin Neurophysiol. 2017b;128(7):1399–405.
45. Steriade M, McCarley RW, SpringerLink (Online service). Brain control of wakefulness and sleep. New York, NY/Boston, MA: Kluwer Academic/Plenum Publishers; 2005.
46. Szentagothai J. Anatomical considerations on monosynaptic reflex arcs. J Neurophysiol. 1948;11(5):445–54.
47. Tellez MJ, Ulktana S, Blitzer A, Sinclair CF. Unearthing a consistent bilateral R1 component of the laryngeal adductor reflex in awake humans. Laryngoscope. 2018;128(11):2581–7.
48. Tellez MJ, Mirallave-Pescador A, Seidel K, Urriza J, Shoakazemi A, Raabe A, Ghatan S, Deletis V, Ulkatan S. Neurophysiological monitoring of the laryngeal adductor refle during cerebellar-pontine angle and brainstem surgery. Clin Neurophysiol. 2021.
49. Ulkatan S, Jaramillo AM, Téllez MJ, Goodman RR, Deletis V. Feasibility of eliciting the H reflex in the masseter muscle in patients under general anesthesia. Clin Neurophysiol. 2017;128(1):123–7.
50. Valls-Solé J. Neurophysiological assessment of trigeminal nerve reflexes in disorders of central and peripheral nervous system. Clin Neurophysiol. 2005;116(10):2255–65.

Part III
Brain Functions: Eloquent Areas

Chapter 13
The Brain Surface

Eduardo Carvalhal Ribas and Guilherme Carvalhal Ribas

Introduction

The encephalon is the part of the central nervous system that lies within the intracranial space. It is divided by the tentorium into an infratentorial compartment, which contains the brainstem and cerebellum, and a supratentorial compartment, which contains the diencephalon and the telencephalon constituted by two cerebral hemispheres separated by the falx. In order to favor its better understanding, organize its nomenclature, and apply this knowledge in clinical practice, the cerebral hemispheres were arbitrarily divided into lobes, regions, and compartments. As these divisions correspond to different concepts and have been created according to different criteria, they partly overlap, are complementary to each other, and are particularly useful for a better understanding of the brain architecture [1]. Among other criteria, the brain can be subdivided according to its sulcal patterns, comparative anatomy, cytoarchitecture, myeloarchitecture, myelogenesis, connectivity, and cerebral functions.

The mean volume of the brain ranges between 440 and 517 cm^3 (females and males, respectively), weighting 1508.91 ± 299.14 g and housing 170.68 ± 13.86 cells, where half are neuronal cells (Table 13.1) [2]. The surface of the brain, also called cortex, is much larger than that of a simple ovoid structure. Due to its convoluted shape, almost two thirds of the human neocortex are hidden away in the depth of the sulci, ranging in total between 1470 and 2275 cm^2.

E. C. Ribas (✉) · G. C. Ribas
Hospital Israelita Albert Einstein, São Paulo, SP, Brazil

University of São Paulo Medical School, São Paulo, SP, Brazil

S. M. Verst et al. (eds.), *Intraoperative Monitoring*,
https://doi.org/10.1007/978-3-030-95730-8_13

Table 13.1 The number of neuronal and nonneuronal cells of the brain [2]

	Whole brain	Telencephalon (gray and white matters)	Cerebellum	Basal ganglia, diencephalon, mesencephalon, and pons
Mass (g)	1508.91 ± 299.14	1232.93 ± 233.68	154.02 ± 19.29	17.66 ± 45.42
All cells (billions)	170.68 ± 13.86	77.18 ± 7.72	85.08 ± 6.92	8.42 ± 1.50
Neuronal cells (billions)	86.06 ± 8.12	16.34 ± 2.17	69.03 ± 6.65	0.69 ± 0.12
Nonneuronal cells (billions)	84.61 ± 9.83	60.84 ± 7.02	16.04 ± 2.17	7.73 ± 1.45
Nonneuronal/ neuronal cells ratio	0.99	3.76	0.23	11.35
Percentage of brain mass	100%	81.8%	10.3%	7.8%
Percentage of brain neurons	100%	19.0%	80.2%	0.8%

Sulcal Pattern

The phylogenetic and embryological development of the brain surface is based on its invagination processes, being the fissures and sulci natural extensions of the subarachnoid space, with depths ranging from 1 to 3 cm approximately and harboring small gyri within its sulcal space, known generically as transverse gyri [3]. Also, the brain undergoes a process of circular curvature, placing each thalamus as the morphological center of each cerebral hemisphere.

These processes led to a typical superficial organization of sulci and gyri. Each mammalian species has a highly characteristic cerebral surface, with humans having a higher complexity. However, there's a considerable intersubject variability if individual sulci are seen in detail. Sulci may be continuous or interrupted, once or at several points, and some sulci may be doubled over a certain part of their trajectory [4]. The sulcal pattern not only varies among individuals but also varies between the two hemispheres of the same individual.

The cerebral gyri constitute a continuum of the cerebral surface, and their appearance as distinct gyri is only superficial since they are continuous along the entire sulcal depth and along its extremities. Also, in humans, almost two thirds of the neocortex are hidden away in the depth of the sulci [5]. Therefore, each gyrus must be understood as a region and not as a well-defined and distinct structure [6].

Currently, the International Anatomical Terminology describes each cerebral hemisphere as being divided into six lobes: frontal, parietal, occipital, temporal, insular, and limbic [7].

The lateral sulcus of the brain, also called the Sylvian fissure, is promptly and easily identifiable. It has a stem, which extends from the carotid cistern to the anterior Sylvian point on the superolateral surface of the brain, and gives rise to three rami: anterior horizontal, anterior ascending, and posterior [8]. The anterior horizontal and anterior ascending rami delineates the *pars triangularis* in the inferior frontal gyrus, having the *pars orbitalis* anterior to the anterior horizontal ramus and the *pars opercularis* posterior to the anterior ascending ramus. The posterior ramus separates the frontal and parietal lobes superiorly from the temporal lobe inferiorly.

The parietotemporal line is an imaginary line, drawn from the upper extremity of the parieto-occipital sulcus on the lateral surface to the preoccipital notch, and constitutes the anterior limit of the occipital lobe. Another imaginary line, drawn as a posterior continuation of the Sylvian fissure to the parietotemporal line, separates the parietal lobe superiorly from the temporal lobe inferiorly. The insula is separated from the other cerebral lobes by its anterior, superior, and inferior limiting sulci; and the limbic lobe is bounded by the cingulate and collateral sulci [9].

Each cerebral hemisphere has three surfaces: superolateral, medial, and basal; three margins: superior, inferior, and medial; and three poles: frontal, temporal, and occipital.

The superolateral surface of the brain, also referred to as cerebral convexity, faces the concave inner surface of the skull (Fig. 13.1a). At this surface, three horizontal gyri (superior, middle, and lower frontal gyri) converge anteriorly to form the frontal pole, three horizontal gyri (upper, middle, and inferior temporal gyri) converge anteriorly to form the temporal pole, and three gyri (superior, middle, and inferior occipital gyri) converge posteriorly to form the occipital pole. Two oblique, ascending gyri are clearly seen: precentral and postcentral gyri. Immediately posteriorly, a quadrangular region called the superior parietal lobule can be noted superiorly, and the inferior parietal lobule inferiorly, formed by two curved gyri: the supramarginal gyrus, which can be seen as the posterior continuation of the superior temporal gyrus and whose trajectory curves over the posterior margin of the Sylvian fissure; and the angular gyrus, which corresponds to a posterior and curvilinear extension of the middle temporal gyrus forming a horse-shoe "C" shape [6].

Although a considerable intersubject variability exists, some uniformity can be noted. The superior frontal and superior temporal sulci are usually continuous, whereas the inferior frontal and inferior temporal sulci are usually interrupted. The pre- and postcentral sulci are always interrupted: the first having interruptions due to the frontal gyri connections to the precentral gyrus and the second having interruptions due to the postcentral gyrus connections with the superior parietal lobule. The intraparietal sulcus separates the superior and inferior parietal lobules and is usually clearly identifiable with an anterior-posterior disposition. The intermediate sulcus of Jensen is located between the supramarginal and angular gyri, and can arise from the intraparietal sulcus, superior temporal sulcus, or both. The occipital gyri have a higher intersubject variability.

The medial surface of the brain lies at the depth of the interhemispheric fissure, where both hemispheres face each other, and is anatomically more constant (Fig. 13.1b). The corpus callosum is placed around its inferior margin with the cingulate gyrus describing an arc around it. Anteriorly and inferiorly, the cingulate

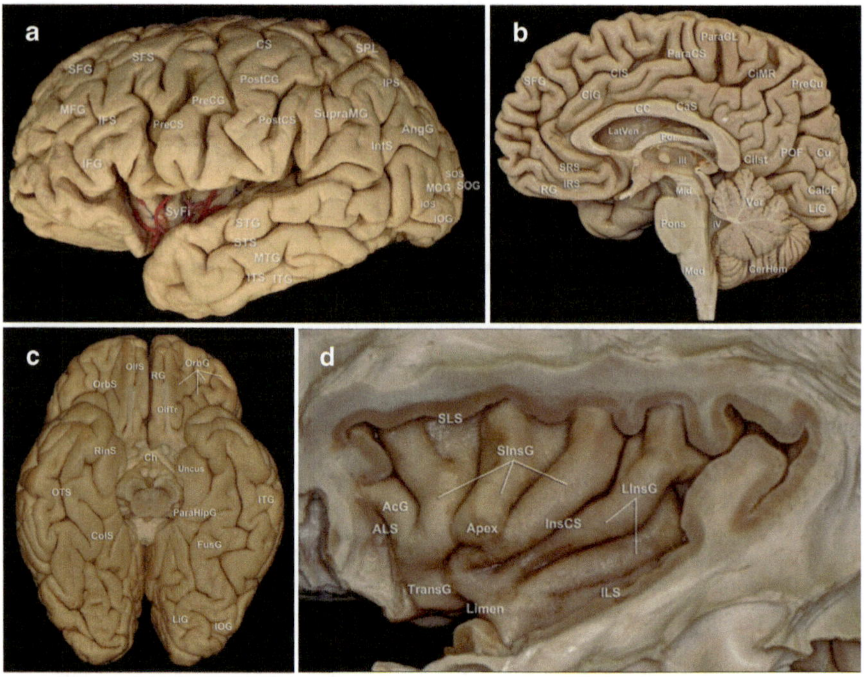

Fig. 13.1 Cortical anatomy of the brain: lateral (**a**), medial (**b**), basal (**c**), and insular (**d**) surfaces. AcG accessory gyrus, ALS anterior limiting sulcus, AngG angular gyrus, CalcF calcarine fissure, CaS callosal sulcus, CC corpus callosum, CerHem cerebellar vermis, Ch optic chiasm, CiG cingulate gyrus, CiIst cingulate isthmus, CiMR cingulate marginal ramus, CiS cingulate sulcus, ColS collateral sulcus, CS central sulcus, Cu cuneus, For fornix, FusG fusiform gyrus, IFG inferior frontal gyrus, IFS inferior frontal sulcus, III third ventricle, ILS inferior limiting Sulcus, InsCS insular central sulcus, IntS intermediate sulcus of Jensen, IOG inferior occipital gyrus, IOS inferior occipital sulcus, IPS intraparietal sulcus, IRS inferior rostral sulcus, ITG inferior occipital gyrus, ITG inferior temporal gyrus, ITS inferior temporal sulcus, IV fourth ventricle, LatVen lateral ventricle, LiG lingual gyrus, LInsG long insular gyri, LInsG long insular gyrus, Med medulla oblongata, MFG middle frontal gyrus, Mid midbrain, MOG middle occipital gyrus, MTG middle temporal gyrus, OffS olfactory sulcus, OlfTr olfactory tract, OrbG orbital gyri, OrbS orbital sulcus, OTS occipito-temporal sulcus, ParaCL paracentral lobule, ParaCS paracentral sulcus, ParaHipG parahippocampal gyrus, POF parieto-occipital fissure, PostCG postcentral gyrus, PostCS postcentral sulcus, PreCG precentral gyrus, PreCS precentral sulcus, PreCu precuneus, RG rectus gyrus, RinS rinal sulcus, SFG superior frontal gyrus, SFS superior frontal sulcus, SInsG short insular gyri, SLS superior limiting sulcus, SOG superior occipital gyrus, SOS superior occipital sulcus, SPL superior parietal lobule, SRS superior rostral sulcus, STG superior temporal gyrus, STS superior temporal sulcus, SupraMG supramarginal gyrus, SyFi sylvian fissure, TransG transverse gyrus, Ver cerebellar vermis

gyrus joins the rectus gyrus forming the cingulate pole. The rectus gyrus harbors the inferior rostral sulcus and is separated from the superior frontal gyrus by the superior rostral gyrus. Three vertical gyri can be identified posterior to the cingulate pole and form the septal region: anterior para-olfactory gyrus, posterior para-olfactory gyrus, and paraterminal gyrus. Posteriorly, the cingulate gyrus presents a narrowing, called the isthmus, which continues with the parahippocampal gyrus.

The superior frontal gyrus curves along the superior cerebral margin, and along the medial surface of brain, it is separated from the cingulate gyrus by the cingulate sulcus. Similarly, the precentral and postcentral gyri also curve along the superior cerebral margin and along the medial surface of brain form together the paracentral lobule. The cingulate sulcus separates the paracentral lobule inferiorly from the cingulate gyrus, and posteriorly curves superiorly to constitute the ascending ramus of the cingulate sulcus separating the paracentral lobule from the pre-cuneus. The paracentral sulcus originates more anteriorly from the cingulate sulcus and separates the superior frontal gyrus from the paracentral lobule. The precuneus has a quadrangular shape, is incompletely separated inferiorly from the cingulate gyrus by the subparietal sulcus rami, and is deeply separated anteriorly from the paracentral lobule by the ascending ramus of the cingulate sulcus and posteriorly from the cuneus by the parieto-occipital fissure. The cuneus has a triangular shape, with its vertex pointing anteriorly, and is separated from the lingual gyrus by the calcarine fissure. The calcarine fissure is divided into two parts by the origin of the parieto-occipital sulcus. While the proximal part supports the isthmus where it is originated and the caudal base of the precuneus, the distal part lies between the cuneus and the lingual gyrus.

The basal surface of the brain lies along the base of the skull (Fig. 13.1c). The anterior fossa supports the fronto-orbital surface, constituted laterally by the orbital gyri (subdivided by the "H"-shaped orbital sulcus into anterior, posterior, lateral, and medial orbital gyri) and medially by the rectus gyrus. The temporo-occipital surface lies over the middle fossa and the tentorium, constituted by three longitudinal gyral strips: (1) laterally is the inferior temporal gyrus that continues posteriorly with the inferior occipital gyrus; (2) medially is the parahippocampal gyrus, which anteriorly curves over itself forming the uncus and posteriorly continues with both the cingulate and lingual gyri; (3) and in between there is the fusiform gyrus. The superior and medial surface of the parahippocampal gyrus, called subiculum, is flat and supports the inferior aspect and pulvinar of the thalamus. This surface is separated laterally by the hippocampal fissure from the dentated gyri, which continues posteriorly as the fasciolar gyri (also known as fasciola cinerea, gyrus of Andreas Retzius, or retrosplenial gyri) circling the splenium, and subsequently as the indusium griseum over the trunk of the corpus callosum. The indusium griseum extends also along the genu and rostrum of the corpus callosum, and finishes within the paraterminal gyrus at the septal region.

The surface of the insula has a triangular shape, with the limen insulae at its anteroinferior vertex, and is separated from the other cerebral lobes by its anterior, superior, and inferior limiting sulci (Fig. 13.1d). It is subdivided by the central sulcus of the insula into an anterior portion, composed of short gyri which usually converge to form an apex, and a posterior portion, formed by long insular gyri. At its anterior and basal aspect, a transverse gyrus can be identified immediately superior to the limen insulae and an accessory gyrus can be identified superiorly to the later [1, 9].

The disposition and arrangement of cerebral lobes can also be understood in relation to the central core of the brain [1]. The concept of central core of the brain is based on the evident anatomical delimitation of a central region within each hemisphere between the brainstem, the ventricular cavities, and the cerebral lobes, and which has important clinical and surgical implications. It is basically composed by the insular surface, basal ganglia, and thalamus, and is connected with the rest of the supratentorial compartment by cerebral isthmi (represented by the continuation of the internal, external, and extreme capsules toward the cerebral lobes). It also houses part of the anterior commissure, amygdalofugal pathways, and the region of the innominate substance. This block is at the morphological center of each cerebral hemisphere and plays an important role in the integration of information, motor and sensory functions, emotion, and cognition. From an anatomical and architectural point of view, the central core is covered laterally by the insula, medially by the supratentorial ventricular surfaces, and embraced by the limbic lobe which describes a "C"-shaped ring around the thalamus. The frontal, parietal, occipital, and temporal lobes are placed anteriorly, superiorly, posteriorly, and inferiorly in relation to the central core, respectively.

Detailed knowledge of the cerebral surface, formed by sulci and turns, is essential for the interpretation of imaging exams and intraoperative guidance. Once identified, the cerebral sulci can be used by the neurosurgeon as landmarks, as microneurosurgical corridors, and also as an aid for cortical mapping techniques in order to identify specific sites related to cortical functions.

Although the sulci and the gyri of the brain are easily identified in standard magnetic ressonance images, their accurate visual transoperative recognition is notoriously difficult because of their common anatomic variations and their arachnoid, cerebrospinal fluid, and vessel coverings. Ribas et al. studied sulcal and gyral key points with more constant anatomical cranial-cerebral relationships, mostly formed by the main sulci extremities and/or intersections, and by the gyral sites that underlie particularly prominent cranial points (Fig. 13.2) [8, 10, 11]. These key points together constitute a neurosurgical anatomic framework that can help in the understanding of other cerebral sulci, lesions, and that can be used to orient the placement of supratentorial craniotomies and to ease the initial transoperative identification of

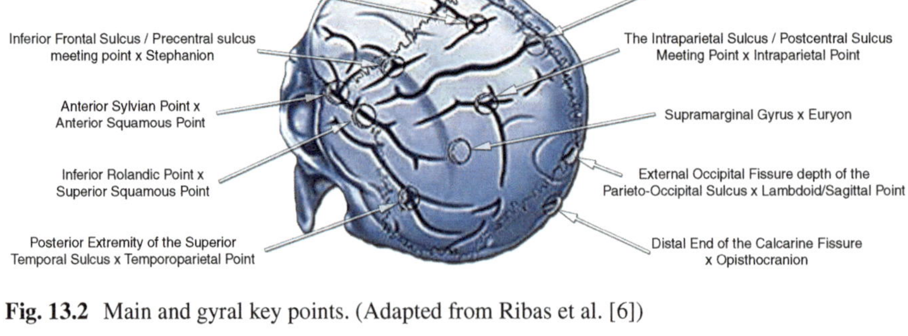

Fig. 13.2 Main and gyral key points. (Adapted from Ribas et al. [6])

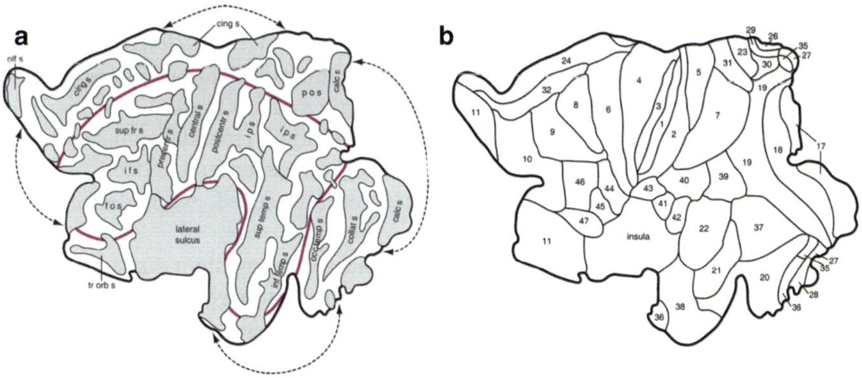

Fig. 13.3 Van Essen's flat maps of the left human cerebral hemisphere surface. (**a**) The sulcal surfaces are shaded in gray and the main sulci are labelled. In order to facilitate orientation, the structures visible at a lateral surface of the hemisphere are present between the red lines, and the medial and basal surfaces are outside the red lines. If the dashed, arrow-headed curves are connected at corresponding points, the flat map can be transformed into a tri-dimensional map. (**b**) The cytoarchitectonic areas of Brodmann can be transferred and depicted onto these flat maps. (Adapted from Drury and Van Essen et al. [12, 13])

brain sulci and gyri. Anatomical landmarks can be used as complementary, and not substitute, stereotactic, and navigation systems when available; and transoperative functional or neurophysiological testing is paramount for eloquent cerebral areas identification.

The "folded" natural surface of the brain buries vast neocortical areas, with two thirds of the neocortex present in the depth of the sulci, and can be a barrier to researches focused on the cortical surface. To address this problem, Van Essen et al. used computerized transformations to "unfold" the entire surface of a cerebral hemisphere into a two-dimensional reconstruction or flat map, where all cortical surface can be represented (Fig. 13.3) [12]. Other cortical information, like Brodmann's areas, can be transferred and depicted onto these flat maps.

Cytoarchitecture

The cerebral cortex is recognized as a laminated structure throughout its extent by using these staining methods. The piriform cortex and hippocampal parts of the paleomammalian cortex have three layers of cells, known as allocortex or paleocortex. The neocortex, also designated as isocortex or homogenetic cortex, represents the vast majority of the cortical area and is formed by six layers of cells, which are (beginning at the surface):

I. Lamina molecularis (or lamina zonalis), made by sparsely scattered horizontal cells of Cajal and the horizontal fibers of pyramidal cells, stellate cells, and cells of Martinotti.

II. Lamina granularis externa, composed of small, densely packed stellate and small pyramidal cells. This area is traversed by vertical fibers from both ascending axons and apical dendrites of large pyramidal cells in lamina V. The ascending axons often synapse with the apical dendrites in this layer.
III. Lamina pyramidalis externa, a thick layer with high pyramidal somata relation and neurons increasing progressively in size from superficial to deep.
IV. Lamina granularis interna, made by small, densely packed, pyramidal, and non-pyramidal somata.
V. Lamina pyramidalis interna, constituted mainly by medium-sized and large, loosely arranged pyramidal somata. It is also characterized by many ascending and descending fibers. A horizontal band of concentrated fibers, the internal band of Baillarger, traverses this layer.
VI. Lamina multiformis, composed of relatively tightly packed, spindle-shaped somata of a variety of morphological type.

The basic laminar pattern is seen at the entire neocortex, but it is not a homogeneous structure. Korbinian Brodmann distinguished 44 sharply delineated areas, although his images show areas numbered up to 52, the areas numbered 13–16, and 48–51 are not shown (Fig. 13.4) [14–16]. Von Economo and Koskinas and Sarkissov distinguished more areas, subdividing several of Brodmann's areas (BA) into smaller ones [13].

Distinct inputs reach the cortex, and each is directed to a different cortical layer:

- Layer I: inputs from intralaminar thalamic nuclei, the reticular formation, and feedback from precursor cortical areas.
- Layers II and IV: intrinsic inputs from the same cortical unit.
- Layers II, III, and IV: feedforward inputs from adjacent cortical regions.
- Layers III and IV: thalamic and commissural inputs.
- Layers V and VI: intrinsic and some thalamic inputs.

Information in layer I is transferred to the intrinsic circuitry of the cortical unit by providing afferent contacts with the apical dendrites of supragranular (layers II and III) and infragranular neurons (layers V and VI). Layers II and IV provide information to the supragranular and infragranular neurons within a cortical module [17].

Efferent fibers arise from the cortical neurons and form three distinct categories: (1) the association fibers, (2) the striatal fibers, and (3) the confluence of fibers (the "cord") that carries the commissural and subcortical fibers. Layers II and III give rise to association and commissural systems, while layers V and VI to subcortical connections. The short association fibers (aka local or U-fibers) are found directly underneath the sixth layer. Neighborhood and long association fibers travel within the central part of the white matter of the core of the gyrus, accompanied in the initial stages by the striatal fibers. The subcortically directed fibers and the commissural fibers travel initially centripetally in the central part of the white matter of the gyrus and form a "cord" formation. These fibers segregate later into commissural fibers and the subcortical bundle, which further divides into fibers destined for thalamus, and those to brainstem and spinal cord in the pontine bundle [17].

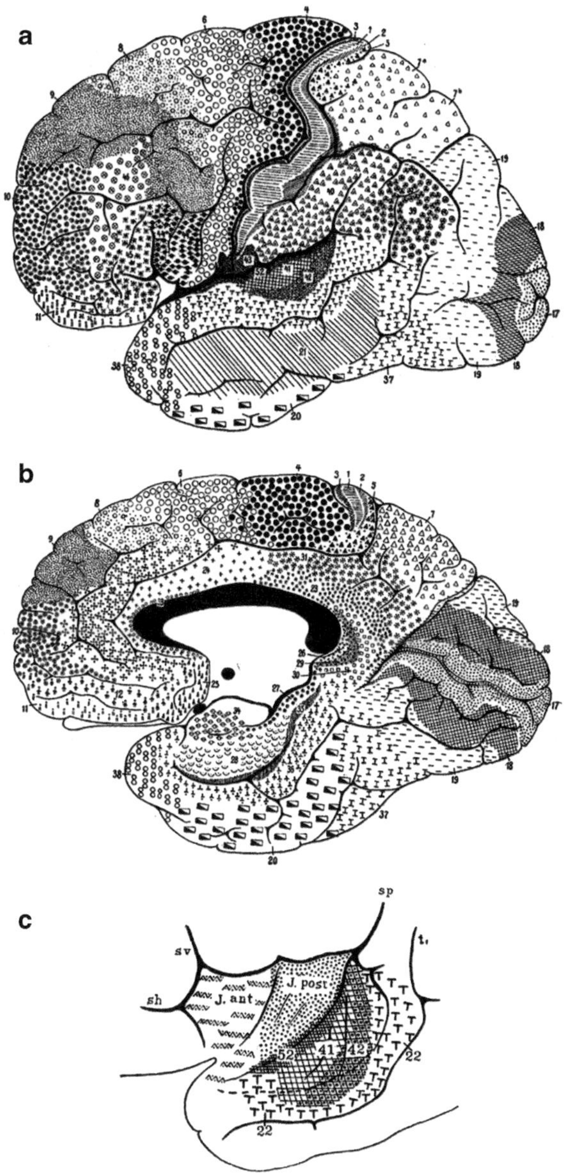

Fig. 13.4 "Cytoarchitectonic cortical areas after Brodmann" (**a**, **b**), as mentioned in the final and modified version of the Brodmann's cortical map, and Brodmann's only map of the insular and adjacent supratemporal cortex (**c**) [16]

Intrinsic Connectivity

Broadly, brain intrinsic connections are separated in thalamocortical and cortico-cortical groups, and distinct areas are related with different connections.

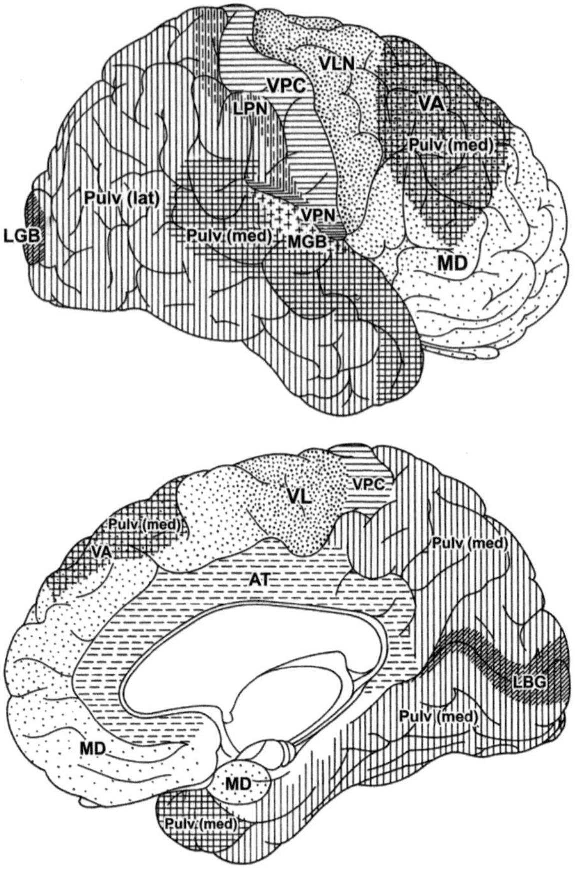

Fig. 13.5 Connections between the thalamic nuclei and the cerebral cortex II: cortical projection areas of the thalamic nuclei. AT anterior thalamic nuclei, CM centromedian nucleus, LGB lateral geniculate body, LP lateral posterior nucleus, MD mediodorsal thalamic nucleus, MGB medial geniculate body, PF parafascicular nucleus, Pulv (ant) pulvinar thalami, anterior part, Pulv (lat) pulvinar thalami, lateral part, Pulv (med) pulvinar thalami, medial part, VA ventral anterior thalamic nucleus, VL ventral lateral nucleus, VMP ventromedial posterior nucleus, VPC ventral posterior complex. (Adapted from Nieuwenhuys et al. [13])

The entire cortex receives thalamic projections, which arise from four main groups of thalamic nuclei (sensory relay, motor relay, limbic, and association nuclei) (Fig. 13.5).

The cortico-cortical connections will spread information from primary areas to association areas. Each primary sensory area is adjoined by a modality-specific sensory association area: somatosensory unimodal association cortex (SA) is located directly behind the primary somatosensory area (BA 3, 1 and 2) and include parts of BA 5 and 7 (at the superior parietal lobule) and parts of BA 40 (at the inferior parietal lobule); visual unimodal association cortex (VA) extends over the occipital lobe and anteriorly into the temporal lobe posterior aspect, including BA 18, 19, 20, 21, and 37; and auditory unimodal association cortex (AA) is around the primary auditory cortex (located in Heschl's gyrus, corresponding BA 41 and 42), and includes the superior temporal gyrus (BA 22). Some areas in the posterior orbitolateral cortex and anterior insula may correspond to the olfactory unimodal association area. Marek-Marsel Mesulam considers the premotor cortex (BA 6, 8, and 44), located anterior to the primary motor, a motor association area (MA), a motor analogue of the modality-specific sensory association areas because it provides the main cortical input to this region.

Human brains have 3 heteromodal association areas (polymodal or supramodal areas), which receive inputs from unimodal areas, other heteromodal areas, and paralimbic areas. A parietotemporal heteromodal association area is located at the superior parietal lobule inferior aspect (BA 7), inferior parietal lobule (BA 39 and 40), and anteriorly into the temporal lobe (BA 21 and 22); a medial temporal heteromodal association area is seen at the perirhinal areas (BA 35 and 36); and a prefrontal heteromodal association area located anterior to the motor association cortex (BA 9, 10, 45, 46, 47 and the anterior aspects of BA 8, 11, and 1).

Cerebral Functions

Several theories and models have been proposed to explain the functional organization of the brain, and can usually be classified into three different concepts: equipotentiality, localizationism, and connectionism.

For historic purposes, interesting to point that the equipotentially theory, or antilocalizationism, believed that the entire brain, or at least one complete hemisphere, is implied in the practice of a functional task.

Localizationism, on the other hand, states that each region of the neocortex is related to complete and distinct function. Franz Joseph Gall (1758–1828) and his collaborator Johann Spurzheim (1758–1832) were pioneers in this concept founding phrenology.

The connectionism theory, or disconnectionism, includes the idea of functional specialized areas, but understands that cognitive functions are best explained as a result from the functional integration of the elementary processing operations occurring in different functional areas, which are interconnected by networks.

Also, the traditional view of brain composed of fixed "eloquent" and "non-eloquent" regions, used respectively to define the regions whose lesion gives rise to major irrevocable neurological deficits and to the regions which lesions would not cause clinical consequences, is challenged by this connectivist view of brain functions. The dogma of a static functional organization of the brain which would not be able to compensate any injury involving these so-called eloquent areas is criticized by the connectivist view by considering cerebral plasticity. The phenomenon of cerebral plasticity which allows cerebral functions remodeling through the recruitment of other preserved cerebral networks constitutes both the basics and the main clinical contribution of this connectivist view.

Marek-Marsel Mesulam postulated that five anatomically defined large-scale networks are most relevant to clinical practice: left-dominant perisylvian network for language, a right-dominant parietofrontal network for spatial cognition, an occipitotemporal network for face and object recognition, a limbic network for retentive memory, and a prefrontal network for attention and behavior. The inner organization of networks may vary from one person to another (as in the case of right versus left handers) and may therefore need to be ascertained individually when the goal is to guide surgical interventions [18, 19].

Functional magnetic resonance imaging (fMRI) and positron emission tomography (PET) are recent advances in functional neuroimaging methods that can detect changes in blood flow or metabolism in specific regions of the brain while human subjects perform various sensory, motor, or cognitive tasks (Fig. 13.6). Since increased blood flow and metabolism reflect changes in neuronal activity, particularly synaptic, these methods can identify which cortical areas are more functionally

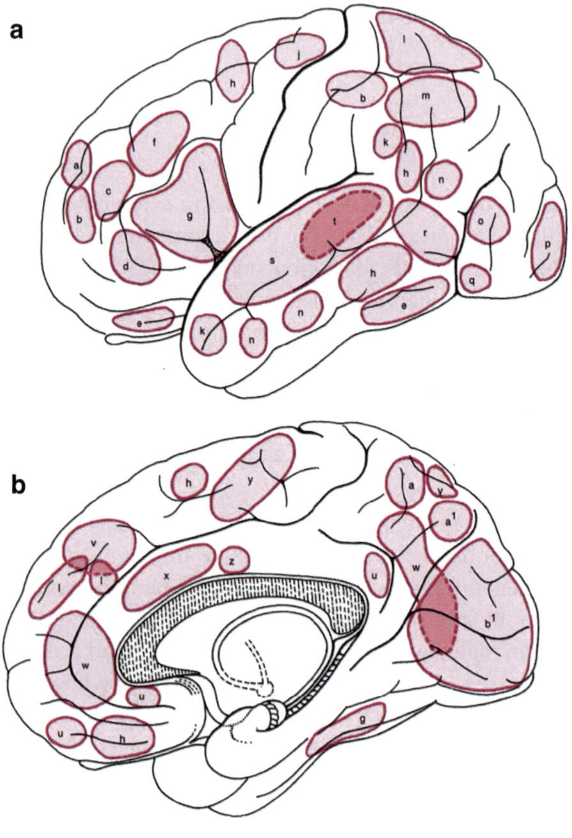

Fig. 13.6 Summary of activation cortical areas from functional imaging experiments, depicted upon the lateral (**a**) and medial (**b**) surface of the brain. a: attention, b: calculation, c: activation arising from a working memory task, d: processing of incorrect arithmetic equations, e: maternal love, f: performance of a verbal working memory task, g: reading aloud irregular words, h: meditative state, j: finger opposition task, k: visual-spatial orienting, l: coherence processes in language comprehension, m: executive function in working memory, n: embarrassment, o: perception of visual motion, p: written sentence comprehension, q: processing of color patterns, r: verb comprehension, s: judgment of the grammaticality of sentences, t: selective auditory attention, u: evaluation of unpleasant, arousing words, v: cross-modal sensory processing, w: error processing, x: categorization of written object descriptions, y: pursuit eye movements, z: painful visceral sensation, a^1: saccades, b^1: visual stimulation. (From Nieuwenhuys et al. [13])

activated during a given brain function. Cortical functional maps based on neuroimaging methods can help in clinical practice to highlight cortical areas related to each brain function, but cannot infer which areas are essential or critical for performing a specific brain function.

Diffusion-weighted imaging (DWI) is a modern MRI technique that can measure the thermal Brownian motion of water molecules and diffusion tensor imaging (DTI) can also detect the more favorable diffusivity direction of these molecules, termed anisotropy. Since water molecules tend to diffuse more freely along the direction of axonal fascicles rather than across them at the subcortical space, tracking and tracing the more favorable trajectory of water molecules allows the 3D reconstruction of white matter tracts, a technique called fiber tractography (FT). The white matter tracts architectural arrangement can now be studied in vivo and individually; however, fiber tractography can still not inform about the function and eloquency of a given tract.

Brain mapping techniques using direct electric stimuli on cortical areas and subcortical white matter are seen as the gold standard for clarifying the function and eloquency of each region and have brought us new insights about the anatomofuncional organization of the brain. More recently, Hugues Duffau, who has worked extensively with brain mapping during awake neurosurgeries with patients affected by gliomas, has contributed enormously by identifying cortical areas and subcortical pathways related to different brain functions. Presurgical understanding of the basic anatomo-functional organization of the brain is crucial to optimize the selection of the most appropriate intraoperative tasks for the patient, given the limited intrasurgical awake time frame. An ideal intraoperative protocol includes essential tasks related to the function of each cerebral region and additional tests that can be chosen on the basis of each patient-specific profile, in order to preserve an optimal quality of life [20].

Duffau et al. also proposed the concept of a "minimal common brain," which is based in connectivism at the expense of cortical localizationism (Fig. 13.7). This work brings a probabilistic postsurgical tumor residue atlas computed on a series of patients who underwent incomplete WHO grade II glioma resection on the basis of intraoperative direct electric stimuli brain mapping, and suggests which cortical areas and subcortical pathways are essential for the basic cognitive functions despite the inter-individual anatomo-functional variability and plastic mechanisms. By relating the high probability of residual tumor to regions in the deep white matter, projection and association axonal pathways seem to play a critical role in the proper functioning of the brain. The functions subserved by long-range axonal pathways seem to be less subject to inter-individual variability and reorganization than cortical sites, and constitute the main obstacle to radical tumor surgical resection. Input and output areas, being respectively the first relay of information entering the brain and the last relay or the fiber tracts sending information, have to be preserved probably due to absence of parallel alternative pathways to restore their function after any damage; examples are projection fibers, primary motor and somatosensory areas. Other essential areas may act as with cortical epicenters or "hubs," connected by U-shaped fibers, associative and commissural pathways, required to allow proper

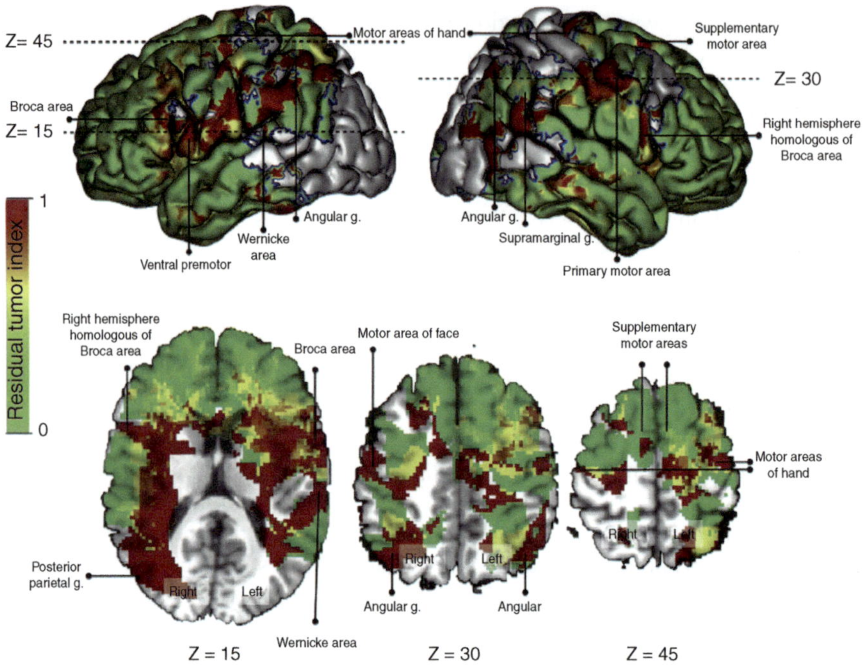

Fig. 13.7 Probabilities of residual WHO grade II glioma after resection under brain mapping (residual tumor index). (From Ius et al. [21])

synchronization between several distant areas or to integrate plurimodal data coming from the unimodal areas, like the posterior part of the left dominant superior temporal gyrus and its junction with the inferior parietal lobule [21].

Multi-modal Parcellation

More recently, researches have used high-quality magnetic resonance imaging (MRI) data provided by the Human Connectome Project, which benefited from major advances in image acquisition and preprocessing, to parcellate cerebral cortical regions by combining cortical architecture, function, connectivity, and/or topography together. Architectural measures of relative cortical myelin content and cortical thickness were derived from T1-weighted and T2-weighted structural images; cortical function was measured using task functional MRI contrasts from seven tasks; functional connectivity and topographic organization were analyzed from resting-state functional MRI (Fig. 13.8) [22, 23].

An objective semi-automated neuroanatomical approach was able to delineate 180 areas per hemisphere, bounded by sharp margins. Interestingly, this method characterized 97 new areas in addition to the 83 areas previously reported using

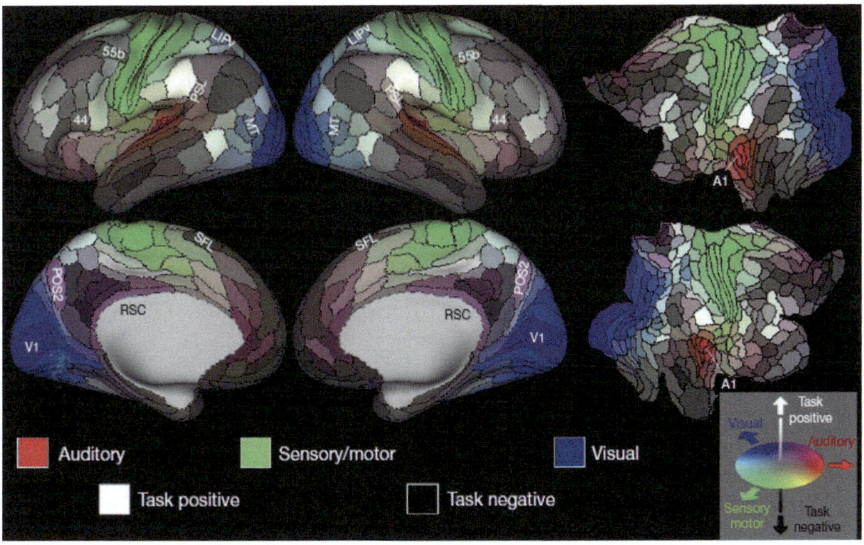

Fig. 13.8 The Human Connectome Project's multi-modal parcellation map, version 1.0. The 180 areas delineated and identified in both left and right hemispheres are displayed on inflated and flattened cortical surfaces. Black outlines indicate areal borders. Colors indicate the extent to which the areas are associated in the resting state with auditory (red), somatosensory (green), visual (blue), task positive (towards white), or task negative (towards black) groups of areas. (Adapted from Glasser et al. [23])

post-mortem microscopy or other specialized methods and could be replicated and validated in other group of subjects [23].

Functionally, less than half of the neocortical sheet appears to be occupied by predominantly unimodal regions, which are divided into five specialized groups of areas. Three are related to the major input streams to the brain (early auditory, early somatosensory/motor, and early visual areas), and two are core groups of cognitive areas (positive network and task negative network, also called the default mode network). Most of the cortex houses bi-modal or multi-modal areas and both hemispheres have a remarkable bilateral functional symmetry, with asymmetries most associated to language-related areas.

References

1. Ribas EC, Yağmurlu K, de Oliveira E, Ribas GC, Rhoton A. Microsurgical anatomy of the central core of the brain. J Neurosurg. 2018;129(3):752–69.
2. Azevedo FAC, Carvalho LRB, Grinberg LT, Farfel JM, Ferretti REL, Leite REP, et al. Equal numbers of neuronal and nonneuronal cells make the human brain an isometrically scaled-up primate brain. J Comp Neurol. 2009;513(5):532–41.
3. Ribas GC. The cerebral sulci and gyri. Neurosurg Focus. 2010;28(2):E2.

4. Ono M, Kubik S, Abernathey CD. Atlas of the cerebral sulci. Stuttgart/New York: G. Thieme Verlag/Thieme Medical Publishers; 1990. 218 p.
5. Braak H. Architectonics of the human telencephalic cortex [Internet]. Berlin, Heidelberg: Springer Berlin Heidelberg; 1980 [cited 2021 Jul 13]. Available from: https://doi.org/10.1007/978-3-642-81522-5.
6. Ribas G. Applied cranial-cerebral anatomy: brain architecture and anatomically oriented microneurosurgery. Cambridge, UK\New York, NY: Cambridge University Press; 2018. 132 p.
7. de Anatomia SB, de Terminologia Anatômica C, da Terminologia Anatômica CF. Terminologia anatômica: terminologia anatômica internacional. São Paulo: Manole; 2001.
8. Ribas GC, Ribas EC, Rodrigues CJ. The anterior sylvian point and the suprasylvian operculum. Neurosurg Focus. 2005;18(6B):E2.
9. Ribas EC, Yagmurlu K, Wen HT, Rhoton AL. Microsurgical anatomy of the inferior limiting insular sulcus and the temporal stem. J Neurosurg. 2015;122(6):1263–73.
10. Ribas GC, Yasuda A, Ribas EC, Nishikuni K, Rodrigues AJ. Surgical anatomy of microneurosurgical sulcal key points. Neurosurgery. 2006;59(4 Suppl 2):ONS177–210; discussion ONS210–211.
11. Ribas GC, Rodrigues AJJ. The suprapetrosal craniotomy. J Neurosurg. 2007;106(3):449–54.
12. Drury HA, Van Essen DC, Anderson CH, Lee CW, Coogan TA, Lewis JW. Computerized mappings of the cerebral cortex: a multiresolution flattening method and a surface-based coordinate system. J Cogn Neurosci. 1996;8(1):1–28.
13. Nieuwenhuys R, Voogd J, van Huijzen C. The human central nervous system. 4th ed. New York: Springer; 2008. p. 967.
14. Brodmann K. Feinere Anatomie des Grosshirns. In: Handbuch der Neurologie, 1 Band: Allgemeine Neurologie. Verlag von Julius Springer, Berlin: Lewandowsky, M.; 1910.
15. Brodmann K. Physiologie des Gehirns. In: Neue Deutsche Chirurgie, 11 Band: Allgemeine Chirurgie der Gehirnkrankheiten. Verlag von Ferdinand Enke, Stuttgart: Von Bruns P; 1914.
16. Judaš M, Cepanec M, Sedmak G. Brodmann's map of the human cerebral cortex — or Brodmann's maps? Transl Neurosci [Internet]. 2012 [cited 2021 Jul 31];3(1). Available from: https://www.degruyter.com/document/doi/10.2478/s13380-012-0009-x/html
17. Schmahmann JD, Pandya DN. Fiber pathways of the brain. Oxford/New York: Oxford University Press; 2006. 654 p.
18. Mesulam MM. Large-scale neurocognitive networks and distributed processing for attention, language, and memory. Ann Neurol. 1990;28(5):597–613.
19. Duffau H, editor. Brain mapping: from neural basis of cognition to surgical applications. Wien/New York: Springer; 2011. 392 p.
20. Coello AF, Moritz-Gasser S, Martino J, Martinoni M, Matsuda R, Duffau H. Selection of intraoperative tasks for awake mapping based on relationships between tumor location and functional networks: a review. JNS. 2013;119(6):1380–94.
21. Ius T, Angelini E, Thiebaut de Schotten M, Mandonnet E, Duffau H. Evidence for potentials and limitations of brain plasticity using an atlas of functional resectability of WHO grade II gliomas: towards a "minimal common brain". NeuroImage. 2011;56(3):992–1000.
22. Van Essen DC, Smith SM, Barch DM, Behrens TEJ, Yacoub E, Ugurbil K, et al. The WU-Minn human connectome project: an overview. NeuroImage. 2013;80:62–79.
23. Glasser MF, Coalson TS, Robinson EC, Hacker CD, Harwell J, Yacoub E, et al. A multi-modal parcellation of human cerebral cortex. Nature. 2016;536(7615):171–8.

Chapter 14
Brain Functions: Eloquent Areas – Motor and Somatosensory

Kathleen Seidel and Marcos Vinicius Calfat Maldaun

Abbreviations

CST	Corticospinal tract
DCS	Direct cortical stimulation
GTR	Gross total resection
M1	Primary motor area
MEP	Motor evoked potential
TES	Transcranial electrical stimulation

The Neuro-oncological Challenge

Minimizing the risk of disabling motor deficits is a main factor during surgery in eloquent motor areas. At the same time, this constitutes the major challenge for the neurosurgeon, who aims to achieve the best possible surgical outcome, such as maximal extent of tumor removal, without compromising the patient's functional status.

Complete removal or gross total resection (GTR) remains the surgical goal for most intracranial tumors including gliomas, and there is increasing evidence that GTR prolongs overall and progression-free survival in lower grade gliomas and

K. Seidel (✉)
Department of Neurosurgery, Inselspital, Bern University Hospital, University of Bern, Bern, Switzerland
e-mail: Kathleen.Seidel@insel.ch

M. V. C. Maldaun
Instituto de Ensino e Pesquisa (Teaching and Research Institute) of Hospital Sirio Libanês, São Paulo, SP, Brazil

Neurosurgery Department, Hospital Sirio Libanês, São Paulo, São Paulo, Brazil

S. M. Verst et al. (eds.), *Intraoperative Monitoring*,
https://doi.org/10.1007/978-3-030-95730-8_14

glioblastomas [1–7]. However, more than 50% of these tumors are judged to be "presumably eloquent" based on the preoperative images [8–10]. Intraoperative neurophysiological mapping can help to verify or falsify intraoperative eloquence and therefore to define "true-eloquence" and non-eloquent areas. Thus, intraoperative mapping may preserve function and increase the extent of tumor resection at the same time [10, 11].

To guide intraoperative decision-making, when to stop and when to continue resection, various neurophysiological methods are available. Continuous monitoring techniques, for example, monitoring of motor evoked potentials (MEPs), enable real-time assessment of the functional integrity of the observed functional system [12–20]. Electrical cortical mapping is the gold standard for localization of eloquent cortex [21–25]. Subcortical mapping is used to localize white matter tracts at different stages of tumor resection [8, 10, 21, 26–34].

The choice of the intraoperative neurophysiological technique may also depend on the intraoperative pathology, which needs to be treated (Fig. 14.1). Extra-axial lesions such as meningioma differ from infiltrative glioma. Brain plasticity and the goal of supra-marginal resection render intraoperative neurophysiological mapping an essential adjunct in the latter case [30, 35]. However, neurophysiological techniques may reassure the surgeon as well during the resection of cavernoma or metastasis by defining safe entry zones and by influencing the speed of tumor resection [11, 18, 36]. Intraoperative neurophysiological techniques should also be adapted to the tumor location. Tumors close to and in the precentral region may need precise and continuous mapping techniques whereas insular tumors may also need monitoring techniques for vascular ischemia [37–41].

Advances in imaging techniques such as functional MRI and fiber tracking algorithms as well as preoperative navigated transcranial magnetic stimulation examinations may help to plan the surgical approach and to prepare for intraoperative pitfalls. However, after opening the dura and especially after corticotomy and tumor debulking, neuronavigation loses accuracy due to brain shift [42]. Therefore, "maximal safe resection" should be guided by intraoperative neurophysiologic monitoring and mapping methods.

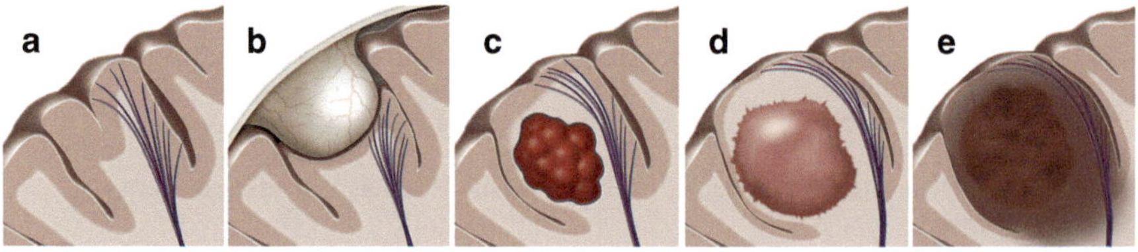

Fig. 14.1 (**a**) Coronar cut illustrating CST fibres originating from M1 in an healthy brain. (**b**) An extra-axial tumor such as an meningioma pushes the whole cortex down and may cover and partially infiltrate eloquent areas. Lesions like a cavernoma (**c**) and a metastasis (**d**) may displace the CST fibres in an unpredicted trajectory. Glioma infiltrate eloquent tracts (**e**), and thus, they render resection particulary challegning. (© Inselspital, Bern University Hospital, Dept. of Neurosurgery)

Monitoring Motor Function

Obviously, mapping only provides information at and distal to the stimulation site. If feedback about the whole integrity of the motor or sensory system in an anesthetized patient is needed, monitoring methods for a continuous assessment are recommended [18, 19, 43]. Thus, remote vascular injury due to coagulation of vessel perforators can only be detected by monitoring methods [15–17].

If MEP monitoring under general anesthesia is performed, some requirements for the anesthesia regime should be considered. The standard recommendation is total intravenous anesthesia, but inhalation agents with a low mean alveolar concentration might be possible in selected circumstances. A short-acting relaxant should be administered for intubation purpose only [44, 45]. Recovery from muscle relaxation could be tested by the use of the "train-of-four" technique involving percutaneous stimulation of median nerve applying 40 mA and a 0.2 ms pulse duration [45]. Under general anesthesia, classical short train technique, also called high-frequency stimulation, is applied. The temporal summation of multiple descending volleys in high-frequent short train stimulation finally triggers a time-locked MEP response [13, 14]. It typically consists of trains with four-to-nine monophasic rectangular electrical pulses of 200–500 μs pulse width with an inter stimulus interval of 2–4 ms (corresponding to 250–500 Hz) [13, 14, 19, 28, 44, 46]. Continuous MEP monitoring is performed either with via scalp electrodes (transcranial electrical stimulation, TES) or electrodes directly placed on the precentral gyrus (direct cortical stimulation, DCS, Fig. 14.2). For further details on MEP for supratentorial approaches, refer to Chap. 9.

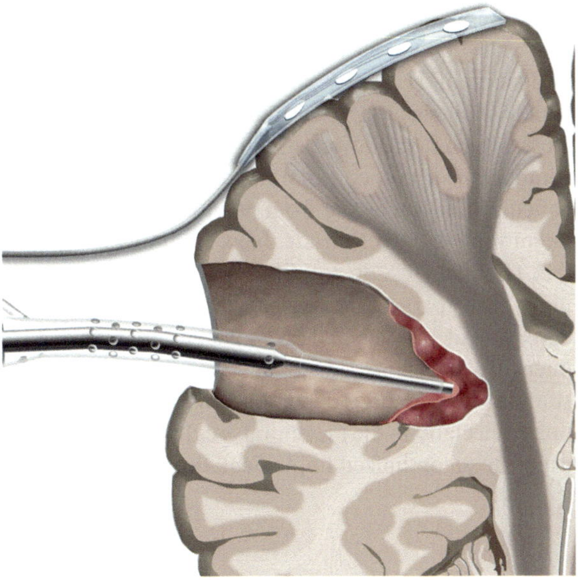

Fig. 14.2 Real-time assessment of direct cortical stimulated MEP via a strip electrode may monitor the functional integrity of M1 and the CST to assess the functional integrity of the primary motor system. Focal cortical stimulation may avoid false-negative results in case of more distal stimulation of the CST to the resection site. MEP will warn for remote vascular injury and help to predict long-term postoperative motor outcome. (© Inselspital, Bern University Hospital, Dept. of Neurosurgery)

MEP warning criteria represent a priori defined parameters. Optimally, they should alert the surgical team and they prompt the implementation of corrective measures [47]. Obviously, a false-negative reassurance will miss the neurological injury; however, a false-positive alarm may also indirectly harm the patient by stopping the surgery too early [47]. The most common proposed MEP alarm criteria include disappearance of MEP signal, amplitude reduction, and stimulation threshold elevation [48]. Disappearance of MEP signal is considered as a major alarming sign that required reassessment of intraoperative settings and adjustment of surgical strategy. Apart from MEP loss, the most commonly used warning criterion is amplitude reduction, and a >50% amplitude reduction is regarded in the vast majority of studies as significant during supratentorial surgery [16, 46, 49, 50]. Threshold cut-off values vary depending on stimulator settings (constant current versus constant voltage stimulation) and electrode montages (TES versus DCS) [51]. Cut-off values that have been used during TES were >100 V or >20 mA and during DCS >3 mA, ≥4 mA, and ≥5 mA.

TES may allow bilateral assessment, and therefore, the non-affected side may serve as control for non-surgical factors, like change in anesthetic depth. Therefore, Abboud et al. [52, 53] introduced a novel threshold criterion and suggested that a TES threshold increase on the affected side of more than 20% beyond the percentage increase on the unaffected side should be considered as a warning sign. The stimulation intensity has special importance when interpreting the amplitude criterion, as MEP exhibits trial-to-trial variability and MEP amplitude alterations may be caused by non-surgical factors [48]. Rothwell et al. [54] stated that strong stimulation currents may activate the CST even at the foramen magnum. Hence, depending on the area of interest, there might be the risk of stimulating the white matter more caudally than the site of neurological damage, leading to a higher rate of false-negative results. A topographic-guided MEP description is detailed in Chap. 9. Furthermore, loss of cerebrospinal fluid after the opening of the dura leads to brain shift and subdural air accumulation. That fact may interfere with the reliability and evaluation of TES-MEP warning criteria. Further, TES may cause a higher rate of patient movement [18]. Because of these drawbacks, many neurosurgeons opt for DCS, which needs lower stimulation intensities and allows a focal and superficial stimulation of corticospinal neurons [18]. Nonetheless, DCS is not applicable in patients with scar tissue from previous operations. It may also interfere with MEP monitoring due to electrode dislocation on the cortex [50]. Szelényi et al. reported that TES and DCS do not differ in their ability to detect an impending neurological injury. Both paradigms may be alternatively applied during the same surgical procedure, provided if lateral TES montages are not used and near-threshold stimulation intensities are applied [55]. However, a more thorough comparison between the two stimulation modalities depending on the type of surgery, pathology, and tumor location (especially in the precentral area) would be clinically meaningful and may contribute to an optimized implementation of warning criteria [47].

Monitoring Sensory Function

For brain tumor surgery, SEP may be used to detect cortical or subcortical ischemia affecting the somatosensory cortex or lemniscal pathways. A well-established relationship between the critical cortical perfusion of brain parenchyma below 15 ml/100 g/min and a decline of SEP amplitudes is described [56]. Recording of the median and tibial nerve cortical potentials of the unaffected hemisphere may serve as systemic controls to detect factors unrelated to the surgical resection such as the level of anesthesia and body temperature. A 50% amplitude decrement and an increment in the latency of the cortical potential are commonly used as warning criteria. However, smaller amplitude decrements may be significant when trial-to-trial reproducibility is high, and disappearance may be needed to detect non-random amplitude reduction when reproducibility is low [57].

A special application is the technique of SEP phase reversal (Fig. 14.3). The phenomenon of recording an inversion of the median nerve cortical SEP polarity between the postcentral and precentral gyri is used to determine the central sulcus [58, 59]. Many surgical teams being very experienced with cortical mapping do not routinely use this methodology as they find that direct cortical mapping provides sufficiently precise information. Nevertheless, SEP phase reversal is an excellent tool considerably helpful in distorted anatomy and inconclusive mapping results [59].

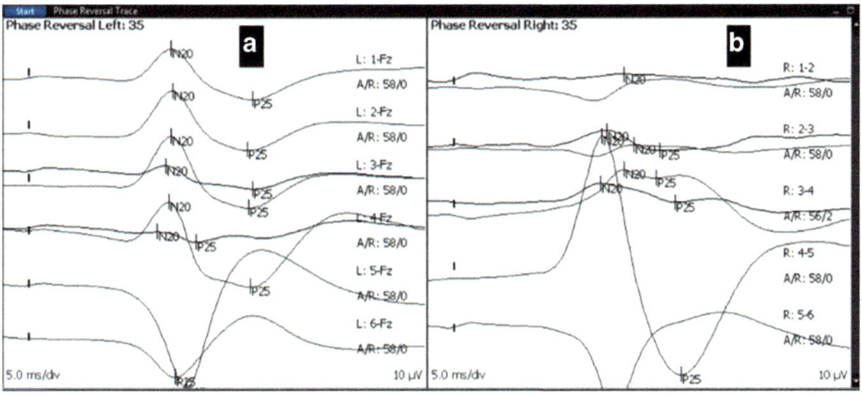

Fig. 14.3 Phase reversal of the ulnar nerve for identification of the central sulcus. (**a**) Referential technique: grid contacts are individually referred to Fz. (**b**) Differential technique: bipolar setup of the grid contacts: 1-2, 2-3, 3-4, 4-5, 5-6. Reversal of N20/P22 is seen between 4 and 5 in both techniques

Subcortical Mapping

Distance Estimation Toward CST

Identification of mapping alarm criteria for impending mechanical damage of the CST remains a challenge to the surgeon and neurophysiologist. During tumor removal, the surgeon needs to know how distant the resection cavity is at a certain point to the CST.

Eliciting an MEP depends on the charge applied to the tissue [28]. The charge density decreases with distance. The higher the charge, the larger the area where MEPs can be generated, and vice versa [18]. This also implies that with higher stimulus intensity or charge a positive stimulation can be found at a greater distance from the CST. This "stimulation-strength-to-CST-distance" relationship has been increasingly investigated by many groups that have correlated the stimulation intensity in mA needed to elicit MEPs with distance in mm to the CST using different pulse durations [60–65].

One of the first correlations was done by Kamada et al. [60] who found a convergent nonlinear correlation of distance and postulated 1.8 mA as the threshold of direct CST contact during monopolar cathodal subcortical stimulation using trains of five 0.2 ms pulses. Nossek et al. [62] compared the thresholds of subcortical monopolar mapping using trains of 5–7 0.5 ms pulses at 300 Hz to navigation with brain shift correction by intraoperative ultrasonography. They showed an approximately linear correlation between MEP thresholds and distance to the CST with a relationship of 0.97 mA for every 1 mm of brain tissue, which corresponds to the "rule-of-thumb" of 1 mA = 1 mm [45]. A linear correlation between stimulus intensity and distance was also postulated in another study by Ohue et al. [64] that used trains of five 0.2 ms pulses at 500 Hz and analyzed the distance of the postoperative resection cavity to the imaged CST in early postoperative diffusion tensor imaging MRI. Maesawa et al. [61] and Prabhu et al. [63] compared subcortical stimulation to intraoperative MRI tractography. Maesawa et al. (bipolar probe, train of 5 stimuli, pulse duration 0.4 ms, 500 Hz) found an approximately linear correlation, whereas Prabhu et al. (monopolar probe, train of 5 stimuli, 0.3–0.5 ms, 500 Hz) described a trend toward worsening neurologic deficits if the distance from the probe to the CST was <5 mm. Shiban et al. [65] marked the intraoperative stimulation site at the end of tumor resection with a titanium clip. At this location, different stimulation paradigms were executed with cathodal or anodal stimulation using pulse durations of 0.3, 0.5, and 0.7 ms. Postoperatively, the distance between the CST as defined by postoperative diffusion tensor imaging fiber tracking and the titanium clip was measured. The correlation between this distance and the subcortical MEP electric charge was calculated. Correlational and regression analyses showed a nonlinear correlation between stimulation intensity and the distance to the CST, and cathodal 0.5 ms pulse duration stimulation appeared best suited for subcortical stimulation.

When comparing these different studies, the applied number of stimuli, pulse duration, polarity, and especially charge might be of importance. Therefore, for subcortical motor mapping, it may be advisable to keep the number of stimuli and pulse duration constant, and to apply constant-current cathodal stimulation [18, 26, 45, 66]. It is important to understand that up to now, no definitive statement on this relationship is possible, but the vague rule of thumb "1 mA correlates to 1 mm" is increasingly being used when performing subcortical short train monopolar stimulation with five 0.5 ms cathodal constant-current pulses.

A consequent question is then what would be a reasonable lowest mapping threshold in mA to stop tumor resection. Several studies have shown that decreasing MEP thresholds correlate with an increasing risk of mechanical injury to the CST [18, 19, 36, 63, 66]. Applying monopolar subcortical cathodal short train stimulation at low stimulation intensities, Seidel et al. [18] demonstrated that motor thresholds correlate with the risk of CST injury. However, it was demonstrated that even mapping thresholds ≤3 mA might be safe if DCS MEP monitoring remains stable at the same time and mapping is repeated frequently [18, 43]. Therefore, a safe mapping corridor for mechanical injury of the CST exists between high and low mapping thresholds, and neither significant signal changes in MEP monitoring nor permanent motor deficits occur before very low subcortical mapping MEP thresholds [18, 43]. However, the stimulation intensity limit during subcortical short train mapping at which tumor removal is supposed to stop depends on various factors like tumor histopathology, planned goal of tumor resection, infiltration of other eloquent areas, or method of hemostasis; and therefore, the internal safety limit varies among surgical centers [18, 19, 26, 27, 36, 62–68].

Continuous Dynamic Mapping

Furthermore, the intermittent technique of conventional mapping with insufficient spatial and temporal coverage of the surgical site may fail to prevent motor deficits despite stopping resection at higher and apparently safe mapping thresholds, such as 3–6 mA applying monopolar short train stimulation [18]. A significant advance would be to apply mapping continuously with the highest possible temporal coverage, and directly at the site of tumor removal. This could be especially important at very low mapping thresholds of ≤3 mA in close proximity to the CST.

In keeping with this concept, Raabe et al. [26] recently described a new mapping protocol and developed a device allowing continuous subcortical stimulation without interrupting the surgical workflow of tumor removal (Fig. 14.4). This was achieved by integrating cathodal high-frequency stimulation (five 0.5 ms pulses, 250 Hz) into the tip of the surgical suction device at a repetition rate of 0.4–2 Hz. Positive MEP responses were coupled with an alarm sound to facilitate real-time feedback to the surgeon. In a proof-of-concept analysis of this continuous "dynamic"

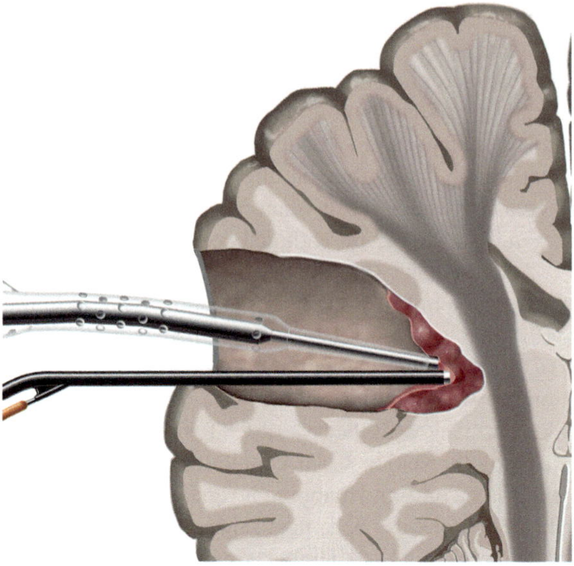

Fig. 14.4 Subcortical mapping may indicate the proximity to eloquent tracts such as the CST. If stimulation is included in the surgical instrument such as the suction device or CUSA, continuous dynamic mapping may be performed without interrupting the surgical workflow and thus continuously. (© Inselspital, Bern University Hospital, Dept. of Neurosurgery)

mapping method, safety was confirmed with a 3% rate of permanent motor deficits (due to remote vascular injury of the CST). In this series, no patient had a permanent motor deficit caused by a mechanical injury of the CST. The intraoperative rate of seizures was 4%, all detected by simultaneous electrocorticography (ECoG) recordings and easily terminated without alteration of the surgical workflow. Applying this continuous dynamic mapping technique to surgery of glioblastoma, Schucht et al. [73] demonstrated complete resection of enhancing tumor in 69% of patients despite high proximity to the CST and a permanent motor deficit rate of 4% (caused by vascular injury). Continuous "dynamic" mapping will not completely avoid so-called "mechanical" injury of the CST; however, allowing mapping during every surgical step at every surgical site increases the mapping coverage and provides real-time feedback [69]. This way, mapping is possible during the whole process of tumor removal and at every site of tumor removal.

Recently, the concept of continuous subcortical stimulation was also applied by stimulating directly via the cavitron ultrasonic surgical aspirator (CUSA) and it was again demonstrated to be a safe method [70, 71]. However, CUSA activity might also interfere with mapping results in rare occasions [72]. Integration of mapping into a standard suction device might be more ergonomic because continuous mapping will be available during all steps of tumor removal including subpial dissection and hemostasis, which may be performed with a variety of instruments [26, 68, 69, 73, 74]. The integration of the stimulation probe into any surgical instrument (CUSA or suction probe) might increase the reliability, surgical acceptance, and clinical handling of subcortical mapping.

Adapting Neurophysiological Tools to the Surgical Context

Achieving a maximal safe resection is a challenging process for both low- and high-grade gliomas. Infiltrative lesions located in the primary motor gyrus and close to the corticospinal tract require a tight symbiotic work between the surgical and neurophysiological team. Important concepts for lesions located in these areas are the following:

A. Beyond the intraoperative decrease of motor response, vascular infarction (causing post-operative MRI DWI alteration) is one of the main causes of permanent motor deficits. It is crucial that the surgeon avoids coagulation of sulcal vessels, truncal arteries, or main draining veins as shown in Fig. 14.5.
B. In our own clinical experience and based on literature, there is no difference in morbidity or extent of resection between proper neurophysiological mapping and monitoring under general anesthesia and performing testing of the patient during awake craniotomy [75].
C. Considering a risk of permanent motor deficits up to 40% during resection of low-grade gliomas in the primary motor gyrus, there is no harm to not achieve a gross total resection to avoid permanent motor deficits as illustrated in Figs. 14.6, 14.7, 14.8, and 14.9.

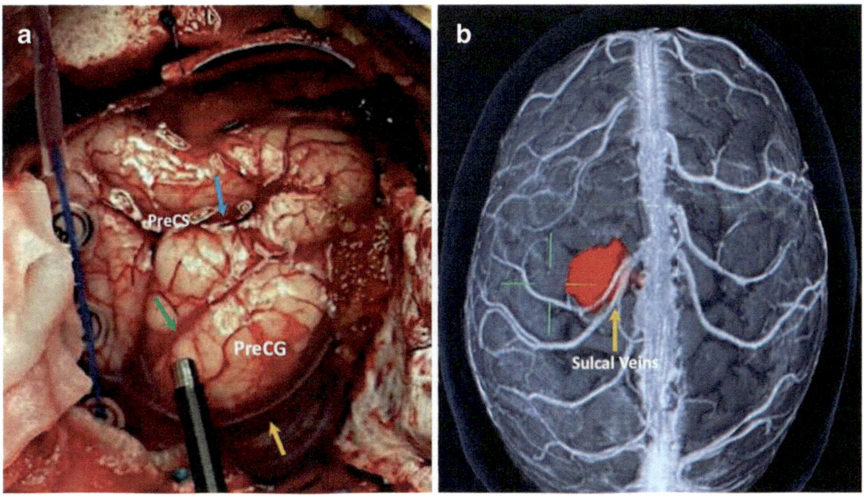

Fig. 14.5 (**a**) Fronto parietal craniotomy with the exposure of the precentral gyrus (PreCG), with a strip electrode positioned crossing the central sulcus (CS). Three critical concerns should be kept in mind during the resection of a lesion in an eloquent gyrus: (1) Avoid coagulating truncal vessels (green arrow); (2) avoid coagulating sulcal vessels, thorough subpial dissection (blue arrow); and (3) avoid coagulating prominent drainage veins (yellow arrow). (**b**) 3D-reconstruction image highlighting the drainage veins related with the tumor (yellow arrow). (© Marcos Maldaun)

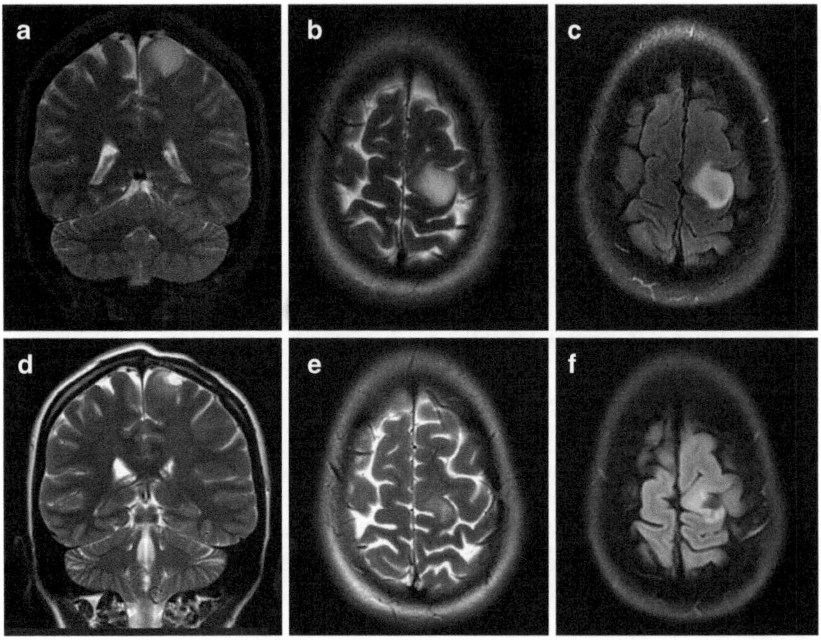

Fig. 14.6 Woman, 24 years old, with a left-sided frontal glioma. Preoperative MRI T2-weighted images, coronal (**a**) and axial (**b**) views, showing a hyperintense lesion in right-side precentral gyrus. On axial T2-FLAIR image (**c**), the tumor also has a homogeneous and strikingly high signal. Postoperative images (**d**–**f**), showing residual lesion adjacent to the surgical lacunae. Surgery was stopped due positive mapping response in right leg. (© Marcos Maldaun)

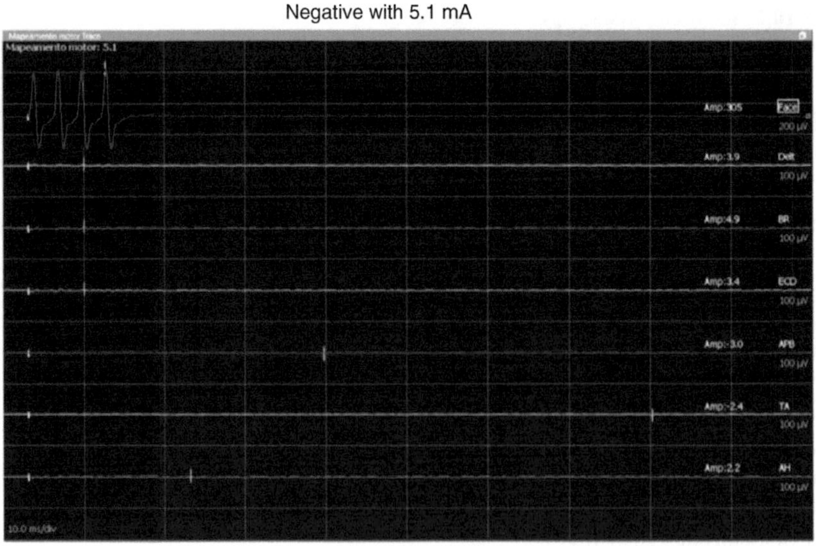

Fig. 14.7 Cortical mapping: anodal stimulation, To4, ISI 4 ms, pulse 500 uS. (© Marcos Maldaun)

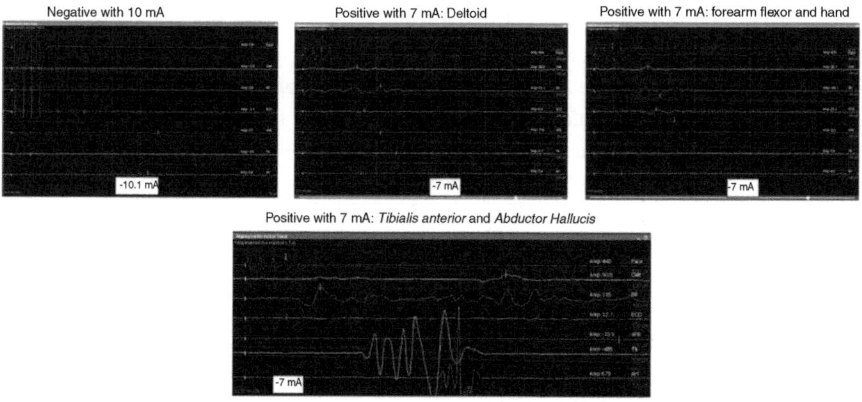

Fig. 14.8 Sequential subcortical mapping: cathodal stimulation, To4, ISI 4 ms, pulse 500 uS. (© Marcos Maldaun)

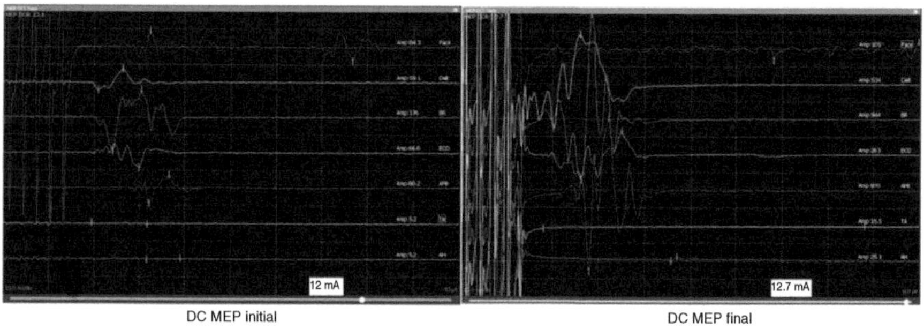

Fig. 14.9 Continuous direct cortical motor evoked potential (DC MEP): To4, ISI 4 ms, pulse 500 uS. (© Marcos Maldaun)

Prediction of Motor Recovery

In supratentorial surgery, intraoperative MEP monitoring indicates the functional integrity of the CST [18, 19, 47]. MEP monitoring is a useful adjunct to cortical and subcortical mapping techniques due to its ability to detect remote vascular injury [17, 18, 76]. Several series have shown a low risk for permanent change in postoperative motor function as long as intraoperative direct cortical stimulated (DCS) MEPs are preserved without alteration [12, 18, 19, 47, 77, 78]. However, permanent neurological deficits may occur after surgery despite extensive intraoperative neurophysiological monitoring and mapping, although at a much lower rate. The uncertainty about whether a limb will recover from paresis is stressful for the patient and the surgeon. Neurological examination may fail to clearly attribute deficits to damage of the primary motor area (M1) or the adjacent supplementary/ventral/dorsal motor area (SMA/VPM/ DPM) [79–81], yet the patient will only recover from the latter [81, 82]. In tumor surgery there might be no isolated lesion to just one classical motor area. More likely, multiple white matter tract connections are involved and, for example, SMA and VPM projections are still unresolved [83–85]. The patient's quality of life and degree of dependency often influences the choice of adjuvant treatment. Ultimately, guidelines recommend reducing adjuvant treatment of high-grade glioma if a certain threshold of day-to-day independence is not reached by the patient, and new postoperative neurological deficits are known to have a negative impact on overall survival [86].

Non-invasive transcranial magnetic stimulation (TMS) testing could indicate which patients would benefit most from intensive postoperative rehabilitation. In patients with hand palsy due to ischemic stroke, TMS 1 day after the event has a high predictive value for motor recovery [87–89]. This aspect becomes even more important in the context of adjuvant neuro-oncological treatment in brain tumor patients. In early postoperative TMS studies, Zentner et al. were able to demonstrate that TMS-elicited MEP amplitudes would correlate with stepwise improvement of motor function [80]. They illustrated that a patient waking up with postoperative hemiplegia presented no TMS-elicited MEPs, but once the patient gradually recovered his motor strength, MEPs could be elicited with higher and higher amplitudes. TMS was thus shown to have a descriptive value but was not able to forecast recovery. A limitation of the study might have been the low excitability of the motor cortex additionally influenced by postoperative scalp edema, air collecting in the surgical resection cavity, and low intensity stimulation. In a single case report, Sala et al. overcame that challenge by applying multi-pulse stimulation with a short train [90]. They performed non-navigated TMS 1 day after surgery in a patient with hemiplegia due to a possible SMA syndrome and recorded TMS-elicited MEP. The patient did recover and had regained full function within a few weeks. Another way to improve the effectiveness in TMS stimulation might be to use navigated TMS, especially as the classical site for the best coil position might be displaced by tumor growth, shift of the primary motor area, and the resection cavity [91]. To overcome these challenges, Takakura et al. used navigated TMS (nTMS) and showed that the presence of a positive hand MEP 1 week after surgery correlated highly with motor recovery [92]. So far, postoperative TMS examinations for lower-extremity deficits have been neglected, as MEPs to the leg are more difficult to elicit than MEPs to the hand [93]. In a recent series Seidel et al. were able to confirm that in a case when MEP were present in postoperative nTMS performed within 14 days, the patient did recover, at least to MRCS 4 within 1 month [94]. Furthermore, they were able to demonstrate this predictive value not only for upper-, but also for lower-extremity deficits. Thus, early postoperative nTMS may reliably predict long-term motor recovery of patients suffering from severe motor deficits immediately after resection of tumors located in motor eloquent areas. In the case of intraoperative alterations of MEP monitoring, early postoperative nTMS may clarify the potential of rehabilitation for motor recovery [94].

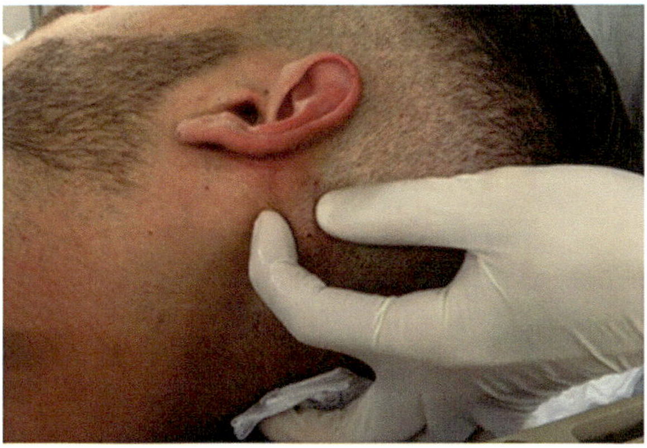

Fig. 15.4 Engorgement confirming the deposit of local anesthetic in the proper pathway (the author's personal file)

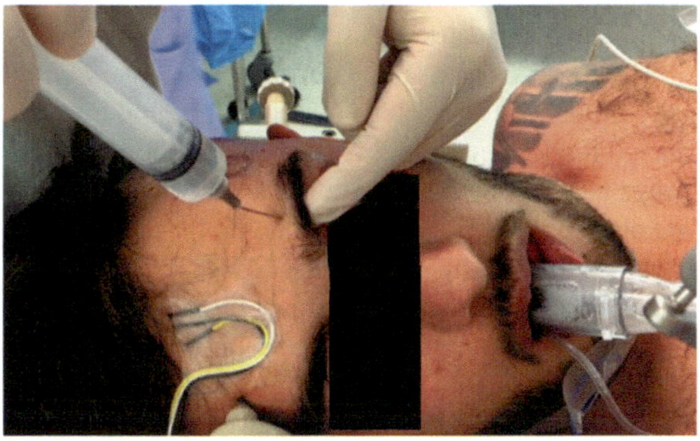

Fig. 15.5 Supra-trochlear and supra-orbital nerve blocks (the author's personal file)

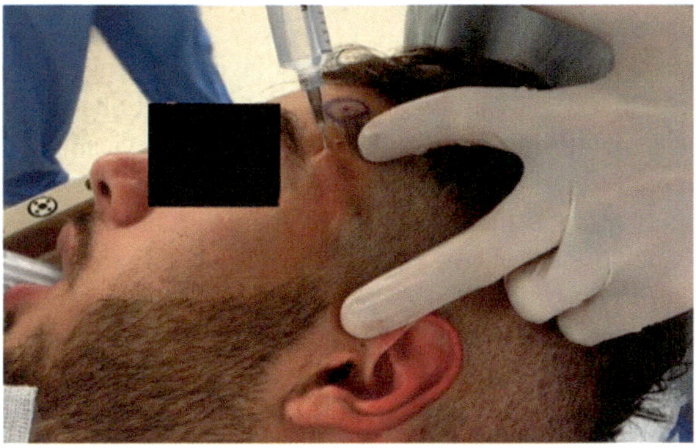

Fig. 15.6 Zygomatic nerve block (the author's personal file)

sequence, the anesthetist must allow the neurophysiologist to place electrodes. In addition, at the time of positioning, there must be a harmonious organization in order for the various electrophysiological monitoring cables not to get tangled with the anesthesiologist's monitoring cables, with the venous hydration lines, with the

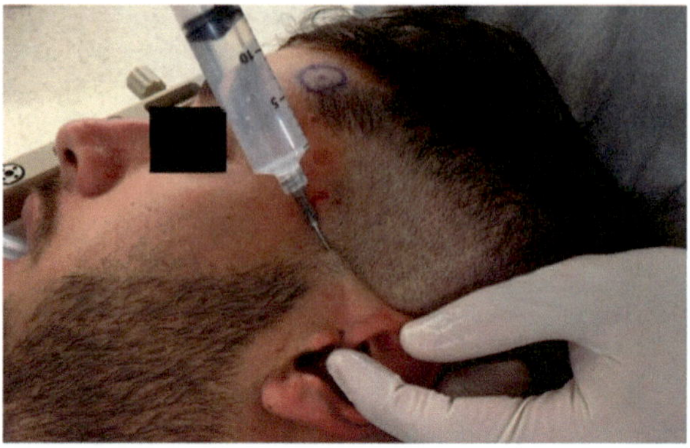

Fig. 15.7 Block of the auriculo-temporal nerve (the author's personal file)

invasive blood pressure monitoring line, or even with the mechanical ventilator tube. Still, we must observe if any of these devices is in contact with the patient's skin, which can cause pressure damage.

Homeostasis is essential during neurosurgery with IOM. Physiologic factors that may influence EPs include temperature, blood pressure, hematocrit, acid-base balance, blood glucose, and oxygen and carbon dioxide tensions. In addition, several drugs can also influence the electrophysiological responses. Thereby, anesthetists are able to support IOM by managing these aspects.

It is noteworthy that bolus doses of anesthetics or sudden and pronounced changes in infusion doses impair monitoring because they cause changes in the recording of potentials and compromise the neurophysiologist's assessment [1].

Pharmacological Effects

Anesthesia involves the choice of favorable drug combination and maintenance of a steady state, avoiding changes in concentration or bolus drug delivery during critical monitoring periods [12]. The effect of anesthetics on synaptic transmission is greater than on axonal conduction [13]. For this reason, responses recorded from polysynaptic pathways (e.g., cortical recordings) are affected by anesthesia to a much greater extent than those recorded from oligosynaptic pathways (e.g., spinal cord and subcortical recordings) [14]. This may explain why inhalational agents produce a dramatic nonlinear, dose-dependent reduction in cortical responses, increasing with the number of synapses involved [15].

It is noteworthy that bolus doses of anesthetics or sudden and pronounced changes in their infusion doses impair monitoring, since they cause alteration of the baseline potentials and compromise the neurophysiologist's evaluation [1].

Inhalational Agents

In general, the inhalational anesthetic agents have the most profound effect on monitoring [16]. All volatile anesthetics produce a dose-dependent increase in SSEP latency, an increase in central conduction time (CCT), and a decrease in amplitude [17, 18]. They may also cause morphologic changes, such as contraction of early cortical waveforms (N-20) into a simple monophasic wave under deep isoflurane [19] or sevoflurane [20] anesthesia. The later cortical waveform components are most sensitive to volatile anesthetics, with marked attenuation at concentrations exceeding 0.5 minimum alveolar concentration (MAC) [19].

How volatile anesthetics differ quantitatively in their effects on the SSEP is not completely settled [1]. Sevoflurane and desflurane are associated with less amplitude reduction than isoflurane at a MAC range of 0.7–1.3 [21]. The newer volatile anesthetics desflurane and sevoflurane affect SSEPs not unlike isoflurane but may permit the use of higher inhaled concentrations [1]. In contrast to their effects on the cortical SSEP, all volatile anesthetics, even at concentrations above 1.0 MAC, only minimally affect the subcortical waveform, resulting in high recordability [21] and reliability. The effect of volatile anesthetics on cortical SSEP amplitude is exacerbated by nitrous oxide [1]. Eliminating nitrous oxide from the background anesthetic has been shown to improve cortical amplitude sufficiently to make IOM more reliable [22].

Potent volatile anesthetics are associated with small increases in BAEP latency but do not affect wave I–V amplitude [23–26]. The prolongation of wave I–V latency and interpeak latency (IPL) reflects the depressant effect of volatile anesthetics on brainstem neuronal activity [26]. In adults, the effect of volatile anesthetics on BAEP latency is dose dependent [27]. In contrast to cortical SSEPs, the action of volatile anesthetics on BAEP latency or amplitude is not affected by 50–70% nitrous oxide [1]. 10–50% nitrous oxide alone also had no effect on the latency, interpeak latency, or amplitude of waves I–V in healthy volunteers [28].

Volatile anesthetic agents produce predictable dose-dependent increases in mid-latency auditory evoked potential (MLAEP) latency and decreases in amplitude [26]. At approximately 1 MAC, MLAEP components are markedly attenuated, indicating suppression of cortical auditory processing such as auditory perception, intraoperative wakefulness, and explicit or implicit recall of intraoperative events [29].

In general, all volatile anesthetics markedly prolong VEP latency and decrease amplitude in a dose-dependent manner [30].

The inhalational agents produce minimal changes in the epidurally recorded D-wave of the MEP with dramatic depression of the compound muscle action potential (CMAP) response [31]. The CMAP response of the MEP appears most easily abolished by low concentrations of halogenated inhalational agents [1]. However, MEP monitoring of neurologically normal individuals undergoing spine surgery can frequently be accomplished with the use of 0.5 MAC of desflurane or sevoflurane [31].

The effects of anesthesia on the EP can be greater in neurologically impaired patients than in patients without preoperative deficits [32]. Several strategies can be used to enhance the amplitude and reproducibility of SSEPs during volatile anesthesia [1]. Technical strategies such as keeping electrode impedance low and using appropriate bandpass filters are important [33]. Increasing the rate of stimulation in patients with normal baseline SSEPs may improve the preservation of SSEP waves, particularly at higher volatile anesthetic concentrations [1].

When IOM is being performed, volatile anesthetics alone at a dose greater than 1 MAC and volatile anesthetics at greater than 0.5 MAC in combination with nitrous oxide should be avoided. Therefore, volatile anesthetics alone at up to 1 MAC can be used, although it is critical to avoid sudden changes in volatile anesthetic depth. However, in general, intravenous anesthetic techniques result in less amplitude and latency perturbation than volatile anesthetics [18].

Intravenous Agents

Total venous anesthesia is preferred during IOM because it influences EPs much less than volatile anesthetics.

Barbiturates produce a dose-dependent increase in latency and decrease in early cortical SSEP amplitude that does not preclude IOM. Even at much higher doses, such as those used for barbiturate coma, barbiturates allow recording of cortical SSEPs [34]. Barbiturates in doses used for the induction of anesthesia do not affect the BAEP [35]. Amplitude was unchanged in doses used for the induction of anesthesia, and BAEP waveforms were easily recorded even in the presence of an isoelectric electroencephalogram [36].

Etomidate dramatically increases cortical SSEP amplitude (N-20), up to 400% above preinduction baseline in some patients [37], with no changes in subcortical and peripheral sensory responses [38].

Propofol is the most commonly used anesthetic in neurosurgery, especially at the IOM context. Induction produces amplitude depression in cortical SSEPs [16], although SSEP waveforms stabilized within 30 min after anesthetic administration and were compatible with IOM [39]. Propofol suppresses EPs less than other anesthetics, mainly when compared with inhaled agents [1]. The rapid propofol metabolism allows quickly adjustments when EPs are affected.

The effects of ketamine on subcortical and peripheral responses are also minimal; it increases the amplitude of the cortical SSEP and MEP CMAP [40]. The use of ketamine with propofol reduces the depressant effect of propofol while providing an enhancement effect on responses.

Benzodiazepines have only mild-to-moderate depressant effects on SSEPs [1] and do not change the amplitude or latency of BAEP [41].

Opioids cause only mild depression of all responses [31], but most authors report clinically unimported changes.

Dexmedetomidine appears to have minimal effects on SSEP responses when combined with opioids [31].

Neuromuscular blocking agents do not directly influence SSEP, BAEP, or VEP [42]. However, depression of the neuromuscular junction impairs MEP and electromyography (EMG) monitoring [31].

Complications

The most common complications are seizure, airway emergence, hypertension, desaturation, nausea and vomiting, cerebral edema, insufficient duration of scalp block, and inability to perform neurofunctional tests.

Failure due to the patient's inability to perform neurofunctional tests is commonly caused by seizure, cerebral edema, dysphasia, and somnolence [43].

Convulsion is an infrequent event. If it occurs, any electrical stimulation should be discontinued, and the surgeon should promptly irrigate the brain tissue with ice-cold saline solution. If it persists, a small dose of propofol is recommended. We should avoid benzodiazepines, as the prolonged effect may make it impossible to continue neurofunctional testing. Fortunately, airway instrumentation is usually not necessary [44].

Emergency airway supplies should always be available. If ventilatory depression occurs, generally placing a Guedel tube and performing manual ventilation with a face mask is successful. In any case, a laryngeal mask should be available if the need arises.

Cerebral edema should be treated by elevating the head, improving ventilation with a consequent reduction in the CO2 level, and controlling blood pressure. The use of hyperosmolar solutions such as mannitol or hypertonic saline may be required. In some situations, these measures may be ineffective, and tumor surgical emptying may be necessary to improve the operative site.

Arterial hypertension is not desirable as it compromises resection. However, vasodilators cause cerebral vasodilation and should be used with caution. In this situation, if there is no contraindication, beta-blockers can be used.

Failure to perform neurofunctional tests requiring conversion to general anesthesia is rare. A meta-analysis showed that both the asleep-awake-asleep technique and the conscious sedation technique are similar in relation to the occurrence of major adverse events [5].

Conclusion

Intraoperative awake craniotomy reduces the length of stay in the hospital, potentially reducing the risk of infection and thromboembolic events, and shortens the interval between surgery and chemotherapy [45].

Accumulating evidence suggests that, compared with surgery under general anesthesia, craniotomy with intraoperative awakening is associated with better outcomes, including greater extent of tumor resection, less subsequent neurological deficit, shorter hospital stay, and increased survival [45].

In this scenario, the decisions made by the anesthesiologist have great influence on the intraoperative success and postoperative clinical outcome.

The anesthesiologist should, to minimize the impact on evoked potentials, preserve adequate homeostasis, use intravenous anesthetics whenever possible, avoid bolus doses or sudden and large changes in infusions, and notify the neurophysiologist whenever any change or modification in the anesthetic regimen occurs.

References

1. Banoub M, Tetzlaff JE, Schubert A. Pharmacologic and physiologic influences affecting sensory evoked potentials: implications for perioperative monitoring. Anesthesiology [Internet]. 2003;99(3):716–37. Available from: https://doi.org/10.1097/00000542-200309000-00029.
2. Tewari A, Francis L, Samy RN, Kurth DC, Castle J, Frye T, et al. Intraoperative neurophysiological monitoring team's communiqué with anesthesia professionals. J Anaesthesiol Clin Pharmacol. 2018;34(1):84–93.
3. Alcaraz García-Tejedor G, Echániz G, Strantzas S, Jalloh I, Rutka J, Drake J, et al. Feasibility of awake craniotomy in the pediatric population. Paediatr Anaesth. 2020;30(4):480–9.
4. Bilotta F, Rosa G. "Anesthesia" for awake neurosurgery. Curr Opin Anaesthesiol. 2009;22(5):560–5.
5. Sewell D, Smith M. Awake craniotomy: anesthetic considerations based on outcome evidence. Curr Opin Anaesthesiol. 2019;32(5):546–52.
6. Hall JE, Uhrich TD, Barney JA, Arain SR, Ebert TJ. Sedative, amnestic, and analgesic properties of small-dose dexmedetomidine infusions. Anesth Analg. 2000;90(3):699–705.
7. Bustillo MA, Lazar RM, Finck AD, Fitzsimmons B, Berman MF, Pile-Spellman J, et al. Dexmedetomidine may impair cognitive testing during endovascular embolization of cerebral arteriovenous malformations: a retrospective case report series. J Neurosurg Anesthesiol. 2002;14(3):209–12.
8. Mack PF, Perrine K, Kobylarz E, Schwartz TH, Lien CA. Dexmedetomidine and neurocognitive testing in awake craniotomy. J Neurosurg Anesthesiol. 2004;16(1):20–5.
9. McAuliffe N, Nicholson S, Rigamonti A, Hare GMT, Cusimano M, Garavaglia M, et al. Awake craniotomy using dexmedetomidine and scalp blocks: a retrospective cohort study. Can J Anaesth. 2018;65(10):1129–37.
10. Goettel N, Bharadwaj S, Venkatraghavan L, Mehta J, Bernstein M, Manninen PH. Dexmedetomidine vs propofol-remifentanil conscious sedation for awake craniotomy: a prospective randomized controlled trial. Br J Anaesth. 2016;116(6):811–21.
11. Guilfoyle MR, Helmy A, Duane D, Hutchinson PJA. Regional scalp block for postcraniotomy analgesia: a systematic review and meta-analysis. Anesth Analg. 2013;116(5):1093–102.
12. Sloan TB. General anesthesia for monitoring. In: Monitoring the nervous system for anesthesiologists and other health care professionals. New York: Springer; 2012. p. 319–35.
13. Richards CD. Actions of general anaesthetics on synaptic transmission in the CNS. Br J Anaesth. 1983;55(3):201–7.
14. Samra SK, Vanderzant CW, Domer PA, Sackellares JC. Differential effects of isoflurane on human median nerve somatosensory evoked potentials. J Am Soc Anesthesiol. 1987;66(1):29–35.

15. Sloan TB, Heyer EJ. Anesthesia for intraoperative neurophysiologic monitoring of the spinal cord. J Clin Neurophysiol. 2002;19(5):430–43.
16. Sloan T, Jameson L, Janik D, Koht A. Evoked potentials. In: Cottrell J, Patel P, editors. Neuroanesthesia. 6th ed. Elsevier; 2017. p. 114–26.
17. Pathak KS, Amaddio MD, Scoles PV, Shaffer JW, Mackay W. Effects of halothane, enflurane, and isoflurane in nitrous oxide on multilevel somatosensory evoked potentials. J Am Soc Anesthesiol. 1989;70(2):207–12.
18. Sebel PS, Ingram DA, Flynn PJ, Rutherfoord CF, Rogers H. Evoked potentials during isoflurane anaesthesia. BJA: Br J Anaesth. 1986;58(6):580–5.
19. Porkkala T, Kaukinen S, Häkkinen V, Jäntti V. Median nerve somatosensory evoked potentials during isoflurane anaesthesia. Can J Anaesth. 1997;44(9):963–8.
20. Rytky S, Huotari AM, Alahuhta S, Remes R, Suominen K, Jäntti V. Tibial nerve somatosensory evoked potentials during EEG suppression in sevoflurane anaesthesia. Clin Neurophysiol. 1999;110(9):1655–8.
21. Rehberg B, Rüschner R, Fischer M, Ebeling BJ, Hoeft A. Concentration-dependent changes in the latency and amplitude of somatosensory-evoked potentials by desflurane, isoflurane and sevoflurane. Anasthesiol Intensivmed Notfallmedizin Schmerztherapie AINS. 1998;33(7):425–9.
22. Porkkala T, Janit V, Kaukinen S, Hakkinen V. Nitrous oxide has different effects on the EEG and somatosensory evoked potentials during isoflurane anaesthesia in patients. Acta Anaesthesiol Scand. 1997;41(4):497–501.
23. Manninen PH, Lam AM, Nicholas JF. The effects of isoflurane and isoflurane-nitrous oxide anesthesia on brainstem auditory evoked potentials in humans. Anesth Analg. 1985;64(1):43–7.
24. Madler C, Keller I, Schwender D, Pöppel E. Sensory information processing during general anaesthesia: effect of isoflurane on auditory evoked neuronal oscillations. Br J Anaesth. 1991;66(1):81–7.
25. Schwender D, Klasing S, Conzen P, Finsterer U, Pöppel E, Peter K. Midlatency auditory evoked potentials during anaesthesia with increasing endexpiratory concentrations of desflurane. Acta Anaesthesiol Scand. 1996;40(2):171–6.
26. Schwender D, Conzen P, Klasing S, Finsterer U, Poppel E, Peter K. The effects of anesthesia with increasing end-expiratory concentrations of sevoflurane on midlatency auditory evoked potentials. Anesth Analg. 1995;81(4):817–22.
27. Thornton C, Heneghan CPH, James MFM, Jones JG. Effects of halothane or enflurane with controlled ventilation on auditory evoked potentials. Br J Anaesth. 1984;56(4):315–23.
28. Sebel PS, Flynn PJ, Ingram DA. Effect of nitrous oxide on visual, auditory and somatosensory evoked potentials. Br J Anaesth. 1984;56(12):1403–7.
29. Schwender D, Klasing S, Madler C, Pöppel E, Peter K. Midlatency auditory evoked potentials and cognitive function during general anesthesia. Int Anesthesiol Clin. 1993;31(4):89–106.
30. Chi OZ, Field C. Effects of isoflurane on visual evoked potentials in humans. Anesthesiology. 1986;65(3):328–30.
31. Edmonds HL Jr. Multi-modality neurophysiologic monitoring for cardiac surgery. Heart Surg Forum. 2002:225–8.
32. Gillerman R, Duncan J, Bolton J. Prolonged somatosensory evoked potential depression following a brief exposure to low concentrations of inhalation anaesthetic in a 3-year-old child. Pediatr Anesth. 2000;10(3):336–8.
33. Kalkman CJ, ten Brink SA, Been HD, Bovill JG. Variability of somatosensory cortical evoked potentials during spinal surgery. Effects of anesthetic technique and high-pass digital filtering. Spine (Phila Pa 1976). 1991;16(8):924–9.
34. Sutton LN, Frewen T, Marsh R, Jaggi J, Bruce DA. The effects of deep barbiturate coma on multimodality evoked potentials. J Neurosurg. 1982;57(2):178–85.
35. Duncan PG, Sanders RA, McCullough DW. Preservation of auditory-evoked brainstem responses in anaesthetized children. Can Anaesth Soc J. 1979;26(6):492–5.

36. Drummond JC, Todd MM, U HS. The effect of high dose sodium thiopental on brain stem auditory and median nerve somatosensory evoked responses in humans. J Am Soc Anesthesiol. 1985;63(3):249–54.
37. McPherson RW, Sell B, Traystman RJ. Effects of thiopental, fentanyl, and etomidate on upper extremity somatosensory evoked potentials in humans. J Am Soc Anesthesiol. The American Society of Anesthesiologists. 1986;65:584–9.
38. Koht A, Schütz W, Schmidt G, Schramm J, Watanabe E. Effects of etomidate, midazolam, and thiopental on median nerve somatosensory evoked potentials and the additive effects of fentanyl and nitrous oxide. Anesth Analg. 1988;67(5):435–41.
39. Borrissov B, Langeron O, Lille F, Gomola A, Saillant G, Riou B, et al. Combination of propofol-sufentanil on somatosensory evoked potentials in surgery of the spine. Ann Fr Anesth Reanim. 1995;14:326–30.
40. Schubert A, Licina MG, Lineberry PJ. The effect of ketamine on human somatosensory evoked potentials and its modification by nitrous oxide. J Am Soc Anesthesiol. 1990;72(1):33–9.
41. Schwender D, Klasing S, Madler C, Pöppel E, Peter K. Effects of benzodiazepines on mid-latency auditory evoked potentials. Can J Anaesth. 1993;40(12):1148–54.
42. Sloan TB. Nondepolarizing neuromuscular blockade does not alter sensory evoked potentials. J Clin Monit. 1994;10(1):4–10.
43. Nossek E, Matot I, Shahar T, Barzilai O, Rapoport Y, Gonen T, et al. Failed awake craniotomy: a retrospective analysis in 424 patients undergoing craniotomy for brain tumor. Clinical article. J Neurosurg. 2013;118(2):243–9.
44. Meng L, McDonagh DL, Berger MS, Gelb AW. Anesthésie pour craniotomie éveillé: guide pratique pour le praticien occasionnel. Can J Anesth. 2017;64(5):517–29.
45. Blanshard HJ, Chung F, Manninen PH, Taylor MD, Bernstein M. Awake craniotomy for removal of intracranial tumor: considerations for early discharge. Anesth Analg. 2001;92(1):89–94.

Chapter 16
Anatomy: Language Network and DTI

João Tiago Alves-Belo

Abbreviations

AF	Arcuate fasciculus
DTI	Diffusion tensor imaging
FAT	Frontal aslant tract
HDFT	High-definition fiber tracking
IFOF	Inferior fronto-occipital fasciculus
ILF	Inferior longitudinal fasciculus
ITG	Inferior temporal gyri
LLG	Low-grade gliomas
MdLF	Middle longitudinal fasciculus
MTG	Middle temporal gyri
pre-SMA	Pre-supplementary motor area
SLF	Superior longitudinal fasciculus
SMA	Supplementary motor area
STG	Superior temporal gyri
UF	Uncinate fasciculus

Introduction

The human language faculty is a cognitive capacity shared by all normal humans but no other species on the planet [1]. Several definitions can be attributed to it, but it is essentially the capacity of human beings to express themselves, allowing us to

J. T. Alves-Belo (✉)
Neurosurgery Department, Hospital Felício Rocho, Belo Horizonte, MG, Brazil

S. M. Verst et al. (eds.), *Intraoperative Monitoring*,
https://doi.org/10.1007/978-3-030-95730-8_16

live in community. Spoken language is an exceedingly complex faculty that allows us to encode, elaborate, and communicate thoughts and experiences by mediating arbitrary symbols known as words [2].

Preserving language is a challenge when we face diseases that involve eloquent brain areas. Several conditions can impair communication, and its treatment may be associated with the risk of permanent deficits, which severely reduces the quality of life of the patients. Low-grade gliomas (LGG), for instance, are typically located within eloquent areas and can involve brain regions related to language in about 50% of the cases [3].

For those who intend to deal with brain lesions related to language, understanding the anatomy and functional basis of the language network is paramount. This chapter aims to review the current language model under an anatomical and functional view based on traditional fiber dissections made as proposed by Klingler [4] and also with the aid of high-definition fiber tracking (HDFT) based on the use of diffusion tensor imaging (DTI) [5].

The Classic Language Model, History, and Evolution

Understanding how the brain can create effective communication has been a challenge for researchers over the centuries. Pierre Broca and Carl Wernicke have a vital contribution in this field. Their work has been applied for several years. Broca did his research through observations of patients who had different lesions affecting the left inferior frontal gyrus. He observed that these patients lost their ability to articulate words, while their "memory of the words" and "action of the nerves and muscles of phonation and articulation" were preserved [6].

Few years after Broca's theory was spread, Wernicke observed that lesions in the posterior superior temporal lobe caused paraphasic errors with impaired naming, repetition, and comprehension. However, the fluency of speech was preserved [7]. He named this region "the area of word images" and further postulated that this region was connected to the inferior frontal region described by Broca. Therefore, Wernicke proposes that the language function was distributed in the two different cortical sites: an anterior frontal cortex involved in motor processing and a posterior temporal cortex performing sensory functions [8]. The arcuate fasciculus would make the connections between these two areas. Wernicke believed that lesions involving this bundle of fibers result in the so-called conduction aphasia, which was subsequently confirmed by Lichtheim in the clinic scenario [9].

In the subsequent decades, this approach to brain function raised a wave of criticisms, and the clinic-anatomical correlation method came under attack by many prominent investigators [2, 8]. On the other hand, the localizationist theories gained strength after the work of Brodmann and Penfield. Brodmann mapped the human cortex in 52 distinct cortical areas based on cytoarchitectonic features. He then postulated that regions with different histologic structures performed different functions [10]. Based on direct electrical stimulation (DES), Penfield, in his turn, mapped the somatosensory and motor cortices of the human brain. He also attributed different manifestations to stimulations of temporal and parietal lobes [11].

The idea that each brain function is rigidly localized in a particular cortical area of the brain and an injury to a specific area of the cortex would lead to a loss of corresponding brain function became prominent. In this view, cortices or cortical areas where neurons are located are more relevant when considering the functional aspects of the brain rather than white matter [12].

This dialectic between the localizationists and their opponents lasted for several decades until the work of Geschwind, in the 1960s, pacified the question through new insights into the functional role of connections and specialized cortical areas [2]. He proposed that disconnections syndromes could be induced by lesions involving the white matter and the association cortex. For language, he argued that the perisylvian cortex acts as a relay station between Wernicke's and Broca's areas. Therefore, conduction aphasia would be generated to either a lesion in the arcuate fasciculus or the association perisylvian cortex, notedly the angular gyrus [13]. These ideas were compiled as the Wernicke-Geschwind language model (Fig. 16.1). In this theory, a sensory word image would be formatted when an individual first heard a word; given the cortico-cortical connections between the two primary language areas, it would precipitate the simultaneous formation of a motor word image [8]. Although these motor and sensitive words were formatted from the same stimulus, they are not equivalent concepts. The sensory word is located at the auditory cortex, and the meaning attributed to it is diffusely spread through connections coming from the two language centers. Therefore, the spontaneous speech production demands "awakening" of the concept (diffusely located) that activates the sensory

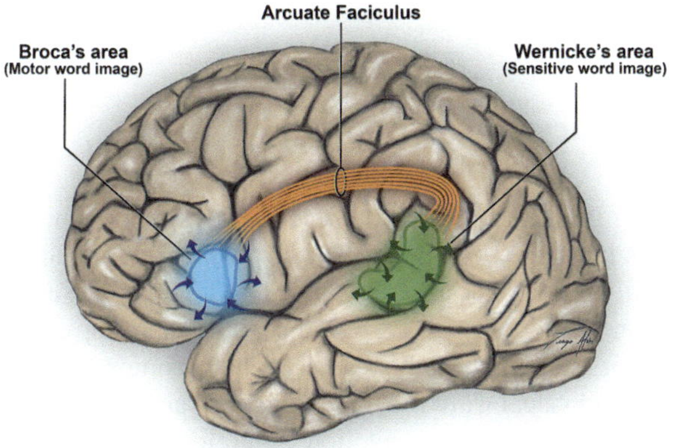

Fig. 16.1 Classical model of language organization proposed based on the Wernicke and Geschwind theory. Broca's area (represented in blue), located in the inferior frontal gyrus, is the motor center of language, and Wernicke's area (represented in green), located in the posterior temporal region, is the sensitive word center. The connection of these two language centers is made through the arcuate fasciculus. Cortico-cortical connections coming from these two areas (blue and green arrows) would be responsible for linking the primary language center and the perisylvian cortex, where the language concepts are located

word yet created (Wernicke's area) and precipitates the selection of the corresponding motor word (Broca's area) [8, 13].

Although the new insights coming from the Geschwind have increased the scope and solved some inconsistencies that were present since the Broca and Wernicke ideas, this classical model still had some inconsistencies that raised doubts. The Wernicke-Geschwind model predicts lesions involving the arcuate fasciculus would generate the same deficit, independent of its segment affected, which is not clinically observed [2]. This model was revealed to be an oversimplification since it could not recognize the complexity of linguistic processing that we now know involve different language domains such as lexical, phonological, and semantic [8, 14]. Even the fundaments of the classical model were in check after the advances in neuroimaging. It is known that Broca's area lesions do not cause the so-called Broca's aphasia; instead, it demands lesions in broader areas such as the precentral gyrus. Lesions limited to the original Broca's area generate a transient deficit or a milder aphasia [8, 12, 15]. In a recent paper, Dronkers et al. submitted the brains used by Broca to fundament his theory to MRI, which revealed that their lesions were not confined to the left inferior frontal gyrus but involved deeper structures such as the superior longitudinal fasciculus [16].

Recent advances in neuroscience have demonstrated that the brain is organized as complex, multimodal, and integrated parallel distributed networks, with cognitive processes consisting of a continuous and often redundant stream of information dynamically modulated by experience and the external environment [12, 17]. Catani introduced the concept of "hodotopy," which gives importance to the cortical epicenters and assumes the relevance of the connectivity of different areas [17, 18]. Under the light of these new neuroscience concepts, the classical language model has been replaced by a new contemporary model.

The Contemporary Language Model

When considering the neural basis of a function or dysfunction, mainly cognitive functions such as language, it is essential to focus not only on cortices but also on both cortices and white matter as a network [12]. Language execution is a higher cognitive function that demands several processes, requiring executive resources and involvement of a range of brain areas. Language comprehension, for example, involves auditory and visual word recognition, lexical and morphological processes, syntactic analysis, conceptual interpretation, and referential processes [7].

In this scenario, the current language model is organized in a dual-stream framework. This model was proposed by Hickok and Poeppel [14, 19, 20] and used similar concepts as used for auditory [21] and visual processes [22] already accepted in modern neuroscience. It is essential to mention that Wernicke initially conceived these general concepts. He was the first who proposed, in 1874, that sensory representations of speech in the left posterior temporal lobe interact with two different systems, a broadly diffused conceptual system for comprehension and the motor system to engage in speech production. Therefore, the recent model's major contribution has been the refinement of anatomical localization, specification of language subprocesses, and confirmation, which demanded the best available evidence provided by modern imaging methods and careful lesion-deficit studies [8].

The Hickok-Poeppel model argues that language processing begins with a spectrotemporal analysis supported by the auditory cortices in both hemispheres. Thus, computed information moves to the phonological network in the middle to a posterior portion of the cortex in and around the superior temporal sulcus; information then moves via the dorsal stream, which is strongly left-lateralized and supports auditory-motor integration in speech processing. At the same time, this information travels through the ventral stream, which is bilateral, with a slight left hemisphere bias, and supports auditory comprehension. The dorsal stream's posterior part involves a segment of the Sylvian fissure at the parietotemporal boundary, supporting the auditory-motor interface. Its anterior portion, in the frontal lobe, includes Broca's area and its surrounding, which, together with its more dorsal premotor component, supports processes relating sound to speech. The ventral stream's posterior portion (posterior middle and inferior portions of the temporal lobes) supports the linking of phonological and semantic information (the lexical interface). In contrast, its more anterior areas support combinatorial semantic processes [7, 19] (Fig. 16.2).

Therefore, this contemporary model assumes that the semantic processing, performed by the ventral stream, is bilaterally located, with a slight left dominance. The speech perception tasks, executed by the dorsal stream, are strongly

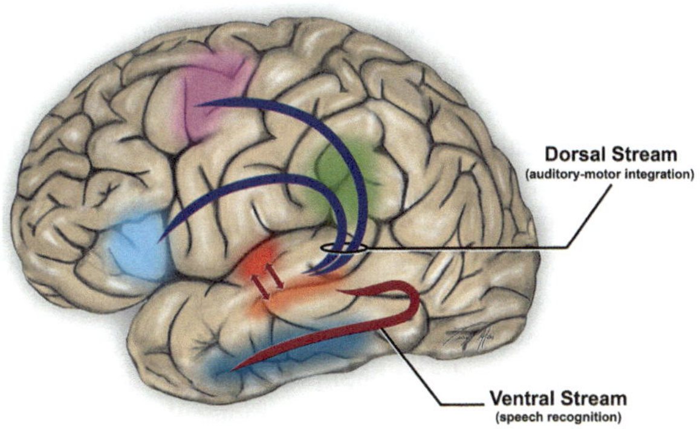

Fig. 16.2 Contemporary dual-stream language model as proposed by Hickok and Poeppel. The language processing begins with a spectrotemporal analysis supported by the auditory cortex (red region); information moves to the phonological network in the middle to a posterior portion of the cortex in and around the superior temporal sulcus (orange region). The information then moves via the dorsal stream (dark blue lines), which supports auditory-motor integration in speech processing, to achieve the premotor cortex (pink region), inferior frontal gyrus (blue region), and parietotemporal boundary region (green region). This information is also carried by the ventral stream (dark red line), which supports auditory comprehension, to achieve the anterior and middle temporal lobe (dark blue region). In this dual-stream model, the dorsal stream is left-lateralized, and the ventral stream is bilateral with a slight left predominance

left-dominant. Unilateral temporal damages will not cause speech recognition deficits, whereas speech production deficits are prominent sequelae of dorsal temporal and frontal lesions in the left hemisphere [19].

Duffau has an extensive work based on DES during awake surgery demonstrating the segmentation of the language subprocess that supports the dual-stream model [23]. DES has demonstrated that the dorsal stream has a phonological function in speech production and is mainly composed of the arcuate fasciculus. In contrast, the main tract of the ventral stream is the inferior fronto-occipital fasciculus, which has a semantic function in language processing [23, 24].

The anatomical description of the main tracts which form the dorsal and ventral streams will be made in the subsequent sections of this text.

Fiber Tracks' Morphology, from Klingler to DTI Tractography

The adoption of the new hodotopic framework gave similar importance to the white matter and cortex. In this way, comprehension of the language network demanded a better understanding of the fiber tracts implicated in language, as this knowledge had been neglected for decades.

Klinger described a technique for fiber dissection based on fixation of the specimen in 5% formalin followed by freezing the brains before dissection [25]. His technique was diffusely spread by anatomists and made possible a systematization of the fiber dissections. The classical Klinger's technique was used for Türe in brilliant papers that brought attention for neurosurgeons to the necessity of understanding the white matter tracts [26, 27].

Although the fiber dissection provides a better understanding of the fiber tracts, it is limited for anatomical purposes since it does not allow in vivo studies. Nowadays, modern neuroradiological studies have allowed a detailed study of the human white matter, especially after the advent of tractography based on diffusion tensor imaging (DTI) [28]. This imaging method utilizes the principles of water molecules' diffusibility to track fiber bundles in the encephalon. Free water molecules move randomly following the principle of the Brownian movement. Therefore, water molecules do not have a directional preference, which is called an isotropic movement. On the other hand, when the water molecules are inside a fiber tract, it will move in the fiber axis, thus having an anisotropic movement (Fig. 16.3).

DTI fiber tracking technique analyzes the diffusion of water molecules in the brain tissue. The direction of the highest diffusivity coincides with the white matter fiber tract axis. Variation of the diffusion along different spatial directions provides information about diffusion anisotropy and, ultimately, tissue architecture [29].

Currently, DTI fiber tracking has been widely utilized in both anatomy studies and surgical planning in neurosurgery [5, 30–33]. In the next section of this chapter,

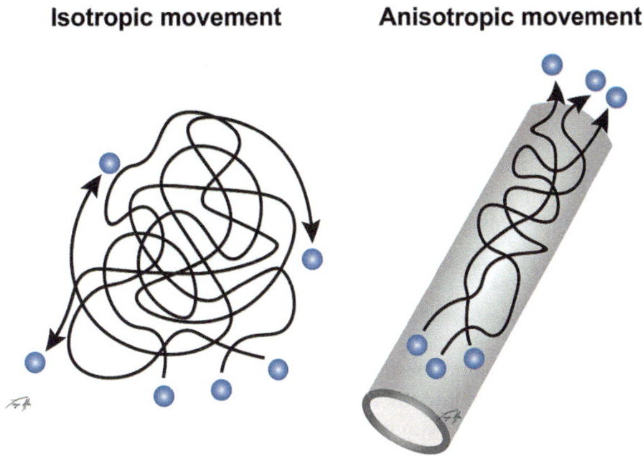

Fig. 16.3 The isotropic movement of free water molecules respects the Brownian movement, where the particles move randomly with no directional preference (left side). When inside a bundle, the water molecules tend to move preferentially in the fiber axis, called an anisotropic movement (right side)

the anatomy of fiber tracks related to language will be discussed. The Klingler technique and DTI fiber tracking were used to delineate the complex architecture of the language network. DTI fiber tracking was made using the DSI studio software (http://dsi-studio.labsolver.org). The three-dimensional reconstruction of fiber tracts on DSI studio followed the general color map, so the green color indicates that a given bundle has an anterior to posterior direction. A fiber orientated in a latero-lateral direction will be represented in red color. The blue color will be used to represent tracts that have superior to inferior direction. Fibers that have oblique direction will be represented in a mix of these three colors proportionally.

The Anatomy of the Language Network

The human language is a higher cognitive function that requires several processes working together, demanding organizational resources, and involving a range of brain areas. The white mater acts providing the complex network of different brain areas that work in conjunction to execute the speech.

A given cortical region can have four main types of connectivity patterns: (1) locoregional connectivity, mediated through short association or U-fibers; (2) subcortical connectivity, which connects different regions of both hemispheres through the long association bundles (horizontal connectivity); (3) interhemispheric connectivity, made by commissural fibers; and (4) the vertical connectivity, mediated by projection fibers and allowing the modulation of cortical processing by deep gray nuclei [17].

The U-fibers are tiny association fibers that connect different gyri in the same hemisphere; they are the most superficial white matter fibers in the human brain and are also called intergyral fibers (Fig. 16.4). As a general principle, deeper tracts used to be longer than superficial ones [34].

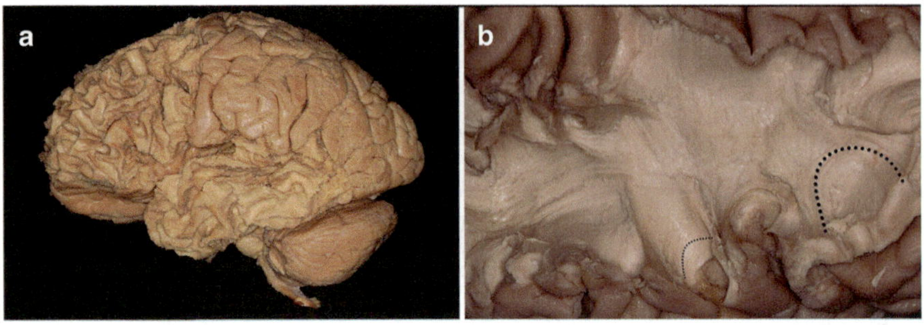

Fig. 16.4 The short association or U-fibers are the most superficial white matter fibers. Located immediately deeper to the cortex, they connect neighboring gyri. (**a**) The cortex of the frontal and temporal lobes has been removed, exposing the U-fibers of these regions. (**b**) Closer view of the U-fibers. The dotted lines represent the trajectory of these fibers

The major tracts of the dorsal stream are the arcuate fasciculus (AF), a frontotemporal connection bundle, and the superior longitudinal fasciculus (SLF), which consists of frontoparietal connection fibers.

Superior Longitudinal Fasciculus

The SLF defines a set of frontoparietal connections which are classically segmented in three separate subcomponents based on a monkey brain study: the most dorsal component of the SLF is the SLF-I, the second branch is SLF-II, and the most ventral branch is SLF-III [35]. These findings were adopted for the human brain after some papers confirming these segmentations [36, 37]. In this way, the SLF-I is located deeply in the superior frontal gyrus. The SLF-II is located more profound in the middle frontal gyrus, and the SLF-III, the shorter and most superficial segment, lies in the deep of the inferior frontal gyrus [34] (Fig. 16.5).

The SLF-III is the shortest segment of the SLF. It is located within the frontoparietal operculum and connects the pars opercularis of the inferior frontal gyrus and the ventral precentral gyrus to the supramarginal gyrus in the inferior parietal lobule. After removing the short association fibers in the middle frontal gyrus, the SLF-II can be found. This segment is located immediately deeper to the SLF-III and is also longer. It courses between the angular and middle frontal gyri at the level of the upper edge of the atrium and the body of the lateral ventricle [34].

The SLF-I is believed to be a connection of the superior frontal gyrus and precuneus region. There are some controversies in the characterization of this tract. Some authors were not able to distinguish these fibers in brain dissections or DTI tractography [26, 38, 39]. As the SLF-I is located deeper to the SLF-II and medial to the corona radiata in a supracingulate region, this bundle should be understood as a segment of the cingulum, reserving the term superior longitudinal fasciculus to the more lateral tracts. In this view, SLF-II would be named as "dorsal SLF," and

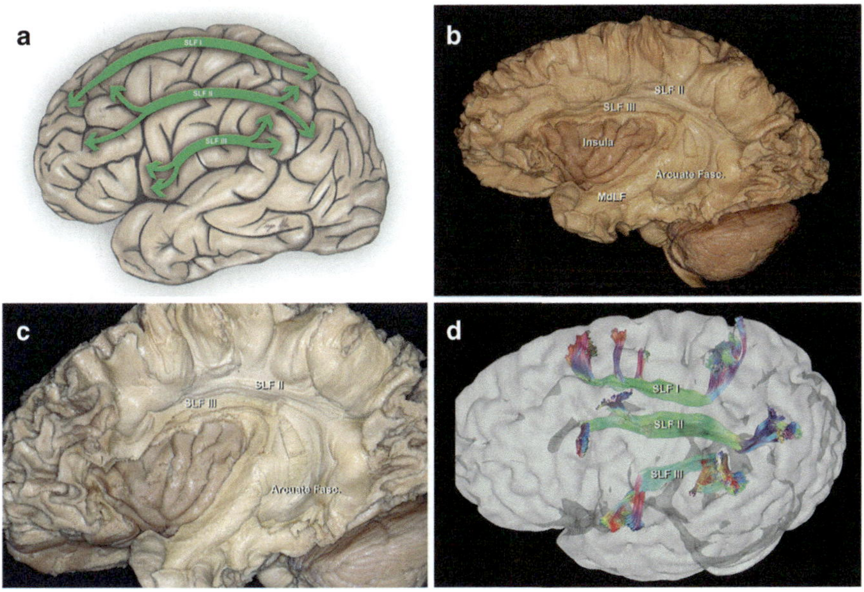

Fig. 16.5 The superior longitudinal fasciculus is a set of fibers connecting the frontal and parietal lobes. It is generally segmented in three different bundles. (**a**) Illustration demonstrating the general arrangement of the SLF segments. The SLF-I is the more profound and more prolonged segment; it is located within the superior frontal gyrus and connects the medial and dorsal parietal cortex and precuneus (BA 5 and 7) to the dorsal and medial part of the frontal lobe (BA 8, BA 9, and BA 32). The SLF-II runs deep in the middle frontal gyrus connecting the inferior parietal region (BA 39) and the posterior regions of the superior and middle frontal gyrus (BA 6, BA 8, and BA 9). The SLF-III, located in the inferior frontal gyrus, connects the inferior parietal lobule to the inferior frontal gyrus (BA 44, 45, 47). (**b**) Fiber dissection of a left hemisphere. The U-fibers of the perisylvian region have been removed, exposing the long association fibers. The SLF-III is the more superficial segment of the SLF situated just lateral to the arcuate fasciculus (AF), located just lateral to the SLF-II, also superiorly situated concerning the AF. (**c**) Closer view of the perisylvian region tracts demonstrating the intimal relations and the relative position between the AF, SLF-II, and SLF-III. (**d**) DTI fiber tracking reconstruction of the SLF components. The SLF-I is located in the superior frontal gyrus connecting the medial portion of the superior parietal lobule and the medial portion of the superior frontal gyrus. The SLF-II is located laterally to the SLF-I, in the interior of the middle frontal gyrus, linking the middle frontal gyrus to the inferior parietal lobule. The SLF-III is the shorter and most superficial segment of the SFL, situated within the inferior frontal gyrus. It connects the posterior portion of the inferior frontal gyrus to the inferior parietal lobule. (**e**) Superior view of the left hemisphere. The SLF-II and SLF-III are exposed as well as the temporal terminations of the AF. The SLF-II is situated superior and medial to the SLF-III and AF. The frontal aslant tract can be seen. It is located medial and crosses the SLF-II inferiorly. The AF turns around the insula to reach the posterior temporal region; the SLF components parallel the superior imitating sulcus of the insula, terminating at the inferior parietal lobule. (**f**) Fiber tract reconstruction of the SLF-II (represented in yellow color), the SLF-III (represented in red color), and the AF (green color) in the lateral surface of the left hemisphere. The AF lies in between the SLF-III, situated laterally, and the SLF-II superior and medially situated

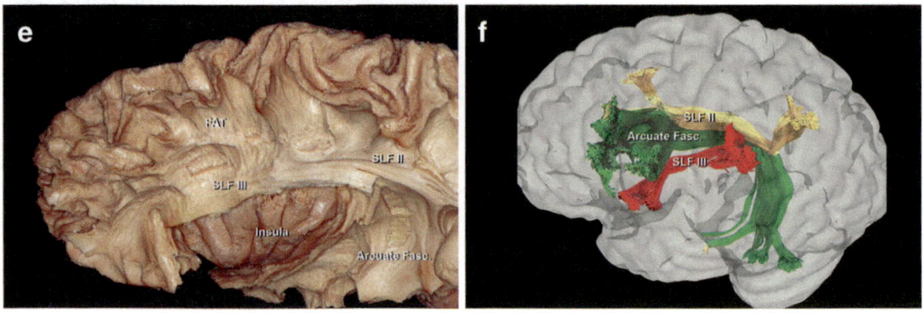

Fig. 16.5 (continued)

SLF-III can be named as "ventral SLF" as proposed by the Fernandez-Miranda group [39].

The SLF-III has a clear role in language, as a component of the dorsal stream. It is involved in decoding visual information to articulation through visuo-phonological conversion in the phonological processing (working memory) [8, 23, 24, 34]. This bundle's DES will elucidate speech arrest, phonemic paraphasia, and articulatory disorders [8, 40]. The SLF-II is also implicated in language, but its role is still unclear. Nevertheless, there are several differences in the architecture of this tract when we compare the left and right sides [39]. In a clinical scenario, DES of the SLF-II generates speech arrest and dysarthria. The current data do not implicate SLF-I on language production.

Arcuate Fasciculus

The AF comprises a set of fibers that connects the inferior frontal gyrus and the posterior temporal regions. Reil was the first to identify a group of fibers in the perisylvian region that connects frontal, inferior parietal, and posterior temporal regions. Burdach, in 1922, detailed this tract and named it *fasciculus arcuatus* [2]. Since then, several descriptions of this tract have been made.

Some authors consider it a segment of the superior longitudinal fasciculus [24, 32, 38]. However, modern descriptions based on DTI and fiber dissection have demonstrated that the AF is a distinct tract [34, 39]. Utilizing high-definition fiber tracking and careful dissection is possible to separate these tracts. Also, based on anatomical principles, the SLF is a tract that connects frontal and parietal lobes; on the other hand, the AF should be understood as a tract that links frontal and temporal lobes [26] (Fig. 16.6).

The AF has a significant dominance in the left hemisphere [37, 41]. There are four different cortical termination of the AF fibers in the frontal region: pars opercularis, pars triangularis, precentral gyrus (ventral portion), and middle frontal gyrus (caudal portion) [41]. In the temporal lobe, the fibers of AF connect to the superior (STG), middle (MTG), and inferior (ITG) temporal gyri. Classically, this

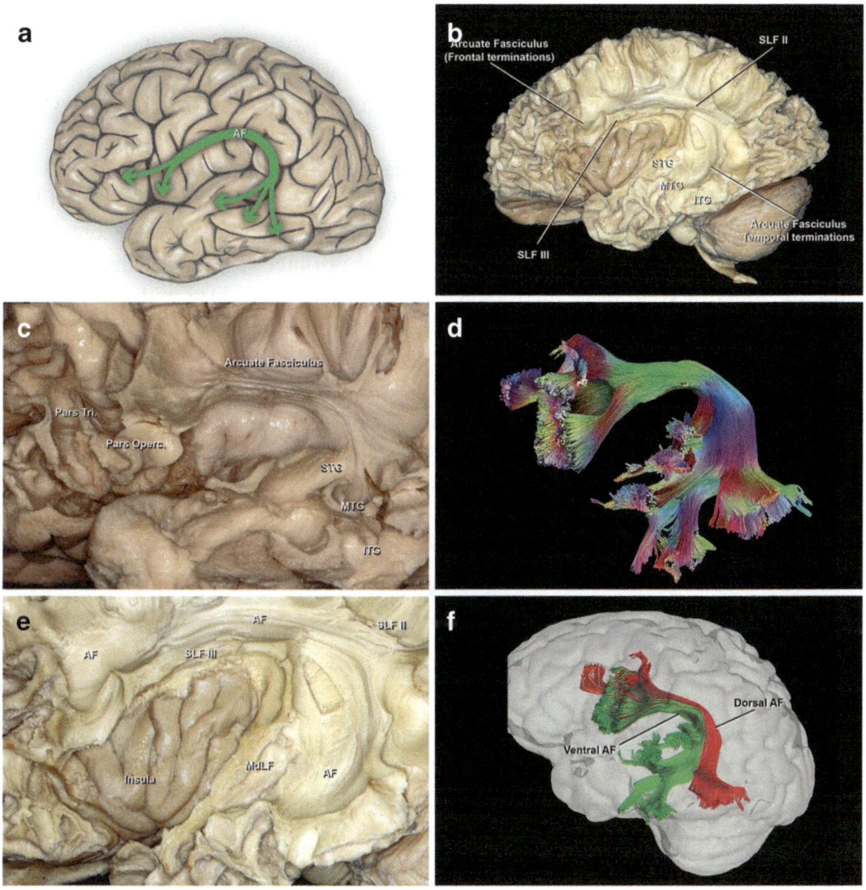

Fig. 16.6 The arcuate fasciculus is a bundle of fibers that connects the inferior frontal region to the posterior portion of the temporal lobe. (**a**) The frontal terminations of the AF include the pars triangularis (BA 45), the pars opercularis (BA 44), the ventral precentral and caudal middle frontal gyri (BA6), and the dorsolateral prefrontal cortex (BA 9). In the temporal lobe, the AF terminates in the middle and posterior portion of the superior temporal gyrus (BA 22 and BA 42), rostral middle temporal gyrus (BA 21), and caudal middle temporal gyrus and inferior temporal gyrus (BA 37). (**b**) Fiber dissection of the left hemisphere demonstrating the AF terminations. The AF begins in the inferior frontal region, turns around the insula, and terminates at the posterior temporal region, reaching the superior, middle, and inferior temporal gyri. The SLF-III lies in the inferior frontal gyrus and is located lateral to the AF. The SLF-II is situated medial and superior to the AF. (**c**) Closer view of the AF. The SLF segments and insular cortex have been removed. The AF has a C-shaped format connecting the inferior frontal and posterior temporal regions. (**d**) DTI reconstruction of the left AF in the directional color map demonstrating its general aspect on MRI fiber tract reconstruction. (**e**) Perisylvian fiber tracts. The SLF-II and SLF-III connect the frontal and inferior parietal regions. The AF turns around the insula connecting the inferior frontal and posterior temporal regions; its temporal terminations are located lateral to the middle longitudinal fasciculus, connecting the superior temporal gyrus with the superior parietal lobule. (**f**) Three-dimensional reconstruction of the subcomponents of the AF. The ventral AF (green) interconnects STG and rostral MTG with the pars opercularis and most ventral premotor cortex. The dorsal AF (red) links ITG and caudal MTG with the ventral precentral and caudal middle frontal gyrus

tract is described as having a direct segment that links the inferior frontal and posterior temporal regions, connecting the primary language areas, and an anterior indirect segment that connects frontal and parietal regions as well as a posterior indirect segment that connects the inferior parietal and posterior temporal regions [2, 42].

More recent studies suggest a different segmentation of the AF. Based on DTI-based tractography and fiber dissections, it was observed that the subset of fibers that comes from the ITG and caudal MTG terminates on the ventral precentral and caudal middle frontal gyrus comprising a dorsal or outer segment of the AF. In its turn, the inner or ventral AF interconnects STG and rostral MTG with pars opercularis and most ventral premotor cortex [41, 43]. In this conception, the anterior and posterior indirect segments described by Catani would be part of the SLF-III and temporoparietal aslant tract, respectively [44]. Functionally, the ventral AF connects the primary language areas being associated with phonological language processing. The dorsal segment interconnects the supplementary language areas associated with lexical and semantic language processing [41, 43].

Stimulation of the AF during awake craniotomies leads to phonemic paraphasias, anomia, and phonological errors [24, 45, 46]. Syntactical errors have also been attributed to the AF based on DTI tractography and subcortical stimulation studies [47, 48].

Frontal Aslant Tract

Recent studies have confirmed the presence of connections between the inferior frontal and medial superior frontal gyrus [49]. Although the term frontal aslant tract (FAT) was used for the first time by Catani in 2012 [50], previous researches had demonstrated the existence of this tract [51, 52]. The FAT connects the pre-supplementary motor area (pre-SMA) and the supplementary motor area (SMA) located in the posterior portion of the superior frontal gyrus to the inferior frontal region, especially the pars triangularis and pars opercularis [53]. This tract has an oblique trajectory and is located just medial to the AF and immediately lateral to the corona radiata (Fig. 16.7).

The FAT is related to both language and motor control. Imaging studies have shown that the left FAT connections are associated with controlled lexical and phonological selection/retrieval in many linguistic domains, including understanding sign language and gesture. It is also related to executive function/inhibitory control [49]. When the left FAT is stimulated during surgery, speech arrest is generated, a symptom also present in patients whit lesions involving the SMA [54].

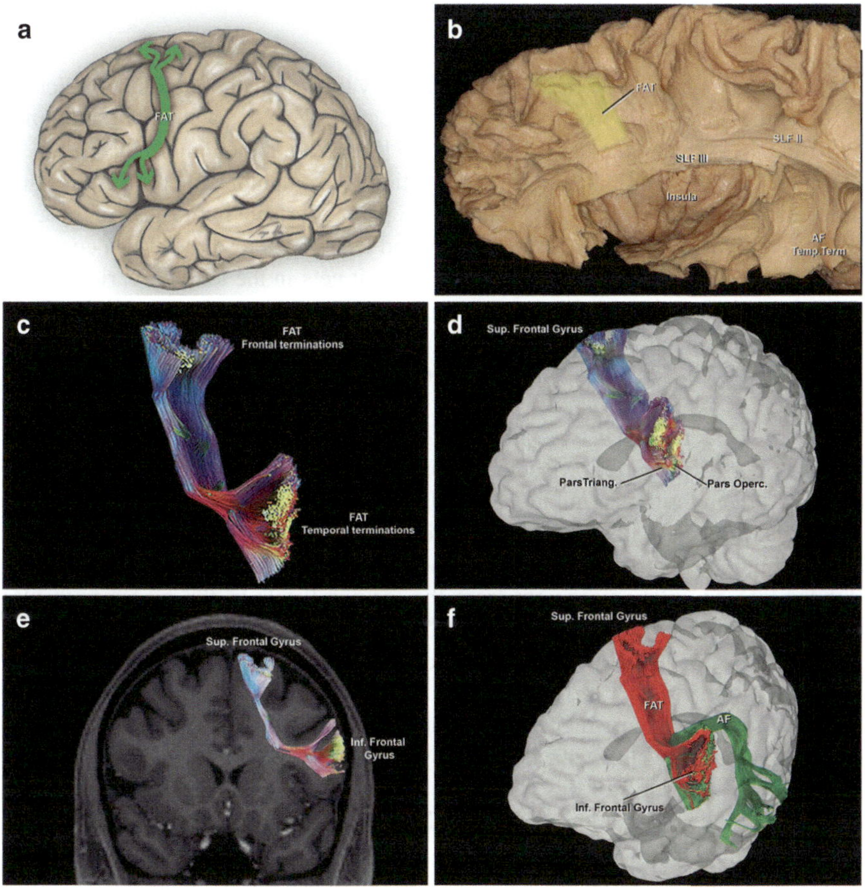

Fig. 16.7 (**a**) The frontal aslant tract (FAT) connects the pre-supplementary motor area (pre-SMA) and supplementary motor area (SMA) (BA 6) in the superior frontal gyrus with the pars triangularis and pars opercularis in the inferior frontal gyrus (BA 44 and 45). (**b**) The FAT has been highlighted in yellow. It has an oblique trajectory from the superior frontal gyrus to the inferior frontal gyrus and passes medially to SLF-II perpendicular to this one. (**c**) DTI 3D reconstruction of the FAT on the directional color map demonstrating its general appearance. (**d**) Reconstruction of the FAT on the left hemisphere. It has an oblique trajectory connecting the posterior aspect of the superior frontal gyrus with the pars triangularis and pars opercularis in the inferior frontal gyrus. (**e**) T1 coronal plane MRI with DTI fiber tracking superposition of the left PAT showing the trajectory of this bundle connection of the SFG and IFG. (**f**) 3D reconstruction of the left hemisphere with the AF (green) and the PAT represented. These two tracts have similar terminations on the IFG

Middle Longitudinal Fasciculus

The temporal pole and parietal lobe are linked by the middle longitudinal fasciculus (MdLF) that lies within the superior temporal gyrus (STG). Some previous studies were unable to isolate the fibers of the MdLF [26, 32], although more recent papers based on DTI tractography and fiber dissections have demonstrated its course and anatomical relationships [34, 55]. The MdLF fibers originate in the STG at the level of the temporal pole and direct posteriorly and laterally. It also receives a contribution from the transverse temporal gyrus. When it gets in the temporoparietal junction, the MdLF makes a wide-angle turn and redirects the trajectory of the fibers from the anterolateral (temporal region) to posteromedial (parietal region) and ascends to reach the superior parietal (precuneus) and occipital regions (cuneus) [55] (Fig. 16.8).

The MdLF is located between the AF terminations on the STG, laterally situated, and the fibers of the inferior fronto-occipital fasciculus, situated just medial to the MdLF. At the inferior parietal lobule level, the MdLF is situated lateral to the claustrocortical projection fibers that form the dorsal external capsule.

The function of the MdLF is still unclear. Some argue that this tract can be divided into an anterior segment from the temporal pole to the posterior insular point and a posterior segment, from the posterior insular point to its terminations in the parietal region [34]. In this view, the posterior segment would be associated with language [56]. However, this bundle does not have a clear left lateralization, a common feature in language-related fiber tracts [56]. Indeed, a study involving eight subjects that underwent awake craniotomy for resection of gliomas involving STG demonstrated that DES of this tract does not induce language impairments during surgery and the resection of parts of the MdLF did not cause permanent language deficits [57]. As the MdLF connects the STG with the superior parietal lobule, a multisensory processing center, it has been proposed that this tract might be involved in auditory processing acting as the "dorsal auditory pathway" or "where pathway" [55] as proposed by the dual-stream auditory model [21, 58].

Inferior Fronto-occipital Fasciculus

Situated medially to the MdLF, the inferior fronto-occipital fasciculus (IFOF) links the frontal lobe to the posterior part of the parietal and occipital lobes. It is a long association fiber tract that forms the ventral external capsule together with the uncinate fasciculus, while the dorsal external capsule is composed of the claustrocortical fibers [32, 34, 59] (Fig. 16.9).

The frontal terminations of the IFOF include the middle part of the middle frontal gyrus (prefrontal cortex), pars orbitalis, and pars triangularis. It then directs posterior and inferiorly, deep to the anterior third of the superior limiting sulcus and the superior half of the anterior limiting sulcus to reach the limen of the insula, where it

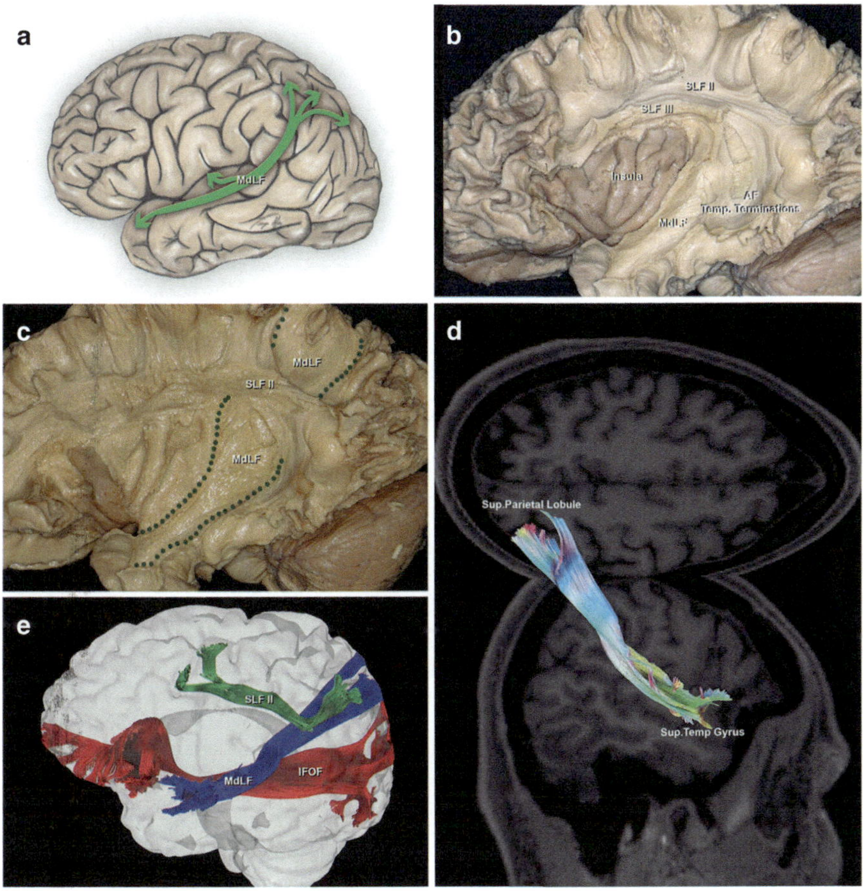

Fig. 16.8 The middle longitudinal fasciculus (MdLF) connects the superior temporal gyrus (STG) with the superior parietal region. (**a**) Illustration demonstrating the connections of the MdLF. This tract connects the superior temporal gyrus (BA 38 and BA 22) with the superior parietal lobule (BA 7) and cuneus (BA 19). (**b**) Fiber dissection of the left hemisphere. The short association fibers of the temporal, parietal, and posterior frontal lobes have been removed, showing the long association fibers. The MdLF can be seen occupying the STG and running posterior and superiorly when it becomes medial to the temporal terminations of the AF and SLF components. (**c**) The AF and insular cortex have been removed, demonstrating the trajectory of the MdLF that crosses the SLF-II, being medial to it in the parietal region, and finally reaches the superior parietal lobule. (**d**) T1 MRI in axial and sagittal planes with superposition of the 3D-reconstructed MdLF showing its terminations on the STG and superior parietal lobule. (**e**) Left hemisphere 3D reconstruction with a representation of the MdLF (blue), SLF-II (green), and IFOF (red). The MdLF is located lateral to the IFOF in the temporal lobe. When it achieves the inferior parietal lobule, it has a superior and medial trajectory passing medial to the SLF-II and finally reaching the superior parietal lobule

has a shorter diameter. It then passes deep to the middle third of the inferior limiting sulcus, getting in the superior and middle temporal gyri. At the middle temporal region level, the IFOF runs in the roof of the temporal horn, superior and lateral to

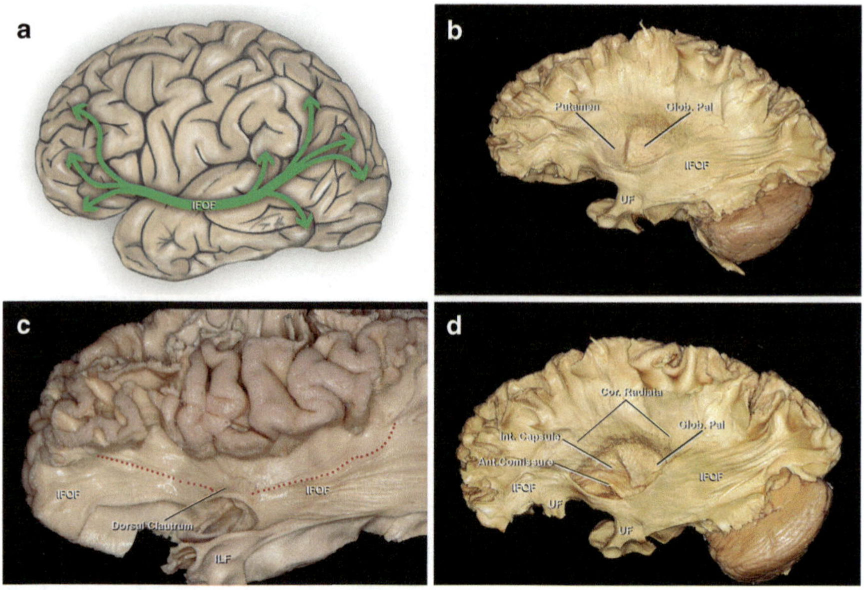

Fig. 16.9 The inferior fronto-occipital fasciculus (IFOF) is a long association fiber tract that connects the frontal lobe to the posterior parietal region and occipital lobe. (**a**) Illustration demonstrating the connections of the IFOF. The frontal connections of the IFOF include the pars opercularis (BA 44), pars triangularis (BA 45), pars orbitalis (BA 47), superior frontal and middle frontal gyri (BA 8, BA 9, BA 10), and orbitofrontal region (BA 11). The posterior terminations of the IFOF include the calcarine sulcus and cuneus (BA 17), superior and middle occipital gyri (BA 19), superior parietal lobule (BA 7), and fusiform gyrus (BA 37). (**b**) Fiber dissection of the left hemisphere, SLF, AF, and MdLF has been removed, exposing the ventral external capsule composed of the IFOF, superiorly, and the uncinate fasciculus (UF) inferiorly. The claustrocortical projection fibers that form the dorsal external capsule were removed, exposing the putamen; the posterior portion of putamen was resected, exposing the globus pallidus. (**c**) Fiber dissection of the left hemisphere in a closer view. The U-fibers and UF have been removed, exposing the terminations of the IFOF in the inferior frontal gyrus. The dorsal claustrum and the dorsal external capsule are viewed superiorly located to the IFOF. In the anterior temporal region, the inferior longitudinal fasciculus (ILF) is exposed. It is laterally located about the IFOF. (**d**) The central core of the left hemisphere has been dissected. The corona radiata fibers are located superiorly to the basal ganglia. The putamen has been removed, and the anterior half of the globus pallidus enables the visualization of the internal capsule fibers. The anterior commissure can be seen. A commissural fiber tract crosses the midline just inferior to the anterior limb of the internal capsule and then gains the temporal lobe, having a medial position to the IFOF. The ventral external capsule is seen. It is formed by the IFOF dorsally and UF ventrally. (**e**) T1 MRI in axial and sagittal planes with DTI fiber tracking of the IFOF superposed demonstrates this tract's regular aspect and its cortical connections. (**f**) 3D reconstruction of the left hemisphere and the subcomponents of the IFOF. The IFOF is segmented in a ventromedial subfascicle (green), a ventrolateral subfascicle (red), and a dorsomedial subfascicle (blue)

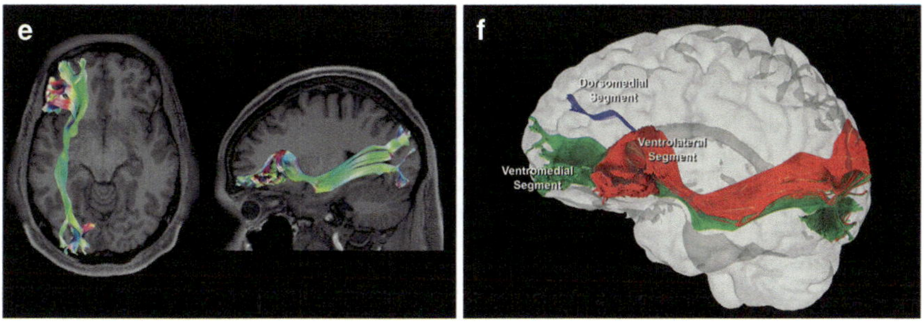

Fig. 16.9 (continued)

the optic radiations and medial to the MdLF and AF. It continues backward, laterally to the lateral surface of the atrium to reach the parietal and occipital lobes [34, 59, 60]. The posterior terminations of the IFOF include the superior parietal lobule, superior and middle occipital gyri, calcarine sulcus, and fusiform gyrus [59, 61].

Based on fiber dissection, Martino et al. argue that the IFOF has a dorsal and superficial segment and a ventral and deeper segment [59]. Indeed, in a posterior study utilizing both fiber dissection and DTI-based tractography, Sarubbo et al. detailed the frontal cortical terminations of these two segments as the dorsal IFOF connects the pars triangularis and opercularis to Wernicke's area, fusiform gyrus, superior parietal lobule, and occipital lobe. The ventral IFOF connects the pars orbitalis, middle temporal gyrus, and dorsolateral prefrontal cortex to the same distal terminations of the dorsal IFOF [62].

Based on a diffusion spectrum imaging-based tractographic study, Panesar et al. proposed that IFOF is divided into three subfascicles according to their spatial orientation within the IFOF bundle:

I. *Ventrolateral*: originating from the pars opercularis, pars triangularis, and pars orbitalis. It remained superficial throughout its course through the external capsule and into the parietooccipital cortex.
II. *Dorsomedial*: originating from the superior frontal and middle frontal gyri, traveling deep to the ventrolateral subfascicle and assuming a fan-like frontal arrangement.
III. *Ventromedial:* originating from the medial, lateral, anterior, and posterior orbital gyri which assumed a deep-and-ventral course in respect to the other subfascicles [61].

The IFOF forms the principal component of the ventral semantic pathway. It has been noted that DES of this tract induces semantic errors during awake craniotomies [60, 62, 63]. Regarding the frontal cortical terminations of the IFOF, stimulation of the pars triangularis and middle and posterior superior temporal gyri induces semantic paraphasia. At the subcortical level, semantic paraphasia was constantly induced when stimulating the course of the IFOF in the posterior orbitofrontal area, at the level of the limen insulae, in the posterior part of the temporal stem, and at the floor of the external capsule [63]. On a lesion-based study, Han et al. conclude that the superficial layer of the IFOF may support bridging the semantic memory with the verbal system. The deep layer of the IFOF may be critical for object semantic processing [64]. Other language functions also have been attributed to the IFOF, such as reading and writing [7]. Also, the right IFOF is involved in non-verbal semantic cognition [65].

Duffau et al. argue that the semantic ventral stream is divided into a direct pathway represented by the IFOF and an indirect pathway, composed of the inferior longitudinal fasciculus (ILF), which relay on the uncinate fasciculus (UF), that, in turn, transmits information from the temporal pole to the inferior frontal region [23]. This theory assumes a degree of subcortical plasticity within the network, as the function of the indirect pathway (ILF and UF) may be compensated by the IFOF in the case of damages to UF or ILF. It is observed in patients that underwent anterior temporal lobectomy during epilepsy surgery [23, 66].

Inferior Longitudinal Fasciculus

The inferior longitudinal fasciculus (ILF) connects the temporal pole to the dorsolateral occipital cortex. It is located mainly within the inferior and middle temporal gyri and runs laterally and inferiorly to the temporal horn of the ventricle. At the level of the paraoccipital notch, it bends upward to be distributed to the dorsolateral occipital cortex, not reaching the calcarine sulcus (Fig. 16.10) [34, 67].

The curse of the ILF is lateral to the IFOF in its anterior part and then directs medially, becoming interconnected with IFOF fibers [32]. Panesar et al., in a recent paper, found that ILF is also divided into two different subfascicles, a dorsal and a ventral one [68]. The authors found that the dorsal subfascicle connects mainly the middle and superior temporal gyri with the superior occipital gyrus. On the other hand, the ventral ILF, a generally less robust bundle, links the superior, middle, and inferior temporal gyri with the lingual gyrus [68].

The ILF is recognized as a multi-functional tract involved in a broad range of brain functions concerning the visual modality, including object, face, and place processing, reading, lexical and semantic processing, emotion processing, and visual memory [69]. Regarding its subcomponents, it is argued that the dorsal ILF subserves both semantic, spatial, and facial recognition tasks and the ventral ILS is involved in visual recognition tasks [68]. ILF, together with the uncinate fascicule, is implicated as part of an indirect semantic pathway. Indeed, electric stimulation of this tract during surgery elucidates semantic paraphasias [23, 67].

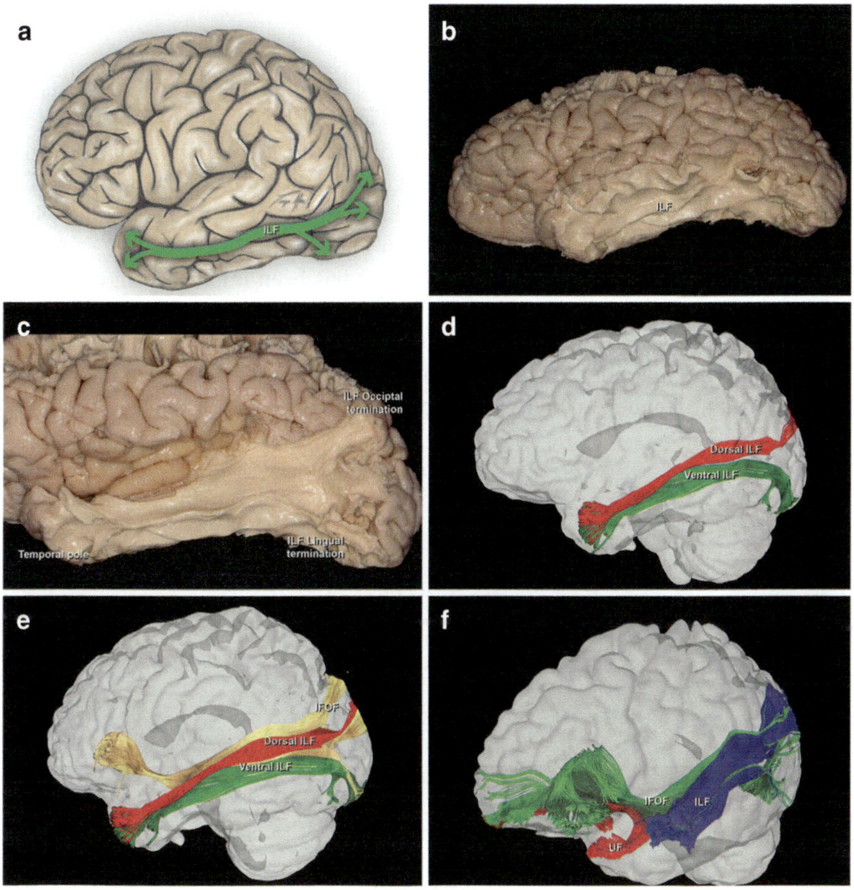

Fig. 16.10 The inferior longitudinal fascicle (ILF) connects the temporal pole to the occipital lobe. (**a**) Illustration demonstrating the inferior cortical connections of the ILF. This tract connects the temporal pole (BA 38) to the occipital region and lingual gyrus (BA 18 and BA 19). (**b**) Fiber dissection of the left hemisphere. The cortex and U-fibers of the basal surface of the temporal lobe have been removed. The terminations of ILF can be seen in the anterior temporal pole and lingual gyrus. (**c**) Lateral view of the ILF. The ILF fibers have an anterior to posterior direction connecting the temporal pole to the superior and middle occipital gyrus and lingual gyrus. (**d**) 3D reconstruction of the left hemisphere and ILF subsegments. The ILF is composed of a dorsal component (red) that connects the temporal pole with the occipital lobe and a ventral segment (green) that mainly finishes at the lingual gyrus. (**e**) 3D reconstruction of the left hemisphere demonstrating the relationship of ILF (green and red bundles) and IFOF (yellow bundle). Both subcomponents of the ILF are laterally located to the IFOF, reaching more superior regions than ILF. (**f**) Oblique view of the left hemisphere on an MRI-based 3D reconstruction. The components of the ventral external capsule were rendered to demonstrate their relationship with ILF. The IFOF (green) connects the frontal lobe with the occipital region, having standard posterior terminations with the ILF. The UF (red) terminates at the temporal pole, medial to the ILF (blue) temporal pole terminations

Uncinate Fasciculus

The uncinate fasciculus (UF) is a frontotemporal association tract as it connects the anterior temporal region with the orbitofrontal area of the inferior frontal gyrus [32, 34]. It runs along the limen of the insula, inferiorly situated to IFOF, and forms with this one the ventral external capsule. After it crosses the limen of the insula, it penetrates in the ventral portion of the temporal stream, which is formed by the white matter of the three temporal gyri [70] (Fig. 16.11).

Given the UF cortical connections, this tract has been implicated in emotional processes. Damages to UF are also related to psychiatric disorders [71, 72]. The role of UF on language is still unclear. Although the DES of this tract during awake craniotomies did not induce language disturbances, and its resection did not implicate permanent language deficits [70], some argue that the UF damage results in

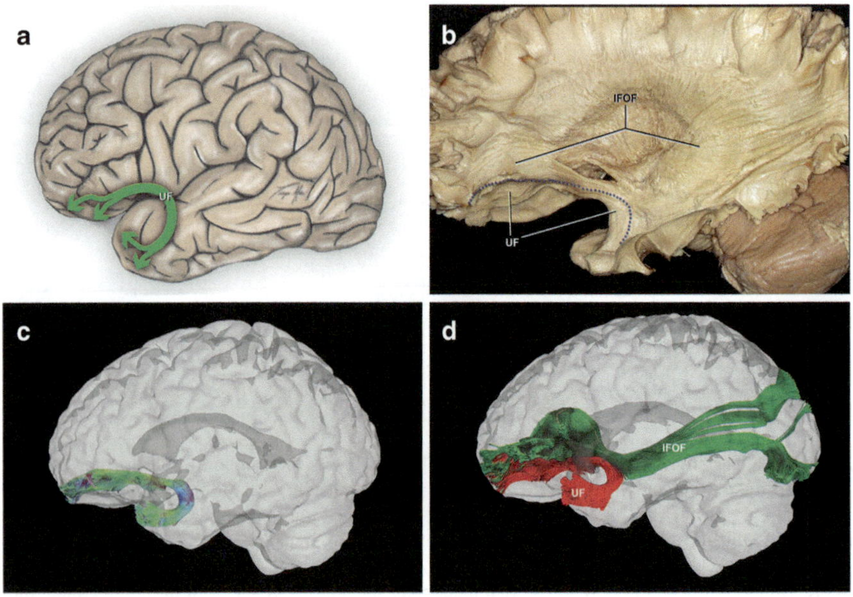

Fig. 16.11 The uncinate fascicle (UF) is a C-shaped fiber tract that connects the inferior frontal lobe with the temporal pole. (**a**) Illustration demonstrating the cortical connectivity of the UF. The UF mainly connects the orbitofrontal region (BA 47) and the temporal pole (BA 38). (**b**) Fiber dissection of the left hemisphere with an emphasis on the ventral internal capsule. The UF is located in the ventral aspect of the IFOF, and its frontal terminations are also inferiorly located to the IFOF frontal terminations. The dotted line separates the fibers of IFOF that have a posterior course from the UF fibers, which have a curved course to reach the temporal pole. (**c**) MRI-based 3D reconstruction of the left hemisphere with a 3D reconstruction of the UF based on DTI fiber tracking. The UF reaches the anterior portion of the orbitofrontal gyrus and the temporal pole. It passes through the ventral portion of the limen of the insula. (**d**) Fiber tracking of the components of the ventral external capsule: IFOF (green) and UF (red), the three-dimensional reconstruction of the left hemisphere was also added to demonstrate the relationship of these tracts with the cortical anatomy

53. Bozkurt B, Yagmurlu K, Middlebrooks EH, Karadag A, Ovalioglu TC, Jagadeesan B, et al. Microsurgical and tractographic anatomy of the supplementary motor area complex in humans. World Neurosurg. 2016;95:99–107.
54. Vassal F, Boutet C, Lemaire J-J, Nuti C. New insights into the functional significance of the frontal aslant tract: an anatomo–functional study using intraoperative electrical stimulations combined with diffusion tensor imaging-based fiber tracking. Br J Neurosurg. 2014;28:685–7.
55. Wang Y, Fernández-Miranda JC, Verstynen T, Pathak S, Schneider W, Yeh F-C. Rethinking the role of the middle longitudinal fascicle in language and auditory pathways. Cereb Cortex. 2013;23:2347–56.
56. Makris N, Papadimitriou GM, Kaiser JR, Sorg S, Kennedy DN, Pandya DN. Delineation of the middle longitudinal fascicle in humans: a quantitative, in vivo, DT-MRI study. Cereb Cortex. 2009;19(4):777–85.
57. De Witt Hamer PC, Moritz-Gasser S, Gatignol P, Duffau H. Is the human left middle longitudinal fascicle essential for language? A brain electrostimulation study. Hum Brain Mapp. 2010;32:962–73.
58. Lomber SG, Malhotra S. Double dissociation of "what" and "where" processing in auditory cortex. Nat Neurosci. 2008;11:609–16.
59. Martino J, Brogna C, Robles SG, Vergani F, Duffau H. Anatomic dissection of the inferior fronto-occipital fasciculus revisited in the lights of brain stimulation data. Cortex. 2010;46(5):691–9.
60. Martino J, Vergani F, Robles SG, Duffau H. New insights into the anatomic dissection of the temporal stem with special emphasis on the inferior fronto-occipital fasciculus: implications in surgical approach to left mesiotemporal and temporoinsular structures. Oper Neurosurg. 2010;66:ons-4–ons-12.
61. Panesar SS, Yeh F-C, Deibert CP, Fernandes-Cabral D, Rowthu V, Celtikci P, et al. A diffusion spectrum imaging-based tractographic study into the anatomical subdivision and cortical connectivity of the ventral external capsule: uncinate and inferior fronto-occipital fascicles. Neuroradiology. 2017;59:971–87.
62. Sarubbo S, De Benedictis A, Maldonado IL, Basso G, Duffau H. Frontal terminations for the inferior fronto-occipital fascicle: anatomical dissection, DTI study and functional considerations on a multi-component bundle. Brain Struct Funct. 2013;218:21–37.
63. Almairac F, Herbet G, Moritz-Gasser S, de Champfleur NM, Duffau H. The left inferior fronto-occipital fasciculus subserves language semantics: a multilevel lesion study. Brain Struct Funct. 2015;220:1983–95.
64. Han Z, Ma Y, Gong G, He Y, Caramazza A, Bi Y. White matter structural connectivity underlying semantic processing: evidence from brain damaged patients. Brain. 2013;136:2952–65.
65. Herbet G, Moritz-Gasser S, Duffau H. Direct evidence for the contributive role of the right inferior fronto-occipital fasciculus in non-verbal semantic cognition. Brain Struct Funct. 2017;222:1597–610.
66. Duffau H, de Schotten MT, Mandonnet E. White matter functional connectivity as an additional landmark for dominant temporal lobectomy. J Neurol Neurosurg Psychiatry. 2008;79:492–5.
67. Mandonnet E, Nouet A, Gatignol P, Capelle L, Duffau H. Does the left inferior longitudinal fasciculus play a role in language? A brain stimulation study. Brain. Oxford Academic. 2007;130:623–9.
68. Panesar SS, Yeh F-C, Jacquesson T, Hula W, Fernandez-Miranda JC. A quantitative tractography study into the connectivity, segmentation and laterality of the human inferior longitudinal fasciculus. Front Neuroanat. 2018;12:47.
69. Herbet G, Zemmoura I, Duffau H. Functional anatomy of the inferior longitudinal fasciculus: from historical reports to current hypotheses. Front Neuroanat. 2018;12:77.
70. Duffau H, Gatignol P, Moritz-Gasser S, Mandonnet E. Is the left uncinate fasciculus essential for language? A cerebral stimulation study. J Neurol. 2009;256:382–9.

71. Kubicki M, Westin C-F, Maier SE, Frumin M, Nestor PG, Salisbury DF, et al. Uncinate fasciculus findings in schizophrenia: a magnetic resonance diffusion tensor imaging study. Am J Psychiatry. 2002;159:813–20.
72. Kubicki M, Park H, Westin CF, Nestor PG, Mulkern RV, Maier SE, et al. DTI and MTR abnormalities in schizophrenia: analysis of white matter integrity. NeuroImage. 2005;26:1109–18.
73. Papagno C. Naming and the role of the uncinate fasciculus in language function. Curr Neurol Neurosci Rep. 2011;11:553–9.
74. De Witt Hamer PC, Robles SG, Zwinderman AH, Duffau H, Berger MS. Impact of intraoperative stimulation brain mapping on glioma surgery outcome: a meta-analysis. J Clin Oncol. 2012;30:2559–65.
75. Desmurget M, Bonnetblanc F, Duffau H. Contrasting acute and slow-growing lesions: a new door to brain plasticity. Brain. 2006;130:898–914.
76. Benzagmout M, Gatignol P, Duffau H. Resection of World Health Organization Grade II gliomas involving Broca's area: methodological and functional considerations. Neurosurgery. 2007;61:741–52; discussion 752–753.
77. François C, Garcia-Alix A, Bosch L, Rodriguez-Fornells A. Signatures of brain plasticity supporting language recovery after perinatal arterial ischemic stroke. Brain Lang. 2021;212:104880.
78. Wang S, Young KM. White matter plasticity in adulthood. Neuroscience. 2014;276:148–60.
79. Duffau H. Does post-lesional subcortical plasticity exist in the human brain? Neurosci Res. 2009;65:131–5.
80. Duffau H. New concepts in surgery of WHO grade II gliomas: functional brain mapping, connectionism and plasticity – a review. J Neuro-Oncol. 2006;79:77–115.

Chapter 17
Awake Surgery: Performing an Awake Craniotomy

Silvia Mazzali Verst, Juliana Ohy, Cleiton Formentin, and Marcos Vinicius Calfat Maldaun

Abbreviations

CC	*Corpus callosum*
CNS	Central nervous system
DES	Direct electrical stimulation
DTI	Tractography
ECoG	Electrocorticography
EOR	Extent of resection
FLAIR	Fluid-attenuated inversion recovery
GBM	Glioblastoma
GTR	Gross total resection
HF	High frequency

Supplementary Information The online version contains supplementary material available at [https://doi.org/10.1007/978-3-030-95730-8_17].

S. M. Verst (✉)
Instituto de Ensino e Pesquisa (Research and Educational Institute) of Sírio Libanês Hospital, São Paulo, Brazil

Brain Spine Neurofisiologia, Jundiaí, SP, Brazil

J. Ohy · C. Formentin
Researcher at Instituto de Ensino e Pesquisa (Teaching and Research Institute) of Hospital Sirio Libanês, São Paulo, SP, Brazil

M. V. C. Maldaun
Instituto de Ensino e Pesquisa (Teaching and Research Institute) of Hospital Sirio Libanês, São Paulo, SP, Brazil

Neurosurgery Department, Hospital Sirio Libanês, São Paulo, São Paulo, Brazil

S. M. Verst et al. (eds.), *Intraoperative Monitoring*,
https://doi.org/10.1007/978-3-030-95730-8_17

HFC	High functional connectivity
IDH	Dehydrogenase gene
iMRI	Intraoperative magnetic resonance imaging
IOM	Intraoperative neurophysiology monitoring
ioUS	Intraoperative ultrasound
LF	Low frequency
LLG	Low-grade glioma
MEG	Magnetoencephalography
MEP	Motor evoked potential
MGMT	O^6-methylguanine-DNA methyltransferase
NF	Neurophysiologist
OMFTCT	Ohy-Maldaun Fast Track Cognitive Test
ON	Object naming
VMLA	Verst-Maldaun Language Assessment

Introduction

Initially, awake craniotomy was planned to help epileptic focus resection in Montreal Neurological Institute and Hospital by Wilder Penfield. Medical search for language function understanding goes back to Broca, who in 1861 showed that a small area of left hemisphere had the power of speech (cited by Penfield [1]). George A. Ojemann developed language tasks to be performed during DES of the brain and standardized the awake approach, being pointed as the father of the modern awake craniotomy. Hugues Duffau extensively investigated intraoperative proper language and cognitive tasks and keeps pushing us forward to new concepts and frontiers in connectivity and neuroplasticity. Unfortunately, it is not the scope of this chapter to commemorate all the incredible researchers of the last century. But we have to mention Brazilian pioneer Professor Raul Marino, who learned directly from Penfield (more details in Chap. 1).

A PubMed search using the terms "language," "brain," and "mapping" comprising the period from January 1, 1959, until May 20, 2021, resulted in 10,710 results. There was a slowly growing curve concerning the amounts of publications in the subject in the first 37 years. It jumped to over 100 papers per year in 1997. And in 2015, a record was achieved with 777 papers on this subject that year. Therefore, since Wilder Penfield mapped the brain using an electrical protocol of 2.5 ms pulse duration at 1 V and 60 pulses per second (60 Hz) in 1959 and found out "an interpretative cortex in temporal lobe" [1], awake craniotomy has evolved greatly. Penfield was a visionary ahead from his time. With brain mapping, he discovered specific brain function in different cortical areas: motor and sensory (1937), language (1949, 1952, and 1959), and supplementary motor area (1951) [2]. Nowadays, awake craniotomy is a complex teamwork that demands proper training.

General Concepts Presented by the Neurosurgeon

Low-Grade Glioma Surgery

Low-grade gliomas (LLGs) are known for their diverse pathology and clinical behavior and account for 17% to 22% of all primary brain tumors [3–5]. The natural growth rate of LGGs is believed to be linear regarding diameter and to progress approximately 4 mm/year [6], ultimately evolving to high-grade glioma. Unlike solid tumors, for which exponential or geometric growth represents expansion of volume, gliomas consist of motile cells that can migrate through white matter pathways as well as proliferate [6]. At an unpredictable point of time, LGG speed of growth increases due to malignant transformation, a key clinical event that leads to increased morbidity and premature death [7].

Recent understandings into the molecular biology of LGG with the discovery of isocitrate dehydrogenase (IDH) gene and 1p19q codeletion and their impact on survival have led to a recent reclassification of gliomas, by incorporating molecular parameters [3]. Median survival for patients with LGG ranges from 5.6 to 13.3 years and is dependent on specific histology and molecular characteristics [8]. Treatment options include surgery, radiotherapy, and chemotherapy. In 2012, a Norwegian study including patients with LGG showed that early surgical resection was associated with better overall survival than biopsy and watchful waiting [9]. Surgical intervention is generally performed with the goal of maximum safe resection and aids in diagnosis by providing tissue for molecular testing [10]. Gross total resection (GTR) is significantly associated with decreased mortality and likelihood of progression at all time points compared to subtotal resection [10].

Moreover, a supratotal resection, i.e., a wide resection with a margin beyond MR imaging abnormalities, ideally with 2 cm of margin around the diffuse LGG visible on MRI, can dramatically change the natural history of LGG by delaying the risk of malignant transformation [11].

Glioblastoma and Extent of Resection

The role of surgery in the treatment of glioblastoma (GBM) has been considerably studied. The concept of resection changed from those arbitrary categories (gross total, subtotal, and partial) into the new model of maximal and safely achievable volumetric resection. A study from the University of Texas on 416 patients with newly diagnosed and recurrent GBM demonstrated that overall survival significantly increases with each unit increase in the extent of resection (EOR), starting from 89%, with the strongest effect of resection on survival being achieved at the 98% threshold [12]. Later, a University of California study including 500 patients with GBM showed a significant survival advantage starting at 78% EOR, and an EOR $\geq$ 95% had the greatest impact on overall survival [13]. However, its already known that GBM is as an invasive tumor and the area outside the contrast-enhanced region on a T1-weighted MRI is usually infiltrated by tumor cells [14]. Fluid-attenuated inversion recovery (FLAIR) images represent these invasive cells. There are some evidence that additional removal of a significant portion of the FLAIR abnormality region, when safely feasible, may result in the extension of survival without significant increases in postoperative morbidity [14]. A recent JAMA study confirms association between maximal EOR and overall survival for the contrast-enhanced tumor in all molecular subgroups, and, in younger patients, the additional maximal resection of non-contrast-enhanced tumor, regardless of IDH and O^6-methylguanine-DNA methyltransferase (MGMT) status [15].

"Safe" Resection

Glioma surgery is a delicate balance between achieving maximal tumor resection and inducing new deficits. Surgically acquired motor and language deficits may have a negative impact on survival and quality of life in GBMs' patients [16]. Those patients were less likely to receive normal-fractioned radiotherapy and chemotherapy [16]. In this context, to maximize contrast-enhanced and non-contrast-enhanced resection, advanced intraoperative imaging methods and fluorescence-based tumor biomarkers can be used, whereas direct electric stimulation (DES) will help to decrease perioperative morbidity.

Considering tumors in apparent functional areas, mapping of language and sensorimotor function is the gold standard to achieve maximal safe resection [17–21]. Since the original description of awake craniotomy by Horsley, this technique has been used for different indications with the predominant aim of improving safety [22]. Different techniques have been described in the literature for the testing and identification of functional sites [23–25]. DES during awake surgery allows the identification of eloquent functional cortex, and it is applicable for lesions arising in different locations in the brain. Indeed, awake craniotomy is associated with low complication and mortality rates, as well as low resource utilization [26–28]. However, it is used in just around 20% of glioma surgeries [18, 29].

A meta-analysis examining the usefulness of DES in glioma surgery revealed that mapping is associated with twofold reduction in late severe neurologic deficits compared to surgery without DES. Yet, there might be an increase in temporary early severe deficits [18, 30].

"Maximal" Resection

The importance of maximal safe resection in gliomas supports the use of different tools to increase the EOR during surgery, like intraoperative magnetic resonance imaging (iMRI), 5-ALA, intraoperative ultrasound (ioUS), and neuronavigation. iMRI has been used for more than a decade intending to accomplish better results in the EOR of gliomas. EOR of contrast-enhancing lesions might be improved by iMRI, since this technique can show contrast-enhancing tumor on the surgical cavity as well as underneath it (T1, T2, and T1 w/ gadolinium). Also, awake craniotomy can be safely performed in a high-field (1.5 T) iMRI suite to maximize tumor resection in eloquent brain areas with an acceptable morbidity profile at 1 month [31]. However, it requires an interruption of the surgery for acquisition of the images, and, therefore, it's a time-consuming method.

5-ALA offers the possibility to detect fluorescent tumor tissue in the cavity through the microscope in a real-time way. The use of 5-ALA has a rational extra cost and is possible without complex equipment. An analysis of residual tumor, total resections, and neurological outcomes comparing iMRI and 5-ALA demonstrated that iMRI may be significantly superior to 5-ALA for GBMs at comparable peri- and postoperative morbidities [32].

ioUS is a compact and portable system, widely available, that can independently provide real-time imaging during brain surgery. It has a significant advantage over the other intraoperative aids for image guidance, especially in terms of cost and adaptability to different clinical scenarios. On the other hand, ioUS is user dependent, with a steep learning curve.

Neuronavigation system is crucial for planning a tailored craniotomy in glioma surgery, whereas shifts in the position of the brain or tumor related to resection may cause critical errors in navigational data [33]. It is recommended to associate neuronavigation to brain mapping techniques, which performs a functional assessment of the exposed tissue.

Case Selection

Suitable patient selection is essential to ensuring intraoperative success with awake mapping. Awake craniotomy should be considered in all patients with supratentorial lesions that are in or adjacent to eloquent areas, although other groups have utilized the technique non-selectively for supratentorial tumors [28].

A full assessment of a patient's clinical history, medical comorbidities, neurological deficits, psychiatric disorders, and seizure frequency should be taken into consideration when formulating the operative plan. In our experience, there are few absolute contraindications to awake craniotomy, as unwillingness of the patient and claustrophobia. We have adopted some maneuvers to alleviate most potential problems: (a) patients with a psychiatric history were treated preoperatively with antidepressant medications; (b) patients with significant mass effect were offered a staged procedure or initial internal debulking, followed by awake mapping; (c) intraoperative seizures were treated with iced saline's solution applied to the cortex during stimulation; and (d) patients with severely impaired preoperative function underwent a staged procedure.

Previous tumor resection limited by positive mapping should not preclude awake surgery, because the adult central nervous system (CNS) reorganizes motor and language areas in patients with glioma. This neural plasticity results in up to 25% of previously identified sites no longer demonstrating eloquence at a repeat surgery [23, 34]. We always should concern that the main principles of modern neurosurgical oncology are (1) accessibility (ability to reach the tumor using anatomical references, navigation, and ioUS); (2) resectability (ability to remove the tumor using microsurgical skills, ioUS, IMRI, and 5-ALA); and (3) preservation of quality of life (improving physical and emotional performance of your patient during adjuvant therapies, like radio- and chemotherapy). To reach these goals, functional-anatomical understanding, awake craniotomy, and intraoperative neurophysiology monitoring (IOM) are crucial.

Perioperative Evaluation

Preoperative imaging includes MRI with and without gadolinium, and diffusion tensor imaging (DTI) for white matter pathways (corticospinal tract, superior longitudinal fasciculus, arcuate fasciculus, uncinate fasciculus, inferior orbitofrontal fasciculus, optic pathways) Functional MRI (fMRI) may be included if available. However, these preoperative imaging techniques are insufficient to accurately exclude function and should therefore not be used to justify asleep surgery [23]. Although useful for determining laterality of language, these techniques are insufficient to determine the exact location of functional areas and may not effectively distinguish between involved and essential language locations. Compared with DES, fMRI had a sensitivity and specificity, respectively, of 91 and 64% in Broca's area, 93 and 18% in Wernicke's area, and 100 and 100% in motor areas [35]. Therefore, DES was significantly more accurate compared with fMRI in demonstrating functional speech areas [35].

Preoperative magnetoencephalography (MEG) measures high functional connectivity (HFC) network sites. Its role in functional language connectivity evaluation is still sparse. Identifying HFC sites might assist with preoperative planning and improve intraoperative safety. Mitchel Berger, 2021, resected DES-negative HFC sites during surgeries for low- and high-grade gliomas. The patients evolved a transient language impairment for naming and syntax that resolved in 6 months. Therefore, MEG seems to be useful regarding patients' counseling about postoperative risk and assisting with preoperative surgical planning [36].

There is an unpredictable shifting of major white matter tracts during surgery. The real position of functional cortex and tracts may differ by more than 1 cm from that predicted by neuronavigation. The use of intraoperative mapping techniques can overcome this situation [37].

Preoperative clinical evaluation includes baseline language and sensorimotor test performed 24–48 hours prior to surgery. Although there is no guideline, preoperative deficits may hinder intraoperative testing if the previous object naming (ON) error rate ranges between 10% and 25% [19]. Pre-op assessment is relevant for obtaining comparative data for the next phases. The patient gains confidence, feeling trained for the intraoperative testing [38]. In addition, it is during this phase that the neuropsychologist creates a bond with the patient and his/her family. Doing so, the next steps will be carried out with greater overall acceptance.

Language assessment is further applied before hospital release and 30 days after release. It allows a more precise estimation of patient's cognitive status and aims to minimize long-term bad outcome [39]. The before-hospital release evaluation takes place usually 3 days after the surgery in non-complicated cases. Due to the fact that the patient is recovering from the surgical procedure, the applied tasks have a lower level of difficulty. Yet, all cognitive functions are tested in the same way as in the preoperative phase. At this point, the diagnosis of patient's cognitive status is important to better understand intraoperative behavior and to plan rehabilitation, if needed.

During the 30th-day follow-up, the patient is checked for any significant cognitive impairment. He/she will receive his/her neuropsychologic discharge or will be referred to continue his/her cognitive rehabilitation.

Language protocols vary among institutions. For perioperative testing, we created Ohy-Maldaun Fast Track Cognitive Test (OMFTCT), already under Portuguese native speakers' validation. It aims to assess patients' cognitive functions completely and briefly, consisting of ten subtests: naming, verbal memory, semantics, calculation, spelling, visual memory, reading, syntax, drawing, and spelling. Each task is composed of 5 items that score 1 point each, with a total score of 50 points. Some cognitive tasks, like calculation and object naming, might be combined with a simultaneous motor test (e.g., static or dynamic body balancing, walking, limb movement), composing a dual task. OMFTCT was created from the database images used by Verst-Maldaun Language Assessment (VMLA) [40], made for intraoperative testing (see details in Chap. 18). In order to universalize testing and to enable access to free language tests, OMFTCT and VMLA can be freely accessed at vemotests.com. Figure 17.1 illustrates a case, showing perioperative scores and intraoperative tasks.

<table>
<tr><th>TEST OHY-MALDAUN</th><th>SCORE PRE-OP</th><th>INTRAOPERATIVE ASSESSMENT</th><th>SCORE AT RELEASE</th><th>SCORE at 30th day follo-up</th></tr>
<tr><td>Object naming</td><td>5/5</td><td rowspan="11"><u>Initial cortical mapping (To4, ISI 2, 0.5ms, 10 mA, 2Hz):</u>
VMLA-ON: with DES: 1 to 22: negative
VMLA-Semantic:_with DES: S1-S19: negative

<u>During resection:</u>
- Repetition of a sequence of 3 words (3-4 syllables): ok
- Sentences formation: ok
- Word formation: ok

<u>Subcortical mapping and resection by pars triangularis and opercularis:</u>
VMLA-ON: with DES: reverberation 4-9, 1-33, 2-37 and 6-2
Without DES:
VMLA- Semantic: S20-S42: hesitation at: S23 and S42
VMLA-ON: 23 objects: no errors</td><td>5/5</td><td>5/5</td></tr>
<tr><td>Verbal memory</td><td>3/5</td><td>5/5</td><td>5/5</td></tr>
<tr><td>Semantics</td><td>5/5</td><td>5/5</td><td>5/5</td></tr>
<tr><td>Calculating</td><td>5/5</td><td>5/5</td><td>5/5</td></tr>
<tr><td>Writing</td><td>5/5</td><td>5/5</td><td>5/5</td></tr>
<tr><td>Visual memory</td><td>4/5</td><td>5/5</td><td>5/5</td></tr>
<tr><td>Reading/ repetition</td><td>5/5</td><td>5/5</td><td>5/5</td></tr>
<tr><td>Syntax</td><td>5/5</td><td>5/5</td><td>5/5</td></tr>
<tr><td>Drawing</td><td>5/5</td><td>5/5</td><td>5/5</td></tr>
<tr><td>Spelling</td><td>5/5</td><td>5/5</td><td>5/5</td></tr>
<tr><td>TOTAL</td><td>47/50</td><td>50/50</td><td>50/5</td></tr>
</table>

Fig. 17.1 Man, 41 years old, left frontal glioma. Complaining from memory impairment. By preoperative Ohy-Maldaun Fast Track Cognitive Test: verbal memory 3/5, a score that precludes intraoperative testing of this function. Patient was mapped and monitored during tumor resection. Initial cortical mapping: negative. Positivity was observed at subcortical level with DES and by resection during object naming and semantics

One of the most helpful features of OMFTCT is that it can be applied during hospitalization by the neuropsychologist, the medical resident, or the neurosurgeon. Application takes no longer than 1 hour, which increases patient compliance. Usually, other standard language tests demand long testing, being stressful and tiring to the patient. OMFTCT is usually effective in most of our cases, but there are patients that need to be submitted to a complete neuropsychological assessment, for more detailed diagnosis.

The combination of intraoperative language tasks will depend on the side and anatomical tumor location and patient's hand dominance. The language network is more complicated and integrated than historically considered, and the location of essential language sites can be extremely variable and difficult to predict preoperatively, far beyond "Broca's" and "Wernicke's" areas [36, 41]. Speech arrest is most frequently evoked in the pars opercularis or precentral gyrus but can also be found throughout the frontal operculum and temporoparietal region [41] (details in Chap. 18).

Awake Surgery: Technical Nuances

A skilled neuroanesthesiologist is paramount for a successful awake craniotomy. We prefer the "asleep-awake" technique (details in Chap. 15).

A craniotomy is performed to expose the cortex corresponding to the tumor area and a limited amount of surrounding tissue. Dural manipulation can be painful, so copious irrigation is required during craniotomy, and a dura mater block is performed using a 30-gauge needle with 1% lidocaine to infiltrate the region around the proposed dural incision. The dura is opened in a manner that best suits an ideal exposure of the lesion. Once the dura mater is opened, the patient is gradually awakened by suspending the administration of all medications. Upon opening the dura, the brain is assessed for swelling, which could be overcome by asking the patient to perform controlled hyperventilation. If an unacceptable degree of brain swelling occurs after durotomy, additional mannitol may be given, the head of the bed raised, and the arachnoid space opened for the release of CSF as additional maneuvers. Mapping begins after patient's wakefulness. Irritation of the middle fossa floor during resection may cause pain or elicit the trigeminocardiac reflex, causing nausea, vomiting, hypotension, and bradycardia [23].

Initial cortical mapping is used to identify negative speech and motor regions, allowing the entrance of the cortical area [42]. Considering the variability across patients, subcortical mapping is virtually always required for safely identification of the language network. DES can detect eloquent structures by inducing a transient virtual lesion based on the inhibition of a circuit, identifying with great accuracy and reproducibility the structures that are crucial for language.

Electrical stimulation (either bipolar or monopolar) is usually applied manually with a handheld probe. Electrocorticography is required to monitor for epileptic events and discharges [23, 43].

Brain Mapping from the Technical Point of View

Language function is based on interaction between different neuronal circuits. Theoretically, a disturbance at any point of a connected cortical-subcortical pathway could manifest clinically as symptom from a related cortical area. This phenomenon is called hodotopy [44, 45] (Fig. 17.2). This feature might be reproduced by DES, in which any focal blockage produced at a point of a tract could interrupt the function at any cortical area related to this point [45]. For instance, a patient with a tumor in the posterior temporal region may have spelling difficulty due to impairment of the U-fibers that connect temporal cortex to inferior parietal gyri.

Preferably, we perform the awake technique only for language mapping demanding cases. In our routine, the neurophysiologist (NF) applies the cognitive tasks and manages the IOM, due to cost optimization. Usually, a technician operates the IOM system.

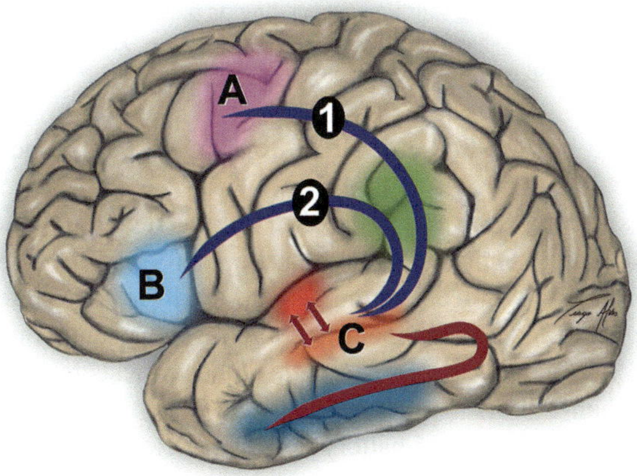

Fig. 17.2 Hodotopy: cortical-subcortical interconnections form an inter-dependent network. It can be disrupted by focal disease or stimulation at subcortical level (points 1 and 2) resulting in the disruption of related cortical function (points A, B, or C). Disconnection syndrome, topographic dysfunction, or both could arise from this focal blockage. (Catani, M and de Schotten, MT 2012; [45])

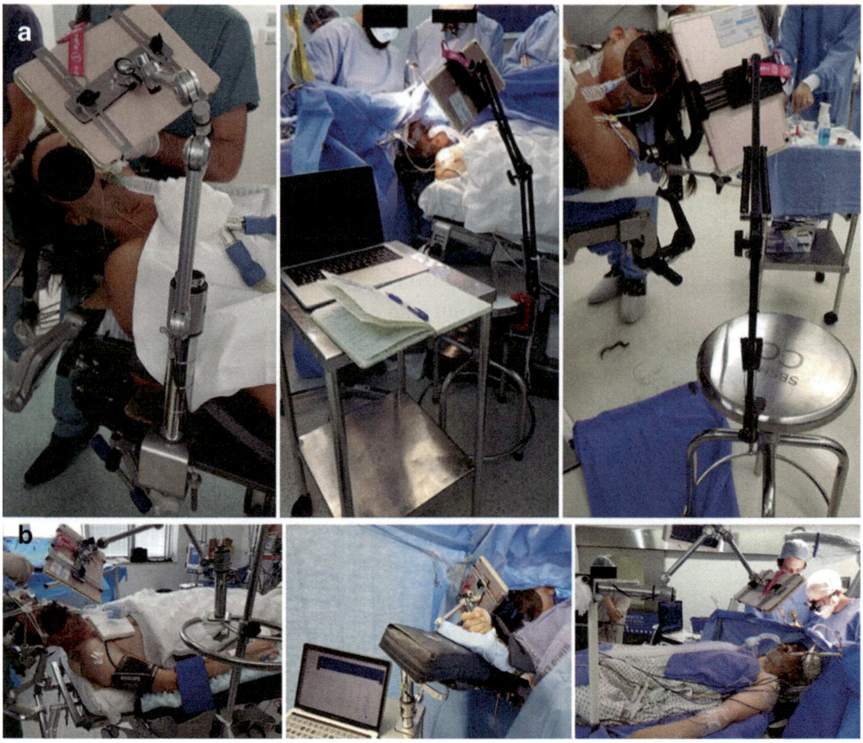

Fig. 17.3 (**a**, **b**) Tablet positioning solutions, depending on patient's face exposure. Positioning of the tablet must attend patients' need of fully watching the screen. The tester must have access for any needed adjustments and to switch between tests

Positioning the patient and the tablet for language task demands all team cooperation.

Figure 17.3 shows possibilities of tablet fixation adapted to patient's face exposure. Usually, the tablet is placed soon after the neuronavigation setup. During the awake phase, the NF sits in front of the patient, to allow better interaction, control unproper movements and quickly identify epileptogenic events' onset, check on the tablet, and perform dual task. Optimizing the choice of tests is critical since testing takes no longer than 2 hours.

Our protocol includes an IOM battery of tests for eloquent area in all patients. It is composed of phase reversal (if the central lobe is reachable), direct cortical motor evoked potential (MEP) using the grid electrode, somatosensory evoked potential of contralateral ulnar and tibial nerves, cortical and subcortical mapping, electromyography, and electrocorticography (ECoG). The reason for the complete IOM protocol relies on the possibility of non-cooperative patient and seizure events that demand sedation. Additionally, preservation of MEP and loss of limb voluntary movement point to a supplementary motor syndrome in frontal approaches. Early identification of epileptogenic events and afterdischarges using ECoG improves patient's management. ECoG should be included in IOM protocol for language and motor cortical and subcortical mapping for safety reasons. Additionally, continuous direct cortical MEP during motor mapping is mandatory.

Language tests are continuously performed during tumor resection, alternating with cortical and subcortical mapping as necessary (Figs. 17.4 and 17.5). Monitoring do not replace mapping. Indeed, they should be performed as a complement to each other. By monitoring while the resection goes on, it is possible to identify areas that

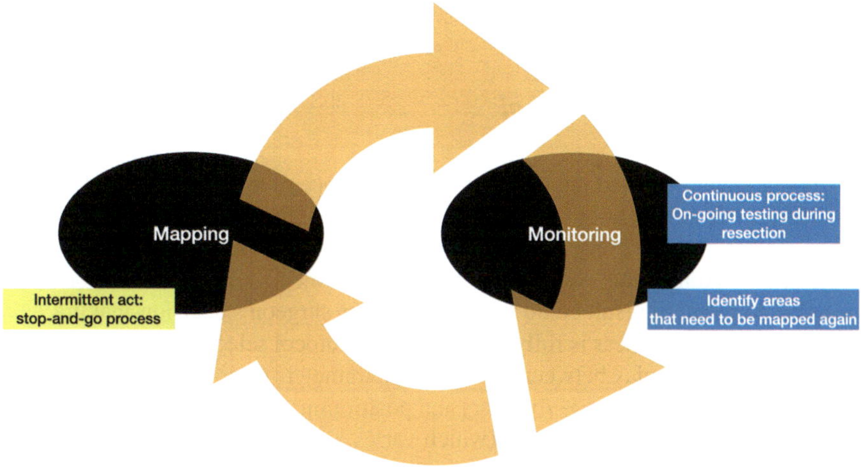

Fig. 17.4 Language mapping and monitoring are complementary to each other and should be interspersed. Ongoing cognitive assessment during resection is monitoring. If positivity starts, for example, hesitation, reverberation, and paraphasia, the surgeon re-maps the area. Interchanging mapping and monitoring improves overall safety

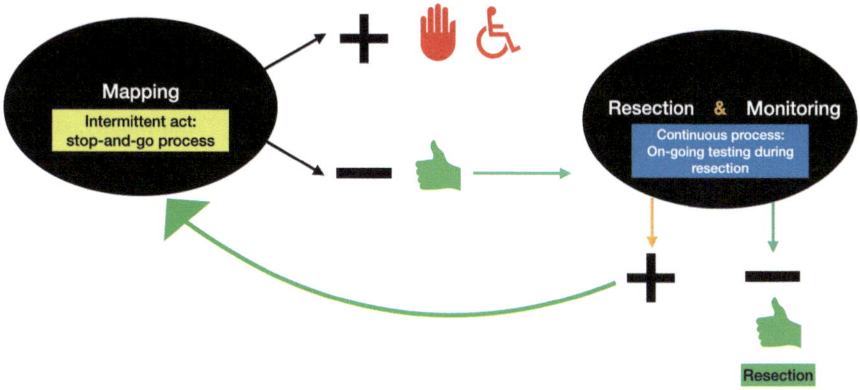

Fig. 17.5 Flowchart on how we perform and react during awake craniotomy. Positive mapping identifies areas that should be preserved, while negative mapping sites to be resected. Ongoing language monitoring improves identification of function disruption or “network instability,” and immediate re-mapping is performed

repeatedly evoke an error, for example, phonemic paraphasia. This situation leads to mapping this area again to identify and preserve eloquent tissue. Assuming the methodology is strictly applied, no false negatives are expected, and brain function will be blocked by DES [46]. This optimal sensitivity justifies why mapping is the gold standard for recognizing reshaped brain modified by slow tumor growth and neuroplasticity. Mapping should not be overlooked.

In our practice, when language areas are identified, the resection margin is maintained 1–2 cm away from those cortical areas. Resection is stopped if speech function deteriorates but is restarted if full recovery occurs within 5 min.

Choosing Stimulus Protocol

Methodological rigor and the meticulous performance of mapping are fundamental to adequate tumor resection and avoidance of permanent neurological deficits [47]. If the principles are strictly observed, the sensitivity of DES for the detection of cortical and axonal eloquent structures is 100% [46]. Any false-positive or false-negative stimulation result could lead to erroneous surgeon's decision-making.

Mapping effectiveness is fully dependent on protocol selection and application. It is a complex interplay between stimulation parameters (rheobase and chronaxie), probe characteristics (mono−/bipolar) and positioning according to the orientation to the fiber, and tissue impedance (which varies according to the illness, whether tumor or epilepsy) [46]. The stimulation aims to block the function which leads to clinical error during the language testing. The clinical error points to underlying eloquent tissue (either cortical or subcortical) that needs to be preserved. Functional disturbances should be analyzed by a dedicated person during the awake craniotomy in order to improve their identification.

Lastly, by language mapping, it is not possible to estimate the distance between the probe and the tract fiber.

Low Frequency (LF) Versus High Frequency (HF)

Low Frequency

In 1986, Ojemann synthesized his methodology:

1. For ON, image was presented every 3 to 4 seconds.
2. Two positive stimulations in three trails meant eloquent area.
3. Current level should be adequate to block the function, without spreading to distant sites and loosing specificity.
4. "The adequate but localized" current level is the highest one that does not result in afterdischarges in ECoG.
5. Biphasic 1ms-pulse at 60 Hz (LF), bipolar 5 mm-apart tips stimulator, 2–8 mA (one to four times cortical motor threshold).

DES suboptimal specificity. It could result in premature interruption of resection to preserve false functional borders [46].

Last but not least, positive mapping could set resection borders of structures whose functions could be compensated. This phenomenon is a result of network reorganization or neuroplasticity, in which the other side could overtake the control of the function [27]. Thus, an essential area at the time of mapping could be not a definitive crucial area in sequential surgeries. Yet, caution should be taken since resecting structures closer to positive mapping areas may result in permanent deficits.

New Concepts and Frontiers

The new concept is that language network is essentially connectivity, overcoming the localizationist models. "The stimulated point (axonal or cortical) is only an input gate into this whole network" [46]. The cortical area connected to the activated axon will receive this propagated upward and downward potential [43, 45]. This hypothesis matches hodotopy and would be translated by blockage of function at any stimulated point of an interconnected system.

Neuroplasticity occurs due to slow tumor growth and after tumor resection. Better understanding the abilities of functional reshaping might enlarge resection borders to a supramaximal functional limit.

Proper parameters for testing more complex language and cognitive tasks intraoperatively should be set, regarding stimulus onset, triggering, and duration of application.

References

1. Penfield W. The interpretive cortex. The stream of consciousness in the human brain can be electrically reactivated. Science. 1959;129:1719–25. https://doi.org/10.1126/science.129.3365.1719.
2. Leblanc R. The white paper: Wilder Penfield, the stream of consciousness, and the physiology of mind. J Hist Neurosci. 2019;28:416–36. https://doi.org/10.1080/0964704X.2019.1651135.
3. Louis DN, Perry A, Reifenberger G, et al. The 2016 World Health Organization classification of tumors of the central nervous system: a summary. Acta Neuropathol (Berl). 2016;131:803–20. https://doi.org/10.1007/s00401-016-1545-1.
4. Ostrom QT, Gittleman H, Liao P, et al. CBTRUS statistical report: primary brain and other central nervous system tumors diagnosed in the United States in 2010-2014. Neuro-Oncol. 2017;19:v1–v88. https://doi.org/10.1093/neuonc/nox158.
5. Recht LD, Bernstein M. Low-grade gliomas. Neurol Clin. 1995;13:847–59. https://doi.org/10.1016/s0733-8619(18)30021-5.
6. Swanson KR, Bridge C, Murray JD, Alvord EC. Virtual and real brain tumors: using mathematical modeling to quantify glioma growth and invasion. J Neurol Sci. 2003;216:1–10. https://doi.org/10.1016/j.jns.2003.06.001.

7. Jakola AS, Bouget D, Reinertsen I, et al. Spatial distribution of malignant transformation in patients with low-grade glioma. J Neuro-Oncol. 2020;146:373–80. https://doi.org/10.1007/s11060-020-03391-1.
8. Buckner JC, Shaw EG, Pugh SL, et al. Radiation plus Procarbazine, CCNU, and vincristine in low-grade glioma. N Engl J Med. 2016;374:1344–55. https://doi.org/10.1056/nejmoa1500925.
9. Jakola AS, Myrmel KS, Kloster R, et al. Comparison of a strategy favoring early surgical resection vs a strategy favoring watchful waiting in low-grade gliomas. JAMA – J Am Med Assoc. 2012;308:1881–8. https://doi.org/10.1001/jama.2012.12807.
10. Brown TJ, Bota DA, Van Den Bent MJ, et al. Management of low-grade glioma: a systematic review and meta-analysis. Neuro-Oncol Pract. 2019;6:249–58. https://doi.org/10.1093/nop/npy034.
11. Duffau H. Long-term outcomes after supratotal resection of diffuse low-grade gliomas: a consecutive series with 11-year follow-up. Acta Neurochir. 2016;158:51–8. https://doi.org/10.1007/s00701-015-2621-3.
12. Lacroix M, Abi-Said D, Fourney DR, et al. A multivariate analysis of 416 patients with glioblastoma multiforme: prognosis, extent of resection, and survival. J Neurosurg. 2001;95:190–8. https://doi.org/10.3171/jns.2001.95.2.0190.
13. Sanai N, Polley MY, McDermott MW, et al. An extent of resection threshold for newly diagnosed glioblastomas: clinical article. J Neurosurg. 2011;115:3–8. https://doi.org/10.3171/2011.2.JNS10998.
14. Li YM, Suki D, Hess K, Sawaya R. The influence of maximum safe resection of glioblastoma on survival in 1229 patients: can we do better than gross-total resection? J Neurosurg. 2016b;124:977–88. https://doi.org/10.3171/2015.5.JNS142087.
15. Molinaro AM, Hervey-Jumper S, Morshed RA, et al. Association of Maximal Extent of resection of contrast-enhanced and non-contrast-enhanced tumor with survival within molecular subgroups of patients with newly diagnosed glioblastoma. JAMA Oncol. 2020;6:495–503. https://doi.org/10.1001/jamaoncol.2019.6143.
16. Gulati S, Jakola AS, Nerland US, et al. The risk of getting worse: surgically acquired deficits, perioperative complications, and functional outcomes after primary resection of glioblastoma. World Neurosurg. 2011;76:572–9. https://doi.org/10.1016/j.wneu.2011.06.014.
17. Beez T, Boge K, Wager M, et al. Tolerance of awake surgery for glioma: a prospective European Low Grade Glioma Network multicenter study. Acta Neurochir. 2013;155:1301–8. https://doi.org/10.1007/s00701-013-1759-0.
18. Hervey-Jumper SL, Li J, Lau D, et al. Awake craniotomy to maximize glioma resection: methods and technical nuances over a 27-year period. J Neurosurg. 2015;123:325–39. https://doi.org/10.3171/2014.10.JNS141520.
19. Morshed RA, Young JS, Lee AT, et al. Clinical pearls and methods for intraoperative awake language mapping. Neurosurgery. 2020;89(2):143–53. https://doi.org/10.1093/neuros/nyaa440.
20. Riva M, Fava E, Gallucci M, et al. Monopolar high-frequency language mapping: can it help in the surgical management of gliomas? A comparative clinical study. J Neurosurg. 2016;124:1479–89. https://doi.org/10.3171/2015.4.JNS14333.
21. So EL, Alwaki A. A guide for cortical electrical stimulation mapping. J Clin Neurophysiol. 2018;35:98–105. https://doi.org/10.1097/WNP.0000000000000435.
22. Horsley V. Remarks on ten consecutive cases of operations upon the brain and cranial cavity to illustrate the details and safety of the method employed (what a table). Br Med J. 1887;1:863–5. https://doi.org/10.1136/bmj.1.1373.863.
23. Gogos AJ, Young JS, Morshed RA, et al. Awake glioma surgery: technical evolution and nuances. J Neuro-Oncol. 2020;147:515–24. https://doi.org/10.1007/s11060-020-03482-z.
24. Ojemann G, Ojemann J, Lettich E, Berger M. Cortical language localization in left, dominant hemisphere. An electrical stimulation mapping investigation in 117 patients. J Neurosurg. 1989;71:316–26. https://doi.org/10.3171/jns.1989.71.3.0316.
25. Penfield W, Boldrey E. Somatic motor and sensory representation in man. Brain. 1937:389–443.
26. Duffau H, Capelle L, Denvil D, et al. Usefulness of intraoperative electrical subcortical mapping during surgery for low-grade gliomas located within eloquent brain regions: functional

results in a consecutive series of 103 patients. J Neurosurg. 2003b;98:764–78. https://doi.org/10.3171/jns.2003.98.4.0764.
27. Duffau H. Brain mapping – from neural basis of cognition to surgical applications. 1st ed. Wien, Austria: Springer; 2011.
28. Serletis D, Bernstein M. Prospective study of awake craniotomy used routinely and nonselectively for supratentorial tumors. J Neurosurg. 2007;107:1–6. https://doi.org/10.3171/JNS-07/07/0001.
29. Chang SM, Parney IF, Huang W, et al. Patterns of care for adults with newly diagnosed malignant glioma. J Am Med Assoc. 2005;293:557–64. https://doi.org/10.1001/jama.293.5.557.
30. De Witt Hamer PC, Robles SG, Zwinderman AH, et al. Impact of intraoperative stimulation brain mapping on glioma surgery outcome: a meta-analysis. J Clin Oncol. 2012;30:2559–65. https://doi.org/10.1200/JCO.2011.38.4818.
31. Maldaun MV, Khawja SN, Levine NB, Rao G, Lang FF, Weinberg JS, Tummala S, Cowles CE, Ferson D, Nguyen AT, Sawaya R, Suki D, Prabhu SS. Awake craniotomy for gliomas in a high-field intraoperative magnetic resonance imaging suite: analysis of 42 cases. J Neurosurg. 2014;121(4):810–7. https://doi.org/10.3171/2014.6.JNS132285. Epub 2014 Aug 8. PMID: 25105702.
32. Roder C, Bisdas S, Ebner FH, et al. Maximizing the extent of resection and survival benefit of patients in glioblastoma surgery: high-field iMRI versus conventional and 5-ALA-assisted surgery. Eur J Surg Oncol. 2014;40:297–304. https://doi.org/10.1016/j.ejso.2013.11.022.
33. Orringer DA, Golby A, Jolesz F. Neuronavigation in the surgical management of brain tumors: current and future trends. Expert Rev Med Devices. 2012;9:491–500. https://doi.org/10.1586/erd.12.42.
34. Southwell DG, Hervey-Jumper SL, Perry DW, Berger MS. Intraoperative mapping during repeat awake craniotomy reveals the functional plasticity of adult cortex. J Neurosurg. 2016;124:1460–9. https://doi.org/10.3171/2015.5.JNS142833.
35. Sawaya R, Prabhu SS. Impact of preoperative functional magnetic resonance imaging during awake craniotomy procedures for intraoperative guidance and complication avoidance. Stereotact Funct Neurosurg. 2014;92(5):315–22. https://doi.org/10.1159/000365224.
36. Lee AT, Faltermeier C, Morshed RA, et al. The impact of high functional connectivity network hub resection on language task performance in adult low- and high-grade glioma. J Neurosurg. 2021a;134:1102–12. https://doi.org/10.3171/2020.1.JNS192267.
37. Nimsky C, Ganslandt O, Hastreiter P, et al. Intraoperative diffusion-tensor MR imaging: shifting of white matter tracts during neurosurgical procedures – initial experience. Radiology. 2005;234:218–25. https://doi.org/10.1148/radiol.2341031984.
38. Bilotta F, Stazi E, Titi L, et al. Diagnostic work up for language testing in patients undergoing awake craniotomy for brain lesions in language areas. Br J Neurosurg. 2014;28:363–7. https://doi.org/10.3109/02688697.2013.854313.
39. Acuña-Padilla Y, Salazar-Villanea M, Vindas-Montoya R, et al. Rol de la Neuropsicologia en la Evaluaci6n y preparación del paciente candidato a craneotomía con paciente despierto. Role of neuropsychology in the evaluation and preparation of the patient who is a candidate for craniotomy with an awake patient O papel da neuropsicologia na avaliação e preparação do paciente candidato a craniotomia em pacientes acordados. Cuad Neuropsicol Panam J Neuropsychol. 2020;14:56–64. https://doi.org/10.7714/CNPS/14.1.207.
40. Verst SM, de Castro I, Scappini-Junior W, et al. Methodology for creating and validating object naming and semantic tests used by Verst-Maldaun language assessment during awake craniotomies. Clin Neurol Neurosurg. 2021;202:106485. https://doi.org/10.1016/j.clineuro.2021.106485.
41. Chang EF, Raygor KP, Berger MS. Contemporary model of language organization: an overview for neurosurgeons. J Neurosurg. 2015;122:250–61. https://doi.org/10.3171/2014.10.JNS132647.Disclosure.
42. Simon MV. Intraoperative neurophysiology – a comprehensive guide to monitoring and mapping. 2nd ed. New York: Demos Medical Publishing; 2019.

43. Ritaccio AL, Brunner P, Schalk G. Electrical stimulation mapping of the brain: basic principles and emerging alternatives. J Clin Neurophysiol. 2018;35:86–97. https://doi.org/10.1097/WNP.0000000000000440.
44. Catani M, de Schotten MT. Atlas of human brain connections. 1st ed. Oxford: Oxford University Press; 2012.
45. Duffau H, Moritz-Gasser S, Mandonnet E. A re-examination of neural basis of language processing: proposal of a dynamic hodotopical model from data provided by brain stimulation mapping during picture naming. Brain Lang. 2014;131:1–10. https://doi.org/10.1016/j.bandl.2013.05.011.
46. Mandonnet E, Sarubbo S, Duffau H. Proposal of an optimized strategy for intraoperative testing of speech and language during awake mapping. Neurosurg Rev. 2017;40:29–35. https://doi.org/10.1007/s10143-016-0723-x.
47. Szelényi A, Bello L, Duffau H, et al. Intraoperative electrical stimulation in awake craniotomy: methodological aspects of current practice. Neurosurg Focus. 2010;28:E7. https://doi.org/10.3171/2009.12.FOCUS09237.
48. Ojemann GA. Mapping of neuropsychological language parameters at surgery. Int Anesthesiol Clin. 1986;24:115–31. https://doi.org/10.1097/00004311-198602430-00011.
49. Taniguchi M, Cedzich C, Taniguchi M, et al. Modification of cortical stimulation for motor evoked potentials under general anesthesia. Neurosurgery. 1993;32:219–26. https://doi.org/10.1227/00006123-199302000-00011.
50. Kombos T, Süss O. Neurophysiological basis of direct cortical stimulation and applied neuroanatomy of the motor cortex: a review. Neurosurg Focus. 2009;27:E3. https://doi.org/10.3171/2009.8.FOCUS09141.
51. Deletis V, Isgum V, Amassian VE. Neurophysiological mechanisms underlying motor evoked potentials in anesthetized humans. Part 1. Recovery time of corticospinal tract direct waves elicited by pairs of transcranial electrical stimuli. Clin Neurophysiol. 2001a;112:438–44.
52. Deletis V, Rodi Z, Amassian VE. Neurophysiological mechanisms underlying motor evoked potentials in anesthetized humans. Part 2. Relationship between epidurally and muscle recorded MEPs in man. Clin Neurophysiol. 2001b;112:445–52.
53. Szentagothai-Schimert J. Die Bedeutung des Faserkalibers und der Markscheidendicke im Zentralnervensystem. Z Fuer Anat Entwicklungsgeschichte. 1942;111:201–23. https://doi.org/10.1007/BF00538084.
54. Tomasch J. Size, distribution, and number of fibres in the human corpus callosum. Anat Rec. 1954;119:119–35. https://doi.org/10.1002/ar.1091190109.
55. Li L, Velumian AA, Samoilova M, Fehlings MG. A novel approach for studying the physiology and pathophysiology of myelinated and non-myelinated axons in the CNS white matter. PLoS One. 2016a;11:e0165637. https://doi.org/10.1371/journal.pone.0165637.
56. Ranck JB. Which elements are excited in electrical stimulation of mammalian central nervous system: a review. Brain Res. 1975;98:417–40. https://doi.org/10.1016/0006-8993(75)90364-9.
57. Abalkhail TM, MacDonald DB, AlThubaiti I, et al. Intraoperative direct cortical stimulation motor evoked potentials: stimulus parameter recommendations based on rheobase and chronaxie. Clin Neurophysiol. 2017;128:2300–8. https://doi.org/10.1016/j.clinph.2017.09.005.
58. Axelson HW, Hesselager G, Flink R. Successful localization of the Broca area with short-train pulses instead of 'Penfield' stimulation. Seizure. 2009;18:374–5. https://doi.org/10.1016/j.seizure.2009.01.005.
59. Verst SM, de Aguiar PHP, Joaquim MAS, et al. Monopolar 250–500 Hz language mapping: results of 41 patients. Clin Neurophysiol Pract. 2019;4:1–8. https://doi.org/10.1016/j.cnp.2018.11.002.
60. Puglisi G, Howells H, Sciortino T, et al. Frontal pathways in cognitive control: direct evidence from intraoperative stimulation and diffusion tractography. Brain. 2019;142:2451–65. https://doi.org/10.1093/brain/awz178.

61. Desmurget M, Richard N, Beuriat P-A, et al. Selective inhibition of volitional hand movements after stimulation of the dorsoposterior parietal cortex in humans. Curr Biol. 2018;28:3303–3309.e3. https://doi.org/10.1016/j.cub.2018.08.027.
62. Puglisi G, Sciortino T, Rossi M, et al. Preserving executive functions in nondominant frontal lobe glioma surgery: an intraoperative tool. J Neurosurg. 2018;131:474–80. https://doi.org/10.3171/2018.4.JNS18393.
63. Baldissera F, Lundberg A, Udo M. Stimulation of pre- and postsynaptic elements in the red nucleus. Exp Brain Res. 1972;15 https://doi.org/10.1007/BF00235579.
64. Hongo T, Jankowska E, Lundberg A. The rubrospinal tract. I. Effects on alpha-motoneurons innervating hindlimb muscles in cats. Exp Brain Res. 1969;7 https://doi.org/10.1007/BF00237320.
65. Rudin DO, Eisenman G. The action potential of spinal axons in vitro. J Gen Physiol. 1954;37:505–38. https://doi.org/10.1085/jgp.37.4.505.
66. Picht T, Kombos T, Gramm HJ, et al. Multimodal protocol for awake craniotomy in language cortex tumour surgery. Acta Neurochir. 2006;148:127–38. https://doi.org/10.1007/s00701-005-0706-0.
67. Jayakar P. Cortical electrical stimulation mapping: special considerations in children. J Clin Neurophysiol. 2018;35:106–9. https://doi.org/10.1097/WNP.0000000000000451.
68. MacDonald DB. Safety of intraoperative transcranial electrical stimulation motor evoked potential monitoring. J Clin Neurophysiol. 2002;19:416–29. https://doi.org/10.1097/00004691-200210000-00005.
69. MacDonald DB, Skinner S, Shils J, Yingling C. Intraoperative motor evoked potential monitoring – a position statement by the American Society of Neurophysiological Monitoring. Clin Neurophysiol. 2013;124:2291–316. https://doi.org/10.1016/j.clinph.2013.07.025.
70. Szelényi A, Kothbauer KF, Deletis V. Transcranial electric stimulation for intraoperative motor evoked potential monitoring: stimulation parameters and electrode montages. Clin Neurophysiol. 2007;118:1586–95. https://doi.org/10.1016/j.clinph.2007.04.008.
71. Ojemann GA, Whitaker HA. Language localization and variability. Brain Lang. 1978;6:239–60. https://doi.org/10.1016/0093-934X(78)90061-5.
72. Pereira LCM, Oliveira KM, L'Abbate GL, et al. Outcome of fully awake craniotomy for lesions near the eloquent cortex: analysis of a prospective surgical series of 79 supratentorial primary brain tumors with long follow-up. Acta Neurochir. 2009;151:1215–30. https://doi.org/10.1007/s00701-009-0363-9.

Chapter 18
Language and Cognitive Tests: A Target-Guided Protocol

Silvia Mazzali Verst, Tatiana Vilasboas Alves, and Leonardo Dornas de Oliveira

Abbreviations

a	Anterior
AF	Arcuate fasciculus
AnG	Angular gyrus
CC	*Corpus callosum*
DES	Direct electrical stimulation
EL	Educational level
FAT	Frontal aslant tract
fMRI	Functional magnetic resonance imaging
GA	Geschwind area
IFG	Inferior frontal gyrus
IFOF	Inferior fronto-occipital fasciculus
ILF	Inferior longitudinal fasciculus

Supplementary Information The online version contains supplementary material available at [https://doi.org/10.1007/978-3-030-95730-8_18].

S. M. Verst (✉)
Instituto de Ensino e Pesquisa (Research and Educational Institute) of Sírio Libanês Hospital, São Paulo, Brazil

Brain Spine Neurofisiologia, Jundiaí, SP, Brazil
e-mail: silvia@brainspine.com.br

T. V. Alves
Neurosurgeon at São Camilo Hospital, Unit Pompéia, São Paulo, Brazil

L. D. de Oliveira
Hospital das Clínicas da Universidade Federal de Minas Gerais, Belo Horizonte, MG, Brazil

S. M. Verst et al. (eds.), *Intraoperative Monitoring*,
https://doi.org/10.1007/978-3-030-95730-8_18

ITG	Inferior temporal gyrus
m	Medial
MFG	Middle frontal gyrus
MTF	Middle temporal gyrus
ON	Object naming
OR	Optic radiation
p	Posterior
PCG	Post-central gyrus
phPRP	Phonological paraphasia
PPTT	Pyramids and Palm Trees Test
RMET	Read the Mind in the Eyes Task
semPRP	Semantic paraphasia
SFG	Superior frontal gyrus
SLF	Superior frontal gyrus
SMA	Supplementary motor area
SMG	Supramarginal gyrus
STG	Superior temporal gyrus
THR	Stimulus threshold
UF	Uncinate fasciculus
VN	Verb naming
VWFA	Visual word form area
WM	Working memory

Introduction

Understanding the reasoning of test selection and interchanging during the awake craniotomy for language and cognitive assessment is fundamental. Any task should be simple enough to be reliably performed in the operating room and to be accomplished by the patient, who usually has the head fixed by a holder [1, 2]. Surgical objectivity and a summarized intraoperative assessment targeted to brain tumor localization are the key [1, 3, 4].

The approach success is fully dependent on teamwork. The surgeon is the manager of the act and needs to interpret intraoperative imaging and surgical field and instruct the tester in the sequence of applied tests. More importantly, neurosurgeons need to be familiarized with them so that the stimulation can be applied according to task particularities. Anesthesia plays an important role in patient wellness and cooperation. Specific details in this matter were in Chap. 15.

Direct electrical stimulation (DES) aims to disrupt a language circuitry, blocking the function. DES threshold (THR) is set by evoking speech arrest, anomia, or motor or sensory response [1]. Motor response after DES can be a contralateral muscle twitch or a recorded motor evoked potential, and a sensitive response is usually referred as dysesthesia. DES-THR can be determined during number counting, object or verbal naming, reading, semantics, and dual task, with great variations

Verbal Naming

Verbal naming (VN) is more a grammatical work within a syntactic structure [10, 22]. Rofes et al. (2015a) [14], pointed that in addition to the language processes involved in ON, VN requires syntactic ability.

To produce functional communication skills, processes of diverse syntactic complexities are involved. To compose a sentence, it is necessary to decide between transitive and intransitive verbs, correlate the subject and verb, and determine the temporal moment of the action. It demands choosing verbs (within our brain glossary) and differing them from similar nouns ("to sit" instead of seat). Hence, VN correlates with language abilities in daily living more strongly than ON itself.

Yet, languages differ in sentence and verb structural complexity, being by Chinese much less complex than by Italian, for example [14]. It is not known its impact on VN testing.

Rofes et al. (2015a) [14], presented VN in different ways:

1. Naming finite verbs: Patients are supposed to compose a sentence with correct inflected verb form using the shown object on screen, like "apple" and "she eats an apple" (Fig. 18.2a).
2. Verb generation: Patients are shown an object on a screen and must name an action that can be performed with the object, using a verb in the infinitival form. For example, a pan, patients are expected to say "to cook" (Fig. 18.2b).
3. Action naming: The patient is exposed to an action on the screen and should name the verb. For example, two boys fighting, and the patient says "to fight" (Fig. 18.2c).

They showed #1 to be more sensitive, due to the fact of needing complex cognitive-linguistic skills [10, 27].

Naming finite verbs is of easy execution using the same figures as to ON (although it is not written he/she above the figure as described by original authors). The patient is asked to compose a sentence with the shown object using "he/she." For example, "she drives the car."

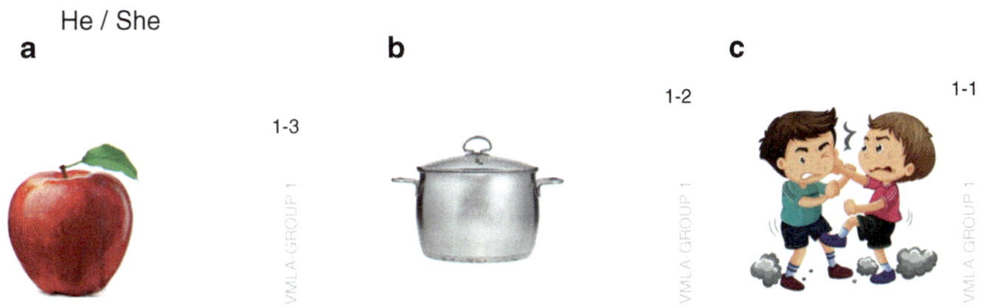

Fig. 18.2 Verbal naming. (**a**) Naming finite verbs. (**b**) Verb generation. (**c**) Action naming

The most probable association of ON and VN can better evaluate language networks.

Target: *left IFG* [27]

Note: can be associated with dual task

Dual Task

The motor test assesses the primary motor cortex in the pre-central motor gyrus, corticospinal pathway, and sensory post-central gyrus, where up to 10% of motor fibers can originate. Short inter-gyrus U-fibers provide a reciprocal integration network between motor and sensory gyri [28]. Awareness and voluntary movement initiation and control depend on a dorsal-medial and lateral pre-motor cortices' network involving the insula, basal ganglia, and supplementary motor area. A complex network of short and mid-range cortico-cortical and cortico-striatal fibers connect these regions, running in the deep frontal lobe white matter, anterior to the pure motor response pyramidal tract [28]. The patient plans the movement using working memory, attention, and executive function skills. To perform dual task, i.e., two tests simultaneously, the superior, middle, and inferior frontal gyri and frontal aslant tract must be accessed [29, 30].

Dual task helps in the differentiation between speech and motor arrest, being very appropriate as the first test for DES threshold setting. Motor arrest corresponds to negative motor area of the tongue or upper or lower limb. Hence, safe identification of speech arrest requires exclusion of motor arrest and after-discharges.

The patient is instructed to continuously flex and extend his forearm, hand, and fingers at a rate of 0.5 Hz [5].

Possible interpretation of dual task during DES of the frontal lobe can be seen in Fig. 18.3 and Video 18.3.

Test simultaneously Counting	UE movement		Type of response	Area name
Stop	Stop		Motor arrest	Total NMA
OK	Stop		Motor arrest	UE NMA
Stop	OK →	Test tongue movement		
		Stop	Motor arrest	Tongue NMA
		OK	Speech arrest	Anarthria area
Test simultaneously Picture-naming "This is a.."	UE movement			
Stop	OK		Anomia	Anomia area

Fig. 18.3 Dual task interpretation for negative motor area (NMA). Inferior frontal area testing with ON or counting (or any other task like VN, reading, or semantics) and simultaneous flexion and extension of the forearm. Stopping of movement and cognitive task points to NMA. (With permission from Mandonnet et al. [5])

Chapter 19
Cranial Nerve Monitoring III to XII

Skull Base Surgery: Part II – Intraoperative Neurophysiology

Silvia Mazzali Verst, Maria Rufina Barros, and Rayssa Addiny Modenesi Lozano

Abbreviations

CMAP	Compound muscle action potential
CMUAP	Compound motor unit action potential
CN	Cranial nerve
CoMEP	Corticonuclear motor evoked potential
CPA	Cerebellopontine angle
CST	Corticospinal tract
CTHY	Cricothyroid muscle
EMG	Electromyography
ETE	Endotracheal tube electrodes
FN	Facial nerve
frEMG	Free-run EMG
HW	Hook wires
IAM	Internal acoustic meatus

S. M. Verst (✉)
Instituto de Ensino e Pesquisa (Research and Educational Institute) of Sírio Libanês Hospital, São Paulo, Brazil

Brain Spine Neurofisiologia, Jundiaí, SP, Brazil

M. R. Barros
Department of Intraoperative Monitoring, Neurological Institute of Espirito Santo, Vitória, ES, Brazil

Department of Neurophysiology, Vitoria Apart Hospital (VAH), Vitória, ES, Brazil

R. A. M. Lozano
Clinical Neurophysiologist at Brain Spine Neurofisiologia, São Paulo, Brazil

S. M. Verst et al. (eds.), *Intraoperative Monitoring*,
https://doi.org/10.1007/978-3-030-95730-8_19

IN	Intermedius nerve
IOM	Intraoperative monitoring
LAR	Laryngeal adductor reflex
MEP	Motor evoked potentials
MU	Motor unit
SSEP	Somatosensory evoked potentials
tEMG	Trigger EMG
TES	Transcranial electrical stimulation
THR	Threshold
HB	House Brackman

Introduction

In surgery for acoustic neuromas, 20–70% of patients suffer from at least transient postoperative facial nerve (FN) deficit without visible anatomical harm during surgery, especially following excision of large tumors [60, 67, 75]. For bulbar IX and X nerves, the risk is even higher, being 76% in large skull base tumors and 84.5% when surgical access is lateral (Deletis 2002). It is a challenging approach for the surgeon since the cerebelum-pontine angle (CPA) area is a small triangular space where CN V to VIII (and just below IX to XII), cerebellar arteries, and petrosal vein belong.

Most lesions result from nervous tissue metabolic alterations, mechanical trauma, coagulator heat, or compression [13]. Stretching, ischemia, and CUSA also play a role on stressing a cranial nerve (CN) [31]. Maneuvers such as irrigation with warm saline solution, release of the traction or compression on the nerve, and changing the operative region could reverse the stress event [1, 17, 26, 84]. The goal is to preserve the integrity of the entire corticonuclear pathway [2, 17, 44, 54].

Intraoperative monitoring (IOM) aims to identify a distorted, dissected, and displaced CN, to recognize risky events to trigger immediate surgeon's reaction, and to predict outcome. Different neurophysiological tests are associated to accomplish the goal, but each of them is somehow tricky. Prognostic parameters conflict with each other, turning IOM into a multi-risk assessment, like in the stock market. Indeed, it remains complex and somewhat limited. Additionally, it demands specialized neurophysiologists with experience and specific skills [35, 89]. They should have a strong understanding of neuroanatomy, neurosurgical steps, and neuroanesthesia [21]. They should be able to anticipate potentially harmful situations and critically analyze multifactorial data, including test interpretation and technical problems, anesthetic events, and surgeon's maneuver. It should take no longer than 3 to 4 minutes to communicate relevant information that might impact patient's outcome. Alert of meaningless events may lead to unnecessary stress of the whole team. The team should be familiar with IOM tests: the surgeon to critically analyze the alerts and the anaestesiologist to correctly select the anesthetic regime.

IOM protocol is multimodal including corticospinal tract MEP, somatosensory evoked potentials, electroencephalography, and train of four. It is advisable to use a 32-channel equipment. This chapter focuses only on the most specific aspects of IOM in skull base approaches. Trigger electromyography (tEMG) results in a *compound muscle action potential (CMAP)* and aims to map the nerve route. Free-run electromyography (frEMG) analyzes spontaneous activity patterns that correlate to outcome. Corticonuclear motor evoked potential (CoMEP) evokes a *compound motor unit action potential (CMUAP)*, which is the result of adequate nucleus activation. The difference between a CMUAP and CMAP is that the first results from the second motor neuron cell body activation, its axon, and its innervated muscle fibers (a motor unit), while CMAP is a product of direct axon stimulation. The abovementioned tests should be performed and interspersed as frequently as possible.

Although we mostly describe FN in this chapter, the concepts apply to IX to XII CNs. There is some uncertainty regarding III, IV, and VI monitoring [31]. Hence, they are more reliably mapped than monitored.

Proper Needling

Correct needling is paramount regarding CN IOM and cannot be overlooked. It includes needle selection and insertion, which directly impacts the techniques in use. A more comprehensive description and an atlas can be accessed at Chap. 3.

The needling of muscle motor unit (MU) point improves greatly CMAP and CMUAP amplitudes, A-train identification, and CN mapping, because it is the point with the largest possible number of active fibers [40]. Indeed, the proximity of the needle tip to the active locus increases the recorded amplitude [38, 40]. Kimura [37], stated that the spatial relationship between the needle and individual muscle fibers and the size of the recording surface play important role in determining the waveform. Arbitrary placement of needles in the recording muscles does not favor robust responses [22]. Special training and care must be taken for needling muscles innervated by CN III, IV, and VI.

The type of needles improves recordings [37, 89]. Bare needles have the advantage of covering a larger number of MUs within the volume-conducting muscle. Insulated needles and hook wires (HW) are preconized to enhance more specific recordings, which may be useful for multiple layers of muscles, like masseter and cricothyroid (CTHY) muscles [10, 14, 15]. HW is Teflon isolated, except for its 2 mm tip that curves to form the hook for anchoring.

Bipolar recordings enhance specificity and attenuate unrelated far-field EMG activity [35]. Recommended distance between needles ranges from 5 to 10 mm for cranial muscles. Needle electrode impedance should be less than 5 Kohms, whereas inter-electrode impedance should be less than 1 Kohm.

Figure 19.1 shows proper needling of CN muscles. Figure 19.2 shows the differences in recordings at the *mentalis* performed in one patient, comparing insulated and bare needles.

Surface electrodes have the largest recording area. Yet, they are more susceptible to artifacts and displacement and less specific regarding recording. Hence, they are not recommended during CPA surgeries [2, 35, 73].

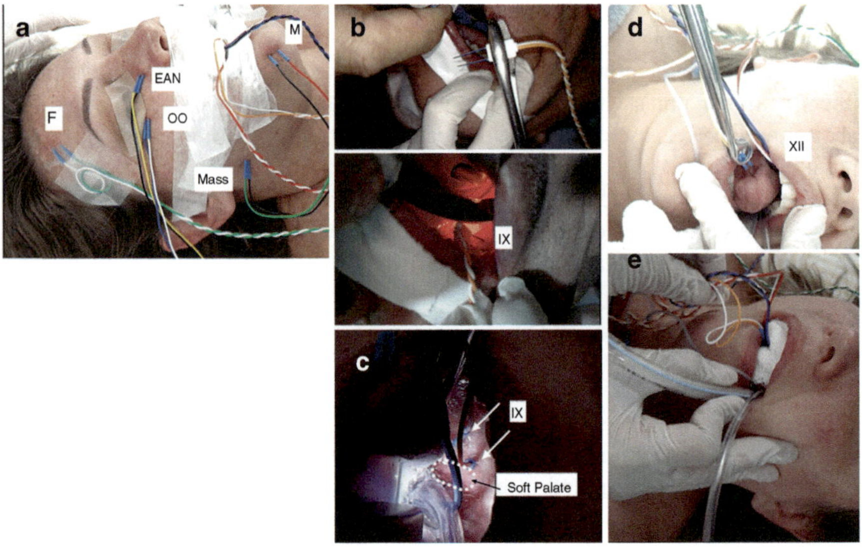

Fig. 19.1 Needling of cranial muscles: (**a**) Trigeminus, mass (masseter), and FN, F (frontalis), OO (oculi), EAN (nasalis), M (mentalis). (**b**) IX: using insulated needles, laterally to soft palate. (**c**) IX: using bare needles, laterally to soft palate. (**d**) Right genioglossus. (**e**) Correct care with cables aiming not to displace needles and organizing them all together at the right side while orotracheal tube is at the left. Gauze is placed inside the mouth and between teeth to avoid bite injury. During all these steps (placement and fixation of cables), electrode impedance is frequently tested

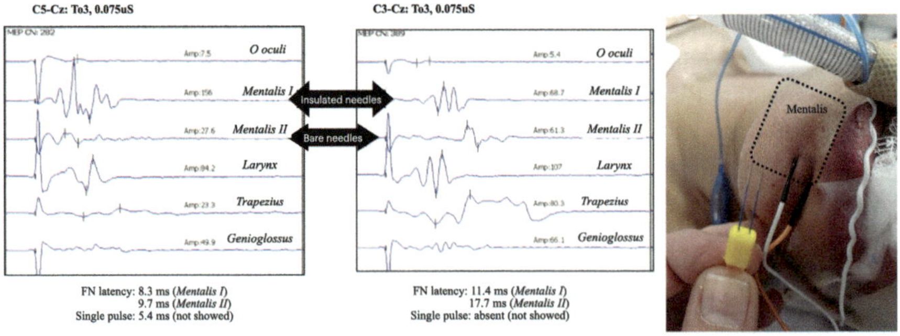

Fig. 19.2 Difference in recordings between insulated needles (mentalis I) and bare needles (mentalis II). Zoomed images for better visualization. Patient was tested for C5-Cz and C3-Cz; a greater and more polyphasic potential was obtained with insulated needles. By C5-Cz, a CMAP was elicited and by C3-Cz a CMUAP

For *vagus* nerve, some questions demand proper attention. Usually, recordings are done using endotracheal tube electrodes (ETE) or HW in the vocal cords, which are innervated by recurrent laryngeal nerve. Bigelow et al. [9], compared both and demonstrated that HW recordings had higher amplitudes, enhancing supra-threshold response registration. Therefore, in cases of previous nerve injury, HW could be an advantage. Additionally, it enables laryngeal adductor reflex (LAR) recordings. HWs reduce vocal cord hematoma risk and improve overall recording selectivity [10, 14].

On the other hand, endotracheal tube must have proper width and should be kept centered for good electrode contact with the vocal cords throughout the surgery. If the contact is lost, invalid recording will ensue [81]. Displacement could occur during setting head position to the Mayfield head holder, for example. Proper bilateral ETE contact with vocal cords can be checked by observing spontaneous waveforms of 30 to 70uV present with respiratory variation and comparison between baselines before and after head positioning [31].

Because we had an event of vocal cord hematoma using bare needles in 2009, we started to needle the lateral larynx wall. The procedure is quite simple: under laryngoscope, using a Magill instrument, we insert two bare needles 2 cm above the vocal cord. Laryngeal muscles are innervated by superior laryngeal nerve [53, 88]. This methodology is not compatible with LAR though.

CTHY recordings could replace vocal cord needling. Of note, it is innervated by superior laryngeal nerve. Yet, CTHY needle placement requires a strict methodology [10, 15] (Fig. 19.3).

Children needling is specially a challenge due to their size and needle characteristics. Adaptations are sometimes necessary, like in the case described in Fig. 19.4.

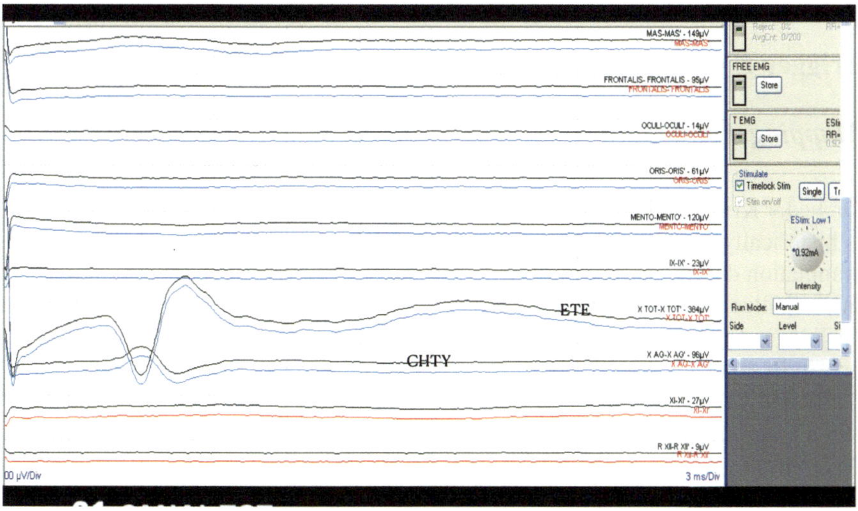

Fig. 19.3 Comparison between ETE and CHTY recordings during tEMG. Both were equally efficient during monopolar stimulation (pulse 0.1 ms, current 0.92 mA). There is no spread of the current or confounding factor from other neck muscles

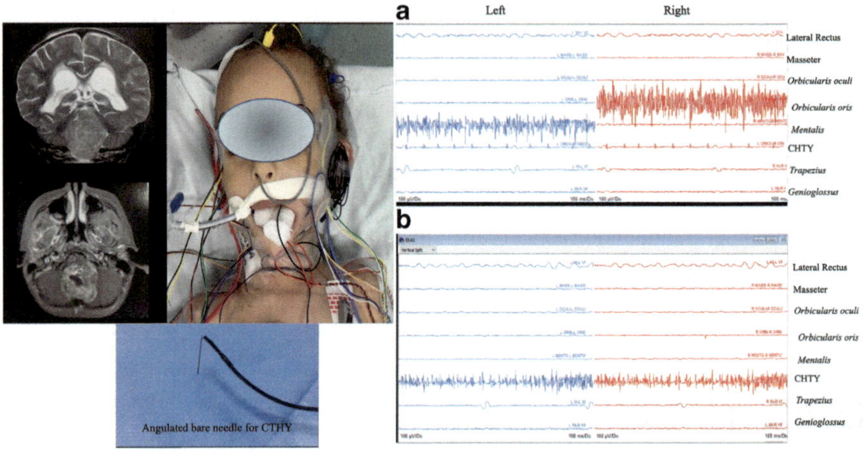

Fig. 19.4 Optimized needle placement due to child's size. Child, 10 months old, tumor located on the floor of the rhomboid fossa: dysphagia. (**a**) A-train in bilateral FN muscles during facial colliculus manipulation using a pair of bare needles per muscle: there is no confounding interference from neighbor muscles. (**b**) A-train in CTHY muscles during manipulation of trigone of the vagus: due to usage of one bare needle per side, responses were recorded bilaterally, not compromising anatomical identification

This child's CHTY was too small for a pair of needles, so we used one needle per side. It did not compromise results since manipulation of the trigone of *vagus* could be easily identified.

Trigger EMG: CN Mapping

Mapping Application

Dr. Fedor Krause (1857–1937), considered the father of German Neurosurgery [12], is historically appointed as the first neurosurgeon to perform intracranial electrical stimulation during surgery [36]. After 110 years, preserving FN remains one of the main challenges in CPA surgeries [33, 39].

Trigger EMG aims to identify, map, and functionally evaluate motor CNs in proximity to or involved in the surgical site of injury [89]. Yet, it is done intermittently and depends on the surgeon's participation [3, 17, 67, 87]. Fundamental is stimulating rostrally to the potential lesional site, to check on functional integrity. Anatomical integrity does not mean functional integrity [55].

Based on tEMG results, the surgeon can change surgical strategy. Mapping should be linked to the main surgical steps to avoid thermal injury and excessive

In monopolar stimulation, the current propagation increases the method's sensitivity during mapping around the tumor in regions free of motor nerve fibers, but this radial current dispersion decreases the mapping specificity when compared to the bipolar technique [32]. The spatial resolution of the monopolar probe is less than 1 mm if the stimulus intensity is kept at an appropriate level and close to the THR [90].

It is possible, and technically feasible, to individualize responses with monopolar stimulation. However, in large lesions, this can be very challenging. Despite the high spread, it has the advantage of reduced shunting and demands less attention concerning positioning. Monopolar probes are the most widely used and commercialized for CN mapping.

Voltage or Current

In the constant voltage system, the final charge changes depending on the resistance of the tissue or the presence of fluid. In the constant current stimulation, the final charge overcome tissue resistance to ensure that a constant current is delivered [77].

The constant current stimulators are mostly used since they provide a consistent response and keep the current charge stable. During the resection of acoustic tumors, current shunting toward blood and cerebral spinal fluid may occur due to their low impedance.

Therefore, the use of isolated "flush tip" probes minimizes shunting and is the most suitable [7]. The level of current shunting may change rapidly, and these unexpected increases in current might be potentially harmful to the nerve. Moller and Jannetta [50], suggested the use of constant voltage probes to avoid these abrupt current oscillations.

Analyzing Threshold and Amplitude

Topsakal et al. [81], defined THR as the intensity of electrical current applied to the nerve, resulting in a CMAP. The main variables that modify the stimulation THR during mapping are:

1. *Stimulator setup – since the intensity required to achieve the THR is inversely proportional to the pulse duration* (Table 19.1). *With 0.2 ms of pulse duration, THR responses are obtained starting at 0.05–0.5 mA of current* [67]. *With a pulse of 0.05–0.1 ms, a higher current of around 1–5 mA is required to elicit a response* [24, 81].
2. *Fiber diameter and preoperative status of the nerve – thinner fibers, previously injured nerves or nerves under regeneration, have higher THRs* [42].
3. *Distance – the greater the distance and the presence or absence of in-between tissue, the higher the stimulation THR, due to higher current demand.*

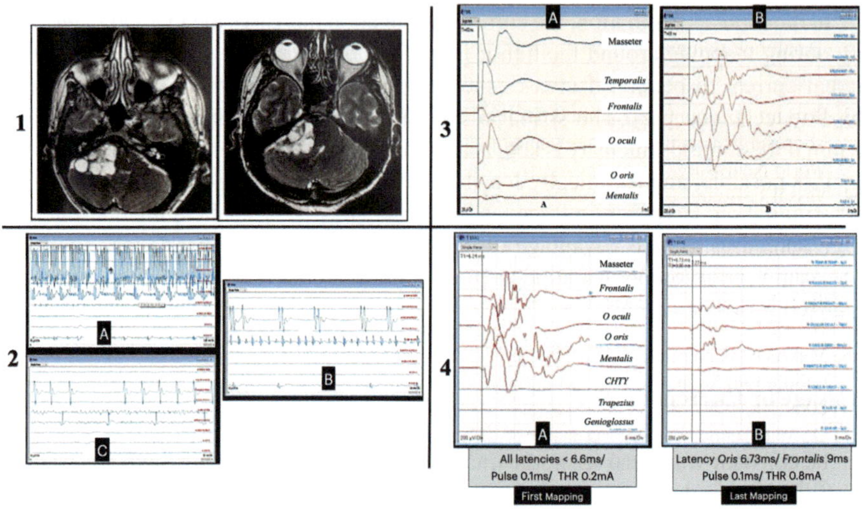

Fig. 19.8 (**1**) Male, 62 years old, right-sided vestibular cystic neurinoma measuring 4.7 × 3.0 cm, House Brackman (HB) 1 preoperatively. The solid-cystic characteristic of the lesion predisposes to an increased inflammatory reaction, attachment of the FN to the tumoral capsule, and hard dissection. In such a case it is recommended to include all branches of the FN aiming to improve tests´ sensitivity. (**2**) Bipolar bare-needle register: different discharge's patterns recorded in frontalis, oculi, oris, mentalis: (**2A**) high frequency and high amplitude discharge, (**2B**) duplet, (**2C**) burst. (**3A**) Conducted volume response recorded in the FN channels with stimulation of the trigeminal nerve, identified by the latency of 4.5 ms (**3B**) Decresing the stimulus to THR intensity allowed a more selective FN activation, with latencies of 6.6 ms. Of note, the morphology of the conducted volume responses is quite different from the true FN CMAPs. **(4A) First Mapping:** a baseline was set as soon as the FN was seen. We set **(4B) Last Mapping:** a four-times increase in THR and CMAP amplitude drop >80% was observed during the surgery. They correlated with a postoperative HB 5, although FN was anatomically intact. CoMEP was tried with C5-Cz, C3+1-Cz and C3-Cz and resulted in extra cranial activation of the FN in all trails

Shunting should be ruled out (Fig. 19.8/3A), before a marked increase in the THR, or CMAP amplitude drop be interpreted as a change in the functional status of the nerve (Fig. 19.8/4B). It is even more important after A-train events [16, 23, 41].

Unusual Responses to Stimulation

Absence of Response to Stimulation

Positive confirmation of stimulation is an important step in any tEMG [41]. False-negative results can lead to disastrous outcomes and must be eliminated. Although the absence of a stimulus artifact indicates an open circuit, its presence is no guarantee of a functioning circuit. Stimulus artifact may be present only if one of the poles is connected [119] (Table 19.2).

Table 19.2 Unexpected absence of a response to stimulation: No Response

Causes		Actions
Nerve damage	Visible injury	Consider repair
	Conduction block	Compare distal and proximal responses
Signal acquisition problems	Nerve more remote than expected	Continue mapping
		Continue surgical exposure
		Increase stimulation current
	Nerve insulated by intervening tissue	Increase stimulation current
	Current shunting	Dry field
		Avoid contact between stimulator and surgical instruments
Technical issues – overall		Obtain control CMAP from adjacent nerve to confirm BOTH stimulation and recording
Technical issues – recording	Drop-out of expected activity	Confirm continued presence of free-run EMG
		Confirm presence of stimulation artifact
		Confirm presence of electrical noise from surgical actions
		Confirm correct volume of audio output
	Configuration of settings	Check electrode inputs
		Check artifact rejection settings
		Check stimulus exclusion settings
		Check filter settings
		Check amplifier gain
	Electrode issue	Check impedances
		Mitigate/eliminate sources of electrical noise
Technical issues – stimulation	Current flow absent	Confirm connection and programming correct
		Replace system components
	Current flow present	consider replacing stimulation system components
Anesthetic issues	Neuromuscular blockade	Reverse neuromuscular blockade
	Local anesthetic on nerve	Appropriate care during administration

Reprinted with permission from *Laryngoscope, 131: S1–S42, 2021- Table V page S33*. Best Practices in Facial Nerve Monitoring. Jack M. Kartush, Kent S. Rice, Robert E. Minahan, Gene K. Balzer, Charles D. Yingling, Christoph N. Seubert
CMAP compound motor action potential

Besides failure by stimulation, absence of response may be due to (1) severe nerve injury preventing depolarization; (2) complete nerve transection; and (3) current shunting through the blood or cerebral spinal fluid, so the stimulating probes must be isolated from any significant volume of fluid [8, 32].

A more detailed and comprehensive description of the variability in the response pattern during the mapping is beyond the scope of this chapter, but we suggest you consult Table 19.3 (with permission from [35]).

Table 19.3 Unexpected responses to stimulation: Atypical Response

Observation	Causes	Actions
Typical response in unexpected location	Atypical location of facial nerve	True positive
	Nerve splayed over tumor	Map surface of tumor
	Abnormal stimulation spread	Dry surgical field
		Reduce stimulation intensity
		Consider bipolar stimulator
Response with atypical latency	Volume conduction	Trigeminal stimulation (latency <5 msec)
	Nervus intermedius response	Latency ~11 msec
Atypical/ inconsistent responses	Misidentification of background free-run EMG activity	CMAPs will repeat with similar latency, activity noted on free-run EMG
	Misidentification of external artifact	CMAPs will repeat with similar latency with each stimulation
	Misidentification of stimulation artifact	Improve recording technique such that stimulation artifact does not contaminate signals with targeted latency

Reprinted with permission from *Laryngoscope, 131: S1–S42, 2021- Table V page S33*. Best Practices in Facial Nerve Monitoring. Jack M. Kartush, Kent S. Rice, Robert E. Minahan, Gene K. Balzer, Charles D. Yingling, Christoph N. Seubert
CMAP compound motor action potentials

If there are doubts about the absence of responses, mapping with higher intensities and consequently a higher current spread (0.5 to 1.0 mA – 0.1 ms pulse duration) should be performed. If no response is detected, the dissection can safely proceed. If CMAPs are recorded, the stimulation intensity should be reduced (0.1 to 0.2 mA – 0.1 ms pulse duration) to reduce the current spread, further allowing more selective responses.

Atypical Responses to Stimulation

An illustrative example is the conducted volume response that can occur between FN and V nerves. Individual stimulation of the V nerve motor fibers produces CMAPs recorded in the masseter and temporalis muscles (Fig. 19.8 3A & 3B). In large tumors, FN can be rostrally displaced, in closer proximity to the V nerve. Hence, the V nerve stimulation may produce a conducted volume response on the face that will also be recorded in the FN channels. In such circumstances, the differentiation is based on their latencies: V nerve latency is around 3–4 ms, while FN latency is of 6–8 ms [6, 47, 48].

Confounding intermedius nerve (IN) response will be discussed in the topic free-run EMG below.

Table 19.3 shows other causes of atypical responses (with permission from [35]).

Continuous Facial Mapping: Ongoing Methodology

Seidel et al. [76], proposed the use of a suction-stimulation probe to continuously map the CN during large vestibular schwannomas (Koos grade III or IV), medial sphenoid wing meningioma, sphenoorbital meningioma, clival chordoma, and surgery of foramen magnum meningioma. It aims to improve CN III to XII distorted course identification. They had already described this monopolar cathode-type stimulator for subcortical motor mapping [63]. It reliably identifies the vicinity of CN depending on stimulus intensity. With the suction device stimulus intensity set at 2 mA, with a 0.3 ms pulse duration, the resulting warning distance is 0.5–1 cm. At 1 mA, neural tissue distance ranges from 0.3 to 0.6 cm [75]. As soon, as the FN is seen at the root entry zone, its THR is determined using a bipolar concentric probe. At normal FN, it usually ranges from 0.05 to 0.1 mA. Suction monopolar intensity is stepwise diminished until 0.25 mA is achieved. This methodology aims to improve gross total resection while diminishing CN impairment. It also has the advantage of avoiding the constant switching of surgical instruments by the surgeon. A disadvantage would be the size in the narrow access route. For Cornelius et al. [11], such a continuous mapping technique identifies early deviated or covered nerves at the surgical site. It is undoubtedly a promising method.

Free-Run Electromyography

Free EMG Patterns

In the 1980s, frEMG with sound feedback was incorporated to FN monitoring [50, 51, 79]. For a detailed historical review about its evolution, we suggest reading Benscoter & Kartush [7]. The rate of anatomical and functional preservation of the FN has significantly improved by providing continuous monitoring, compensating intermittent tEMG [19, 27, 60, 67, 89].

frEMG can identify disturbances in neural structures through the spontaneous firing of MUs. Based on Prass et al. [58], five nomenclature patterns were described: spikes, bursts, and trains A, B, and C (Fig. 19.9). Spikes reflect the

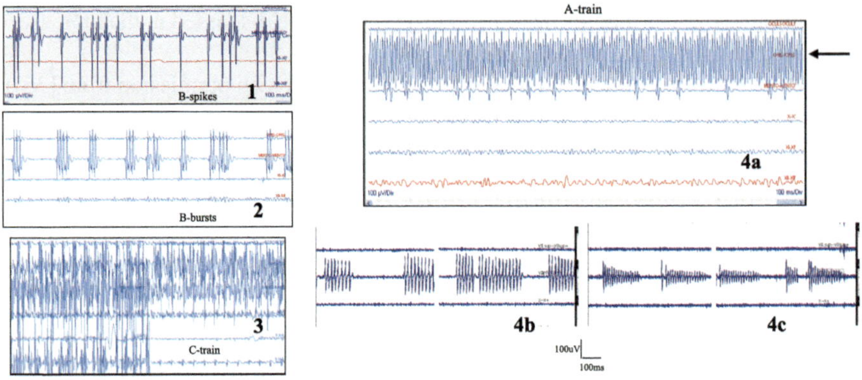

Fig. 19.9 Different patterns of frEMG spontaneous activity. (1) B-spikes: a single MUP depolarization. Differences in amplitude may represent the distance from the firing unit to the recording needle. (2) B-bursts: superimposed MUP activation, building a polyphasic potential (burst). Bursts present different morphologies and firing rates. (3) C-train: great irregular MUP activity with saline irrigation. (4a) A-train: sinusoidal waveform pattern >60 Hz. (4b and 4c) A-train: myokymic pattern

firing of one axon, eliciting a single MU potential, whereas bursts originate from multiple MU activation [35]. Romstöck et al. [67], called them B-spikes and B-bursts. Kimura [37], pointed that "one fiber in the repetitive complex serve as a pacemaker, initiating the burst and driving other fibers ephaptically. Eventually, surrounding muscle fibers re-excite the pacemaker in repetitive cycles, until it blocks." The resulting activity is called "train." If it exceeds 30 Hz, it is called "neurotonic train" [35].

A-train is characterized by a monomorphic sinusoidal wave pattern, with high frequency (60–210 Hz); amplitudes of 100 to 200uV, never exceeding 500uV; and duration of milliseconds to several seconds [60, 67]. It could present a myokymic pattern with small repetitive groups of high-frequency discharges [35]. A-train appears only after dura opening and is always associated with FN manipulation [61, 67]. Yingling & Ashram [89], proposed that A-trains could follow mechanical trauma, irrigation, electrocautery, and traction. Prell et al. [60], stated that A-train may occur exclusively during a moderate gradual trauma.

Trains B and C have amplitude from 20 to 500uV. B-trains are regular or irregular sequences of spikes or bursts. It is advisable, depending on the surgical context, to consider long lasting B-bursts as neurotonic discharges and warning of imminent risk. It should be communicated to the surgeon in order to promote corrective maneuvers.

C-train is characterized by continuous irregular EMG responses [89]. Romstöck et al. [67], found B- and C-trains most frequently in the pharyngeal muscles.

A-Train Intraoperative Interpretation

Prell et al. [60], studied the correlation between A-train duration and FN outcome. Independent of previous FN impairment, the presence and duration of A-train greater than 10 seconds were related to two HB degrees of deterioration in the early postoperative period. Yet, they reported a total of 23% false-negative and two false-positive cases, with A-train lasting up to 209.48 seconds and no clinical worsening. The intriguing false-positive cases arouse the hypothesis of limited acquisition fields and unknown distribution of electrical activity in the facial muscles.

Rampp et al. [64], studied the optimization in the number of electrodes and channels for detecting A-train in an attempt to minimize false-negative cases. Results suggested that more electrodes resulted in earlier detection of A-train. They defined "hot spot channels," that is, a single channel corresponding to more than one third of all total A-train activity. They proposed that MUs can exhibit different degrees of involvement and multichannel capture could increase the sensitivity of frEMG. Accordingly, Ashram showed that more channels enhance the identification of EMG events [6].

Rampp et al. [65], analyzed A-train duration in a cohort of patients with previous radiosurgery, fractionated radiotherapy, or vestibular surgery. A-train duration were longer and without clear correlation with outcome. Therefore, they suggested caution to interpret A-train in this population. The explanation could be that previous treatments impaired microvascular supply and Na+/K+ ATPase activity. Higher extracellular K+ concentrations led to Schwann cell membrane hyperexcitability, resulting in longer A-trains.

Controversies About A-Train

How Many 10s A-Train Events Are Necessary as a Positive Predictive Value (PPV)?

The parameter of 10-second A-train duration as indicative of poor outcome raises some questions: (1) Is only one event or several repeated events necessary for poor outcome? (2) Would only one 10-second A-train be enough to compromise the FN in a surgery lasting many hours? (3) How many 10-second A-trains would be necessary to abort surgery? It does not seem reasonable to base such an important decision-making on just one parameter.

These questions were partially answered by Prell et al. [61]. They addressed the question of false-positive cases, comparing an automatized system with visual analysis of A-train time. The results showed that the greater the number of A-train events, the greater the chance of developing postoperative clinical worsening, in both automatic and visual analysis. They concluded that in cases of impressive amounts of A-trains, far beyond an isolated 10-second event, a poor outcome may be expected. Unfortunately, the need of a specific software and after-surgery analysis are major limitations for its application [25].

Yet, false positivity may occur even in cases with a substantial amount of A-train activity [60, 64]. Therefore, reported train-time PPV was no higher than 64%, matching PPV for CoMEP, in the range of 53–61% and for tEMG at 46% [61, 62]. Frigeni et al. [19], reported PPV for A-trains ranging from 40 to 60%, respectively, for postoperative HB 1–2 and HB 3–5.

Verst [84], in a multimodal prospective cohort showed that A-train as a single parameter during IOM resulted in a PPV of merely 25%, sensitivity of 7%, and specificity of 67% [84, 86].

Aiming to better explain this issue, Prell et al. [61, 62], proposed that long-lasting FN compression could lead to different behaviors among patients. FN could be more prone to elicit A-trains in some cases than in others. This phenomenon could come from alteration in neural metabolism with consequences in neural conduction.

Romstöck et al. [86], found no correlation between A-trains' amplitude and outcome. Lastly, Rampp et al. [66], proposed that A-train time and A-train clusters are more prone to occur in larger tumors and with a separate intermedius nerve (IN), being related to false-positive analysis.

A-Train: A Localized or a Spread Muscle Event?

As A-train is related to nerve injury, it is worth remembering the nerve structure. A nerve is divided into fascicles, which contain bundles, that are constituted by different amounts of axons. The FN is often dissected by the tumor and subdivided into several fascicles, which are interspersed or stick to the tumor and/or to the capsule. Therefore, A-train may reflect the involvement of different amounts of axons.

Prell et al. [60], stated that "It seems possible that a pattern as subtle as the A-train might have a rather small radius of geometrical spread within the facial muscle tissue". Therefore A-train would partially activate nerve bundles. Romstöck et al. [64], proposed a limited spatial extent of A-trains even within a single muscle.

We believe that injury to a fascicle or bundle could depolarize a varying number of axons and consequently MUs. In general, it should be expected that the amplitude of recorded activity relates to the number of muscle fibers that are activated together [40]. Long-lasting FN compression could result in different degrees of fascicles and axon deterioration. This damage could lead to less or more reactivity to intraoperative trauma. Therefore, A-train could represent a greater or a smaller number of muscle fiber activation, directly impacting its behavior [89]. If a great number of MUs are activated, a widespread phenomenon would lead to a great number of muscle fiber firing [35] and A-train of larger amplitudes (500uV). Usually, it hinders CMAP and CMUAP analysis from the same muscles by "polluting" the recording line (Fig. 19.5). We consider that this rampant activity translates an event of higher risk. Conversely, small amplitude and short duration A-train could be associated with a limited amount of MU recruitment, hence a lower predictive value in a previous healthy FN. In such a context, it should be used as an alert for the neurophysiologist to perform CoMEP more frequently. Yet, small amplitude A-train in a context of previous damaged FN could translate activity of the few remaining axons.

Limitations of the Reports

Most of the abovementioned concepts originate from a sole German medical group and need to be validated by other groups [70]. Other authors showed no linear correlation between A-trains and FN outcome [2, 25, 84].

Of important concern, the German group identified a frEMG pattern of risk: A-train. Yet, they analyzed frEMG as a single parameter. Moreover, they reported a rate of 23% of false negatives [60], which was partially improved by the addition of more recording channels [64].

Finally, their samples comprised 30 and 40 patients, respectively, in 2000 and 2007, when they described the correlation of A-train duration with outcome. The small cohort may have played a decisive role in the conclusion. Of note, from 2012 to 2015 and in 2019, the retrospectively analyzed population had little variation, with addition of patients to the same sample.

A-Train: Pitfalls to Interpretation

frEMG activity predictive value remains controversial nowadays [3, 10, 17, 20, 25, 46, 84, 89]. Paradoxically, mild or no frEMG activity can be observed after complete section of a nerve [17, 27, 59]. Mild frEMG or no activity may follow FN section (Fig. 19.10). Yet, the distal stump can still be activated and generate A-trains, giving false impression of nerve continuity [27].

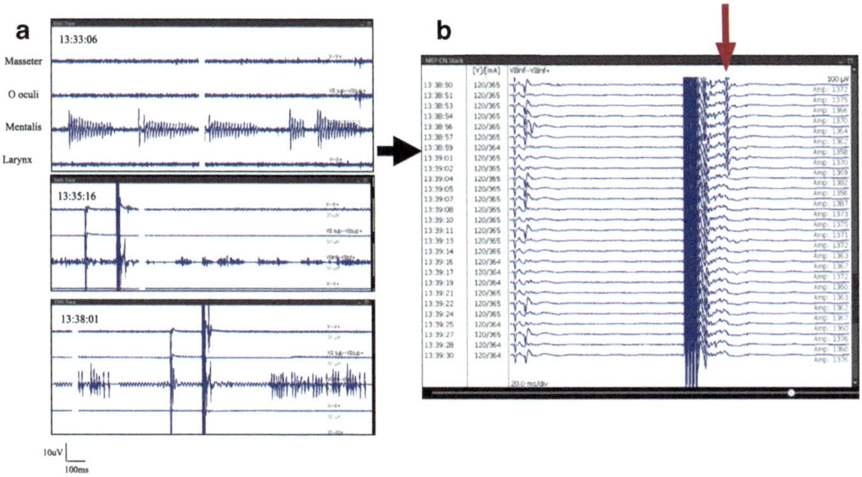

Fig. 19.10 Rare event registration of FN section (same patient of Fig. 19.14). Man, 45 years old. Left CPA schwannoma. FN HB 1 + Deafness. CoMEP: C6-Cz and C4-Cz double-train technique showed peripheral FN response and was not performed during the approach. In such a situation, cranial nerve IOM relies on tEMG and frEMG. (**a**) frEMG was silent for FN except for three brief bursts of A-train starting at 13:33:06. This moment coincided with capsule manipulation and the surgeon's announcement that he had sectioned FN. (**b**) We rechecked CoMEP and the response that was earlier present by multipulse stimulation had also disappeared. Immediate postoperative HB 6. Patient was later submitted to a massetero-facial anastomosis

Karakis & Simon [31] stated that we should expect different behaviors of the FN depending on its previous condition: a) previous healthy FN may endure longer A-train events and may present lower risk to intraoperative damage; b) previous injured FN would present more frequent and abrupt A-train events and less tolerance to stress. Conversely, Yingling [89] had stated that injured axons are less responsive and less capable of generating frEMG activity despite significant manipulation. The controversy exists among other authors: a) absence of A-train may indicate either inability of the FN to react to surgical or electrical stimuli or no trauma at all [27, 59], b) A-trains can be elicited simply by irrigating with cold saline and by many non-injurious maneuvers [17, 35, 70]. Kartush et al. [35], stated that frEMG activity unrelated to ongoing surgical actions is often less concerning.

Yet, frEMG activity plays an indispensable role in CPA approaches as part of a multimodal protocol [1, 20, 46, 84]. If technical limitations prevent CoMEP (as will be discussed below), frEMG gains relevance in intraoperative risk analysis and the surgeon's strategy.

There is still not enough data on the clinical correlation between frEMG activity and prognosis for CN III, IV, VI, and lower CN [31, 70, 81]. However, it seems that A-trains at VI CN correlate to damage [31].

What Is the Role of Intermedius Nerve in FN Monitoring?

IN is usually known as a sensitive and autonomic nerve, responsible for taste, lacrimation, and sensibility of external auditory meatus [5, 29, 53, 71, 88]. Ashram et al. [5], demonstrated the presence of a recordable potential of longer latency (11 ms) and smaller amplitude on perioral muscles after IN stimulation. They argued that the underlying mechanism could not originate in ephaptic cross-transmission with FN, because of the delayed IN response. Ephactic transmission is expected to be extremely rapid. They supposed it could come from (1) antidromic conduction through sensory fibers or (2) orthodromic potentials traveling in the preganglionic parasympathetic fibers.

Prell et al. [62], stated that the potential recorded after IN stimulation was a motor potential. Their previous report by Alfieri et al. [4], had studied IN under electron microscopy and found that 86.45% of its fibers were myelinated. Of those, 0.5% presented a diameter > 12 μ compatible with motor fibers. These fibers would innervate the *levator anguli oris* muscle.

Interestingly, previous report by Youssef & Downes [91], had found IN to have the amount of 3000 myelinated fibers with a diameter of 9 μ [5, 91]. Additionally, Youssef & Downes [91], confirmed previous publications from other authors and reported FN to have 10,000 to 11,000 myelinated fibers much thicker than IN. Moreover, they reported differences in amounts of myelinated fibers depending on the FN segment. In tympanic segment, they found 1,800 more fibers than in cisternal segment. Rhoton et al. [68], had described that the IN can be composed of two or more filaments, more easily identified when they joined the FN motor fibers.

Yet, Prell et al. [62], attributed to around 150 IN motor fibers (0.5% of 3,000) the origin of confounding A-trains in perioral muscles. Although these A-trains had little clinical relevance, they stated these A-trains represented a confounding factor, interfering with correct frEMG interpretation [62]. The proposal that needles placed in the orbicularis oris or mentalis would register A-trains in the neighboring levator anguli oris requires further evidence. It should be taken into consideration Youssef & Downes and Rhoton et al. findings to explain how A-trains are more easily evoked while manipulating intra-meatal FN segment, (where the FN lies just by the neighboring IN).

Corticonuclear Motor Evoked Potentials (CoMEP)

Choosing Between Different Assemblies

CoMEP aims to activate the corticonuclear motor pathway rostrally to the site of the lesion and microsurgical manipulation. It enables monitoring of FN and lower CNs (IX to XII) before their visualization and throughout the surgical procedure [1, 3, 17, 20, 84, 85]. Nerves III, IV, and VI are not amenable to transcranial electrical stimulation (TES) [10]. Yet, CoMEP is the most complex among all MEPs [20]. Anatomical peculiarities influence the results. The CN nuclei may have unilateral or bilateral afferents; muscles are small and overlapped or close to muscles receiving different innervation. Additionally, the proximity of the nuclei to the stimulus source leads to big artifacts [20, 26]. CoMEP was described during TIVA anesthesia, using mainly propofol and opioids. Described alert criteria may differ during inhalational regime, so it is strictly not recommended. Akagami et al. [3] and Dong et al. [17] (from the same group), reported successful CoMEP from VII to XII muscles after contralateral TES. The former used electrodes placed at C3/C4 to Cz and the latter used M3/M4 to Cz (anode-cathode). Although it could be possible to produce CN-CMUAP using interhemispheric C1–C2 or C3–C4, it usually resulted in a high rate of technical failure, overwhelming stimulus artifact and patient disturbing movements [1, 3, 17, 84, 85].

Execution of double train (multipulse + single pulse) is paramount and excludes peripheral CN activation [3, 10, 15, 17]. The explanation is that corticonuclear neurons depend on temporal summation of descending volleys to be activated [10, 13]. By double-train technique, the inter-train interval is set at 70–80 ms, and total sweep is usually kept at 100 ms, so that delayed peripheral CN latencies can be identified. Healthy ipsilateral FN peripheral latency is 5 ms [3, 82] and by intracranial proximal stimulation is about 6–7 ms [17, 35, 82]. It differs from the latency of corticonuclear CMUAP, which is above 10 ms. Double train should be carried out throughout the IOM.

Verst et al. [85], proposed C5/C6 to Cz (Table 19.4). Due to greater facial motor cortex proximity, it usually needs half the intensity used with C3/C4-Cz and results in less neck movements [20, 31, 84, 85]. Consequently, C5/C6 to Cz usually allows

Table 19.4 CoMEP: assemblies and results

Authors, year	Montage (anode to cathode)/ success rate	Technique	Recording muscles and latency	Sensitivity/ specificity	CMUAP loss versus FN outcome
Akagami et al. [3][a]	C3/C4 to Cz 88%	To3 to To5 ISI 1–3 ms Pulse duration: 50uV	*O oris* 12 to 16 ms	S 90%/Sp 89%	>50%
Dong et al. [17][a]	M3/M4 to Mz 92.1%	To3 to To4, ISI 2 ms Pulse duration: 50uS or 500 uS	*O oris* 10.9 to 15.1 ms	>50% S 100% >65%: S 91%/Sp 97%	>50%: Mild >65%: Moderate 100%: Severe
Acioly et al. [1][a]	C3/C4 to Cz 85–86.7%	To3 to To5, ISI 2 ms Pulse duration: 50uS	*OO: 10 to 24.5 ms* O oris: 10 to 23.4 ms	[a]S 53.8/Sp 100%	>20% for OO >65% for O oris[a]
Verst et al. [85, 86][a]	C3/C4 to Cz 82.6% C5/C6 to Cz 86.9%	To3 or To4 ISI 2 ms Pulse duration: 500uS 0.5 to 2 Hz	*OO, M* >10 ms	>50%: S 92.8%/Sp 66% >60%: Not informed	>50% mild >65% moderate to severe
Rufina's experience	M3 or M4 + 1 cm lateral to Cz	To3 to To4 ISI 2 ms Pulse duration: 50 to 75uS	*F, OO, N, O oris*	Not informed	>50% mild >65% moderate to severe
Deletis group	C3/C4 to Cz	To3 to To5 ISI 2 to 4 ms Pulse duration: 500uS 2 to 3 Hz	*OO, N, O. oris, M* Vocal cord CHTY	Not informed	>80%: Mild to moderate Loss: Permanent
Karakis and Simon [31]	C3/C4 + 2 cm lateral and inferior to Cz	To3 to To4 ISI 2 ms Pulse duration: 500uS	F, OO, *O oris*, M	Not informed	>50%
Hiruta et al. [26]	C3/C4 to Cz 84.9%	To5 to To8 ISI 1.4–1.6 ms Biphasic pulse 400uS Double train (ITI 50–100 ms)	*O oris* Latency not informed	Recovery value <35% S 91% Sp 95%	Recovery value <35% for good late outcome

All used TIVA. Matthies et al. [46], did not inform
Constant current stimulator: Rufina Barros (personal experience), Deletis group, and Hiruta et al. [26]
[a] Constant voltage stimulator
Supramaximal CMUAP: all, except Rufina
F frontal, *OO* orbicularis oculi, *N* nasalis, *O* oris orbicularis oris, *M* mentalis
S sensibility, *Sp* specificity

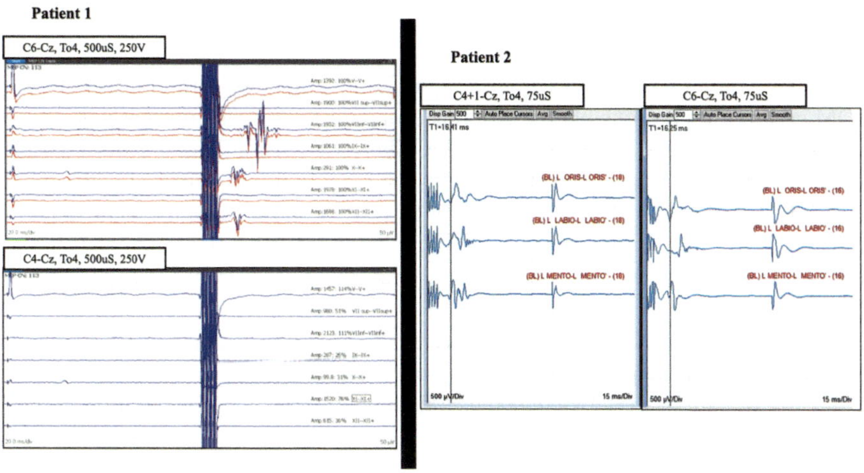

Fig. 19.11 CoMEP of two different patients showing: Patient 1: only C6-Cz technique resulted in CMUAP (Medtronic System, SMV** recordings). Patient 2: C4 + 1*-Cz and C6-Cz resulted in CMUAP. The neurophysiologist chose C4 + 1-Cz because the resulting CMUAP was more polyphasic (Cadwell System, MRB*** recordings). *C4 + 1 = 1 cm lateral to C4. **Silvia Mazzali-Verst. ***Maria Rufina Barros

for continuous stimulation at low train frequencies of 0.5 to 0.8 Hz. Theoretically, less neck movements could have the additional advantage of less muscle confounding factor described by Deletis group by C3/C4-Cz and X-CN recordings [10, 14, 15].

Conversely, Karakis & Simon [31], found more frequent peripheral CN activation by C3/C4-Cz, due to higher stimulus intensity.

CoMEP assembly success ranges from 75% to 92% [1, 3, 17, 25, 26, 76, 85]. Verst et al. [85], compared C3/C4-Cz with C5/C6-Cz in the same patient and concluded that there are patients that have CMUAP with both assemblies, with either one and with neither of them (Figs. 19.2 and 19.11). Therefore, it is an advantage to set up at least two different assemblies. In our practice, if both montages evoke CMUAP(+)/CMAP(−), we choose the one that results in greater supramaximal amplitude and polyphasia and the lowest charge. Conejero [10], pointed out the CoMEP technique difficulties as she stated that (1) by C5/C6-Cz, there is a slightly higher chance of activating extracranial FN and (2) by C3/C4-Cz, there is a greater chance of activation of corticonuclear tract deep in the brainstem or foramen magnum.

Stimulus Parameters

Table 19.4 shows the diversity in techniques and parameters. Differences between IOM systems are responsible for differences in pulse duration, constant voltage, or constant current and fast or slow charge. Shorter pulse duration favors D wave recovery, allowing usage of ISI below 2 ms [49]. Yet, it is compensated with higher intensity, balancing final charge. Hiruta et al. [26], proposed a biphasic pulse duration since it could reduce stimulus artifact. Yet, biphasic pulse interchanges the anode with the cathode, eliciting a response rather different from the expected one [47, 48].

Constant current stimulator overcomes electric resistance changes, like cerebral spinal fluid leak or hypothermia, keeping the charge uniform. Conversely, constant voltage stimulation overlooks impedance fluctuations, resulting in variation of final electric charge [26, 45], directly impacting recorded CMUAP. Fast charge stimulator seems more effective, since it requires 35% less total charge to get the same response [49].

Pulse number and ISI should be adjusted on an individual basis [1, 84, 85]. Dong et al. [17], reported no compromise in efficacy concerning pulse duration differences and usage of constant current or constant voltage stimulator.

Recording Parameters

The number of recording channels impacts CN-IOM [64, 84]. The greater the number of FN branches represented in IOM channels, the greater the chance to map and monitor dissected fascicules and identify risky events [59, 64]. For FN, an optimal record should include one muscle per branch. For lower CNs, muscles are shown in Table 19.5.

Filtering is an important issue regarding CoMEP success. Usual MEP filters range from 30 to 1500 Hz [13]. Low bandpass of 150 to 300 Hz allows a better definition of the onset of FN CMUAP, especially in the *orbicularis oculi and frontalis* [1, 17, 26, 84, 85]. Since there is a direct influence between the filter band and the MEP amplitude, the narrower the band, the smaller the amounts of axons visualized within the potential. This may be an additional factor that impacts the occurrence of false positives in the evaluation of the CoMEP (see below). Additionally, digital filtering may prevent CoMEP acquisition (Fig. 19.12).

Yet, large stimulus artifacts might prevent accurate CMUAP definition. It can be particularly challenging for *orbicularis oculi* recording [2, 20, 26, 46]. Using insulated Mayfield head holder or titan pins [46], shorter ISI [46, 85] or an extra grounding electrode at the frontal area (Rufina Barros personal statement, [47, 48]) might overcome this problem.

Vagus nerve MEPs, [14], can be successfully elicited after hemispheric TES, and recording with a pair of HW at the vocal cord. Latencies range from 9 to

Table 19.5 Cranial nerves at risk at the CPA tumor resection approach: muscle innervation, cortex representation, and remarks

CN	Muscle	Remarks
V	Masseter and temporalis	Bilateral motor cortex
VII	*Temporal branch*: Frontalis*orbicularis oculi* *Zygomatic branch*: Nasalis** *Buccal branch*: Orbicular oris** *Mandibular branch*: Mentalis** *Cervical branch*: Platysma**	*Bilateral motor cortex **Only contralateral motor cortex
IX	Stylopharyngeus muscle (not accessible for needling) Recording from retropharynx or soft palate	Bilateral motor cortex *Jugular foramen* Related to bradycardia and hypotension
X	Constrictor muscles of the pharynx*, palate*, and intrinsic muscles of the larynx CTHY* Larynx lateral wall (above vocal cord) * Vocal cord**	Bilateral motor cortex Vagal trigone: Floor of the IV ventricle *Jugular foramen* Special attention to bradycardia *Superior laryngeal nerve **Recurrent laryngeal nerve
XI	Trapezius (additional cervical motor roots C3–C4) Sternocleidomastoid	Bilateral motor cortex (there is some controversy) *Jugular foramen*
XII	Genioglossus	Bilateral motor cortex

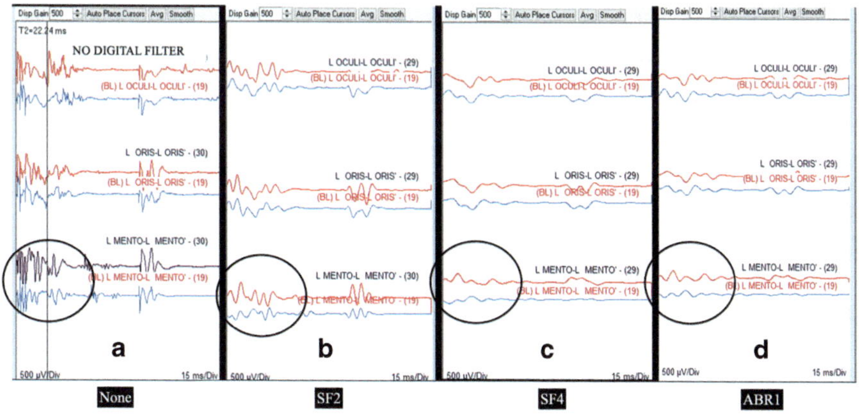

Fig. 19.12 Behavior of CMUAP with different setting of digital filters (**b–d**) using a Cadwell system. The resulting potential (circle) is strongly affected and virtually disappears depending on the digital filtering. We recommend not using digital filters in this system in order to obtain a polyphasic MEP (**a**)

20.9 ms. Deletis et al. [15], proposed CTHY CMUAP, aiming to extend monitoring of the *vagus* nerve to superior laryngeal nerve. The combination of vocal cord and CHTY CMUAP might maximize monitoring results.

We insert needles on lateral laryngeal wall for *vagus* nerve monitoring. Yet, there is no significant rate of false-negative results, meaning there are few, if any, confounding registration from neighbor neck muscles. Our methodology demands a trained neurophysiologist or anesthesiologist, though. For LAR, we use two channels ETE. Deterioration of 50% CMUAP is related to postoperative dysphasia and hoarseness [30].

Ongoing CoMEP Evaluation and Prognostic Scores

Besides an interindividual variability in CMUAP amplitude, a random trial-to-trial amplitude variability is a hallmark of TES MEP [13, 17, 26]. Baseline should reflect it and be chosen after several recordings rather than a single trial. It is set after dura opening [3, 17, 25, 26, 84]. If for any reason there is a delay between dura opening and tumor resection start, a new baseline should be set immediately before microdissection.

During tumor resection, regular CoMEP stimulation optimizes variability measurement. It is recommended to perform as frequently as possible, upon surgeon's request or after A-train registration [17, 25, 84]. Accordingly, significant changes should be reproduced in a couple of trials, and clinical and pharmacological events excluded, before alerting the surgeon. Keep in mind that patients with previous deficits are more prone to greater intraoperative CMUAP fluctuations, because of previous axonal damage or block.

There is a relation between final-to-baseline ratio of CMUAP amplitude drop and severity of immediate postoperative HB (Fig. 19.13) [1, 3, 17, 46, 69, 84, 86]. The amount of acceptable CMUAP deterioration is a matter of debate (Table 19.4). CMUAP disappearance is the major criteria [1, 10, 17].

Dong et al. [17], and others have related 50% loss to mild deficit, 65% loss to moderate to higher risk of deterioration, and 100% loss to HB 3–6 [1, 84, 86]. Conejero [10], relates >80% CMUAP deterioration to mild to moderate FN impairment. The absence of final CMUAP deterioration has shown a negative predictive value of 100% [1, 3, 10, 17, 46, 86].

As preservation of motor function is the main goal, amplitude loss of 30% or more should be alerted to trigger surgeon´s reaction and enable fast recovery ([1, 46], Rufina Barros personal statement).

Analysis of THR parameter for eliciting CMUAP is still controversial. Goto et al. [20], proposed a THR increase above 100 mA with poor FN function (using C3′/C4′ to Cz, To4 or 5, pulse duration 0.2–0.3 ms). Hendriks et al. [25],

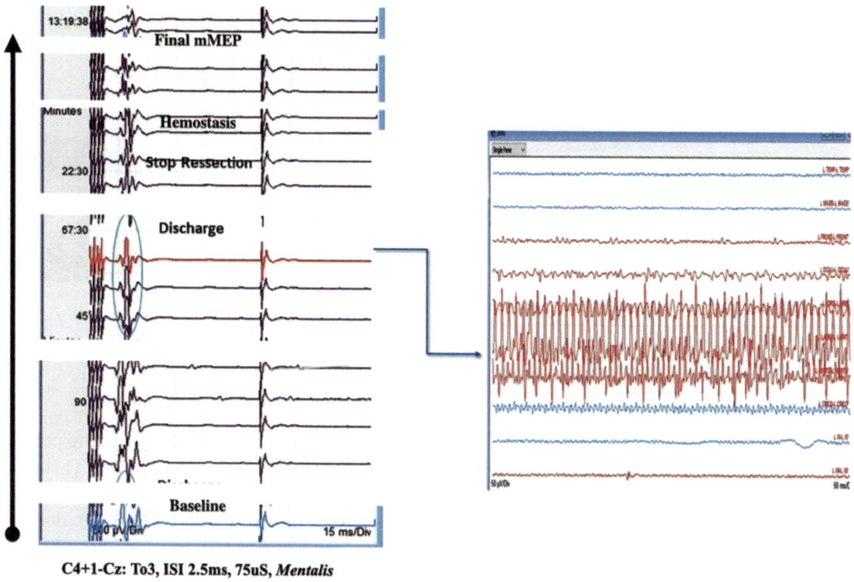

Fig. 19.13 Woman, 56 years old. Left CPA schwannoma. FN HB 1 + Hypoacusia + tinnitus. CoMEP shows deterioration of CMUAP after A-train event, and surgeon ended resection. Final CMUAP with >80% deterioration. Patient's immediate HB was 4

managed to record THR-CMUAP in 90% of their sample and related an increase <20 mA with good prognosis. Verst [84], could not relate THR increase to FN outcome.

"Compound" CMUAP

Matthies et al. [46], showed a case of peripheral CMAP and central CMUAP combining in one sole potential. In our experience, there are situations where CoMEP technique generates what seems to be a combined CMAP and a CMUAP, resulting in a "compound potential." These potentials may be clearly defined and easily recognized, each of them with proper latency (Fig. 19.14). However, this phenomenon might result from sub-threshold peripheral nerve activation by short trains of TES [10, 80, 83]. The resulting polyphasic CMAP is a confounding factor in CoMEP analysis. Indeed, it might be expected that long-lasting compression disturbed the nerve sheath, resulting in increased CMAP and CMUAP latencies (Fig. 19.6). Matthies et al. [46], pointed a direct relation between FN CMUAP latency and tumor extension, due to nerve elongation. Classically, in the presence of CMAP, CoMEP technique has failed. In this situation, IOM relies on frEMG and tEMG.

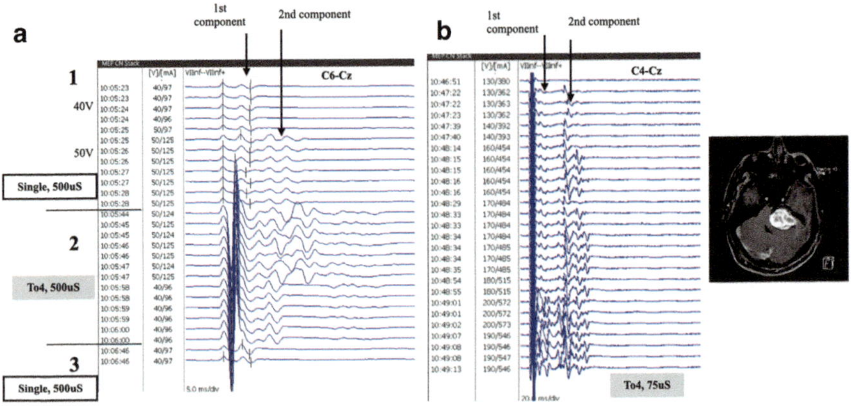

Fig. 19.14 Man, 45 years old. Left CPA schwannoma. FN HB 1 + deafness. Confounding peripheral FN activation related to increase in stimulus intensity and multipulse stimulation. This phenomenon might result from sub-threshold peripheral nerve activation by short trains of TES. (**a**) We applied a single stimulus (A1 and 3) and a short train of electrical stimuli (A2 and B) (double-train technique during CoMEP C6-Cz). (A1) By single stimulus, increase in intensity from 40 V to 50 V, resulted in a second component. (A2) When we switched to To4 at 50 V, this second component looked very similar to a CMUAP. The potential lost phases by To4/40 V. (A3) by single stimulation, it turned to an expected CMAP (**b**) zoom window for the To4 technique with increasing intensities from 130 to 190V. The second component really resembled a CMUAP. Care must be taken to avoid misinterpretation. CoMEP failed to evoke a central potential

CoMEP Limitations

CoMEP is a product of an intra-axial pathway activation and a peripheral nerve component. Each of them may limit somehow its accuracy. As an important remark, corticonuclear motor pathways innervate bilateral CN nuclei [53, 56, 88] (Table 19.5). The reason is that bilateral control is functionally necessary to better coordinate simultaneous movements of the head and neck. The facial motor nucleus is an exception because lower facial muscles are innervated solely by contralateral cortex. Some controversy exists regarding the XI CN nucleus receiving bilateral cortical afferents. Yet, there might be slight predominance from the contralateral hemisphere [56].

Dong et al. [17], pointed that CMUAP correspond to one-fifth of an intracranial FN CMAP. Therefore, CMUAP probably originates from partial neuron activation. During tumor resection, it is possible that axonal damage be not homogeneously distributed, so that CMUAP could miss or overinterpret this injury. This phenomenon is shown in CMUAP amplitude drop versus outcome analysis. Preservation of 50% of CMUAP might correspond to a more pronounced deficit, if a more severe injury has occurred in axons not included in CMUAP. Similarly, the injury could predominate in the axons represented in the CMUAP, undermining its amplitude, but without significant deficit [17]. During CMUAP analysis, special attention should be paid to rule out anesthesia bolus or fading, deep anesthesia level, hypothermia and hypotension, intracranial air, scalp edema, CSF leak, and equipment failure [1, 3, 26]. These conditions would change both CoMEP and extremities-MEP. Additionally, initial CMUAP could already be small due to previous nerve impairment and a reduction in active axons [46].

Decrease in CMUAP amplitude translates events affecting the nerve itself rather than the nuclei. It is conceivable that intraoperative damage to FN axons can be due to a combination of varying degrees of severity and extent of injury to the neural components [26]. Nerve injury severity could present as neurapraxia, axonotmesis, or neurotmesis, as classified by Seddon [74].

The abovementioned features, i.e., partial central motor pathway activation, bilateral nuclei cortical innervation, and extent of peripheral nerve injury phenomenon, directly impact CMUAP deterioration analysis.

Final Statements

In the perfect scenario, changes should be analyzed associating tEMG, frEMG, and CoMEP. The overall variation in these parameters will certainly impact the outcome. In critical situations, when no reliable CoMEP can be recorded, relying on FN-THR and CMAP amplitude index can indicate changes in FN functional status. We present such a case, where four-times increase in THR and 80% CMAP loss were the sole alert landmarks for the bad outcome (Fig. 19.8). The combined analysis of these parameters becomes relevant, especially when it is necessary to decide on early FN reconstruction.

Conclusion

There are many variables acting on IOM for skull base surgeries. They rely on the CN physiological behavior caused by the slowing tumor growth. Conflicting information points to lesser or greater FN reaction to intraoperative stress. Most likely, the FN will react differently among different individuals. Therefore, we should keep in mind a wide range of behavioral possibilities while performing intraoperative evaluation.

Motor CN V, IX, X, XI, and XII might resemble FN in many aspects and should be evaluated with the same methodology. Future studies might indicate singularities for each. III, IV, and VI CN are amenable to mapping by direct stimulation and to monitoring by frEMG. Future cohorts might identify particularities.

Most probably, an association of tests might give us a three-dimensional assessment of the situation. Hence, multimodal monitoring improves safety and recognition of dangerous events. It should always include frEMG, tEMG, and CoMEP. Each of them has its merits and demerits. Superiority of one test over the others is yet to be determined.

References

1. Acioly MA, Liebsch M, Carvalho CH, Gharabaghi A, Tatagiba M. Transcranial electrocortical stimulation to monitor the facial nerve motor function during cerebellopontine angle surgery. Neurosurgery. 2010;66(2):354–62.
2. Acioly MA, Liebsch M, de Aguiar PH, Tatagiba M. Facial nerve monitoring during cerebellopontine angle and skull base tumor surgery: a systematic review from description to current success on function prediction. World Neurosurg. 2013;80(6):271–300.
3. Akagami R, Dong CCJ, Westerberg BD. Localized transcranial electrical motor evoked potentials for monitoring cranial nerves in cranial base surgery. Neurosurgery. 2005;57(1):78–85.
4. Alfieri A, Rampp S, Strauss C, Julius F, Rachinger J, Scheller C, Prell J. The relationship between nervus intermedius anatomy, ultrastructure, electrophysiology, and clinical function. Usefulness in cerebellopontine microsurgery. Acta Neurochir. 2014;156:403–8.
5. Ashram YA, Jackler RK, Pitts LH, Yingling CD. Intraoperative Electrophysiologic identification of the Nervus intermedius. Otol Neurotol. 2005;26:274–9.
6. Ashram YA, Badr-El-Dine MMK. Multichannel facial nerve monitoring: value in detection of mechanically elicited electromyographic activity and prediction of postoperative outcome. Otolol Neurotol. 2014;35:1290–7.
7. Benscoter BJ, Kartush JM. Intraoperative facial nerve monitoring. In book: Facial nerve disorders and diseases: diagnosis and management; Guntinas-Lichius and Schaitkin, Facial Nerve Disorders and Diseases: Diagnosis and Management (ISBN 978-3-13-175181-2), copyright © 2016 Georg Thieme Verlag All rights reserved. 2016. p. 200–12.
8. Bernat I, Grayeli AB, Esquia G, Zhang Z, Kalamarides M, Sterkers O. Intraoperative electromyography and surgical observations as predictive factors of facial nerve outcome in vestibular schwannoma surgery. Otol Neurotol. 2010;31:306–12.
9. Bigelow DC, Patterson T, Weber R, Stecker MM, Judy K. Comparison of endotrachial tube and hookwire electrodes for monitoring the vagus nerve. J Clin Monit. 2002;17:217–20.
10. Conejero IF. Chapter 10: corticobulbar motor evoked potentials in skull base surgery. In: Deletis V, Shils J, Sala F, Seidel K, editors. Neurophysiology in neurosurgery. A modern approach. 2nd ed. London, UK: Academic Press; 2020.
11. Cornelius JF, Schipper J, Tortora A, Krause-Molle Z, Smuga M, Petridis AK, Steiger HJ. Continuous and dynamic facial nerve mapping during surgery of cerebello-pontine angle tumors: clinical pilot series. World Neurosurg. 2018;119:855–63.
12. Costea CF, Turliuc DM, Sava A, Dumitrescu GG, Cucu AI, Patraşcanu E, Trandafir D, Turliuc S, Krause F. (1857–1937): the father of German neurosurgery. Romanian Neurosurg. 2016;XXX 2:241–7.
13. Deletis V, Shils JL. Neurophysiology in neurosurgery. A modern intraoperative approach. 1st ed. California: Elsevier; 2002.
14. Deletis D, Conejero IF, Ulkatan S, Costantino P. Methodology for intraoperatively eliciting motor evoked potentials in the vocal muscles by electrical stimulation of the corticobulbar tract. Clin Neurophysiol. 2009;120(2):336–41.
15. Deletis V, Conejero IF, Ulkatan S, Rogic M, Carb EL, Hiltzik D. Methodology for intraoperative recording of the corticobulbar motor evoked potentials from cricothyroid muscles. Clin Neurophysiol. 2011;122(9):1883–9.
16. Delgado TE, Buchheit WA, Rosenholtz HR, Chrissian S. Intraoperative monitoring of facial muscle evoked responses obtained by intracranial stimulation of the facial nerve. Neurosurgery. 1979;4(5):418–21.
17. Dong CCJ, MacDonald DB, Akagami R, Westerberg B, AlKhani A, Kanaan I, Hassounah M. Intraoperative facial motor evoked potential monitoring with transcranial electrical stimulation during skull base surgery. Clin Neurophysiol. 2005;116(3):588–96.
18. DeMonte, F., Warf, P., and Al-Mefty, O. (1994). Intraoperative mapping of the lower cranial nerves during surgery of the jugular foramen and lower clivus. In Intraoperative Monitoring

Techniques in Neurosurgery, ed. C.M. Loftus and V.C. Traynelis. New York: McGraw-Hill, pp.205–12.
19. Frigeni B, Bivona R, Foresti C, Guazzo E, Danesi G. Predictive value of preoperative and intraoperative neurophysiology in evaluating long-term facial function outcome in acoustic neuroma surgery. Otol Neurotol. 2020;41(4):530–6.
20. Goto T, Muraoka H, Kodama K, Hara Y, Yako T, Hongo K. Intraoperative monitoring of motor evoked potential for the facial nerve using a cranial peg-screw electrode and a "threshold-level" stimulation method. Skull Base. 2010;20(6):429–34.
21. Guerit J. Neuromonitoring in the operating room: why, when, and how to monitor? Electroencephalogr Clin Neurophysiol. 1998;106(1):1–21.
22. Guo L, Jasiukaitis P, Pitts LH, Cheung SW. Optimal placement of recording electrodes for quantifying facial nerve compound muscle action potential. Otol Neurotol. 2008;29(5):710–3.
23. Harner SG, Daube JR, Beatty CW, Ebersold MJ. Intraoperative monitoring of the facial nerve. Laryngoscope. 1988;98(2):209–12.
24. Harpcr CM. Intraoperative cranial nerve monitoring. Muscle Nerve. 2004;29:339–51.
25. Hendriks T, Kunst HPM, Huppelschoten M, Doorduin J, Laan MT. TcMEP threshold change is superior to A-train detection when predicting facial nerve outcome in CPA tumour surgery. Acta Neurochir. 2020;162:1197–203.
26. Hiruta R, Sato T, Itakura T, Fujii M, Sakuma J, Bakhit M, Kojima T, Ichikawa M, Iwatate K, Saito K. Intraoperative transcranial facial motor evoked potential monitoring in surgery of cerebellopontine angle tumors predicts early and late postoperative facial nerve function. Clin Neurophysiol. 2021;132(4):864–71.
27. Holland NR. Intraoperative electromyography. J Clin Neurophysiol. 2002;19(5):444–53.
28. Husain, A. M, Wright, D.R., Stolp, B. W., Friedman, A. H., and Keifer, J.C. (2008). Neurophysiological intraoperative monitoring of glossopharyngeal nerve: technical case report. Neurosurgery, 63: 277–78.
29. Irving RM, Viani L, Hardy DG, Baguley DM, Moffat DA. Nervus intermedius function after vestibular schwannoma removal: clinical features and pathophysiological mechanisms. Laryngoscope. 1995;105(8 Pt 1):809–13.
30. Ito E, Ichikawa M, Itakura T, Ando H, Matsumoto Y, Oda K, Sato T, Watanabe T, Sakima J, Saito K. Motor evoked potential monitoring of the vagus nerve with transcranial electrical stimulation during skull base surgery. Clinical article. J Neurosurg. 2013;118(1):195–201.
31. Karakis I, Simon MV. Neurophysiologic mapping and monitoring of cranial nerves and brainstem. In: Intraoperative neurophysiology. A comprehensive guide to monitoring and mapping. 2nd ed. Springer Publishing Company; 2019.
32. Kartush JM, Niparko JK, Bledsoe SC, Graham MD, Kemink JL. Intraoperative facial nerve monitoring. Laryngoscope. 1985;95(12):1536–40.
33. Kartush JM. Electroneurography and intraoperative facial nerve monitoring in contemporary neurotology. Otolaryngol Head Neck Surg. 1989;101:496–503.
34. Kartush JM, Lundy LB. Facial nerve outcome in acoustic neuroma surgery. Otolaryngol Clin N Am. 1992;25:623–47.
35. Kartush JM, Rice KS, Minahan RE, Balzer GK, Yingling CD, Seubert CN. Best practices in facial nerve monitoring. Laryngoscope. 2021;131:S1–S42.
36. Krause F. Surgery of the brain and spinal cord, based on personal experiences. New York: Rebman; 1912. p. 738–43.
37. Kimura J. Electrodiagnosis in diseases of nerve and muscle: principles and practice. 2nd ed. Philadelphia: F.A. Davis Company; 1989.
38. Kohara N, Kaji R, Kimura J. Comparison of recording characteristics of monopolar and concentric needle electrodes. Electroencephalogr Clin Neurophysiol. 1993;89(4):242–6.
39. Lalwani AK, Butt FY, Jackler RK, Pitts LH, Yingling CD. Facial nerve outcome after acoustic neuroma surgery: a study from the era of cranial nerve monitoring. Otolaryngol Head Neck Surg. 1994;111(5):561–70.

40. Landau WM. Comparison of different needle leads in EMG recording from a single site. Electroencephalogr Clin Neurophysiol. 1951;3(2):163–8.
41. Liu S, Jiang W, Zhang H, Li X, Wan X, Emmanuel B, et al. Intraoperative neuromonitoring for removal of large vestibular schwannoma: facial nerve outcome and predictive factors. Clin Neurol Neurosurg. 2015;133:83–9.
42. Lopez JR. Cranial nerve monitoring. In: Galloway GM, editor. Cranial nerve monitoring. Intraoperative neurophysiologic monitoring. New York: Cambridge University Press; 2010. p. 109–41.
43. MacDonald DB. Intraoperative motor evoked potentials monitoring: overview and update. J Clin Monit Computing. 2006;20(5):347–77.
44. MacDonald DB. Intraoperative facial motor evoked potentials? J Neurosurg. 2007;106: 517–20.
45. Macdonald DB, Skinner S, Shils J, Yingling C. Intraoperative motor evoked potential monitoring – a position statement by the American Society of Neurophysiological Monitoring. Clin Neurophysiol. 2013;124(12):2291–316.
46. Matthies C, Raslan F, Schweitzer T, Hagen R, Roosen K, Reiners K. Facial motor evoked potentials in cerebellopontine angle surgery: technique, pitfalls and predictive value. Clin Neurol Neurosurg. 2011;113(10):872–9.
47. Moller AR. Monitoring of motor nerves. In: Moller AR, editor. Intraoperative neurophysiologic monitoring. Sydney., pp. 173–21omment 863: Harwood Academic Publishers; 1995a. https://doi.org/10.1227/00006123-199305000-00025.
48. Moller AR. Chapter 8: Practical aspects of eletrophysiologic recording in the operating room. In: Intraoperative neurophysiologic monitoring. 1st ed. Luxembourg: Harwood Academic Publishers GmbH; 1995b. p. 249–75.
49. Moller AR. Chapter 10: Practical aspects of monitoring spinal motor systems. In: Intraoperative neurophysiological monitoring. 2nd ed. New Jersey: Human Press; 2006. p. 179–96.
50. Moller AR, Jannetta PJ. Preservation of facial function during removal of acoustic neuromas. Use of monopolar constant-voltage stimulation and EMG. J Neurosurg. 1984;61:757–60.
51. Moller AR, Jannetta PJ. Monitoring of facial nerve function during removal of acoustic tumor. Am J Otol. 1985;Suppl:27–9.
52. Møller AR. Intraoperative neurophysiological monitoring. 3rd ed. New York: Springer; 2011.
53. Netter FH. The Ciba collection of medical illustrations. Volume 1 nervous system. Part I anatomy and physiology. 3rd ed. USA: Pharmaceuticals Division. Ciba-Geigy Corporation; 1991. Section V: page 102
54. Neuloh G, Bogucki J, Schramm J. Intraoperative preservation of corticospinal function in the brainstem. J Neurol Neurosurg Psychiatry. 2009;80(4):417–22.
55. Nielsen A. Acoustic tumors. Ann Surg. 1942;115(5):849–63.
56. Nolte J. The human brain: an introduction to its functional anatomy. 6th ed. Philadelphia: Mosby Elsevier; 2009.
57. Prass RL, Lüders H. Acoustic (loudspeaker) facial electromyographic monitoring: Part 1. Evoked electromyographic activity during acoustic neuroma resection. Neurosurgery. 1986;19:392–400.
58. Prass RL, Kinney SE, Hardy RW, Hahn JF, Luders H. Acoustic (loudspeaker) facial EMG monitoring: II. Use of evoked EMG activity during acoustic neuroma resection. Otolaryngol Head Neck Surg. 1987;97:541–51.
59. Prass RL. Iatrogenic facial nerve injury: the role of facial nerve monitoring. Otolaryngol Clin North Am. 1996;29(2):265–75.
60. Prell J, Rampp S, Romstock J, Fahlbusch R, Strauss C. Train time as a quantitative electromyographic parameter for facial nerve function in patients undergoing surgery for vestibular schwannoma. J Neurosurg. 2007;106:826–32.
61. Prell J, Strauss C, Rachinger J, Alfieri C, Scheller C, Herfurth K, Rampp S. Facial nerve palsy after vestibular schwannoma surgery: dynamic risk-stratification based on continuous EMG-monitoring. Clin Neurophysiol. 2014;125:415–21.

62. Prell J, Strauss C, Rachinger J, Scheller C, Alfieri A, Herfurth K, Rampp S. The intermedius nerve as a confounding variable for monitoring of the free-running electromyogram. Clin Neurophysiol. 2015;126:1833–9.
63. Raabe A, Beck J, Schucht P, Seidel K. Continuous dynamic mapping of the corticospinal tract during surgery of motor eloquent brain tumors: evaluation of a new method. J Neurosurg. 2014;120:1015–24.
64. Rampp S, Rachinger J, Scheller C, Alfieri A, Strauss C, Prell J. How many electromyography channels do we need for facial nerve monitoring? J Clin Neurophysiol. 2012;29: 226–9.
65. Rampp S, Strauss C, Scheller C, Rachinger J, Prell J. A-trains for intraoperative monitoring in patients with recurrent vestibular schwannoma. Acta Neurochir. 2013;155:2273–9.
66. Rampp S, Illert J, Krempler K, Strauss C, Prell J. A-train clusters and the intermedius nerve in vestibular schwannoma patients. Clin Neurophysiol. 2019;130:722–6.
67. Romstöck J, Strauss C, Fahlbusch R. Continuous electromyography monitoring of motor cranial nerves during cerebellopontine angle surgery. J Neurosurg. 2000;93:586–93.
68. Rhoton AL Jr, Kobayashi S, Hollinshead WH. Nervus intermedius. J Neurosurg. 1968;29(6):609–17.
69. Sala F, Manganotti P, Tramontano V, Bricolo A, Gerosa M. Monitoring of motor pathways during brain stem surgery: what we have achieved and what we still miss? Clin Neurophysiol. 2007;37:399–406.
70. Sala F. Take the a train. Clin Neurophysiol. 2015;126(9):1647–9.
71. Scheller C, Rachinger J, Prell J, Kornhuber M, Strauss C. Schwannoma of the intermediate nerve. J Neurosurg. 2008;109(1):144–8.
72. Schlake HP, Goldbrunner RH, Milewski C, Krauss J, Trautner H, Behr R, et al. Intraoperative electromyographic monitoring of the lower cranial motor nerves (LCN IX–XII) in skull base surgery. Clin Neurol Neurosurg. 2001;103:72–82.
73. Sclabassi RJ, Kalia KK, Sekhar L, Jannetta PJ. Assessing brain stem function. Neurosurg Clin N Am. 1993;4:415–31.
74. Seddon HJ. A classification of nerve injuries. Br Med J. 1942;2:237–9.
75. Seidel K, Biner MS, Zubak I, Rychen J, Beck J, Raabe A. Continuous dynamic mapping to avoid accidental injury of the facial nerve during surgery for large vestibular schwannomas. Neurosurg Rev. 2018;43(1):241–8.
76. Seidel K, Zubak I, Raabe A. Chapter 23: continuous dynamic mapping during surgery of large vestibular schwannoma. In: Deletis V, Shils J, Sala F, Seidel K, editors. Neurophysiology in neurosurgery. A modern approach. London, UK: Academic Press; 2020.
77. Selesnick SH, Carew JF, Victor JD, Heise CW, Levine J. Predictive value of facial nerve electrophysiologic stimulation thresholds in cerebellopontine-angle surgery. Laryngoscope. 1996;106(5):633–8.
78. Sobottka SB, Schackert G, May SA, Wiegleb M, Reiss G. Intraoperative facial nerve monitoring (IFNM) predicts facial nerve outcome after resection of vestibular schwannoma. Acta Neurochir. 1998;140(3):235–43.
79. Sugita K, Kobayashi S. Technical and instrumental improvements in the surgical treatment of acoustic neurinomas. J Neurosurg. 1982;57:747–52.
80. Téllez MJ, Ulkatan S, Urriza J, Arranz-Arranz B, Deletis V. Neurophysiological mechanism of possibly confounding peripheral activation of the facial nerve during corticobulbar tract monitoring. Clin Neurophysiol. 2016;127(2):1710–6.
81. Topsakal C, Al-Mefty O, Bulsara KR, Williford VS. Intraoperative monitoring of lower cranial nerves in skull base surgery: technical report and review of 123 monitored cases. Neurosurg Rev. 2008;31(1):45–53.
82. Ulkatan S, Deletis V, Fernandez-Conejero I. Central or peripheral activations of the facial nerve? J Neurosurg. 2007;106:519–20.
83. Urriza J, Arranz-Arranz B, Ulkatan S, Téllez MJ, Deletis V. Integrative action of axonal membrane explored by trains of subthreshold stimuli applied to the peripheral nerve. Clin Neurophysiol. 2016;127(2):1707–9.

84. Verst SM. Monitoração neurofisiológica intraoperatória em tumores de ângulo pontocerebelar: papel de parâmetros distintos na predição do resultado funcional do nervo facial. Faculdade de Medicina da Universidade de São Paulo, 2011. https://www.teses.usp.br/teses/disponiveis/5/5138/tde-27072011-171947/publico/SilviaMazzaliVerst.pdf. Accessed 1st March, 2021.
85. Verst SM, Maldaun MVC, Chung TM, Caivano AS, Aguiar PHP. Comparison between the C5 or C6-Cz electrode assembly and C3 or C4-Cz assembly for transcranial electric motor activation of muscular response of the contralateral facial nerve. Acta Neurochir. 2012;12(154):2229–35.
86. Verst SM, Sucena AC, Maldaun MVC, Aguiar PHP. Effectiveness of C5 or C6-Cz assembly in predicting immediate postoperative facial nerve deficit. Acta Neurochir. 2013;155(10):1863–9. https://doi.org/10.1007/s00701-013-1806-x.
87. Vivas EX, Carlson ML, Neff BA, Shepard NT, McCracken DJ, Sweeney AD, Olson JJ. Congress of neurological surgeon systematic review and evidence-based guidelines on intraoperative cranial nerve monitoring in vestibular schwannoma surgery. Neurosurgery. 2018;82:E44–6.
88. Wilson-Pauwels L, Akesson EJ, Stewart PA, Spacey SD. Cranial nerves in health and disease. 2nd ed. Canada: BC Decker Inc.; 2002.
89. Yingling CD, Ashram YA. Intraoperative monitoring of cranial nerves in skull base surgery. In: Jackler R, Brackmann DE, editors. Neurotology. 2nd ed. Philadelphia: Elsevier; 2005. p. 958.
90. Yingling CD, Gardi JN. Intraoperative monitoring of facial and cochlear nerves during acoustic neuroma surgery. Neurosurg Clin N Am. 2008;19(2):289–315.
91. Ylikoski J, Savolainen S, Sjoback DB. The human facial nerve: quantitative features. Acta Otolaryngol. 1982;386(Suppl):258–61.

Chapter 20
Fourth Ventricle's Floor Mapping

Kathleen Seidel and Andreas Raabe

Abbreviations

BR	blink reflex
CMAP	compound muscle action potential
CN	cranial nerve
LAR	adductor laryngeal reflex
MEP	motor evoked potential
SEP	somatosensory evoked potential

Oncological and Surgical Considerations

The complex anatomy renders surgical approaches and resection of brainstem lesions a challenge. If not well prepared, surgery may result in a high postoperative morbidity. Thus, resection of brainstem lesions requires not only extraordinary expertise in microsurgical techniques but also critical support from other technological advances. Image guidance combined with intraoperative neurophysiological mapping and monitoring may help to achieve the surgical goal. Especially in tumors, where adjuvant radiosurgery/radiotherapy is available, the main goal is to prevent neurological deficits and to preserve the patient's quality of life. In this regard,

K. Seidel (✉) · A. Raabe
Department of Neurosurgery, Inselspital, Bern University Hospital, University of Bern, Bern, Switzerland
e-mail: Kathleen.Seidel@insel.ch; Andreas.Raabe@insel.ch

S. M. Verst et al. (eds.), *Intraoperative Monitoring*,
https://doi.org/10.1007/978-3-030-95730-8_20

surgical tumor resection should be paused when neurophysiological techniques detect signs of an impending nerve injury [1]. On the other side, neurophysiological methods may help to increase the extent of tumor resection and simultaneously preserve neurological function similar to supratentorial surgery for gliomas [2].

Diffuse intrinsic brainstem gliomas are treated by biopsy only, followed by observational repetitive MRI scans or different oncological and radiooncological protocols depending on histopathology, molecular markers, and symptoms of the patient. However, focal and especially exophytic brainstem gliomas may be approached by surgical resection, implying functional guidance with multimodal neurophysiological techniques. Preservation of function overweighs the goal of complete resection, following the strategy of "maximal safe" tumor resection.

Further important groups of pathologies, which may infiltrate the floor of the fourth ventricle, are ependymoma and medulloblastoma, the latter being highly frequent in children. For both pathologies, first-line treatment is surgical resection as the extent of resection affects significantly the prognosis of the patient. However, in case of infiltration of eloquent nuclei, radiosurgery/radiotherapy might be an alternative or adjuvant option. Even with all advances in intraoperative imaging techniques, only identification of eloquent tissue by mapping may define safe borders and may help to decide when to stop and when to continue with surgery. Therefore, neurophysiological mapping techniques and monitoring modalities to assess the functional integrity of the patients affect those surgeries significantly.

An additional brainstem pathology, which may require surgical treatment, is brainstem cavernoma. Compared to other locations, brainstem cavernoma present a high rate of bleeding (up to 5–30% per year) which is more likely to result in neurological deficits, and they present a higher incidence of recurrent hemorrhage [3]. Expert opinion varies regarding indication and timing of surgery, but in the case of hemorrhage with worsening of neurological deficits, the surgical resection is recommended [4]. Generally, the clinical symptoms of the patient are the main indications for surgery. During the past two decades, waiting 4–6 weeks after hemorrhage was recommended with the intention to stabilize the patient's condition and to wait for hematoma organization. Recently, the paradigm seems to shift more toward resection in the subacute phase. Anyhow, complete removal of the cavernoma is essential to prevent re-bleeding. Truly, cavernoma themselves contain non-functional tissue; however, most of them are surrounded by a hallow of hemosiderin infiltrating eloquent tissue. Thus, some centers wait until the bleeding reaches the surface as then the lesion itself defines the surgical entry zone. However, due to advances in neurosurgical techniques, brainstem cavernomas beneath the pia are resected as first-line management in specialized centers around the world [5].

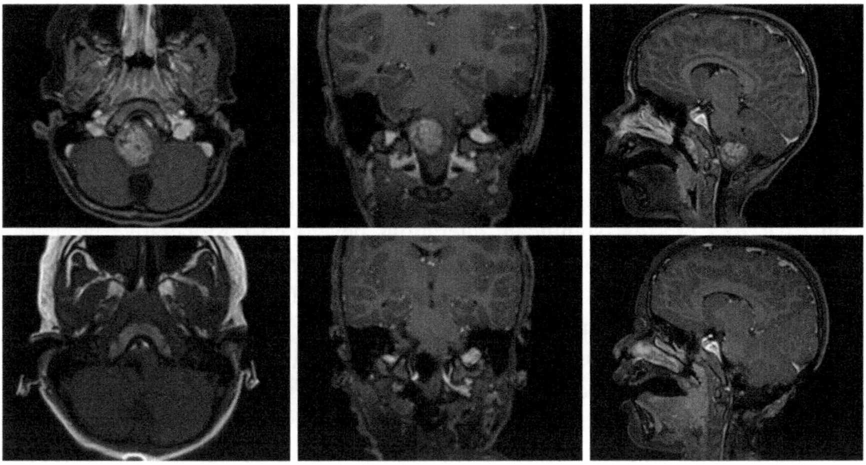

Fig. 20.4 Upper row: preoperative axial, corner, and sagittal T1 gadolinium MRI slice illustrating an intra-axial contrast-enhancing tumor involving the caudal pons and medulla oblongata. Lower row: postoperative MRI, which illustrates gross total resection after surgery under advanced neurophysiological monitoring and mapping (for further details, see case discussion). (© Inselspital, Bern University Hospital, Dept. of Neurosurgery)

technique might be beneficial not only in complex skull base surgery [15] but also when entering the brainstem and resecting intra-axial lesions. In the latter case, the stimulation paradigm has to be switched from single pulse stimulation (to identify nuclei and peripheral cranial nerves) to the short train stimulation paradigm (5 monophasic pulses of 200–500 μs pulse width with an interstimulus interval of 2–4 msec) to activate the corticobulbar tract (Fig. 20.4).

Advanced Techniques Besides Mapping

Monitoring MEPs of the corticobulbar muscles was initially introduced for the facial nerve and later for all motor cranial nerves [1, 8, 18–21]. Deletis et al. suggested applying a single stimulus 90 ms after delivering a short train of stimuli [1, 8]. The rationale for this kind of stimulation is that only a short train of stimuli can elicit "central" responses (activation of the corticobulbar tract for the cranial nerves) elicited from the motor cortex under general anesthesia. If a single stimulus elicits a response, this should be considered a "peripheral" response due to the spreading of current distally and activation of the cranial nerve directly. Beside intraoperative monitoring of corticobulbar MEP (Chap. 21), SEP (Chap. 8), and BAEP (Chap. 6), which will be discussed in different chapters, monitoring of reflexes may increase the safety during brainstem surgery (Chap. 12). Recently, the blink reflex (BR) [22], masseter H reflex [23], and adductor laryngeal reflex (LAR) have been introduced to neurosurgery [24].

Intraoperative injury to the vagus nerve and its reflexive pathways may induce swallowing deficits, aspiration, and pneumonia. In a multi-center study, Tellez et al. monitored 53 patients during skull base and brainstem surgeries [24]. LAR was recorded from an endotracheal tube with imbedded electrodes or hook wire electrodes. A LAR significant change (LAR-SC) was defined as ≥50% amplitude decrement or loss. By the end of the surgery, it was classified as either transient or permanent injury to the vagus nerve or medullary pathways. Patients with permanent LAR loss or LAR-significant alterations developed postoperative laryngeal dysfunction such as aspiration or pneumonia and permanent swallowing deficits. All patients with transient LAR-SC or loss, which could be reverted by changing the surgical approach, did not present a permanent deficit. Thus, permanent significant amplitude decrement or loss of the laryngeal adductor reflex correlated with postoperative laryngeal dysfunction. LAR predicted not only motor but also sensory dysfunction of the vagus nerve and reflexive medullary pathways. In contrast, a LAR-SC or loss, averted by a timely surgical adjustment, prevented irreversible damage. This might imply that monitoring of the LAR may enhance safety to resect complex lower brainstem lesions. Further, LAR monitoring offers the opportunity to assess sensory function of the vagus nerve and its reflexive pathways.

Illustrative Case

This 5-year-old girl presented with vomiting and headache but no neurological deficits. Imaging revealed an intra-axial contrast-enhancing tumor raising from the caudal floor of the fourth ventricle involving the medulla oblongata and caudal pons (Fig. 20.4, upper row). Surgery was performed under intraoperative neurophysiological monitoring of SEP, BAER, and MEP including corticobulbar MEP for CN VI, VII, IX, X, XI, and XII. Additionally, monitoring of the LAR was done. To define a safe entry site, mapping of brainstem nuclei was performed. Later during resection, continuous dynamic mapping for the corticobulbar tracts and cranial nerve trajectories was performed. Surgery was stopped when bilateral responses for the tongue were observed with low stimulation intensities in the caudal anterior resection border. Beside loss of the right tibial SEP, no significant changes of the neurophysiological recordings had been occurred. The girl did wake up with a severe ataxia of the right leg which completely recovered within 1 month; she did not present any other neurological deficits especially intact swallowing and caudal cranial nerve functions. Gross total resection was achieved, and the postoperative MRI showed a minor remnant at the anterior-inferior border (Fig. 20.4, lower row). Histopathology confirmed a pilocytic astrocytoma, and thus, no adjuvant treatment but sequential follow-up MR images were recommended.

Conclusion

If not well prepared, surgery near the floor of the fourth ventricle and especially surgery of intra-axial brainstem lesions might be associated with significant perioperative morbidity. Neurophysiological guidance can significantly impact those high-risk procedures. Mapping helps to identify eloquent nuclei, nerves, and tracts, and continuous dynamic mapping methods may provide real-time feedback. Thus, even in distorted anatomy, safe surgical corridors can be identified. Monitoring methods provide the assessment of the functional integrity of important structures, and recently, the introduction of intraoperative reflex monitoring may further improve patient safety.

References

1. Sala F, Manganotti P, Tramontano V, Bricolo A, Gerosa M. Monitoring of motor pathways during brain stem surgery: what we have achieved and what we still miss? Neurophysiol Clin. 2007;37(6):399–406.
2. De Witt Hamer PC, Robles SG, Zwinderman AH, Duffau H, Berger MS. Impact of intraoperative stimulation brain mapping on glioma surgery outcome: a meta-analysis. J Clin Oncol. 2012;30(20):2559–65.
3. Porter RW, Detwiler PW, Spetzler RF, Lawton MT, Baskin JJ, Derksen PT, et al. Cavernous malformations of the brainstem: experience with 100 patients. J Neurosurg. 1999;90(1):50–8.
4. Bozinov O, Hatano T, Sarnthein J, Burkhardt JK, Bertalanffy H. Current clinical management of brainstem cavernomas. Swiss Med Wkly. 2010;140:w13120.
5. Lawton MT, Lang MJ. The future of open vascular neurosurgery: perspectives on cavernous malformations, AVMs, and bypasses for complex aneurysms. J Neurosurg. 2019;130(5):1409–25.
6. Kyoshima K, Kobayashi S, Gibo H, Kuroyanagi T. A study of safe entry zones via the floor of the fourth ventricle for brain-stem lesions. Report of three cases. J Neurosurg. 1993;78(6):987–93.
7. Yang Y, van Niftrik B, Ma X, Velz J, Wang S, Regli L, et al. Analysis of safe entry zones into the brainstem. Neurosurg Rev. 2019;42(3):721–9.
8. Deletis V, Fernandez-Conejero I. Intraoperative monitoring and mapping of the functional integrity of the brainstem. J Clin Neurol. 2016;12(3):262–73.
9. Strauss C, Romstock J, Nimsky C, Fahlbusch R. Intraoperative identification of motor areas of the rhomboid fossa using direct stimulation. J Neurosurg. 1993;79(3):393–9.
10. Morota N, Deletis V, Lee M, Epstein FJ. Functional anatomic relationship between brain-stem tumors and cranial motor nuclei. Neurosurgery. 1996;39(4):787–93; discussion 93-4.
11. Bertalanffy H, Tissira N, Krayenbuhl N, Bozinov O, Sarnthein J. Inter- and intrapatient variability of facial nerve response areas in the floor of the fourth ventricle. Neurosurgery. 2011;68(1 Suppl Operative):23–31; discussion
12. Morota N, Ihara S, Deletis V. Intraoperative neurophysiology for surgery in and around the brainstem: role of brainstem mapping and corticobulbar tract motor-evoked potential monitoring. Childs Nerv Syst. 2010;26(4):513–21.
13. Sala F, Lanteri P. Brain surgery in motor areas: the invaluable assistance of intraoperative neurophysiological monitoring. J Neurosurg Sci. 2003;47(2):79–88.

14. Schucht P, Seidel K, Jilch A, Beck J, Raabe A. A review of monopolar motor mapping and a comprehensive guide to continuous dynamic motor mapping for resection of motor eloquent brain tumors. Neuro-Chirurgie. 2017;63(3):175–80.
15. Seidel K, Biner MS, Zubak I, Rychen J, Beck J, Raabe A. Continuous dynamic mapping to avoid accidental injury of the facial nerve during surgery for large vestibular schwannomas. Neurosurg Rev. 2020;43(1):241–8.
16. Raabe A, Beck J, Schucht P, Seidel K. Continuous dynamic mapping of the corticospinal tract during surgery of motor eloquent brain tumors: evaluation of a new method. J Neurosurg. 2014;120(5):1015–24.
17. Seidel K, Schucht P, Beck J, Raabe A. Continuous dynamic mapping to identify the corticospinal tract in motor eloquent brain tumors: an update. J Neurol Surg A Cent Eur Neurosurg. 2020;81(2):105–10.
18. Dong CC, Macdonald DB, Akagami R, Westerberg B, Alkhani A, Kanaan I, et al. Intraoperative facial motor evoked potential monitoring with transcranial electrical stimulation during skull base surgery. Clin Neurophysiol. 2005;116(3):588–96.
19. Sarnthein J, Bozinov O, Melone AG, Bertalanffy H. Motor-evoked potentials (MEP) during brainstem surgery to preserve corticospinal function. Acta Neurochir. 2011;153(9):1753–9.
20. Sala F, Krzan MJ, Deletis V. Intraoperative neurophysiological monitoring in pediatric neurosurgery: why, when, how? Childs Nerv Syst. 2002;18(6–7):264–87.
21. Macdonald DB, Skinner S, Shils J, Yingling C. Intraoperative motor evoked potential monitoring – a position statement by the American Society of Neurophysiological Monitoring. Clin Neurophysiol. 2013;124(12):2291–316.
22. Deletis V, Urriza J, Ulkatan S, Fernandez-Conejero I, Lesser J, Misita D. The feasibility of recording blink reflexes under general anesthesia. Muscle Nerve. 2009;39(5):642–6.
23. Ulkatan S, Jaramillo AM, Tellez MJ, Goodman RR, Deletis V. Feasibility of eliciting the H reflex in the masseter muscle in patients under general anesthesia. Clin Neurophysiol. 2017;128(1):123–7.
24. Tellez MJ, Mirallave-Pescador A, Seidel K, Urriza J, Shoakazemi A, Raabe A, et al. Neurophysiological monitoring of the laryngeal adductor reflex during cerebellar-pontine angle and brainstem surgery. Clin Neurophysiol. 2021;132(2):622–31.

Chapter 21
Microvascular Decompression

Jamison Beiriger, Varun Shandal, Josh Sunderlin, and Parthasarathy D. Thirumala

MVD: Their Indications, Clinical Presentation, and Pathophysiology

Microvascular decompression (MVD) is a minimally invasive surgical technique that relieves symptoms of cranial nerve disorders by alleviating the compression by vascular structures. Common indications for MVD include trigeminal neuralgia (TN), glossopharyngeal neuralgia (GPN), and hemifacial spasm (HFS). TN has an incidence of 12.6/100,000 people per year [1]. There are three classifications of TN: classic, atypical, and mixed. TN is classic when no cause other than nerve compression has been identified [2]. Classic TN presents with sharp, shooting pain, while atypical TN presents with constant aching, numbness, or burning [3, 4]. Mixed TN

J. Beiriger
School of Medicine, Drexel University, Philadelphia, PA, USA
e-mail: jcb362@drexel.edu

V. Shandal
Department of Neurological Surgery, Center for Clinical Neurophysiology, University of Pittsburgh, Pittsburgh, PA, USA
e-mail: shandalv@upmc.edu

J. Sunderlin
Procirca, Clinical Neurophysiology, University of Pittsburgh Medical Center, Pittsburgh, PA, USA
e-mail: sunderlinrj2@upmc.edu

P. D. Thirumala (✉)
Department of Neurological Surgery and Neurology, University of Pittsburgh, Pittsburgh, PA, USA
e-mail: thirumalapd@upmc.edu

S. M. Verst et al. (eds.), *Intraoperative Monitoring*,
https://doi.org/10.1007/978-3-030-95730-8_21

involves a combination of classic and atypical symptoms [5]. GPN is rare with an incidence of 0.2/100,000 people per year [6–9]. This is only 1.3% of the incidence of TN, so there are relatively fewer studies examining the effectiveness of MVD [10]. MVD for GPN accounted for only 2% of MVD surgery in the United States between 1996 and 2000 [11, 12]. With an incidence of 0.77/100,000, HFS is less common than TN and more common than GPN [13, 14]. The purpose of MVD is to part the vessel and nerve, eliminating the compression and subsequently relieving symptoms.

Surgical Techniques

The procedure involves an elliptical (2 cm × 3 cm) post-auricular craniectomy just caudal to the asterion for entry and visualization of cranial nerves in the area of the brainstem. The surgeon explores the area to identify the vessel(s) compressing the nerve, ensuring visualization of all potential offending vessels [15]. Clinical presentation and imaging indicate likely areas of compression, which guides the surgery. Once an offending vessel is detected, the surgeon carefully retracts the artery, or less commonly the vein, from the nerve. A Teflon pillow, nonstick PTFE (polytetrafluoroethylene), is placed between the separated vessel and nerve to prevent contact with the nerve [16]. Oxidized cellulose and bioglue slings are also used to retain retraction of the vessels [15, 17–19]. Neither the artery nor the spacing agent should be contacting the nerve at the end of the procedure [15]. Outcomes of MVD vary by presenting syndrome.

Outcomes of MVD

Trigeminal Neuralgia

Microvascular decompression is an option for the treatment of medication refractory TN. This technique is very effective for treating classic TN with 70–96.7% of patients experiencing complete pain relief with no reoccurrence [4, 20–22]. MVD leads to decreased pain recurrence and decreased need for additional treatment compared to other common therapies such as radiofrequency, rhizotomy, and stereotactic radiosurgery [23, 24]. Results can change postoperatively, as 13% of patients without postoperative pain relief experience a delayed cure, while 17% of cured patients have pain recurrence [25]. For patients with atypical TN, MVD is slightly less effective with postoperative pain relief between 79% and 88%, yet only 54% remain pain-free after 5 years without medication [4, 26]. Like atypical TN, mixed TN has similar postoperative pain relief to classic TN (91.8%) and much lower long-term relief (39.7%) with no reoccurrence [5]. Additionally, atypical symptoms reoccur much more than classic symptoms in mixed TN [4]. Classic TN symptoms, identification of compression on imaging, and clear nerve compression intraoperatively are recognized as predictors of long-term pain relief [5, 26].

additional neuromuscular blockers during the procedure. The neuromuscular junction blockade should be tested with a train of four standard twitches.

Facial Motor Evoked Potentials

Anesthesia can suppress facial motor evoked potentials (FMEPs), potentially affecting the accuracy of IONM of FMEPs. Centrally acting anesthetic agents such as desflurane can diminish MEPs. In patients under anesthesia, multi-pulse stimulation is generally required for the generation of MEPs. In HFS, single-pulse stimulation is often sufficient on the spasm side. Interestingly, the effects of anesthetic are significantly greater on the non-spasm side. While anesthesia effects may be reduced in HFS, it is recommended to incorporate less than 0.5 MAC of desflurane into the anesthetic regimen [81]. Optimal anesthesia for MEP monitoring includes intravenous agents such as propofol and opioids [68]. Anesthetic treatment should be accounted for in the interpretation of MEPs.

IONM Modalities Used in MVD

Brainstem Auditory Evoked Potentials

Purpose

During MVD, IONM of BAEPs is useful for indicating early signs of potential hearing loss, warning the surgeon to exercise caution and allowing correction of the maneuver [82–87]. Intraoperative monitoring of BAEPs is an accurate and reliable predictor of hearing loss in MVD for HFS [84, 88].

Hearing impairment is significantly reduced in procedures utilizing intraoperative monitoring of BAEPs, which takes under 10 s [87, 89]. Almost a complete reduction in the hearing loss rate of MVD was achieved after the introduction of BAEPs [22, 90–92]. While intraoperative monitoring of BAEPs is helpful in MVD for HFS [82–86] and GPN [12], its importance is controversial in MVD for TN [87, 90, 93–97]. BAEP monitoring is useful in MVD for TN for identifying maneuvers harmful to cochlear nerve function while the surgeon is learning the procedure, but not necessary after [87, 94]. IOM of BAEPs during MVD is an effective way to reduce hearing loss and could be improved with enhanced alarm criteria [69, 82, 98].

Technique

BAEPs are electric signals produced by the auditory pathway in response to peripheral acoustic stimuli [99, 100]. An auditory stimulus is generated with clicks at a certain frequency and intensity, and the resulting signal is measured [101]. The waveform produced consists of five to seven vertex-positive peaks. Peaks I, III, and V are most commonly assessed as they are the most stable within and across subjects. These signals are generally anesthesia resistant, so they are useful for intraoperative monitoring of the auditory pathway [69, 76]. Refer to Chap. 6 for more information regarding BAEP technique.

There are a few causes of BAEP loss during MVD. Excessive retraction of CNVIII, blood flow changes in the brainstem or CNVIII, and direct trauma to the nerve result in loss of BAEP response. Excessive retraction of CNVIII may cause a transient loss of BAEPs, while the other causes can result in quicker, irreversible injuries. Not every loss of BAEP signal correlates with hearing loss, and not every case of hearing loss is preceded by loss of BAEPs. However, patients who lost their hearing were nine times more likely to have significant change or loss of BAEP response intraoperatively [88].

Technical Considerations

Generating a Reliable Response

Measuring BAEPs has certain challenges to consider. One challenge is that BAEPs are far-field responses with low amplitudes since they are measured by electrodes on the scalp. This results in difficulty distinguishing signals with background electrical noise. Filtering, amplification, and signal averaging are necessary to record the signals. There are specific guidelines about filtering, amplification, and averaging that need to be followed to improve signal detection and reduce the possibility for errors. The time required to produce a reliable signal varies from less than 10 s to 2 min based on the filter settings, amplifier quality, extraneous noise level, and amplitude of the evoked potential [101].

Temperature Considerations

Body temperature should also be a consideration when monitoring BAEPs. Drop in core body temperature below 35 °C results in the prolongation of latencies and interpeak intervals with decrease in amplitude. One technique to reduce anesthesia and temperature effects is to measure baseline BAEPs intraoperatively rather than using potentials measured before anesthetic induction. Baseline potentials should be obtained after anesthesia, but before major surgical procedures such as opening the dura [102]. This confers a higher sensitivity for hearing outcomes.

Operative Considerations

Certain techniques and occurrences throughout the surgery can artificially alter BAEPs. Drilling the skull during surgery masks acoustic stimulation by creating bone-conducted noise. Monitoring should not be relied upon during drilling to avoid misinterpretation due to resulting inaccurate and variable signals. Cerebellar retraction is another surgical technique that may alter auditory evoked potentials. Retraction can cause temporal dispersion and loss of amplitude. While these changes are reversible in some cases [88], retraction is correlated with permanent hearing loss in MVD for HFS [103]. Transient nerve stretch due to retraction may be the underlying mechanism for hearing preservation following loss of BAEPs [88].

Alarm Criteria

The American Clinical Neurophysiology Society (ACNS) recommends a prolonged wave V latency of >1.0 ms or a decrease in amplitude of ≥50% as the alarm criteria for IONM of BAEP [101, 104]. BAEP signals meeting these criteria are termed significant changes. Some physicians support a >0.5 ms latency delay, 50% decrease in amplitude, and/or a 10% increase in latency for any evoked potential as their alarm criteria, although the prognostic value is unclear [68]. An analysis of the ACNS criteria demonstrated increased prevention of hearing loss when significant changes and loss of response are monitored as compared to solely loss of response. However, loss of response alone is better at predicting postoperative deficits [88].

Intraoperative Changes

There are five possible BAEP outcomes, each of which has a specific implication in relation to hearing loss:

1. No Change

   Consistent BAEPs are the desired signal response during surgery. No change in signaling indicates the auditory pathway remains intact. Hearing loss has been reported in cases with no change; however, this is the outcome with the least reported hearing loss at 1.8% [88].
2. Reversible Significant Change

   Significant change in BAEPs can be either reversible or irreversible. The purpose of using alarm criteria is to notify the surgeon of significant changes in an effort to reverse significant changes. For significant change, IONM of BAEPs has sensitivity, specificity, and diagnostic odds ratio of 0.88. 0.63, and 0.09, respectively [88]. One possible explanation for the low sensitivity is that rate of change rather than absolute change in latency is a better predictor of postoperative hearing loss [98, 105].
3. Irreversible Significant Change

   Despite the alarm, some cases of significant change are unable to be reversed. Postoperative hearing loss occurs in 8.97% of cases with intraoperative BAEP significant changes [88].
4. Reversible Loss of Response

   Loss of response can also be either reversible or irreversible. For loss of response, IONM of BAEPs has sensitivity, specificity, and diagnostic odds ratio of 0.74, 0.98, and 0.69, respectively. Reversible loss of response can occur due to transient stretching of CNVIII during retraction. If the stretch is reversible, BAEP response could return without lasting damage [88]. However, the delayed recovery may not be apparent during surgery [106, 107].

5. Irreversible Loss of Response

   In some cases, loss of response is irreversible. Irreversible loss of response is the worst BAEP outcome during surgery. Permanent BAEP loss can be caused by excessive nerve stretching, lack of blood flow to the brainstem or CNVIII, or trauma to the nerve [108–111]. Hearing loss occurs in 31.14% of patients with loss of response [88].

Hearing loss occurs in 15.01% of patients with any significant change or loss of response. Please refer to Figs. 21.1 and 21.2 for examples of monitored BAEPs during MVD.

Limitations

There are some limitations to monitoring of BAEPs. Despite drastically limiting hearing loss during MVD, BAEPs do not completely eliminate this adverse outcome. Sudden loss of BAEPs, such as injury to a perforator, cannot be prevented by monitoring. Permanent damage occurs before there is a chance for reversal. Additionally, hearing loss may still occur in cases with no changes in BAEPs. This may involve other unknown mechanisms of hearing loss.

Electromyography

Purpose

IOM of EMG is a proven technique with the capability to prevent facial palsies [112–118], dysphonia, and dysphagia [12, 114, 117, 119–121]. It is commonly used in MVD for HFS [64, 84, 85, 122–128] and improves outcomes [129]. The sensitivity, specificity, and accuracy of facial nerve EMG during MVD for HFS have been calculated as high as 0.97, 1, and 0.97, respectively [84]. EMG is also useful in limiting complications of MVD for TN and GPN although not as well studied [8, 9, 12, 27, 35, 87, 130–132]. While complications are reduced, improvement of EMG techniques and research into specific criteria for the injury threshold could enhance the effectiveness of this monitoring modality [12, 129].

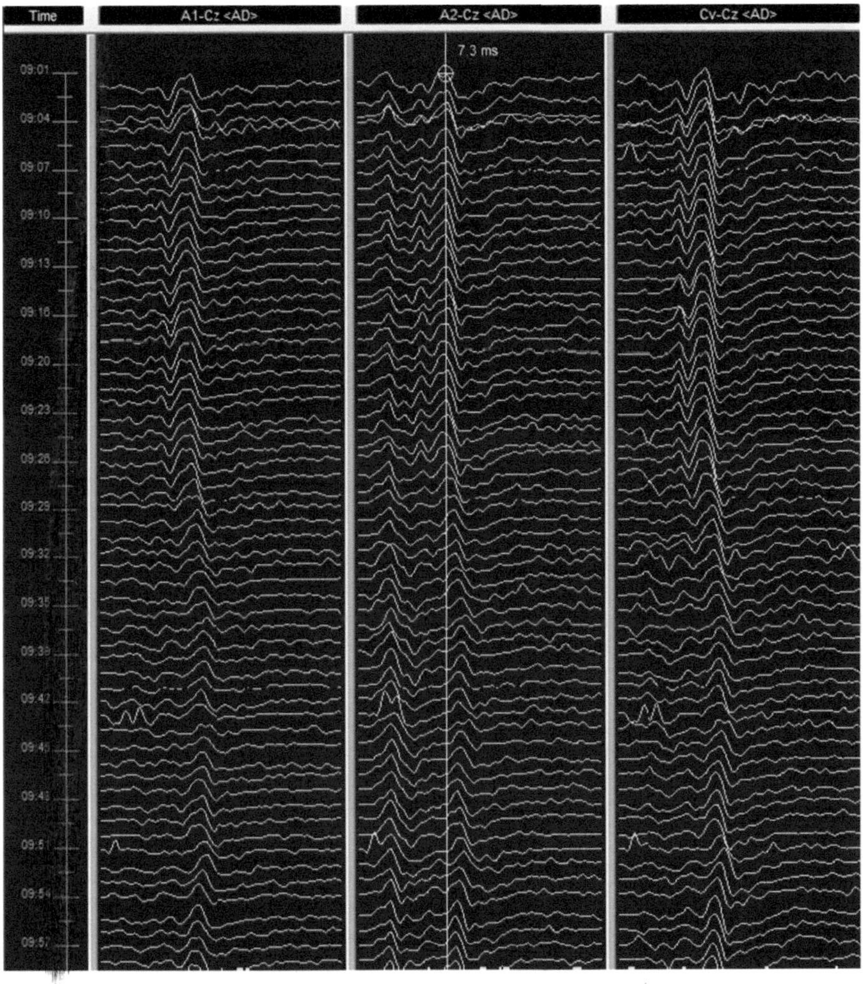

Fig. 21.1 "Waterfall" view of the BAEP data for about 1 h showing BAEP changes during a microvascular decompression of the right facial nerve for hemifacial spasm. From 09:26 through 09:48, the surgeon actively isolated the facial nerve for decompression while retracting the cerebellum causing stretching of vestibular-cochlear nerve. The latency of waves 2–5 of the BAEP shifts out, and some amplitude loss is appreciated. Once the decompression is complete and pressure no longer applied to the vestibular-cochlear nerve, the latency and amplitude begin to improve toward baseline values. Timely alerts from the neuromonitoring team can guide the surgeon during this critical point in the procedure and prevent over-stretching of the vestibular-cochlear nerve during the decompression. Once a sudden BAEP latency shift and/or an acute amplitude loss has been reported, the surgeon may opt to take time to allow for some recovery of the waveform toward baseline value before making another attempt to decompress the facial nerve

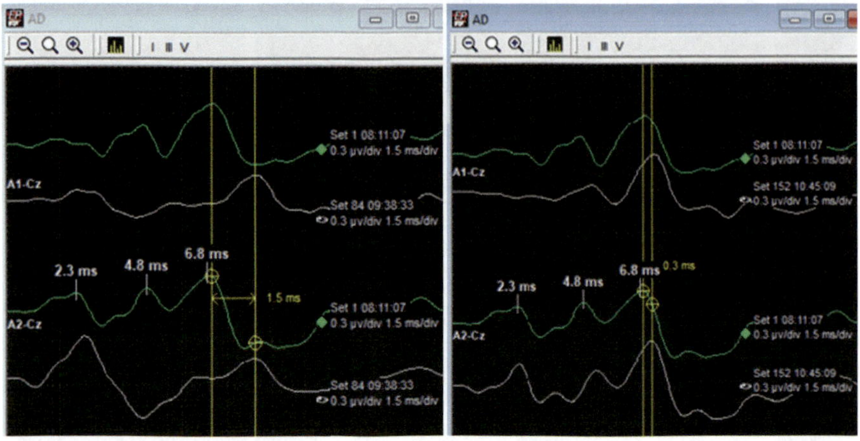

Fig. 21.2 (LEFT) A single set of data (white) compared to the baseline (green) captured while the surgeon was actively decompressing the facial nerve in a microvascular decompression procedure. The latency shift of wave V reached a maximum of 1.5 ms from baseline value (6.8 ms), while the amplitude of wave V reduced to nearly 50% of baseline. (RIGHT) shows data from the same procedure an hour later (during closure) demonstrating a near-complete recovery of BAEP amplitude and latency. Patient suffered no discernable hearing loss after the procedure

Technique

EMG is the measurement of electrical activity produced by skeletal muscles. Free-running EMG (frEMG), triggered EMG (tEMG), and intraoperative nerve conduction studies (NCS) are some common techniques [69]. Free-running EMG is a continuous recording of innervated muscles to detect changes representing nerve irritation. Phasic activation indicates mechanical irritation, while tonic activation indicates traction, heat, or irrigation damage [69, 116, 133]. Triggered EMG and NCS involve intentionally stimulating the nerve and observing potentials in the innervated muscle. This technique can elucidate damage to a nerve or improper placement of surgical material [69, 76].

Both frEMG and tEMG are used to measure facial nerve response in MVD. To measure frEMG for a cranial nerve, subdermal needle electrodes are inserted into muscles innervated by the nerve. Each muscle being monitored needs two electrodes. During the surgery, surgeons slowly inject saline into the root exit zone of the monitored cranial nerve, and the response is recorded from the electrodes. This is done once before surgery and once after surgery, and the values are compared in a ratio of postoperative response to preoperative response [134]. Triggered EMG also utilizes two needle electrodes in each muscle; however, instead of initiating nerve conduction with saline, direct electrical stimulation is applied. Compound muscle action potentials (CMAPs) are recorded from the muscles. CMAP amplitude, stimulation threshold, and onset latency serve as indicators of facial nerve function [78].

Technical Considerations

Procedural Considerations

Various solutions can provoke responses in frEMG, but saline is optimal for intraoperative monitoring during MVD as it induces the highest nerve activity. When using saline, ratios of frEMG post-MVD to pre-MVD greater than 50% trend toward a correlation with persistence of spasm. Other solutions are unable to produce large enough EMG responses to confirm quantifiable differences between pre- and postoperative measurements [134]. Determining which muscles to monitor is also a consideration. For the trigeminal nerve, the masseter and temporalis can be monitored, and for the facial nerve, the frontalis, orbicularis oculi, orbicularis oris, and mentalis can all be monitored.

Alarm Criteria

EMG monitoring is used to ensure proper nerve conduction. Appropriate nerve conduction is characterized by quantifiable tEMG responses at stimulation currents of 0.5 mA or lower. In order to ensure prevention of injury, some physicians have used responses at as low as 0.025 mA for alarm criteria. Lack of response at 0.5 mA signals a loss of proper conduction [78]. Free-running EMG alarm criteria is to alert the surgeon with any spontaneous activity. Baseline is characterized by no spontaneous activity [79]. Spontaneous activity and exaggerated responses to saline in frEMG may reflect facial nerve irritation or injury [134].

Intraoperative Changes

Triggered EMG

The goal for tEMG during MVD is to maintain responsiveness to stimulation by currents 0.5 mA or lower. Nerve damage is indicated by decreased or diminished tEMG response to stimulation. Signals of nerve damage can warn the surgeon that the nerve is at risk for complications including persistence of spasm or facial paralysis [78].

Free-Running EMG

Intraoperative change in free-running EMG can help with ensuring adequate decompression and maintaining proper nerve conduction. The goal for frEMG recording is no spontaneous stimulation and more than 50% reduction in saline stimulation intensity from pre-surgery to post-surgery [134]. In patients with HFS, saline-mediated frEMG overactivity suggests facial nerve irritability as a result of vascular compression. This makes it a great indicator of sufficient decompression. Spontaneous activation during frEMG is not desirable but may not always reflect injury to the facial nerve. Still, all cases of spontaneous stimulation should be recorded as significant events [79].

Limitations

EMG monitoring has several limitations. Free-running and triggered EMG are well studied for intraoperative monitoring of the facial nerve, but not other cranial nerves. This means EMG usefulness is limited in MVD for TN or GPN. Caution is required when observing the EMG and stimulation parameters. Sudden nerve transection does not result in any EMG responses making it difficult to monitor. Disappearance of abnormal muscle response (AMR), measured by frEMG, can occur without postoperative reduction of HFS in some patients [127]. This points to the likelihood of delayed normalization of hyperactivity in the facial nerve. Reduction in frEMG does not always translate to initial recovery [134]. In addition, EMG is useful in alleviating cases of persistent spasm immediately after surgery, but not delayed recurrence of spasm. Delayed facial palsy may be a result of herpes simplex virus or varicella zoster virus reactivation [135].

Lateral Spread Response

Purpose

LSR, an example of stimulated EMG, is used to measure AMR [136–138]. In HFS, an AMR is always observed [129]. A nerve is considered adequately decompressed with elimination of LSR [62–64]. Disappearance of AMR, as measured by LSR, during MVD for HFS is well correlated with resolution of HFS [139–141], yet predictive value is limited [127, 139, 141]. EMG monitoring of LSR has a high specificity but modest sensitivity for predicting clinical outcome after surgery [61]. A new method of LSR using preoperative mapping and intraoperative centrifugal stimulation of the facial nerve improves prognostic value with disappearance of AMR [142]. After adequate decompression of HFS, residual LSR amplitude does not predict long-term spasm relief, despite a correlation with initial spasm relief [143]. The lack of significant difference in long-term spasm relief is mostly explained by pain remission in patients without initial spasm rather than pain recurrence in the pain-free patients [143, 144]. Without adequate decompression, persistence of spasms is high risk [61].

Technique

LSR works by stimulating one branch of the facial nerve and monitoring activity by a muscle supplied by a different branch. Excitation of a muscle innervated by a different branch indicates an abnormal response [145]. For example, an AMR in HFS can be detected as an impulse in the *orbicularis oris* after stimulation of the zygomatic nerve, as the trigemino-facial reflex should only involve the *orbicularis oculi* [129]. Other popular options include recording the *mentalis* muscle after stimulation of the temporal branch of the facial nerve or the *orbicularis oculi* after stimulation of the marginal mandibular branch [138]. Please refer to Fig. 21.3 for a sample recording of an LSR.

Alarm Criteria

No alarm criteria are necessary since LSR is primarily useful in determining adequate decompression and not involved in the safety of the procedure. Presence of LSR after attempted decompression can aid the surgeon to find additional sites of nerve compression. Elimination of LSR is the desired response.

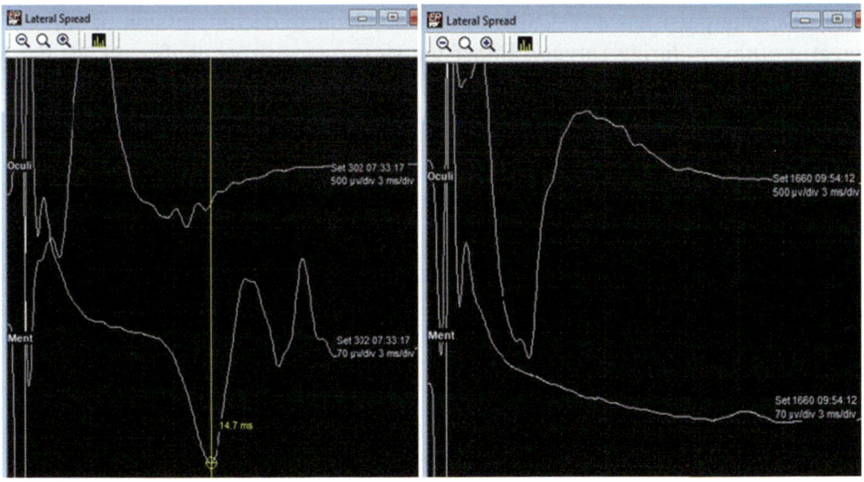

Fig. 21.3 (LEFT) Lateral spread response (LSR) recorded from mentalis at a latency of 14.7 ms (10–15 mA stim at zygomatic arch) in a patient undergoing microvascular decompression of the facial nerve for hemifacial spasm. (RIGHT) Near-complete abolishment of LSR after successful microvascular decompression of the facial nerve. The patient was discharged 2 days after surgery without experiencing any postoperative facial spasm

Intraoperative Changes

There are two outcomes in IONM of LSR. The optimum outcome is elimination of LSR which correlates with immediate postoperative spasm relief. Despite this immediate effect, elimination of LSR in patients with HFS has not been correlated with success at long-term follow-up [143]. The other scenario is residual LSR after surgery. Adequate decompression with persistence of LSR is linked with worse immediate but on par long-term outcomes as LSR elimination [143]. In some patients, hyperexcitability of the facial motor nucleus takes months or years to regress to a normal state after decompression [146]. Some patients may have a residual LSR after adequate decompression, but persistence of LSR can also indicate inadequate decompression. With persistence of LSR, the neurophysiologist and the neurosurgeon should communicate to determine if adequate decompression has been achieved [146].

Limitations

During the MVD, LSR is only useful for HFS. Adequate decompression in MVD for TN or GPN cannot be monitored with LSR. Practical value of LSR in determining sufficient decompression during MVD for HFS is also controversial [143, 147, 148]. Despite persistence of LSR in cases of adequate decompression, it still has great usefulness during surgery. Either the surgeon can have confirmed adequate decompression with loss of LSR or can be extra sure to decompress the nerve with residual LSR [146]. Additionally, a new method of LSR monitoring with centrifugal stimulation of the facial nerve demonstrates significantly lower risk of residual LSR after MVD [142].

Facial Motor Evoked Potentials

Purpose

FMEP monitoring allows the surgeon to assess facial nerve function intraoperatively and predict facial nerve outcome [65–68]. The ratio of the final FMEP amplitude to baseline amplitude can be a prognostic measure for surgery success during MVD [149, 150]. FMEP corresponds with LSR monitoring and gives another measure for surgical success [151]. Effectiveness of monitoring of FMEP has been well documented in HFS [65–68, 150–152], and it has also been shown to reduce complication rates in GPN and TN. MEPs can determine integrity of nerve function in lower cranial nerves often damaged by MVD for GPN [93] and TN [151]. MVD for TN and GPN should not result in the same decrease in amplitude observed in HFS [93, 151]. Coupled with free-running EMG, MEPs can provide reliable, timely indications of lower cranial nerve damage during MVD [93].

Technique

FMEP monitoring requires electrodes inserted into muscles innervated by cranial nerves similar to EMG. Corkscrew electrodes placed between C3' and C4' deliver shocks to the facial motor cortex. Repeat transcranial electrical stimulation of the facial nerves results in muscle responses of corticobulbar pathway origin that are measured as MEPs [65]. FMEP amplitude is measured as the range from maximum positive and negative peaks. Stimulation intensity is increased until FMEP amplitude plateaus before surgery and remains at that voltage during surgery, with alterations in amplitude constantly being monitored during the procedure [153–156]. HFS is characterized by a hyperexcitable state, suggesting the need for a decreased amplitude [149]. See Chap. 21 for more details on FMEP technique.

Technical Considerations

Proximity Interference

Measuring the FMEP is more challenging than measuring MEPs in extremities. The close proximity of the stimulation site to the recording site can distort the recorded MEPs. Transcranial stimulation intended for the nerve can result in direct electrical stimulation of the temporalis muscle. Peripheral portions of the facial nerve can also be stimulated leading to premature excitation without traversing the central motor pathway from the cortex. These potential deviations must be taken into account when monitoring FMEPs [157].

Alarm Criteria

FMEPs are generated when nerve conduction is intact. The alarm threshold for FMEP is decrease in amplitude of 50% or more. In the case of HFS, the non-spasm side should be used as baseline [158]. Disappearance is a major warning signal [68]. Decrease or disappearance of MEPs indicates impaired facial nerve function – the surgeon is subsequently notified and may decide to alter the procedure [153–156].

Intraoperative Changes

The facial nerve in HFS is in a hyperexcitable state with initial spasm side FMEPs of higher amplitude and duration than contralateral FMEPs. IONM of FMEPs allows the surgical team to monitor correction of this hyperexcitable state. In HFS, there should be some decrease in MEP without elimination of response. Maintaining the FMEP amplitude above 50% of baseline is correlated with reduction in both short- and long-term deficits [67]. In cases of HFS, the contralateral MEP should be used as a control to allow for necessary signal reduction without concern for damage. No reduction in hyperexcitable state is correlated with persistence of spasm. Correction of the vascular compression with MVD results in the elimination of this state with a return to baseline. Lack of adequate decompression is evidenced by a maintained hyperexcitable state [158].

Limitations

Intraoperative monitoring of FMEPs has a few limitations. Prognostic value for measuring FMEPs for HFS has been clearly demonstrated, but usefulness in MVD for TN and GPN is less clear. Monitoring of FMEPs in TN and GPN may preserve integrity of nerve function but is unable to indicate adequate decompression. The responses should not be reduced as in HFS. Additionally, monitoring of FMEPs is affected more than other monitoring techniques by anesthesia. Centrally acting inhaled agents can disrupt the response, creating false alarms. Proximity interference can also produce false results due to reception of the stimulus by the receiving electrodes or peripheral portions of the nerve. The responses must be monitored closely to ensure proper stimulation and signal reception.

References

1. Koopman JSHA, Dieleman JP, Huygen FJ, de Mos M, Martin CGM, Sturkenboom MCJM. Incidence of facial pain in the general population. Pain. 2009;147(1–3):122–7.
2. Igarashi H. The international classification of headache disorders. 2nd ed. Neuro-Ophthalmology Japan; 2007.
3. Eller JL, Raslan AM, Burchiel KJ. Trigeminal neuralgia: definition and classification. Neurosurg Focus. 2005;18(5):E3.
4. Tyler-Kabara EC, Kassam AB, Horowitz MH, Urgo L, Hadjipanayis C, Levy EI, et al. Predictors of outcome in surgically managed patients with typical and atypical trigeminal neuralgia: comparison of results following microvascular decompression. J Neurosurg. 2002;96(3):527–31.
5. Wu A, Doshi T, Hung A, Garzon-Muvdi T, Bender MT, Bettegowda C, et al. Immediate and long-term outcomes of microvascular decompression for mixed trigeminal neuralgia. World Neurosurg. 2018;117:e300–7. https://doi.org/10.1016/j.wneu.2018.06.016.
6. Yomo S, Arkha Y, Donnet A, Régis J. Gamma knife surgery for glossopharyngeal neuralgia: report of 2 cases. J Neurosurg. 2009;110(3):559–63.
7. Kawashima M, Matsushima T, Inoue T, Mineta T, Masuoka J, Hirakawa N. Microvascular decompression for glossopharyngeal neuralgia through the transcondylar fossa (supracondylar transjugular tubercle) approach. Oper Neurosurg. 2010;66(suppl_2):ons275-80.
8. Resnick DK, Jannetta PJ, Bissonnette D, Jho HD, Lanzino G. Microvascular decompression for glossopharyngeal neuralgia. Neurosurgery. 1995;36(1):64–9.
9. Kondo A. Follow-up results of using microvascular decompression for treatment of glossopharyngeal neuralgia. J Neurosurg. 1998;88(2):221–5.
10. Kim MK, Park JS, Ahn YH. Microvascular decompression for glossopharyngeal neuralgia: clinical analyses of 30 cases. J Korean Neurosurg Soc. 2017;60(6):738–48.

11. Kalkanis SN, Eskandar EN, Carter BS, Barker FG, Bricolo A, Casey KF, et al. Microvascular decompression surgery in the United States, 1996 to 2000: mortality rates, morbidity rates, and the effects of hospital and surgeon volumes. Neurosurgery. 2003;52(6):1251–61.
12. Habeych ME, Crammond DJ, Gardner P, Thirumala PD, Horowitz MB, Balzer JR. Intraoperative neurophysiological monitoring of microvascular decompression for glossopharyngeal neuralgia. J Clin Neurophysiol. 2014;31(4):337–43.
13. Auger RG, Whisnant JP. Hemifacial spasm in Rochester and Olmsted County, Minnesota, 1960 to 1984. Arch Neurol. 1990;47(11):1233–4.
14. Haller S, Etienne L, Kövari E, Varoquaux AD, Urbach H, Becker M. Imaging of neurovascular compression syndromes: trigeminal neuralgia, Hemifacial spasm, vestibular Paroxysmia, and glossopharyngeal neuralgia. Am J Neuroradiol. 2016;37(8):1384–92.
15. Broggi G, Broggi M, Ferroli P, Franzini A. Surgical technique for trigeminal microvascular decompression. Acta Neurochir. 2012;154(6):1089–95.
16. Jannetta PJ, Mclaughlin MR, Casey KF. Technique of microvascular decompression. Neurosurg Focus. 2005;18(5):E5.
17. Yang D, Tao C, Zhou S, Wang Z. The outcome of sling retraction technique in microvascular decompression for hemifacial spasm. J Craniofac Surg. 2018;29(8):e764–7. Available from: https://journals.lww.com/jcraniofacialsurgery/Fulltext/2018/11000/The_Outcome_of_Sling_Retraction_Technique_in.95.aspx
18. Tandon A, Chandela S, Langer D, Sen C. A novel sling technique for microvascular decompression of a rare anomalous vertebral artery causing cervical radiculopathy. Neurosurg Focus. 2013;35(3):E2.
19. Lee SH, Park JS, Ahn YH. Bioglue-coated Teflon sling technique in microvascular decompression for Hemifacial spasm involving the vertebral artery. J Korean Neurosurg Soc. 2016;59(5):505–11.
20. Xia L, Zhong J, Zhu J, Wang Y-N, Dou N-N, Liu M-X, et al. Effectiveness and safety of microvascular decompression surgery for treatment of trigeminal neuralgia: a systematic review. J Craniofac Surg. 2014;25(4):1413–7.
21. Kondo A. Follow-up results of microvascular decompression in trigeminal neuralgia and hemifacial spasm. Neurosurgery. 1997;40(1):42–6.
22. Barker FG, Jannetta PJ, Bissonette DJ, Larkins MV, Jho HD. The long-term outcome of microvascular decompression for trigeminal neuralgia. N Engl J Med. 1996;334(17):1077–83.
23. Hitchon PW, Holland M, Noeller J, Smith MC, Moritani T, Jerath N, et al. Options in treating trigeminal neuralgia: experience with 195 patients. Clin Neurol Neurosurg. 2016;149:166–70. https://doi.org/10.1016/j.clineuro.2016.08.016.
24. Spatz AL, Zakrzewska JM, Kay EJ. Decision analysis of medical and surgical treatments for trigeminal neuralgia: how patient evaluations of benefits and risks affect the utility of treatment decisions. Pain. 2007;131(3):302–10.
25. Sindou M, Leston J, Howeidy T, Decullier E, Chapuis F. Micro-vascular decompression for primary trigeminal neuralgia (typical or atypical). Long-term effectiveness on pain; prospective study with survival analysis in a consecutive series of 362 patients. Acta Neurochir. 2006;148(12):1235–45.
26. Zhang H, Lei D, You C, Mao B-Y, Wu B, Fang Y. The long-term outcome predictors of pure microvascular decompression for primary trigeminal neuralgia. World Neurosurg. 2013;79(5–6):756–62.
27. Sampson JH, Grossi PM, Asaoka K, Fukushima T. Microvascular decompression for glossopharyngeal neuralgia: long-term effectiveness and complication avoidance. Neurosurgery. 2004;54(4):884–90.
28. Ferroli P, Fioravanti A, Schiariti M, Tringali G, Franzini A, Calbucci F, et al. Microvascular decompression for glossopharyngeal neuralgia: a long-term retrospectic review of the Milan-Bologna experience in 31 consecutive cases. Acta Neurochir. 2009;151(10):1245–50.

29. Zheng X, Wei X-Y, Zhu J, Yuan Y, Ying T-T, Li S-T. Microvascular decompression alone without rhizotomy is an effective way of treating glossopharyngeal neuralgia: clinical analysis of 46 cases. Stereotact Funct Neurosurg. 2020;98(2):129–35. Available from: https://www.karger.com/DOI/10.1159/000505712
30. Zhao H, Zhang X, Zhu J, Tang Y, Li S-T. Microvascular decompression for glossopharyngeal neuralgia: long-term follow-up. World Neurosurg. 2017;102:151–6.
31. Xia L, Li Y-S, Liu M-X, Zhong J, Dou N-N, Li B, et al. Microvascular decompression for glossopharyngeal neuralgia: a retrospective analysis of 228 cases. Acta Neurochir. 2018;160(1):117–23.
32. Owler BK, Johnston I, Kennedy M. Late recurrence of glossopharyngeal neuralgia after IXth and partial Xth nerve rhizotomy: treatment by microvascular decompression. J Neurol Neurosurg Psychiatry. 2000;69(6):834–5.
33. Kano H, Urgosik D, Liscak R, Pollock BE, Cohen-Inbar O, Sheehan JP, et al. Stereotactic radiosurgery for idiopathic glossopharyngeal neuralgia: an international multicenter study. J Neurosurg. 2016;125(Suppl 1):147–53.
34. Wang J, Yu R, Qu C, Jiang J, Wang C, Meng Q, et al. Does glossopharyngeal neuralgia need rhizotomy in neurovascular decompression surgery? J Craniofac Surg. 2018;29(8):2192–4.
35. Patel A, Kassam A, Horowitz M, Chang Y-F. Microvascular decompression in the management of glossopharyngeal neuralgia: analysis of 217 cases. Neurosurgery. 2002;50(4):701–5.
36. Rosenstengel C, Matthes M, Baldauf J, Fleck S, Schroeder H. Hemifacial spasm-conservative and surgical treatment options. Dtsch Arztebl Int. 2012;109(41):667–73.
37. Lu AY, Yeung JT, Gerrard JL, Michaelides EM, Sekula RF, Bulsara KR. Hemifacial spasm and neurovascular compression. Sci World J. 2014;2014:349319.
38. Miller LE, Miller VM. Safety and effectiveness of microvascular decompression for treatment of hemifacial spasm: a systematic review. Br J Neurosurg. 2012;26(4):438–44.
39. Wang X, Thirumala PD, Shah A, Gardner P, Habeych M, Crammond D, et al. Microvascular decompression for hemifacial spasm: focus on late reoperation. Neurosurg Rev. 2013;36(4):637–43.
40. Liu MX, Xia L, Zhong J, Li B, Dou NN, Li ST. What should we do for those hemifacial spasm patients without efficacy following microvascular decompression: expectation of delayed relief or early reoperation? World Neurosurg. 2018;110:e897–900.
41. Wang X, Thirumala PD, Shah A, Gardner P, Habeych M, Crammond DJ, et al. Effect of previous botulinum neurotoxin treatment on microvascular decompression for hemifacial spasm. Neurosurg Focus. 2013;34(3):E3.
42. Zhao H, Li G, et al. Long-term efficacy of initial microvascular decompression versus subsequent microvascular decompression for idiopathic hemifacial spasm. World Neurosurg. 2018;109:e778–82.
43. Cote DJ, Dasenbrock HH, Gormley WB, Smith TR, Dunn IF. Adverse events after microvascular decompression: a National Surgical Quality Improvement Program Analysis. World Neurosurg. 2019;128:e884–94.
44. Gubian A, Rosahl SK. Meta-analysis on safety and efficacy of microsurgical and radiosurgical treatment of trigeminal neuralgia. World Neurosurg. 2017;103:757–67.
45. Hanakita J, Kondo A. Serious complications of microvascular decompression operations for trigeminal neuralgia and hemifacial spasm. Neurosurgery. 1988;22(2):348–52.
46. Cohen-Gadol AA. Microvascular decompression surgery for trigeminal neuralgia and hemifacial spasm: nuances of the technique based on experiences with 100 patients and review of the literature. Clin Neurol Neurosurg. 2011;113(10):844–53.
47. Bederson JB, Wilson CB. Evaluation of microvascular decompression and partial sensory rhizotomy in 252 cases of trigeminal neuralgia. J Neurosurg. 1989;71(3):359–67.
48. Bick SK, Huie D, Sneh G, Eskandar EN. Older patients have better pain outcomes following microvascular decompression for trigeminal neuralgia. Clin Neurosurg. 2019;84(1):116–22.
49. Phan K, Rao PJ, Dexter M. Microvascular decompression for elderly patients with trigeminal neuralgia. J Clin Neurosci. 2016;29:7–14.

50. Bick SK, Huie D, Eskandar EN. 192 older patients have greater improvements in pain score following microvascular decompression. Neurosurgery. 2016;63(Suppl):169.
51. Rughani AI, Dumont TM, Lin CT, Tranmer BI, Horgan MA. Safety of microvascular decompression for trigeminal neuralgia in the elderly: clinical article. J Neurosurg. 2011;115(2):202–9.
52. Bahgat D, Ray DK, Raslan AM, McCartney S, Burchiel KJ. Trigeminal neuralgia in young adults. J Neurosurg. 2011;114(5):1306–11.
53. Günther T, Gerganov VM, Stieglitz L, Ludemann W, Samii A, Samii M. Microvascular decompression for trigeminal neuralgia in the elderly: long-term treatment outcome and comparison with younger patients. Neurosurgery. 2009;65(3):477–82.
54. Lu VM, Goyal A, Graffeo CS, Perry A, Jonker BP, Link MJ. Glossopharyngeal neuralgia treatment outcomes after nerve section, microvascular decompression, or stereotactic radiosurgery: a systematic review and meta-analysis. World Neurosurg. 2018;120:572–82.
55. Zhao H, Zhang X, da Tang Y, Zhang Y, Ying T, et al. Operative complications of microvascular decompression for hemifacial spasm: experience of 1548 cases. World Neurosurg. 2017;107:559–64.
56. Hyun SJ, Kong DS, Park K. Microvascular decompression for treating hemifacial spasm: lessons learned from a prospective study of 1,174 operations. Neurosurg Rev. 2010;33(3):325–34.
57. Lee MH, Jee TK, Lee JA, Park K. Postoperative complications of microvascular decompression for hemifacial spasm: lessons from experience of 2040 cases. Neurosurg Rev. 2016;39(1):151–8.
58. Lovely TJ, Getch CC, Jannetta PJ. Delayed facial weakness after microvascular decompression of cranial nerve VII. Surg Neurol. 1998;50(5):449–52.
59. Hirata S, Kobayashi M, Wakiya K, Fujimaki T. Preservation of the lesser occipital nerve prevents occipital sensory disturbance after microvascular decompression: long-term results. World Neurosurg. 2020;136:e126–31.
60. Montava M, Rossi V, Curto Fais CL, Mancini J, Lavieille JP. Long-term surgical results in microvascular decompression for hemifacial spasm: efficacy, morbidity and quality of life. Acta Otorhinolaryngol Ital. 2016;36(3):220–7.
61. Thirumala PD, Altibi AM, Chang R, Saca EE, Iyengar P, Reddy R, et al. The utility of intraoperative lateral spread recording in microvascular decompression for hemifacial spasm: a systematic review and meta-analysis. Neurosurgery. 2020;87(4):E473–84.
62. Kim HR, Rhee DJ, Kong DS, Park K. Prognostic factors of hemifacial spasm after microvascular decompression. J Korean Neurosurg Soc. 2009;45(6):336–40.
63. Ishikawa M, Ohira T, Namiki J, Kobayashi M, Takase M, Kawase T, et al. Electrophysiological investigation of hemifacial spasm after microvascular decompression: F waves of the facial muscles, blink reflexes, and abnormal muscle responses. J Neurosurg. 1997;86(4):654–61.
64. Hatem J, Sindou M, Vial C. Intraoperative monitoring of facial EMG-responses during microvascular decompression for hemifacial spasm. Prognostic value for long-term outcome: a study in a 33-patient series. Br J Neurosurg. 2001;15(6):496–9.
65. Dong CCJ, MacDonald DB, Akagami R, Westerberg B, AlKhani A, Kanaan I, et al. Intraoperative facial motor evoked potential monitoring with transcranial electrical stimulation during skull base surgery. Clin Neurophysiol. 2005;116(3):588–96.
66. Fukuda M, Oishi M, Saito A, Takao T, Fujii Y. Facial nerve motor evoked potentials elicited by transcranial electrical stimulation for intraoperative monitoring. No Shinkei Geka. 2008;36(4):315–21.
67. Fukuda M, Oishi M, Hiraishi T, Saito A, Fujii Y. Intraoperative facial nerve motor evoked potential monitoring during skull base surgery predicts long-term facial nerve function outcomes. Neurol Res. 2011;33(6):578–82.
68. MacDonald DB, Skinner S, Shils J, Yingling C. Intraoperative motor evoked potential monitoring – a position statement by the American Society of Neurophysiological Monitoring. Clin Neurophysiol. 2013;124(12):2291–316.

69. Kim SM, Kim SH, Seo DW, Lee KW. Intraoperative neurophysiologic monitoring: basic principles and recent update. J Korean Med Sci. 2013;28(9):1261–9.
70. Thirumala PD, Kassasm AB, Habeych M, Wichman K, Chang YF, Gardner P, et al. Somatosensory evoked potential monitoring during endoscopic endonasal approach to skull base surgery: analysis of observed changes. Neurosurgery. 2011;69(1 Suppl Operative):ons64-76.
71. Nuwer MR, Packwood JW. Intraoperative monitoring of neural function. Amsterdam: Elsevier; 2008.
72. Scheufler KM, Zentner J. Total intravenous anesthesia for intraoperative monitoring of the motor pathways: an integral view combining clinical and experimental data. J Neurosurg. 2002;96(3):571–9.
73. Huotari AM, Koskinen M, Suominen K, Alahuhta S, Remes R, Hartikainen KM, et al. Evoked EEG patterns during burst suppression with propofol. Br J Anaesth. 2004;92(1):18–24.
74. Sloan TB, Heyer EJ. Anesthesia for intraoperative neurophysiologic monitoring of the spinal cord. J Clin Neurophysiol. 2002;19(5):430–43.
75. Schubert A, Licina MG, Lineberry PJ. The effect of ketamine on human somatosensory evoked potentials and its modification by nitrous oxide. Anesthesiology. 1990;72(1):33–9.
76. Grundy BL, Jannetta PJ, Procopio PT, Lina A, Boston JR, Doyle E. Intraoperative monitoring of brain-stem auditory evoked potentials. J Neurosurg. 1982;19(5):396–408.
77. Saito T, Yamamoto I, Huang XL, Yukawa N, Osawa M, Takeichi S. Effects of muscle relaxants on EEG, ABR and EMG in rabbits. Hum Exp Toxicol. 1999;18(12):718–23.
78. Feroze RA, Mcdowell MM, Balzer J, Crammond DJ, Thirumala P, Sekula RF. Estimation of intraoperative stimulation threshold of the facial nerve in patients undergoing microvascular decompression. J Neurol Surg B Skull Base. 2019;80(6):599–603.
79. Thirumala PD, Mohanraj SK, Habeych M, Wichman K, Chang YF, Gardner P, et al. Value of free-run electromyographic monitoring of lower cranial nerves in endoscopic endonasal approach to skull base surgeries. J Neurol Surg B Skull Base. 2012;73(4):236–44.
80. Fang Y, Zhang H, Liu W, Li Y. A comparison of three induction regimens using succinylcholine, vecuronium, or no muscle relaxant: impact on the intraoperative monitoring of the lateral spread response in hemifacial spasm surgery: study protocol for a randomised controlled trial. Trials. 2012;13:160.
81. Wilkinson MF, Chowdhury T, Mutch WA, Kaufmann AM. Analysis of facial motor evoked potentials for assessing a central mechanism in hemifacial spasm. J Neurosurg. 2017;126(2):379–85.
82. Polo G, Fischer C, Sindou MP, Marneffe V, Bricolo A, Sala F, et al. Brainstem auditory evoked potential monitoring during microvascular decompression for hemifacial spasm: intraoperative brainstem auditory evoked potential changes and warning values to prevent hearing loss – prospective study in a consecutive series of 84. Neurosurgery. 2004;54(1):97–104.
83. Polo G, Fischer C. Intraoperative monitoring of brainstem auditory evoked potentials during microvascular decompression of cranial nerves in cerebellopontine angle. Neurochirurgie. 2009;55(2):152–7.
84. Huang BR, Chang CN, Hsu JC. Intraoperative electrophysiological monitoring in microvascular decompression for hemifacial spasm. J Clin Neurosci. 2009;16(2):209–13.
85. Sindou MP. Microvascular decompression for primary hemifacial spasm. Importance of intraoperative neurophysiological monitoring. Acta Neurochir. 2005;147(10):1019–26.
86. Park SK, Joo BE, Lee S, Lee JA, Hwang JH, Kong DS, et al. The critical warning sign of real-time brainstem auditory evoked potentials during microvascular decompression for hemifacial spasm. Clin Neurophysiol. 2018;129(5):1097–102.
87. Brock S, Scaioli V, Ferroli P, Broggi G. Neurovascular decompression in trigeminal neuralgia: role of intraoperative neurophysiological monitoring in the learning period. Stereotact Funct Neurosurg. 2004;82(5-6):199–206.

88. Thirumala PD, Carnovale G, Loke Y, Habeych ME, Crammond DJ, Balzer JR, et al. Brainstem auditory evoked potentials' diagnostic accuracy for hearing loss: systematic review and meta-analysis. J Neurol Surg B Skull Base. 2017;78(1):43–51.
89. Joo BE, Park SK, Cho KR, Kong DS, Seo DW, Park K. Real-time intraoperative monitoring of brainstem auditory evoked potentials during microvascular decompression for hemifacial spasm. J Neurosurg. 2016;125(5):1061–7.
90. Radtke RA, Erwin CW, Wilkins RH. Intraoperative brainstem auditory evoked potentials: significant decrease in postoperative morbidity. Neurology. 1989;39(2 Pt 1):187–91.
91. Simon MV. Neurophysiologic intraoperative monitoring of the vestibulocochlear nerve. J Clin Neurophysiol. 2011;28(6):566–81.
92. Moller AR, Moller MB. Does intraoperative monitoring of auditory evoked potentials reduce incidence of hearing loss as a complication of microvascular decompression of cranial nerves? Neurosurgery. 1989;24(2):257–63.
93. Motoyama Y, Nakagawa I, Takatani T, Park HS, Kotani Y, Tanaka Y, et al. Microvascular decompression for glossopharyngeal neuralgia using intraoperative neurophysiological monitoring: technical case report. Surg Neurol Int. 2016;7(Suppl 2):S28–35.
94. Thirumala P, Meigh K, Dasyam N, Shankar P, Sarma KRK, Sarma DRK, et al. The incidence of high-frequency hearing loss after microvascular decompression for trigeminal neuralgia, glossopharyngeal neuralgia, or geniculate neuralgia. J Neurosurg. 2015;123(6):1500–6.
95. Lee CC, Liao CH, Lin CF, Yang TF, Hsu SPC, Yen YS, et al. Brainstem auditory evoked potential monitoring and neuro-endoscopy: two tools to ensure hearing preservation and surgical success during microvascular decompression. J Chin Med Assoc. 2014;77(6):308–16.
96. He X, Li N, Liang J, Wang Y, Cao W, Qu Y, et al. Alarming effect of intraoperative neuroelectrophysiological monitoring in microvascular decompression for primary trigeminal neuralgia. Zhonghua Yi Xue Za Zhi. 2015;95(21):1651–4.
97. Wilkins RH, Radtke RA, Erwin CW. Value of intraoperative brainstem auditory evoked potential monitoring in reducing the auditory morbidity associated with microvascular decompression of cranial nerves. Skull Base Surg. 1991;1(2):106–9.
98. Ying T, Thirumala P, Chang Y, Habeych M, Crammond D, Balzer J. Empirical factors associated with brainstem auditory evoked potential monitoring during microvascular decompression for hemifacial spasm and its correlation to hearing loss. Acta Neurochir. 2014;156(3):571–5.
99. Legatt AD. Brainstem auditory evoked potentials (BAEPs). In: Encyclopedia of the neurological sciences. Elsevier Inc; 2014. p. 505–8.
100. Legatt AD, Pedley TA, Emerson RG, Stein BM, Abramson M. Normal brain-stem auditory evoked potentials with abnormal latency-intensity studies in patients with acoustic neuromas. Arch Neurol. 1988;45(12):1326–30.
101. Martin WH, Stecker MM. ASNM position statement: intraoperative monitoring of auditory evoked potentials. J Clin Monit Comput. 2008;22(1):75–85.
102. Mohanraj SK, Thirumala PD, Habeych ME, Crammond DJ, Balzer JR. Appropriate time to establish baseline responses for brain stem auditory evoked potentials during microvascular decompression for hemifacial spasm. J Clin Neurophysiol. 2014;31(5):500–4.
103. Lee MH, Lee HS, Jee TK, Il JK, Kong DS, Lee JA, et al. Cerebellar retraction and hearing loss after microvascular decompression for hemifacial spasm. Acta Neurochir. 2015;57(2):337–43.
104. American Clinical Neurophysiology Society. Guideline eleven: guidelines for intraoperative monitoring of sensory evoked potentials. J Clin Neurophysiol. 1994;11:77–87.
105. Thirumala PD, Ilangovan P, Habeych M, Crammond DJ, Balzer J. Analysis of interpeak latencies of brainstem auditory evoked potential waveforms during microvascular decompression of cranial nerve VII for hemifacial spasm. Neurosurg Focus. 2013;34(3):E6.
106. Harner SG, Michel Harper C, Beatty CW, Litchy WJ, Ebersold MJ. Far-field auditory brainstem response in neurotologic surgery. Am J Otol. 1996;17(1):150–3.

107. Nadol JB, Chiong CM, Ojemann RG, McKenna MJ, Martuza RL, Montgomery WW, et al. Preservation of hearing and facial nerve function in resection of acoustic neuroma. Laryngoscope. 1992;102(10):1153–8.
108. Der LC, Wei IH, Tsai MH, Kao MC, Lai CH, Hsu CJ, et al. Changes in guinea pig cochlea after transient cochlear ischemia. Neuroreport. 2010;21(15):968–75.
109. Ogata K, Naito M. Blood flow of peripheral nerve effects of dissection stretching and compression. J Hand Surg Am. 1986;11(1):10–4.
110. Baik MW, Branston NM, Bentivoglio P, Symon L. The effects of experimental brain-stem ischaemia on brain-stem auditory evoked potentials in primates. Electroencephalogr Clin Neurophysiol. 1990;75(5):433–43.
111. Wall EJ, Massie JB, Kwan MK, Rydevik BL, Myers RR, Garfin SR. Experimental stretch neuropathy: changes in nerve conduction under tension. J Bone Joint Surg Br. 1992;74(1):126–9.
112. Harner SG, Daube JR, Ebersold MJ. Electrophysiologic monitoring of facial nerve during. Laryngoscope. 1986;32(3):399–405.
113. Harper CM. Intraoperative cranial nerve monitoring. Muscle Nerve. 2004;29(3):339–51.
114. Kartush JM, LaRouere MJ, Graham MD, Bouchard KR, Audet BV. Intraoperative cranial nerve monitoring during posterior. Skull Base Surg. 1991;1(2):85–92.
115. Minahan RE, Mandir AS. Neurophysiologic intraoperative monitoring of trigeminal and facial nerves. J Clin Neurophysiol. 2011;28(6):551–65.
116. Prass RL, Luders H. Acoustic (loudspeaker) facial electromyographic monitoring: part 1. Evoked electromyographic activity during acoustic neuroma resection. Neurosurgery. 1986;19(3):392–400.
117. Schlake HP, Goldbrunner R, Milewski C, Siebert M, Behr R, Riemann R, et al. Technical developments in intra-operative monitoring for the preservation of cranial motor nerves and hearing in skull base surgery. Neurol Res. 1999;21(1):11–24.
118. Moller AR, Jannetta PJ. Preservation of facial function during removal of acoustic neuromas. Use of monopolar constant-voltage stimulation and EMG. J Neurosurg. 1984;61(4):757–60.
119. Tracy Mishler E, Smith PG. Technical aspects of intraoperative monitoring of lower cranial nerve function. Skull Base Surg. 1995;5(4):245–50.
120. Singh R, Husain AM. Neurophysiologic intraoperative monitoring of the glossopharyngeal and vagus nerves. J Clin Neurophysiol. 2011;28(6):582–6.
121. Taha JM, Tew JM, Keith RW, Payner TD. Intraoperative monitoring of the vagus nerve during intracranial glossopharyngeal and upper vagal rhizotomy: technical note. Neurosurgery. 1994;35(4):775–7.
122. Møller AR, Jannetta PJ. Hemifacial spasm: results of electrophysiologic recording during microvascular decompression operations. Neurology. 1985;35(7):969–74.
123. Mooij JJA, Mustafa MK, Van Weerden TW, Barker FG, Møller AR, Barrow DL, et al. Hemifacial spasm: intraoperative electromyographic monitoring as a guide for microvascular decompression. Neurosurgery. 2001;49(6):1365–70.
124. Shin JC, Chung UH, Kim YC. Prospective study of microvascular decompression in hemifacial spasm. Neurosurgery. 1997;88(4):730–4.
125. Yamashita S, Kawaguchi T, Fukuda M, Watanabe M, Tanaka R, Kameyama S. Abnormal muscle response monitoring during microvascular decompression for hemifacial spasm. Acta Neurochir. 2005;9(4):347–51.
126. Dannenbaum M, Lega BC, Suki D, Harper RL, Yoshor D. Microvascular decompression for hemifacial spasm: long-term results from 114 operations performed without neurophysiological monitoring. J Neurosurg. 2008;109(3):410–5.
127. Il JW, Lee KJ, Park HK, Chough CK, Rha HK. Prognostic value of intra-operative lateral spread response monitoring during microvascular decompression in patients with hemifacial spasm. J Clin Neurosci. 2008;106(3):384–7.
128. Kiya N, Bannur U, Yamauchi A, Yoshida K, Kato Y, Kanno T. Monitoring of facial evoked EMG for hemifacial spasm: a critical analysis of its prognostic value. Acta Neurochir. 2001;143(4):365–8.

129. Sekula RF, Bhatia S, Frederickson AM, Jannetta PJ, Quigley MR, Small GA, et al. Utility of intraoperative electromyography in microvascular decompression for hemifacial spasm: a meta-analysis. Neurosurg Focus. 2009;27(4):E10.
130. Donna Jacobs R EEG T CN. A practical approach to neurophysiologic intraoperative monitoring. J Neurol Neurophysiol. 2014;56(1):48.
131. Kandan SR, Khan S, Jeyaretna DS, Lhatoo S, Patel NK, Coakham HB. Neuralgia of the glossopharyngeal and vagal nerves: long-term outcome following surgical treatment and literature review. Br J Neurosurg. 2010;24(4):441–6.
132. Xiong NX, Zhao HY, Zhang FC, Liu RE. Vagoglossopharyngeal neuralgia treated by microvascular decompression and glossopharyngeal rhizotomy: clinical results of 21 cases. Stereotact Funct Neurosurg. 2012;90(1):45–50.
133. Yingling CD, Ashram YA. Intraoperative monitoring of cranial nerves in skull base surgery. Neurotology. 2005;5(3):958–93.
134. Fukuda M, Takao T, Hiraishi T, Fujii Y. Free-running EMG monitoring during microvascular decompression for hemifacial spasm. Acta Neurochir. 2015;157(9):1505–12.
135. Lakshmi Prasad G, Kumar V, Menon G. Delayed facial palsy after microvascular decompression: report of two cases. J Neurosci Rural Pract. 2017;8(3):461–5.
136. Moller AR, Jannetta PJ. Microvascular decompression in hemifacial spasm: intraoperative electrophysiological observations. Neurosurgery. 1985;16(5):612–8.
137. Moller AR, Jannetta PJ. Monitoring facial EMG responses during microvascular decompression operations for hemifacial spasm. J Neurosurg. 1987;15(6):496–9.
138. Yamashita S, Kawaguchi T, Fukuda M, Suzuki K, Watanabe M, Tanaka R, et al. Lateral spread response elicited by double stimulation in patients with hemifacial spasm. Muscle Nerve. 2002;25(6):845–9.
139. von Eckardstein K, Link M. The significance of intraoperative electromyographic "lateral spread" in predicting outcome of microvascular decompression for hemifacial spasm. J Neurol Surg B Skull Base. 2012;75(3):198–203.
140. Neves DO, Lefaucheur JP, Ciampi De Andrade D, Hattou M, Ahdab R, Ayache SS, et al. A reappraisal of the value of lateral spread response monitoring in the treatment of hemifacial spasm by microvascular decompression. J Neurol Neurosurg Psychiatry. 2009;80(12):1375–80.
141. Kong DS, Park K, Shin BG, Jeong AL, Eum DO. Prognostic value of the lateral spread response for intraoperative electromyography monitoring of the facial musculature during microvascular decompression for hemifacial spasm. J Neurosurg. 2007;106(3):384–7.
142. Lee S, Park SK, Lee JA, Joo BE, Kong DS, Seo DW, et al. A new method for monitoring abnormal muscle response in hemifacial spasm: a prospective study. Clin Neurophysiol. 2018;129(7):1490–5.
143. Thirumala PD, Wang X, Shah A, Habeych M, Crammond D, Balzer JR, et al. Clinical impact of residual lateral spread response after adequate microvascular decompression for hemifacial spasm: a retrospective analysis. Br J Neurosurg. 2015;29(6):818–22.
144. Thirumala PD, Shah AC, Nikonow TN, Habeych ME, Balzer JR, Crammond DJ, et al. Microvascular decompression for hemifacial spasm: evaluating outcome prognosticators including the value of intraoperative lateral spread response monitoring and clinical characteristics in 293 patients. J Clin Neurophysiol. 2011;28(1):56–66.
145. Nielsen VK. Electrophysiology of the facial nerve in hemifacial spasm: ectopic/ephaptic excitation. Muscle Nerve. 1985;8(7):545–55.
146. Park S-K, Joo B-E, Park K. Intraoperative neurophysiological monitoring during microvascular decompression surgery for hemifacial spasm. J Korean Neurosurg Soc. 2019;62(4):367–75. Available from: https://pubmed.ncbi.nlm.nih.gov/31290293
147. Tobishima H, Hatayama T, Ohkuma H. Relation between the persistence of an abnormal muscle response and the long-term clinical course after microvascular decompression for hemifacial spasm. Neurol Med Chir (Tokyo). 2014;54(6):474–82.
148. Xu XL, Zhen XK, Yuan Y, Liu HJ, Liu J, Xu J, et al. Long-term outcome of repeat microvascular decompression for hemifacial spasm. World Neurosurg. 2018;110:e989–97.

149. Fukuda M, Oishi M, Takao T, Hiraishi T, Sato Y, Fujii Y. Monitoring of abnormal muscle response and facial motor evoked potential during microvascular decompression for hemifacial spasm. Surg Neurol Int. 2012;3:118.
150. Park JS, Lee S, Park SK, Lee JA, Park K. Facial motor evoked potential with paired transcranial magnetic stimulation: prognostic value following microvascular decompression for hemifacial spasm. J Neurosurg. 2019;131(6):1780–7.
151. Wilkinson MF, Kaufmann AM. Monitoring of facial muscle motor evoked potentials during microvascular decompression for hemifacial spasm: evidence of changes in motor neuron excitability. J Neurosurg. 2005;103(1):64–9.
152. Fernández-Conejero I, Ulkatan S, Sen C, Deletis V. Intra-operative neurophysiology during microvascular decompression for hemifacial spasm. Clin Neurophysiol. 2012;123(1):78–83.
153. Fukuda M, Oishi M, Takao T, Saito A, Fujii Y. Facial nerve motor-evoked potential monitoring during skull base surgery predicts facial nerve outcome. J Neurol Neurosurg Psychiatry. 2008;79(9):1066–70.
154. MacDonald DB. When to warn – update on interpretation of MEP. Clin Neurophysiol. 2016;127(3):e50.
155. Liu Q, Wang Q, Liu H, Wu WKK, Chan MTV. Warning criteria for intraoperative neurophysiologic monitoring. Curr Opin Anaesthesiol. 2017;30(5):557–62.
156. MacDonald DB. Overview on criteria for MEP monitoring. J Clin Neurophysiol. 2017;34(1):4–11.
157. Goto T, Muraoka H, Kodama K, Hara Y, Yako T, Hongo K. Intraoperative monitoring of motor evoked potential for the facial nerve using a cranial peg-screw electrode and a "threshold-level" stimulation method. Skull Base. 2010;20(6):429–34.
158. Kaufmann A. Microvascular decompression surgery for hemifacial spasm. In: Schmidek & sweet operative neurosurgical techniques: indications, methods, and results. 5th ed; 2006. p. 1473–90.

Part V
Spine and Spinal Cord Surgery

Chapter 22
Spinal Deformity Surgery

Ricardo José Rodriguez Ferreira, Emília Caram Bordini, André Cleriston J. dos Santos, Roberto Waldesmand Farias Pontes, Paulo Tadeu Maia Cavali, and Tiago Bertacini Gonzaga

Abbreviations

BIS	Bispectral index
EMG	Electromyography
EMG-fr	Electromyography free running
EMG-tg	Electromyography triggered
IONM	Intraoperative neurophysiological monitoring
MAP	Mean arterial pressure
MEP	Motor evoked potential
MEP-CM	Cortical-myogenic motor evoked potential

R. J. R. Ferreira (✉) · E. C. Bordini
AACD - Disabled Child Care Association, São Paulo, SP, Brazil

Dr Ricardo Ferreira Clinic, São Paulo, SP, Brazil

Spine Surgery Department at Orthopedics and Trauma Institute of Clinical Hospital of the University of São Paulo Medical School, São Paulo, SP, Brazil

A. C. J. dos Santos · R. W. F. Pontes
Neurology and Neurophysiology Department, Ribeirão Preto Medical School of the, University of São Paulo, Ribeirão Preto, SP, Brazil

P. T. M. Cavali
Scoliosis Group, AACD - Disabled Child Care, Association, São Paulo, SP, Brazil

Scoliosis Department at Sirio Libanês Hospital, São Paulo, SP, Brazil

T. B. Gonzaga
Anesthesiology Department, AACD - Child Care Association, São Paulo, SP, Brazil

S. M. Verst et al. (eds.), *Intraoperative Monitoring*,
https://doi.org/10.1007/978-3-030-95730-8_22

MEP-CS	Cortical-spinal motor evoked potential (D-wave)
SSEP	Somatosensory evoked potential
Tc-MEP	Transcranial motor evoked potential
TIVA	Total venous anesthesia
TOF	Train of four

Surgeon's Point of View

Surgical treatment of spinal deformities has greatly evolved in the last 20 years, making possible the corrections of very accentuated and rigid curves. The most pronounced and rigid deformities are those with the highest risk for neurological complications, especially cases of congenital kyphosis, acute angle kyphosis, kyphosis secondary to achondroplasia, scoliosis above 100° cobb, and scoliosis due to neurofibromatosis. Yet, there has been an increase in efficiency and safety, especially regarding the risks of neurological lesions.

This evolution encloses anesthesia, analgesic medications, drugs that reduce intraoperative bleeding, technological development inside the operating room, intraoperative 3D imaging devices such as the O-Arm, virtual navigation, and robotics. Three specific factors should be emphasized:

1. Evolution of implants and instruments
2. New techniques of leading with the flexibility of the sharp and rigid curves such as the development of new osteotomies and vertebrectomies
3. Advent of multimodal intraoperative neurophysiological monitoring (IONM)

It is important to point out that the implants, such as the pedicle screws, and the instruments for fixation and correction of the spinal deformities are not the same ones used for the fixations of spinal surgeries in general, such as trauma surgeries, spinal degenerative diseases, tumor surgeries, etc. Implants and instruments for deformity correction surgery are specific because they are extremely powerful forceps that act in several planes: coronal, sagittal, and axial. They are offered in several models: multiplanar or polyaxial, uniplanar or monoaxial, the flexible sublaminar bands, and different types of hooks and cages for anterior support. They match specially designed instruments, improving versatility and the grade of correction.

The risks of a traumatic neurological injury produced by instruments, such as Kerrison, high rotation or ultrasonic drill, curette, or osteotomes, during osteotomy always exist. These procedures must be performed by trained and experienced surgeons, with the use of adequate materials and specific instruments, and under the continuous control of IONM.

Although improvement in the degree of correction is desirable, the currently main limiting factors for correction became bone quality and the patient's neurological status during the act of "reduction" (correction) of the deformity. If the surgeon underestimates these limiting factors, there may be neurological damage triggered by pulling out or loosening of the implants, bone fractures, migration of the implants into the spinal canal or foramen, or even an abrupt and exaggerated correction of the deformity that causes spinal ischemia.

Ponte's osteotomy, pedicle subtraction osteotomy, and posterior approach vertebrectomy are techniques for making the spine more flexible to allow greater correction of very sharp and rigid curves. These techniques are based on the removal of anatomical structures, that is, the removal of bony and ligamentous parts of the vertebrae, "destabilizing" them to increase vertebral motility in the osteotomized segment.

In Ponte's osteotomy, the anatomical structures of the posterior arch are removed, such as spinous apophysis, lamina, intra-articular pars, and facets. In the pedicle subtraction osteotomy, besides all the structures of the posterior arch, the pedicles are totally resected, and a wedge or "V"-shaped osteotomy is performed on the posterior aspect of the vertebral body. In the vertebral resection or total vertebrectomy, the entire vertebra is removed posteriorly, in addition to the respective superior and inferior intervertebral discs.

Thus, the greater the removal of parts of vertebral structure, the greater the destabilization and therefore the correction of deformities. Yet, it increases intraoperative neurological-related risks. The relationship of the potential correction of an osteotomy to the potential risk of neurological injury is directly proportional.

These osteotomies are "holes" or "gaps" created in the osteotomized segments that must be closed during the reduction maneuver for curve correction. In these closing movements of the osteotomies or wedges, the anteroposterior or laterolateral translation movement of the osteotomized upper segment over the lower segment must be avoided. It is related to "pinching" or stretching of the spinal cord or its roots, resulting in severe neurological injury. Yet, angular movements and the shortening of the osteotomized segment are strongly recommended, always keeping the congruence of the upper and lower extremities of the osteotomy.

IONM has been used routinely in spinal deformity surgeries since the late 1990s. We have been using IONM in our institution for the last 20 years, performing over 3600 scoliosis corrections. We followed the development in this area, from the use of somatosensory evoked potential as a sole technique to the current use of multimodal IONM. The new generation of scoliosis surgeons, anesthesiologists, and neurophysiologists should keep in mind that IONM is a real-time procedure. Therefore, a constant multidisciplinary understanding and communication between the team members are cornerstones. It is a sine qua non condition for the efficiency of IONM. One should understand exactly what role each member plays.

The use of 3D images through the O-Arm, navigation, and robotics has significantly increased the accuracy in the positioning of pedicle screws, drastically reducing the incidence of medullary and root lesions by invasion of the medullary canal and foramen, respectively. Yet, they do not replace IONM during deformity surgery. IONM performs real-time assessment of positioning, osteotomy performance, corrective maneuvers of compressions, rotations, and translations of the implants under the rods. Therefore, it is possible the immediate recognition of migration or loosening of material and bone fractures. Additionally, IONM can detect neural suffering in evolution during vertebral derotation, and position of the implant, whether it is caudal, cranial, lateral, or intracanal [19].

IONM starts before the surgery and immediately after the patient is anesthetized. At this moment, a complete IONM analysis is performed to determine the patient's basal data. Similarly, after the surgery and still inside the operating room, new data can diagnose any compromise of neurological functions. During the surgery, any IONM alteration should trigger a neurophysiological checklist, including blood pressure, bolus of anesthetic drugs, SO2, or technical failure of the equipment and electrodes. Exclusion of external sources directs attention to surgeon last maneuvers. Surgeon should consider reverting them and wait for IONM signal recovery. Stopping the surgery and removing all implants should be considered if there is a complete loss of neurological functional responses, and a wake-up test can be done to check on active lower limb movements.

Brief History

Historically, the detection of spinal cord injury during spinal surgical procedures was limited to the so-called wake-up test or Stagnara test, which was published in 1973 by Vauzelle, Stagnara, and Jouvinroux. The authors reported a case series describing what has become the first clinical intraoperative neurological test in scoliosis surgery.

The wake-up test was performed after preoperative orientation of the patient and anesthetic planning, so that after the deformity correction maneuvers (instrumentation, osteotomies, and rod implantation), the patient was awakened (still in the surgical position) and was asked to perform voluntary movements of the upper limbs (which served as a control, showing that the patient is understanding the commands) followed by moving the lower limbs. In the presence of upper limb movements and absence of lower limb movements, the test was considered positive. Appropriate measures were taken in an attempt to reverse the causes of paraplegia [68].

In the 1970s, somatosensory evoked potentials (SEP) [15] during scoliosis surgery began, followed by single-pulse stimulated electromyography (EMG-ST) to test the implantation of pedicle screws [6]. Motor evoked potentials (MEP) were added late in the 1990s [47]. In Brazil, IONM for scoliosis surgery started in AACD performed by the main author. More details on the history in Brazil and Latin America, refer to Chap. 1.

Introduction

Surgery for spinal deformity, even under the most experienced and skilled teams, brings risk to the neural structures [21, 23]. A careful control of the patient's hemodynamic and clinical parameters by the anesthesiologist is recommended since medullar hypoperfusion, added to surgical trauma, can cause neurological deficit.

Frequently, in neuromuscular scoliosis, patients present paraplegia and may have spasticity related to their underlying pathology. Even so, IONM is justified since additional injury associated with wrong implantation of pedicle screws may worsen the degree of spasticity. Moreover, many of those patients have functional control of sphincter, which must be continuously evaluated during surgery.

In patients in whom scoliosis is secondary, preoperative magnetic resonance (MRI) of the neuroaxis should evaluate the presence of coexistent spinal dysraphisms, especially tethered cord [17], syringomyelia, and intracanal neurofibroma. If those pathologies are not properly diagnosed and previously treated, at spinal cord stretching during correction of the deformity, irreversible neural damage may occur.

Today, multimodal intraoperative neurophysiological monitoring (IONM) (Fig. 22.1) is considered a "standard modality" during spinal deformity correction surgeries by the Scoliosis Research Society (2020) [22].

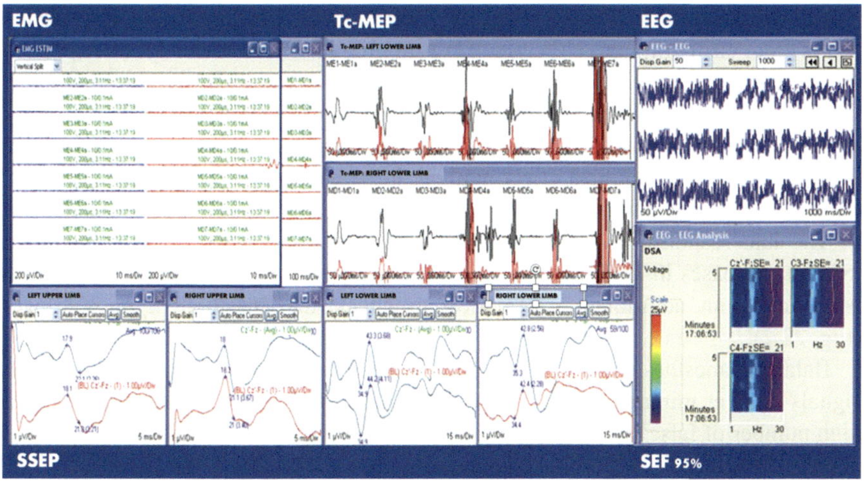

Fig. 22.1 **Multimodal IONM**

The most critical steps in deformity corrective surgeries are (1) instrumentation with pedicle screws, pedicle/facet hooks, sublaminar bands, or steel wires, (2) osteotomies, and (3) the correction of the deformity.

Anesthesia in Deformity Surgeries

Modern anesthesiology goes beyond the limits of the operating room, and its actions have repercussions from preparation to long-term postoperative prognosis [14, 71]. From this perspective, the anesthetic act must be planned and synchronized to IONM.

Thus, emphasis should be given to the use of drugs and techniques that have minimal interference in the register of neurophysiological signals or even facilitate their acquisition. Besides, the drugs should promote effective pain control, rapid recovery with less repercussions on the respiratory and hemodynamic systems, and hematimetric, cardiocirculatory, and thermal control.

In a surgical scenario, the anesthesiologist should be aware that most of his drugs may interfere with the generation of IONM signals, out mostly resulting in misinterpretation of signal deterioration. Therefore, he should avoid large fluctuations in the anesthetic plan [74]. Fast titrating drugs that allow changes in the anesthetic plan and recovery of the neurological status should always be preferred. Chapter 5 brings detailed information on general anesthesia.

Anesthetic Technique

Recent data supports total venous anesthesia (TIVA) as the main anesthetic option in spinal deformity surgeries using IONM ([51] [38] [34] Lo et al. 2006). TIVA allows a better balancing of the dose-dependent drug regime, facilitating neurophysiological signal recordings, especially regarding motor evoked potential (MEP), and is more easily titrated. However, TIVA in high doses decreases MEP amplitude in a dose-dependent manner [42].

The hypnotic-level monitoring using bispectral index (BIS) or SEF-95 entropy allows for a more rational and balanced use of anesthetic agents, at the lowest possible doses for the desired clinical effect, without large fluctuations in plasma concentrations. Consequently, it enhances the generation and interpretation of IONM signals.

The late response (N2) of the tibial nerve somatosensory evoked potentials (SSEP) decreases in amplitude with increasing hypnosis [61]. This parameter can be used as an additional information to check the anesthetic/hypnosis level (Fig. 22.2).

Balanced anesthesia using halogenated, despite easy titration, can suppress MEP signals even at minimal alveolar concentrations (MAC) such as 0.5, leading to a high number of false positives [71].

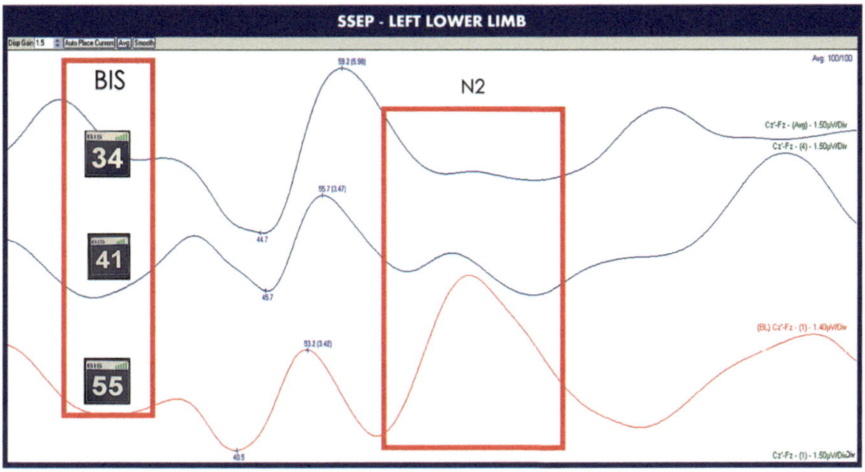

Fig. 22.2 Tibial nerve SSEP late responses and its relation with de bispectral index (BIS). The left red rectangle shows the BIS values; the right red rectangle shows the appearance and increasing of the N2 response as the BIS values gets higher

Multimodal Analgesia

Through the synergism of different analgesic effects of several drugs, multimodal analgesic therapy plays an important role in nociceptive inhibition in spinal deformity surgeries. It reduces the administration of opioids and, consequently, their adverse effects, prevents hyperalgesia and pain chronicity, and reduces postoperative systemic inflammatory status. Understanding the characteristics of these drugs is fundamental to know which and when to use them in spinal surgeries with IONM.

Lidocaine

Lidocaine promotes analgesia, both peripherally and centrally, by reducing the neuronal response to pain. A meta-analysis that included 2802 surgical patients demonstrated that continuous intravenous lidocaine infusion initiated before the surgical incision promoted reduction in pain scores for up to 24 h postoperatively [57]. For patients undergoing spinal surgery, evidence suggests a reduction in opioid consumption from the intraoperative period up to 48 h postoperatively [3], with emphasis on the first 6 h (with a reduction in consumption at the range of 30%). Lidocaine has an anti-inflammatory effect with diminishing serum levels of pro-inflammatory markers.

Besides not having a direct adverse effect on IONM, when used intraoperatively as part of the TIVA regimen, lidocaine improves neurophysiological signals by reducing the consumption of propofol and opioids (Seki 2018).

Ketamine

Because of its minimal effect on IONM responses and its analgesic effect, ketamine is considered the main adjunct of TIVA regimen for spinal deformity surgery [71]. Its analgesic effect, even in subdoses, makes it an essential component of multimodal analgesia and is particularly useful in controlling pain chronicity.

A recent meta-analysis demonstrated that the perioperative use of ketamine decreased postoperative pain intensity and morphine consumption, without increasing the incidence of adverse effects, in several types of surgery (Seki 2019).

Ketamine may even increase the amplitude of SSEP and MEP responses. This effect may be beneficial, especially for patients with preoperative neurological deficits.

Alpha-Agonists

Alpha-agonists may be used as part of multimodal analgesia regimens during several types of surgeries (Seki 2018).

In spinal deformity surgeries, they seem to be related to lower postoperative pain scores, with reduced opioid consumption throughout the perioperative period [24]. At low doses, they do not demonstrate major interference with IONM. However, at higher doses, or through synergism with propofol, they can dramatically reduce recorded neurophysiological responses [1, 2, 24]. Attention should be given to the difficulty of titration and its great sedative power.

Due to their beneficial analgesic effect, they can be used at low doses or soon after the last IONM responses are obtained.

Magnesium Sulfate

Anesthetic adjuvant used for many decades, magnesium exhibits curare-like effects by antagonizing acetylcholine in neuromuscular transmission, acting as a synergist with inhaled anesthetic drugs and neuromuscular blockers in muscle relaxation.

It causes bronchodilation and is particularly useful in the anesthetic management of patients with asthma and other lung pathologies. It is a useful drug in the multimodal analgesic regimen by acting and amplifying the effects of NMDA receptor antagonism.

During spinal deformity surgery, magnesium has a deleterious effect on the of myogenic responses (Tc-MEP and EMG), and therefore its use should be avoided.

Neuromuscular Blockers

It is usually assumed that neuromuscular blockers should not be used in spinal deformity surgeries with IONM. However, our protocol includes them at strategic moments of the surgery, as long as they can be quickly reversed to allow proper analysis of the MEP and EMG during critical steps of the approach.

Succinylcholine, a depolarizing neuromuscular blocker, is commonly used to facilitate orotracheal intubation. It has a short-life action. In addition, its administration avoids very deep initial anesthetic plans, which enhances IONM first recordings.

Some depolarizing neuromuscular blockers of intermediate duration, such as rocuronium, can be used in this surgical scenario since its specific reversal agent, Sugammadex®, is available.

Hemodynamic Control

Reduction in blood pressure levels diminishes cerebral and spinal cord blood flow, but autoregulation mechanisms maintain their perfusion pressures. However, in the perioperative period, especially for patients with previous neurological deficits, these reductions in blood pressure may add risk [70, 77].

In an ideal scenario, pressure anesthetic management should aim to maintain the same baseline values or at least mean arterial pressure around 80–85 mmHg [71, 77]. Induced hypotension should await the IONM baseline recordings and may be restricted to the paravertebral muscles' dissection period, aiming to avoid excessive bleeding in this phase. Proper blood mean pressure levels should be reestablished at the time of surgical instrumentation [74].

Special attention must be given to large variations and pressure liabilities during surgery, because they cause confusion in the interpretation of neurophysiological signals, generating false positives. By IONM, signal deterioration is indicated to raise the mean arterial pressure above 85mmhg. This measure can solve, on average, 20% of cases [74].

Hematimetric Control

As in the general perioperative context, there is no ideal numerical value for hemoglobin and hematocrit in spinal deformity surgeries. However, evidence points to a direct association between spinal cord ischemia and low hemoglobin levels. This event can be proven by deterioration of Tc-MEP and SSEP signals, when facing a hypovolemic shock.

Decrease in hemoglobin levels diminishes arterial oxygen content. In addition, large blood volume losses raise the serum levels of anesthetic drugs, both culminating in neurophysiological signal deterioration. It may cause false-positive results [33]. Safe levels of hemoglobin, both for medullary protection and for the correct interpretation of IONM, are around 9–10 g/dL [73].

The intraoperative use of antifibrinolytic agents allows greater hematimeter control in these surgeries, avoiding massive transfusions of blood products [27]. Tranexamic acid is the most used drug during spinal deformity surgery. Its main adverse effects are thromboembolic events and seizures, which are not usual by 50 mg/kg of weight and maintenance doses of 5–10 mg/kg/h [26].

Thermal Control

Maintaining normothermia is important in the perioperative period because it maintains enzymatic functions and homeostasis. In addition, it is associated with lower rates of infection due to the implant of synthesis material.

Hypothermia and, especially, abrupt temperature variations in the intraoperative period reduce the amplitude of Tc-MEP and increase the latency of SSEP. Another deleterious effect of hypothermia is the possibility of elevating the plasma levels of drugs [45].

Anesthesia Positioning Care

After introducing bite blockers inside the mouth, it is time to promote the ventral positioning. Care should be taken to avoid peripheral neural compressions. The placement of the cushions should result in adequate venous return; otherwise, it may generate decreased blood flow. These events could interfere with IONM recordings.

The head should be properly positioned, with attention to the degree of cervical flexion and absence of ocular compression (MacDonald et al. 2013).

IONM Protocol in Deformity Surgeries

Surgeries to correct deformity are performed with the patient in ventral decubitus. There are rare cases in which a lateral approach may be necessary, to perform discectomies or even corpectomies, aiming to turn rigid curvatures more flexible.

Preoperative

Anesthesia

TIVA protocol and the correct placement of anti-bite guards are recommended.

Nursing

- Bladder catheterization. In female patients, when the electrodes have already been applied, as a form of protection, it is suggested that the neurophysiologist assist in the patient's leg opening, as well as, at the end of the catheterization, to put the lower limbs back in the proper position.
- Skin protection on bony prominences, avoiding the occurrence of pressure ulcers, with adhesives. It is suggested that the neurophysiologist insert the electrodes before this nursing step.
- Anti-thromboembolic event protocol. When possible, it is suggested to avoid the use of elastic stockings, as these can promote the modification or loosening of the electrodes in the lower limbs. Crepe bandages can be used instead. If indicated, pneumatic compressors can be used.

Neurophysiology

Preparation

With the patient already anesthetized, proceed to apply the needle and surface electrodes. Corkscrew needle electrodes adapted to the scalp for both SSEP and MEP according to the 10/20 or 10/10 EMG system.

SSEP

Stimulation
We stimulate the ulnar and tibial nerves with surface electrodes. In specific cases, such as the presence of edema of the extremities or morbid obesity, subdermal needle electrodes can be used.

In the upper limbs, it is also possible to use the median nerve, but our preference for the ulnar nerve is due to the following factors:

A. Analysis of the complete posterior cervical spinal cord pathway from C8 to T1
B. Evaluation of upper limb positioning, especially elbows
C. Better position of the electrodes on the wrist, leaving the lateral edge free for radial artery puncture

Recording

C3′/C4′ (upper limbs), Cz′/Fz (lower limbs). To analyze segments of the sensory pathway, other electrodes may be added: Erb's point for upper limbs (N9) and popliteal fossa (N8) for lower limbs. Segmentation is recommended because it can serve as a sentinel.

Tc-MEP and EMG

Tc-MEP Stimulation Corkscrew electrodes should be inserted at positions C3/C4 or C1/C2. These electrodes can also be inserted up to cm anterior to these positions.

Recording

Deformity surgeries should have muscle recording according to Table 22.1.

Pitfalls

A. *Importance of Using the Complete Protocol*

We recommend the recording of all myotomes abovementioned because it enables correct data interpretation during the "Transpedicular Neurophysiological Navigation" (detailed below).

The same applies to Tc-MEP. It is known that the most robust Tc-MEP responses are usually obtained in the more distal muscles, due to their representation in the motor cortex [49]. Although some protocols include only tibialis anterior and abductor hallucis muscles, it may induce misinterpretation and make it impossible to diagnose sentinel events during the surgery, such as femoral nerve compression by positioning and sciatic nerve stretching by skeletal traction in the lower limb.

Table 22.1 Recording myotomes suggested for the IONM in deformity spine surgerie. Corresponding muscle atlas is available in Chap. 3

Myotome	Nerve root	Nerve
Abductor digiti minimi	**C8–T1**	Ulnar
Intercostalis	T2–T5	Intercostal
Rectus abdominis	T6–T12	Intercostal
Iliopsoas	**L1–L2**	Femoral
Rectus femoris	L2–**L3**–L4	Femoral
Tibialis anterior	**L4**–S1	Deep fibular
Fibularis longus	**L5**–S1	Superficial fibular
Gastrocnemius	L5–**S1**	Tibial
Abductor hallucis	S1–**S2**	Medial plantar
External anal sphincter	**S2–S3–S4**	Pudendal

In addition, in neuromuscular scoliosis, numerous underlying pathologies are observed. The distal responses may be more compromised than the proximal ones, for example, in patients with associated hereditary polyneuropathies.

B. *External Anal Sphincter*

We emphasize that in all surgeries involving pedicle instrumentation in lumbosacral territory, and in cases of neuromuscular scoliosis, S2–S4 (external anal sphincter) root recording is mandatory. In the latter group, this is often the only response obtained by Tc-MEP.

C. *Femoral Nerve: Iliopsoas and Quadriceps*

Since the surgery is performed with the patient in ventral decubitus, supported by cushions placed in the hip region, femoral nerve may get compressed. Hence, MEP and EMG monitoring of muscles innervated by the femoral nerve is mandatory. It allows identification of the event and repositioning of the cushions, at the level of the anterosuperior iliac spines, with recovery of the potentials (Fig. 22.3). The misinterpretation as spinal cord suffering could lead to unnecessary interruption of the surgery, causing stress to the surgical team and undermining the credibility of the IONM.

Another particularity of the femoral and sciatic territories is during the intraoperative cranial and/or transfemoral traction. During this maneuver, there is a risk of excessive stretching of the spinal cord, roots, and peripheral nerves. Tc-MEP should be performed before the traction and repeated after load placement. If a significant deterioration (amplitude drop >50%) is observed, it is recommended to reduce the load until parameters return to baseline. The main mechanism of injury is vascular, and therefore, the alterations may not be immediate. Thus, surveillance with Tc-MEP must last at least 10 min after the traction.

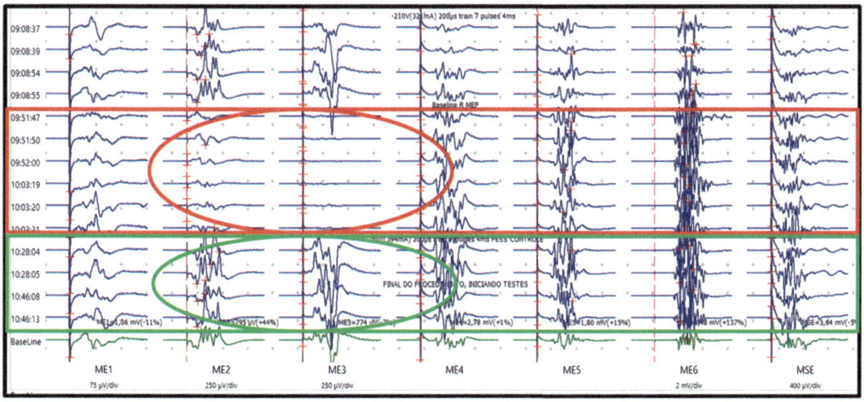

Fig. 22.3 Tc-MEP responses of the left lower limb: transient amplitude drop in the femoral nerve territory. Red circle: Tc-MEP amplitude drop in the iliopsoas and quadriceps muscles; Green circle: Tc-MEP amplitude recovery after repositioning the cushions at the level of the anterosuperior iliac spines

D. *Muscle Recording*

Muscle recordings, mandatorily, must be done with recording and reference electrodes inserted in the SAME muscle. This information may seem obvious, but it is not uncommon to observe the so-called hybrid recording in some protocols. We emphasize that in deformity correction surgeries, the segmentation of root territories is of particular importance for accurate diagnosis, in both EMG-ST and Tc-MEP.

Positioning

After the patient is transferred to the ventral decubitus, the neurophysiological tests should be repeated and compared with the baselines previously recorded in dorsal decubitus. It allows technical and anesthesiologic checklist. Moreover, the baseline in dorsal decubitus can identify previous neurological deficits.

Intraoperative

Deformity correction surgery has main steps, and IONM should follow each one. Therefore, a step-by-step IONM protocol is proposed below.

Step-by-Step IONM Protocol

1. Exposure of anatomical planes – EMG-fr, Tc-MEP, and SSEP
2. Instrumentation – pedicle screws: EMG-ST, Tc-MEP, and SSEP
3. Instrumentation – sublaminar bands or hooks: EMG-fr, Tc-MEP, and SSEP
4. Osteotomies – EMG-fr, Tc-MEP, and SSEP
5. Placement of rods – Tc-MEP and SSEP
6. Deformity correction – Tc-MEP and SSEP
7. Closure by planes – Tc-MEP and SSEP

Considerations

- *Step 1*: After MEP baselines in ventral position, neuromuscular blockade with rocuronium may be done, as described under the topic 4.2. If used, Sugammadex® should be administered before the next step.
- *Step 2*: During the pedicle screw instrumentation, there is the risk of direct lesion of the medulla (thoracic screws) or cauda equina (lumbosacral screws), in the case of medialization of the screw and rupture of the medial wall of the pedicle. Special attention should be given to the proximity of the spinal cord to the pedi-

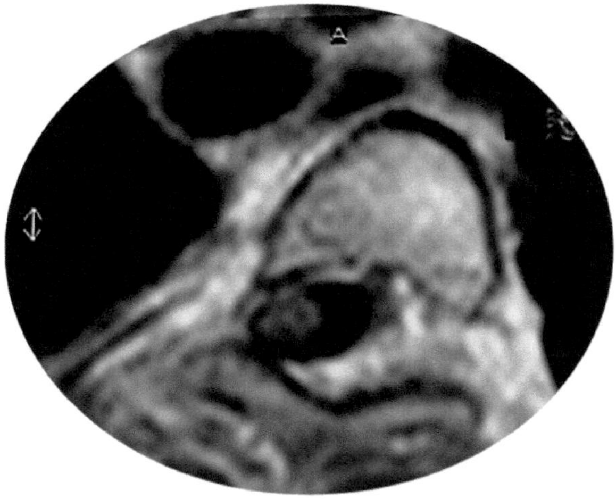

Fig. 22.4 MRI: Apex of the concavity curve. This shows the proximity of the spinal cord to the pedicle vertebra in the concavity of the curve

cle vertebra in the concavity of the curve (Fig. 22.4). Additionally, the perforation and transfixation of any pedicle cortical (superior, inferior, lateral, or medial) may result in radicular lesion.

- Therefore, EMG-ST and Tc-MEP and SEP should be performed. During thoracic instrumentation, Tc-MEP should be performed intermittently after each pedicle instrumentation, interspersed with EMG-ST.
- The particularities of EMG-ST at this stage will be addressed in the topic "Transpedicular Neurophysiological Navigation" (section "Pedicle Instrumentation").
- *Step 3*: Sublaminar bands and hooks can serve as a supporting element for the corrective rods. They can cause direct injury to the neural tissue, which can be identified by SSEP because of injury to the dorsal column of the spinal cord (Fig. 22.5). Interspersing EMG-ST with EMG-fr and Tc-MEP allows prompt identification of adverse events and reversal of the maneuver.
- *Step 4*: Osteotomies are critical steps with a high risk of spinal cord injury. Ponte's osteotomy approach is the most used. Indeed, the greater the resection of vertebral elements in an osteotomy, the greater the exposure of the spinal cord and, consequently, the greater the risk of inadvertent percussion by the instruments. Thus, continuous monitoring with EMG-fr, Tc-MEP, and SEP is paramount.
- The presence of neurotonic discharges in EMG-fr is suggestive of neural insult, which is checked with Tc-MEP, and, if necessary, a pause in the maneuvers to await recovery is requested (Fig. 22.6).
- Usually, the direct spinal MEP (D-wave) has no indication in deformity surgeries because the instrumentation generally extends to the lumbar levels. However, our protocol includes D-wave in very particular cases, such as in acute angle congenital kyphoscoliosis involving hemivertebrae or vertebral fusions in the thoracic territory. In our experience, during the osteotomy phase at the apex of the deformity, or even during spinal decompression in cases of stenosis, D-wave

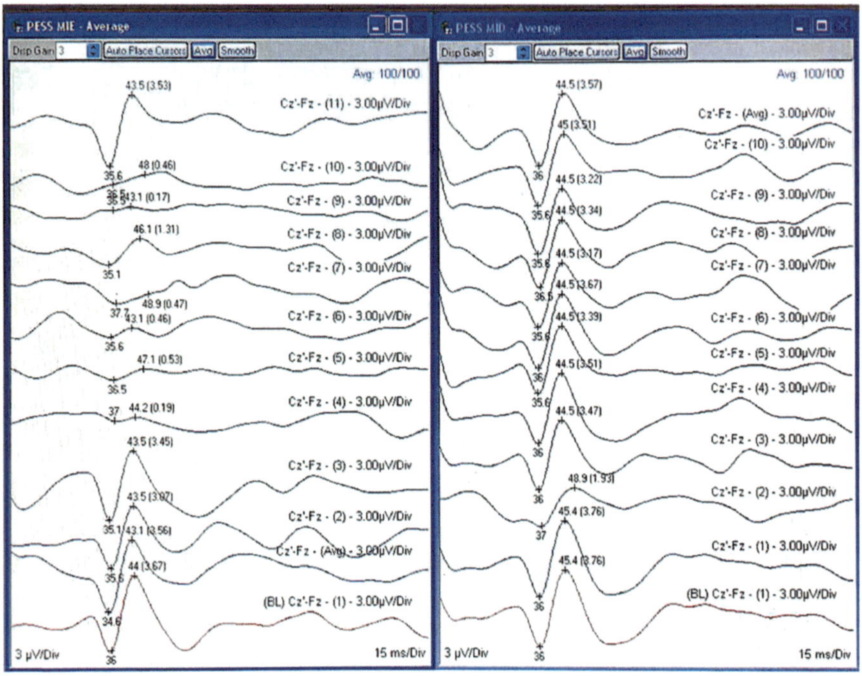

Fig. 22.5 Tibial nerve SSEP responses during the placement of sublaminar bands in the left T8 vertebra. In the left lower limb (left responses), a transient amplitude drop was observed during this surgical step. The surgeon was alerted and stopped the maneuver; after that, the responses recovered

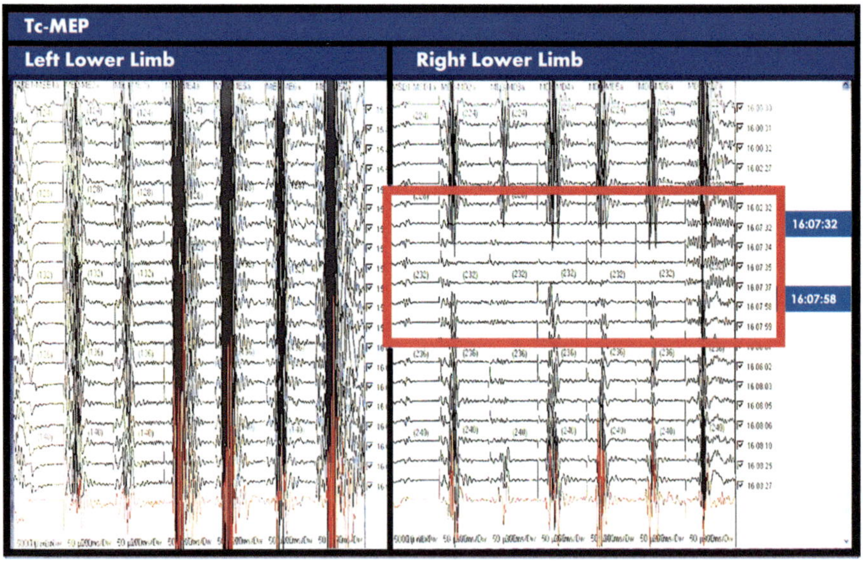

Fig. 22.6 Tc-MEP amplitude drop during osteotomy of right T6 level. The surgical team was alerted and the responses showed a recovery, after a brief pause of the maneuver

may act as an additional parameter to control the integrity of the motor pathways, enabling the surgery to proceed, even if there is a drop or loss of Tc-MEP responses (*Note of the editors: exclusively reflects the experience of the authors*).

- *Step 5*: The rod placement step is generally harmless to neural structures. However, the exception is in the correction of kyphosis when the cantilever maneuver is applied. In this situation, correction of the curve occurs simultaneously with rod placement. Tc-MEP and SSEP tests should be performed.
- *Step 6: Curve correction*: IONM improved safety during rotation and translation of the vertebrae, allowing more aggressive corrections. Strict control with Tc-MEP and SEP must be done. Additionally, it is particularly important to control physiological anesthetic, hemodynamic, and hematimetric parameters because the greatest risk is vascular injury and spinal cord ischemia.
- If IONM points to neurological dysfunction, the corrective maneuver should be reversed, and a less aggressive correction should be considered.
- *Step 7*: Final neurophysiological tests.

Pedicle Instrumentation

During pedicle instrumentation, EMG-ST has major importance. The goal is to map the neural structures near the instruments and screws used. The EMG-ST is performed using a monopolar stimulator probe (cathode -) and a subdermal needle electrode (anode +). The needle is inserted in the contralateral paravertebral musculature at the same level being tested. To minimize the risk of nerve injury, our protocol includes stimulating during the following steps:

1. Facet joint
2. Punctor
3. Pedicle finder
4. Pedicle tap
5. Ball tip probe
6. Screw placement
7. Pedicle screw head

Performing EMG-ST at each step is important since an early detection of incorrect path allows for prompt re-evaluation of the technique. Consequently, it avoids multiple path attempts at the pedicle, which could ultimately culminate in cortical violation and/or fracture and inability to instrument the desired level.

Calibrations

Intensity (I) the depolarization threshold can be determined pedicle by pedicle. We start with 7 mA for thoracic pedicles and 10 mA for lumbar pedicles, using a single pulse of 200 uS or 0.2 mS for the massif screws and 50% more intensity when the screws are cannulated. The intensity may be adjusted if a response is present on the facet joint, indicating the need to reduce the stimulus to adequate values.

Duration (D) the total energy charge in microcoulombs (*C*) is calculated by the formula:

$$C = I \times D\left(\text{intensity} \times \text{duration}\right)$$

Therefore, as important as the intensity of the pulse is its duration. In our protocol, we use a duration of 200 μS or 0.2 mS.

To exemplify: 10 mA × 100 μS: 1000 μC; 10 mA × 200 μS: 2000 μC; and 10 mA × 300 μS: 3000 μC. Thus, pulses of the same intensity with different duration will have very different final energy charges.

We highlighted this concept because threshold vary among IONM groups and the surgical team should be aware of the concept of total load, and whenever they ask about intensity, they should also ask about duration. Using total load parameter enhances patient's safety despite the differences between stimulation protocols.

Frequency for *lumbar screws*, simple pulse is used, once the structures at risk are peripheral nerves (spinal nerve roots or lumbosacral plexus). For *thoracic screws*, a train of pulses is used, because they facilitate the depolarization of the spinal cord, in the case of the medialization of the screw. The recommended configuration is 4 pulses of 0.2 ms duration with an interstimulus interval (ISI) of 2 ms (Calancie et al. 1990) [6, 8, 9].

Pedicle Depolarization Threshold

In scoliosis, the surgeon sometimes leads with hypoplastic or even virtual pedicles, especially in the concavity of the curve [69]. In these cases, it becomes even more important to determine the pedicle depolarization threshold by stimulating the facet of the vertebra of the level being instrumented.

Lumbar vertebra: start with an intensity of 10 mA and a pulse duration of 200 μs. If there is a response in the EMG-ST, the intensity of the stimulus should be progressively reduced until no more response is obtained. This value is considered the depolarization threshold of this pedicle and is used as a parameter for instrumentation. The cutoff point (lower limit) is a total charge of 1400 μC, that is, intensity of 7.0 mA. If stimulation is positive below 7 mA, which is the minimum acceptable safety value, the pedicle path is considered unproper according to the neurophysiological parameter. In this situation, the surgical team performs careful radiological control, visualization, and palpation of the pedicle to decide about redoing the path or not.

Thoracic vertebra: the technique recommended by Calancie (2014) [8, 9] consists of using the four-pulse train, ISI of 2 ms, duration of 0.2 ms, frequency of 3 Hz, and intensity of 10–15 mA (screw path) – total load from 2000 to 3000 μC/pulse. However, especially in cases of children's scoliosis and underweight adolescents, in which there is a higher prevalence of narrow pedicles, this proposed total load can generate false positivity. Thus, in our practice, we use all the parameters mentioned above, except for intensity; the threshold used in our protocol is 7–10 mA (total load: 1400–2000 μC/pulse), and the cutoff is 7 mA. We recommend reading the original paper of Calancie (2014) [8, 9] for a more comprehensive understanding. *(Note of the editors: exclusively reflects the experience of the authors. However, they have been performing IOM in disable children for the last 27 years).*

Discarding the False Negatives

In the absence of a myotomal response with EMG-ST, a quick checklist should be performed to avoid false negatives. This checklist is composed of three main factors, according to their potential source of error: stimulator, patient, and screw.

Regarding the stimulator:

1. Is the subdermal needle (anode) inserted into the paravertebral muscle and does it contract rhythmically? This is a practical way to check if the stimulus is being applied.
2. Is the needle/anode placed at the same level as the screw to be stimulated? It is necessary for focal stimulation and to avoid "spread." When the anode is kept "stationary," far from the cathode (stimulator), false results may occur, including responses in myotomes far away from the pedicle level being instrumented.
3. Is the tip of stimulator being properly applied? The shafts are covered with electrical insulation, and the surgeon should be aware of that (Fig. 22.7).
4. Is the stimulator turned on and properly charged? Always evaluate if the electrical circuit is closed.

Regarding the patient:

1. Is the patient under the effect of pharmacological neuromuscular blockers? To answer this question, apply the train of four (TOF) test. Of note, the reversal of neuromuscular blockade does not occur at the same time in all four limbs after administration of the antagonist. Lower limbs may take longer to reverse neuromuscular blockade compared to upper limbs [4].
2. Does the patient have polyneuropathy or chronic radiculopathy? In these cases, the depolarization threshold may be higher than normal [67].

Regarding the screw:

1. Is it massif or cannulated? The cannulated screw has a higher depolarization threshold. In our protocol, we increase the intensity of the stimulus by 50% compared to the massif screw, with a safety margin above what has been performed by other groups [72]. It is important to stimulate the guide wire of the cannulated screw and then the head of the screw already positioned.
2. Is the screw covered with hydroxyapatite? In this case, the inside hole of the probe should be stimulated, because the screw itself is totally isolated to the passage of electric pulses.

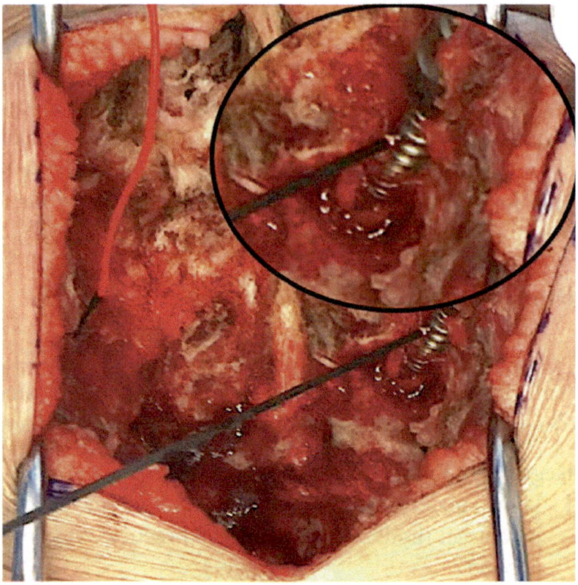

Fig. 22.7 Correct use of the stimulator probe electrode. Only the tip of the probe is uncovered; the shaft is covered with electrical insulation

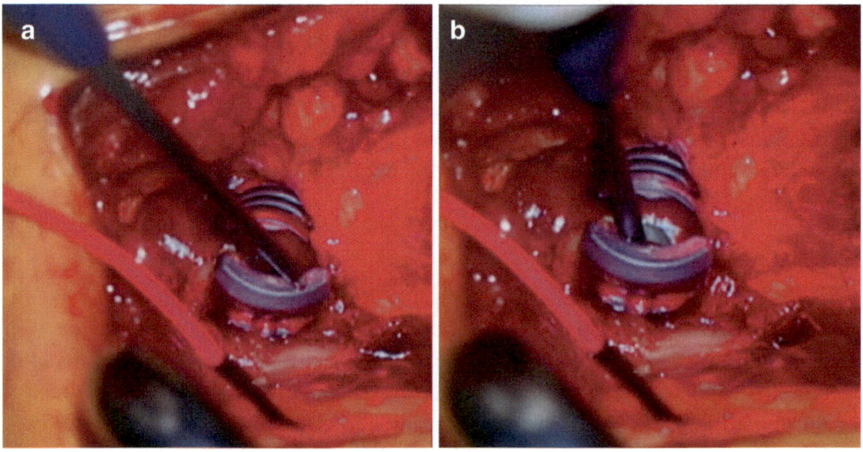

Fig. 22.8 Coaxial screw – head stimulation. (**a**) Incorrect: stimulation in the screw crown and (**b**) Correct: stimulation directly in the screw

3. Is the screw made of metallic materials of different conductance? The polyaxial screws, after being introduced, should be stimulated inside the crown where the screw is. The reason is that they are materials of different compositions, not maintaining perfect contact with the screw, until it is coupled to the rod and connector (Fig. 22.8).

After the checklist, the negative response can be taken as a true negative. Yet, it may not be anatomically well positioned in the image, because it may be in the intervertebral disc space or on the side of the vertebral body, without proximity to any neural structure.

Discarding the False Positives

In the case where there is a response on the EMG-ST, a checklist of two factors must be performed: stimulator and patient.

Regarding the stimulator
Is there no coherence of the response in the EMG-ST with the instrumented level? In some cases, a more cranial response is generated at a non-adjacent level. For example, the surgeon is instrumenting the pedicle of L5, and a response is observed at L1/2. In these cases, it is important to observe if the needle (anode) is correctly placed at the same stimulated level.

Regarding the patient

1. Does the patient have osteoporosis? Bone porosity can allow the stimulus to spread through the wall of the pedicle, lowering the depolarization threshold. In this case, testing the depolarization threshold of the pedicle through the facet joint is an important step.
2. Does the patient have vertebral canal or intervertebral foraminal stenosis (more frequent in adult scoliosis)? Root proximity to the cortical of the pedicle can also facilitate the "spread." Often, in cases of stenosis, even with imaging showing adequate implant location, the EMG-ST evokes persistent responses that usually disappear after decompression – simply because of increasing the distance between the root and the pedicle.
3. Is there a fracture in an adjacent or underlying vertebra? Some fractures in the wall of these pedicles may be imperceptible by surgical palpation or on imaging exams. This fracture may spread electrical stimulus and elicit responses on EMG-ST.
4. Is the pedicle too narrow? Sometimes the same vertebra can have pedicles of different diameters and shapes, and the depolarization threshold of each one should be determined (Fig. 22.9).

After this checklist has been run out, a positive response to stimulation means the screw is "functionally" misplaced and repositioning must be considered (Fig. 22.10).

Conversely, this does not mean that it will be inadequate in the image. Fluoroscopy does not have a three-dimensional image, and the parallax phenomenon can lead to misinterpretation. Despite the 3D O-Arm^R facilitation of pedicle instrumentation, errors are still possible since it is a mathematical model image.

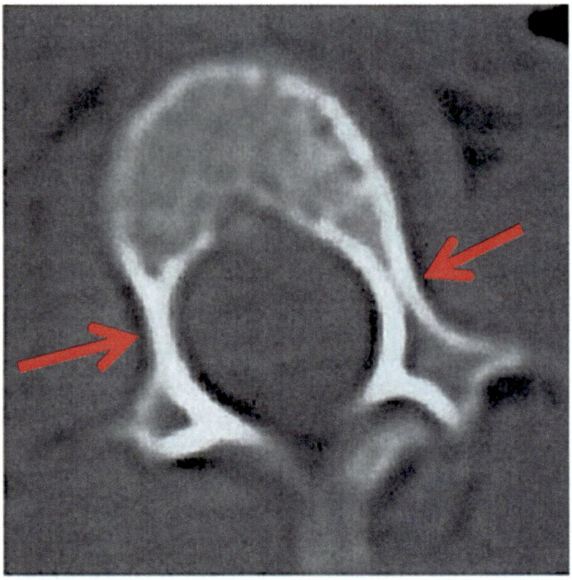

Fig. 22.9 **Pedicle assimetry in the same vertebra**

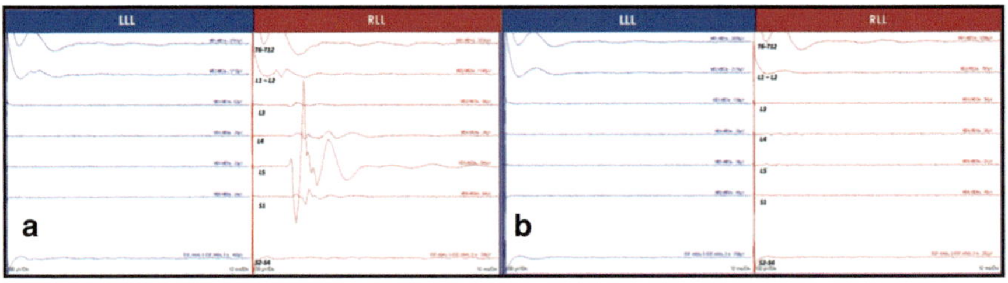

Fig. 22.10 **EMG-St responses during lumbar right L5 pedicle instrumentation.** (**a**) Presence of response in screw stimulation; (**b**) After screw repositioning, no response to stimulation is seem

Transpedicular Neurophysiological Navigation

One of the techniques used for pedicle screw insertion is the "freehand technique" [10]. With the EMG-ST, we can perform what we call "transpedicular neurophysiologic navigation," during the freehand technique, which is the stimulation of all steps of the pedicle instrumentation. This information is continuously communicated to the surgeon, who makes the proper correlation with the surgical step and, if necessary, performs the immediate correction of the implant trajectory (introductory probes and/or screw). Thus, deviations of the path while perforating the pedicle can be promptly identified; even at the early phase of the pedicle finder use, promoting the recognition of the direction the cortical invasion is likely to be.

An additional advantage is that these steps can be performed without the concomitant use of radioscopy, which reduces operative time and exposure to radiation.

For a better understanding of this technique, we cite some examples of its application.

Transpedicular Neurophysiological Navigation: Example L4 Pedicle (Fig. 22.11)

1. Presence of responses in the myotome of L3: interpret as cranial or lateral course of the screw, since this root emerges in the immediately superior foramen and passes laterally and juxtaposed to the pedicle.
2. Presence of responses in the myotome of L4: interpret as the caudal trajectory of the screw since this root emerges from the inferior foramen to this pedicle.
3. Presence of responses in the myotome of L5 and/or multirooted: interpret as a medial route of the screw.

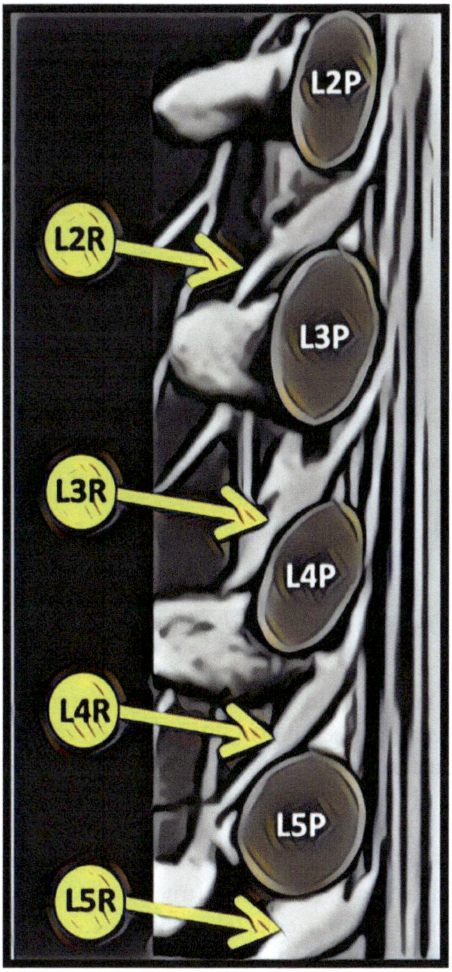

Fig. 22.11 Transpedicular neurophysiological navigation: schematic figure of the lumbar vertebral pedicles and their correlation with the nerve roots

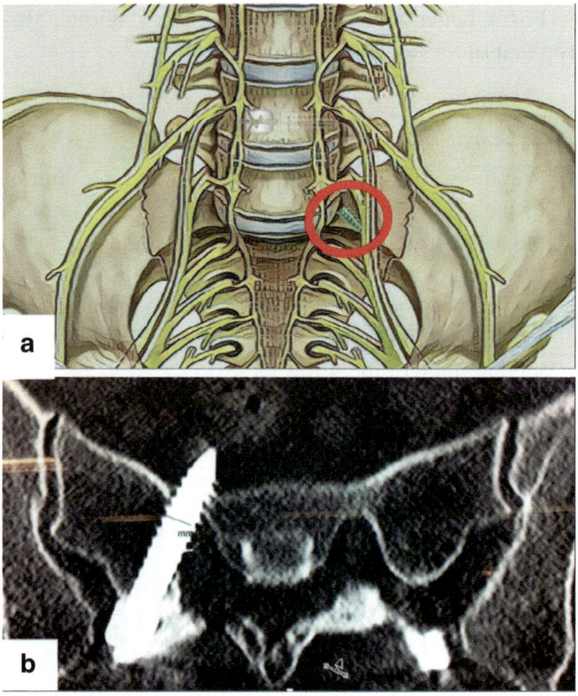

Fig. 22.12 Bicorticalization of the S1 screw. (**a**) Anatomical diagram demonstrating the proximity of the lumbosacral plexus in the anterior position of the S1 vertebra. (Courtesy of Moura Filho, JP and Bordalo-Rodrigues et al. 2020 [39]). (**b**) Bicorticalization of an S1 screw on CT

Transpedicular Neurophysiological Navigation: Other Examples

1. Multi-radicular responses: these responses are usually present when there is medialization of the screw, in both the lumbar and thoracic pedicles.
2. Pedicle of S1: when there is bicorticalization of the screw, EMG-ST may show responses in the L5 root or in multiple root levels, due to the anatomical disposition of the roots and lumbosacral plexus in the anterior portion of this vertebra (Fig. 22.12).

Decision-Making Algorithm Based on Alarm Signals

The prompt identification of a potential neural insult and its cause leads the surgical team to react to avoid tissue injury and its sequelae (definitive or transitory) if the maneuver allows reversibility. Thus, a management algorithm should be established and followed when facing alarm signals.

The importance of checklists in times of stress in the operating room has been developed and suggests a decrease in the incidence of errors [75]. In addition to the detection of real events (true positives), it is part of the skills of the neurophysiologist to minimize the false-positive rate as much as possible, thus improving the positive predictive value of the test. A false-positive event generates unnecessary interruption, increases the stress of the surgical team, and brings IONM into discredit.

Although there are alarm criteria recommended for each test (EMG-fr, SSEP, and Tc-MEP), the algorithm is exclusively based on alterations of Tc-MEP. The reason is that MEP is more susceptible to ischemia, being the one that changes the earliest in cases of spinal cord injury [55]. Additionally, MEP is the first to return to basal levels after the appropriate interventions are made.

Alarm Signals: Tc-MEP

Alarm parameters diverge in the literature [7, 28–30, 32, 48, 53, 54, 56, 60, 70, 76]. The main ones are summarized in Table 22.2.

In daily practice, these parameters are valued with caution (Fig. 22.13). Indeed, a reduction in the number of phases and a 50% drop in the amplitude of responses should be correlated to the moment of the surgery and precipitate exclusion of confounding factors (neurophysiological and anesthesiologic checklist). In deformity surgeries, drops of up to 80% of the Tc-MEP can be tolerated [30].

Table 22.2 Mostly recommended Tc-MEP alarm signals

Alarm criteria	Analysis	Author	Characteristic
Major	"All or nothing"	Kothbauer et al. [28]	Presence or absence of response
Minor/ moderate	Amplitude	Langeloo et al. [30]	Reduction – amplitude of responses (80%)
	Threshold	Calancie et al. [7]	Increase in response strength at 100 V
	Morphology	Quinones-Hinojosa et al. [54]	Reduction in the number of phases
	Mixed index	Segura et al. [56]	Index of latency, amplitude, duration, and area

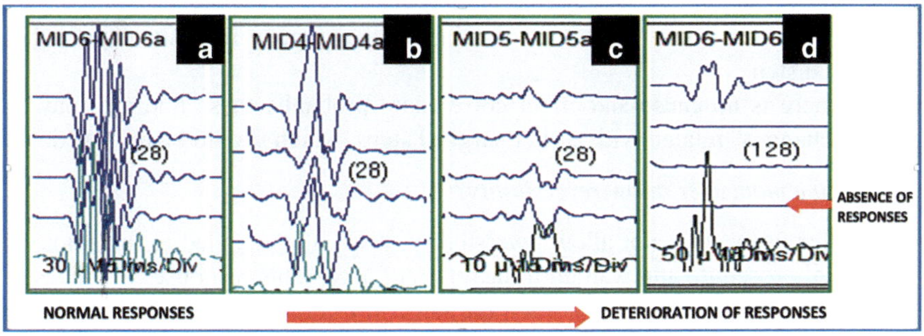

Fig. 22.13 Examples of deterioration of Tc-MEP responses. (**a**) Normal response; (**b**) Reduction in the number of Tc-MEP phases; (**c**) Decrease in amplitude; (**d**) Absence of responses; (Images: courtesy of Maria Lúcia Mendonça, MD)

Based on these algorithms and guidelines, and our clinical experience, we developed our protocol [20].

Alarm signal: Tc-MEP amplitude drop >50% – decision-making
Perform neurophysiological and anesthesiologic checklist before alerting the surgical team:

- Neurophysiological checklist: check the condition and impedance of recording and stimulator electrodes, output current, amplifier setup input, and stimulation parameters.
- Anesthesiology checklist: check on which drugs are being used (attention to inhalation anesthetics), their doses, and if a bolus has been administered. It is important to pay attention to the level of hypnosis through the BIS, which should be >45, MAP >85 mmHg, temperature > 36.0 °C, and HB > 10 g/dl.

After performing these checklists, any mistakes were found?

- *NO*, no mistakes were noted on the checklists: this is a *true positive*; the surgeon will be communicated.
- *YES*, there was an error in the checklists: make the appropriate correction of the inadequate parameter.

Once the appropriate correction of the anesthesiological or neurophysiological factors has been made, have the responses returned to the previous parameters?

- *YES*, the responses return to previous parameters: considered false positive, it is not necessary to communicate the surgical team. The surgery may continue.
- *NO*, the responses remain altered, maintaining the amplitude drop: considered true positive, the surgeon should be notified.

Communicating a true positive
The surgeon evaluates if there is a cause-and-effect correlation between the reported alarm signal and the surgical time:

- *YES*, there is a cause-and-effect correlation: the surgeon reviews only the last surgical step.
- *NO*, there is no cause-and-effect correlation: probably, these findings may be "late changes" related with earlier surgical steps, which should be reviewed.

Does the maneuver allow reversibility?

- *NO*, this event does not allow reversibility: it is recommended to interrupt the surgical procedure and wait until the return of acceptable responses in the tests.
- *YES*, this event allows reversibility: the surgeon will take appropriate actions and observe if IONM signals recover.

Did the result of the reversibility maneuver or the waiting period led to recovery of the responses?

- *YES*, there was recovery between 40% and 60% of the values from the last baseline, updated immediately after these maneuvers: continue the surgery.
- *YES*, however, with poor recovery of responses (less than 40%) after all facilitating maneuvers (MAP increase, hypnosis with BIS >45, temperature > 36 °C, and Hb >10 g/dL): perform the wake-up test. Depending on the surgery, the hypothesis of suspending the surgery should be considered, with a second approach later to finish the procedure.
- *NO*, the responses do not recover, are still below 20%, or are absent: perform the wake-up test.

Wake-up test: voluntary and active movement of the lower limbs was observed?

- *YES*, the patient presents voluntary and active movement in the lower limbs: continue the surgery.
- *NO*, the patient does not present voluntary and active movement of the lower limbs, and it proves the findings of the IONM: the correct conduct is the immediate suspension of the surgery, with removal of all implant materials. In cases of wide osteotomies, the maintenance of some support rod can be considered.

Note: while waiting for the patient to wake up, Tc-MEP continues to be performed. If acceptable Tc-MEP responses (up to 40–60% reduction from baseline) recover within this period, due to simple suspension of anesthetic drugs and reduction of hypnosis, the wake-up test can be canceled, and surgery continued.

Postoperative Guidance and Clinical Monitoring

During postoperative care after surgery for deformity correction, it is advisable to refer the patient to the ICU and maintain MAP above 85 mmHg and Hb > 10 g/dL, mainly in the first 48 h. Also, it is recommended to perform a basic neurological examination to check active movement of the lower limbs, every hour.

Careful motor evaluation is important, as it can diagnose the occurrence of late neurological deficits, secondary to hematoma formation, implant displacement, or even bone spicules due to intracanal or foraminal osteotomies.

False Positives and False Negatives

False positives or negatives in IONM should be analyzed in relation to the neural pathway versus test performed. In older reports, SSEP was the only test performed during spinal deformity surgeries. Therefore, SSEP changes were erroneously correlated to the postoperative *motor* status [35]. Careful methodological analysis should always be done because conclusions could have originated from mistaken assumptions. Of note, SSEP assesses the proprioceptive pathways of the dorsal column of the spinal cord, and Tc-MEP assesses the motor pathways of the spinal cord.

False-negative SSEP can only be so-called if no change in the sensory potentials was recorded and there is a clinically detectable postoperative proprioception deficit.

False-positive SSEP, on the other hand, occurs if significant and persistent changes in SSEP are registered but with no postoperative proprioception impairment.

Statements about motor impairment based solely on SSEP are inaccurate. Tc-MEP checks on motor pathway and should be performed throughout the surgery.

Lastly, sensibility impairment of the lower limbs results in gait disability justifying the absolute necessity of SSEP in the spinal approaches. Thus, the tendency to use only Tc-MEP to the detriment of SSEP is a mistake: both must be used concomitantly.

Usually, the term *true positive* is used to describe an abnormality in IONM followed by a new deficit. However, such nomenclature is misleading in terms of evaluating the performance of IONM. The purpose of the IONM is not simply to predict postoperative neurological status, but rather to alert the surgical team of possible neurological damaging events during a particular maneuver, in time to avoid the injury. Neurophysiological changes, when detected, allow a revision of the procedure by the surgeon to completely reverse or at least reduce the severity of the lesion.

Therefore, when transient alteration occurs in IONM and technical/anesthetic/systemic reasons have been excluded, it means that this patient had a real (true positive) but reversible neurophysiological dysfunction, having a positive result during IONM but no postoperative neurological deficit at the outcome. This finding is commonly, but mistakenly, called false positive, suggesting that abnormal IONM signals during the intraoperative period occurred but without actual neurological injury at the outcome. Yet, they should be considered as true positives, even if they have been correctly reversed by surgical team, either by interrupting the adopted maneuver or by reversing it.

Based on these facts, we disagree that the IONM has its importance or "evidence" only related to the "outcome." The correct intervention of the surgical team facing the neurophysiological alarms allows the performance of reversing maneuvers. Thus, it prevents neurological injury and reverses a true positive to normality, modifying the outcome.

Evidence Level

IONM has been used in spinal deformity surgery since the 1970s [41]. Early descriptions consisted of technical notes, case reports, and case series using SSEP. Nuwer and Cols (1995) [44] conducted a pioneering study with surgeons from the Scoliosis Research Society (SRS) and the European Spine Deformity Society (ESDS), evaluating the role of SSEPs in spine surgeries, and concluded that there had been a significant reduction of neurological lesions. However, the number of false-negative cases was still great. Indeed, it could have been expected since SSEP evaluates solely the sensory pathways of the posterior horn of the spinal cord and cannot predict lesions in the corticospinal tracts. After the association of MEPs in spinal surgery, subsequent studies demonstrated greater sensitivity and specificity in detecting lesions in the motor pathway [36, 37, 62].

Systematic reviews have demonstrated the role of multimodal IONM in spinal deformity surgeries [63, 65]. Fehlings et al. [16] performed a meta-analysis of 32 studies (out of 103 evaluated) and concluded that there is strong evidence that IONM is sensitive and specific in detecting intraoperative neurological lesions, and its use is recommended in spine surgeries where there is a risk of spinal cord or radicular injury. Thirumala et al. [63] evaluated 3284 patients with idiopathic scoliosis, submitted to surgical correction, showing that IONM had a sensitivity of 76.5% and specificity of 95.1% in detecting neurological lesions. Patients who had a new deficit postoperatively were 79.4 times more likely to have had significant changes in SSEP and/or MEP during corrective procedures. Other studies with large cohorts of patients have shown similar results, but all showing very high sensitivity (99.6–100%) and specificity (91.5–99.3%) [50, 52, 55, 64, 65]. These results show that IONM is very sensitive in detecting new deficits and the occurrence of false-negative cases (presence of neurological lesion with normal IONM) is very rare. The slightly lower specificity means that an IONM change does not result in neurological deficits (false positive) but has originated from external factors like use of muscle relaxants, volatile anesthetics, dexmedetomidine, clonidine, hypovolemia, hypotension, hypothermia, and finally technical problems.

In addition to detecting impending neurological damage, IONM has been shown to provide surgeons with real-time information needed to make intraoperative decisions that preserve neural function. Schwartz et al. [55], in a multicenter study evaluating 1121 patients operated on for adolescent idiopathic scoliosis, showed a postoperative neurological deficit rate of 0.8%. Thirty-eight patients (3.4%) had significant changes in IONM (SSEP and/or MEP), and of those, 29 (2.6% of the total) were attributed to specific intraoperative maneuvers (mostly by application of corrective forces and by clamping of segmental vessels). Of these patients who had a drop in evoked potentials, 88% responded to the measures adopted by the surgical team, with improved responses. This favorable result was due to the rapid response to the changes observed in the IONM, being responsible for the decrease in the presence of neurological deficit in 1.2% of all patients. In a study evaluating patients undergoing high-risk deformity surgery requiring three-spine osteotomy (osteotomy with pedicle subtraction, spine resection, and partial spine resection), Jarvis et al. [25] described that the adoption of corrective measures in cases where there were significant changes in the IONM led to a 14% reduction in postoperative neurological deficits, which recovered in approximately 1 month, with no permanent lesions observed. Other studies were also conclusive in demonstrating the facilitating role of early and effective IONM interventions [22, 36, 50].

To avoid permanent neurological damage and rule out false-positive cases as much as possible, studies have been conducted with algorithm and checklists to be followed in cases in which there are significant changes in the IONM. Vitale et al. [70] published guidelines based on a consensus of 21 surgeons specialized in spinal deformities in adults and children and on previous SRS and American Association of Neuromuscular and Electrodiagnostic Medicine (AANEM) guidelines. These guidelines have served as a model for several algorithm published in subsequent years and for use in daily practice. Other recent studies with large numbers of patients with spinal deformities have also suggested similar algorithms [5, 65].

The common principles among these guidelines are good communication between the surgical team (comprising the surgeon, anesthesiologist, and clinical neurophysiologist), confirmation that real alarm events exist (with the exclusion of systemic and technical confounders), consideration of performing the Stagnara wake-up test, and taking effective intraoperative measures to reverse the observed warning signs and preserve neurological function. Our algorithm, presented earlier in this chapter, follows these general principles, coupled with our clinical experience [18].

In addition to the risks from maneuvers with corrective forces (distraction, contraction, and rotation) and osteotomies, there is a considerable risk of myelopathy in instrumentation of pedicle screws in the thoracic spine. Calancie et al. [8, 9] published, in two parts, an elegant study in which they demonstrated the importance of EMG-ST in detecting medial malposition of pedicle screws in the thoracic spine. It was the first blinded and randomized study to implement a new IONM technique that, besides identifying a clinically relevant alteration with high sensitivity, also proved to be effective in providing actions to reverse the problems identified.

Surgeries to correct spinal deformities are the procedures in which the role of the IONM has been studied the most. They also have the strongest evidence and recommendations. The latest SRS statement states that in surgery for spinal deformities, "intraoperative neurophysiological monitoring of the spinal cord is no longer investigational (as it was defined in the last consensus of 2009), but rather a 'standard of care' modality when there is a risk of spinal cord injury" [22]. Numerous studies have conclusively demonstrated that IONM is important in detecting impending spinal cord injury and facilitates early interventions for the purpose of functional preservation [11–13, 31, 40, 43, 46, 54, 58].

Conclusion

Even in the hands of the most experienced and skilled surgeons, scoliosis correction surgery carries risk to the neural structures. The main critical steps from a neurological point of view are instrumentation with pedicle screws, pedicle, or facet hooks, sublaminar bands or wires, osteotomies, and the correction of the deformity.

There is a triad in the operating room, surgeon, anesthesiologist, and neurophysiologist, and the communication between them should be continuous and fluent. This interaction avoids false results and neural lesion.

The anesthesiologist is responsible for meticulous control of the hemodynamic and physiological parameters, ensuring adequate spinal cord perfusion, and avoiding clinical fluctuations.

The neurophysiologist is not a passive observer of signals on a screen but rather an active team member. He should provide IONM as an useful tool for the surgeon

evoked potential intraoperative monitoring in patients with idiopathic scoliosis. Spine. 2016;41(19):1177–84.
64. Thuet ED, Winscher JC, Padberg AM, Bridwell KH, Lenke LG, Dobbs MB, et al. Validity and reliability of intraoperative monitoring in pediatric spinal deformity surgery: a 23-year experience of 3436 surgical cases. Spine. 2010;35(20):1880–6.
65. Tsikiros AI, Duckworth AD, Henderson LE, Michaelson C. Multimodal intraoperative spinal cord monitoring during spinal deformity surgery: efficacy, diagnostic characteristics, and algorithm development. Med Princ Pract. 2020;29:6–17.
66. Turner JD, Eastlack RK, Mirzadeh Z, Nguyen S, et al. Fluctuations in spinal cord perfusion during adult spinal deformity correction identify neurologic changes: proof of concept. World Neurosurg. 2016;85(365):6–80.
67. Uncini A, Santoro L. The electrophysiology of axonal neuropathies: more than just evidence of axonal loss. Clin Neurophysiol. 2020;131(10):2367–74. PMID: 32828039. [cited 2020 Aug 10]. Available from: https://doi.org/10.1016/j.clinph.2020.07.014.
68. Vauzelle C, Stagnara P, Jouvinroux P. Functional monitoring of spinal cord activity during spinal surgery. Clin Orthop Relat Res. 1973;9:173–8. PMID: 4146655. Available from: https://doi.org/10.1097/00003086-197306000-00017.
69. Villas C, Barrios RH. Congenital absence of the pedicles and the neural arch of L2. Eur Spine J. 1997;6(5):354–6. PMID: 9391810; PMCID: PMC3454610. Available from: https://doi.org/10.1007/BF01142686.
70. Vitale MG, Skaggs DL, Pace GI, Wright ML, Matsumoto H, Anderson RCE, et al. Best practices in intraoperative neuromonitoring in spine deformity surgery: development of an intraoperative checklist to optimize response. Spine Deform. 2014;2(5):333–9. PMID: 27927330. [cited 2014 Aug 27]. Available from: https://doi.org/10.1016/j.jspd.2014.05.003.
71. Walker CT, et al. Neuroanesthesia guidelines for optimizing transcranial motor evoked potential neuromonitoring during deformity and complex spinal surgery: a Delphi consensus study. Spine. 2020;45(13):911–20.
72. Wu Y, Cohen D, Tellez MJ, DiGiacinto GV, Barquero AV, Ulkatan S. Application of different thresholds for instrumentation device testing in minimally invasive lumbosacral spine fixation. J Clin Neurosci. 2020;72:224–8. PMID: 31866354. [cited 2019 Dec 19]. Available from: https://doi.org/10.1016/j.jocn.2019.11.036.
73. Xue L, Luo S, Ding H, Zhu Y, Liu Y, Huang W, et al. Risk of spinal cord ischemia after thoracic endovascular aortic repair. J Thorac Dis. 2018;10(11):6088–96. PMID: 30622780 [cited 2018 Nov]. Available from: https://doi.org/10.21037/jtd.2018.10.99.
74. Yang J, Skaggs DL, Chan P, Shah SA, Vitale MG, Neiss G, et al. Raising mean arterial pressure alone restores 20% of intraoperative neuromonitoring losses. Spine. 2018;43(13):890–4. PMID: 29049087. Available from: https://doi.org/10.1097/BRS.0000000000002461.
75. Ziewacz JE, Arriaga AF, Bader AM, Berry WR, Edmondson L, Wong JM, et al. Crisis checklists for the operating room: development and pilot testing. J Am Coll Surg. 2011;213(2):212–7. Erratum in: J Am Coll Surg. 2012;215(2):310. Dosage error in article text. PMID: 21658974. [cited 2011 Jun 11]. Available from: https://doi.org/10.1016/j.jamcollsurg.2011.04.031.
76. Ziewacz JE, Berven SH, Mummaneni VP, Tu TH, Akinbo OC, Lyon R, et al. The design, development, and implementation of a checklist for intraoperative neuromonitoring changes. Neurosurg Focus. 2012;33(5):11. PMID: 23116091. Available from: https://doi.org/10.3171/2012.9.FOCUS12263.
77. Zuckerman SL, Forbes JA, Mistry AM, Krishnamoorthi H, Weaver S, Mathews L, et al. Electrophysiologic deterioration in surgery for thoracic disc herniation: impact of mean arterial pressures on surgical outcome. Eur Spine J. 2014;23:2279–90.

Chapter 23
Lumbar Interbody Fusion Surgeries: LIFS

Ricardo José Rodriguez Ferreira, Marcus Vinícius Magno Gonçalves, Emília Caram Bordini, and Alexandre Fogaça Cristante

Abbreviations

ALIF	Anterior Interbody Fusion
EMG	Electromyography
EMGfr	Electromyography Free Running
EMGst	Electromyography Stimulated
EMGtg	Electromyography Triggered
IONM	Intraoperative Neurophysiological Monitoring
IONMm	Multimodal Intraoperative Neurophysiological Monitoring
IONMu	Unimodal Intraoperative Neurophysiological Monitoring
LIF	Lumbar Interbody Fusion

R. J. R. Ferreira (✉) · E. C. Bordini
AACD - Disabled Child Care Association, São Paulo, SP, Brazil

Dr Ricardo Ferreira Clinic, São Paulo, SP, Brazil

Spine Surgery Department at Orthopedics and Trauma Institute of Clinical Hospital of the University of São Paulo Medical School, São Paulo, SP, Brazil

M. V. M. Gonçalves
Neurologist and Neurophysiologist, Neurology at the University of the Region of Joinville (UNIVILLE), Joinville, Brazil

A. F. Cristante
Spine Surgery Department at Orthopedics and Trauma Institute of Clinical Hospital of the University of São Paulo Medical School, São Paulo, SP, Brazil

S. M. Verst et al. (eds.), *Intraoperative Monitoring*,
https://doi.org/10.1007/978-3-030-95730-8_23

LLIF	Lateral Interbody Fusion
OLIF	Oblique Lumbar Interbody Fusion
PLIF	Posterior Lumbar Interbody Fusion
SEP	Somatosensory Evoked Potentials
TcMEP	Transcranial Motor Evoked Potentials
TLIF	Transforaminal Lumbar Interbody Fusion

Surgeon's Point of View

Lumbar interbody fusion (isolated or associated with posterior arthrodesis) may be indicated for the treatment of various pathologies, including traumatic, neoplasic, and degenerative in origin. Several surgical access techniques have been developed over time to minimize complications and increase the fusion success rate, the main ones being:

- ALIF (former lumbar interbody fusion)
- OLIF (oblique lumbar interbody fusion)
- LLIF – XLIF (lateral lumbar interbody fusion/extreme lateral interbody fusion)
- TLIF (transforaminal lumbar interbody fusion)
- PLIF (posterior lumbar posterior lumbar interbody fusion)

The choice of technique to be used must take into account the surgeon's experience, the underlying disease that leads to the treatment, as well as the lumbar level to be operated.

The anatomical structures at risk vary considerably between each surgical access, and the main complications could be:

- ALIF: vascular injury (mainly iliac vein) and superior hypogastric plexus injury (leading to premature ejaculation in men)
- OLIF: excessive psoas muscle retraction (leading to thigh paresthesia and hip flexion weakness)
- LLIF: lumbar plexus injury (usually temporary symptoms) through the psoas muscle
- TLIF: damage to the dural sac and nerve roots (smaller compared to PLIF due to less distance)
- PLIF: lesion of the dural sac and nerve roots (greater distance for disc space access)

The use of IONM allows increasing the neurological safety of spinal column procedures. The evaluation during the passage of the pedicle screws gives the surgeon a functional parameter of good positioning, thus reducing the risk of neurological damage. Continuous assessment during the manipulation of neurological structures (dural sac and/or nerve root in the case of TLIF/PLIF, or lumbar plexus in the case of XLIF/LLIF) allows the surgeon to minimize actions that could result in further neurological damage.

Effective communication between neurophysiologist and surgeon is very important for quick decision-making during surgery and can change the outcome of neurological status. Therefore, from the surgeon's point of view, IONM is a great ally for the success of lumbar interbody fusion procedures and should, whenever possible, be used.

Intraoperative Neurophysiological Monitoring to LLIF Techniques

The surgical techniques known as LIF (lumbar interbody fusion), LLIF (lateral), ALIF (anterior), OLIF (Oblique), PLIF (posterior), and TLIF (transforaminal) (Figs. 23.1 and 23.2) consist of minimally invasive procedures. The LLIF techniques consist of surgical instrumentation through a direct lateral retroperitoneal approach, used as an alternative to traditional open surgeries.

Numerous advantages are recognized for minimally invasive techniques, but neurological complications arising from this type of surgical procedure have been reported in several studies [1–7]. The neuroanatomical proximity of the lumbar plexus in relation to the iliopsoas muscle, used as one of the access pathways, increases the risk of secondary neurological complications when using this technique [1]. Le et al. [2] found the prevalence of 10.7–26.1% for immediate postoperative paresthesia and 54.9% for ipsilateral weakness of muscles innervated by the femoral nerve. One of the possible causes for the high frequency of neurological lesions is due to the variability of lumbar plexus topography [3], shown using the neurography (tractography) technique through a nuclear magnetic resonance of the lumbar plexus [4].

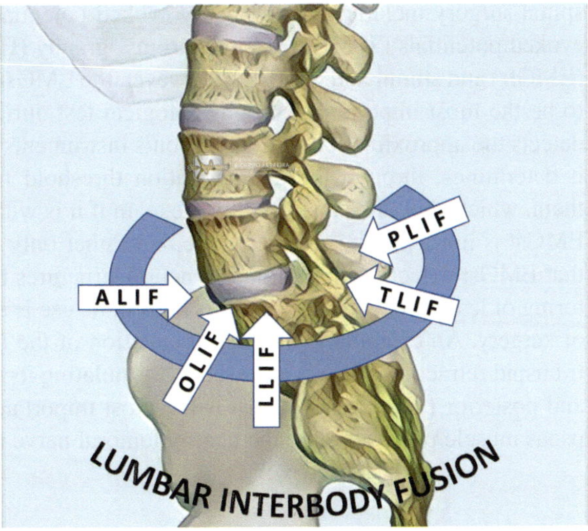

Fig. 23.1 Surgical approaches to the lumbar spine for interbody fusion techniques. The five approaches are shown schematically

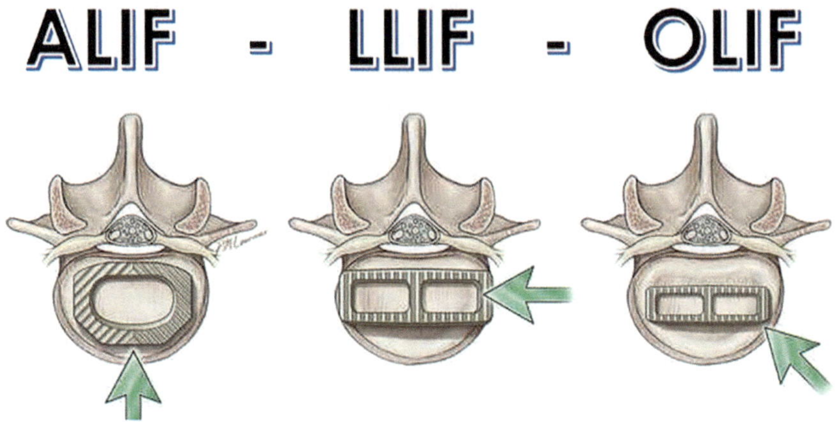

Fig. 23.2 Anterior, lateral, and oblique lumbar interbody fusion

Multimodal IONM (IONMm), by means of its two stages of mapping and monitoring, should yield precise information to the surgeon about the functioning of the peripheral and central nervous systems involved with this access pathway. The real-time feedback lets surgeons correlate their actions at a given surgical step to the IONM findings, allowing them to interrupt maneuvers, retreat, and, with this, prevent neurological lesions. This type of information is supplied to the surgical team throughout all stages of the procedure, including the positioning of both upper and lower limbs of the patient, opening of the transpsoas access, introduction of the first dilators, opening and maintenance of the tricuspid retractor, discectomies, and, lastly, placement of the proof and definitive cage.

Moreover, the safety profile, the efficacy, and the cost-effectiveness of IONM must be taken into consideration [5]. The most used modalities in IONM during spinal surgery include somatosensory evoked potentials (SEP), transcranial motor evoked potentials (TcMEP), and electromyography (EMG), which can be free run (EMGfr) and stimulated (EMGst). However, the EMGst technique, which is claimed to be the most important neurophysiological test during the access pathway, only detects the approximation of the surgeon's instruments to neural structures. Indeed, it determines, through the depolarization threshold found, the distance between them, which should be analyzed by the team if it is within a safety range. However, EMGst is not a monitoring technique, but rather only a mapping tool. This means that EMGst detects the proximity to neural structures but does not allow the monitoring of lesions occurrence. For this reason, its use is restricted to the first moment of surgery. An example is by the implantation of the first dilators followed by the tricuspid retractor, which is assessed by stimulating its three blades: cranial, caudal, and posterior (the latter of which is the most important). The advance through the psoas muscle poses a risk to the nearby femoral nerve (Fig. 23.3).

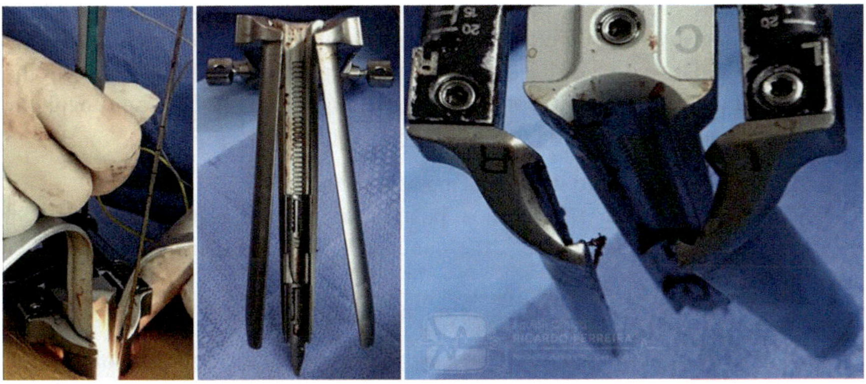

Fig. 23.3 EMG-st: stimulation of the tricuspid retractor in LLIF surgeries

Given these facts, we highlight that unimodal IONM (IONMu) is incomplete to diagnose most lesions that could occur in this pathway. Thus, it is essential to additionally monitor using the evoked potentials above mentioned (IONMm).

Riley et al. [6] published a non-randomized retrospective analysis of 479 procedures operated using the LLIF technique. The group that used TcMEP presented lower rates of immediate postoperative neurologic deficit (22.3%), including sensory and motor deficits, when compared to the group that used EMG alone, with 40.4% of complications. The prevalence of immediate motor deficit was 5.7% in the group that used TcMEP versus 17.1% in the group that used EMG alone, and the rate of irreversible motor deficit was significantly lower in the group that used TcMEP (6.9%) versus the group that used EMG alone (11.0%). The authors concluded that TcMEP seems to be the most effective monitoring modality to prevent permanent neurological lesions in the LLIF approach [6].

Sutter et al. [7] compared the different methods described previously in IONM regarding the detection of neurological complications during spinal surgery in 2728 patients that underwent LLIF. The sensitivity and specificity of IONMm were 93.0% and 99.1%, respectively. For IONMu, sensitivity rates ranged between 13% and 81% to detect neurological complications. The authors concluded that IONMm was more effective and precise in the neurophysiological assessment during spinal surgery for reducing neurological complications, in comparison to the IONMu. We recommend that IONMm be conducted in all orthopedic surgeries, including those applying LLIF techniques. Thus, the TcMEP and SEP modalities should always be used, routinely, to reduce the risk of reversible and irreversible neurological damage.

Hence, in face of this context, we suggest the adoption of seven fundamental steps for IONMm of surgeries using the LLIF technique:

1. The patient is correctly positioned with table folds aiming to vertebral level optimized access. Through radioscopy, the surgeon chooses the adequate location to transverse the psoas muscle. Initially, using a stimulator probe measuring 25 cm in length, the surgeon introduces the probe to map and locate nerves, especially

those that are most exposed: genitofemoral and femoral nerves. Then, surgical reamers (usually three) are introduced and stimulated, applying pulses lasting 0.1 ms/100 us. We use EMGst to correlate the intensity of stimulation with the distance between the stimulator/reamers to neural structures. In our protocol, the decision-making is based on the following parameters (Fig. 23.4):

- Green: ≥10 mA: Safe, not requiring repositioning.
- Yellow: 5.0–10 mA: Caution, repositioning is decided by the surgeon in agreement with images and the concrete possibility of achieving a better position.
- Red: ≤5.0 mA: Danger, we recommend reposition.

It should be considered that polyneuropathies may have higher depolarization thresholds in EMGst. This can lead to false negatives, due to the difficulty in determining the exact distance between the instrument and the nerves and may result in lesions still during the first stage of surgery.

Therefore, we suggest a change of paradigm that has not yet been proposed in the current literature, but that is necessary for a more adequate neurophysiological mapping study. The stimulator probe must be thin and with adequate length (25 cm) and should be the first instrument to be introduced in the psoas muscle. The probe will carry out the mapping through direct stimulation of the lumbar plexus nerves, reducing the occurrence of false results that can be generated through indirect stimulation from the dilators. Of note, the genitofemoral nerve is superficial to the psoas muscle.

2. TcMEP of the muscles innervated by the lumbar plexus nerves, namely, genitofemoral (cremaster muscle), obturator (adductor magnus muscle), and femoral (iliopsoas and quadriceps muscles) should be performed throughout the intraoperative period. It aims to diagnose neurological lesion due to rupture, ischemia, or traction. As previously mentioned, lesions cannot be identified by EMGst because it is solely a mapping/locator tool. Therefore, if a lesion is caused during the introduction of any instrument, EMGfr may show signs of mechanical depolarization; however, to diagnose the lesion, and to determine if it was partial or complete, MEPs are necessary. Of note, a muscle atlas is available in Chap. 3.
3. Add TcMEP of the muscles innervated by the external and internal branches of the sciatic nerve, bilaterally, since there is a great risk of lesion, due to the

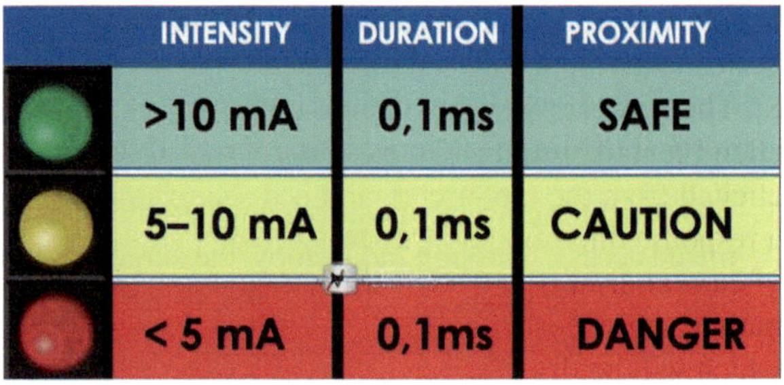

Fig. 23.4 EMG-ST responses schematically grouped by color. Green: Safe, Yellow: Caution, Red: Danger

prolonged hold on lateral position. In this type of surgery, special attention on the consequences of the patient's position is necessary because the lower limbs are routinely fixed with bandages to maintain perfect lateralization of the patient on the surgical table. Additionally, exaggerated traction can occur over the nerves if the table is folded incorrectly, meaning that the table fold should occur ideally at the level of the femoral trochanter. If there is an excessive slope in this fold, greater risk is posed on the lumbosacral plexus.

With the experience acquired with IONMm during transpsoas lateral pathway access, we have frequently observed deterioration in TcMEP potentials not only in the territory of lumbar plexus nerves, but also in the territory of sacral plexus nerves (Fig. 23.5). In practice, we occasionally suggest to the surgeon a decrease in the angle of the table folding, especially in cases where this angle must be increased to move the iliac wing away from the surgical access. Indeed, in this situation, neurophysiological alterations may be seen in the external portion of the sciatic nerve.

4. TcMEP should be carried out every 5 min after the tricuspid retractor is opened. Closing the retractor is recommended if TcMEP presents a significant amplitude reduction greater than 50% in the muscles of the lumbar plexus territory. It is known that after 20–25 min of the opening of the tricuspid retractor, motor responses begin to decrease, regardless of the lack of activity in EMGfr. Thus, in our protocol 20–25 min should be the maximum time for the retractor to remain open. The surgeon may need more time, depending on his learning curve. Therefore, the greater the experience of the surgeon, the shorter the time in which the retractor remains open, with consequent reduction of the risks.

   This time is also correlated with the previous status of the peripheral nerves. In other words, similar to what was mentioned regarding the EMGst, patients with polyneuropathies require closer attention during this stage, since there may be a decrease in time length for MEP alterations to emerge. Thus, in this specific group of patients, it may eventually be necessary to close the tricuspid before reaching 20–25 min, as established for the general population (Figs. 23.6 and 23.7).
5. Routine SEP of the saphenous nerves bilaterally should be performed since it provides sensitive information on the femoral territory. Indeed, the most common sensitive lesion in the LLIF technique is the femoral nerve lesion [2].
6. Carrying out TcMEP and SEP of bilateral ulnar nerve territory is imperative due to the risks posed by prolonged lateral patient's decubitus. The compromise may occur at the elbow, brachial plexus, or cervical roots, due to the maintenance of the patient's head position in lateral rotation.
7. We recommend *femoral nerve H Reflex* with stimulation in the inguinal region and recording in the rectus femoris muscle. The reason is that the sensory loop of the H reflex is shorter, and it does not need the averaging used in the SEPs (Fig. 23.8). Yet, it may be difficult to obtain the H reflex due to the amplitude of the response. To overcome this problem, we increase the distance of the recording electrodes [8].

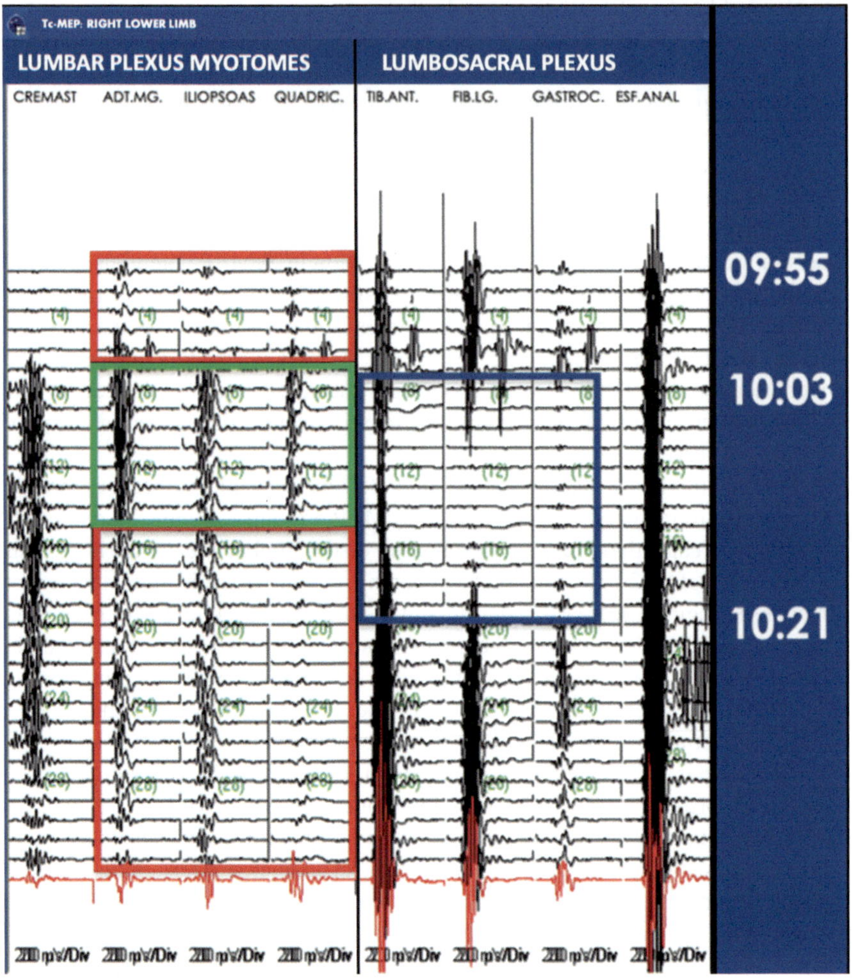

Fig. 23.5 Tc-MEP during LLIF surgery. (**a**) Red squares: amplitude drop of the Tc-MEP in the femoral territory; (**b**) green square: recovery of Tc-MEP responses in the femoral territory; (**c**) blue square: amplitude drop of the Tc-MEP in the lombossacral plexus territory

The Increase of the Inter-electrode Distance in the Quadriceps Femoris Technique [8]

The TcMEP responses of the proximal muscles are reduced in amplitude when compared to the distal muscles [9–13]. This is due to three factors: (1) less representation in the cortex and corticospinal motor tract [9, 13, 14]; (2) greater inhibitory action on the motor neurons of the proximal muscles [14, 15], and (3) greater number of muscle fibers per motor unit in the proximal muscles [16, 17].

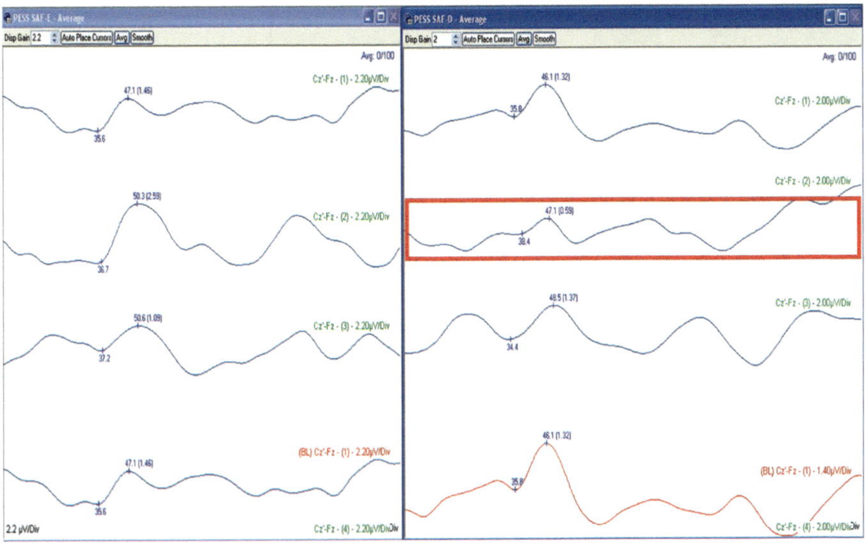

Fig. 23.6 Saphenous nerve – SSEP. Transient amplitude drop during LLIF surgery

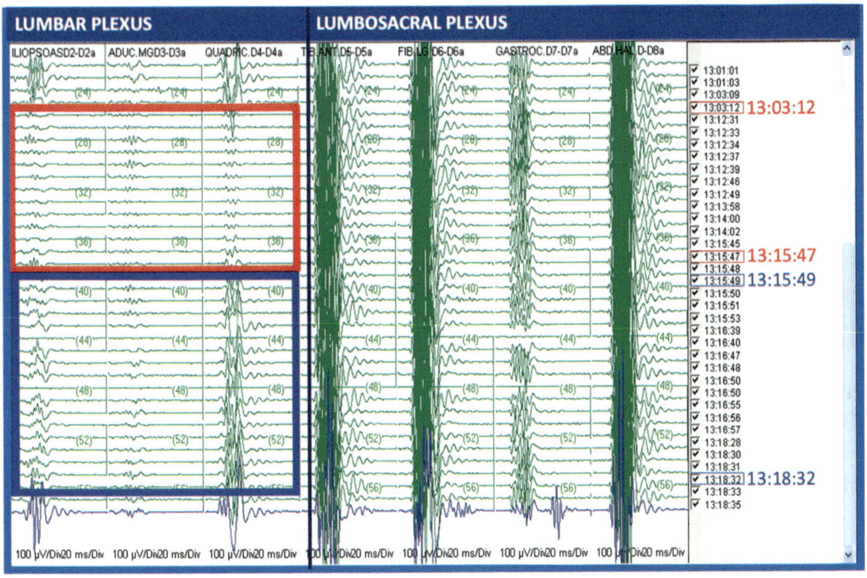

Fig. 23.7 Tc-MEP during LLIF surgeries. (**a**) Red square: transient drop of amplitude responses in the femoral nerve territory (muscles: iliopsoas, rectus femoris, adductor magnus); (**b**) blue square: gradual improvement of Tc-MEP responses of the femoral nerve after releasing the retractor

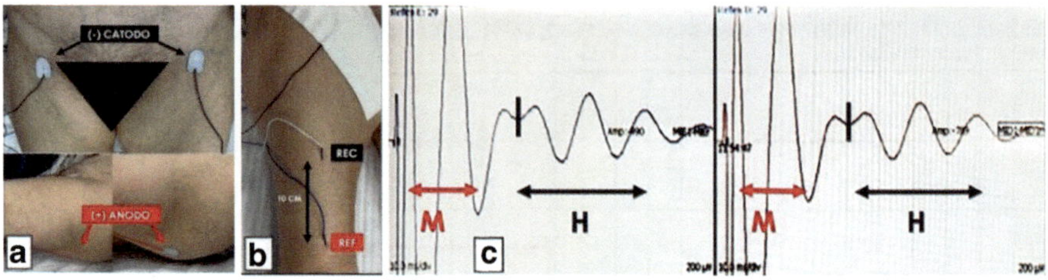

Fig. 23.8 H reflex – femoral nerve. (**a**) Stimulus electrodes; (**b**) recording electrodes in the rectus femoris muscle; (**c**) H reflex of the femoral nerve, left and right. In the picture, it is possible to visualize the M and H responses

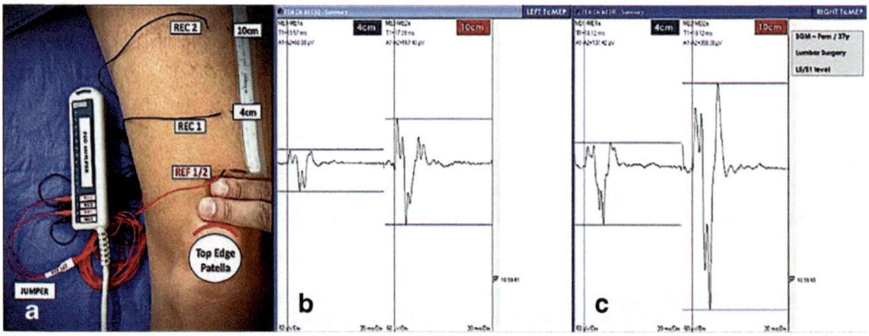

Fig. 23.9 Increase of the inter-electrode distance in the quadriceps femoris technique. (**a**) Myotome recording montage, with 4 cm (REC 1) and 10 cm (REC 2) distance. (**b**) and (**c**) Tc-MEP responses, left and right lower limb, respectively. The responses are significantly greater in amplitude with 10 cm of inter-electrode distance

Parikh et al. [16] found similar results in the study of the TcMEPS and electrical stimulation of lower limbs [12]. Also, based on electroneuromyography studies of sensory and motor conduction, it is known that an increase in the distance between electrodes leads to an increase in the amplitude of the responses [17–20].

Recently, we addressed this issue regarding TcMEP of quadriceps [8], by analyzing 106 patients (212 limbs). The increase in the inter-electrode distance from 4 to 10 cm showed an increase in the Tc-MEP amplitude in all cases evaluated (Fig. 23.9). For this reason, we successfully applied this concept for the intraoperative femoral H reflex.

Prone Position for LLIF

A new positioning technique for performing LLIF surgeries called "prone position" has recently been described. The benefits would be a better anatomical position of the psoas muscle and lumbar plexus, consequently with enhanced safety regarding neurological injuries related to LLIF instrumentation. Additionally, if a posterior approach is needed, the patient is already positioned [21].

Intraoperative Neurophysiological Monitoring to ALIF Techniques

The anterior approach of the lumbar spine (ALIF) for decompression and implantation of lumbar prosthesis or cage is used for the treatment of the lumbosacral spine. Both implants aim to improve and maintain the intervertebral space. The prosthesis maintains mobility in the treated segment and the cage acts as an element for arthrodesis. The anterior approach is made through an abdominal incision, which can be median longitudinal or transverse suprapubic (Fig. 23.10). The main advantages of this approach are the greater spine exposure and direct access to the intervertebral disc, reduced muscle retraction, less blood loss, and reduced intraoperative time [22–25].

One of the major concerns regarding ALIF is the risk to the intraperitoneal and retroperitoneal vessels and to other structures (Fig. 23.11), which may need to be

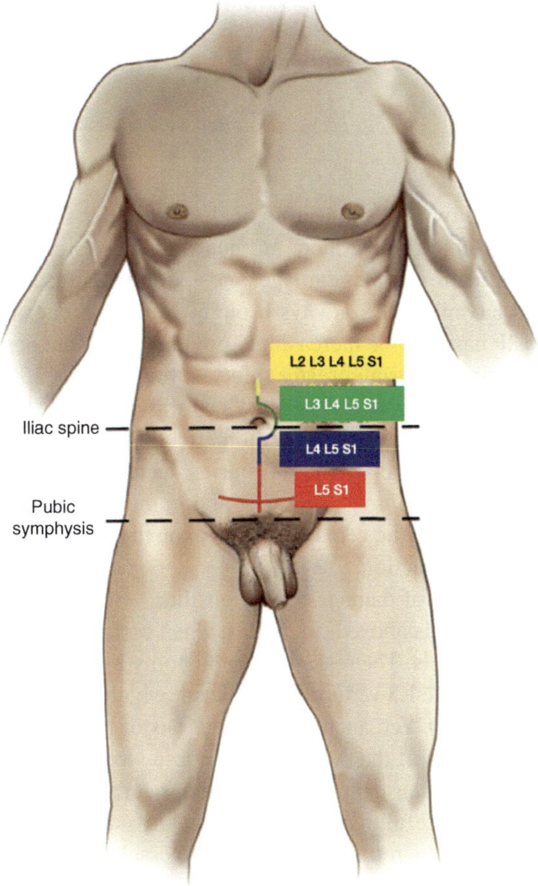

Fig. 23.10 Abdominal incisions in the anterior approach of the lumbar spine surgery. The types of incisions and the level of interest of the surgery are shown schematically. (Image: Courtesy of Aecio Rubens Dias Pereira Filho, MD [11])

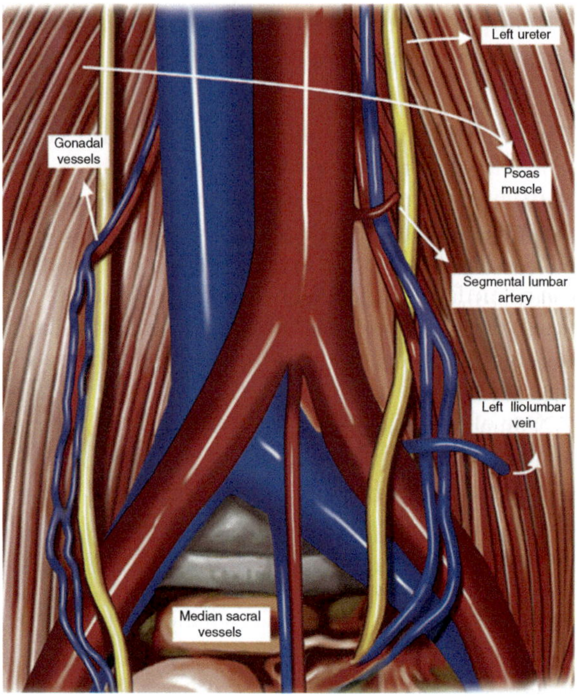

Fig. 23.11 Vessels and retroperitoneal structures. (Image: Courtesy of Aecio Rubens Dias Pereira Filho, MD [11])

repaired by a general, urological, or vascular surgeon on short notice [22]. Among the adverse events, there are neurological lesions, retrograde ejaculation, surgical site infection, ureter damage, and abdominal muscle injury [22–28]. For this reason, this technique has always brought some apprehension to the spine surgeons. Yet, ALIF has become increasingly popular due to the possibility of the aid of an "access surgeon," ensuring greater safety to the surgery [23, 24].

Even so, there are still risks in this approach like vascular injury up to 18.1% [27]. Most frequently laceration affects the left common iliac vein during the vascular retraction step. Arterial injuries occur in 0.45% of the cases, far less frequently than venous injuries [28]. The abdominal arteries are more elastic and more easily movable than the veins; for this reason they are less likely to be injured by mobilization and retraction.

The risk of damage to the left iliac vein is higher in surgeries performed in the lumbar levels above L5 [27, 28], when compared to surgeries performed at the lower lumbar levels. The reason is the anatomy of the iliac vein confluence, which usually occurs at the L5 vertebral body level, which makes the L5-S1 level safer [23, 29, 30] (Fig. 23.12). Yet, anatomical variations of the iliac arteries and veins, including different levels of the bifurcation of these vessels [23, 29], may lead to greater risks of vascular impairment, even in surgeries at the L5-S1 level. For this reason, sometimes it may be useful to perform a preoperative angiographic exam before the ALIF [30].

During the retraction of the iliac vessels, venous congestion may occur, resulting in an increased endoneural pressure [31]. Both arterial insufficiency and venous stasis can lead to ischemia of peripheral nerves and consequent neurophysiological

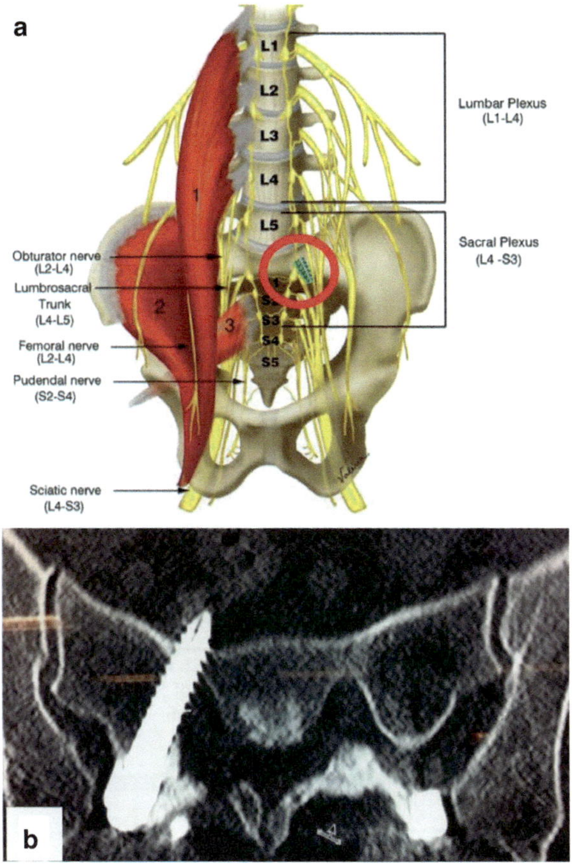

Fig. 23.12 Anterior access of the lumbosacral spine and its correlation with the iliac vessels. In this schematic figure, the greatest technical difficulty can be seen, with the need for greater vessel retraction when approaching the superior levels of lumbassacral spine (L2/L3, L3/L4, and L4/L5). The L5/S1 level is most often located at the confluence of the veins/bifurcation of the iliac arteries; therefore, it needs little or no retraction. (Image: Courtesy of Aecio Rubens Dias Pereira Filho, MD [11])

alteration. The sensory axons are more susceptible to hemodynamic changes than the motor axons [32, 33]. Consequently, changes in SEP precede (Fig. 23.13) changes in the TcMEP responses (Fig. 23.14). Hence, IONMm should always be performed since it allows the early diagnosis of vascular impairment and may lead to vessel retraction removal. The return of responses to baseline levels (reversibility maneuver) proves that IONM changes are "true-positive" findings. It aims to prevent the development of more severe vascular impairment and neurological injuries.

Accordingly, we suggest the adoption of fundamental steps for IONMm for surgeries using the ALIF technique:

1. Patient should be prepared while in dorsal decubitus, with the upper limbs crossed over the chest. The myotomes of choice will depend on the lumbar levels to be treated and the external anal sphincter monitoring is mandatory.
2. Record SEP and MEP baselines from the four limbs.
3. Next, the anesthetist may use neuromuscular blockers during the exposure of the abdominal field because of the difficulties in accessing the peritoneum in unrelaxed patients. It is suggested to control the neuromuscular blockage with the use of TOF (Train of Four), with a target of 50%.

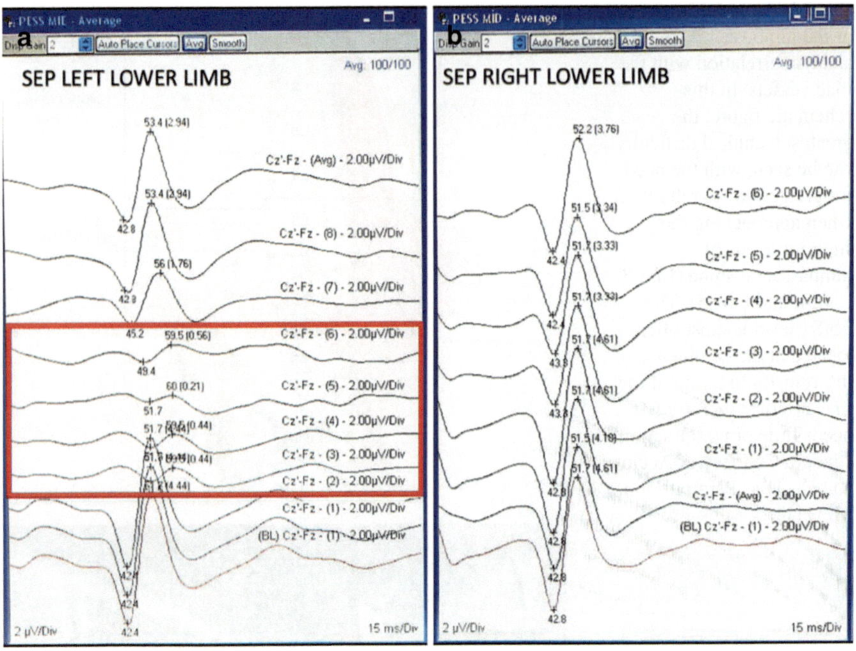

Fig. 23.13 SEP: transient amplitude drop of SEP cortical responses during the ALIF procedure. The amplitude drop is seen in both lower limbs, but is more pronounced in the left lower limb

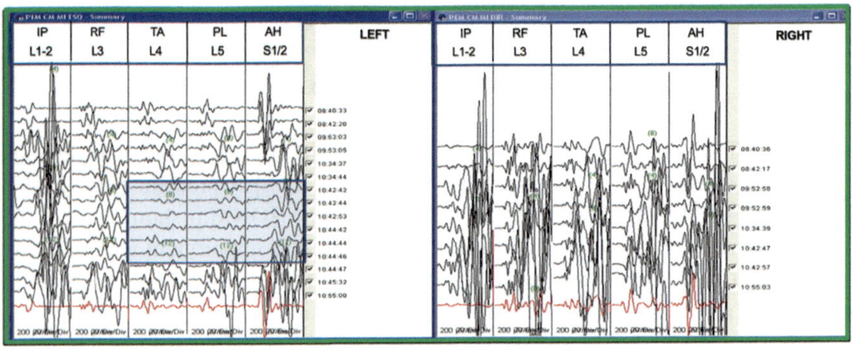

Fig. 23.14 Tc-MEP: transient amplitude drop of Tc-MEP responses during the ALIF procedure. The amplitude drop is shown in the myotomes in the left sciatic nerve territory

4. During the vertebral approach, IONM should be continuously performed and EMGfr should be interspersed with SEP and Tc-MEP.
5. Tc-MEP and SEP should be recorded after implant (cage or disc prosthesis) placement.
6. Tc-MEP changes, with amplitude deterioration greater than 50%, if considered true positives, should be valued. If secondary to vascular etiology, they may be

reversed by releasing the iliac vessel retractors. However, they may be due to direct neural tissue injury (during discectomy) or indirect injury (due to over distraction of the implant).

Usually, concerning the L5-S1 level approach procedures, if at the end of the surgery the Tc-MEP changes remain, it may be secondary to check on the L5 root. The occurrence of posterior foraminal compression by the superior articular process of the inferior vertebra must be evaluated [34] (Fig. 23.15). In these situations, posterior decompression may be considered (Fig. 23.16).

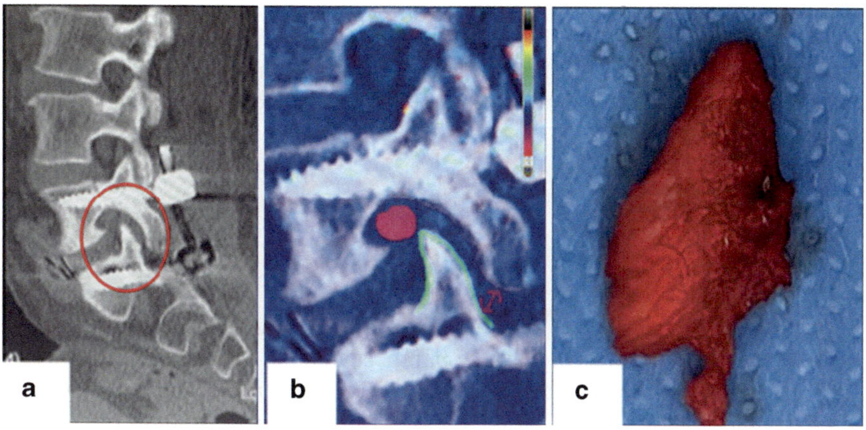

Fig. 23.15 Superior articular process of the inferior vertebra. (**a**) and (**b**) Radiological confirmation and (**c**) anatomical component, surgically resected

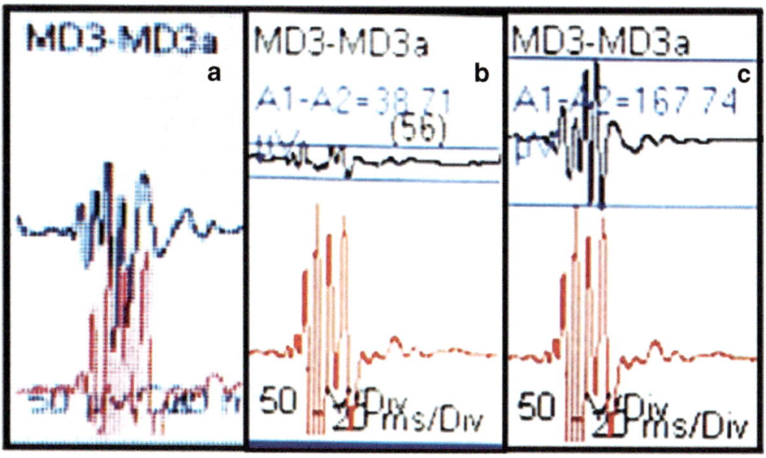

Fig. 23.16 Tc-MEP response changes in the right L5 root ("MD3") during lumbar surgery with the anterior and posterior approach. (**a**) Tc-MEP responses at the end of the anterior approach. (**b**) Significant amplitude deterioration in Tc-MEP responses, at the beginning of the posterior approach. (**c**) Improved Tc-MEP responses after posterior decompression

Final Statements

The use of multimodal IONM is the most adequate protocol to monitor neural integrity [6], but unfortunately, they are not widely used during surgeries applying the LLIF/ALIF techniques. We recommend the use of IONMm in all spinal surgeries.

From a legal aspect in Brazil as in other countries, IONM must be conducted by a physician with adequate training to carry out the procedure. Indeed, in Brazil, non-compliance with this law incurs an illegal practice of medicine, which can lead to legal issues to the surgical team and hospital managers [35].

Remote monitoring, as practiced in several countries, is not permitted according to Brazilian laws. Therefore, it is mandatory that an in-site trained physician perform the IONM. The surgeon, his assistants, and the anesthesiologist are not allowed to perform concomitant neurophysiology monitoring. More details in this subject were detailed in Chap. 2.

Conclusion

Despite the many advantages of minimally invasive surgery, many studies report neurological complications in this type of procedure.

For this reason, the use of multimodal IONM is recommended in all LIF surgeries. The objective of multimodal IONM is to guarantee and assure to the surgical team a reduced rate of partial or permanent neurological complications [36].

References

1. Kepler CK, Bogner EA, Herzog RJ, et al. Anatomy of the psoas muscle and lumbar plexus with respect to the surgical approach for lateral transpsoas interbody fusion. Eur Spine J. 2011;20(4):550–6.
2. Le TV, Burkett CJ, Deukmedjian AR, et al. Postoperative lumbar plexus injury after lumbar retroperitoneal transpsoas minimally invasive lateral interbody fusion. Spine (Phila Pa 1976). 2013;38(1):E13–20.
3. He L, Dong J, Liu B, et al. A MRI study of lumbar plexus in patients with degenerative lumbar scoliosis after extreme lateral interbody fusion. Zhonghua Yi Xue Za Zhi. 2014;94(3):178–81. Published Online First: 2014/04/16.
4. Quinn JC, Fruauff K, Lebl DR, et al. Magnetic resonance neurography of the lumbar plexus at the L4-L5 disc: development of a preoperative surgical planning tool for lateral lumbar transpsoas interbody fusion (LLIF). Spine (Phila Pa 1976). 2015;40(12):942–7.
5. Laratta JL, Shillingford JN, Ha A, et al. Utilization of intraoperative neuromonitoring throughout the United States over a recent decade: an analysis of the nationwide inpatient sample. J Spine Surg. 2018;4(2):211–9.
6. Riley MR, Doan AT, Vogel RW, et al. Use of motor evoked potentials during lateral lumbar interbody fusion reduces postoperative deficits. Spine J. 2018;18(10):1763–78.

7. Sutter M, Eggspuehler A, Jeszenszky D, et al. The impact and value of uni- and multimodal intraoperative neurophysiological monitoring (IONM) on neurological complications during spine surgery: a prospective study of 2728 patients. Eur Spine J. 2019;28(3):599–610.
8. Bordini EC, Ferreira RJR, Germano CSB, Barretto LS, et al. Significant improvement in Tc-MEP responses in quadriceps femoris muscles by the simple increase of the inter-electrode distance: solving a long time problem. Poster session. 2020 American Clinical Neurophysiology Society (ACNS) Annual Meeting. J Clin Neurophysiol. 2020;37(4):310–72. https://doi.org/10.1097/WNP.0000000000000698.
9. Palmer E, Ashby P. Corticospinal projections to upper limb motoneurones in humans. J Physiol. 1992;448:397–412.
10. Lemon RN, Mantel GW, Muir RB. Corticospinal facilitation of hand muscles during voluntary movement in the conscious monkey. J Physiol. 1986;381:497–527.
11. Phillips CG, Porter R. The pyramidal projection to motoneurones of some muscle groups of the baboon's forelimb. Prog Brain Res. 1964;12:222–45.
12. Bernhard CG, Bohm E. Cortical representation and functional significance of the corticomotoneuronal system. AMA Arch Neurol Psychiatry. 1954;72(4):473–502.
13. Buchthal F, Schmalbruch H. Motor unit of mammalian muscle. Physiol Rev. 1980;60(1):90–142.
14. Rothwell JC, Thompson PD, Day BL, et al. Motor cortex stimulation in intact man. General characteristics of EMG responses in different muscles. Brain. 1987;110(Pt 5):1173–90.
15. Wassermann EM, McShane LM, Hallett M, Cohen LG. Noninvasive mapping of muscle representations in human motor cortex. Electroencephalogr Clin Neurophysiol. 1992;85(1):1–8.
16. Parikh P, Cheongsiatmoy J, Shilian P, Gonzalez AA. Differences in the transcranial motor evoked potentials between proximal and distal lower extremity muscles. J Clin Neurophysiol. 2018;35(2):155–8.
17. Zipp P. Effect of electrode geometry on the selectivity of myoelectric recordings with surface electrodes. Eur J Appl Physiol. 1982;50:35–40.
18. Eduardo E, Burke D. The optimal recording electrode configuration for compound sensory action potentials. J Neurol Neurosurg Psychiatry. 1988;51(5):684–7.
19. Evanoff Jr V, Buschbacher RM. Optimal interelectrode distance in sensory and mixed compound nerve action potentials: 3- versus 4-centimeter bar electrodes. Arch Phys Med Rehabil. 2004;85(3):405–8.
20. Jonas D, Bischoff C, Conrad B. Influence of different types of surface electrodes on amplitude, area and duration of the compound muscle action potential. Clin Neurophysiol. 1999;110(12):2171–5.
21. Pimenta L, Amaral R, Taylor W, Tohmeh A, Pokorny G, Rodrigues R, Arnoni D, Guirelli T, Batista M. The prone transpsoas technique: preliminary radiographic results of a multicenter experience. Eur Spine J. 2021;30(1):108–13. https://doi.org/10.1007/s00586-020-06471-y. Epub 2020 May 29. Erratum in: Eur Spine J. 2020.
22. Than KD, et al. Complication avoidance and management in anterior lumbarinterbody fusion. Neurosurg Focus. 2011;31(4):E6.
23. Pereira Filho ARD. Technique for exposing lumbar discs in anterior approach using Steinmann wires: arthroplasties or arthrodesis. World Neurosurg. 2021;148:189–95.
24. Jarrett CD, et al. Anterior exposure of the lumbar spine with and without an "access surgeon": morbidity analysis of 265 consecutive cases. J Spinal Disord Tech. 2009;22(8):559–64.
25. Tropiano P, et al. Surgical techniques for lumbo-sacral fusion. Orthop Traumatol Surg Res. 2017;103:S151–9.
26. Reddy D, et al. Extensive deep venous thrombosis resulting from anterior lumbar spine surgery in a patient with iliac vein compression syndrome: a case report and literature review. Global Spine J. 2015;5:e22–7.
27. Inamasu J, et al. Review article. Vascular injury and complication in neurosurgical spine surgery. Acta Neurochir. 2006;48:375–87.
28. Brau SA, et al. Vascular injury during anterior lumbar surgery. Spine J. 2004;4(4):409–12.

29. Jasani V, et al. The anatomy of the iliolumbar vein. A cadaver study. J Bone Joint Surg Br. 2002;84:1046–9.
30. Inamasu J, et al. Three-dimensional computed tomographic anatomy of the abdominal great vessels pertinente to L4-L5 anterior lumbar interbody fusion. Minim Invasive Neurosurg. 2005;48:127–31.
31. Rydevik BL, et al. The effects of compression on the physiology nerve roots. J Manip Physiol Ther. 1992;15(1):62–6.
32. Bostcock H. Differences in behaviour of sensory and motor axons following release of ischaemia. Brain. 1994;117(Pt 2):225–34.
33. Brau SA, et al. Nerve monitoring changes related to iliac artery compression during anterior lumbar spine surgery. Spine J. 2003;3(5):351–5.
34. Neal MT, Kalani MA, Lyons MK. A technical nuance to avoid lumbar five radiculopathy with anterior lumbar fusion and posterior instrumentation. Case Rep Orthop. 2021;2021:5514720. https://doi.org/10.1155/2021/5514720.
35. Brazilian Federal Council of Medicine. Resoluction number 2.136/2015. Official Diary of the Union; 2016. Section 1, p. 71.
36. Shilian P, et al. Overview of intraoperative neurophysiological monitoring during spine surgery. J Clin Neurophysiol. 2016;33(4):333–9.

Chapter 24
Cervical Spinal Surgery

Ricardo José Rodriguez Ferreira, Patrícia Toscano, Emília Caram Bordini, and Arthur Werner Poetscher

Abbreviations

BIS	Bispectral Indicis
DWILT	D-Wave Interspinous Ligament Technique
EMG	Electromyography
EMG-fr	Electromyography Free Run
EMG-st	Electromyography Triggered
IONM	Intraoperative Neurophysiological Monitoring

R. J. R. Ferreira (✉) · E. C. Bordini
AACD - Disabled Child Care Association, São Paulo, SP, Brazil

Dr Ricardo Ferreira Clinic, São Paulo, SP, Brazil

Spine Surgery Department at Orthopedics and Trauma Institute of Clinical Hospital of the University of São Paulo Medical School, São Paulo, SP, Brazil

P. Toscano
Neurology Department, Ribeirão Preto Medical School of the University of São Paulo, Ribeirão Preto, SP, Brazil

A. W. Poetscher
Neurosurgery Department at Hospital Israelita Albert Einstein, São Paulo, SP, Brazil

S. M. Verst et al. (eds.), *Intraoperative Monitoring*,
https://doi.org/10.1007/978-3-030-95730-8_24

MAP	Mean Arterial Pressure
MEP	Motor Evoked Potential
mMEP	Muscle Motor Evoked potential
MUAP	Motor Unit Action Potential
SSEP	Somatosensory Evoked Potential
Tc-MEP	Transcranial Motor Evoked Potential
TOF	Train of Four

Surgeon's Point of View

IONM has become an essential tool in cervical spine decompression surgery. Although some controversy regarding the use of IOM for specific procedures may persist, tools that improve patient safety should not be dismissed.

The spinal cord and cervical spine nerve roots are always at risk during cervical spine surgery. Damage to spinal nerve roots can lead to weakness of specific muscles in arms and hands, as well as hypoesthesia and neuropathic pain in correspondent dermatomes. Cervical spinal cord injury may cause a variety of syndromes, including tetraplegia and loss of sphincter control.

Cervical spine approaches can be classified into anterior and posterior.

When compression originates from anterior elements, such as intervertebral disc, osteophytes, posterior longitudinal ligament, and normal cervical lordosis is compromised, surgery is usually performed using an anterior approach. Posterior compression caused by ligamentum flavum hypertrophy or multilevel canal stenosis is commonly treated with posterior approaches.

Spinal nerve impingements are often treated by anterior approaches, although for specific compressions a posterior foraminotomy may be the best option.

Intraoperative monitoring should begin before the patient is positioned. Flexion or extension of the neck when positioning can worsen the compression on the spinal cord and cause catastrophic damage.

During an anterior approach, the recurrent laryngeal nerve can also be monitored with an electrode at the endotracheal tube, reducing the risk of injury and hoarseness after surgery. During decompression, when removing the disc or perforating the bone near the dura, injury to the spinal cord or spinal nerve roots can occur. The next step, placing the cage or graft, can also be critical, as improper positioning can cause compression.

The critical times for later approaches are decompression and screw placement. Decompression can be performed by removing small amounts of bone each time with the use of rongeurs or a drill. Some surgeons prefer to perform a laminotomy by cutting the laminae with a drill and removing the posterior elements *en bloc*. When a posterior decompression is associated with a posterior arthrodesis, each screw placement must be carefully monitored to avoid spinal nerve injury. Some patients may wake up with deltoid weakness, the so-called C5 syndrome. This is probably caused by stretching of the nerve root that can occur after decompression. Therefore, C5 should always be monitored.

Cervical compressive myelopathy is a very fragile condition. Minor surgical trauma can lead to dramatic neurological worsening. The IONM team's warnings should always be heeded. Surgery should be paused, the operative field reviewed, and anesthetic parameters checked.

Introduction

One of the main applications of multimodal intraoperative neurophysiological monitoring (IONM) in spine surgery is cervical spine surgery. Its importance begins in the preoperative period, with the evaluation of the correct positioning of the patient, both in anterior and posterior approaches. Motor deficits may arise from positioning in a patient with vertebral canal stenosis associated or not with cervical myelopathy.

In addition, IONM can detect pre-existing neurological deficits, prevent central and peripheral nervous system injuries, and prove successful decompression maneuvers.

Specifically in the anterior approach of cervical spine surgeries, there is a need for additional evaluation of the recurrent laryngeal nerve and/or superior laryngeal nerve structures that may be at risk of injury in the exposure phase [1].

The effectiveness of somatosensory evoked potential (SSEP) and motor evoked potential (MEP) techniques and electromyography (EMG), individually and in combination, provide greater sensitivity for early detection of clinically significant neurological impairment [2, 4, 5].

The incidence of neurological deficits in cervical spine surgery has been relatively low, ranging from 0.2% to 3.2% [6]. Several groups have set out to study the events that determine truly positive neurological outcomes [7, 8].

Main Pathologies of the Cervical Spine

Cervical spine can be approached by both anterior and posterior approaches, and the indications are numerous:

1. Degenerative diseases: herniated discs, arthrosis (osteophytosis), listhesis, vertebral canal stenosis, rheumatologic diseases (ankylosing spondylitis), myelopathy, radiculopathy
2. Trauma: fracture, dislocation, traumatic listhesis, whiplash injury with posterior ligament rupture
3. Vertebral and neuraxial tumors
4. Deformity: cervical kyphosis
5. Congenital: Arnold-Chiari
6. Chronic pain

Approaches

Cervical spine can be approached by an anterior approach, a posterior approach, or both at the same surgical time. Posterior approaches can be performed in open surgeries or minimally invasive (endoscopic) surgeries.

The anterior approach, transoral or latero-anterior cervical, is indicated for:

1. Decompression – discectomy, osteophytes and intracanal fragments resection, corpectomy
2. Arthrodesis – graft, disc cage, body cage
3. Arthroplasty – disk prosthesis

In the posterior approach, the main indications are:

1. Decompression – single or multiple laminotomy or laminectomy
2. Arthrodesis – in situ, lateral mass screw, pedicle screws, sublaminar bands or wires
3. Endoscopic

Anterior Approach

Advantage The main advantage of the anterior approach versus the posterior approach is the possibility of better exposure of the vertebral body, disc space, posterior ligament, and access to the anterior portion of the spinal cord, allowing decompression and arthrodesis with minimal manipulation of the neurological structures.

Disadvantage Possible injuries by withdrawal and even direct trauma to vascular, neural, tracheal, and esophageal structures due to the approach route. These sentinel events are potentially catastrophic [9].

Preoperative

Preparation The patient is transferred from the transport stretcher to the operating table where he will be prepared by the anesthesiologist, neurophysiologist, and nurse.

Anesthesia
Orotracheal tube: Set the gauge to be used so that the neurophysiologist applies the adhesive electrode on the tube.

Tube adhesive electrode: Adhesive electrodes should have two channels and the appropriate width for the chosen tube. If there is excess adhesive that could cover the electrode contacts, this excess part must be cut off (Fig. 24.1).

Anesthetic protocol: Totally intravenous anesthesia is recommended, considering the preoperative neurophysiological tests with the patient at rest. Only after these tests and depending on the responses found is the patient's definitive positioning performed. For more details on general anesthesia, refer to Chap. 5.

Curarization: If necessary, the neuromuscular blockade should be done with succinylcholine, due to the rapidity of its elimination, or even rocuronium, which is rapidly reversed by Sugammadex®, in a few minutes.

Bite protection: After intubation, the neurophysiologist does the bite protection with a specific bite-block device, like Tongard® – Healthnology [10] – Fig. 24.2 – or with gauze cushions, placed bilaterally between the molars, thus avoiding lesions to the tongue, cheek, lips, teeth, and the bite of the orotracheal tube itself.

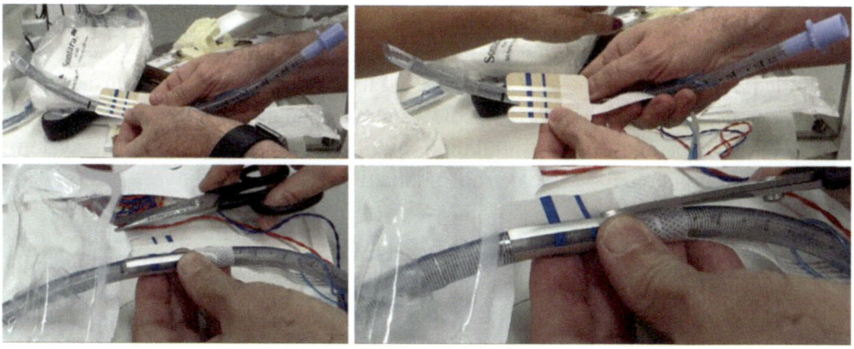

Fig. 24.1 Demonstration of the application of adhesive laryngeal electrode to the orotracheal tube. Eventually, it is necessary to cut an excess adhesive of the electrode

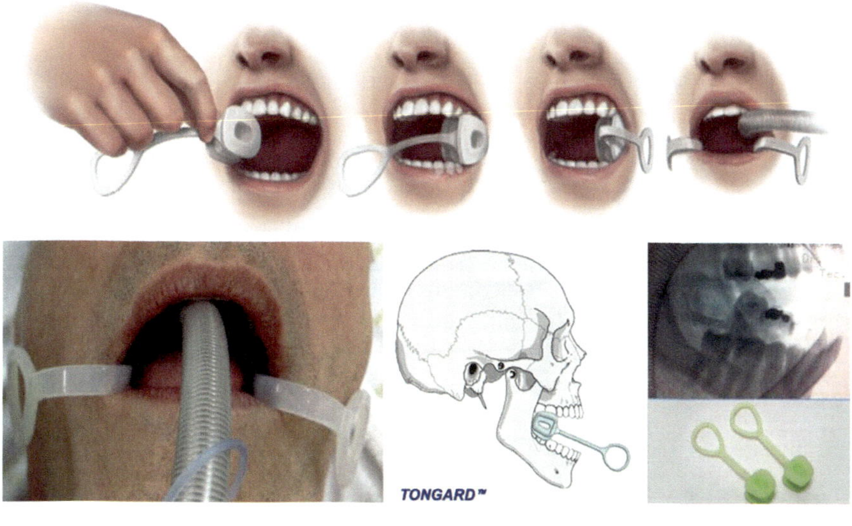

Fig. 24.2 Tongard^{R} Healthnology – bite-block device

Neurophysiology

Tests

- SSEP: Ulnar and median nerves MMSS; tibial nerve MMII at ankle level.
- MEP/EMG: Myotomes of interest according to the level or levels to be addressed. Usually, the upper trapezius (C3/4), deltoid (C5), biceps (C6), triceps (C7) and fifth finger abductor (C8/T1), tibialis anterior (L4), and abductor hallucis (S2) muscles are used. It is also possible to evaluate the recurrent laryngeal nerve (vocal cords), especially when approaching lower levels – C5/C6/C7, or the superior laryngeal nerve (cricothyroid m. – Fig. 24.3), important in surgery of higher levels – C3/C4/C5. In specific cases, external anal sphincter recording (S2-S4) may be considered.
- MEP – D-wave (in cases of the transoral route). (*Note of the editors: exclusively authors' experience*).

Preparation

With the patient already anesthetized, proceed to apply the needle and surface electrodes on the patient. Corkscrew needle electrodes adapted to the scalp for both SSEP recordings and MEP stimulation by the 10/20 or 10/10 EEG system. Orotracheal tube already with electrode adapted as mentioned above.

Positioning

Upper limbs positioning: Position the patient with arms along the body, making sure the thumbs are facing up. This confers the anatomical resting position of the shoulders and prevents postoperative pain related to prolonged inadequate positioning (in internal or external rotation). Also, check on arms position to avoid ulnar or radial nerves compression.

Definitive positioning: After performing the neurophysiological tests at rest and analyzing the responses, agree with the surgical team to place the cushion under the

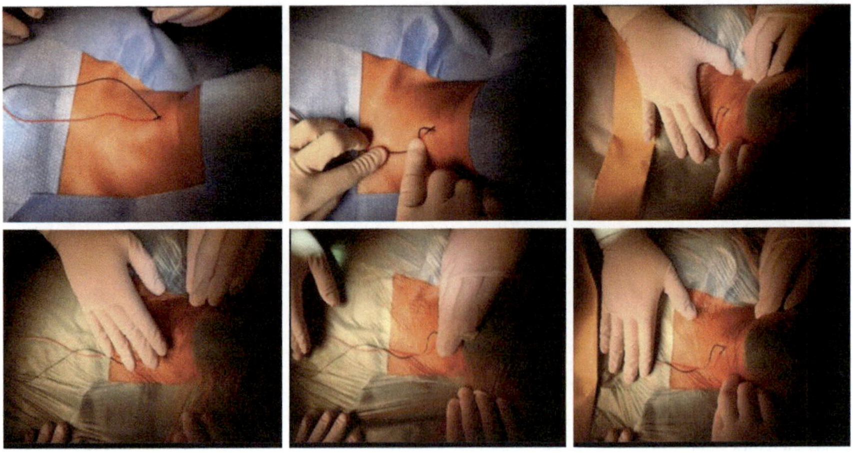

Fig. 24.3 Technique for capturing the cricothyroid muscle with needle electrodes. The neurophysiologist inserts the electrodes, after proper degermation and skin preparation by the surgeon

scapular waist and to perform shoulder traction with adhesive tape. It is important to note that excessive traction on the shoulders can cause brachial plexus injury [11]. Check on fibular nerve at the fibular head.

This positioning allows, preoperatively, the radioscopic evaluation and localization of the correct level to be treated; intraoperatively, a surgical field that is more favorable for direct macro- or microscopic visualization and better evaluation of the vertebral levels on radioscopy, especially the more caudal ones such as C6/C7.

Post-positioning

Repeat the neurophysiological tests and compare with the results obtained at rest.

Tests without deficit change: Authorizing the beginning of surgery.

Tests with some deficient alteration: Neurophysiological and anesthetic checklist: In neurophysiological tests, check electrode connections and if stimulation parameters are correct. In the anesthetic tests, check mainly if decurarization is complete by train of four – TOF and if mean arterial pressure – MAP and hypnosis are at adequate levels, the latter with a bispectral indicis – BIS measurement greater than 45%. If any of these parameters is inadequate, correct and repeat the tests. If the neurophysiological and anesthetic checklist is adequate, it is a true positive, the surgical team must be informed, and the patient repositioned.

Tests now without deficit change or <50% drop: Authorizing the beginning of surgery.

Tests remain with deficit alteration >50%: It is our protocol to consider >50% the major criterion of warning, although others would consider deterioration >80% or loss of MEP [11]. In our institution, the start of surgery should be suspended until the tests return to baseline. If no return of responses to baseline or acceptable levels is observed (a drop of less than 50%), the procedure should be suspended.

In severe cervical myelopathies, in walking patients, simple positioning in cervical extension may lead to loss of caudal responses at the level of compression or myelomalacia. In some cases, deterioration or loss of responses are observed exclusively for the lower limbs. Even reducing the extension caused by positioning, it is possible that the responses do not return to baseline. In these cases, the most prudent decision is to suspend the procedure.

It is worth noting that in some cases, especially in myelopathies, positioning may exert deleterious effects on motor and/or sensory pathways insidiously. Thus, there may be a delayed decline in IONM responses [12]. In these situations, positioning should be reevaluated, possibly with the need to reduce cervical extension.

Thus, given this context, we suggest the adoption of nine key steps for neurophysiological monitoring of anterior approach cervical spine surgeries.

Intraoperative: Step by Step

- Step 1: Exposure by anatomical planes – free run electromyography (EMG-fr)
- Step 2: Pre-positioning of the caspar retractor – muscle MEP (mMEP)
- Step 3: Post-placing and opening caspar – mMEP

- Step 4: Discectomy and decompression – EMG-fr
- Step 5: Cage tester placement – mMEP
- Step 6: Cage placement – mMEP and SSEP
- Step 7: Caspar removal – mMEP and SSEP
- Step 8: Plate placement (if cage is not "stand alone" type) – mMEP and SSEP
- Step 9: Closure by planes – mMEP and SSEP

Considerations

- *Step 1*: Watch out for the occurrence of neurotonic discharges in the EMG-fr in the territory of the recurrent laryngeal/superior laryngeal nerves. If such discharges are observed, control mMEP of the laryngeal nerve should be performed (Fig. 24.4). If the mMEP responses are maintained, such discharges only mean nerve manipulation, and it is suggested to reduce the traction used in the soft tissue retractors.
- *Step 2*: Perform an update of the baseline, prior to the opening of the caspar distractor. This confirms that the positioning (cervical extension) remains adequate, as well as the anesthetic protocol.
- *Step 3*: This is the first *maneuver* of higher risk for spinal cord involvement, by indirect mechanism (distraction). In most cases, after the distraction, transient drops in mMEP/SSEP responses may be seen. If these changes remain or show drops >50%, it should be suggested that the distraction be reduced or the caspar retractor temporarily removed.
- *Step 4*: This is the first *step* that can generate direct spinal cord or radicular trauma. If neurotonic discharges occur in the EMG-fr, they should be reported and, depending on their intensity, control with MEP should be performed.
- *Steps 5 and 6*: These steps can generate direct and indirect trauma to the spinal cord. In this phase, the same phenomenon occurs as reported in step 3 (opening of the caspar and distraction); that is, a transient drop in responses is expected, and if it is not intense or permanent, there is no need for alarm. However, if there is a marked reduction in responses, the surgical team should be notified, and

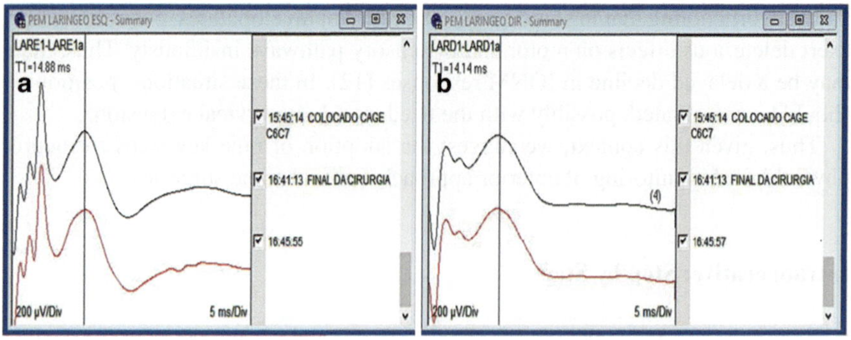

Fig. 24.4 Tc-MEP of the recurrent laryngeal nerve. (**a**) and (**b**) left and right sides, respectively

removal of the disc cage/prosthesis is suggested. Reducing the height of the disc cage/prosthesis may be considered if these changes persist.

It is worth noting that the transient changes reported in steps 3, 5, and 6 occur frequently, and not knowing about them can generate false alarms, causing stress on the surgical team and impacting the neurophysiologist's credibility.

- *Steps 7, 8, and 9*: Observe the responses obtained in the continuous IONM. If a reduction in responses is visualized, inform the surgical team, and suggest a review of the last maneuvers performed.

Posterior Approach

Advantage Posterior approach allows a wide view to spinal cord decompression in severe multi-segmental stenosis. It is also the option of choice when the anterior approach presents significant neurological risks.

Disadvantages It does not address pathologies involving the anterior compartment of the cervical spine; the dreaded C5 palsy occurs more commonly with posterior approach decompressions [13].

Preoperative

Preparation The patient is prepared on the transport stretcher, in dorsal decubitus, by the anesthesiologist, neurophysiologist, and nurse.

Anesthesia The same protocol is recommended as for the anterior approach, except for the monitoring of the recurrent/superior laryngeal nerve (not necessary in this approach).

Neurophysiology
Tests

- SEP, mMEP, and EMG: Follow the same protocol cited for the anterior approach; in this case, the preoperative tests at rest will be on the transport stretcher in dorsal decubitus, and the post-positioning will be in ventral decubitus on the operating table.
- MEP: *It is our opinion* that in cases of severe vertebral canal compromise, such as stenosis, myelopathies, and fractures, the use of the D-wave along with mMEP may be of great use in posterior approach cervical surgeries since there may be a reduction or absence of mMEP responses. The presence of a stable D-wave may allow the continuity of the surgical procedure. *D-wave recording needs to be validated by other groups though.*

Positioning
Definitive positioning: After performing the neurophysiological tests at rest in dorsal decubitus and analyzing the responses, agree with the surgical team to change the decubitus from dorsal to ventral. The positioning is done with the patient supporting the head on a cushion or coupled to a standard cranial stabilization system (Mayfield).

Upper limbs positioning: The upper limbs will be along the body, observing that the thumbs are turned downwards. As mentioned in the anterior approach, but in opposite way, this gives the anatomical resting position of the shoulders and avoids postoperative pain related to prolonged, inadequate positioning. In some cases, the shoulders can be pulled with adhesive tape by the surgical team. This positioning allows, preoperatively, the radioscopic evaluation and localization of the correct level to be treated; intraoperatively, it maintains a surgical field more proper to direct visualization (macro or microscopic) and better evaluation of the vertebral levels in the radioscopy, especially those more caudal such as C6/7.

Post final positioning
Repeat the neurophysiological tests and then compare with the results obtained when resting in the dorsal decubitus position.

Tests without deficient alteration: Authorizing the beginning of surgery.

Tests with some deficient alteration: Neurophysiological and anesthetic checklist, as cited above. If the neurophysiological and anesthetic checklist is adequate, it is a true positive, the surgical team must be informed, and the patient repositioned.

Tests now without deficit change or <50% drop: Authorizing the beginning of surgery.

Tests remain with deficit alteration >50%: It attests that the repositioning did not have the expected effect. In this situation, the start of surgery should be suspended until the tests return to baseline. If no return of responses to baseline or acceptable levels are observed (a drop of less than 50%), the procedure must be stopped, the patient returned to supine position on the transport stretcher, and the tests repeated. As mentioned above, this protocol is performed in our institution (see section "Anterior Approach").

As a protocol, we suggest the recording with the same myotomes recommended for the anterior approach. In addition, because the surgery is performed in ventral decubitus, it is mandatory to include the quadriceps femoris due to the use of cushion in the anterosuperior iliac spines, preventing positioning injuries.

Thus, we suggest the following fundamental steps for neurophysiological monitoring of posterior approach cervical spine surgeries.

Intraoperative: Step by Step

- Step 1: Exposure by anatomical planes – EMG-fr, mMEP, and SSEP
- Step 2: Lateral mass screws and/or pedicle screws – mMEP and SSEP
- Step 3: Laminectomy/decompression – EMG-fr, mMEP, and SSEP
- Step 4: Rods placement – mMEP and SSEP
- Step 5: Closure by planes – mMEP and SSEP

Considerations

- *Step 1*: At this stage, pay attention to any changes in basal tests, as they may be secondary to positioning.
- *Step 2*: The lateral mass screws do not need stimulation (EMGst), because their risk is exclusively vascular (vertebral artery). The pedicle screws, when present (usually C2 and C7), could be stimulated with the same technique as the thoracic screws (EMGst: train of 4 pulses, ISI 2 ms, duration 0.2 ms or 200 μs and intensity 7 mA or determined by the threshold of the instrumented pedicle). Both cases should be monitored with mMEP and SEP.
- *Step 3*: At this stage it is critical to evaluate the dorsal column, with SSEP, as this is the main structure at risk.

  In our institution, if D-wave is indicated, the epidural catheter should be inserted after laminectomy. *Specific authors' experience.*

  A careful evaluation of the mMEP is also important. In cases of multi-laminectomies or multi-laminotomies, a greater possibility of C5 palsy is described [13, 14]. If C5 palsy occurs, it can be diagnosed by abruptly falling mMEP responses in this territory, immediately after laminectomy or a few minutes after decompression.
- *Steps 4 and 5*: Maintaining continuous monitoring with mMEP and SSEP. If changes are observed, the last surgical step performed should always be reviewed.

Endoscopic Approach

There is popularization and increasing expansion of endoscopic and minimally invasive surgeries for the treatment of cervical disc herniations and stenosis, with the advantages of minimal tissue damage, less blood loss, rapid recovery, and early hospital discharge. IONM plays an important role in preventing nerve injury.

Endoscopic cervical surgery can present some technical difficulties, such as the restriction of visualization of the operative field with the inherent risks to neural tissue, and it requires a learning curve for the use of the endoscope.

Some surgeons recommend using local anesthetics or regional anesthesia, keeping the patient awake. This option is more attractive to patients, who are discharged earlier from the hospital. However, this practice is controversial. The development of safer, modern general anesthesia techniques proves that the method is superior or similar to local anesthesia and that surgeons feel more comfortable operating on a sleeping patient [15]. In 2016, Ruetten corroborated these aspects by pointing out that general anesthesia allows for better positioning and clinical stability during the procedure, facilitating more complex maneuvers in the spinal canal [16]. Furthermore, local anesthesia is more frequently associated to respiratory depression, with the need for changing from prone to supine position and from local to general anesthetic regimen – with a consequent need of intubation [17].

The access approaches in endoscopic surgery are: transforaminal and interlaminar [18]. In interlaminar surgeries, IONM is already considered paramount, since, mandatorily, the patient will be under general anesthesia.

IONM in endoscopic surgeries follows the same multimodal protocol, with EMG-fr and EMG-st, monitoring with SSEP and mMEP, and EEG to follow the level of hypnosis. Preoperatively, IONM can detect prior neurological impairment, providing an accurate diagnosis, as mentioned in the other avenues of approach. EMG-fr allows triggering of minimal instrument contact alerts with neural structures and mMEP demonstrates the effectiveness of decompression as well as the occurrence of neural damage.

Thus, the general anesthesia protocol coupled with IONM offers a faster and safer procedure. The awake patient may present more discomfort and problems with positioning, leading to legal issues [19].

In the endoscopic approach, the preoperative care, positioning, and post-positioning follow the same parameters cited for the posterior approach, since the patient is positioned in ventral decubitus.

Thus, the main intraoperative steps in endoscopic surgeries (transforaminal or interlaminar route) are suggested:

Intraoperative: step by step

- Step 1: Introduction of the endoscopic cannula – EMG-fr
- Step 2: Drilling of the foramen and/or lamina – EMG-fr, EMG-st, mMEP, SSEP
- Step 3: Discectomy/decompression – EMG-fr, EMG-st, mMEP, SSEP
- Step 4: End of decompression and removal of instruments – EMG-fr, EMG-st, mMEP, SSEP

Considerations

- *Step 1*: Assess the occurrence of neurotonic discharges by the proximity of neural tissue.
- *Step 2 and 3*: In addition to evaluating the EMG-fr, similarly, to step 1, mapping of neural structures can be done with EMG-st. For this, the surgeon should be offered a long stimulating probe, with a length above 40 cm (average size of endoscopic cannulas). SSEP and mMEP should also be performed intermittently, to diagnose potential neural lesions early.
- *Stage 4*: At this stage, it is particularly important to perform mMEP for final recordings.

IONM Tests Applied to Cervical Spine Surgeries

Motor Evoked Potential

mMEP

mMEP is obtained by transcranial electrical stimulation through corkscrew-type electrodes inserted in the scalp at C3/C4, C3/Cz, C4/Cz, and the combination of other positions in the quadripolar technique (international system 10–20), with slight anteriorization from 2 to 4 cm. Recording is done in the myotomes pertinent to each case, as mentioned in topic 1. In mMEP, the technique used is a train of 5–9 pulses, with a pulse duration ranging from 50 us/0.05 ms to 500 us/0.5 ms (depending on the equipment); the intensity is varied and generally high, from 200 to 1000 V. We recommend the use of supra-maximal intensity because it makes it easier to observe changes in the amplitude of the responses, both decreases and increases. The polarity should be anodic, as it facilitates cortical depolarization. More details on MEP refer to Chap. 9.

There is some controversy in the literature regarding the alarm signs for mMEP [11, 23] These criteria should not be evaluated in isolation, but together [11, 23–27].

Specifically for cervical surgeries, mMEP deterioration may be secondary to positioning alone, even if it occurs later. In these situations, the degree of cervical flexion/extension should always be reassessed, resulting in recovery of responses in most cases. Of note, in posterior approach for cervical kyphosis, improvement is commonly seen by reducing cervical flexion [20].

Motor Evoked Potential: D-Wave (*Note of the editors: this section translates exclusively authors' experience. It is not routinely included in commonsense protocols. Further evidences would be advisable*)

D-wave recording is done by placing an epidural catheter distally to the manipulated level (for monitoring), and another proximally placed catheter (sentinel) [21–23]. The catheter must be placed by the surgeon himself, after the laminectomy. It can also be inserted percutaneously, like an epidural anesthesia; however, this option makes the process more invasive, and with greater risks, it is generally not recommended. D-wave was initially idealized for intramedullary spinal cord tumor surgeries (this theme is detailed in Chap. 28). However, because it is useful in the evaluation of pathologies that involve the first motor neuron, we extended its application to posterior cervical myelopathy surgeries, cervical or thoracic vertebral fractures and tumors, and thoracic disc herniations. The catheter must be placed over the spinal cord in the epidural space; for this reason, this test is restricted to spinal surgeries that extend to T9-T10 at the most.

Transcranial electrical stimulation using a single stimulus results in D-wave (direct) and I-wave (indirect), the most important being the monosynaptic called "D-wave." The stimulating electrodes can be placed at Cz/Cz + 6 cm as described in the original technique by Deletis et al. [21, 22]. However, to be able to observe side-to-side amplitude discrepancies, which could not be visualized in the original technique, we suggest positioning the stimulating electrodes at C1/C2 or C3/C4.

Traditionally, the D-wave alarm signal occurs if an amplitude deterioration greater than 50% occurs [22], indicating real motor pathway injury and poor neurological prognosis. However, in our clinical practice, we suggest a more conservative approach and earlier warning signs, in agreement with other authors [28, 29]. We alert the surgeon when there is a 20–30% decrement in D-wave amplitude, allowing reversibility maneuvers to be performed when possible.

The main difficulties in performing D-Wave are: (1) surgeries that do not require laminectomy (e.g., endoscopic surgeries and cervical surgeries with anterior approach); (2) risks of percutaneous insertion of the epidural catheter; (3) unavailability of the specific epidural catheter. To overcome them, we developed a specific technique, with D-Wave recording with subdermal needles inserted into the interspinous ligaments of two adjacent vertebral spaces: *D-Wave Interspinous Ligament Technique (DWILT)* (Fig. 24.5).

The stimulation parameters traditionally recommended for obtaining the D-wave were maintained (single pulse stimulus), since the stimulation with a train of multipulses could contaminate the D-wave responses (DWILT) with myogenic components of the paravertebral muscles (Fig. 24.6).

Somatosensory Evoked Potentials: SSEPs

SSEPs will be recorded with corkscrew electrodes inserted at C3/C4 (upper limbs), Cz′/Fz (lower limbs), according to the 10/10 or 10/20 EEG system. Fractionating the sensory pathway, and adding recording electrodes, is suggested. For this purpose, additional sites are supraclavicular Erb's point for upper limbs and popliteal fossa for lower limbs. They serve as a sentinel, proving the depolarization wave ascendency. More details on SSEP can be read in Chap. 8.

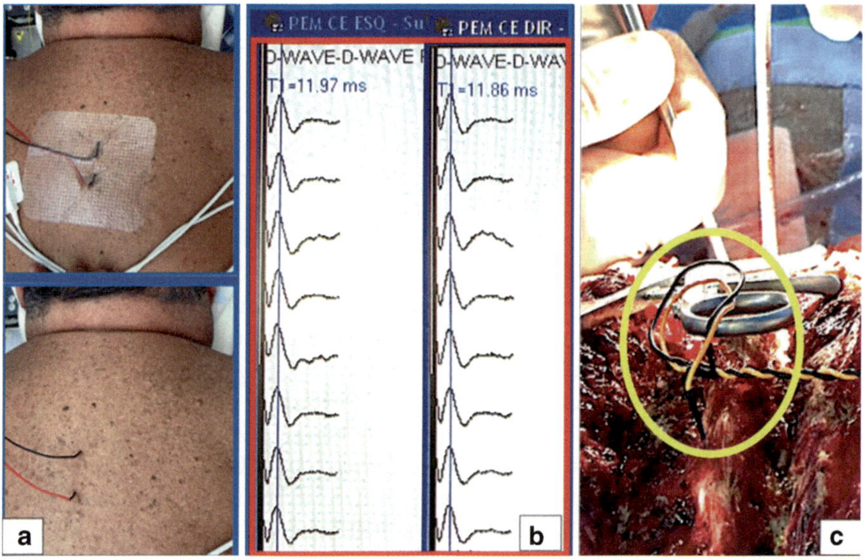

Fig. 24.5 D-Wave Interspinous Ligament Technique – DWILT. (**a**) Subdermal straight twist needles inserted percutaneously. (**b**) Responses with D-wave bilaterally. (**c**) Subdermal needles inserted directly into the surgical field. (*Editors' note: Exclusively authors' personal experience. Careful interpretation should be considered, since replication by other groups is recommended*)

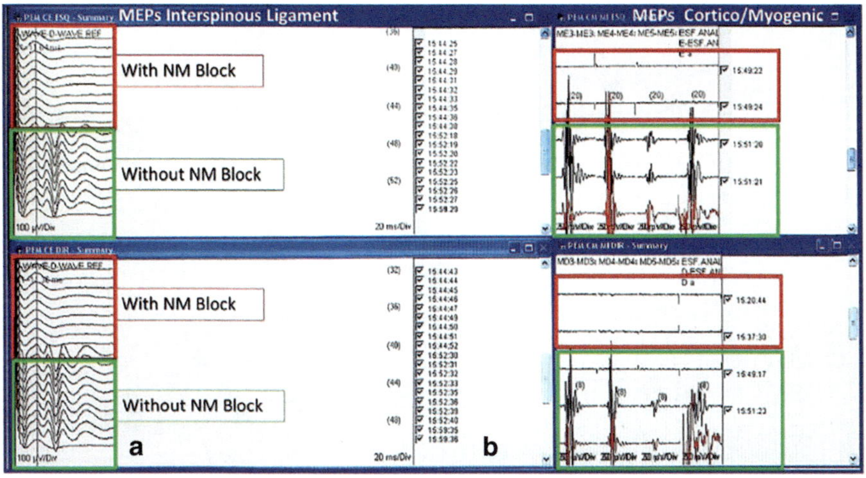

Fig. 24.6 D-Wave Interspinous Ligament Technique – DWILT. D-Wave and Tc-MEP responses, both with multipulse train stimulus technique. Red squares: a patient with neuromuscular block (curarized). Green squares: a patient decurarized. (**a**) Red square: isolated D-wave responses; green square: D-wave responses with an overlap of myogenic components of the paravertebral musculature (multifidus). (**b**) Tc-MEP responses, to confirm the patient's degree of curarization. (*Note of the editors*: DWILT *corresponds exclusively to authors' personal experience. Careful interpretation should be considered before adoption, since validation by other groups is highly recommended*)

The stimuli to obtain SSEPs are performed on mixed peripheral nerves, pure sensory or corresponding dermatomes. The stimulation is done with supramaximal intensity, from 30 to 60 mA, frequency of 3.7 or 4.1 Hz and duration of 200 us/0.2 ms, preferably in the ulnar nerves (upper limbs) and tibial nerves (lower limbs). In upper limbs, it is also possible to use the median nerve, but our preference for the ulnar nerve is due to the following factors: (1) analysis of the complete posterior cervical spinal cord pathway, from C8-T1; (2) evaluation of upper limb positioning; and (3) better position of the electrodes medially at the wrist, leaving the lateral portion free for anesthetic procedures, such as puncture of the radial artery (Fig. 24.7).

Continuous recording of SSEPs and mMEPs is difficult or even impossible during the entire surgical procedure. However, it is important to ask the surgeon to pause occasionally so that SSEPs and mMEPs can be checked. The goal is to avoid large gaps between two consecutive recordings and, during the opening phase, to update the baselines before the main surgical times.

The recommended SSEP alarm signals are a 10% increase in latency and/or a reduction in amplitude greater than 50% [30]. The procedure should restart after a return of the potentials to at least 50% of baselines in less than 10 min. Changes that do not recover after 10 min are critical and may indicate posterior cord dysfunction. As highlighted for mMEP, altered SSEP responses in cervical spine surgeries may be secondary to positioning and this should be reevaluated.

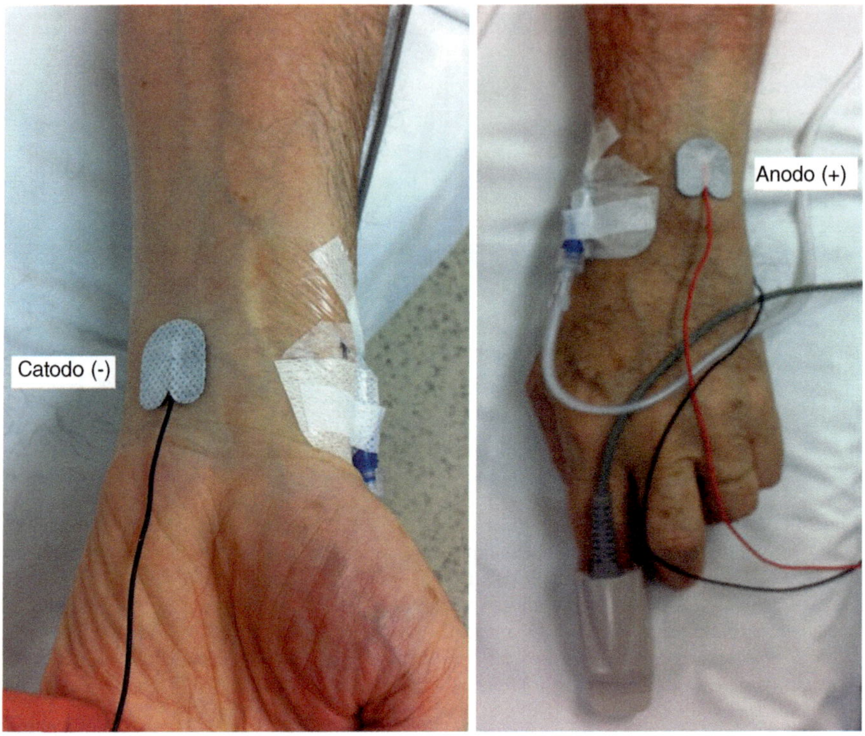

Fig. 24.7 Position of the electrodes on the wrist for SSEP stimulation – ulnar nerve. The electrodes are placed medially at the wrist, enabling the puncture of the radial artery in the lateral portion of the wrist

Electromyography: EMG

EMG is the capture of the Motor Unit Action Potential (MUAP). The capture is done indirectly (involuntary) or directly (voluntary), through electrical stimulation, performed with the assistance of the surgical team. The patient cannot be curarized, which can be confirmed by TOF.

EMG-fr

EMG-fr is performed to detect spontaneous activity caused by mechanical stimulation or by neural dysfunctional discharges. The sources may be a dissection instrumental trauma or a compression or decompression maneuver.

The neurophysiologist should carefully follow each step of the surgery to make the proper correlation of his tests with surgeon maneuvers. Inadequate alerts frequently derive from the following: (1) the neurophysiologist is not following the surgery step by step, or (2) he is using an incomplete protocol ("short protocol"), with recording electrodes in few myotomes. Both situations result in more risks than benefits to the patient.

Neurotonic discharges should be communicated to the surgical team, as they alert to the proximity of neural tissue, and this can prevent the occurrence of injuries. The occurrence in multiple myotomes is possibility due to spinal cord percussion. Although we suggest the communication of every neurotonic discharge, the degree of insult to the neural tissue is mainly related to the constant presence of these discharges, during manipulation or persistent even after the surgeon has interrupted the maneuver.

Neurotonic discharges may be present during manipulation of the dorsal column. In this situation, neurotonic discharges can arise from the reflex arc. Additionally, it is important to make the differential diagnosis with extracellular potassium deposition after neural tissue manipulation. For this purpose, the surgical field must be irrigated with warm serum, washing the extracellular potassium. If even after this maneuver the discharges remain, we consider a "true-positive" sign, and the probability of a neural insult must be considered. In this case, a control with mMEP must be performed, because depending on the degree of insult, this test may prove or discard the installation of motor impairment.

It is worth emphasizing the difference in the analysis of neurotonic discharges in spinal surgeries, when compared to surgeries involving cranial nerves, especially the facial nerve. This is because, in spine surgeries, depolarization takes a longer and more complex pathway, starting in the first motor neuron, and following nerve roots, plexuses and, finally, differentiation into the various peripheral nerves, and its myotomes. Detailed analysis of neurotonic activity in cranial nerves is discussed in Chap. 21.

Thus, we suggest that the alarm signals for EMG-fr are persistent neurotonic discharges during spinal and/or radicular surgical manipulation since the occurrence of these discharges in a severe form may be associated with reduced mMEP responses [30]. Also, neurotonic discharges can be visualized in all access routes in the cervical spine, including endoscopically (Fig. 24.8).

EMG: Triggered (EMG-tg)

The EMG-st is performed by the surgical team with the aid of a stimulator applied to the instruments, guides, and screws. The stimulation is performed by a monopolar electrode probe (cathode -) and a straight subdermal needle as (anode +). This technique is also useful for mapping neural structures in the operative field. As the stimulus is applied by the surgical team, not by the neurophysiologist, it is necessary to teach and guide the proper way to apply the stimulator (cathode) and position the reference needle (anode).

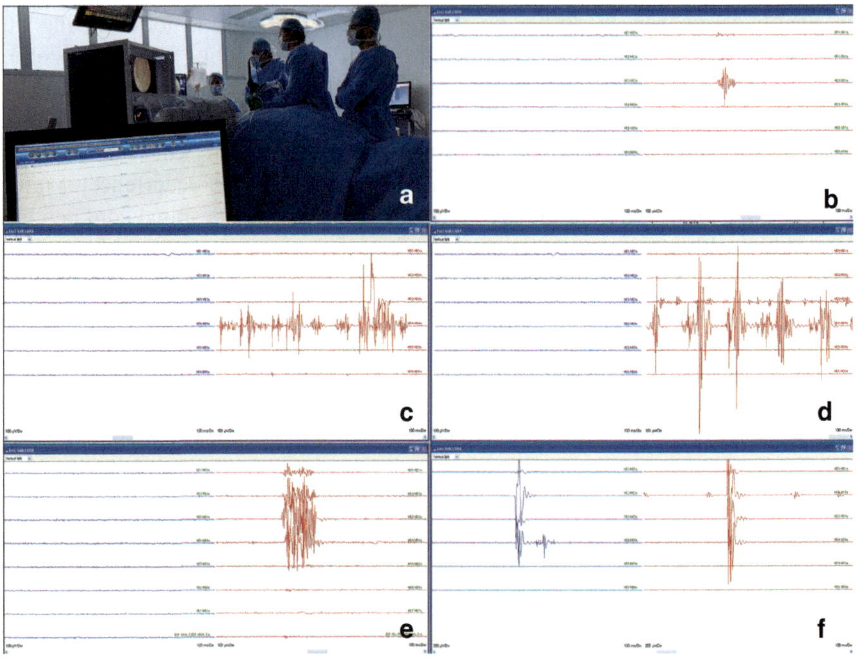

Fig. 24.8 Examples of neurotonic discharges visualized in EMG-fr. (**a**) Neurophysiological monitoring during an endoscopic surgery. (**b–e**) Neurotonic discharges on the right upper limb, in the ascending order of intensity. (**f**) Presence of neurotonic discharges bilaterally

Discussion

IONM During Cervical Spine Surgeries: Evidence

IONM is indicated in several spinal surgeries with risk of iatrogenic injury and neurological deficit, like deformity correction surgeries and intramedullary tumors. In this context, cervical surgeries in all their approach routes have shown increasing benefits with IONM, due to their high risk of neural injury [24].

Multimodal monitoring with a combination of mMEP, SSEP, and EMG tests is currently recommended for all spine surgeries, including cervical, due to its higher sensitivity, and positive and negative predictive values [3, 31, 32]. IONM has evidence of high sensitivity and specificity for intraoperative detection of neurological injury during spinal approaches, as demonstrated by Fehlings et al. [35]. In addition, multimodal IONM can provide instant alerts to the surgical team in the occurrence of surgical insults [33–35].

Wiedemayer et al. [36] compared the rate of new neurological deficits between cases in which the surgeon reacted to an IONM alert and performed some intervention, versus those in which the surgeon did not react to the IONM alert. The authors concluded that IONM prevented the occurrence of postoperative deficit in 5.2% of the monitored cases. Similarly, Hilibrand et al. [33] described 12 patients with the loss of mMEPs responses, from whom 10 achieved complete reversal after the

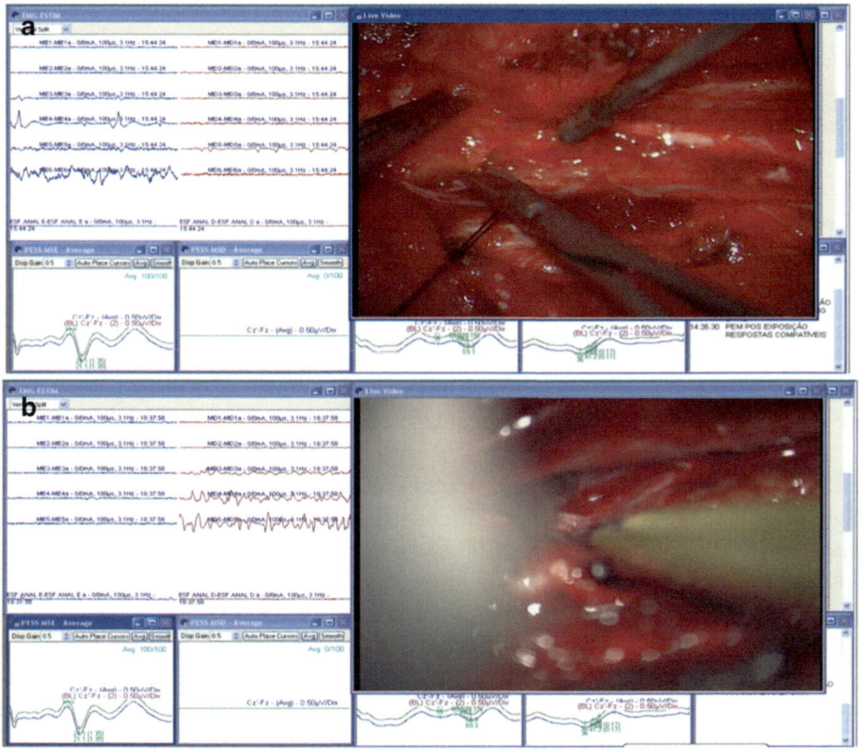

Fig. 25.6 Abnormal f EMG discharges recording during resection of retethered spinal cord by a lipoma. The treatment of a retethered spinal cord is a neurosurgical and neurophysiologist challenge, as nerve tissues are damaged, sometimes to the limit of their resistance. Panel (**a**): Left side (blue color) shows mechanical irritation of motor fibers, duration resection of lipoma, in tibialis anterior, abductor hallucis, and gastrocnemius medial; Panel (**b**): Right side (red color) shows mechanical irritation of motor fibers, duration resection of lipoma, in tibialis anterior, abductor hallucis, and gastrocnemius medial muscle

Several types of electrodes can be used to record muscle activity, but subdermal needle electrodes are used more frequently. Bipolar recording is carried out with a pair of needle electrodes inserted transcutaneously into the motor area of each selected muscle. Our protocol includes bilateral muscle recordings from abductor pollicis brevis (as control), iliopsoas, quadriceps, tibialis anterior, medial gastrocnemius, peroneus longus, abductor hallucis, and anal sphincter (Table 25.1). During TSC approach, due to an increased risk of damaging the motor roots of the bowel and bladder, it is essential to monitor the anal and urethral sphincter muscles [18, 19]. Other muscles can also be used if necessary.

The following settings are used: a time window from 100 to 200 ms/div. Low-frequency filters and high-frequency filters are set between 10 Hz and 2–5 kHz [20]. The appropriate sensitivity settings are 50 uV to 2 mV, which can be adjusted according to the amplitude of the recorded muscle activity.

Table 25.1 Muscles commonly used in IONM in TCS

Muscle	Roots
Iliopsoas	L2–L3–L4
Quadriceps femoris	L2–L3–L4
Tibialis anterior	L4–L5
Peroneus longus	L5–S1–S2
Gastrocnemius (lateral or median heads)	S1–S2
Abductor hallucis	S1–S2
Anal sphincter	S2–S3–S4

Neurotonic discharges are spontaneous potentials that occur in response to mechanical, thermal, or metabolic irritation of the ventral root. The surgeon should be alerted in order to prevent neural damage.

Important aspects should be taken into account to avoid misinterpreting fEMG. Usually, cases of sudden nerve transection or vascular injury may not originate neurotonic activity. Moreover, mechanical activation of the distal stump of a sectioned nerve can also produce EMG activity in the corresponding muscle, thus giving the false impression that the injured nerve is still intact. Conversely, a previously damaged motor root can express decreased excitability and, therefore, low probability of presenting neurotonic activity due to mechanical manipulation.

In order not to alert the surgeon unnecessarily, the spontaneous motor unit discharges that occur in cases of "light anesthesia" should be distinguished from abnormal discharges. During "light anesthesia," motor unit potentials (from several different myotomes) may fire randomly, while stressful events are commonly more focused in the myotome under irritation.

The irritative activity on the fEMG has a high degree of sensitivity to predict new deficits but a low degree of specificity [21]. Gunnarsson et al. [22] showed that neurotonic discharges are frequent in certain spinal surgeries but that they do not always signalize nerve root damage. Robust criteria for interpreting fEMG changes during TCS surgery still need to be defined.

Triggered EMG (tEMG) for Motor Root Mapping

Triggered EMG is a reliable method for identifying functional neural tissue [23]. The surgeon performs direct electrical stimulation on the structures of interest with a handheld probe stimulator, to identify motor nerve roots and distinguish them from fibrous tissue. The resulting compound motor action potential (CMAP) is recorded in the muscles of the lower limbs, anal sphincters, and, if possible, urethral sphincters [24, 25].

We use bipolar stimulation, which allows a more focal current distribution. Monopolar stimulation results in a general current spread in the surgical field. When the anatomy is very distorted, we start with monopolar stimulation to find nerve structures within the tissue and then shift to bipolar stimulation, for a more precise location. In very young children, a small concentric bipolar stimulator may be used, as double-tip bipolar stimulator can cause significant current spread in this age group.

Sala et al. [26] suggest a protocol using (1) constant current with a pulse duration of 200 μs, slowly increasing the intensity from of 0.01 mA up to 3 mA, at 1 Hz frequency until a CMAP response is elicited, (2) sensitivity settings of 50 uV, (3) filters and muscle recordings as already described in section "Free-Running Spontaneous EMG (fEMG)", and (4) time window of 5 ms/division. Unlike them, we use a shorter pulse duration of 100 μs because the threshold for evoking a CMAP of a normal motor root is about 0.2–1.0 mA. Sensory roots require a higher stimulus intensity, of approximately 1.0–2.0 mA, with the same pulse duration. Shorter charges reduce electrical spread (Figs. 25.7, 25.8, and 25.9).

De Almeida et al. [27] suggest that for young children, due to lack of complete myelin development, a higher threshold may be necessary. Conversely, young children's ventral roots are generally of smaller diameters than adults', thus the stimulation threshold can be lower, ranging between 0.5 and 1.5 mA, for a pulse duration of 200 μs. Husain et al. [28] describe that a voltage intensity up to 1 V (in children) and up to 7 V (in adults) is needed to generate a response from nerve roots. Kothbauer et al. [29] suggested that normal nerve roots often require less than 1 V for activation, whereas spinal cord stimulation usually requires about 10 V.

There are two possibilities in cases of no CMAP response after stimulation. Assuming that the stimulation and anesthesia parameters are adequate, either the stimulus intensity is below the threshold, or the stimulated structure is not a motor root. For better checking it out, the stimulus intensity should be gradually increased

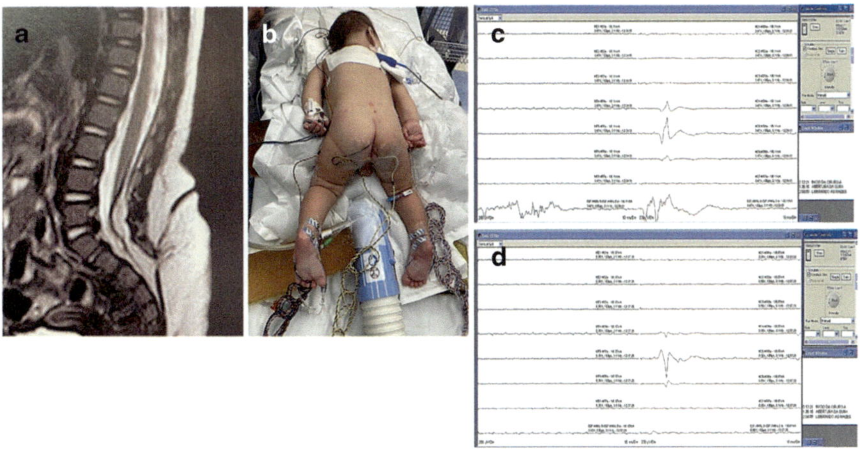

Fig. 25.7 TSC in a 6-month-old boy. Panel (**a**): Preoperative sagittal T2 weight MRI scan demonstrate TSC associated with sinus dermal and filum terminale lipoma. Panel (**b**): Multimodal IONM monitoring in closed spinal dysraphisms with cutaneous stigmas. Panel (**c**): T-EMG – using bipolar handheld stimulator: CMAPs recorded in left L5 (peroneus longus and anterior tibialis) and spread for S1 and anal sphincter with 1.3 mA (0.1 ms duration). Panel (**d**): After reduction the stimulus intensity for 1.0 mA the CMAP: selective recordings at L5 muscles. The lack of response in the abductor hallucis corroborates the selectivity L5 stimulation

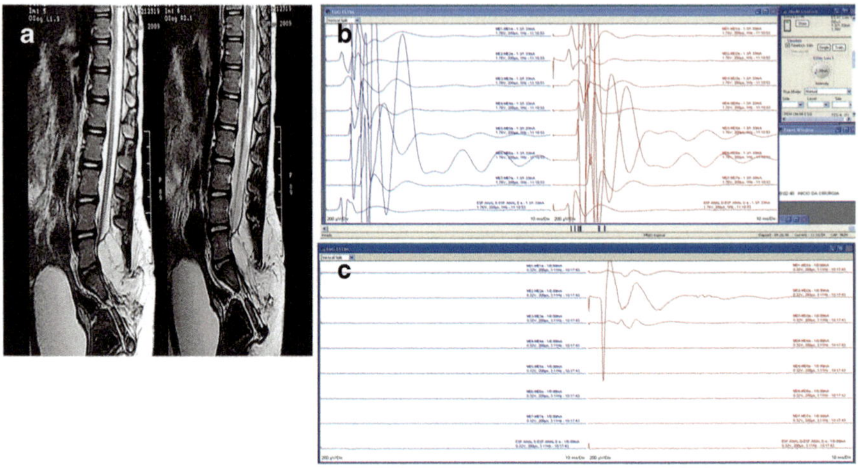

Fig. 25.8 Panel (**a**): Preoperative sagittal T2 weight MRI scan demonstrate TSC associated with lipomeningocele. Panel (**b**): T-EMG using bipolar handheld stimulator elicits CMAPs bilaterally with 1.3 mA (0.1 ms): spread of stimulus through cauda equina at the beginning of the procedure. Bilateral response is also seen with placode stimulation. Panel (**c**): T-EMG, performed during separation of roots from placode, showed CMAPs in the most proximal muscle (iliopsoas and quadriceps) at the right side (red)

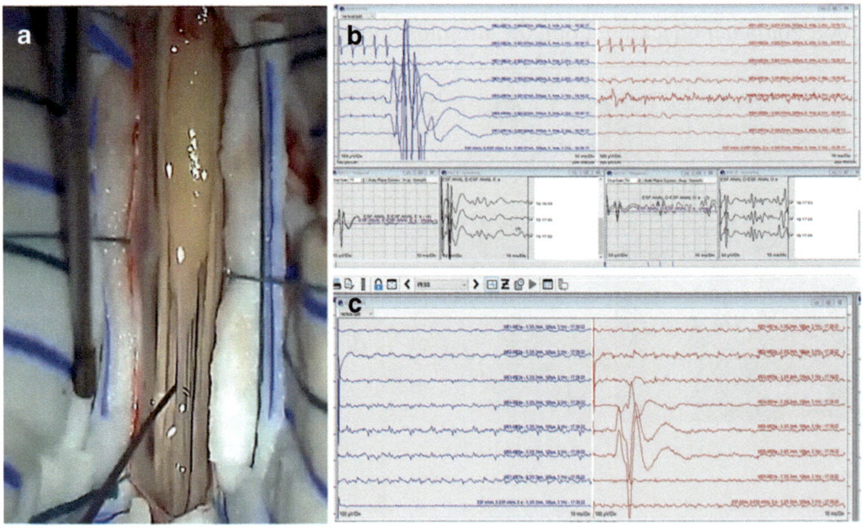

Fig. 25.9 Panel (**a**): TSC and filum terminale lipoma. Panel (**b**): T-EMG – Stimulation with bipolar handheld stimulator triggers CMAPs in left side (blue) in peroneus longus, anterior tibialis, abductor hallucis, and gastrocnemius medial muscle. Panel (**c**): T-EMG – Stimulation with bipolar handheld stimulator triggers CMAPs in right side (red) in peroneus longus, anterior tibialis, abductor hallucis, and gastrocnemius medial muscle

up to 6 mA (100 μs), which should elicit a response from a normal motor root. Thus, a nonresponsive structure at 6 mA can be taken as nonneural and be sacrificed. The identified stimulus threshold can be further used to distinguish functional neural structures that should be preserved from nonfunctional vestigial roots or fibrous bands that can be cut to release the spinal cord. Yet, the presence of injured motor roots may require a higher stimulation threshold.

The surgeon must understand the importance of threshold stimulation. Increasing the stimulus intensity above the threshold can spread the current and thus reduce specificity. The threshold has additional prognostic value, as it can predict the postoperative outcome. The motor roots are stimulated at the same location and with the same stimulus intensity, before and after spinal cord/roots release. If there is no injury during the resection process, the final-to-baseline CMAPs threshold keeps even. However, damage during manipulation can be due to stretching, partial section, and ischemic events, resulting in higher final threshold. It may indicate postoperative worsening of the neurological function. Similarly, a lower threshold after release usually represents a better prognosis [30].

Stimulation of single motor roots is difficult, as the roots are usually clustered, and the surgical field is relatively small. Therefore, most elicited responses are often in all muscles on the left or right side (Fig. 25.9b, c). If the response is bilateral, a current spread has most likely occurred, and the stimulus intensity should be reduced. Stimulation of the placode will also evoke bilateral responses (Fig. 25.8b). For more selective responses in the sacral roots, it is ideal to stimulate more distally, with the assumption that more proximal lumbar roots have already left the spinal canal. Furthermore, as the goal of tEMG is to identify all nerve roots for additional protection, eliciting individualized CMAPs is not fundamental.

Regarding stimulation of the filum terminale (which generally has no neural elements), we believe that a maximum current intensity of 10 mA and 100 us of pulse duration is sufficient in most cases. If CMAPs is not elicited at this intensity, we recommend cutting the filum. Yet, Quiñones-Hinojosa et al. [31] advocate that safe identification of the filum terminale may require stimulus intensities much higher than threshold (up to 100 V).

It must be pinpointed that stimulation of the filum terminale even at a low intensity (at the range used to evoke CMAPs of normal ventral roots) can evoke a motor response. Positive mapping warrants further investigation, as filum terminale stimulation should not evoke CMAPs. In this case, the surgeon should inspect its ventral aspect since a small root can be adhered to it, usually S4. After separating the root, the stimulation should be repeated, to ensure that no other roots are attached to the filum terminale. If no CMAP is evoked, the filum can be safely cut (Fig. 25.10).

Caution should be taken during stimulation, as current spread through the CSF or meninges can be a confounding factor and trigger muscle responses in nonfunctional structures. The surgeon should ensure to have a dry surgical field and that the stimulator probe is selectively placed, and not in contact with adjacent nerve roots.

In TCS, safely sectioning fibrous bands or nonfunctional radicles or rootlets has a significant impact on the degree of spinal cord release, and IONM is critical for optimizing surgical outcomes.

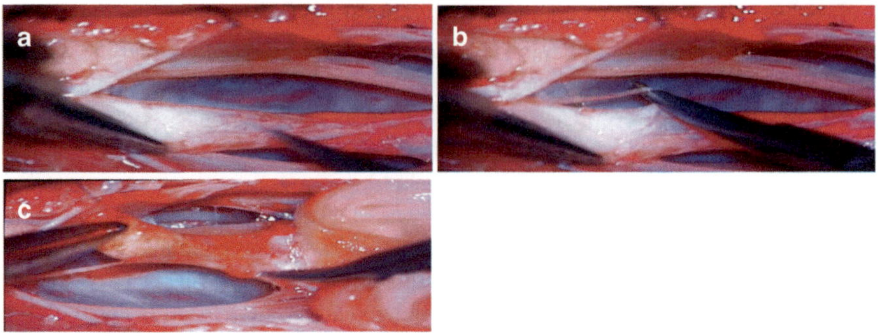

Fig. 25.10 Stimulation of the filum terminale at a low intensity (at the range used to evoked CMAPs of normal ventral roots) can evoke a response. Positive mapping warrants further investigation, as filum terminale stimulation should not evoke CMAPs. Panel (**a**): Shows the filum terminale. Panel (**b**): Surgeon inspect the ventral aspect the filum and found a small, adhered root, usually S4. Panel (**c**): After separating the root, the stimulation should be repeated, to ensure that no other roots are attached to the filum. If no CMAP is evoked, the filum terminale can be safely cut

Motor Evoked Potential

The functional integrity of motoneurons is assessed by activating the motor cortex by transcranial electrical stimulation (TES). The electrodes that are preferably used during this procedure are corkscrew electrodes. They have low impedance and provide a more reliable fixation to the patient's scalp. Some centers choose to use subdermal needle electrodes especially for small children. Great care must be taken in newborns and children who still have open fontanels and in those with a ventriculoperitoneal shunt so that the electrode does not penetrate the fontanel or valve/shunt. EEG electrodes should be preferred in these patients [32].

Lieberman [33] showed that TES motor thresholds are negatively correlated with age, with a higher threshold in younger children, considering other stimulus variables to be even (pulse duration and interstimulus interval).

The selection of the site for placing the stimulating electrodes is crucial for obtaining MEPs with maximum amplitude, using the lowest possible intensity, aiming to reduce patient's movements. Therefore, we suggest the following sites: C4, C3, C1, and C2, with C1 and C2 situated midway between C3–Cz and C4–Cz, respectively (according to the international 10/20 EEG system). C3 and C4 are considered close to the motor area of the arm/hand. C1 and C2 are located closer to the midline and to the motor regions of the legs. In most cases, we obtain responses in both upper and lower limbs with the C1/C2 setup. More details on MEP can be read in Chap. 9.

Stimulus parameters include trains of 5–7 stimulus, with a pulse duration of 0.5–0.75 μs and an interstimulus interval of 3–4 ms. The intensity usually does not exceed 200 mA. Lower limb MEPs may be recorded in neurologically intact children with stimulus intensities as low as 60–70 mA. The C1/C2 and C3/C4 setup evoke MEPs from right-side muscles, while the C2/C1 and C4/C3 evoke responses from left-side muscles. To selectively evoke lower limb MEPs, Cz′ (placed 1 cm behind the typical Cz setup) to Cz + 6 cm is sometimes preferred, since this setup has the advantage of inducing less neck muscle contraction [25, 26, 34].

The needle electrodes for MEP recording are inserted bilaterally into the muscles, as shown in Table 25.1. To monitor the integrity of the pudendal nerve and for pyramidal motor fibers (for volitional control of the anal sphincter), the needle electrodes are inserted bilaterally into the external anal sphincter. Upper limb MEPs are used only as a control to check on anesthetic interference and rule out problems not related to surgery. It is important to mention that the location of the motor cortex in relation to the coronal suture changes during development. Rivet [35] showed that the distance from the coronal suture to the primary motor cortex increased 1.5 mm per year between the ages of 2 months and 8.6 years. Moreover, the distance from the coronal suture to the motor cortex was <3 cm in all patients younger than 6 years. This information has clear implications for the location of the stimulation electrodes for MEPs in young children and infants, when a more efficient stimulation of the primary motor cortex can be obtained at the FC3/FC4 sites (located midway between F3–C3 and F4–C4, respectively, instead of C1/C2) [36].

Suess [37] demonstrated the role of MEPs in lipoma removal during TCS. In this study, patients who had an irreversible decrease in the MEP amplitude (more than 80%) showed deterioration of the motor status that did not improve after months. Conversely, patients with no changes in the MEPs or with reversible changes during surgery had better outcomes, with temporary motor impairment in the immediate postoperative period (with complete resolutions over time) or no clinical worsening. An improvement in lower limb MEPs was observed in some cases after spinal cord release, which was sometimes accompanied by a decrease in the stimulus threshold required to evoke CMAPs.

The presence of MEPs correlates with motor control preservation in all instances. Therefore, it is crucial to preserve MEPs throughout the procedure.

Lower Limb Somatosensory Evoked Potentials

SSEPs allow continuous monitoring of the dorsal column pathways. This method records the sensory response in the scalp (Cz′–Fz and C3′–C4′) or directly from the spinal cord with an epidural electrode, following stimulation of peripheral nerves [38].

They are evoked by stimulation of the posterior tibial nerve at the ankle or at the popliteal fossa with an intensity of 20–40 mA, pulse duration of 200–250 μs, and frequency of 2.79–3.11 Hz. As already described in Chap. 8, a reduction of more than 50% in cortical response amplitude and/or a 10% prolongation in latency is considered significant for an increased risk of injuries in the dorsal roots or dorsal column pathway. In this case, the surgeon should be alerted.

Some authors suggest that monitoring with fEMG and SSEP should be carried out during TCS surgeries and that the methods have a complementary role [22, 36].

Suess [37] reported that tibial nerve SSEPs may have a limited role in some cases, in which the tumor involves the nerve root exit. Dermatomal sensory deficits have been reported, despite unchanged tibial nerve SSEPs. Hence, dermatomal SSEP would be a useful tool to monitor a single sensory root.

Pudendal Nerve Somatosensory Evoked Potential (pSSEP)

Intraoperative pudendal nerve SSEP was shown to be feasible under anesthesia [39, 40]. The pSSEP assesses both sensory roots of the S2–S4 sacral nerve and the dorsal conus medullaris. SSEPs of perineal nerve branches (the pudendal nerve branch) have also been used during TCS surgery to minimize the risk of urinary or sexual dysfunction. The sacral function is effectively monitored by the BCR and the external anal sphincter (EAS) MEP. The BCR covers both motor and sensory nerves and the pathway at the sacral roots and conus, while EAS MEPs represents motor pathway to the sacral roots. In cases in which the BCR is compromised, the EAS MEP or the pSSEP can determine if there is a motor or a sensory impairment. Alternatively, if the BCR or the EAS MEP is unreliable or not obtained at baseline, the pSSEP can be useful for interpreting sacral monitoring.

Cortical and subcortical responses are recorded with the same electrodes used to record tibial SSEPs, with needle electrodes in the CPz–Fz channels and stimulus electrodes placed in the pudendal nerve area. In men, surface electrodes are used to stimulate the dorsal nerve of the penis, with the cathode placed in the proximal region (base) and the anode 1 cm away from the cathode. In women, needle electrodes stimulate the dorsal nerve of the clitoris, with the cathode inserted proximally in the infrapubic area and the anode in the labia majora. The cortical potential latency is approximately 35–40 ms, and the wave is polyphasic [39]. A first small positive wave precedes a large negative peak, followed by positive, negative, and positive waves, in that order.

According to Yang and Kromm [41], the first positive wave recorded in CPz–Fz is the most important component for its reliability and low variability [41].

Yet, the pSSEP also has significant inter-individual variability and a small amplitude. They are generally less reliable and tend to fluctuate during surgery. Therefore, they often require more averaging and time to report any changes to the surgeon [42]. In general, anesthesia and the young age lead to reduced pSSEP monitoring, so surgical decisions are not based on pSSEP monitoring alone [32, 43].

Bulbocavernosus Reflex (BCR)

The BCR is useful for monitoring the functional integrity of the sensory and motor sacral nerve roots as well as the S2–S4 spinal cord segments during TCS surgeries. Monitoring with BCR is important, as iatrogenic damage to S2 to S4 roots represents a significant morbidity that leads to fecal or urinary incontinence. An advantage of BCR is that the surgeon gets immediate feedback.

It was initially thought that EAS monitoring alone was sufficient to assess the integrity of both sphincters. Gunnarsson et al. [22] stated that the two sphincters are innervated by different branches of the pudendal nerve, so they can be damaged separately, and, therefore, individual monitoring of each sphincter is safer. Krassioukov et al. [44] suggested that both sphincters should be monitored to avoid fecal and urinary incontinence. We agree that the best option to avoid fecal and urinary incontinence is monitoring both sphincters. Intraoperative usefulness of BCR for preserving lower sacral nerve structures is well established [45, 46].

Sensory nerve fibers of the pudendal nerve compose the afferent portion of the reflex pathway, while the efferent portion is composed of motor fibers to the pelvic floor, levator ani, and external anal sphincter (inferior rectal nerve, which receives contributions from S2 to S4 sacral roots). The sacral nerves innervate the bladder, urethra, and anal sphincter. The reflex response of the perineal muscles, including the external anal sphincter, following stimulation of the dorsal nerve of the penis or clitoris demonstrates the integrity of the afferent and efferent pathways of the S2 to S4 sacral segments [24, 26, 47].

The BCR is a polysynaptic reflex that is sensitive to various anesthetic agents. Specifically, muscle relaxants and halogenated agents should be avoided. BCR monitoring is technically easy to perform in men, but the responses are less satisfactory in women [48]. Stimulation sites for men and women were described in section "Pudendal Nerve Somatosensory-Evoked Potential (pSSEP)". For the recording, needle electrodes are used inserted in the external anal sphincter muscle with a bilateral arrangement [45] (Fig. 25.11a, b). For the stimulation, we recommend the multipulse technique.

Our parameters consist of a train stimulation of 4 pulses with a duration of 500 μs, an interpulse interval of 2 ms, and a stimulus intensity of up to 30–60 mA. The low-frequency filter is set to 20 Hz and the high-frequency filter to 2000 Hz. The gain is 20–50 uv/div, and the scanning speed is 10–20 ms/day. Deletis and Vodusek [6] suggested a train stimulation of 2–5 pulses, duration of 500 μs, interpulse interval of 3 ms, and stimulus intensity of 5–40 mA. A prior neurological deficit may interfere with responses, and higher stimulus intensity or more pulses may be required to elicit the reflex. To improve the response, double-train stimulation and some averaging may be required.

There are so far no consensual alarm criteria for intraoperative BCR. Most authors consider loss of BCR as an indication of cauda equina or sacral segments of the spinal cord damage, with transient or permanent postoperative fecal and urinary incontinence [49].

This reflex can be extremely sensitive to anesthesia and difficult to interpret in children who have not yet achieved sphincter control and may disappear due to manipulation without a clear clinical correlation (Fig. 25.12). However, if the BCR is preserved, sphincter function is generally preserved.

We recommend that BCR (Fig. 25.11) be routinely included in the IONM protocol during TCS surgeries.

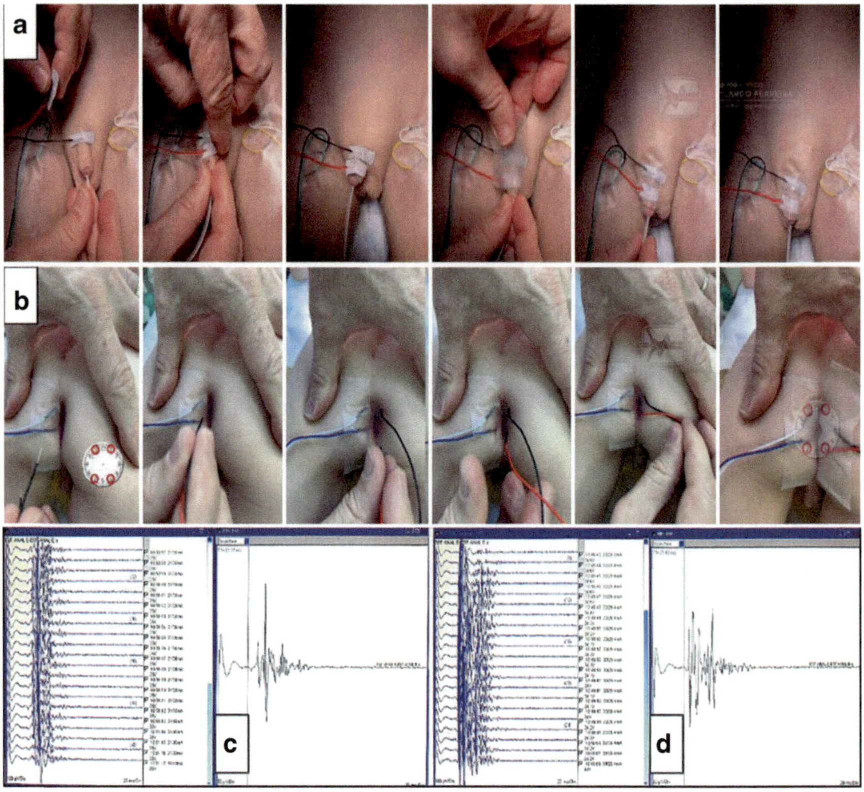

Fig. 25.11 Bulbocavernosus reflex. Panel (**a**): Placement of the electrodes for pudendal nerve stimulation. In males, surface electrodes are used to stimulate the dorsal nerve of the penis, with the cathode placed in the proximal region (base) and the anode 1 cm away from the cathode. (**b**): External anal sphincter recordings – Subdermal needles should be placed in analogue clock positions: Right: 01:00 and 05:00 Left: 07:00 and 11:00 (**c**, **d**): left and right BCR

Hoffmann Reflex

The use of the H reflex in TCS surgeries is an additional method for assessing the functional integrity of the S1 root and the portion of the conus medullaris at this level. This reflex provides immediate feedback to the surgeon, as it is based on a single recording. It can also be monitored in patients in whom SSEPs and MEPs cannot be recorded, due to pre-existing neurological deficits.

Detailed techniques for recording the H reflex can be found in neurophysiology textbooks [50, 51]. The technique involves stimulation of the tibial nerve in the popliteal fossa with surface or subdermal needle electrodes. The anode is placed in the medial and distal portions, and the cathode is placed in the lateral and proximal portions. The active electrode is inserted at the motor point, and the reference

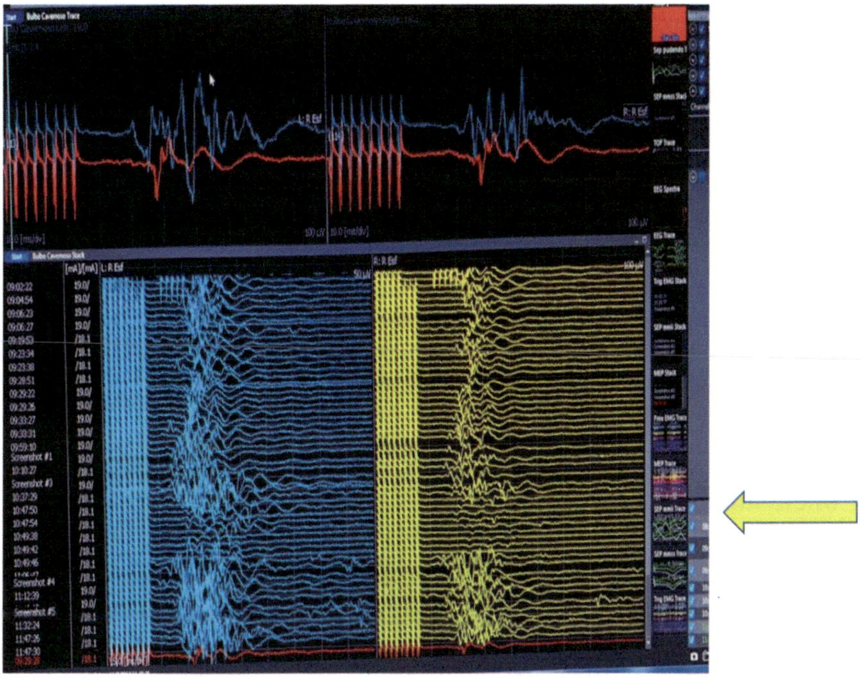

Fig. 25.12 Bulbocavernosus reflex: BCR disappearance (yellow arrow) during manipulation without a clear surgical correlation. Anesthesia was stable without drugs change. Surgeon was notified and irrigated with warm saline. BCR appeared approximately 2 min later. If the BCR is preserved, sphincter function is generally preserved. Patient woke up with no new deficit

electrode is inserted over tendon or bone, at the calf muscles (gastrocnemius or soleus), using surface or subdermal needle electrodes.

Our intraoperative protocol includes constant current, pulse of 500 us, 10–20 ms/div, gain of 50–100 uV, frequency of 2.1–3.1 Hz, 100–500 Hz LFF, and 1000–1500 Hz HFF. A biphasic pulse can also be used. It is possible to use multipulses with four pulses per train, a duration of 500 us, and a stimulus intensity of 10 mA. The stimulus intensity is progressively increased, and the H reflex is typically obtained between 8 and 16 mA. Increasing the stimulus intensity leads to the loss of the H reflex and generation of F-waves.

Intraoperative normal parameters have not been established. Normal parameters established for clinical studies may serve as a guide for intraoperative studies. The gastrocnemius H reflex latency varies with leg length but is usually less than 35 ms. The gastrocnemius or soleus H reflex amplitude and latency are evaluated. A decrease of 50% in the baseline amplitude can be used as an indication of possible neural dysfunction. However, this criterion can only be used if the anesthetic conditions are stable [52].

Anesthesia

Although the rationale for using anesthesia in pediatric patients is similar to the approach in adults, there are some considerations that should be noted. Due to the immaturity of the pediatric central nervous system compared to adults, the anesthetic drugs generally have stronger and more prolonged effects. Particularly with halogenated anesthetic agents (even at lower doses), cortical potentials can be more dramatically attenuated in children. Both amplitude and latency are affected in a dose-dependent manner with inhalation anesthetics, and this is particularly true under the age of 3 years. Similarly, inhalation anesthetics affect MEPs, with loss of amplitude and failure to elicit reliable responses. For most surgeries, unless contraindicated, the use of total intravenous anesthesia allows successful pediatric IONM [43]. For more details in anesthesia protocol, refer to Chap. 5.

Conclusion

TCS surgeries present a challenge for the entire team, particularly when associated with lipomas or in cases of spinal cord retethering. A mutual understanding between the neurosurgeon, the anesthesiologist, and the neurophysiologist is necessary for minimizing postoperative deficits. Multimodal IONM is mandatory.

References

1. Tu A, Steinbok P. Occult tethered cord syndrome: a review. Childs Nerv Syst. 2013;29(9):1635–40. https://doi.org/10.1007/s00381-013-2129-1. Epub 2013 Sep 7. PMID: 24013333 Review.
2. Kamalammal R, Lingappa SM, Rajalu P. Cervical meningocele with tethered cord. Int J Contemp Pediatr. 2016;3(3):1132–4. https://doi.org/10.18203/2349-3291.ijcp20162410.
3. Salomao JF, et al. Cystic spinal dysraphism of the cervical and upper thoracic region. Childs Nerv Syst. 2006;22(3):234–42. https://doi.org/10.1007/s00381-005-1161-1. Epub 2005 Jun 4.
4. Milani HJF, et al. Measurement of the area and circumference of the leg: preliminary results of a new method for estimating leg muscle trophism in fetuses with open lumbosacral spina bifida. J Ultrasound Med. 2022;41(2):377–88.
5. Adzick NS, et al. A randomized trial of prenatal versus postnatal repair of myelomeningocele. N Engl J Med. 2011;364(11):993–1004.
6. Pang D, Zovickian J, Oviedo A. Long-term outcome of total and near-total resection of spinal cord lipomas and radical reconstruction of the neural placode: part I—Surgical technique. Neurosurgery. 2009;65(3):511–29. Available from: https://doi.org/10.1227/01.NEU.0000350879.02128.80.
7. Boor R, et al. Tethered cord after spina bifida aperta: a longitudinal study of somatosensory evoked potentials. Childs Nerv Syst. 1993;9:328–30.
8. Roy MW, Gilmore R, Walsh JW. Evaluation of children and young adults with tethered spinal cord syndrome. Surg Neurol. 1986;26:241–8.

9. Begeer JH, et al. Progressive neurological deficit in children with spina bifida aperta. Z Kinderchir. 1986;41(Suppl I):13–5.
10. Oi S, Yamada H, Matsumoto S. Tethered cord syndrome versus low-placed conus medullaris in an over-distended spinal cord following initial repair for myelodysplasia. Childs Nerv Syst. 1990;6:264–9.
11. Tamaki N, et al. Tethered cord syndrome of delayed onset following repair of myelomeningocele. J Neurosurg. 1988;69:393–8.
12. Mazur JM, et al. Hand function in patients with spina bifida cystica. J Pediatr Orthop. 1986;6:442–7.
13. Drake JM. Occult tethered cord syndrome: not an indication for surgery. J Neurosurg. 2006;104:305–8.
14. Komagata M, et al. Management of tight filum terminale. Minim Invasive Neurosurg. 2004;47:49–53.
15. Metcalfe PD, et al. Treatment of the occult tethered spinal cord for neuropathic bladder: results of sectioning the filum terminale. J Urol. 2006;176:1826–9, discussion 1830.
16. Pang D, Zovickian J, Oviedo A. Long-term outcome of total and near-total resection of spinal cord lipomas and radical reconstruction of the neural placode, part II: outcome analysis and preoperative profiling. Neurosurgery. 2010;66:253–73. Available from: https://doi.org/10.1227/01.NEU.0000363598.81101.7B.
17. Walker CT, et al. Human amniotic membrane for the prevention of intradural spinal cord adhesions: retrospective review of its novel use in a case series of 14 patients. Neurosurgery. 2018;83:989–96.
18. James HE, et al. Use of anal sphincter electromyography during operations on the conus medullaris and sacral nerve roots. Neurosurgery. 1979;4(6):521–3. https://doi.org/10.1097/00006123-197906000-00005.
19. Owen JH, et al. The use of mechanically elicited electromyograms to protect nerve roots during surgery for spinal degeneration. Spine. 1994;19(15):1704–10. https://doi.org/10.1097/00007632-199408000-00009.
20. Minahan RE, Mandir AS. Basic neurophysiologic intraoperative monitoring techniques. In: Husain AM, editor. A practical approach to neurophysiologic intraoperative monitoring. New York: Demos; 2008. p. 21–44.
21. Paradiso G, et al. Multimodality intraoperative neurophysiologic monitoring findings during surgery for adult tethered cord syndrome: analysis of a series of 44 patients with long-term follow-up. Spine. 2006;31(18):2095–102. https://doi.org/10.1097/01.brs.0000231687.02271.b6.
22. Gunnarsson T, et al. Real-time continuous intraoperative electromyographic and somatosensory evoked potential recordings in spinal surgery: correlation of clinical and electrophysiologic findings in a prospective, consecutive series of 213 cases. Spine. 2004;29(6):677–84. https://doi.org/10.1097/01.brs.0000115144.30607.e9.
23. Pasquali C, Tramontano V, Sala F. Intraoperative neurophysiological monitoring in tethered cord surgery. In: Deletis V, Shils J, Sala F, Kathleen S, editors. Neurophysiology in neurosurgery: a modern intraoperative approach. 2nd ed. San Diego: Academic Press; 2020. p. 365–77.
24. Kothbauer KF, Deletis V. Intraoperative neurophysiology of the conus medullaris and cauda equina. Childs Nerv Syst. 2010;26(2):247–53. Available from: https://doi.org/10.1007/s00381-009-1020-6.
25. Sala F, Krzan MJ, Deletis V. Intraoperative neurophysiological monitoring in pediatric neurosurgery: why, when, how? Childs Nerv Syst. 2002;18:262–87.
26. Sala F, et al. Intraoperative neurophysiology in tethered cord surgery: techniques and results. Childs Nerv Syst. 2013;29:1611–24. Available from: https://doi.org/10.1007/s00381-013-2188-3.
27. De Almeida KT, Shin J, Simon MV. Intradural extramedullary spinal cord resection. In: Simon MV, editor. Intraoperator neurophysiology: a comprehensive guide to monitoring and mapping. 2nd ed. New York: Demos Medial Publishing; 2019. p. 426–56.

28. Hussain AM, et al. Tethered cord surgery. In: Husain AM, editor. A practical approach to neurophysiologic intraoperative monitoring. New York: Demos Medical; 2015. p. 142–55.
29. Kothbauer KF, et al. Intraoperative motor and sensory monitoring of the cauda equina. Neurosurgery. 1994;34(4):702–7. https://doi.org/10.1227/00006123-199404000-00020.
30. Husain AM, Shah D. Prognostic value of neurophysiologic intraoperative monitoring in tethered cord syndrome surgery. J Clin Neurophysiol. 2009;26:244–7. https://doi.org/10.1097/WNP.0b013e3181b2edae.
31. Quinones H, et al. Neurophysiological monitoring for safe surgical tethered cord syndrome release in adults. Surg Neurol. 2004;62(2):127–33, discussion 133–5.
32. Sala F, Manganotti P, Grossauer S, et al. Intraoperative neurophysiology of the motor system in children: a tailored approach. Childs Nerv Syst. 2010;26:473–49.
33. Lieberman JA. The effect of age on motor evoked potentials in children under propofol/isoflurane anesthesia. Anesth Analg. 2006;103:316–21. https://doi.org/10.1213/01.ane.0000226142.15746.b2.
34. Sala F, et al. Neurophysiology of complex spinal cord untethering. J Clin Neurophysiol. 2014;31:326–36.
35. Rivet DJ. Distance of the motor cortex from the coronal suture as a function of age. Pediatr Neurosurg. 2004;40:215–9. https://doi.org/10.1159/000082294.
36. Simon MV. Intraoperative neurophysiology. A comprehensive guide to monitoring and mapping. 2nd ed. New York: Demos Medial Publishing; 2019.
37. Suess O. The value of intraoperative neurophysiological monitoring for microsurgical removal of conus medullaris lipomas: a 12-year retrospective cohort study. Patient Saf Surg. 2014;8:35. https://doi.org/10.1186/s13037-014-0035-4.
38. Deletis V, et al. Neurophysiology in neurosurgery: a modern intraoperative approach. 2nd ed. San Diego: Academic Press; 2020.
39. Cohen BA, Major MR, Huizenga BA. Pudendal nerve evoked potential monitoring in procedures involving low sacral fixation. Spine. 1991;16:S375–8. https://doi.org/10.1097/00007632-199108001-00014.
40. Vodušek DB, Deletis V. Sacral roots and nerves, and monitoring for neuro-urologic procedures. In: Nuwer MR, editor. Intraoperative monitoring of neural function handbook of clinical neurophysiology, vol. 8. Amsterdam: Elsevier; 2008. p. 423–33.
41. Yang CC, Kromm BG. New techniques in female pudendal somatosensory evoked potential testing. Somatosens Mot Res. 2004;21(1):9–14. https://doi.org/10.1080/0899022042000201254.
42. Kothbauer KF, Novak K. Intraoperative monitoring for tethered cord surgery: an update. Neurosurg Focus. 2004;16(2):E8. https://doi.org/10.3171/foc.2004.16.2.1.
43. Sloan T. Anesthesia and intraoperative neurophysiological monitoring in children. Childs Nerv Syst. 2010;26(2):22735. Available from: https://doi.org/10.1007/s00381-009-1023-3/.
44. Krassioukov AV, et al. Multimodality intraoperative monitoring during complex lumbosacral procedures: indications, techniques, and long-term follow-up review of 61 consecutive cases. J Neurosurg Spine. 2004;1(3):243–53. https://doi.org/10.3171/spi.2004.1.3.0243.
45. Deletis V, Vodusek D. Intraoperative recording of the bulbocavernosus reflex. Neurosurgery. 1997;40:88–92. Available from: https://doi.org/10.1097/WNP.0000000000000054.
46. Skinner SA, Vodusek DB. Intraoperative recording of the bulbocavernosus reflex. J Clin Neurophysiol. 2014;31(4):31322. Available from: https://doi.org/10.1097/WNP.0000000000000054.
47. Fulkerson DH, et al. Intraoperative neurophysiology of the conus medullaris and cauda equina. Childs Nerv Syst. 2010;29(4):13744. Available from: https://doi.org/10.3171/2014.1.peds11336.
48. Rodi Z, Vodusek DB. Intraoperative monitoring of the bulbocavernosus reflex: the method and its problems. Clin Neurophysiol. 2001;112:879–83. https://doi.org/10.1016/S1388-2457(01)00500-4.

49. Khealani B, Husain AM. Neurophysiologic intraoperative monitoring during surgery for tethered cord syndrome. J Clin Neurophysiol. 2009;2009(26):76–81. https://doi.org/10.1097/WNP.0b013e31819f9067.
50. Delisa J, et al. Somatosensory evoked potentials. In: Manual of nerve conduction velocity and clinical neurophysiology. 3rd ed. New York: Raven Press; 1994. p. 195–274.
51. Kimura J. Electrodiagnosis in diseases of nerve and muscle: principles and practice. 2nd ed. Philadelphia: F.A. Davis; 1989.
52. Zhou HH, et al. Suppression of spinal cord motoneuron excitability correlates with surgical immobility during isoflurane anesthesia. Anesthesiology. 1998;88(4):955–61.

Chapter 26
Selective Dorsal Rhizotomy and Intraoperative Neurophysiological Monitoring: Theory to Practice

Carlo Domênico Marrone, André Bedin, Ana Maria Hoppe, Cristiane Soveral D'Aviz, and Jorge Wladimir Junqueira Bizzi

Abbreviations

BCR	Bulbocavernosus reflex
EEG	Electroencephalography
EMG	Electromyography
fEMG	Free EMG
GMFMS	Gross Motor Function Measure Score
IONM	Intraoperative neurophysiological monitoring

C. D. Marrone (✉)
Brazilian Clinical Neurophysiology Society, Porto Alegre, RS, Brazil

Intraoperative Neurophysiological Monitoring, Department Coordinator of Hospital da Criança Santo Antônio, Porto Alegre, RS, Brazil

Universidade Federal de Ciências da Saúde de Porto Alegre - UFCSPA, Porto Alegre, RS, Brazil

Clínica Marrone, Clinical Neurophysiology, Porto Alegre, RS, Brazil
e-mail: drmarrone@clinicamarrone.com.br

A. Bedin
Brazilian Society of Pediatric Surgery, Porto Alegre, RS, Brazil

A. M. Hoppe
Department of Neurophysiology, Santa Casa de Misericórdia de Porto Alegre, Porto Alegre, RS, Brazil

C. S. D'Aviz
Department of Neurophysiology – Santa Casa de Misericórdia de Porto Alegre/RS, Porto Alegre, RS, Brazil

J. W. J. Bizzi
Pediatric Neurosurgery Department, Clinical Hospital of the Medical School of the University of Rio Grande do Sul, Porto Alegre, RS, Brazil

S. M. Verst et al. (eds.), *Intraoperative Monitoring*,
https://doi.org/10.1007/978-3-030-95730-8_26

MEP	Motor evoked potential
MRI	Magnetic resonance imaging
SDR	Selective dorsal rhizotomy
SSEP	Somatosensory evoked potential
tEMG	Stimulus-triggered EMG

Neurophysiology of Muscle Tonus and Spasticity

The tonus is the involuntary state of natural contraction of the body muscles. It is responsible for making muscles come into action whenever requested. It is also a protective mechanism against stretching, as it depends on the muscle's own elasticity, as well as the strength with which the muscle resists increasing in size [1]. Muscle tonus disorders may be related to motor system injuries, especially those that interfere with descending motor pathways, which can lead to spasticity [2].

Spasticity is a very common neurological phenomenon in medical practice and results in varying degrees of mobility loss and motor dysfunction, in addition to pain and muscle spasms. This condition significantly interferes with the quality of life of patients, their families, and caregivers [3, 4]. It is a set of signs and symptoms that clinically manifest as clonus, hyperactive deep tendon reflexes, resistance to passive movement, and the clasp-knife phenomenon – an exaggerated reflex response to velocity-dependent muscle stretching [5].

An increase in resistance to passive movement is another possible definition for spasticity, secondary to a change in the threshold of tonic and phasic stretch reflexes. Latent myotatic reflexes become obvious, the reflex response to the stretched muscle is increased, and other muscle groups in addition to the stimulated one also respond. These findings are all part of the so-called upper motor neuron syndrome [3, 4].

Spasticity arises in several clinical conditions such as cerebral palsy, multiple sclerosis, stroke, and spinal cord disorders, among others. The mechanism can be explained by two interlinked concepts: the functioning of the motor neuron at the spinal level and its supraspinal and suprasegmental controls [3, 6].

The supraspinal motor control system includes the primary motor area (pyramidal corticospinal pathways) and the supplementary and prefrontal motor cortex, which aids in planning and initiating motor tasks. Subcortical and brainstem nuclei contribute to postural control pathways and circuits, both reflex and repetitive [3]. There are extremely coordinated and complex facilitating and inhibitory pathways and mechanisms.

The spinal cord, besides being the final common pathway of motor execution (alpha motoneuron), has its own circuitry and reflexes that increase coordinated movement and motor skills. Spinal cord motor functions depend on muscle receptors (spindles) and muscle reflexes, interneurons activity, inhibitory and excitatory controls (type I and II sensory fibers), and presynaptic inhibition.

to the end of the conus medullaris, which had been previously visualized by neuroimaging and the L1 neural foramen. The incision, usually 5 cm long, is then made at this level [22].

For adequate exposure of the conus, a laminectomy of L1 and part of the upper and lower lamina is performed, as needed. After the dural and arachnoid opening, the L1 root is identified in its corresponding foramen. The end of the cone, the filum terminale, and the fine sacral roots S3 to S5 are identified, which are left intact. Next to them is located S2, which is bulkier. The clotting of any artery adjacent to the roots or conus is avoided as much as possible [23].

With a lateral angulation of the microscope, it is possible to easily visualize the entry zone of the dorsal roots and their separation in relation to the ventral roots. After careful dissection, a small 5-mm-wide glove strip is pulled through this interspace separating the ventral and dorsal roots from S2 to L2 [24].

Then individual separation of the roots is performed using some anatomical repairs and dissection: L2 toward its vertebral foramen and S2 as a single fascicle laterally to the thin roots of S3–S5. Precise separation of roots is sometimes not possible, but this is not critical for performing SDR using this method, since, in these patients, the motor innervation comes from several segments.

Each dorsal root is then subdivided into three to five parts (rootlets), which are shifted by electrodes and tested individually. The rootlets with abnormal responses (grades 3 and 4) are sectioned, attempting to preserve at least 1/3 of each posterior root. This process is conducted from L2 to S2, bilaterally. Fifty percent of the dorsal root of L1 is sectioned sometimes without using EMG, to reduce hypertonia in the hip flexors [21] (Fig. 26.1).

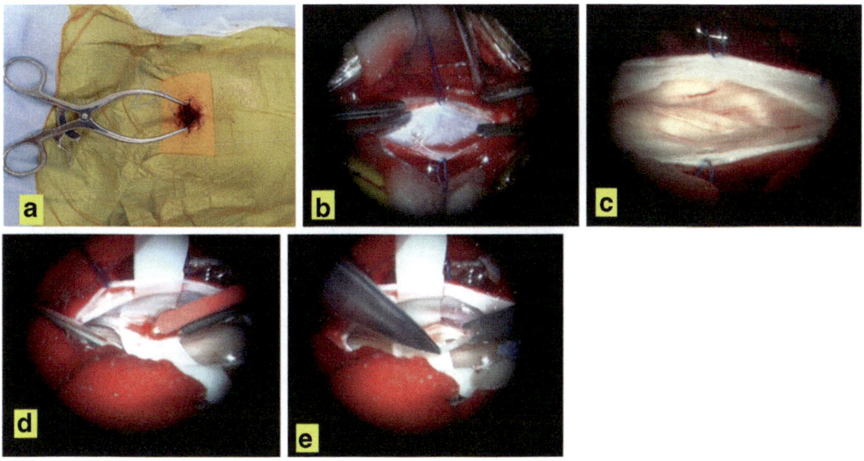

Fig. 26.1 Minimally invasive technique in the conus medullaris. (**a**) Opening, (**b**) exposure of the dura mater, (**c**) exposure of the conus/roots, (**d**) small glove strip separating the ventral and dorsal roots and stimulation by bipolar electrodes, (**e**) section rootlets. (Courtesy Paulo Francheschini, MD)

Conventional Laminotomy Technique

The conventional surgery is more extensive and, in general, involves laminotomy from L1 to L5 with laminectomy of S1 and S2 as proposed by Peacock et al. [25].

SDR is a conventional surgery performed under general anesthesia. The cauda equina is exposed by lumbar laminotomy, exposing the dural sac (Fig. 26.2a). The dorsal sensory roots from S1 to L2 are bilaterally identified (Fig. 26.2b), which is confirmed after neural stimuli with the interposition of material isolating the root to be studied (Figs. 26.1c, d, and 26.2c).

A lesion comprising about 30% of its diameter is performed on each root (Fig. 26.2d) depending on the previous clinical spasticity. The effect achieved is, in general, a decrease of two levels on the Ashworth scale in the spastic muscle group of the lower limbs. In about 50% of children, this effect also extends to the upper limbs.

The goals of the procedure are functional improvement and better quality of life. As to the latter, several factors are considered:

- Child's physical comfort
- Decreased pain, improved positioning, and facilitated or fully functional genital, axillary, and cervical hygiene
- Improvement in caregiver functions: transport, positioning, and hygiene
- Contribution to the prophylaxis of physical complications: bedsores, dislocations, scoliosis, and deformities [26]

Regarding complications in the spine after the multilevel laminectomy technique, Steinbok and colleagues found scoliosis in 55% and 6% of patients with

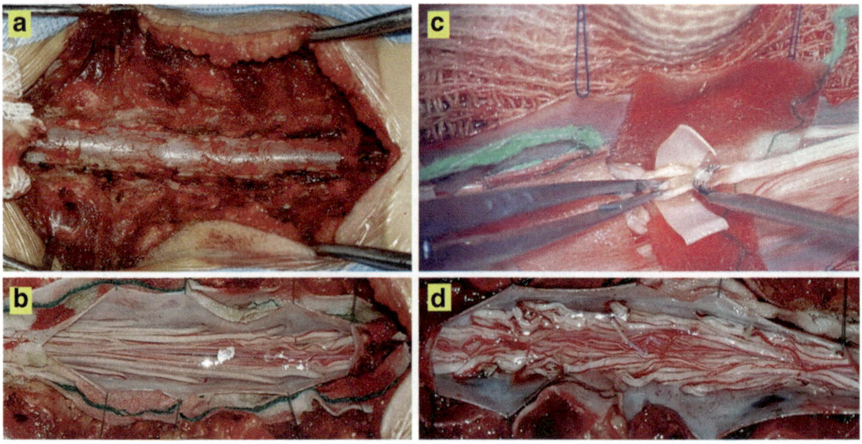

Fig. 26.2 Selective dorsal rhizotomy sequence. (**a**) Laminotomy with exposure of the dural sac, retracted on, without removal of the spine, which will later be repositioned. (**b**) Opening of the dural sac with root exposure from L2 to S2, bilaterally. (**c**) Rootlet isolation and root cell stimulation with hook electrode. (**d**) Rootlet appearance after rhizotomy

curves greater than 35% [27]. In a review between 17 and 26 years after SDR, the South Africans found, except for spondylolisthesis, that deformities appear with the progression of time but are not marked and develop mild scoliosis (less than 30%). With the evolution of laminectomy for laminotomy, vertebral abnormalities have been reduced in this type of technique [9, 28].

Intraoperative Neurophysiological Monitoring (IONM)

In general, IONM for SDR consists of two mapping techniques. The single stimulus (threshold stimulation) aims to identify the ventral (motor) and dorsal roots (sensory) at the lumbosacral level, myotomes, and root laterality. Next, using the tetanic technique at 50 Hz, each one of the three to ten rootlets (previously separated and belonging to each dorsal root) should be tested and sectioned according to their contribution to spasticity, the neurophysiological response, and previous clinical examination [29].

Anesthesia

To perform neurophysiological assessment through electromyography (EMG) alone, either free or stimulated with a single stimulus or in train, continuous inhalation anesthesia, for instance, Sevorane, with fast-acting muscle relaxant only for intubation can be used. However, if IONM is performed in a multimodal way, total intravenous anesthesia should be preferred, such as propofol and remifentanil, with use of myorelaxants (short action only for intubation). In cases of noncooperative children in whom IONM will be used, anesthesia with inhaled agents can be done for the purpose of orotracheal intubation. After adequate venous access is obtained, it is recommended to switch to total venous anesthesia. See Chap. 5 for further information on anesthesia.

Equipment Setup

For the basic electromyographic (EMG) evaluation, we recommend a device with at least 16 channels, band-pass filters of 30–3000 Hz, and notch filter (50–60 Hz) on, 30–75 ms/div sweep length; and 200–500 mV/div.

In multimodal neurophysiological approach, each test must be set up according to proper parameters. These parameters shall be adjusted as needed, as they can vary depending on the interference of the operating room and other endogenous and exogenous conditions. It is of utmost importance to master knowledge on safety and troubleshooting (more details in Chap. 4).

Recording and Stimulator Probes and Anodal or Cathodal Stimulation

Muscle recording must be done with a pair of subdermal needles with a separation of 2–4 cm between them to reduce the effect of volume conduction from neighboring muscles, which may interfere with the interpretation of the findings. The use of surface recording electrodes is not indicated because they provide less selectivity and precision.

Stimulation probes can be either monopolar (a pair of probes placed 1 cm apart by the surgeon) or bipolar with hook-shaped or straight tips (with tips 3–5 mm apart) (Fig. 26.3).

Usually, it would make sense to stimulate the sensory rootlets in ascending (orthodromic) orientation, that is, proximal-cathodal (toward the medullary cone) and distal-anodal (toward the foraminal outlet). It is the way it is done for neural conduction tests during electroneuromyography or electrodes positioning for somatosensory evoked potential [29, 30]. However, a systematic study of the cathode-anode/anode-cathode position for orthodromic stimulation of the rootlets attributed no importance to the tip position [27]. Yet, a lower threshold response may be verified when the cathode is placed proximally, with no other difference in the nature of the responses [27]. The authors state that it is acceptable to perform cathodal-proximal and anodal-distal placement if a pair of monopolar probes with a distance of at least 1 cm between them is used. On the other hand, if bipolar probes are used with a tip distance of a few millimeters, there is no need to follow this positioning.

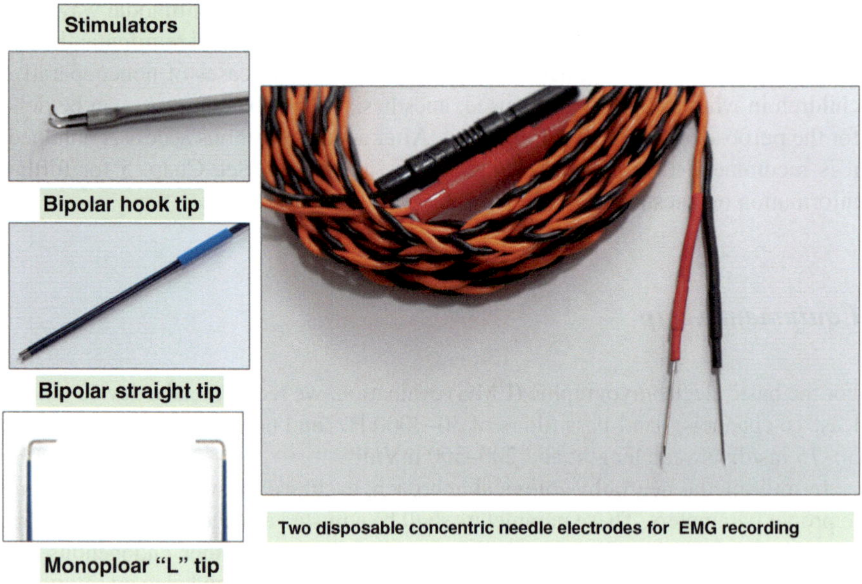

Fig. 26.3 Types of stimulators and recording electrodes

Recording Myotomes

Continuous free-run EMG activity and triggered EMG recorded from lower limb muscles and anal sphincter, according to maps that reveal the correlation between roots, muscles, and their respective actions. There may be discrete interindividual variations (muscles innervated by more than one root and vice versa), or among clinicians' interpretation. Thus, for instance, team members may consider that the thigh adductor could be L2, L1–L2, or L2–L3. These maps are the basis for interpretation and vary among institutions [6, 12, 29] (Table 26.2). It is important to remember that the preoperative assessment of muscle strength, tonus/spasticity, reflexes, and especially the clonus guides the neurosurgeon's decisions regarding the percentage and which rootlet should be sectioned and the neurophysiology as an adjuvant.

Free Electromyography

During the entire approach, especially while rootlets are being separated, it is vitally important to perform free-run EMG, as traction disturbances may be recognized, thus alerting surgeons. In addition, these disturbances may impact irritability and responsiveness to the slightest touch, which may, in turn, influence in threshold and tetanic stimulation excitability [12].

Threshold Stimulation

After exposure of the nerve roots, single pulse triggered EMG is always used as the first step of the neurophysiological protocol. It differentiates motor (ventral) from sensory (dorsal) roots. Additionally, it shows which root level is being stimulated for further subdivision into rootlets and sectioning selection.

Table 26.2 Action, roots, and muscles

Action	Roots/muscle
Hip flexion	L1–2 (iliopsoas)
Thigh adduction	L2 (adductors)
Extended knee	L3–L4 (quadriceps)
Ankle dorsiflexion	L4–L5 (tibialis anterior)
Hip extension	L4–L5[a] (medial hamstring)
Knee flexion	L5 (lateral hamstrings)
Plantar flexion (foot equinism)	S1 (gastrocnemius) S1/S2 (abductor hallux)
Bladder, lower bowel, anal sphincter control	S2–S4

[a]OBS: L5 – fibularis longus

The trigger threshold of the motor nerve roots is much smaller than that of the sensitive ones. It is typically accepted that the sensory threshold is at least three times higher than the motor [6, 31], but usually bigger differences can be seen (sometimes five to ten times more).

The stimulation parameters vary among institutions. A square pulse of 0.1 ms (100 us) duration with a constant current with a low intensity of 0.1 mA (100 uA) is used to start. It usually results in a good muscle response, both clinically and by EMG recordings, when stimulating the ventral root. In normal situations, the motor threshold is around 50 uA (0.05 mA). Therefore, by starting with 0.1 mA and reaching up to 0.2 mA, the ventral root trigger level is mostly reached, reducing the risk of scattering the current to other roots [12]. Regarding the stimulus frequency, 0.5–1.0 Hz is enough. When the motor threshold is reached, the recorded potential shows which root and side it belongs to. Next, stimulation of the corresponding dorsal root will need at least three times the stimulus intensity. The identified dorsal root threshold will be used for the subsequent tetanic stimulation at 50 Hz.

This type of stimulation is performed with the neurosurgeon gently suspending the root with the stimulation electrode itself, with the interposition of a tape or glove finger to separate the root to be studied, making it as isolated as possible. Furthermore, there can be no liquid or other nearby roots to avoid current spreading and misinterpretation of the analyzed myotomes (Figs. 26.1d, e and 26.2c) [29].

From an anatomical point of view, when a laminotomy is used, which exposes a large part of the medullary-radicular region, the entry of the nerve roots into the respective foramens helps to locate which root is being handled. Root S1 is visually located first since it is the largest and thickest and then confirmed by electrical stimulation. Conversely, if a focal exposure of the cauda equina is performed, the foramen visualization is reduced, and the proximal roots L1–L2 can be seen. This focal procedure offers a more difficult anatomic position due to the little foraminal exposure. In both techniques it is necessary to perform electrical stimulation of the roots to locate and differentiate ventral (motor) from dorsal (sensitive) roots, as under no circumstances should motor roots be sectioned. Moreover, roots that innervate sphincters, including sensitive roots, should be spared from sectioning at all costs.

The numerous maps of roots-myotomes-muscles show intertwining and heterogeneity between the close roots, e.g., L3–L4 and L4–L5, but not between L2 and S1 obviously. It may cause confusion in some situations because the muscles of the lower limbs are innervated by several root segments [21]. In our service, when doubts arise about the root map, (a) we review the interposition of tape/glove finger that prevents contact between the stimulator and adjacent roots; (b) we dry the field well, preventing liquids from being in contact with the stimulator so as not to unnecessarily spread the stimulus; (c) we stimulate with as little load as possible (duration × intensity); and (d) we stimulate each of the adjacent roots and check on the recorded responses, comparing with the root in question. We check on latencies and amplitudes of the potentials, that is, the one with shorter latency and greater amplitude possibly designates the root that is being stimulated [32].

At some moments, it is difficult to differentiate the motor roots among each other, especially if the sensitive roots are severely affected [29]. If impossible to differentiate, it is assumed that this ventral root is innervating more myotomes than usual.

If the threshold for the dorsal root is low or close to that of the ventral root, one should consider the possibility of it being part of the anterior root. Hence, the root anatomy should be checked once again, as well as a 50 Hz stimulus may be applied to verify any important and marked spreading. If spreading exists, it must be a dorsal root. This is because the ventral (motor) roots do not show intense spreading, even though they can spread this type of stimulus. In this case, spreading may be either due to secondary sensitization of sensitive muscle afferents or stimulation of afferent fibers within the motor root [12]. Another possibility to distinguish the sensory root causing spasticity from the motor root would be to perform root stimulation while monitoring the somatosensory evoked potential in the scalp and electromyography. If the somatosensory evoked potential is captured in that stimulated root, one may assume it to be the dorsal root and may evaluate if it should be sectioned or not [33].

Tetanic Stimulation

The loss of descending inhibition of spinal segmental synapses causes an increase in reflex responses resulting from the sensory stimuli of the gamma system, that is, an increase in muscle tonus and motor response, which results in spasticity. Therefore, if one of these pathways is interrupted, for example, by sectioning the sensory roots, more specifically some sensory roots that contribute most to spasticity, a reduction in the inflows of the ascending pathway that perpetuates spastic symptoms takes place, without compromising the motor and sphincter portion.

Therefore, after differentiating between the ventral-dorsal root and its location (threshold stimulation), the dorsal root should be separated into rootlets (between 3 and 10, usually around 4–8). Interpretation should concern on which rootlets contribute the most to spasticity.

This interpretation is performed during a 1 s tetanic stimulation at 50 Hz using, at most, the amperage that elucidated the sensory root. Stimulation with higher currents should be avoided so as not to cause propagation or exacerbation of responses, which could lead to misinterpretation. Roots should be carefully isolated from the cerebrospinal fluid to avoid current dispersion (Fig. 26.1d, e and 26.2c). The further parameters described in the threshold stimulation are maintained, using the neurophysiological criteria to identify the peripheral component of the spastic pathological circuit and thus proceed with the root section. These criteria, as shown below, were elaborated based on the authors' experience throughout time, initially based on Fasano's proposal, evolving to the more complex and far-fetched method used by Peacock and finally to the technique most frequently used developed by Phillips

(Table 26.3) [18, 25, 34]. Our team uses the criteria established by Phillips as a basis, together with the need to adapt to each patient's spastic condition, analogous to the characterization of myotatic reflexes in the neurological clinic (Table 26.4) [34, 35].

The secondary criteria for abnormality during the tetanic test of the rootlets must include a response with a low threshold and/or abrupt or irregular responses during a stimulus not considered high, according to individual criteria of each patient. Importantly, roots associated with anal sphincter responses at the S2 level should be spared, even those predominantly at the S1 level, thus preventing sphincter dysfunction.

Table 26.3 Sectioned rootlets – neurophysiological techniques and criteria to 50 Hz stimulation evolution, as per Phillips classification

Fasano	Peacock	Phillips[a]
Normal	Decremental	0 – unstained discharge or a single discharge to train of stimuli (ipsilateral)
Abnormal – spread	Squared	1 – sustained response only at stimulated segmental level (ipsilateral)
	Decremental – squared	2 – sustained response at level of stimulation and spread within one adjacent segmental level (ipsilateral)
	Incremental	3 – sustained response at level of stimulation with spread ipsilaterally >1 segmental level (ipsilateral)
	Multiphasic	4 – sustained response involving multiple segmental levels and spread to the contralateral leg
	Clonic	
	Irregular	
	Sustained	

[a]Our protocol

Table 26.4 Similar classification of EMG response and myotatic reflex

SDR reflex grading	EMG response	Myotatic reflex grading (/+4)	Response
0	Unsustained discharge or a single discharge to train of stimuli (ipsilateral)	0/+4	No contraction
1	Sustained response only at stimulated segmental level (ipsilateral)	+/+4	Weak, slight response
2	Sustained response at level of stimulation and spread within one adjacent segmental level (ipsilateral)	++/+4	Brisk reflex
3	Sustained response at level of stimulation with spread ipsilaterally >1 segmental level (ipsilateral)	+++/+4	Increased, greater than brisk response, with the absence of clonus
4	Sustained response involving multiple segmental levels and spread to the contralateral leg	++++/+4	Elicitation of clonus and same times contralateral brisk response

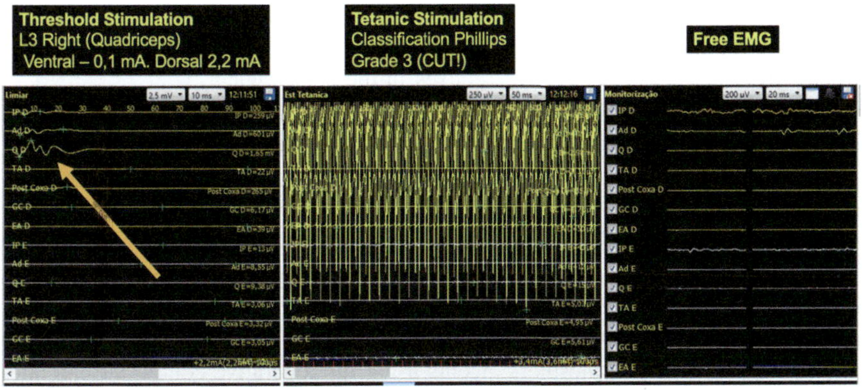

Fig. 26.4 Graphic stimulation threshold (ventral 0,1 mA and dorsal 2,2 mA), tetanic (Phillips classification grade 3 – "sustained" as per Peacock) and *free* EMG

Although Peacock described several patterns of recognizable neurophysiological abnormalities in the muscles when the dorsal rootlets are stimulated, some of them have no further practical validity [21]. Some patterns, however, could help secondarily in the classification of "normal" or "abnormal" and are worth mentioning. Decremental responses in amplitude, particularly when located in the myotomes corresponding to the stimulation, are considered normal. On the other hand, incremental responses in amplitude and/or sustained responses are considered abnormal mainly if dispersed from the stimulated myotomes [30]. When the Phillips classification is also used, the criteria become clearer (Fig. 26.4).

As seen in the descriptions above, this idea has existed since the end of the nineteenth century. It has been progressively improved during the twentieth century to surgically reduce spasticity. Indeed, the use of this type of ablative functional neurosurgery technique has proven effective in combating to spastic sequelae [7, 14–19, 21].

From Fasano on, the quantitative methodology gave way to the functional approach, based on EMG for the transection of the sick rootlets, introducing electrophysiological recordings [7, 18, 19, 21]. In the Fasano's primordial works, the muscles of the upper limbs, neck, and face were also monitored, with a spread of discharges captured by EMG being found in these muscles when certain lumbar rootlets were stimulated. This suggested that the presence of this contralateral spread, as well as spread for the upper portions of the body, would be a valid criterion to define that this rootlet is "acting beyond" the medullary-spinal circuit and maintaining spasticity [18, 36, 37].

When analyzing children without spasticity who underwent laminectomy for other situations using electrical stimulation of the posterior root at 50 Hz, Steinbok found 1 of 11 roots with contralateral spread to the muscles of the lower limbs and even to the upper limbs, neck, and face yet minimal and with a nonincreasing pattern, suggesting normality. In turn, in spastic children, this spread was seen more frequently (76%) [27, 30]. In other words, contralateral spreading is an important factor in judging the rootlet to be sectioned. Nevertheless, it is important to bear in mind that children without spasticity could present spreading, although less frequently.

The neurophysiological criteria for sectioning the rootlets include as an unequivocal "go/cut" responses to tetanic stimulation with Phillips grades 3 and 4. Yet, grades 0–2 mean "spare." Between 50% and 75% of the rootlets shall be sectioned, ranging from 20% to 80% depending on the clinical behavior for that root [29] (Figs. 26.4 and 26.5).

The responses to stimulation are not absolute, clearly, as there is subjectivity to a greater or lesser degree depending on the patient and the "feeling" of the surgeon and team. Depending on the frequency of stimuli, root refractoriness, or suppression of spinal reflexes to the anesthetic agents used, intraoperative conditions can alter motor responses. Electrophysiological responses, however, are reliable enough to represent a safe indication regarding spasticity and strength preservation. Clinical judgment must still prevail, and special care must be taken when deciding the degree

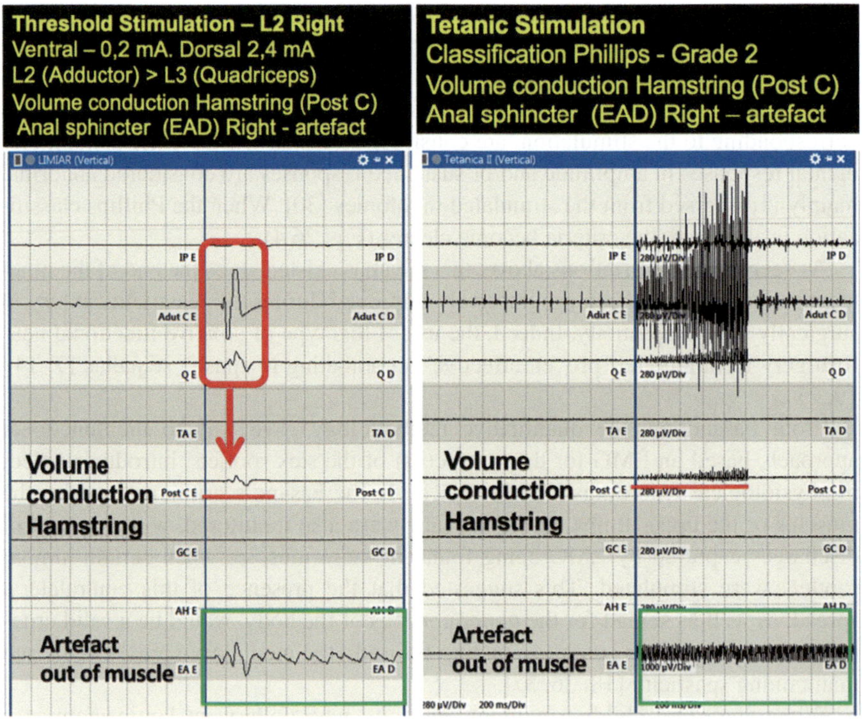

Fig. 26.5 Graphic. Stimulation L2 Right: Threshold (Ventral 0,2 mA and Dorsal 2,4 mA), L2 (adductor) > L3 (quadriceps), conduction volume in Hamstring, artefact (out of muscle) Anal Sphincter and Tetanic (Phillips Classification grade 2 – "Incremental" as per Peacock). To section or not would depend on the clinical map and on the "incremental" waveform. In this case it was sectioned

of injury at S2 for bladder function and whether larger or smaller sections at L4 for knee stability should be made (see below).

Consequently, it is extremely important to know in advance the clinical presentation and act on a given root under the anatomical (neurosurgical) and neurophysiological perspective but always correlating with individual patient's status.

Recording of Threshold and Tetanic Stimulations

Each institution has its own method of recording single pulse (threshold) and pulse train (tetanic) stimulations. Ours is shown in Table 26.5.

Root Excitability

In relation to the excitability of the dorsal roots, the L2–L3 roots have a modest excitability, and the L4–L5–S1 roots have a high excitability. The manipulation of the roots, either by stretching them when suspending them, or when dissecting them, impacts in a lower responsiveness. It can be a confounding factor when judging the degree of contribution to spasticity considering the Phillips criteria (Tables 26.3 and 26.4) [34].

Table 26.5 Recording of threshold and tetanic stimulations

Right				Left		
Threshold	Ventral	Dorsal	L1	Threshold	Ventral	Dorsal
Tetanic grade		%Cut		Tetanic grade		%Cut
Threshold	Ventral	Dorsal	L2	Threshold	Ventral	Dorsal
Tetanic grade		%Cut		Tetanic grade		%Cut
Threshold	Ventral	Dorsal	L3	Threshold	Ventral	Dorsal
Tetanic grade		%Cut		Tetanic grade		%Cut
Threshold	Ventral	Dorsal	L4	Threshold	Ventral	Dorsal
Tetanic grade		%Cut		Tetanic grade		%Cut
Threshold	Ventral	Dorsal	L5	Threshold	Ventral	Dorsal
Tetanic grade		%Cut		Tetanic grade		%Cut
Threshold	Ventral	Dorsal	S1	Threshold	Ventral	Dorsal
Tetanic grade		%Cut		Tetanic grade		%Cut
Threshold	Ventral	Dorsal	S2	Threshold	Ventral	Dorsal
Tetanic grade		%Cut		Tetanic grade		%Cut

L4 and L5 Roots Sectioning

Since Foester, the section of L4 and L5 roots has been discussed due to the antigravity function of L4 and the pelvic stability of L5, and, in our view, it should be closely linked to the analysis of the patient's clinical condition in relation to spasticity and weakness in this region. The assessment should be conducted by a multidisciplinary team, including physiotherapists. The benefit in the specific eligible cases is for ambulation improvement, which should guide the degree of sectioning of the roots [15, 16, 34] (see Tables 26.3 and 26.4).

EMG Artifacts/Pitfalls

Artifacts are frequently found and need to be differentiated from activity in response to electrical stimulus. Stimulus artifact is found during simple pulse stimuli (threshold stimulation) and train stimulus (tetanic stimulation). For tetanic stimulation, the artifact appears as a series of individual, thin, equally spaced responses of equal amplitude. The amplitude is proportional to the intensity of the stimulus. This type of artifact is usually greater in channels close to the stimulation site, and usually the impedance is greater in those recording channels.

The movement artifact shows a low-frequency oscillation in the recording channels occurring during the movement of the legs or of the electrodes themselves. They may also occur due to electrode displacement (Fig. 26.5).

The muscle groups that are most affected by spasticity on clinical examination may present motor unit potentials with a continuous firing pattern around 10–20 Hz (interferential pattern), which hinders the identification of responses to stimulation. This activity can be observed more frequently after stimulation of the roots or rootlets during intraoperative individualization.

Flowchart: Our Routine

To carry out neurophysiology in SDR, we must keep in mind what resources we have at our disposal. The minimum to be performed is free-run EMG (fEMG), triggered EMG (tEMG) with threshold, and tetanic stimulation. However, the use of several established intraoperative neurophysiological techniques brings greater safety to the procedure, as recommended for a long time by Dr. Ricardo Ferreira (personal communication) and his team. Flowchart 26.1 shows their assembly.

The stability of the transcranial motor evoked potentials (MEP) that are being recorded in the same muscles evaluated by EMG enhances safety. Additionally, the bulbocavernosus reflex (BCR) in conjunction with MEP of the anal sphincter improves the assessment of the sensory and motor pathways of this reflex arc. The

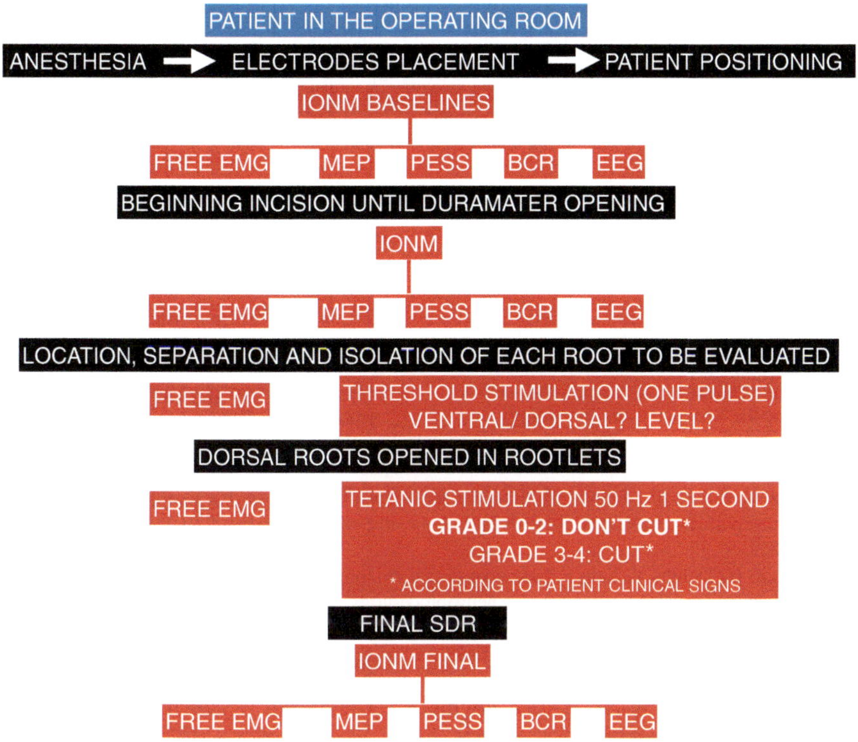

Flowchart 26.1 Intraoperative neurophysiological monitoring and SDR

electroencephalogram (EEG) helps to check on the anesthetic level, and the somatosensory evoked potential (SSEP) can assess part of the sensitive pathway and even help to compare the ventral or dorsal root. Usually, SSEP is limited in this type of surgery because it is restricted to tibial nerves, identifying compromise focused on the ascending pathways of S1.

Note: The abovementioned multimodal techniques are routinely used in IOM and were detailed in the corresponding chapters in this book.

Conclusion

SDR is an important part of the therapeutic arsenal available for the treatment of spasticity, especially for children with cerebral palsy. It aims to improve locomotion in cases of ambulatory patients, or to ease the performing of hygiene and comfort care, reducing or removing addictive positions, enabling passive stretching and comfort, and stopping the evolution of deformities. To more objectively perform SDR, the use of neurophysiology through free-run and triggered electromyography brings important benefits to the patient. The use of neurophysiological multimodality including MEP, SSEP, BCR, and EEG improves the accuracy of functional assessment. Teamwork enhances patient safety and outcome.

References

1. Kandel ER, Schwartz JH, Jessel TM. Princípios da Neurociência. 4th ed. São Paulo: Manole Ltda; 2003. p. 713–35.
2. Decq P. Physiopathologie De La Spasticité. Neurochirurgie. 2003;49:163–84, 2.
3. Mukherjee A, Chakravarty A. Spasticity mechanisms – for the clinician. Front Neurol. 2010;1:149. https://doi.org/10.3389/fneur.2010.00149. PMID: 21206767; PMCID: PMC3009478.
4. Bishop B. Spasticity: its physiology and management. Part II. Neurophysiology of spasticity: current concepts. Phys Ther. 1977;57(4):377–84. https://doi.org/10.1093/ptj/57.4.377. PMID: 139621.
5. Abbott R, Forem SL, Johann M. Selective posterior rhizotomy for the treatment of spasticity: a review. Childs Nerv Syst. 1989;5(6):337–46. https://doi.org/10.1007/BF00271889. PMID: 2692811.
6. Pasquali C, Deletis V, Sala F. Selective dorsal rhizotomy: functional anatomy of the conus-cauda and essentials of intraoperative neurophysiology. Childs Nerv Syst. 2020;36(9):1907–18. https://doi.org/10.1007/s00381-020-04746-9. Epub 2020 Jul 7. PMID: 32638074.
7. Peacock WJ, Arens LJ. Selective posterior rhizotomy for the relief of spasticity in cerebral palsy. S Afr Med J. 1982;62(4):119–24. PMID: 7089801.
8. Haberl H. Chapter 39 – Selective dorsal rhizotomy. In: Deletis V, Shils JL, Sala F, Seidel K, editors. Neurophysiology in neurosurgery. 2nd ed. Academic Press; 2020. p. 551–64. https://doi.org/10.1016/B978-0-12-815000-9.00039-3. ISBN 9780128150009.
9. Enslin JMN, Langgerak NG, Fieggen AG. The evolution of selective dorsal rhizotomy for the management of spasticity. Neurotherapeutics. 2019;16:3–8. https://doi.org/10.1007/s13311-018-00690-40.
10. Nicolini-Panisson RD'A, et al. Rizotomia dorsal seletiva na paralisia cerebral: critérios de indicação e protocolos de reabilitação fisioterapêutica pós-operatória. Rev Paul Pediatr. 2018;36(1):100–8. https://doi.org/10.1590/1984-0462. Epub 15 Jan 2018. ISSN 1984-0462.
11. Palisano R, Rosenbaum P, Walter S, Russell D, Wood E, Galuppi B. Development and reliability of a system to classify gross motor function in children with cerebral palsy. Dev Med Child Neurol. 1997;39(4):214–23.
12. Georgoulis G, Brînzeu A, Sindou M. Dorsal rhizotomy for children with spastic diplegia of cerebral palsy origin: usefulness of intraoperative monitoring. J Neurosurg Pediatr. 2018;22(1):89–101. https://doi.org/10.3171/2018.1.PEDS17577. Epub 2018 Apr 13. PMID: 29652243.
13. Michael P. Powell, Sir Victor Horsley at the birth of neurosurgery. Brain. 2016;139(2):631–4. https://doi.org/10.1093/brain/awv345.
14. Sherrington CS. Decerebrate rigidity, and reflex coordination of movements. J Physiol. 1898;22(4):319–32. https://doi.org/10.1113/jphysiol.1898.sp000697. PMID: 16992412; PMCID: PMC1513016.
15. Foerster O. Resection of the posterior spinal nerve-roots in the treatment of gastric crises and spastic paralysis. SAGE Publications; 1911.
16. Foerster O. On the indication and results of the excision of posterior roots in men. Surg Gynecol Obstet. 1913;16:463–75.
17. Gros C, Ouaknine G, Vlahovitch B, Frerebeau P. La radicotomie sélective postérieure dans le traitement neuro- chirurgical de l'hypertonie pyramidale. Neurochirurgie. 1967;13:505–18.
18. Fasano VA, Barolat-Romana G, Ivaldi A, Sguazzi A. La radicotomie postérieure fonctionnelle dans le traitement de la spasticité cérébrale Premieres observations sur la stimulation

électrique peropératoire des racines postérieures, et leur utilisation dans le choix des racines à sectionner. Neurochirurgie. 1976;22(1):23–4.
19. Park TS, Gaffney PE, Kaufman BA, Molleston MC. Selective lumbosacral dorsal rhizotomy immediately caudal to the conus medullaris for cerebral palsy spasticity. Neurosurgery. 1993;33:92933.
20. Funk JF, Haberl H. Monosegmental laminoplasty for selective dorsal rhizotomy—operative technique and influence on the development of scoliosis in ambulatory children with cerebral palsy. Childs Nerv Syst. 2016;32(5):81925. Available from: https://doi.org/10.1007/s00381-016-3016-3. Epub 2016 Jan 13.
21. Park TS, Johnston JM. Surgical techniques of selective dorsal rhizotomy for spastic cerebral palsy. Technical note. Neurosurg Focus. 2006;21(2):e7.
22. Meythaler JM. Concept of spastic hypertonia. Phys Med Rehabil Clin N Am. 2001;12(4):725–32.
23. Abbott R. Complications with selective posterior rhizotomy. Pediatr Neurosurg. 1992;18(1):43–7.
24. Farmer JP, Sabbagh AJ. Selective dorsal rhizotomies in the treatment of spasticity related to cerebral palsy. Childs Nerv Syst. 2007;23(9):991–1002.
25. Peacock WJ, Arens LJ, Berman B. Cerebral palsy spasticity. Selective posterior rhizotomy. Pediatr Neurosci. 1987;13(2):61–6.
26. Drazin D, Auguste K. Contemporary dorsal rhizotomy surgery for the treatment of spasticity in childhood. In: Quinones-Hinojosa A, editor. Schmidek & sweet operative neurosurgical techniques: indications, methods and results. Philadelphia: Elsevier/Saunders; 2012. p. 753–8. Selective.
27. Steinbok P, Hicdonmez T, Sawatzky B, Beauchamp R, Wickenheiser D. Spinal deformities after selective dorsal rhizotomy for spastic cerebral palsy. J Neurosurg Pediatr. 2005;102:363–3730.
28. Langerak NG, Vaughan CL, Hoffman EB, et al. Incidence of spinal abnormalities in patients with spastic diplegia 17 to 26 years after selective dorsal rhizotomy. Childs Nerv Syst. 2009;25:1593–603. https://doi.org/10.1007/s00381-009-0993-5.
29. Turner RP. Neurophysiologic intraoperative monitoring during selective dorsal rhizotomy. J Clin Neurophysiol. 2009;26(2):82–4. https://doi.org/10.1097/WNP.0b013e31819f9077. PMID: 19279497.
30. Hays MH, McLaughlin JF, Bjornson KF, Stephen K, Roberts TS, Price R. Electrophysiological monitoring during selective dorsal rhizotomy, and spasticity and GMFM performance. Dev Med Child Neurol. 1998;40:233–8.
31. Vaughan CL, Berman B, Peacock WJ. Cerebral palsy and rhizotomy. A 3-year follow-up evaluation with gait analysis. J Neurosurg. 1991;74(2):178–84. https://doi.org/10.3171/jns.1991.74.2.0178. PMID: 1988585.
32. Clinical practice guidelines for intraoperative neurophysiological monitoring: 2020 update. Special Article. Ann Clin Neurophysiol. 2021;23(1):35–45. https://doi.org/10.14253/acn.2021.23.1.35. Published online: April 29, 2021.
33. Song Y, Ferri SA, Kobylarz EJ, Thomas Jr GP, Bauer DF. Advances in neurophysiological intraoperative monitoring during selective dorsal rhizotomy. http://www.asnm.org/resource/resmgr/Events/2018/Annual/2018_Eposters/5._Song_-_Advances_in_Neurop.pdf.
34. Phillips LH, Park TS. Electrophysiologic studies of selective posterior rhizotomy patients. In: Park TS, Phillips LH, Peacock WJ, editors. Management of spasticity in cerebral palsy and spinal cord injury. Philadelphia: Hanley and Belfus Inc; 1989. p. 459–69. Neurosurgery: State of the Art Reviews; Vol. 4, No. 2.
35. Dolbow J, Throckmorton Z. Neuroanatomy, spinal cord myotatic reflex. [Updated 2020 Sept 19]. In: StatPearls [Internet]. Treasure Island: StatPearls Publishing; 2021. Available from: https://www.ncbi.nlm.nih.gov/books/NBK551629/.
36. Fasano VA, Broggi G, Zeme S. Intraoperative electrical stimulation for functional posterior rhizotomy. Scand J Rehabil Med Suppl. 1988;17:149–54. PMID: 3165207.
37. Steinbok P, Langill L, Cochrane DD, Keyes R. Observations on electrical stimulation of lumbosacral nerve roots in children with and without lower limb spasticity. Childs Nerv Syst. 1992;8(7):376–82. https://doi.org/10.1007/BF00304784. PMID: 1458494.

Chapter 27
Intramedullary Spinal Cord Tumors

Andreya Fonseca Cardoso Cavalcanti, Karina Maria Alécio de Oliveira, Monica Nascimento de Melo, and Silvia Mazzali Verst

Abbreviations

CST	Corticospinal tract
DC	Dorsal column
DREZ	Dorsal root entry zone
D-wave	Direct wave
EMG	Electromyography
IMSCT	Intramedullary spinal cord tumor
IOM	Intraoperative monitoring
ITI	Inter-train interval
L	Lumbar
MEP	Motor evoked potential

Supplementary Information The online version contains supplementary material available at [https://doi.org/10.1007/978-3-030-95730-8_27].

A. F. C. Cavalcanti (✉)
Department of Neurology and Neurophysiology, Neurocol Neurofisiologia Avançada, São Paulo, SP, Brazil
e-mail: andreya@neurocol.com.br

K. M. A. de Oliveira
Department of Neurology and Neurophysiology, Clinica Stela de Monitoramento Clínico e Cirúrgico em Neurologia, Brasília, DF, Brazil

M. N. de Melo
Department of Neurophysiology, Integrated Neuroscience Institute, Goiânia, GO, Brazil

S. M. Verst
Instituto de Ensino e Pesquisa (Research and Educational Institute) of Sírio Libanês Hospital, São Paulo, Brazil

Brain Spine Neurofisiologia, Jundiaí, SP, Brazil

S. M. Verst et al. (eds.), *Intraoperative Monitoring*,
https://doi.org/10.1007/978-3-030-95730-8_27

mMEP	Muscle motor evoked potential
NAP	Nerve action potential
PT	Posterior tibial (nerve)
SC	Spinal cord
SCT	Spinal cord tumors
SEP	Somatosensory evoked potential
TES	Transcranial electrical stimulation
Th	Thoracic

Introduction

Spinal cord tumors (SCT) can be classified based on the location of the tumor as intradural intramedullary, intradural extramedullary, or extradural.

The majority of spinal tumors are extradural, accounting for 60% of SCT, and are frequently metastatic lesions. The most common intradural extramedullary lesions are meningioma and schwannoma [1].

Extramedullary intraspinal tumors (intra- or extradural) represent another category of spinal tumors. Some neurophysiological techniques of intraoperative monitoring (IOM) of these pathologies (such as nerve root mapping and bulbocavernosus reflex) have already been covered in Chap. 26. In this chapter, we will address intradural intramedullary tumors and the particularities of their IOM.

Intramedullary spinal cord tumors (IMSCT) are rare pathologies. They correspond to 2–4% of central nervous system tumors [2] and 10% of spinal tumors [3], with ependymomas (60–70%), astrocytomas (30–40%), and hemangioblastomas (3–8%) being the most frequent histological types [2, 4–7].

SCT often present first with progressive local or radicular pain, and then other symptoms appear, including weakness, generalized numbness, paresthesias, loss of proprioception, gait imbalance, and sphincter dysfunction [8].

Surgical resection continues to be the most effective treatment modality for most intramedullary tumors, with gross total resection aiming to preserve neurological function and improve survival [9].

However, surgical treatment is often difficult and carries significant risk of postoperative neurological complications. IOM has been shown to be of clinical importance in the surgical resection of IMSCT [10].

The neurophysiological strategy in IMSCT resection surgeries must take into account five fundamental points: (1) the anatomical landmarks of the spinal cord (Fig. 27.1); (2) the safe entry zones; (3) the surgical strategy; (4) the oncological strategy; and (5) the expectation of the functional outcome [11].

There are different aspects related to the pathology of IMSCT that will determine different surgical and neurophysiological strategies. The approach is largely dependent on tumor histology and patient functionality [11].

Tumors that are well demarcated (e.g., ependymomas, hemangioblastomas) can be resected for cure, while more infiltrative tumors (e.g., high-grade astrocytomas)

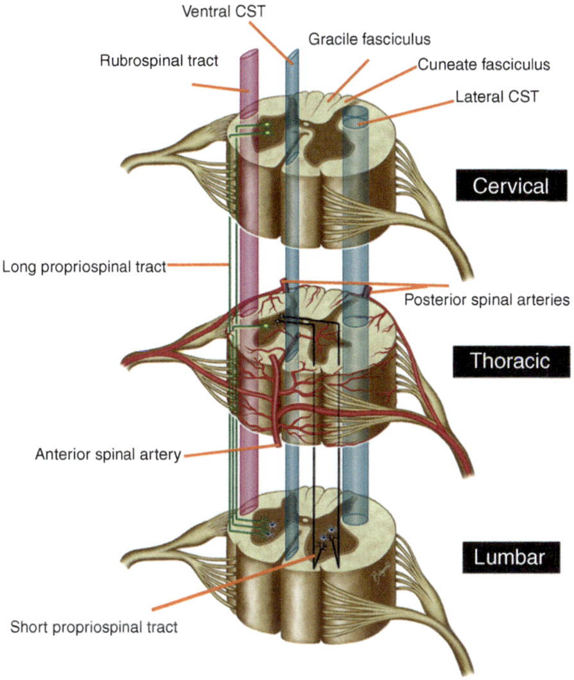

Fig. 27.1 Cervical, thoracic, and lumbar spinal cord segmentation. Lateral CST carries 85% of all fibers, mainly fast synchronized fibers, and is analyzed by D-wave. Ventral CST carries about 10–15% of total fibers. Both end at the second motor neuron at the anterior horn, mostly through interneurons connections. Short propriospinal tract connects up to six spinal segments, while long propriospinal tract connects cervical to lumbar segments. Anterior spinal artery irrigates anterior two thirds of the spinal cord. Thus, its ischemia or spasm is translated by motor deficit. There are two posterior spinal arteries responsible for irrigation of the posterior third spine. At the posterior funiculus, *gracilis* and cuneiform tracts transit, medially and laterally, respectively. (@ copyright from Silvia Mazzali-Verst (editor))

are typically managed with biopsies or limited resections in order to minimize the significant risk of damage to the spinal cord (SC) [12].

The use of IOM and the choice of appropriate neurophysiological techniques may help guide the extent of surgery while minimizing damage to normal tissue [10, 11].

IOM Modalities Applicable in IMSCT Resection Surgeries

IOM of the functional integrity of SC pathways is crucial to prevent and limit surgically induced injury [10, 13–16].

The available methods can be divided into monitoring and mapping techniques.

Motor evoked potentials (MEPs), including the D-wave recording, and somatosensory evoked potentials (SEPs) with established interpretation and warning criteria are used for the purpose of monitoring [17, 18].

However, monitoring only provides information about integrity, not about the location and somatotopy of long tracts. Mapping methods are able to identify SC structures [15, 19].

Three methods have been described to map the dorsal column (DC): (1) peripheral nerve stimulation and SEPs recording over the DC using a miniature multi-contact electrode [15, 20, 21]; (2) DC stimulation and phase reversal SEPs recording over the scalp [22]; and (3) DC stimulation and antidromic responses recording over peripheral nerves [23].

Three methods have also been reported to map the corticospinal tract (CST) in the SC: (1) the D-wave collision technique [20, 24]; (2) the evocation of muscle responses in the limbs after direct SC stimulation [24–28]; and (3) a more refined and selective stimulation through the double-train stimulation technique [29, 30].

Methodology

SEPs Monitoring

The stimulation and recording methodology for obtaining SEPs has already been well detailed (see Chap. 8).

Posterior tibial (PT) SEPs monitoring is important during an IMSCT resection, due to the high risk of the *gracilis* tracts damage during myelotomy and tumor dissection. In cases of cervical tumors, the upper limb SEPs should be added.

Most patients with IMSCT already have an impaired large fiber sensory system, resulting in lower limb basal SEPs with small amplitudes, increased latencies, and poor morphology. Therefore, an effort should be made to obtain reliable baselines.

Muscle MEPs Monitoring

The stimulation and recording methodology for obtaining muscle MEPs (mMEPs) has also been well detailed in another chapter, including the transcranial electrical stimulation (TES) facilitation techniques to try to optimize the baselines, often difficult to record in symptomatic patients (see Chap. 9).

The extent of the myotomes sampling should be individualized to the level of surgery (see Chap. 3) and also to the patient's preoperative neurological status. The greater the number of muscle channels used, the greater the possibility of obtaining reproducible and reliable baselines. The tumor growth can cause dispersion of the fibers of the CST, and the limited number of monitored muscles can lead to false negative results (see Chap. 9).

Therefore, for high cervical injuries, it is recommended to record all cervical innervation myotomes and at least two or three more muscles of each lower limb (see the suggested myotomes sampling for cervical spine surgeries in Chap. 25). For lesions below Th1, it is recommended to record all lumbosacral myotomes, including the anal sphincter (see the suggested myotomes sampling for thoracic spine surgeries in Chap. 23).

D-Wave Monitoring

Direct (D) corticospinal tract (CST) discharges are descending volleys registered on the first motor neuron axon within SC. Mostly, D-wave is the potential of CST fast-conducting fibers of lateral funiculus. Several D-waves are generated after short train stimulation of motor cortex, and they will be responsible for second motor neuron activation and consequent mMEP. Conversely, in order to intraoperatively evaluate D- wave, single anodic pulse is used through TES [31].

An extensive and detailed explanation about D-wave anatomical bases and its methodology was covered in the chapter about motor evoked potential (see Chap. 9). Here we will review the key points about stimulation and recording and practical tips to improve D-wave acquisition.

Anatomical and functional basis of SC sources for D-wave and mMEP are different. CST originates from premotor frontal lobe, postcentral, and precentral gyrus. The latter counts for approximately 80% of its origin. Around 85% of CST fibers decussates at the pyramids and runs at SC lateral funiculus. They are the ticker myelinated synchronized fibers of the motor tract and are mostly related to fine coordinated movements [10, 15, 32].

A small percentage connects directly to the second motor neuron, while the remaining fibers terminate on propriospinal interneurons. In fact, most input to alpha motor neurons originates in interneurons, building a complex network of connections. This neural network links somatosensory and proprioceptive information with motor control. Long and short propriospinal tracts integrate multiple spinal segments [32, 33] (Fig. 27.1).

D-wave corresponds to direct recording of the descending volley at the lateral funiculus, while mMEP is a product of alpha motor neuron activation and motor units' depolarization (see Chap. 9). Combining the use of D-wave and mMEPs provides the most comprehensive assessment of the SC motor tracts' functional integrity during surgery for IMSCT [15]. It is considered the gold standard.

For D-wave recording, the catheter electrode (Fig. 27.2) may be sited both rostrally (as a reference) and caudally (as active electrode) to the tumor, at the epidural or subdural space. Once placed, the best combination between two of the electrode tips 1, 2, and 3 is tested to ensure the highest possible D-wave amplitude. D-wave is usually recorded in 20 ms epochs and amplified 10.000 times with filter settings of 1.5 ± 1700 Hz [31]. Low impedance values improve quality of recordings. The most efficient pulse duration is 0.5 ms because it allows for the quicker recovery of each

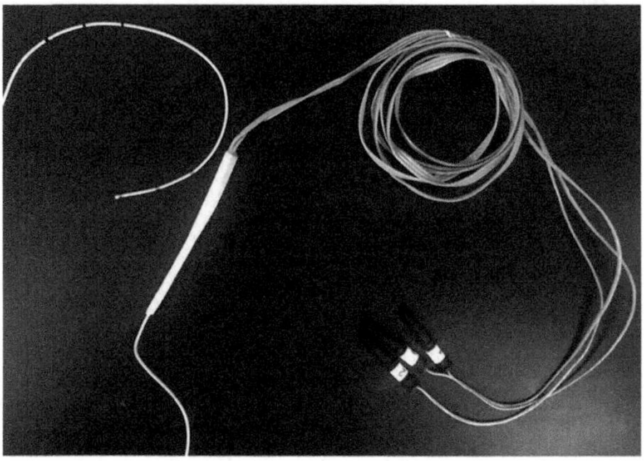

Fig. 27.2 D-wave catheter

Table 27.1 Summary of the stimulation and recording methodology for obtaining the D-wave

	Stimulation	Recording
Site	Scalp Montage: C1/C2, 6 cm/Cz or C3/C4	Epidural or subdural space (below the lesion)
Electrodes	Corkscrew electrodes	D-wave catheter
Parameters	Anodic single pulse Duration: 0.5–1.0 ms Frequency: 0.5–2.0 Hz	Screen: 30 μV/div and 1–6 ms/div Sweeps: 20 ms Filter settings: 1.5 ± 1700 Hz

consecutive D-wave amplitude [15]. The choice for scalp electrodes montage remains of some debate. Either montage C1–C2 or C3–C4 will work fine. Choose the one that results in less neck movement, so that it allows for continuous D-wave monitoring at a rate of 0.5–2 Hz. The stimulation and recording methodology of the D-wave monitoring technique [31, 34] is summarized in Table 27.1.

D-wave amplitude reaches approximately 80 μV at cervical region (Fig. 27.3) and half this amplitude by lumbar spinal cord (at the vertebral level of Th10) [15]. Below Th10 there is a small amount of recordable CST running to conus medullaris at L1. D-wave is quite unrecordable [35]. Amplitude variation from trial to trial of 10% is acceptable. Expected latencies increase when the recording site is moved caudally. Reference values are 3–6 ms at cervical region and 6–9 ms at thoracic region [34, 35].

D-waves can be evaluated during intra-axial supratentorial, cervical-bulbar, and SC approaches. During mid-low cervical IMSCT resections, the electrode is located below vertebra C7, and it will record thoracic and lower limbs CST only. For upper cervical SC level surgery, electrode may be placed at lower cervical levels. In conclusion, D-wave translates the CST running along the surgical field but not of the segmental spinal cord.

Hence, selection of segmental muscles to record from is an important issue in the monitoring of mMEPs in order to ensure selectivity. Additionally, selection of the atrophied muscles is nonoptimal and hinders monitorability. Taking care to needling the muscle motor point is standard of care (more details in Chap. 3).

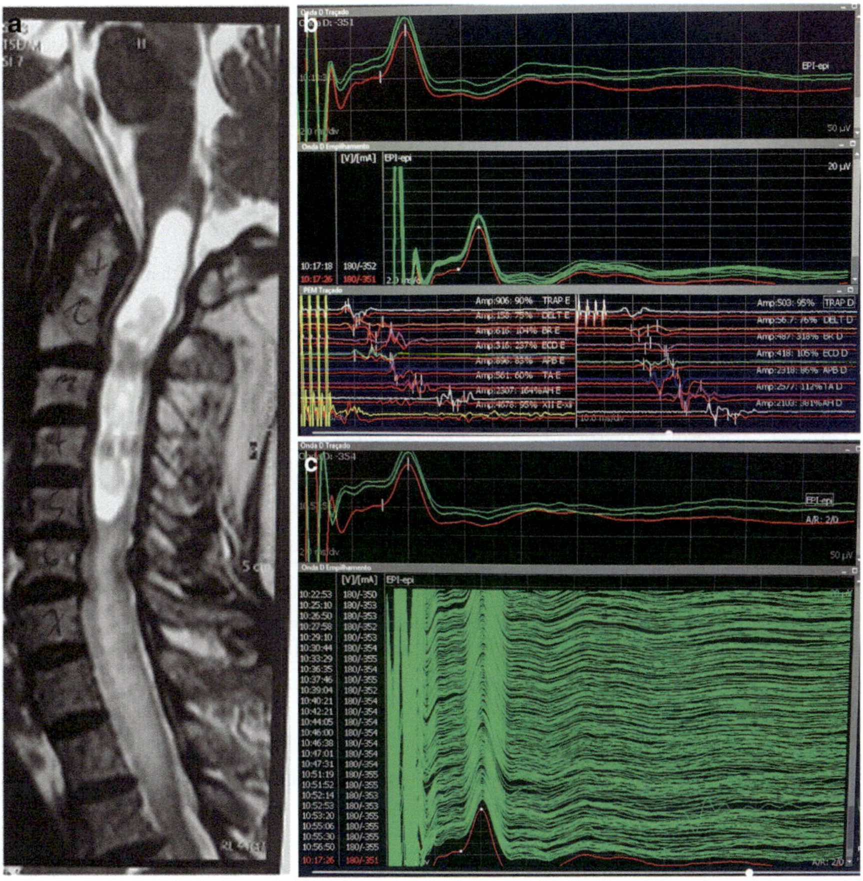

Fig. 27.3 Muscle MEPs and D-waves recordings in a 65-year-old woman who underwent resection of a C1–C5 ependymoma. (**a**) Preoperative MRI. (**b**) Basal mMEPs (lower image) and D-waves (upper image). (**c**) Continuous D-wave monitoring. Total tumor resection without intraoperative neurophysiological changes (stable mMEPs and D-waves). Postoperative outcome without new neurological deficit. The traces in red color correspond to baselines. E, left; *TRAP, trapezius; DELT, deltoid; BR, brachioradialis; ECD, extensor digitorum; APB, abductor pollicis brevis; TA, tibialis anterior; AH, abductor hallux; XII, genioglossus*

Motor outcome prognosis during IMSCT resection can be predicted by IOM changes. Fundamentally, a combination of D-wave and mMEP is analyzed (Table 27.2). Physiological basis for understanding this behavior lies on SC functional architecture. mMEP is dependent on the positive and negative inputs to the alpha motor neuron, through interneurons and originating from different tracts. Intramedullary manipulation during tumor resection may result in disorganization of this system and mMEP deterioration or loss. Yet, postoperative neuroplasticity is mostly related to propriospinal tracts, due to their greatly innate regenerative capacity [33]. Conversely, D-wave deterioration means axonal loss and there is less room for recovery. Thus, the long-term postoperative

Table 27.2 Using the mMEP and D-wave data to guide surgery and predict outcome

mMEPs	D-wave amplitude	Surgeon response	Postoperative motor function
No change	No change	None	Same as preoperative
↓ Amplitude ↑ Threshold	No change or >80% of baseline	*Tip*: Time/break Irrigation Pressure improvement Use of papaverine	Same as preoperative or transient deficit
Lost	No change or >80% of baseline	*Tip*: Time/break Irrigation Pressure improvement Use of papaverine	New deficit that often improves
Lost	*Reaching 80% of baseline*	*Proceed with caution* *Consider Stop*	*High risk for permanent deficit*
Lost	*Below 50% of baseline*	***Stop***	*Permanent new deficit; possible plegia*

Source: Reproduced from Sala et al. [36] (with permission)

motor prognosis is highly dependent on the stability of the D-wave amplitude (Fig. 27.4) during the intraoperative period (preservation of at least 50% of D-wave amplitude) [10, 15, 32, 37].

D-wave is recordable in two thirds of the patients [38]. Failure is believed to be related to desynchronization of the wave if motor status is preserved.

Free Electromyography Monitoring

After the description by Skinner et al. in 2009 on the correlation of suprasegmental electromyography (EMG) discharges and mechanical irritation of CST fibers [39], several other authors began to value free-run EMG recordings during surgeries for resection of brain and SC tumors [40].

In this context, the presence of EMG discharges may alert to the need to intensify surveillance in the MEP (see Chap. 11).

Dorsal Column Mapping Techniques

Retrograde Recording of Posterior Tibial Nerve Action Potentials (NAPs)

The recording of the posterior tibial (PT) NAP after DC stimulation with bipolar handheld electrode is a time-consuming and poorly reproducible antidromic technique for mapping the DC.

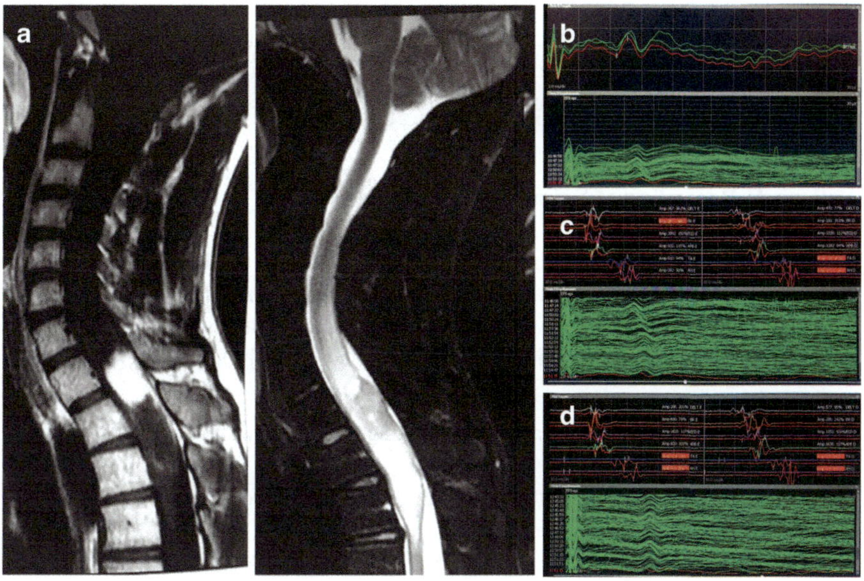

Fig. 27.4 Muscle MEPs and D-waves recordings in a 25-year-old man undergoing resection of a cervicothoracic astrocytoma. (**a**) Preoperative MRI. (**b**) Continuous and stable D-wave monitoring. (**c**) Preserved D-wave amplitude (lower image) and an important drop in the amplitudes of the lower right limb mMEPs (upper image). The slight delay in D-wave latency may be related to a small displacement of the catheter. (**d**) Complete disappearance of lower limb mMEPs (upper image), maintaining amplitude stability of D-wave (lower image). Total tumor resection without D-wave changes. Immediate postoperative status was paraplegia. After 3 months of motor rehabilitation, patient showed complete neurological recovery. IOM mMEPs disappearance led to a transient paraplegia. The traces in red color correspond to baselines. E, left; *TRAP, trapezius; DELT, deltoid; BR, brachioradialis; ECD, extensor digitorum; APB, abductor pollicis brevis; TA, tibialis anterior; AH, abductor hallux*

The method was described by Quinones-Hinojosa et al. in 2002, who suggested its use in identifying the median raphe for performing midline myelotomy in IMSCT resection surgeries [23].

The stimulator probe should be positioned with the cathode tip pointing distally to the longitudinal axis of the spinal cord, starting 2 mm lateral to the presumed midline. As the PT NAPs appear after at least about 50 averages, the probe should be moved 1 mm lateral to the presumed midline, and a new attempt at stimulation should be performed, comparing the amplitudes of the NAPs according to the displacement of the stimulator.

This procedure is repeated on the contralateral side of the presumed midline. The region of complete absence of response or lowest amplitude is assumed to be the region with the fewest number of axons (functional midline).

When it is not possible to visualize any anatomical outline of the midline (in cases of distortion of the fibers of the DC by the tumor), a good alternative is to perform the stimulation by moving the probe several times every 1 mm from the extreme left to the extreme right (or vice versa) in the dorsal aspect of the SC. The disappearance of the NAP will indicate the location of the median raphe.

The stimulation and recording methodology of this retrograde recording of PT NAPs technique [23] is summarized in Table 27.3.

Antegrade Recording of Spinal SEPs

The principle of this method is based on the fact that at the level of the *gracilis* tracts, the recorded electrical volleys triggered by peripheral stimulation of the ipsilateral posterior tibial nerve will have the highest amplitudes, thus enabling the identification of the neurophysiologic midline (median raphe) [18, 41].

Table 27.3 Summary of the stimulation and recording methodology of the three dorsal column mapping techniques

Technique	Retrograde recording of PT NAP		Antegrade recording of spinal SEPs		Phase reversal technique	
	Stimulation	Recording	Stimulation	Recording	Stimulation	Recording
Site	Spinal cord (DC) Parallel to the spine axis Cathode pointing distally	Posterior tibial nerves: Ankle (medial malleolus) Popliteal fossa	Posterior tibial nerves: Ankle (medial malleolus)	Spinal cord (DC) Perpendicular to the spine axis Equidistant referential recording	Spinal cord (DC) Parallel to the spine axis Cathode pointing proximal	Scalp recording: CP3–CP4 CPz–Fz
Electrode	Bipolar handheld electrode 2–3 mm between the tips	A pair of electrodes: Subdermal needle	A pair of electrodes	8-contact microelectrode Referential recording: Subdermal needle	Bipolar handheld electrode 2–3 mm between the tips	Corkscrew electrodes
Parameters	Pulse duration: 0.2 ms Intensity: 3–8 mA Frequency: 9.1 Hz 50–100 trials	Sensitivity: 1–5 μV Time base: 100 ms Bandpass: 30–300 Hz	Identical to those used for the SEPs monitoring technique (see Chap. 8) Pulse duration: 0.2 ms Intensity: 40 mA Frequency: 13.3 Hz 100–200 averages	Sensitivity: 10–50 μV Time base: 50 ms Bandpass: 50–1700 Hz	Pulse duration: 0.2–0.3 ms Intensity: 0.2–0.5 mA Maximum intensity: 1 mA Frequency: 3.17 Hz 10–20 trials	Sensitivity: 1–5 μV Time base: 50 ms Bandpass: 30–300 Hz

Later, Gandhi et al., using the same Penfield paradigm, expanded muscle sampling and used a concentric bipolar stimulator. Thus, they were able to provide a more delicate and more selective stimulation of the CST fibers [25].

As with subcortical motor mapping of the CST in supratentorial surgery (see Chaps. 14 and 17), some authors [28, 40] have been successfully using high-frequency cathodal monopolar stimulation to map the CST at the cord level. It consists in applying repetitive trains at 1–2 Hz, with 4–6 pulses/train, and a pulse duration of 0.5 ms. It can also be applied continuously, with the cavitronic ultrasonic surgical aspirator (CUSA), allowing simultaneous mapping and resection of the tumor [28]. In this case, it is recommended to use a short train of cathodal pulses (3 pulses, 0.2 ms pulse duration, interstimulus interval 3 ms) with an intensity ranging from 0.5 to 2 mA and recordings from limb muscles [28].

However, stimulation of cord tissue can be non-focal, resulting in confusing interpretation. Despite the limitation of this direct SC stimulation technique, it has its benefits mainly in cases of absence of basal D-wave recordings.

Double-Train Stimulation Technique

The main problem related to proposed techniques for mapping the CST in the SC is related to the lack of selectivity of the motor response obtained. Responses recorded from limb muscles after stimulation of the exposed SC can also be obtained by stimulation of the DC and not exclusively by stimulation of the CST [29, 30].

Deletis et al. demonstrated that muscle responses after CST or DC stimulation have distinguishable features if double-train stimulation is used [30].

The spinal interneurons targeted by CST fibers have a much shorter recovery time than 60 ms (see Chap. 9). Meanwhile, the spinal interneurons targeted by branches of DC fibers ending up to the alpha motoneurons as a part of reflex arc have a recovery time significantly longer than 60 ms [50].

It is expected that CST stimulation with 60 ms inter-train interval (ITI) would generate a response after the second train, whereas stimulation of the DC would not do so. Therefore, mapping of the exposed SC can be performed with a double-train stimulation paradigm [30]. If a response in a limb muscle appears after the first as well as after the second stimulus train, this indicates that the stimulating electrode is in close proximity to the CST. If there is no response to the second train of stimuli, this indicates that the electrode is in close proximity to the DC, because interneurons targeted by DC fibers are still in the refractory period (Fig. 27.7).

This concept might improve the intraoperative SC mapping especially in tumors with infiltrative margins such as astrocytoma, where it is difficult to establish a clear resection plane.

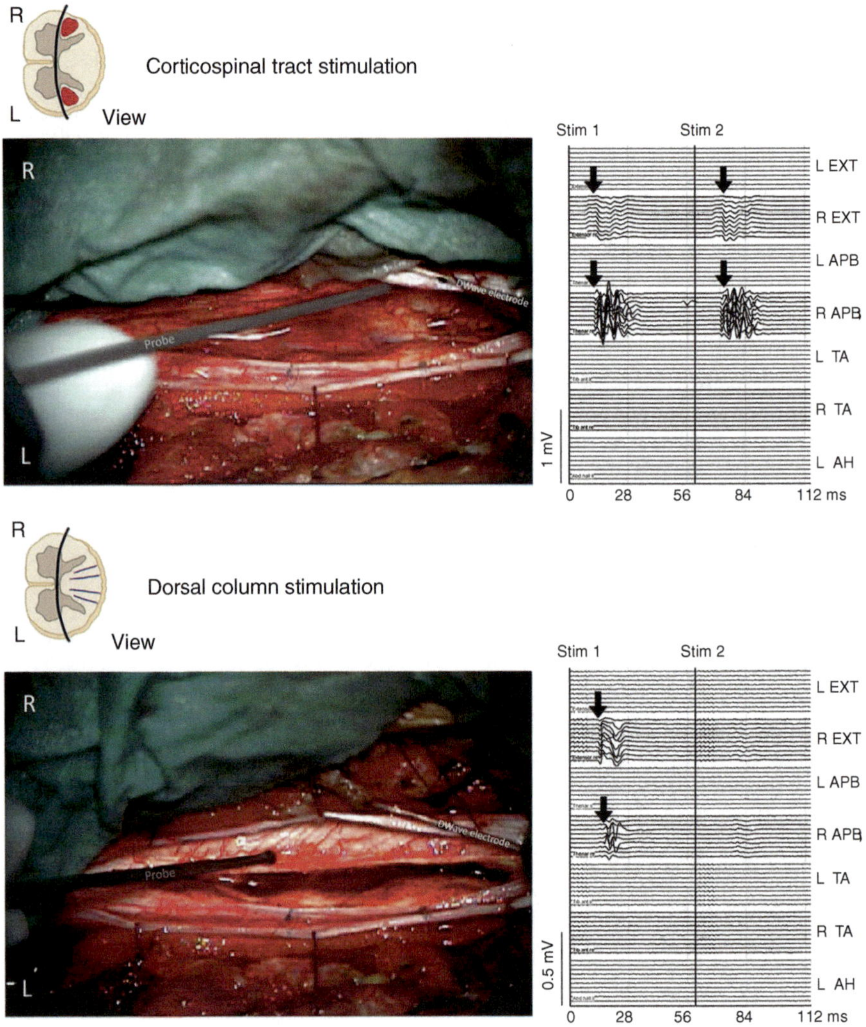

Fig. 27.7 Consecutive trials of double-train stimulation (stim) of SCT and DC with an inter-train interval of 60 ms and muscle recordings. Patient with an intramedullary pilocytic astrocytoma at the C2–Th1 level. Stimulation of the SCT with double trains of stimuli elicited identical double responses in the resection cavity (upper image). Stimulation of the DC elicited only one response after the first train, but no response after the second train (lower image). Identification of both tracts guided surgery with continuous mapping during tumor removal providing real-time neurophysiological feedback of the location of those tracts. *AH, abductor hallucis; APB, abductor pollicis brevis; EXT, extensor digitorum; TA, tibialis anterior.* Probe indicates the stimulating probe. (*Source*: Reproduced from Deletis et al. [30] (with permission))

Critical Surgical Times and Neurophysiological Techniques

Table 27.4 systematizes the neurophysiological modalities that should be applied in each of the different surgical steps of SCT resection surgery.

Interpretation

SEPs and MEPs monitoring are important during an IMSCT resection, due to the high risk of the *gracilis* tracts and CST damage during myelotomy and tumor dissection. However, the primary objective of IOM in SCT resection surgeries is to preserve the CST and distal motor function. And the gold standard is through continuous and combined monitoring of mMEPs and D-waves.

Muscle MEPs are the result of depolarization of the alpha motor neuron, not only by the CST but also by other descending tracts, such as the propriospinal tract, which could be injured during myelotomy and tumor resection. Their injury causes immediate significant but not selective changes or disappearance of the mMEPs. Additionally, desynchronized electrical volleys on CST primary axons may not contribute to D-wave amplitudes. Thus, their damage may not be detected by changes in D-wave amplitudes.

To detect early injury to the CST in SCT surgeries, the recommended alarm criteria are based on the combined information of mMEP and D-wave monitoring, and

Table 27.4 Proposed neurophysiological monitoring protocol for each of the surgical steps for intramedullary tumor resection

Anesthesia	Placement of electrodes SEPs and mMEPs baselines
Positioning, opening and dissection of muscle planes, laminectomy to dura opening	SEPs and mMEPs
Immediately before and during dura opening	New SEPs and mMEPs baselines Add D-wave recording (with epidural catheter placement)
Immediately after dura opening	SEPs, mMEPs, and D-wave (now with subdural catheter placement)
Immediately before the myelotomy (to identify median raphe)	DC mapping (with the technique with which you have more experience) New SEPs, mMEPs, and D-wave baselines
During myelotomy	SEPs and D-wave
During tumor resection	SEPs, mMEPs, and D-wave
Advancing in tumor resection	Pause for mapping the SCT (if the surgeon deems to do so)
End of tumor resection until closing	Last record of the D-wave Catheter removal SEPs and mMEPs to skin suture

mostly on the measurement of the D-wave amplitude [14, 15, 37]. Yet, there is still controversy in relation to a strictly numerical "cut-off" of the D-wave amplitude drop. Controversy includes also disappearance of mMEPs as superior to its amplitude drop or stimulation threshold increase [40].

Alarm criteria for mMEP changes differ depending upon the type of surgery and the mechanism of injury (see Chap. 9) [51]. If there is a significant reduction in mMep amplitude, the neurophysiological recommendation is to immediately stop the surgical manipulation for at least 30 min or until recovery, irrigate the surgical field with warm saline including papaverine, and elevate mean arterial blood pressure [36]. The decision to continue or discontinue the procedure will depend on the recovery level of the mMEPs and the amplitude status of the D-wave [37] (Fig. 27.8).

In general, patients who experience a complete loss of mMEP, but D-wave amplitude preserved to at least 50% of baseline, would sustain only a transient new motor deficit [14, 36, 52]. However, some authors reported new and irreversible postoperative motor deficit in this situation [40, 53]. Thus, Mirela et al.

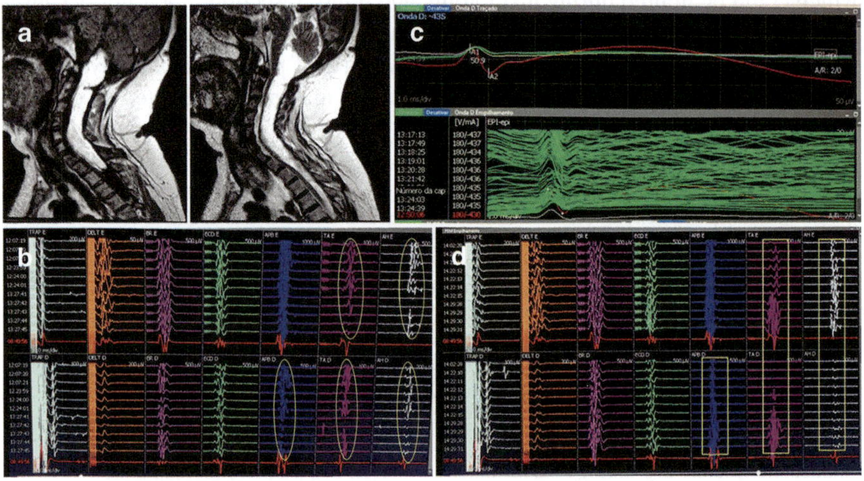

Fig. 27.8 Female, 52 years old, evolving with asymmetric tetraparesis and gait ataxia due to extensive cervical intradural and intramedullary lipoma (C1–Th1). There was drop in the mMEP and D-wave amplitudes during the surgical manipulation. It was followed by a complete improvement in the D-wave and almost complete improvement in the mMEPs. Subtotal tumor resection and C3 to Th4 arthrodesis were performed. Immediate postoperative: worsening of tetraparesis. After 6 months of follow-up, patient recovered to initial preoperative clinical tetraparesis. (**a**) Preoperative MRI. (**b**) Onset of instability and drop in amplitude of mMEPs. (**c**) 50% drop in the D-wave amplitude. (**d**) Partial recovery of mMEPs. (**e**) Full recovery of D-wave. (**f**) Final mMEPs (partial recovery, no return to baseline status). (**g**) Pre-tumor resection and post-arthrodesis surgical image. (**h**) Surgical image after tumor resection. The traces in red color correspond to baselines. E, left; *TRAP, trapezius; DELT, deltoid; BR, brachioradialis; ECD, extensor digitorum; APB, abductor pollicis brevis; TA, tibialis anterior; AH, abductor hallux.* (*Source* (**g**) and (**h**): Courtesy of neurosurgeons Chrystiano Fonseca Cardoso, MD, and Alessandro Fonseca Cardoso, MD. Unpublished personal data (with permission))

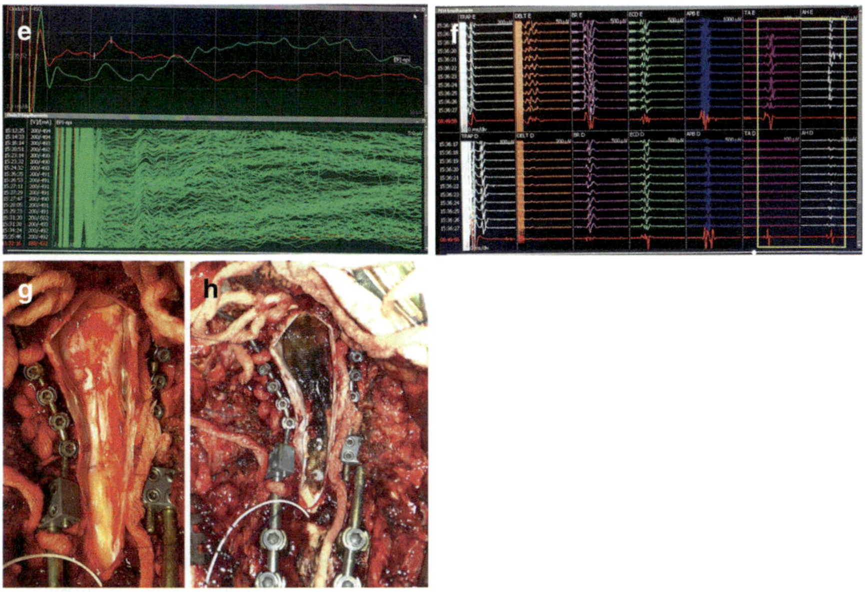

Fig. 27.8 (continued)

recommended a more conservative approach: in the case of total loss of mMEPs, the resection can be safely continued only if D-wave remains at least 80% of baseline (very close to baseline). Mirela et al. agree that a drop in the averaged D-wave recordings of more than 20% from baseline should be considered a warning sign.

Table 27.2 summarizes the correlation that should be made between the interpretation of neurophysiological changes and the surgical approach to be taken, as well as the expected postoperative neurological functional outcome.

Conclusion

Surgical approach remains the main way of treatment for patients with IMSCT. The goal is achieving maximum safe tumor resection, maintaining functional neurological viability. IOM is responsible for revisiting old paradigms in IMSCT treatment, such as that they are synonymous of inoperable injuries. Choosing appropriate neurophysiological techniques can help to guide the extent of surgery, minimizing damage to normal tissue.

IOM techniques have greatly evolved in recent years beyond the continuous monitoring of the long pathways through SEPs, mMEPs, and D-waves. DC mapping has become a reliable technique and the CST mapping is just a step ahead.

Currently, the refinement of these alarm criteria has contributed to improve the neurological outcome.

References

1. Kim TE, Nechtman CM, Hsu W. Chapter 8 – Imaging of spinal lesions. In: Strowd RE, editor. Neuro-oncology for the clinical neurologist. Elsevier; 2021. p. 93–103.
2. Clemenceau S, Lopez M. Intramedullary tumors. Rev Prat. 2001;51:1206–10.
3. Naidu MR, Dinakar I. Intramedullary mass lesions of the spinal cord. Clin Neurol Neurosurg. 1989;91:135–8.
4. Fornari M, Pluchino F, Solero CL, et al. Microsurgical treatment of intramedullary spinal cord tumors. Acta Neurochir. 1988;43(Suppl):3–8.
5. Fischer G, Brotchi J. Results. In: Fischer G, Brotchi J, editors. Intramedullary spinal cord tumors. New York: Thieme; 1996. p. 85–104.
6. Houten JK, Weiner HL. Pediatric intramedullary spinal cord tumors: special considerations. J Neuro-Oncol. 2000;47:225–30.
7. Miller DC. Surgical pathology of intramedullary spinal cord neoplasms. J Neuro-Oncol. 2000;47:198–4.
8. Vaillant B, Loghin M. Treatment of spinal cord tumors. Curr Treat Options Neurol. 2009;11(4):315–24. https://doi.org/10.1007/s11940-009-0035-3. PMID: 19523357.
9. Verla T, Fridley JS, Khan AB, Mayer RR, Omeis I. Neuromonitoring for intramedullary spinal cord tumor surgery. World Neurosurg. 2016;95:108–16. https://doi.org/10.1016/j.wneu.2016.07.066. Epub 2016 Jul 26. PMID: 27474459.
10. Sala F, Palandri G, Basso E, et al. Motor evoked potential monitoring improves outcome after surgery for intramedullary spinal cord tumors: a historical control study. Neurosurgery. 2006;58:1129–43. discussion 1129-1143.
11. Seidel K. ISIN Spring Virtual Course 2021; WEBINAR Intrinsic spinal cord tumors. 1st June.
12. Juthani RG, Bilsky MH, Vogelbaum MA. Current management and treatment modalities for intramedullary spinal cord tumors. Curr Treat Options in Oncol. 2015;16(8):39. https://doi.org/10.1007/s11864-015-0358-0. PMID: 26143269.
13. Kothbauer K, Deletis V, Epstein FJ. Intraoperative spinal cord monitoring for intramedullary surgery: an essential adjunct. Pediatr Neurosurg. 1997;26:247–54.
14. Kothbauer KF, Deletis V, Epstein FJ. Motor-evoked potential monitoring for intramedullary spinal cord tumor surgery: correlation of clinical and neurophysiological data in a series of 100 consecutive procedures. Neurosurg Focus. 1998;4:e1.
15. Deletis V, Sala F. Intraoperative neurophysiological monitoring of the spinal cord during spinal cord and spine surgery: a review focus on the corticospinal tracts. Clin Neurophysiol. 2008;119:248–64.
16. Scibilia A, Terranova C, Rizzo V, et al. Intraoperative neurophysiological mapping and monitoring in spinal tumor surgery: sirens or indispensable tools? Neurosurg Focus. 2016;41:E18.
17. Deletis V. Evoked potentials. Clinical monitoring for anesthesia and critical care. W.B. Saunders Company; 1994. p. 282–314.
18. Kothbauer S. Intraoperative neurophysiological monitoring during surgery for intramedullary spinal cord tumors. In: Nuwer MR, editor. Intraoperative monitoring of neural function. Amsterdam: Elsevier; 2008. p. 632–50.
19. Sala F, Krzan MJ, Deletis V. Intraoperative neurophysiological monitoring in pediatric neurosurgery: why, when, how? Childs Nerv Syst. 2002;18:264–87.
20. Deletis V, Bueno De Camargo A. Interventional neurophysiological mapping during spinal cord procedures. Stereotact Funct Neurosurg. 2001;77:25–8.
21. Yanni DS, Ulkatan S, Deletis V, Barrenechea IJ, Sen C, Perin NI. Utility of neurophysiological monitoring using dorsal column mapping in intramedullary spinal cord surgery. J Neurosurg Spine. 2010;12:623–8.
22. Nair D, Kumaraswamy VM, Braver D, Kilbride RD, Borges LF, Simon MV. Dorsal column mapping via phase reversal method: the refined technique and clinical applications. Neurosurgery. 2014;74:437–46. discussion 446.

23. Quinones-Hinojosa A, Gulati M, Lyon R, Gupta N, Yingling C. Spinal cord mapping as an adjunct for resection of intramedullary tumors: surgical technique with case illustrations. Neurosurgery. 2002;51:1199–206. discussion 1206-1197.
24. Deletis V. Intraoperative neurophysiology of the corticospinal tract of the spinal cord. In: Barber C, Tsuji S, Tobimatsu S, Uozumi T, Akamatsu N, Eisen A, editors. Functional neuroscience: evoked potentials and related techniques. (Suppl. To clinical neurophysiology), vol. 59. Elsevier; 2006. p. 105–9.
25. Gandhi R, Curtis CM, Cohen-Gadol AA. High-resolution direct microstimulation mapping of spinal cord motor pathways during resection of an intramedullary tumor. J Neurosurg Spine. 2015;22:205–10.
26. Duffau H, Lopes M, Sichez JP, Bitar A, Capelle L. A new device for electrical stimulation mapping of the brainstem and spinal cord. Minim Invasive Neurosurg. 2003;46:61–4.
27. Duffau H, Capelle L, Sichez J. Direct spinal cord electrical stimulations during surgery of intramedullary tumoral and vascular lesions. Stereotact Funct Neurosurg. 1998;71:180–9.
28. Barzilai O, Lidar Z, Constantini S, Salame K, Bitan-Talmor Y, Korn A. Continuous mapping of the corticospinal tracts in intramedullary spinal cord tumor surgery using an electrified ultrasonic aspirator. J Neurosurg Spine. 2017;27:161–8.
29. Deletis V, Kothbauer KF, Sala F, Seidel K. Letter to the editor: electrical activity in limb muscles after spinal cord stimulation is not specific for the corticospinal tract. J Neurosurg Spine. 2017;26:267–9.
30. Deletis V, Seidel K, Sala F, Raabe A, Chudy D, Beck J, et al. Intraoperative identification of the corticospinal tract and dorsal column of the spinal cord by electrical stimulation. J Neurol Neurosurg Psychiatry. 2018;89(7):754–61.
31. Deletis V, Rodi Z, Amassian VE. Neurophysiological mechanisms underlying motor evoked potentials in anesthetized humans. Part 2. Relationship between epidurally and muscle recorded MEPs in man. Clin Neurophysiol. 2001;112:445–52.
32. Moller AR. Intraoperative neurophysiological monitoring. 2nd ed. New Jersey: Humana Press Inc.; 2006.
33. Deng LX, Walker C, Xu XM. Schwann cell transplantation and descending propriospinal regeneration after spinal cord injury. Brain Res. 2015;1619:104–14.
34. Seidel K. ISIN Spring Virtual Course 2021; Scientific Session (1st Part); Recipes: D-wave. 5th June.
35. Simon MV. Intraoperative neurophysiology. A comprehensive guide to monitoring and mapping. 1st ed. New York: Demos Medical Publishing; 2010.
36. Sala F, Bricolo A, Faccioli F, Lanteri P, Gerosa M. Surgery for intramedullary spinal cord tumors: the role of intraoperative (neurophysiological) monitoring. Eur Spine J. 2007;16(Suppl. 2):S130–9. https://doi.org/10.1007/s00586-007-0423-x.
37. Macdonald DB, Skinner S, Shils J, Yingling C, American Society of Neurophysiological Monitoring. Intraoperative motor evoked potential monitoring – a position statement by the American Society of Neurophysiological Monitoring. Clin Neurophysiol. 2013;124(12):2291–316. https://doi.org/10.1016/j.clinph.2013.07.025. Epub 2013 Sep 18. PMID: 24055297.
38. Deletis V, Shils JL. Neurophysiology in neurosurgery. A modern intraoperative approach. 1st ed. San Diego: Academic Press; 2002.
39. Skinner SA, Transfeldt EE, Mehbod AA, Mullan JC, Perra JH. Electromyography detects mechanically-induced suprasegmental spinal motor tract injury: review of decompression at spinal cord level. Clin Neurophysiol. 2009;120(4):754–64. https://doi.org/10.1016/j.clinph.2008.11.030.
40. Simon MV. Intraoperative neurophysiology: a comprehensive guide to monitoring and mapping. 2nd ed. New York: Demos Medical Publishing; 2019.
41. Krzan M, Deletis V, Isgum V. Intraoperative neurophysiological mapping of dorsal columns. A new tool in prevention of surgically induced sensory deficit? Electroencephalogr Clin Neurophysiol. 1996;102:37P. https://doi.org/10.1016/S0921-884X(97)85317-9.

42. Jeanmonod D, Sindou M, Mauguiere F. Three transverse dipolar generators in the human cervical and lumbo-sacral dorsal horn: evidence from direct intraoperative recordings on the spinal cord surface. Electroencephalogr Clin Neurophysiol. 1989;74:236–40.
43. Jeanmonod D, Sindou M, Mauguiere F. The human cervical and lumbo-sacral evoked electrospinogram. Data from intra-operative spinal cord surface recordings. Electroencephalogr Clin Neurophysiol. 1991;80:477–89.
44. Turano G, SMaMF. Spinal cord evoked potential monitoring during spinal surgery for pain and spasticity. In: Halter DA, editor. Atlas of human spinal cord evoked potential. Butterworth-Heinemann; 1995. p. 107–22.
45. Campbell JA, Miles J. Evoked potentials as an aid to lesion making in the dorsal root entry zone. Neurosurgery. 1984;15:951–2.
46. Nashold BS Jr, Ovelmen-Levitt J, Sharpe R, Higgins AC. Intraoperative evoked potentials recorded in man directly from dorsal roots and spinal cord. J Neurosurg. 1985;62:680–93.
47. Berić A, Dimitrijević MR, Sharkey PC, Sherwood AM. Cortical potentials evoked by epidural stimulation of the cervical and thoracic spinal cord in man. Electroencephalogr Clin Neurophysiol. 1986;65(2):102–10. https://doi.org/10.1016/0168-5597(86)90042-0.
48. North RB, Drenger B, Beattie C, McPherson RW, Parker S, Reitz BA, Williams MG. Monitoring of spinal cord stimulation evoked potentials during thoracoabdominal aneurysm surgery. Neurosurgery. 1991;28(2):325–30. https://doi.org/10.1227/00006123-199102000-00027.
49. Simon MV, Chiappa KH, Borges LF. Phase reversal of somatosensory evoked potentials triggered by gracilis tract stimulation: case report of a new technique for neurophysiologic dorsal column mapping. Neurosurgery. 2012;70:E783–8.
50. Shils JL, Arle JE. Intraoperative neurophysiologic methods for spinal cord stimulator placement under general anesthesia. Neuromodulation. 2012;15:560–71. discussion 571–562.
51. MacDonald DB. Overview on criteria for MEP monitoring. J Clin Neurophysiol. 2017;34(1):4–11. https://doi.org/10.1097/WNP.0000000000000302.
52. Morota N, Deletis V, Constantini S, Kofler M, Cohen H, Epstein FJ. The role of motor evoked potentials during surgery for intramedullary spinal cord tumors. Neurosurgery. 1997;41:1327–36. https://doi.org/10.1097/00006123-199712000-00017.
53. Burke D, Hicks RG. Surgical monitoring of motor pathways. J Clin Neurophysiol. 1998;15(3):194–205. https://doi.org/10.1097/00004691-199805000-00003.

Part VI
Vascular Surgery

Chapter 28
Intraoperative Neurophysiologic Monitoring of Cerebrovascular Disorders

Jaime R. López and Felix W. Chang

Abbreviations

ACA	Anterior cerebral artery
APB	Abductor pollicis brevis
AVMs	Arteriovenous malformations
BAEP	Brainstem auditory evoked potential
CCT	Central conduction time
CDSA	Color density spectral array
CI	Confidence interval
CTA	Computed tomography angiogram
dcMEP	Direct cortical motor evoked potential
DSA	Density spectral array
EC-IC	Extracranial-intracranial
EEG	Electroencephalography
EMG	Electromyography
FDI	First dorsal interosseous
ICA	Internal carotid artery
INR	Interventional neuroradiology

J. R. López (✉)
Department of Neurology and Neurological Sciences, Stanford University, Stanford, CA, USA

Department of Neurosurgery (Courtesy), Stanford University, Stanford, CA, USA
e-mail: lopezjr@stanford.edu

F. W. Chang
Department of Neurology and Neurological Sciences, Stanford University, Stanford, CA, USA

S. M. Verst et al. (eds.), *Intraoperative Monitoring*,
https://doi.org/10.1007/978-3-030-95730-8_28

IONM	Intraoperative neurophysiologic monitoring
mA	Milliamps
MAP	Mean arterial pressure
MCA	Middle cerebral artery
MEP	Motor evoked potential
mRS	Modified Rankin score
mTICI	Modified thrombolysis in cerebral infarction grading
NIRS	Near-infrared spectroscopy
OR	Odds ratio
OR	Operating room
qEEG	Quantitative EEG
rCBF	Regional cerebral blood flow
rSO_2	Regional saturation of oxygen
SSEP	Somatosensory evoked potentials
STA	Superior temporal artery
TCD	Transcranial Doppler
TcMEP	Transcranial motor evoked potential

Introduction

Intraoperative neurophysiologic monitoring (IONM), the use of neurophysiologic testing intraoperatively to monitor the integrity of neural structures, has seen increasingly widespread use in a variety of procedures over the last several decades. The surgical and endovascular treatment of cerebrovascular disorders is an area where IONM has seen great growth, and in some institutions, it now plays the role of an indispensable adjunct for these procedures. IONM is able to identify cerebral ischemia, one of the most feared complications of these types of procedures. It can also indirectly identify hemorrhage, another potential complication. The ability to identify and reverse cerebral ischemia using different techniques is important in increasing the safety of cerebrovascular procedures.

There are several electrophysiologic techniques which have been demonstrated to be useful for the purpose of improving neurologic outcomes by identifying and potentially reversing intraoperative cerebral ischemia. The goals of this chapter are to discuss the types of cerebrovascular procedures in which IONM is utilized, the different IONM techniques that can be used in monitoring these procedures, the physiologic rationale for why these techniques can be used, and the expected types of changes in response to cerebral ischemia in these techniques.

Cerebrovascular Procedures Where IONM Is Commonly Utilized

There are a variety of cerebrovascular disorders which are approached both surgically and endovascularly. The most common of these disorders in which IONM is utilized are the following:

1. High-grade carotid artery stenosis
2. Cerebral aneurysms
3. Cerebral arteriovenous malformations (AVMs)
4. Cerebral cavernous malformations
5. Vascular occlusive disorders, e.g., moyamoya disease

Effect of Regional Cerebral Blood Flow on Electrophysiologic Studies

Cerebrovascular procedures carry the risk of cerebral infarction as they involve the manipulation of the cerebrovascular system, which can cause a number of complications, including thromboses, emboli, vasospasm, vascular occlusion, and hemorrhage. Before discussing specific surgeries, it is important to understand the physiologic basis on which electrophysiologic studies are able to detect ischemia. Electroencephalography (EEG) and somatosensory evoked potentials (SSEPs) have been extensively studied in this context and can indirectly detect cerebral ischemia before it progresses to a cerebral infarct. Their utility for this purpose was established by a series of human and animal studies in the 1970s and 1980s which separately showed a strong correlation between regional cerebral blood flow (rCBF) and changes in EEG and/or SSEP.

Several primate studies showed the relationship of rCBF with SSEP amplitude. In Branston et al. [13], they showed that that cortical SSEPs remained present when rCBF was ≥16 ml/100 g/min and became absent at <12 ml/100 g/min and between 14 and 16 ml/100 g/min a sharp decline in SSEP amplitude was seen. Branson et al. [14] and Symon [125] showed that a 50% SSEP amplitude reduction corresponded to rCBF of 16 ml/100 g/min.

Similar results were seen in humans around the same time period. Sharbrough et al. [116], Sundt et al. [123, 124], and Trojaborg and Boysen [133] showed that in patients undergoing carotid endarterectomy (CEA) at rCBF <10 ml/100 g/min, "major" EEG changes were seen. Normal EEG was seen above 18 ml/100 g/min and increasing severity of EEG changes below this level. A critical level was defined at 15 ml/100 g/min. Regional CBF was determined in Sharbrough et al. [116] by measuring the clearance of intra-arterially injected Xenon-133 with measurements taken prior to cross-clamp, during cross-clamp, after cross-clamp, and during shunting if applicable.

Central conduction time (CCT) measured by SSEPs similarly becomes prolonged in response to ischemia, with a threshold of rCBF 15 ml/100 g/min, as measured in baboons and cats [51, 65]. This rCBF level is similar to that detected for the SSEP loss and major EEG changes mentioned earlier. From these multiple studies, it is evident that electrical failure occurs at a threshold rCBF level. This failure is mediated by cellular dysfunction, and experimental evidence in baboons also showed that cellular membrane failure occurs at a threshold level of rCBF [8, 125].

Branston et al. [14] showed in baboon work that at rCBF of 12–16 ml/100 g/min, where the SSEP was abolished, there was small, limited extracellular K^+ efflux. At 8–11 ml/100 g/min, a large efflux of K^+ was seen and was associated with structural changes of infarction, indicating that at those levels the cell was no longer able to maintain its sodium-potassium pumps and would proceed to cell death.

Animal studies have also identified the rCBF threshold level that results in cerebral infarction. In baboon stroke models, cerebral infarction was seen with rCBF less than 10 ml/100 g/min [125, 126]. In macaques, infarcts occurred when rCBF was less than or equal to 12 ml/100 g/min [56, 83]. Not all tissue is equally susceptible to ischemia. Branston et al. [15] looked at subcortical components of the SSEPs in baboons and found that there was no change in electrophysiologic function at the brainstem and spinal cord levels at systemic hypotension levels that resulted in changes in the cortical SSEP signals. This work established the concept of electrical failure (loss of SSEP) preceding pump failure and is why SSEPs can be used for detecting ischemia before permanent injury occurs.

From these studies we can reasonably conclude that:

1. Cerebral infarction is associated with rCBF less than a level of 10–12 ml/100 g/min
2. A 50% amplitude reduction of the cortical SSEP is seen around 14–16 ml/100 g/min and therefore implies cerebral ischemia is present
3. Major EEG changes occur when rCBF is less than 10 ml/100 g/min, with lesser changes occurring between 10 and 18 ml/100 g/min and with a critical level seen at around 15 ml/100 g/min
4. The rCBF level at which EEG changes and "critical" SSEP changes (50% amplitude reduction) occur is likely above the rCBF level associated with cerebral infarction (10–12 ml/100 g/min)
5. Increasing rCBF to >16 ml/100 g/min may reverse changes caused by cerebral ischemia

In addition to sensory evoked potentials, transcranial motor evoked potentials (TcMEPs) are now routinely used to assess cerebral ischemia [49, 54, 76, 111, 128]. However, a literature search did not yield any similar experimental or animal studies, as those done with SEPs and EEG, looking at the relationship between MEPs and rCBF. It is reasonable to assume that there exists a similar rCBF threshold which will cause the abolishment or alteration of the MEP. However, what this level is remains unknown at this time. Future studies on this relationship would greatly enhance our understanding of how MEPs change in relation to cerebral ischemia. Based on our experience in using MEPs for monitoring cerebrovascular disorders, it appears that the level of ischemia required to abolish MEPs is similar to that necessary to cause SSEP and EEG changes. We have also found that TcMEPs can identify reversible subcortical focal ischemia affecting the corticospinal pathways but sparing the somatosensory pathways (see section "Case Example 2"). MEPs must be used more carefully however, as overstimulation may cause activation of subcortical structures distal to the area of ischemia and result in lack of MEP changes while monitoring for cortical ischemia (see section "Case Example 3"). Therefore, it is imperative that multimodality IONM, using SSEPs, EEG, and MEPs, when appropriate, be performed when monitoring cerebral function and the potential occurrence of cerebral ischemia.

High-Grade Carotid Artery Stenosis

CEA was first described in the 1950s [26, 34]. Despite initial negative results from randomized trials, the procedure became increasingly popular in the 1980s, growing from 15,000 cases in 1961 to 107,000 in 1985 [38, 101, 117]. In 1991, the results from the North American Symptomatic Carotid Endarterectomy Trial (NASCET) were published and unequivocally showed that CEA was superior to medical management for patients with symptomatic high-grade carotid stenosis [90]. In 1995, a modest benefit was also found for CEA over medical management in patients with asymptomatic high-grade carotid stenosis [36]. The NASCET authors also emphasized that the benefit of CEA was based on maintaining a low perioperative complication rate. In the trial the risk of major stroke and death was 2.1%; if complication rates approach 10%, the benefit of CEA over medical therapy is eliminated. In addition to CEA, high-grade carotid artery stenosis is now also treated with carotid stent placement (either transfemorally or with transcarotid revascularization) and carotid angioplasty [28, 62, 84].

IONM of Surgical and Endovascular Procedures of the Carotid Artery

In comparison to other procedures, the perceived risk of cerebral ischemia is higher in surgical and endovascular procedures involving the carotid artery as these often require transient occlusion of the carotid artery. In CEAs, it is common practice to cross-clamp the common, internal, and external carotid arteries. If the patient does not have adequate intracranial collateral cerebral blood flow from their circle of Willis, they will develop ipsilateral hemispheric ischemia. Similarly, in carotid stenting, there is transient occlusion of the internal carotid artery during stent deployment, which also carries the risk of transient cerebral ischemia.

Many techniques have been investigated specifically for CEA to identify cerebral ischemia. These techniques are divided into two main categories. The first category includes techniques that measure the function of the cerebrovascular system, with emphasis on the vascular system. These include transcranial Doppler (TCD), near-infrared (NIR) spectroscopy, radionuclide cerebral blood flow measurements, and stump pressure measurements. The second category includes electrophysiologic techniques that measure cerebral function and are indirect measures of cerebral ischemia. These include techniques such as EEG, SSEPs, MEPs, and brainstem auditory evoked potentials (BAEPs). We will discuss the use of these techniques in more detail in the following sections.

If cerebral ischemia is detected, there are a few measures which can be taken. The mean arterial pressure can be increased as the increase in systemic blood pressure should also cause an increase in cerebral blood flow. In CEA, an intraluminal carotid shunt can be placed to enhance blood flow to the ipsilateral internal carotid artery. There is no clear consensus on the optimal usage of shunts, and surgeons tend to fall into one of the three categories regarding shunts: selectively shunt, always shunt, and never shunt [39, 69]. Despite the advantage of potentially eliminating ischemic time during CEA, shunts possess a few disadvantages. They can cause arterial damage, create emboli resulting in stroke, or may malfunction [40, 50, 67, 70, 137]. A meta-analysis in 2011 by AbuRahma et al. [1] compared routine, selective, and no shunting and showed similar stroke rates between the groups: 2% in routine non-shunt; 1.4% in routine shunting; 1.6% for selective shunting with EEG; 1.8% for selective shunting with SSEP; 4.8% for selective shunting with TCD; and 1.6% for selective shunting with stump pressure measurement. Their conclusion was that surgeons should select the method with which they were most comfortable. It is difficult to draw a specific conclusion about the use of different modalities in selective shunting from this meta-analysis, as methods used in EEG and SSEP monitoring may be variable. The analysis did not specify details of EEG monitoring such as how many channels were used, use of quantitative EEG, type of montage used in each study, or type of person interpreting the EEG. Differences in the methods can cause great variability in the quality of EEG monitoring.

Selective shunting relies on IONM techniques for decision-making. If IONM techniques do not indicate the presence of cerebral ischemia, it is assumed that there is adequate cerebral perfusion, due to sufficient collateral circulation, and that surgery can proceed without a shunt. In this strategy, that patient is only exposed to the potential risks of shunting if they demonstrate that carotid occlusion leads to cerebral ischemia. Although IONM will usually identify large cerebral territory ischemia (ICA, ACA, and MCA territories), the spatial resolution of current techniques is insufficient to consistently detect small focal areas of ischemia/infarct.

Continuous EEG Monitoring

EEG monitoring has a long history of use in monitoring of carotid surgeries and was first reported in CEA by Perez-Borja and Meyer in 1965. Compared to evoked potentials, an advantage of EEG is that the signal being analyzed is constantly and spontaneously being generated by the cerebral tissue, in addition to being relatively easy to record. Thanks to relative familiarity with EEG, ease of setup, availability of equipment, and reliability in determining ischemia related to cross-clamping, EEG is a popular IONM technique for monitoring cerebral ischemia in carotid procedures. Several studies showed that CEA patients with EEG changes suggestive of ischemia had higher incidences of stroke compared to patients without changes, demonstrating that EEG is able to identify ischemia and predict neurologic deficit [21, 116, 124, 136].

In Zampella et al. [141], 43 of 59 (72%) CEA patients had EEG changes, with 10 of 59 (17%) developing postoperative complications. Redekop and Ferguson [104] found in their series of 293 patients major EEG changes in 22 of 293 patients (7%), with a higher proportion of changes occurring in patients with accompanying contralateral carotid stenosis. Immediate postoperative deficit occurred in 4 of 22 of patients (18%) with major EEG changes compared to 5 of 271 (1.8%) without. Sundt [122] stated in their study of 1145 consecutive CEAs that they "never had a patient emerge from anesthesia with a new deficit that was not predicted by the EEG." These studies show the sensitivity of EEG changes in predicting in stroke. Additionally, studies have shown that EEG monitoring in CEA is associated with improved neurologic outcomes, as well as reduced the frequency of carotid shunts [21, 136]. A recent meta-analysis of 10,672 patients showed that intraoperative EEG changes had a sensitivity of 46% (95% CI 38–54%) and a specificity of 86% (95% CI 83–88%) for perioperative stroke within 30 days of CEA and that 92.4% of EEG changes were reversible [19]. Additionally, the authors calculated the diagnostic odds ratio for reversible and irreversible EEG changes to be 8.25 and 70.84, respectively. Sensitivity ranged from 10% to 92% in the analyzed studies. A similar sensitivity of 52% and specificity of 84% in a meta-analysis of 8765 cases were reported by Thirumala et al. [130, 131]. In both these studies, true positives were defined as intraoperative EEG change with perioperative stroke, which might partially explain the poor sensitivity. If ischemia is reversed and stroke averted, although EEG may have correctly identified ischemia, this would be counted as a "false positive" rather than true positive. Thus, using this logic, one can make the case that this is precisely what IONM is designed to do: identify reversible ischemia (EEG/SSEP change; "true positive"), followed by an effective intraoperative intervention that reverses the ischemia (improved EEG/SSEP), resulting in the patient not having any new postoperative neurologic deficits (so-called false positive). Reducing the total number of true positives compared to false negatives would decrease the sensitivity.

Interpreting Intraoperative EEG Changes

There are many patterns of EEG changes that can be seen intraoperatively. It is important to recognize which of these changes are associated with ischemia and which are not.

Ischemia

Quickly and accurately recognizing EEG patterns associated with ischemia are key in monitoring cerebrovascular procedures, in which signals may change rapidly. The major changes are outlined as follows:

(a) Typical: generalized slowing and decreased amplitude in the ischemic hemisphere, which is usually ipsilateral to cross-clamping [99, 133]
(b) Common: attenuation of faster beta rhythms associated with anesthetic agents [20]
(c) Uncommon: bilateral EEG changes which can occur in patients with suboptimal collateral circulation [20]

It should also be noted that unusual and unexpected patterns of EEG changes such as bilateral, contralateral, and unilateral can be seen if the patient's MAP falls below a critical level related to their baseline blood pressure (personal observation). These types of changes are likely related to patients with bilateral carotid disease and/or intracranial tandem lesions.

Several predictors for intraoperative EEG changes have been identified: abnormal preoperative EEG, preoperative neurologic symptoms, >70% stenosis in the contralateral carotid, and bilateral vertebral stenosis [32, 119, 124]. Interestingly, after controlling for other factors, >70% stenosis in the ipsilateral carotid decreased the odds of EEG changes (OR 0.43), likely reflecting the patient had developed sufficient collateral circulation in chronic carotid stenosis [119].

Anesthesia

Anesthetic agents can have a multitude of effects on the EEG, ranging from electrocerebral inactivity, mild slowing, to increasing the frequency. The effects of anesthesia on EEG are typically bilateral and symmetric, which is important in differentiating anesthetic effects from hemispheric ischemia. If the patient has a previous cerebral insult, increased prominence of a previous focal abnormality is possible in response to anesthesia. It is good practice to periodically have the anesthetic levels noted to assess their relation to the EEG. It is common to see increased rhythmic beta (12–18 Hz) activity following induction. This is typically over the anterior hemispheres. As the procedure progresses, and the patient reaches a lighter steady state compared to induction, the amplitude of the EEG typically increases and slows to 8–14 Hz. Intermittent delta activity can be seen anteriorly in this state. At high enough levels of inhaled or intravenous anesthetics, burst suppression and electrocerebral silence can be seen on the EEG. Boluses of narcotics can sometimes induce burst suppression as well (personal observation).

Technical Factors

Ensuring proper electrode placement, intact electrodes, low electrode impedances, and isolation of any ambient electrical noise is important in ensuring a good-quality EEG recording. Knowing how to efficiently troubleshoot to find the technical factors which are interfering with the recording is essential. If these factors are not present, the interpretation of the EEG will be difficult.

Critical Intraoperative EEG Changes

The most critical point of a CEA occurs at the time of cross-clamping the carotid. If there are ipsilateral EEG changes following cross-clamping, this indicates the presence of cerebral ischemia. To reverse ischemia, cerebral blood flow to the ipsilateral hemisphere must be increased, usually through carotid shunting. Surgeons who are selective shunters and utilize IONM services will typically shunt following major EEG changes. If the EEG changes are mild, raising the MAP prior to shunting may optimize ipsilateral cerebral blood flow to the point where the EEG improves, and shunting is not needed. Of course, the EEG will need to be carefully monitored during the remainder of the shunt period in case evidence of ischemia arise anew. If needed, carotid shunting can be done during any stage of the cross-clamp period.

Quantitative EEG

Quantitative EEG (qEEG) refers to any mathematical processing of conventional EEG. Conventional EEG may also be referred to as raw EEG, unprocessed EEG, or EEG. There are many different techniques and tools that can be used to analyze the EEG. qEEG in the operating room dates back to the 1970s [20, 87]. As a technique, it has gained increasing popularity as it has become more accessible. In a review of qEEG outside of the OR, Gavvala et al. [44] reported that 52% of neurophysiologists were using qEEG. EEG data is normally viewed in the time domain. The most used qEEG techniques use Fourier analysis to translate the EEG to the frequency domain. The most common way to represent this is the density spectral array (DSA) or color density spectral array (CDSA) [66]. The DSA displays time on the horizontal axis and frequency on the vertical axis and uses color to code the power.

Ischemic changes, which include slowing and attenuation of faster frequencies, are visually represented by a change in color (change in power) and downward shift of the main frequency bands. Visually, these are easier to interpret than the same changes would be on the unprocessed/raw EEG (see Fig. 28.1).

There have been several studies that have shown the usefulness of qEEG in identifying ischemia and predicting neurologic outcome in CEA, with some authors reporting that they find qEEG more useful than raw EEG [2, 20, 103].

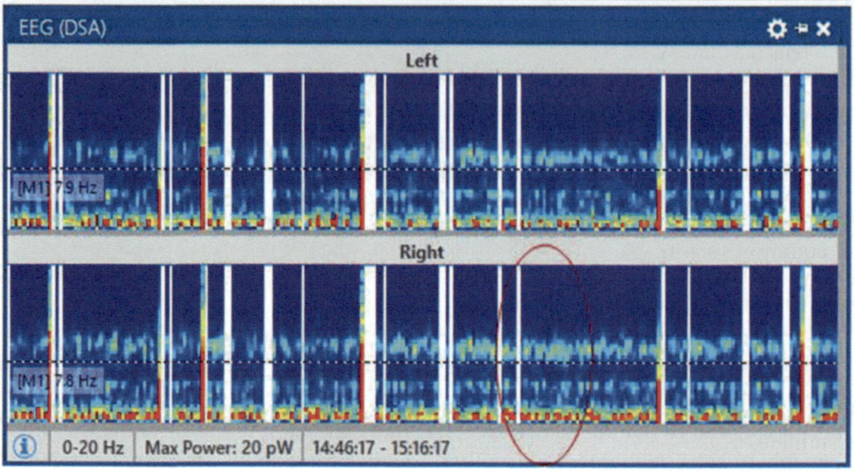

Fig. 28.1 This figure demonstrates mild hemispheric slowing during a right-sided CEA on DSA. The left and right hemispheres are shown. The *y*-axis is frequency; the *x*-axis is time. Low power is shown in cool colors and high power in warm colors. The dotted line is a frequency marker placed to help better visualize changes in frequency. White bars that take up the whole frequency spectrum are times where electrosurgery is occurring and the program has automatically excluded the resulting high amplitude EEG artifact from analysis. A 30-min segment is shown here. A small downward shift in the dominant frequency band of the right hemisphere can be seen in the area highlighted by the red circle. At the same time, a 30% decrease in the amplitude of the left median nerve cortical SSEP also occurred. Both changes resolved when the carotid was unclamped

qEEG is a powerful tool when used correctly but has limitations. It should not be thought of as a replacement for the raw EEG but rather an adjunct. The main advantages of qEEG lie in the ability to see trends develop over longer time scale and scan larger time periods quickly. It is important to confirm any suspected findings on qEEG with the raw EEG. Rhythmic artifacts, common in the OR, can frequently mimic the appearance of physiologic signals on DSA. DSA is well-suited for purposes such as assessing the change in depth of anesthesia over the course of the case. In the context of IONM, it may be easier to observe subtle ischemia on qEEG than raw EEG, as one can more easily detect smaller changes in frequencies. As monitoring of simultaneous cases continues to grow, the advantage in time may also become more important. Looking at the DSA provides less real-time information than the unprocessed EEG. This is because Fourier analysis is performed on discrete time epochs, often around 8 s in length. It likely will take several epochs before a trend becomes apparent on the DSA, which can represent a lag of 30 s or more from when a change might first be apparent on unprocessed EEG. For critical time points, such as cross-clamping, this may not be ideal.

In Kearse et al. [61], a prospective study of 103 CEA patients, EEG and DSA were used together, and it was found that the two observers using DSA, respectively, identified 61% and 18% of mild unprocessed EEG changes, 70% and 71% of moderate changes, and 95% of severe changes. This was limited however, as it was based on two observers. There was also a significant difference in performance between the two observers on the mild EEG change task. We can at least conclude that mild EEG changes on DSA are more difficult to detect. There have not been any similar studies looking at DSA performance in the context of CEA. For non-OR EEG interpretation, Moura et al. [86] analyzed performance by three neurophysiologists on 2094 h of EEG review, and DSA showed sensitivities of 98.7% for focal slowing and 100% for generalized slowing. Although there are differences between OR and non-OR interpretation (retrospective vs real-time interpretation; proportion of sedated patients), this shows that DSA potentially can perform as well as view unprocessed EEG for certain tasks.

There are many qEEG measures under investigation in CEA. Kamitaki et al. [59] looked at many different measures (alpha, beta, theta, delta power; alpha-delta ratio; beta-delta ratio; amplitude-integrated EEG; spectral edge frequency) in 118 CEA cases and found that in patients with ischemia following clamping, all qEEG measures were found to be significantly decreased compared to post-clamp values. Although quantitative EEG is quickly growing in applications in non-OR settings, its role for monitoring CEA has not been extensively investigated. Its usefulness may depend on the interpreter's experience in using unprocessed and quantitative EEG, as well as number of monitored cases.

SSEP Monitoring

SSEPs are used widely in IONM. Due to the strong correlation between SSEPs and cerebral ischemia, as discussed earlier, SSEPs are now commonly used as intraoperative surrogates for cerebral ischemia. In CEAs, the cerebrovascular territories at risk include the ipsilateral ICA, and more specifically the middle cerebral artery (MCA) territories. The anterior cerebral artery (ACA) territory tends to be less at risk than the MCA as it receives more collateral flow from the anterior communicating artery than the MCA. To monitor these territories, an appropriate neurophysiological signal that is generated from structures in these territories must be selected. The SSEP signal is generated from the somatosensory cortex in the parietal lobe. The primary hand sensory areas are included in the MCA territory and the primary leg sensory areas in the ACA territory. The median or ulnar nerve SSEP, which results in a hand sensory area cortical signal, is therefore a good marker of functional status and ischemia in the MCA territory. Compared to EEG, SSEPs are more resistant to anesthesia, require fewer electrodes, and are easier to interpret/report and easier to compare over time [79].

SSEPs have been well studied in CEA. Their use in CEA was first reported in 1982 by Moorthy et al. [82]. Another early case series of 38 patients (28 with regional anesthesia) was Markand et al. [80], where 4 patients had SSEP changes following cross-clamping reversed by shunting. There subsequently were many studies that supported the reliability and accuracy of SSEPs in CEA [5, 45, 52, 60, 114, 132].

The sensitivity of SSEPs was found to be 100% with a specificity of 86.5% in a study of 196 patients [97]. False negative and false negative rates were reported as relatively low in multiple studies, with the false negative rate of 0–3.5 in one review [5, 63, 78, 139]. A more recent meta-analysis of SSEP in CEA of 4557 patients showed a sensitivity of 58%, a specificity of 91%, and a false negative rate of 0.96% [91]. True positives were defined as SSEP changes with a new postoperative deficit for this review, which may lower sensitivity, as mentioned in the EEG monitoring section. Lam et al. [63] reviewed six studies and found sensitivities ranging from 83% to 100% and specificities from 83% to 99%. They also concluded that EEG and SSEP monitoring had similar sensitivity/specificity. Fisher et al. [39] performed a meta-analysis of 3028 patients and found SSEP changes in 5.6% of cases, with 20% of patients with SSEP changes developing a postoperative deficit.

Though most studies have reported good performance of SSEPs, there are some studies that have raised concerns that SSEPs are not sensitive enough for cerebral ischemia and unreliably predict neurologic outcome [63, 139]. In Lam et al. [63], SSEPs were compared to EEG, and the authors reported that there was prolongation of the central conduction time in 10 of 23 patients with EEG evidence of ischemia but a SSEP amplitude reduction of >50% in only 1 of 23 patients. Based on these results, they felt that these specific criteria were not sensitive enough to detect cerebral ischemia.

In Wöber et al. [139], 32 patients were evaluated, and it was found that between shunted and non-shunted patients, there were no differences in the cortical SSEP amplitudes and latencies. They also conducted a meta-analysis of 15 studies and found no improvement in neurologic outcome with selective shunting and SSEP monitoring. This meta-analysis was limited by several factors; the authors noted these to be that transient neurologic deficits may have been underestimated or not reported in some studies, possible discrepancies in data in some studies, and inclusion of multiple serial series by the same groups. Additionally, there were no uniform criteria for shunt placement between studies and there were differing definitions of critical SSEP changes.

A differing view was presented in Amantini et al. [5], which concluded that EEG monitoring had a high incidence of false positives compared to SSEPs because there is less agreement on what constitutes a significant EEG changes compared to an SSEP change. Most studies have found a 50% amplitude reduction of the cortical SSEP (N19/P24), or a 1 ms delay of the central conduction time correlates best with the development of postoperative neurologic deficits [16, 25, 45, 52, 60, 61, 114].

A 50% reduction in SSEPs has also been associated with worsened performance on neuropsychological testing performed pre- and postoperatively [16]. Other than immediate postoperative deficits, there is some suggestion that SSEP and EEG changes might also predict long-term stroke. In Domenick Sridharan et al. [31], follow-up of 853 consecutive patients showed that patients with SSEP or EEG changes compared to those without had a stroke-free survival rate of 88.2% vs 94.7% at 5 years and 78% vs 86.1% at 10 years. There was no difference in overall survival at 10 years.

EEG and SSEP have been frequently combined for monitoring of CEA as well. Thiagarajan et al. [129] performed a meta-analysis which found that using EEG and SSEP together was 1.32 times more sensitive than EEG alone and 1.26 times more sensitive than SSEP alone. Overall, we can conclude that SSEP monitoring for CEA is a reliable modality for identifying intraoperative ischemia.

MEP Monitoring

Since their introduction, MEPs have quickly expanded in use in IONM and are well established for monitoring spinal surgeries. There remain more questions on their use and interpretation in cerebrovascular disorders. Many of these questions arise from the lack of similar studies regarding impact of rCBF on MEPs in comparison to literature evidence for the utility of EEG and SSEP. Despite this, there are many studies on their use for monitoring in this context. In our institution, TcMEPs are a standard part of our multimodality monitoring approach to cerebrovascular disorders.

There have been several studies that have used the combination of SSEP, TcMEP, and EEG together for monitoring CEAs. The addition of TcMEPs can potentially identify pure motor subcortical ischemia, which monitoring with only SSEP and EEG would likely not detect [49]. In Malcharek et al. [73], 9 of 600 patients (1.5%) undergoing CEA were shown to have isolated transient MEP changes thought to be due to subcortical ischemia. Three of those patients developed postoperative motor deficits. In a follow-up, Malcharek et al. [74, 75] found a 0.4% false negative rate for multimodal monitoring with MEPs, with MEP changes in 32 patients (12.1%), 11 patients (4.2%) with transient motor deficits, and 1 patient (0.4%) with permanent motor deficits. Isolated motor changes were not seen in Alcantara et al. [4], with 11 of 181 patients (6%) with reported changes during IONM, all with SSEP changes and 6 also with MEP changes. Interestingly, Malcharek et al. [74, 75] compared outcomes in awake CEA versus multimodal monitoring and found similar motor outcomes (postoperative deficits of 4.9% vs 4.3%), with less technical failures (defined as not being able to record either SSEPs or MEPs for the general anesthesia group and as not being able to perform a clinical neurological evaluation in the regional anesthesia group) in the multimodal monitoring group. Overall, these studies show that the addition of MEP monitoring provides added benefit in the monitoring of CEAs.

The technical setup of these studies was similar, typically sampling a hand and foot muscle bilaterally, as these areas have large cortical representation. Our institutional practice is to sample the hand (APB-FDI), tibialis anterior (TA), and adductor hallucis (AH) while primarily tracking the stimulation threshold for the hand only, and the threshold required to elicit the hand together with either the TA or AH. There is no consensus on the alarm criteria to be used in monitoring MEPs [72]. The previously mentioned studies on MEP monitoring in CEA tended to use MEP loss as their criteria, with threshold level MEP responses used.

A large concern in using MEPs for cerebrovascular monitoring is overstimulation. As stimulation increases above threshold, the probability of directly activating deep subcortical motor pathways, and thus undercutting the cortex, increases. If this occurs, there can be false negative monitoring for cortical ischemia. SSEPs do not have the same concern, as the near-field scalp evoked potential is generated at the cortex. Using close to motor threshold stimulation minimizes the risk of this occurring [49]. It is important to ensure there is no crossover (simultaneous MEPs recorded from ipsilateral limbs) present when obtaining MEPs in this context. The presence of any ipsilateral response is a sign that deeper motor pathways are being activated. Direct cortical MEPs (dcMEPs) can potentially avoid the issue of deep subcortical stimulation but are more common when the intracranial space is already being accessed such as in cerebral aneurysm clipping. However, studies of MEPs and CEA only included utilization of TcMEPs.

Malcharek et al. [76] retrospectively looked at different MEP warning criteria in 571 patients. They found that that using criteria of a 50% reduction in MEP amplitude and area under the curve resulted in false-positive rates of 24% and 29%, respectively, and concluded that using such criteria was likely not useful. Currently, based on the literature, using MEP loss is the preferred method in CEA monitoring. That amplitude criteria are not as useful in this scenario does not seem surprising. At close to threshold levels used in cerebrovascular monitoring, MEPs exhibit greater trial to trial variability than at suprathreshold levels [58]. It is possible that monitoring changes in threshold MEP level may be useful, but these have not been studied in this context yet. Overall, these studies show that the addition of MEP monitoring provides added benefit in the monitoring of CEAs.

Transcranial Doppler (TCD)

Transcranial Doppler approaches cerebral ischemia from a different perspective. While EEG, SSEP, and MEPs focus on measuring cerebral function as a surrogate for ischemia, TCD focuses on measuring cerebral blood velocity and detection of embolic events. EEG and evoked potentials can miss smaller embolic events. If an embolus occurs outside of the pathway that generates the evoked potential signal, then no change will be detected as EEG is limited to the evaluation of subcortical ischemia.

TCD is able to measure the blood flow velocity in large intracranial arteries like the ICA, MCA, ACA, and basilar and vertebral arteries. The technique is based on the Doppler effect. The TCD probe emits ultrasound waves which reflect off moving red blood cells. Due to the Doppler effect, the reflected waves will be of a slower frequency. The difference in emitted and reflected frequency is proportional to velocity and can be used to calculate the blood flow velocity. Blood flow velocity in turn can provide useful clinical information on intracranial vascular abnormalities. Vessel stenosis can result in an increase in blood flow velocity. Additionally, if fluctuations in arterial blood pressure and CO_2 remain small, then changes in blood flow velocity are felt to be reflective of cerebral blood flow. A reduction in mean flow velocities or slow flow acceleration is thought to occur in the setting of hemodynamic compromise [120]. TCD is able to detect microscopic emboli, which have characteristic changes.

In IONM, TCD has seen variable use and is utilized more often in specific centers. It tends to be less common than EEG or SSEP and is mostly limited to CEA. There are several technical factors that limit more widespread use. These include lack of an adequate acoustic window in a significant number of patients; the probe becoming dislocated, as it is relatively close to the surgical field; and the requirement of personnel specifically trained in its use.

Despite its limitations, TCD has been well studied in the context of monitoring CEAs. Halsey [50] conducted a multicenter, retrospective trial of 1495 patients. Ischemia was classified based on reduction in mean velocity with 16–40% of preclamp velocity classified as mild and 0–15% as severe. These cut-offs were based on other studies that correlated ischemia using EEG and rCBF [9, 57, 81, 121]. Major findings of this trial included that in patients with no evidence of ischemia (mean velocity remained >40% of baseline), the risk of stroke was higher in the shunt group than the no shunt group (4.4% vs 0.7%) and 7.2% of cases had severe ischemia. In these severe ischemia cases, ischemia resolved spontaneously in half. In patients where severe ischemia did not spontaneously resolve, the rate of stroke was high, with shunting protective against stroke. Six of 13 patients with severe ischemia and no shunt developed stroke, though 1/3 of these severe strokes were hemorrhagic stroke or carotid thrombosis. In the mild ischemia group, stroke rates were 3.9% vs 0.6% in the shunt vs no shunt groups.

Bornstein et al. [12] looked at velocity changes in 50 consecutive CEA patients performed under regional anesthesia with TCD monitoring. They found that the velocity changes seen were similar in patients with and without complications and concluded that TCD was not useful in deciding whether to shunt in CEA. Another study in CEA under regional anesthesia was performed by Moritz et al. [85]. This was a study of 48 patients and compared TCD, stump pressure measurement, near-infrared spectroscopy, and SSEPs. They found that all techniques were able to detect ischemia; however SSEPs had the lowest accuracy. In this study, SSEPs were performed with a stimulation intensity of 10 milliamps (mA), likely to avoid patient discomfort, as the patient was awake. At this intensity level, it is unlikely that a supramaximal SSEP signal, as is usually desired, was obtained, which may explain why the SSEP performance in this study was worse. TCDs were not able to be recorded in 21% of patients due to technical difficulties.

EEG, SSEP, and TCD were compared by Rowed et al. [109]. One hundred fifty-six patients were monitored with SSEPs and EEG, and TCD monitoring was attempted in 91 patients. TCD monitoring was only technically successful throughout the procedure in 63% of patients. EEG yielded one false negative, no false positives. SSEP had no false negatives or positives. None of the TCD emboli detections were associated with postoperative deficits.

A larger recent meta-analysis looked at TCD monitoring in 4705 patients [134]. They found that TCD monitoring of cerebral microembolic signals and MCA velocity yielded a sensitivity of 56.1% and a specificity of 72.7% for perioperative stroke. MCA velocity changes alone had a sensitivity of 49.7% and specificity of 84.1%. The authors stated they did not find studies where TCD was combined with SSEP and EEG, so they were not able to perform a comparison. A limitation of this study is the pooled studies used differing standards for critical MCA velocity or microembolic signal changes, as there is no agreed upon critical value.

Overall, TCDs do show utility in monitoring CEA but are more limited compared to other modalities due to technical difficulties and due to the ability to only monitor one intracranial vessel. There have not been many studies comparing them directly to SSEP or EEG, but in the existing studies, it did not clearly appear to be superior.

Near-Infrared Spectroscopy (NIRS)

NIRS, sometimes referred to as cerebral oximetry, is a noninvasive technique for assessing cerebral oxygenation. The technique depends on light in the near-infrared range to evaluate cerebral oxygenation [120]. Beer-Lambert law states that the amount of light transmission through a solution is a function of the concentration of the absorbing molecules in the solution and the length of the path [135]. Oxygenated and deoxygenated blood have characteristic and distinct absorbance spectra [24]. By using this characteristic of oxygenated blood, it is possible to use near-infrared light to determine the level of oxygenated blood cerebrally. Additionally, an advantage of the near-infrared spectrum of light is that skin, skull, and other biological tissue are relatively transparent to this wavelength. This allows blood in the brain to be analyzed.

There are a number of commercially available cerebral oximeters available for use in the United States presently. These include the INVOS (Somanetics/Covidien, Boulder, CO), ForeSight (CAS Medical Systems, Branford, CN), EQUANOX (Nonin Medical, Plymouth, MN), CerOx (Ornim Medical, Lod, Israel), NIRO (Hamamatsu Photonics, Hamamatsu City, Japan), TOS-96 (Tostec, Tokyo, Japan), and Root with O3 Regional Oximetry (Masimo, Irvine, CA). These devices work by measuring the ratio of hemoglobin to oxyhemoglobin using a single light-emitting diode with near-infrared light transmitted with a wavelength of 724 and 810 nm and recorded with two photodiodes [24]. One can refer to the excellent reviews by Wahr et al. [135] and Davies and Janelle [24] for a more detailed review of the technology underlying cerebral oximetry, which is beyond the scope of this chapter.

There have been many studies looking at the performance of NIRS in CEA. As mentioned in the previous section, Moritz et al. [85] compared NIRS, TCD, EEG, and SSEP in CEA under regional anesthesia and found that all of the techniques were able to identify cerebral ischemia but that NIRS and stump pressure measurement had the highest accuracy, as compared to clinical deterioration which was described as the gold standard. Clinical deterioration was defined as any new neurologic deficit occurring, such as speech abnormalities, motor weakness, or impaired consciousness. The patient's clinical exam was assessed every 30 s during surgery, with orientation, command following, and handgrip assessed by the anesthetist. In Beese et al. [10], NIRS and SSEP were compared in 317 CEA patients. SSEPs were stable in 287 of 317 patients, and none of these patients developed postoperative deficits. Twenty-seven of 317 patients (9%) had flattening of the SSEP during cross-clamping. These patients had the regional cerebral saturation (rSO_2) before cross-clamping and the trough level after cross-clamping recorded. It was found that a statistically significant decrease of rSO2 was seen in patients both with (65.8% vs 56.1%) and without (63.9% vs 60.9%) SSEP changes. Substantial interindividual variability and change of rSO_2 did not allow them to definc a threshold value. From this they concluded that without a threshold rSO_2 value for cerebral ischemia, interventions based on cerebral oximetry were not justified.

Rigamonti et al. [106] attempted to establish a threshold in a prospective study of 50 CEA patients with regional anesthesia. They monitored clinical signs, EEG, and NIRS. Patients who had clinical or EEG changes and required shunt showed a 16% decrease in rSO2 vs 8% in non-shunted patients ($p = .01$). A decrease of 15% in rSO2 had an odds ratio of 20 for severe cerebral ischemia. The same decrease of 15% had a sensitivity of 55% and specificity of 82%. The authors concluded that although NIRS could correlate with cerebral ischemia, they were not able to identify a threshold that could be used alone for prediction of shunt placement due to poor sensitivity and specificity. A literature review by Pennekamp et al. [98] had similar conclusions that, although NIRS correlated with TCD and EEG, a threshold was unable to be determined for selective shunting or cerebral ischemia.

Poor sensitivity and specificity were similarly seen in a more recent meta-analysis of 1237 NIRS in CEA under regional anesthesia [33]. In that study, summary sensitivity was found to be 72% with a specificity of 84.1%. The authors concluded that NIRS could not be used alone to monitor CEA under regional anesthesia, and the threshold for ischemia remains poorly defined. In that meta-analysis, 8 of the 11 studies reported a relative decrease of around 15–20%. A Cochrane review of NIRS for perioperative monitoring (including non-CEA surgeries) concluded that it was unclear whether NIRS had an effect on postoperative stroke due to wide confidence intervals and a low number of events in published studies [140].

The technical setup of NIRS is relatively straightforward compared to other monitoring modalities, similar to applying pulse oximetry. Some of technical factors that can affect its signals include lack of correlation and agreement between different NIRS devices, vulnerability to light and movement artifacts (such as overhead surgical lights), and the ability to only detect regional oxygenation (usually in the frontal lobes, as this is the hair follicle-free skin area that overlies the brain) [115]. NIRS should probably not be used as the sole modality for monitoring CEA. Its exact role in CEA monitoring is not completely clear.

Monitoring Intracranial Cerebrovascular Disorders

The rationale and basis of IONM for CEA also translates similarly to intracranial cerebrovascular disorders. IONM may be useful in patients undergoing surgical or endovascular treatment of cerebral aneurysms, cerebral arteriovenous malformations (AVMs), cerebral cavernous malformations, intracranial vascular occlusive disorders, and deliberate cerebral vessel occlusion.

Cerebral Aneurysm Surgery

Due to the strong correlation between SSEPs and cerebral ischemia seen experimentally, these modalities naturally became adopted for the monitoring of cerebral aneurysm surgery. Besides being able to monitor for cortical ischemia, SSEPs also are able to provide functional information about the integrity of the cortical and subcortical somatosensory pathways. This is an advantage over EEG, which also provides information on cortical structures. In intracranial non-epilepsy surgery, EEG is more limited in its use of detecting cerebral ischemia as EEG recording is interfered with by the introduction of airspace between the dura and arachnoid mater that occur from craniotomy and brain relaxation [35]. It has been shown that median nerve SSEPs also provide information on thalamic activity supplied by the posterior cerebral artery [17]. As previously mentioned, the cortical generator of the median or ulnar nerve SSEP lies in the parietal cortex in primary sensory cortex representing the hand, located in the MCA territory, while the cortical generator of the posterior tibial nerve SSEP lies parasagitally in the primary sensory cortex, in the ACA territory.

Our typical setup for aneurysm and AVM surgery varies depending on the cerebrovascular territory that is felt to be most at risk. We will include EEG, median/ulnar nerve SSEP, posterior tibial nerve SSEP, and TcMEPs (sampling the hand (FDI-APB), TA, AH) for all territories. For vertebrobasilar cases we will include BAEPs and sometimes free-running cranial nerve EMG. For ACA territory procedures, we will include additional centrally located stimulation electrodes (e.g., at Cz) to better isolate leg MEP responses.

Earlier studies of IONM in aneurysm surgery involve a combination of EEG, SSEP, and BAEP. Palatinsky et al. [93] reported the outcomes of ten studies of MCA aneurysm and found median nerve SSEPs were 78–100% reliable in predicting clinical outcome. Friedman et al. [43] found a decrease or disappearance in the cortical SSEP accurately predicted postoperative deficits. In López et al. [71], 70 aneurysm cases monitored with SSEP, EEG, and or BAEP were evaluated. The authors found that 26% of patients had transient SSEP changes and 4% with transient BAEP changes. Aneurysm clip placement caused IONM changes in 9 of 70 cases, with removal or adjustment of the clip resolving changes in all cases. Other changes were caused by transient hypotension and retractors. Two patients had persistent IONM changes, one developed a new deficit post-op, and one died. Manninen et al. [77] reported SSEP and BAEP use in posterior fossa aneurysm surgery. They found that 10 of 67 patients showed BAEP changes, with 6 developing a postoperative neurologic deficit. The false negative rate of SSEP/BAEP was 20%.

Friedman et al. [42] reported the results of 53 patients undergoing MCA aneurysm surgery. New postoperative deficits were seen in four patients with persistent SSEP changes, while one of five patients with a transient SSEP change developed a postoperative deficit. There was one false negative case. SSEPs were also able to identify a case of peripheral ischemia in this series, as in one patient a malfunctioning blood pressure cuff caused limb ischemia. Schramm et al. [113] looked at 134 aneurysm cases and found alteration of surgical course in 15 of 17 instances of SSEP changes.

Using multimodality monitoring can be useful in identifying focal or regional ischemia, which is of importance in intracranial aneurysm surgery, where the vascular territories involved are more variable compared to those in carotid surgery. Multimodal monitoring has been reported in an increasing number of studies in cerebral aneurysm surgery. Quiñones-Hinojosa et al. [102] reported a series of 30 patients undergoing basilar artery aneurysm clipping performed with monitoring of SSEP, EEG, and MEP. Changes occurred in 10 of 30 patients, with 6 caused by temporary clipping, 3 by permanent clipping, and 1 by retraction. Isolated TcMEP changes occurred in five patients, with four patients having changes in both TcMEPs and SSEPs and a single patient with isolated SSEP changes. All changes were transient after corrective measures. They felt that the results suggested that TcMEPs may be more sensitive than SSEPs for basilar artery procedures. Horiuchi et al. [54] looked at dcMEPs and SSEPs in MCA aneurysm surgery in 53 patients. Nine patients had transient dcMEP changes, with five of those being isolated MEP changes of which three had transient motor deficits. One patient had persistent dcMEP loss and developed postoperative hemiparesis, with imaging showing a subcortical infarct.

Sasaki et al. [111] analyzed cerebral infarction of perforating artery territories in 1043 patients who had underwent aneurysm surgery. They found that intraoperative microscopic inspection was not able to determine the patency of perforating arteries, but MEPs were able to detect disturbances in blood flow in several perforating arteries (anterior choroidal artery, lenticulostriate arteries), whereas SSEPs were less useful for this purpose. Infarct was related to aneurysmal neck clipping, temporary occlusion of the parent artery, direct injury, retraction, and trapping of the parent artery. Similarly, Neuloh and Schramm [88] also found that TcMEPs were better than other modalities at detecting subcortical ischemia.

There are now several large studies reviewing the performance of different IONM modalities in aneurysmal surgery. In Thirumala et al. [130, 131], a meta-analysis of 2015 patients was performed. They found that SSEP changes had a sensitivity of 56.8% and a specificity of 84.5%. SSEP sensitivity may be lower here, as the analysis included anterior and posterior circulation aneurysms. In general, SSEPs appear less sensitive to brainstem infarcts. Sahaya et al. [110] reported their experience with 470 procedures with SSEP and EEG in endovascular and surgical aneurysm repair. They found that IONM changes demonstrated a sensitivity of 90%, a specificity of 98%, and a negative predictive value of 99.78%. For multimodal monitoring, a systematic review and meta-analysis by Zhu et al. [142] looked at SSEP and MEP in 4011 patients in 35 studies. The pooled sensitivity and specificity were as follows: SSEP 59% and 86%; MEP 81% and 90%; and MEP and SSEP 92% and 88%. The analysis was limited by modest quality and high heterogeneity of the primary studies. Park et al. [95] compared aneurysm clipping with and without IONM (MEP/SSEP) in 545 procedures. Procedures without IONM all occurred prior to procedures with IONM in this study. IONM changes had a sensitivity of 90%, a specificity of 94%, and a negative predictive value of 99.7%. The rate of postoperative neurologic deficits in the non-IONM group was 6.7% compared to 3.1% in the group with IONM. Additionally, patients with IONM had lower rates of sustained postoperative neurologic deficits (odds ratio = 0.36), ischemic complications (odds ratio = 0.39), and radiologic complications (odds ratio = 0.4). Overall, from these studies, we can see that using a multimodality IONM approach effectively identifies cerebral and brainstem ischemia.

Cerebral AVMs

The number of studies on the use of IONM in monitoring AVM surgery is much less than that of aneurysms but also supports the use of IONM in this context. Chang et al. [18] looked at 56 cases of vascular malformation resection. SSEPs were monitored in 96% of these cases and BAEPs in 30%. Five of 54 patients (9%) had SSEP changes, with 4 patients with transient changes and 4 patients who developed new transient postoperative deficits. In those patients with transient SSEP changes, adjustment or removal of clips or increasing MAP resolved the changes. There were one false negative in the BAEP group and one change with associated permanent deficit. The overall sensitivity for SSEP and BAEP was 86% and specificity was 98%.

Ichikawa et al. [55] also described the use of MEPs in AVM resection in a series of 21 patients. Selected patients had lesions where motor cortex or corticospinal pathways were felt to be directly at-risk during resection. Either dcMEPs or TcMEPs were used, with dcMEPs used if motor cortex was exposed. The warning criteria consisted of MEP disappearance and/or a decrease in amplitude of 50% or more. Five of 21 patients showed MEP changes, with 4 transient changes and 1 persistent loss. Two of these patients developed transient motor deficits and two developed permanent motor deficits. Causes of changes included temporary occlusion of a feeding artery, venous infarction, coagulation of a capillary network, and AVM bleeding. The authors felt that monitoring using MEP was useful in differentiating passing arteries from feeding arteries.

Extracranial-Intracranial (EC-IC) Bypass

The goal of EC-IC bypass surgery is revascularization and involves taking an extracranial artery branch and anastomosing it into the intracranial vasculature, bypassing a stenotic or occluded proximal vessel. The most common EC-IC bypass is the superior temporal artery-middle cerebral artery (STA-MCA) bypass. EC-IC bypass has been used to treat a variety of conditions: moyamoya disease, symptomatic vascular stenosis, aneurysm, and tumors requiring vascular sacrifice [105]. In STA-MCA bypass, the STA is grafted to a branch of the MCA. While anastomosis of the STA to the MCA is occurring, the MCA must be occluded, and there is a risk of cerebral ischemia.

In what appears to be the only published study on IONM in EC-IC bypass, Dengler et al. [27] described the use of TcMEP monitoring in EC-IC bypass in 32 cases with SSEP used as a backup if TcMEPs were not able to be monitored. They observed 14 reversible TcMEP changes, with 1 patient developing a transient postoperative deficit, and 1 irreversible TcMEP change associated with a permanent neurologic deficit. Reasons for reversible changes included temporary occlusion of the recipient vessel (leading to a more distal bypass site being chosen), the occurrence of bypass anastomosis (reversed with MAP increase or after anastomosis is complete), temporary aneurysm clipping (leading to repositioning of the clip), and others. There were no false negative events. Warning criteria used in this study were a reduction of TcMEP amplitude of more than 50% or an increase of TcMEP peak latency >10%. MEPs were obtained at a near-threshold level. The use of 50% amplitude reduction criteria might explain the relatively high number of changes in this study (15 of 32 cases). In our institution, the practice is typically to obtain near-threshold MEPs and use an 80% reduction in MEP amplitude as warning criteria. As detailed in the section on MEP monitoring in CEAs, variability of MEPs at near-threshold levels may make following complete MEP loss a preferable warning criterion in cerebrovascular monitoring. Due to this risk of cerebral ischemia, IONM can potentially play a role in monitoring these surgeries, using a combination of EEG, SSEP, and MEP.

Interventional Neuroradiologic Procedures

Interventional neuroradiologic (INR) procedures have rapidly expanded in volume and are now a routine occurrence in many institutions. Diseases previously treated surgically can now often be treated endovascularly. The potential risk of cerebral ischemia present in open surgical cerebrovascular cases remains in endovascular procedures. The use of IONM in these procedures has grown, as evidenced by an increase in the number of reports on IONM in INR procedures in the last decade. EEG, MEP, SSEP, and BAEP can equally be applied in the endovascular suite to monitor selected procedures. The most common of these include carotid artery angioplasty, deliberate arterial occlusion of extra- and intracranial arteries, coiling of cerebral aneurysms, placement of flow-diverting stents for aneurysms, and glue embolization of cerebral AVMs. The exact modalities chosen to monitor these procedures depend on the cerebrovascular territory that will be at risk and whether the patient will be under general anesthesia or awake during the procedure.

The IONM setup and recording for INR procedures is similar to surgical cases. There are a few small differences. We do not use corkscrew EEG electrodes, as the artifact associated with these can obscure imaging. For patients being stented and on dual antiplatelet therapy, we use cup electrodes rather than needle electrodes, as we have observed cases of extensive subdermal hematoma with needle electrodes.

Paulsen et al. [96] reported using SSEPs in 23 rolandic AVM embolizations. During amobarbital sodium testing, one awake case showed a SSEP change with associated transient neurologic deficit, and a second general anesthesia case showed a SSEP change. The authors felt that SSEPs and clinical neurological examination were useful tools in this context. Paiva et al. [92] used EEG monitoring in AVM embolization and found focal or diffuse low-frequency abnormalities were followed by clinical hazards in 3 of 11 cases. Positive amobarbital testing in this study caused ipsilateral focal slowing. Liu et al. [68] also report the use of IONM in 35 patients, with management altered in 5 of 35 patients.

Dietz et al. [30] looked at 17 patients undergoing balloon test occlusion of the ICA (due to tumor infiltrating the area). These patients were monitored using clinical exam, SSEP, TcMEPs, and TCDs. Balloon test occlusion is performed when a vessel, such as the ICA, needs to be sacrificed. It involves temporarily inflating a balloon in the ICA and looking for changes in the patient's neurological exam or neurophysiologic indices to determine if the vessel can be safely sacrificed. Their conclusion was monitoring was important in predicting outcome from permanent occlusion of the ICA. Cloughesy et al. [23] used clinical exam, EEG, and qEEG for monitoring balloon test occlusions. They found 4 of 17 cases with changes. These changes were as follows: increased slowing and clinical changes; attenuation of the alpha band, but no clinical change; and clinical change without EEG change.

More recently, Takamura et al. [127] compared the performance of preoperative balloon test occlusion done awake with intraoperative findings. Patients underwent a standard balloon test occlusion prior to their surgery. The systolic blood pressure was kept under 140 mmHg, and tests were considered negative if there were no changes after 20 min of occlusion. During this period, patients underwent continuous neurological evaluation, not further specified in the study. The majority of surgeries following balloon test occlusion were CEAs (28 of 32). Any change during cross-clamping was noted. The accuracy of multimodality monitoring was compared to BTO. MEPs were performed at an intensity of 20% higher than threshold level. They found that a >80% amplitude reduction in MEPs resulted in a sensitivity and specificity of 100% for a positive balloon test occlusion. They found that in this comparison MEPs performed better than EEG and SSEP in accuracy. This study is similar to studies comparing modalities in CEA done under regional anesthesia, but the clinical exam for balloon test occlusion may be more accurate, as the patient is on minimal anesthetics for balloon test occlusion compared to CEA.

Pandey et al. [94] looked at the use of BAEP in six patients undergoing vertebrobasilar stenting and angioplasty. They found that one patient had a 1 ms increase in wave V latency during angioplasty, and the patient developed post-procedural hemiplegia.

There have now been several larger studies on the use of IONM in INR. Phillips et al. [100] looked at 873 patients undergoing INR procedures who were monitored with SSEP. They found 52 of 873 patients with SSEP changes. Twenty-four of these were reversible and 28 patients had persistent changes. The negative predictive value of reversible SSEP changes for postoperative stroke was 83%. It does not appear there was false negative SSEP monitoring. Sensitivity and specificity of unstratified SSEP changes were not calculated. Ares et al. [7] looked at 888 cases of SSEP monitoring in endovascular aneurysm cases. They found SSEP changes occurred in 8.6% of cases with 3.1% of patients developing new postoperative deficits. A transient or persistent total loss of SSEP had an odds ratio of 267 for development of a new deficit. A 50–99% loss in SSEP amplitude was associated with an odds ratio of 18.4 for a new deficit. False negative rate, sensitivity, nor specificity was specifically reported.

Lee et al. [64] reported SSEP and MEP monitoring in 578 patients undergoing INR procedures. SSEP changes occurred in 1% of patients, and MEP changes in 1.2%. Postoperative deficits developed in 0.7% of patients. They determined a sensitivity and specificity of SSEPs to be 100%, and 50% and 99.5% for MEPs. The sensitivity and specificity in this study were limited by the occurrence of relatively few postoperative deficits.

Similar performance is seen for IONM in AVM embolization. Church et al. [22] looked at 173 embolizations monitored with SSEP and EEG and found a negative predictive value of 90%. They also noted that their overall complication rate (1.3%) was among the lowest reported in the literature for this indication, which suggests IONM may improve outcomes. In a large study, Wilent et al. [138] analyzed 2278 INR cases where SSEP, MEP, and EEG monitoring were used. Seven hundred and sixty-three of the 2278 cases used MEPs; the rest did not. They had an overall incidence of postoperative deficit of 1.2%. In cases with IONM changes, 20% of these patients developed a deficit, while 0.09% of cases without a change developed a deficit. Complete signal loss had an odds ratio of 1437 for a postoperative deficit. Cases with MEP monitoring had a sensitivity of 92.3% compared to 85.7% without, and a specificity of 96.7% vs 98.2%. There are many studies that support the use of multimodality IONM in interventional neuroradiologic procedures.

In addition to monitoring procedures, provocative testing can also be performed. At our institution, endovascular treatment of AVMs typically involves provocative testing. This involves superselective intra-arterial injection of an agent, usually 50 mg of amobarbital sodium (methohexital, propofol, pentobarbital, and etomidate have also been described) into the pedicle that will be embolized or the vessel that will be embolized. If there is a significant change in the patient's EEG, evoked potentials, or clinical exam, this suggests that the vessel likely supplies blood flow to normal cerebral tissue and should not be embolized. Instead, a different or more distal vessel can be tested. If no change occurs, then embolization will proceed.

Bican et al. [11] detail the use of provocative testing in awake patients and patients under general anesthesia. This was a series of 63 cases, with 9 awake and the rest under general anesthesia. There were no instances of new neurologic deficits. Provocative testing was positive in two patients and results were comparable between general anesthesia and awake groups. Specificity of testing was reported as 100%. Provocative testing can also be used for spinal lesions, such as spinal dural arteriovenous fistulas; this will be covered in the chapter on monitoring spinal cord ischemia.

There are relatively few studies on how IONM affects cost. Feng et al. [37] looked at patients undergoing AVM embolization in a large database. They found that in patients who underwent embolization with IONM, length of stay was shorter (2.72 vs 4.92 days), complication rates were lower (0% vs 1.88%), and total payment was lower (40,179$ vs 50,844$). As with database studies, there may be many potential confounders in these results, such as hospitals with IONM services for embolization being more likely to be larger centers with more experience.

Mechanical Thrombectomy for Acute Stroke

In the last decade, mechanical thrombectomy for the treatment of large vessel occlusions in acute stroke has gone from experimental to standard of care [3, 41, 46, 47, 89]. Mechanical thrombectomy is an interventional neuroradiologic procedure where an acute thrombus of a large cerebral blood vessel, most often the ICA or M1 segment of the MCA, is removed with a stent-retriever device. With this type of treatment, many patients are able to walk away from previously devastating strokes with minimal deficits. In SWIFT PRIME 60% of patients receiving thrombectomy had a 90-day modified Rankin score (mRS) of 0–2 vs 35% of the control group [112]. While it is not the current practice at our institution to monitor mechanical thrombectomy, there are other centers where it is common.

The ideal IONM setup for these procedures is not clear yet. Greve et al. [48] employed a single modality, MEPs recorded at the bilateral adductor pollicis brevis. Only monitoring MEPs may provide an advantage in decreased setup time and may be appropriate if the goal is to only provide prognostic information. Compared to other procedures, shorter setup time is more important in thrombectomy. The American Heart Association stroke center goals for thrombectomy are a door-to-device time in 50% of transfer patients of 60 and 90 min in directly arriving patients, door being defined as arrival into the hospital [6]. Another logistical concern is that many of these procedures are performed under moderate sedation, which may limit the use of needle electrodes and further increase setup time. Additionally, if the patient is not deeply sedated, it may be possible to follow the clinical exam instead.

There is not yet much literature on the use of IONM in mechanical thrombectomy. The use of IONM in thrombectomy differs from many other procedures in that the neurologic deficit has already occurred prior to the start of monitoring.

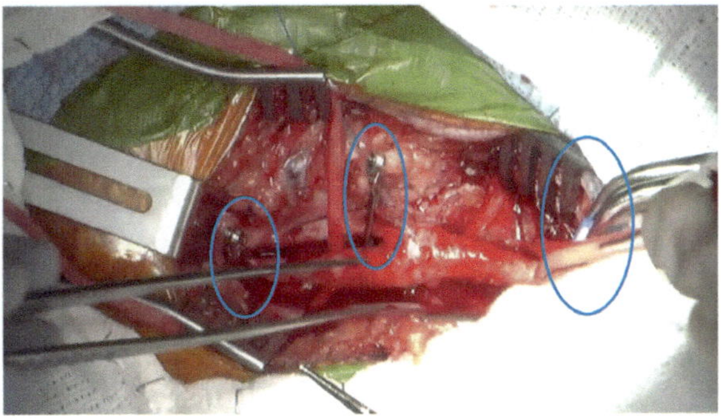

Fig. 28.5 Case Example 1: Shown here is the carotid bifurcation during a CEA. The common carotid is to the right, and the internal and external carotids are on the left. The blue circles highlight the cross-clamps over each of the vessels

There are a few interesting occurrences in this case. The propofol bolus causes an increase in the amplitude of the SSEP due to the change in morphology or by improving signal to noise ratio by decreasing spontaneous EMG. The left median SSEP initially decreases in amplitude immediately upon cross-clamping but soon recovers. It may have also been warranted to proceed with a shunt at that point. This case also illustrates the potential added value of MEPs, as there was loss of the hand MEP before there was a critical change in the amplitude of the left median SSEP. Although we would expect that primary sensory and motor cortex would be equally affected by carotid clamping, the signals may not respond equally fast to ischemia, and having redundant coverage can increase the sensitivity. Motor evoked potentials do not have to be averaged, so a change can potentially be detected faster if those are run frequently. Additionally, if there was subcortical ischemia causing pure motor deficits, SSEPs would be insensitive to this. It should also be noted that as the patient was in burst suppression during cross-clamping, making it difficult to rely on the EEG for detecting ischemia, there is increased importance in the inclusion of the other modalities.

Case Example 2

A 67-year-old woman presented with recent worsening of chronic headaches and was diagnosed with a 4 mm left M1 MCA aneurysm with secondary subarachnoid hemorrhage. Physical exam showed no preoperative sensorimotor deficits. She underwent a left frontotemporal craniotomy for clipping of the aneurysm using IONM. IONM was performed with upper and lower SSEPs, TcMEPs, and two channels of EEG. Figures 28.6, 28.7, 28.8, and 28.9 summarize the relevant IONM events.

After recovery of the TcMEP, the aneurysm was successfully clipped using two different clips, and there were no further IONM changes during the remainder of the case. The patient awoke with mild right arm weakness that resolved within minutes after being fully awake, and she had no other deficits during her hospitalization.

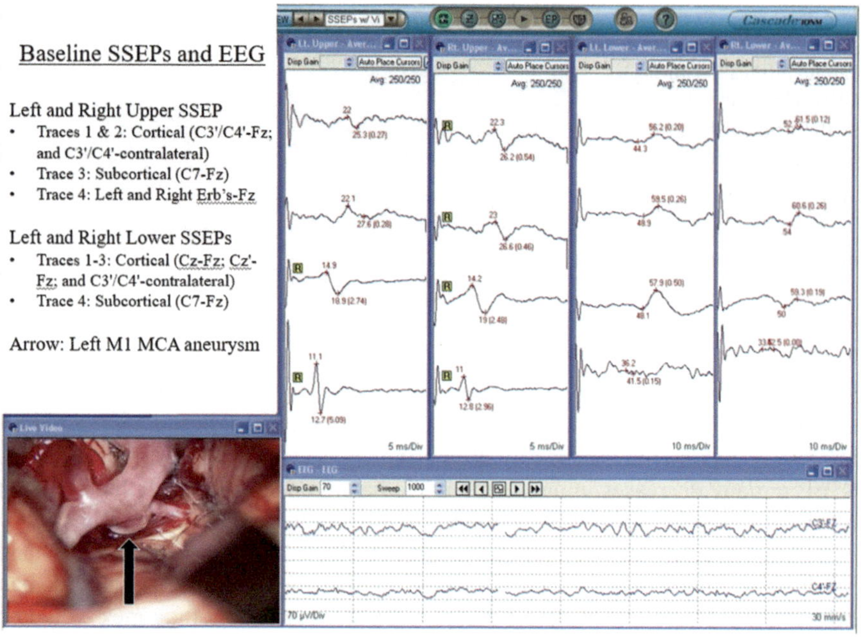

Fig. 28.6 Case Example 2: The baseline SSEPs and EEG are shown

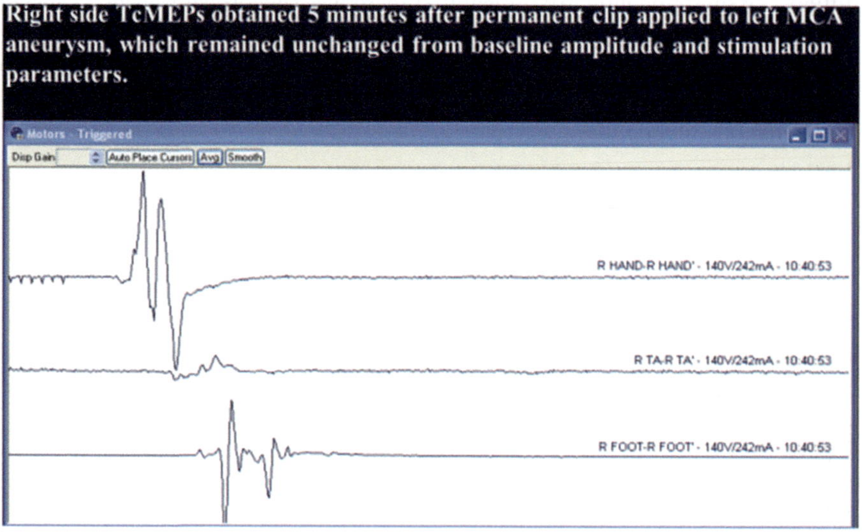

Fig. 28.7 Case Example 2: TcMEPs obtained 5 min after permanent clip application remain unchanged from baseline

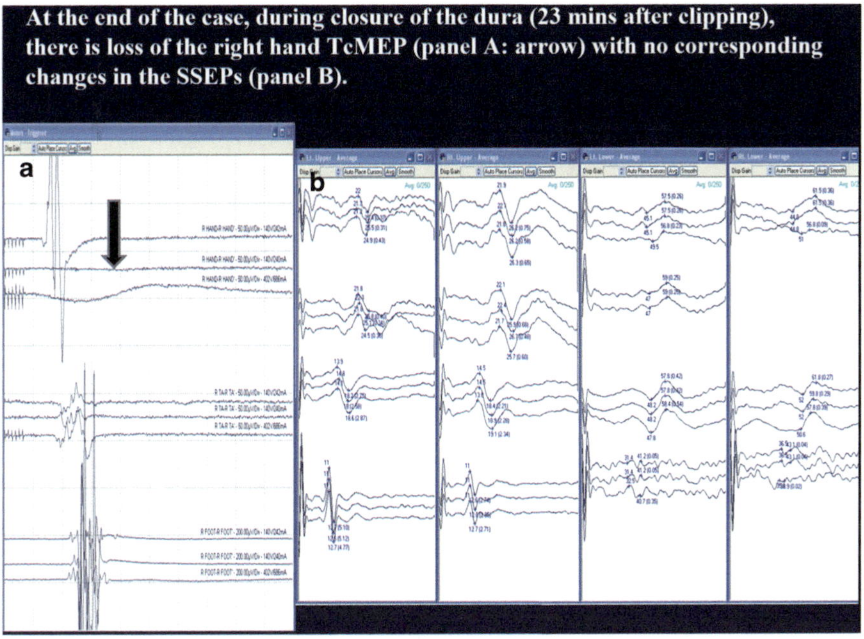

Fig. 28.8 Case Example 2: Loss of the right-hand TcMEP during dural closure, 23 min following clipping of the aneurysm, with no associated SSEP change

Case Example 3

A 64-year-old male was incidentally found to have 10 mm anterior communicating artery (ACOM) aneurysm while being staged for bladder cancer. Because of the size of the aneurysm and associated risk for hemorrhage, surgical clipping was recommended (Fig. 28.10, arrow). A left craniotomy for clipping of the aneurysm under mild hypothermia and IONM was performed. IONM was done using upper and lower SSEPs and TcMEPs and two channels of EEG.

Figure 28.11 shows SSEPs obtained during the case. As indicated above each panel, the left-to-right panels show cortical SSEPs over a period of 90 min from left and right median and left and right posterior tibial nerve stimulation, respectively. Down arrows indicate baseline lower extremity (LE) SSEPs, and the right arrow points to loss of bilateral LE SSEPs, which occurred during temporary occlusion of bilateral A1 arteries and before placing the permanent clip. The surgeon was informed of the LE SSEP change, and the patient's MAP was increased to >90 mm Hg. Major LE SSEP changes lasted approximately 25 min. During this time, the temporary clips were briefly removed on two occasions to provide vessel reperfusion. A permanent clip was successfully placed and complete SSEP recovery occurred 35 min after the initial change. The up arrow shows recovery to baseline levels of the LE SSEP. Note that there are no changes in the upper extremity (UE) SSEPs.

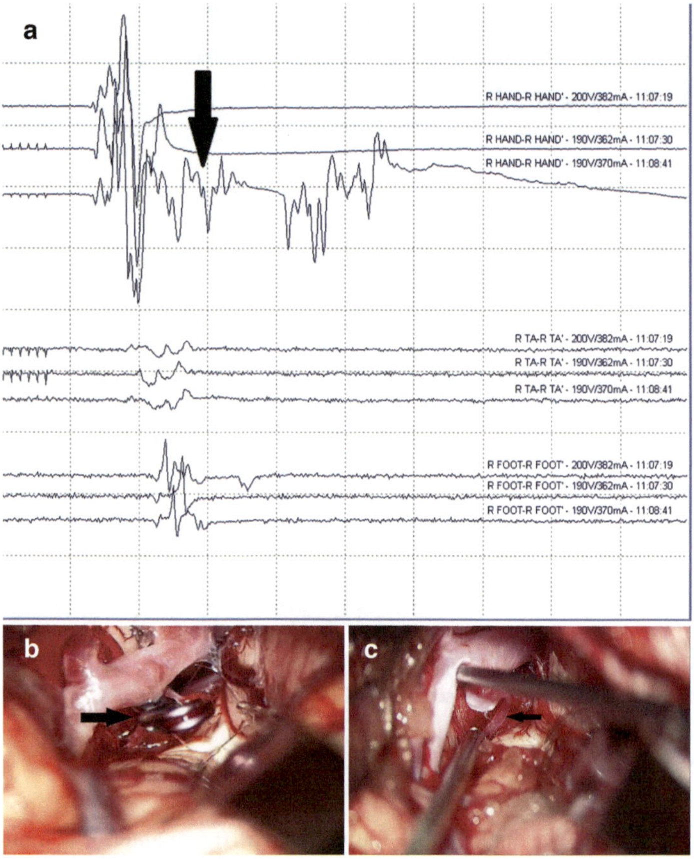

Fig. 28.9 Case Example 2: The surgeon was notified of the change, the dura was reopened and the clip was removed. (**a**) Removal of the permanent clip resulted in the right-hand TcMEP returning to baseline levels (arrow). (**b**) Position of the permanent clip (arrow) prior to removal. (**c**) A small vessel (arrow) was noted behind the aneurysm, which likely became occluded during closure due to clip migration

Fig. 28.10 Case Example 3: Computed tomography angiography with 3D reconstruction showing ACOM aneurysm (arrow)

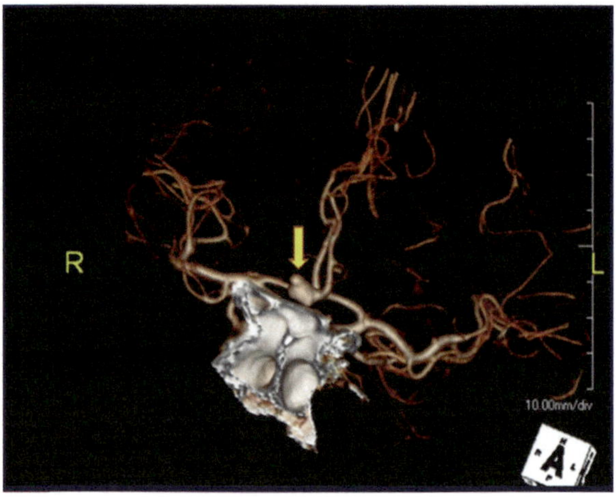

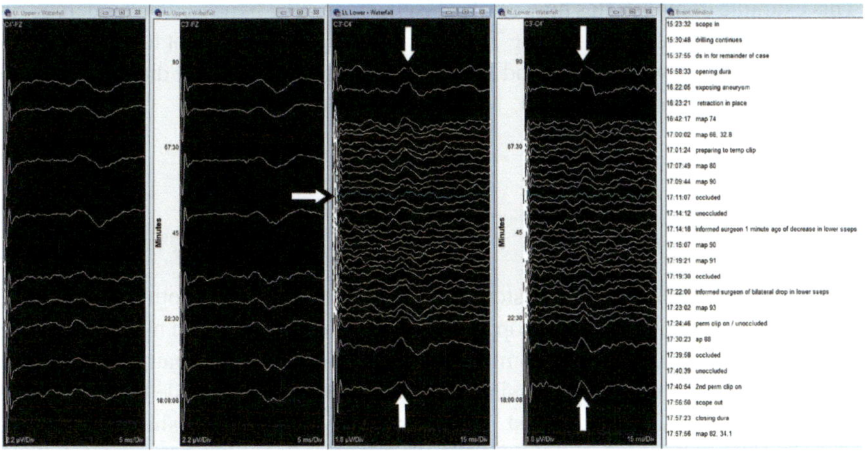

Fig. 28.11 Case Example 3: Cortical SSEPs from all four limbs

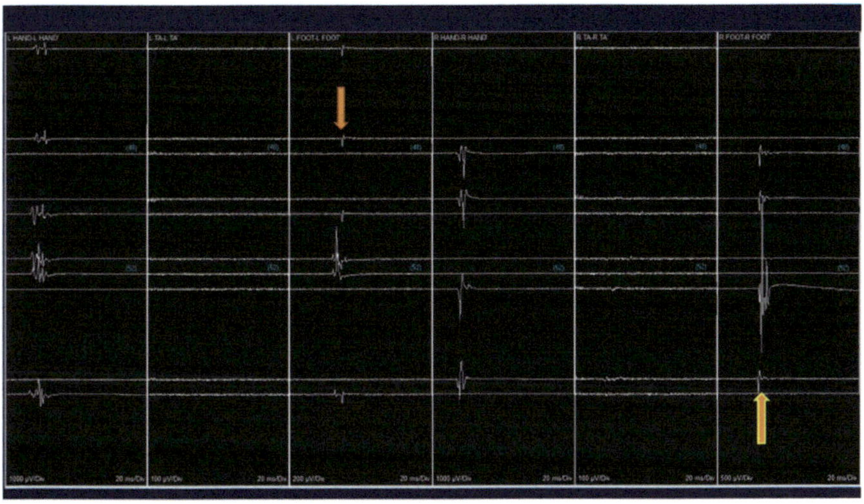

Fig. 28.12 Case Example 3: TcMEPs obtained during the period of temporary bilateral A1 artery occlusion

Figure 28.12 shows the TcMEPs obtained during the period of temporary bilateral A1 artery occlusion. TcMEPs were performed using threshold stimulation intensity levels required to elicit only contralateral LE TcMEPs to reduce the likelihood of activating deep subcortical corticospinal pathways. Note that each stimulation session activates TcMEPs only from one side, never from both. Down arrow points to the presence of left foot (AH) TcMEPs while the up arrow to those from the right foot. These did not change from baseline at any point during the case.

This example demonstrates how cerebral ischemia can be bypassed or "undercut" in certain circumstances when using TcMEPs and why it is important to use multimodality monitoring with SSEPs and EEG. The patient did well and did not have any postoperative neurologic deficits.

Case Example 4

A 69-year-old female with history of hypertension and hypothyroidism who 4 months prior to presentation stopped taking her antihypertensive medications due to side effects. A day prior to admission, she felt dizzy, and her gait was unsteady. She rested but her symptoms persisted. She was taken to an outside hospital where a brain CT scan without contrast demonstrated 2 cm × 1.3 cm slightly irregular, global mass, ventral and slightly superior to the medulla, causing local mass effect. Further evaluation revealed a giant basilar artery aneurysm (Fig. 28.13). Neurologic exam was notable for moderate anxiety but was otherwise normal.

In the ICU, the patient experienced an episode of acute faintness associated with bradycardia to the 30s and MAPs in the 40s. She subsequently rapidly recovered to her baseline. This was felt likely to be an effect of midbrain compression caused by the aneurysm.

Due to the surgically inaccessible location of the aneurysm and the limited endovascular options, she was treated with a novel stent system and IONM.

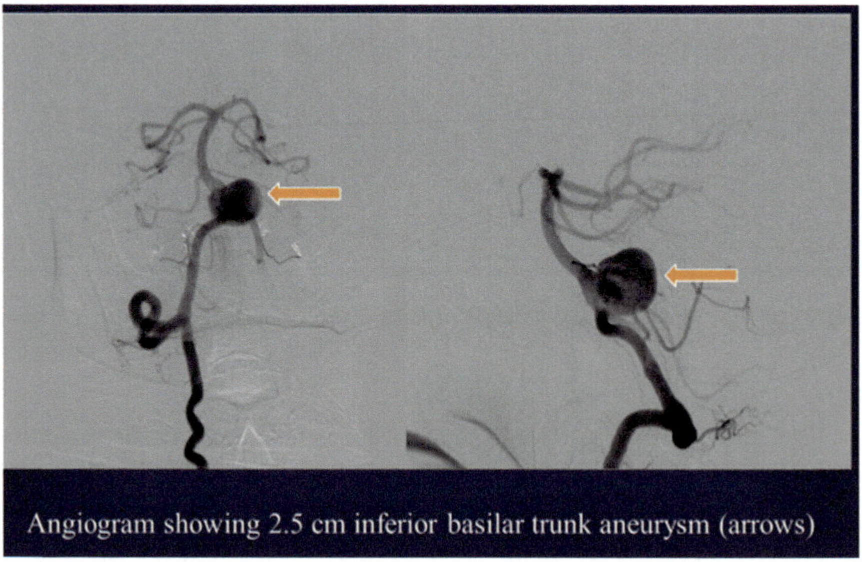

Fig. 28.13 Case Example 4: Angiogram showing a 2.5 cm inferior basilar trunk aneurysm

IONM was performed using UE and LE SSEPs and BAEPs. The surgeon requested the use of neuromuscular blocking agents during the case to avoid any movement due to the high risk for aneurysm rupture, so TcMEPs were not used.

Figure 28.14 shows the baseline SSEPs and BAEPs. Panel A shows left median nerve SSEPs; top two traces are cortical scalp recordings; third trace is C7–Fz; fourth trace is Erb's point–Fz. Panel B shows right median nerve SSEP, with similar montages as in A. Panels C and D are left and right posterior tibial nerve SSEPs, respectively. The top three traces are all cortical scalp recordings, Cz–Fz, Cz′–Fz, and C3′/C4′ contralateral; and the bottom trace is C7–Fz. Left BAEP montage is Cz–A1 and the right BAEP is Cz–A2.

Figure 28.15 shows amplitude reduction of the right BAEP (arrow) after placement of the microcatheter in the right vertebral artery. This worsens several minutes later as shown in Fig. 28.16 by loss of the right BAEP (arrow). Note that there are no changes in the SEPs or the left BAEP. The surgeon was alerted after the initial BAEP amplitude reduction and the microcatheter was removed. Upon removal of the microcatheter, the right BAEP quickly recovered (Fig. 28.17, arrow). These changes occurred during the two periods, 6 and 11 min, respectively, when the microcatheter was in the right vertebral artery placing the stents. There were no further changes noted after the placement of three stents from her right vertebral artery into her basilar artery. Her left vertebral artery was then occluded using coils. She woke from the procedure without any neurologic deficits, and she was discharged 3 days later. Her postoperative day 6 CT angiography shows normal posterior circulation blood flow and minimal residual aneurysm (Fig. 28.18).

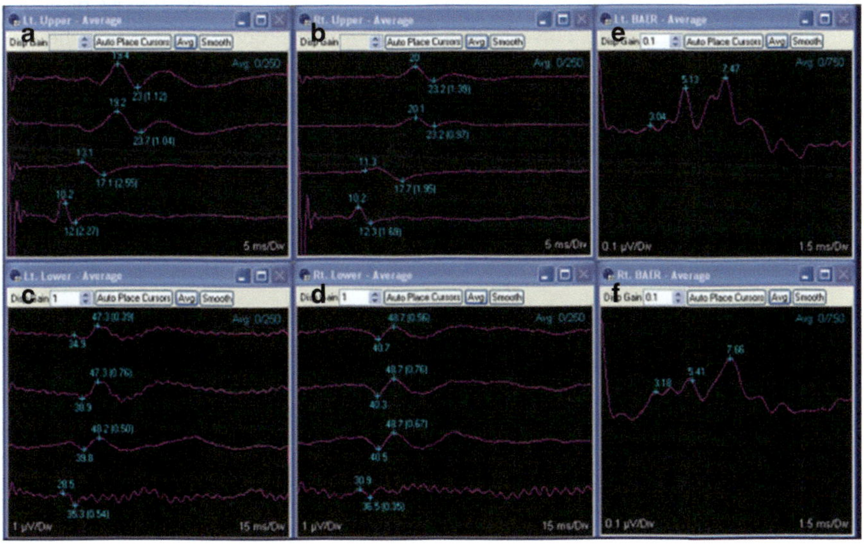

Fig. 28.14 Case Example 4: Baseline SSEPs and BAEPs. (**a**) Baseline left median nerve SSEP (**b**) Baseline right median nerve SSEP (**c**) Baseline left posterior tibial nerve SSEP (**d**) Baseline right posterior tibial nerve SSEP (**e**) Baseline left BAEP (**f**) Baseline right BAEP. The montages used for each evoked potential are further described in the corresponding section of the case description

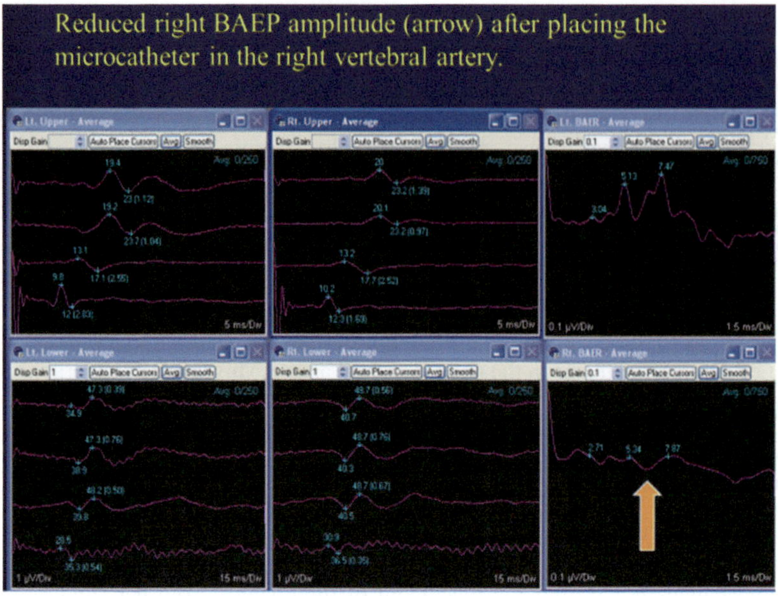

Fig. 28.15 Case Example 4: Reduction in the amplitude of the right BAEP following placement of the microcatheter in the right vertebral artery

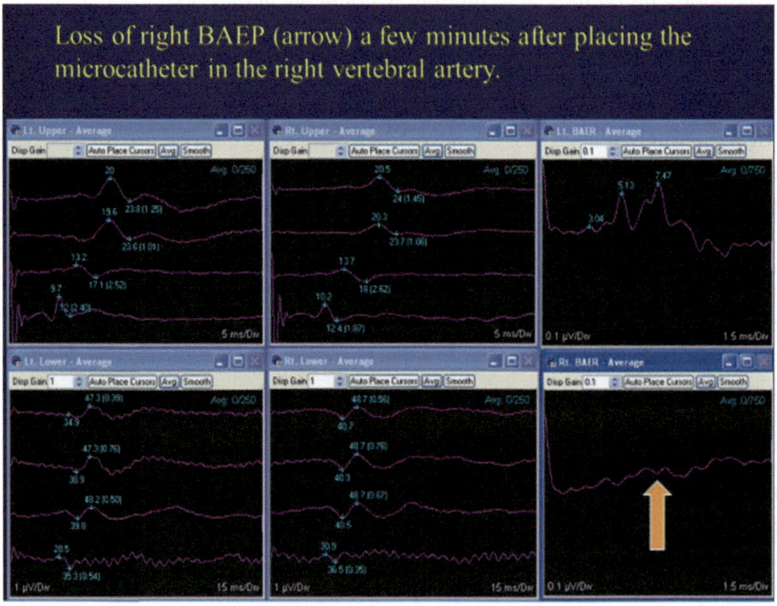

Fig. 28.16 Case Example 4: Loss of the right BAEP following placement of the microcatheter in the right vertebral artery

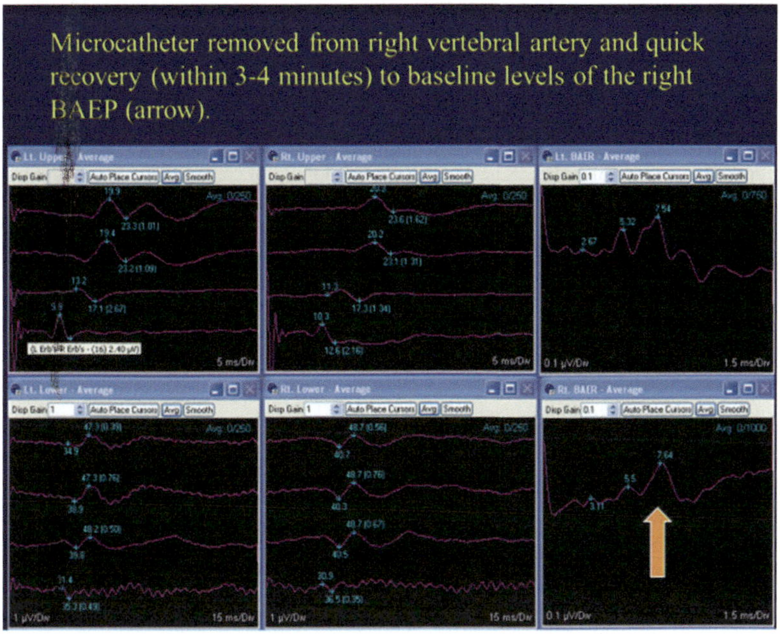

Fig. 28.17 Case Example 4: Recovery of the right BAEP within several minutes of removal of the microcatheter from the right vertebral artery

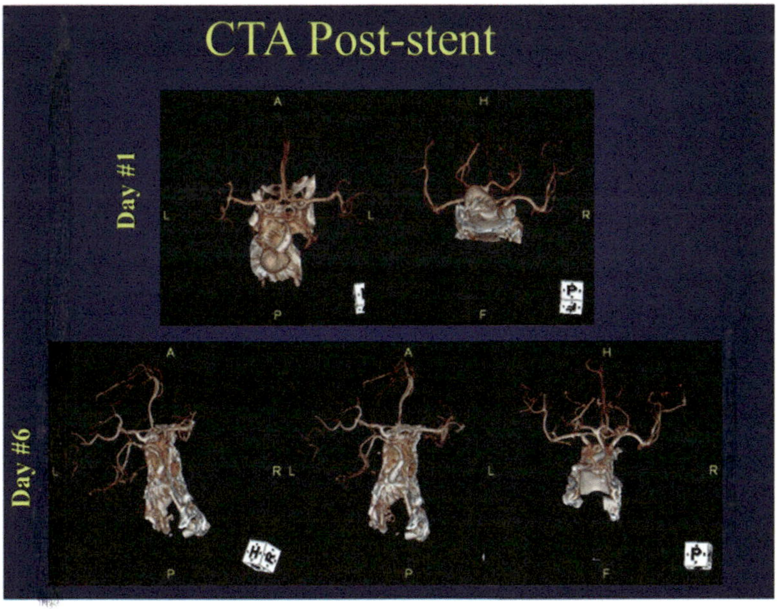

Fig. 28.18 Case Example 4: CT angiography of the head shows normal posterior circulation blood flow and minimal residual aneurysm post-procedurally

References

1. AbuRahma AF, Mousa AY, Stone PA. Shunting during carotid endarterectomy. J Vasc Surg. 2011;54(5):1502–10.
2. Ahn S, Jordan SE, Nuwer MR, Marcus DR, Moore WS. Computed electroencephalographic topographic brain mapping. A new and accurate monitor of cerebral circulation and function for patients having carotid endarterectomy. J Vasc Surg. 1988;8(3):247.
3. Albers GW, Marks MP, Kemp S, Christensen S, Tsai JP, Ortega-Gutierrez S, et al. Thrombectomy for stroke at 6 to 16 hours with selection by perfusion imaging. N Engl J Med. 2018;378(8):708–18.
4. Alcantara SD, Wuamett JC, Lantis JC, Ulkatan S, Bamberger P, Mendes D, et al. Outcomes of combined somatosensory evoked potential, motor evoked potential, and electroencephalography monitoring during carotid endarterectomy. Ann Vasc Surg. 2014;28(3):665–72.
5. Amantini A, Bartelli M, de Scisciolo G. Monitoring of somatosensory evoked potentials during carotid endarterectomy. J Neurol. 1992;239:241.
6. American Heart Association. Introducing target: stroke phase III [Internet]. [cited 2021 Jul 31]. Available from: https://www.heart.org/en/professional/quality-improvement/target-stroke/introducing-target-stroke-phase-iii.
7. Ares WJ, Grandhi RM, Panczykowski DM, Weiner GM, Thirumala P, Habeych ME, et al. Diagnostic accuracy of somatosensory evoked potential monitoring in evaluating neurological complications during endovascular aneurysm treatment. Oper Neurosurg. 2018;14(2):151–6.
8. Astrup J. Energy-requiring cell functions in the ischemic brain: their critical supply and possible inhibition in protective therapy. J Neurosurg. 1982;56(4):482.
9. Bass A, Krupski WC, Schneider PA, Otis SM, Dilley RB, Bernstein EF. Intraoperative transcranial Doppler: limitations of the method. J Vasc Surg. 1989;10(5):0549–53.
10. Beese U, Langer H, Lang W, Dinkel M. Comparison of near-infrared spectroscopy and somatosensory evoked potentials for the detection of cerebral ischemia during carotid endarterectomy. Stroke. 1998;29(10):2032.
11. Bican O, Cho C, Suarez-Roman A, Nguyen V, Lee L, Le S, et al. Superselective methohexital challenge prior to intracranial endovascular embolization. J Clin Neurosci. 2019;63:68–71.
12. Bornstein NM, Rossi GB, Treves TA, Shifrin EG. Is transcranial Doppler effective in avoiding the hazards of carotid surgery? Cardiovasc Surg. 1996;4(3):335.
13. Branston NM, Symon L, Crockard HA, Pasztor E. Relationship between the cortical evoked potential and local cortical blood flow following acute middle cerebral artery occlusion in the baboon. Exp Neurol. 1974;45(2):195.
14. Branston NM, Strong AJ, Symon L. Extracellular potassium activity, evoked potential and tissue blood flow: relationships during progressive ischaemia in baboon cerebral cortex. J Neurol Sci. 1977;32(3):305.
15. Branston NM, Ladds A, Symon L, Wang AD. Comparison of the effects of ischaemia on early components of the somatosensory evoked potential in brainstem, thalamus, and cerebral cortex. J Cereb Blood Flow Metab. 1984;4(1):68.
16. Brinkman SD, Braun P, Ganji S, Morrell RM, Jacobs LA. Neuropsychological performance one week after carotid endarterectomy reflects intraoperative ischemia. Stroke. 1984;15(3):497.
17. Buchtal A, Belopavlovic M. Somatosensory evoked potentials in cerebral aneurysm surgery. Eur J Anaesthesiol. 1992;9:493.
18. Chang SD, López JR, Steinberg GK. The usefulness of electrophysiological monitoring during resection of central nervous system vascular malformations. J Stroke Cerebrovasc Dis. 1999;8(6):412.
19. Chang R, Reddy RP, Sudadi S, Balzer J, Crammond DJ, Anetakis K, et al. Diagnostic accuracy of various EEG changes during carotid endarterectomy to detect 30-day perioperative stroke: a systematic review. Clin Neurophysiol. 2020;131(7):1508–16.

20. Chiappa KH, Burke SR, Young RR. Results of electroencephalogram monitoring during 367 carotid endarterectomies: use of a dedicated minicomputer. Stroke. 1979;10(4):381.
21. Cho I, Smullens SN, Streletz LJ, Fariello RG. The value of intraoperative EEG monitoring during carotid endarterectomy. Ann Neurol. 1986;20(4):508.
22. Church EW, Rohatgi P, Feidt AE, Kalapos P, Cockroft KM. Neurophysiological monitoring during arteriovenous malformation embolization. Oper Neurosurg. 2019;17(5):503–8.
23. Cloughesy TF, Nuwer MR, Hoch D. Monitoring carotid test occlusions with continuous EEG and clinical examination. J Clin Neurophysiol. 1993;10(3):363.
24. Davies LK, Janelle GM. Conclusion: all cardiac surgical patients should not have intraoperative cerebral oxygenation monitoring. J Cardiothorac Vasc Anesth. 2006;20(3):450.
25. De Vleeschauwer P, Horsch S, Matamoros R. Monitoring of somatosensory evoked potentials in carotid surgery: results, usefulness and limitations of the method. Ann Vasc Surg. 1988;2(1):63.
26. Debakey ME. Successful carotid endarterectomy for cerebrovascular insufficiency: nineteen-year follow-up. JAMA. 1975;233(10):1083–5.
27. Dengler J, Cabraja M, Faust K, Picht T, Kombos T, Vajkoczy P. Intraoperative neurophysiological monitoring of extracranial-intracranial bypass procedures: clinical article. J Neurosurg. 2013;119(1):207–14.
28. Diao Z, Jia G, Wu W, Wang C. Carotid endarterectomy versus carotid angioplasty for stroke prevention: a systematic review and meta-analysis. J Cardiothorac Surg. 2016;11(1):142.
29. Dickey AS, Mitsias PD, Olango WM, Agan MC, Roche WP, Thomas JR, et al. The prognostic value of quantitative EEG in patients undergoing mechanical thrombectomy for acute ischemic stroke. J Clin Neurophysiol. 2020; https://doi.org/10.1097/WNP.0000000000000769.
30. Dietz A, Von Kummer R, Adams HP, Kneip M, Galito P, Maier H. Balloon occlusion test of the internal carotid artery to examine the resectability in vascular infiltrating cervical metastasising of advanced head and neck carcinomas – experiences collected in Heidelberg. Laryngorhinootologie. 1993;72(11):558–67.
31. Domenick Sridharan N, Chaer RA, Thirumala PD, Balzer J, Long B, Tzeng E, et al. Somatosensory evoked potentials and electroencephalography during carotid endarterectomy predict late stroke but not death. Ann Vasc Surg. 2017;38:105–12.
32. Domenick Sridharan N, Thirumala P, Chaer R, Balzer J, Long B, Crammond D, et al. Predictors of cross-clamp-induced intraoperative monitoring changes during carotid endarterectomy using both electroencephalography and somatosensory evoked potentials. J Vasc Surg. 2018;67(1):191–8.
33. Duarte-Gamas L, Pereira-Neves A, Sousa J, Sousa-Pinto B, Rocha-Neves J. The diagnostic accuracy of intra-operative near infrared spectroscopy in carotid artery endarterectomy under regional anaesthesia: systematic review and meta-analysis. Eur J Vasc Endovasc Surg. 2021;62(4):522–31.
34. Eastcott HHG, Pickering GW, Rob CG. Reconstruction of internal carotid artery in a patient with intermittent attacks of hemiplegia. Lancet. 1954;264(6846):994–6.
35. Emerson RG, Turner CA. Monitoring during supratentorial surgery. J Clin Neurophysiol. 1993;10(4):404.
36. Executive Committee for the Asymptomatic Carotid Atherosclerosis Study, Marler JR, Goldstein M, Grady PA, Toole JF, Baker WH, et al. Endarterectomy for asymptomatic carotid artery stenosis. JAMA. 1995;273(18):1421–8.
37. Feng AY, Sussman ES, Jin MC, Wong S, Lopez J, Pulli B, et al. Intraoperative neuromonitoring for cerebral arteriovenous malformation embolization: a propensity-score matched retrospective database study. Cureus. 2021;13(1):e12946.
38. Fields WS, Maslenikov V, Meyer JS, Hass WK, Remington RD, Macdonald M. Joint study of extracranial arterial occlusion: V. Progress report of prognosis following surgery or nonsurgical treatment for transient cerebral ischemic attacks and cervical carotid artery lesions. JAMA. 1970;211(12):1993–2003.

39. Fisher RS, Raudzens P, Nunemacher M. Efficacy of intraoperative neurophysiological monitoring. J Clin Neurophysiol. 1995;12:97.
40. Fode NC, Sundt TM, Robertson JT, Peerless SJ, Shields CB. Multicenter retrospective review of results and complications of carotid endarterectomy in 1981. Stroke. 1986;17(3):370.
41. Fransen PSS, Beumer D, Berkhemer OA, van den Berg LA, Lingsma H, van der Lugt A, et al. MR CLEAN, a multicenter randomized clinical trial of endovascular treatment for acute ischemic stroke in the Netherlands: study protocol for a randomized controlled trial. Trials. 2014;15(1):343.
42. Friedman WA, Kaplan BL, Day AL, Sypert GW, Curran MT. Evoked potential monitoring during aneurysm operation: observations after 50 cases. Neurosurgery. 1987;20(5):678.
43. Friedman WA, Chadwick MA, Verhoeven FJ, Mahla M, Day AL. Monitoring of somatosensory evoked potentials during surgery for middle cerebral artery aneurysms. Neurosurgery. 1991;29(1):83.
44. Gavvala J, Abend N, LaRoche S, Hahn C, Herman ST, Claassen J, et al. Continuous EEG monitoring: a survey of neurophysiologists and neurointensivists. Epilepsia. 2014;55(11):1864–71.
45. Gigli GL, Caramia M, Marciani MG. Monitoring of subcortical and cortical somatosensory evoked potentials during carotid endarterectomy: comparison with stump pressure levels. Electroencephalogr Clin Neurophysiol. 1987;68(6):424.
46. Goyal M, Demchuk AM, Menon BK, Eesa M, Rempel JL, Thornton J, et al. Randomized assessment of rapid endovascular treatment of ischemic stroke. N Engl J Med. 2015;372(11):1019–30.
47. Goyal M, Menon BK, Van Zwam WH, Dippel DWJ, Mitchell PJ, Demchuk AM, et al. Endovascular thrombectomy after large-vessel ischaemic stroke: a meta-analysis of individual patient data from five randomised trials. Lancet. 2016;387(10029):1723–31.
48. Greve T, Wagner A, Ille S, Wunderlich S, Ikenberg B, Meyer B, et al. Motor evoked potentials during revascularization in ischemic stroke predict motor pathway ischemia and clinical outcome. Clin Neurophysiol. 2020;131(9):2307–14.
49. Guo LJ, Gelb AW. The use of motor evoked potential monitoring during cerebral aneurysm surgery to predict pure motor deficits due to subcortical ischemia. Clin Neurophysiol. 2011;122:648–55.
50. Halsey JH. Risks and benefits of shunting in carotid endarterectomy. Stroke. 1992;23(11):1583.
51. Hargadine JR, Branston NM, Symon L. Central conduction time in primate brain ischemia – a study in baboons. Stroke. 1980;11(6):637.
52. Haupt WF, Horsch S. Evoked potential monitoring in carotid surgery: a review of 994 cases. Neurology. 1992;42(4):835.
53. Hiramatsu R, Furuse M, Yagi R, Ohnishi H, Ikeda N, Nonoguchi N, et al. Limit of intraoperative near-infrared spectroscopy monitoring during endovascular thrombectomy in acute ischemic stroke. Interv Neuroradiol. 2018;24(1):57–63.
54. Horiuchi K, Suzuki K, Sasaki T. Intraoperative monitoring of blood flow insufficiency during surgery of middle cerebral artery aneurysms. J Neurosurg. 2005;103(2):275.
55. Ichikawa T, Suzuki K, Sasaki T, Matsumoto M, Sakuma J, Oinuma M, et al. Utility and the limit of motor evoked potential monitoring for preventing complications in surgery for cerebral arteriovenous malformation. Neurosurgery. 2010;67(Suppl. 1):ons222–8.
56. Jones TH, Morawetz RB, Crowell RM. Thresholds of focal ischemia in awake monkeys. J Neurosurg. 1981;54(6):773.
57. Jorgensen LG, Schroeder TV. Transcranial Doppler for detection of cerebral ischaemia during carotid endarterectomy. Eur J Vasc Surg. 1992;6(2):142–7.
58. Journée HL, Berends HI, Kruyt MC. The percentage of amplitude decrease warning criteria for transcranial MEP monitoring. J Clin Neurophysiol. 2017;34:22–31.
59. Kamitaki BK, Tu B, Wong S, Mendiratta A, Choi H. Quantitative EEG changes correlate with post-clamp ischemia during carotid endarterectomy. J Clin Neurophysiol. 2021;38(3):213–20.

60. Kearse LA, Brown EN, McPeck K. Somatosensory evoked potential sensitivity relative to electroencephalography for cerebral ischemia during carotid endarterectomy. Stroke. 1992;23(4):498.
61. Kearse LA, Martin D, McPeck K, Lopez-Breshnahan M. Computer-derived density spectral array in detection of mild analog electroencephalographic ischemic pattern changes during carotid endarterectomy. J Neurosurg. 1993;78(6):884.
62. Kwolek CJ, Jaff MR, Leal JI, Hopkins LN, Shah RM, Hanover TM, et al. Results of the ROADSTER multicenter trial of transcarotid stenting with dynamic flow reversal Presented at the Late Breaking Clinical Trials Session at Vascular Interventional Advances (VIVA) 2014, November 4–7, 2014. J Vasc Surg. 2015;62:1227–1234.e1.
63. Lam AM, Manninen PH, Ferguson GG, Nantua W. Monitoring electrophysiologic function during carotid endarterectomy: a comparison of somatosensory evoked potentials and conventional electroencephalogram. Anesthesiology. 1991;75(1):15.
64. Lee S, Kim DY, Bin KS, Kim W, Kang MR, Kim HJ, et al. Predictive value of neurophysiologic monitoring during neurovascular intervention for postoperative new neurologic deficits. Neuroradiology. 2019;61(2):207–15.
65. Lesnick JE, Michele JJ, Simeone FA, DeFeo S, Welsh FA. Alteration of somatosensory evoked potentials in response to global ischemia. J Neurosurg. 1984;60(3):490.
66. Levy WJ, Shapiro HM, Maruchak G, Meathe E. Automated EEG processing for intraoperative monitoring: a comparison of techniques. Anesthesiology. 1980;53(3):223.
67. Lindsey RL. A simple solution for determining shunt flow during carotid endarterectomy. Anesthesiology. 1984;61(2):215.
68. Liu AY, López JR, Do HM. Neurophysiological monitoring in the endovascular therapy of aneurysms. Am J Neuroradiol. 2003;24:1520.
69. Loftus CM, Quest DO. Technical issues in carotid artery surgery 1995. Neurosurgery. 1995;36(4):629.
70. Loftus CM, Dyste GN, Reinarz SJ, Hingtgen WL. Distal cervical carotid dissection after carotid endarterectomy: a complication of indwelling shunt? Neurosurgery. 1986;19(3):441.
71. López JR, Chang SD, Steinberg GK. The use of electrophysiological monitoring in the interoperative management of intracranial aneurysms. J Neurol Neurosurg Psychiatry. 1999;66(2):189.
72. MacDonald DB. Overview on criteria for MEP monitoring. J Clin Neurophysiol. 2017;34:4–11.
73. Malcharek MJ, Ulkatan S, Marinò V, Geyer M, Lladó-Carbó E, Perez-Fajardo G, et al. Intraoperative monitoring of carotid endarterectomy by transcranial motor evoked potential: a multicenter study of 600 patients. Clin Neurophysiol. 2013;124(5):1025–30.
74. Malcharek MJ, Herbst V, Bartz GJ, Manceur AM, Gille J, Hennig G, et al. Multimodal evoked potential monitoring in asleep patients versus neurological evaluation in awake patients during carotid endarterectomy: a single-centre retrospective trial of 651 patients. Minerva Anestesiol. 2015;81(10):1070–8.
75. Malcharek MJ, Kulpok A, Deletis V, Ulkatan S, Sablotzki A, Hennig G, et al. Intraoperative multimodal evoked potential monitoring during carotid endarterectomy: a retrospective study of 264 patients. Anesth Analg. 2015;120(6):1352–60.
76. Malcharek MJ, Hesse J, Hesselbarth K, Thoma K, Wegner C, Sablotzki A, et al. Warning criteria for MEP monitoring during carotid endarterectomy: a retrospective study of 571 patients. J Clin Monit Comput. 2020;34(3):589–95.
77. Manninen PH, Patterson S, Lam AM, Gelb AW, Nantua WE. Evoked potential monitoring during posterior fossa aneurysm surgery: a comparison of two modalities. Can J Anaesth. 1994;41(2):92.
78. Manninen P, Tan T, Sarjeant RM. Somatosensory evoked potential monitoring during carotid endarterectomy in patients with a stroke. Anesth Analg. 2001;93(1):39.

79. Markand ON. Continuous assessment of cerebral function with EEG and somatosensory evoked potential techniques during extracranial vascular reconstruction. In: Intraoperative monitoring techniques in neurosurgery. McGraw-Hill; 1994. p. 19.
80. Markand ON, Dilley RS, Moorthy S, Warren C. Monitoring of somatosensory evoked responses during carotid endarterectomy. Arch Neurol. 1984;41(4):375.
81. McDowell HA, Gross GM, Halsey JH. Carotid endarterectomy monitored with transcranial Doppler. Ann Surg. 1992;215:514–9.
82. Moorthy SS, Markand ON, Dilley RS, McCammon R, Warren CH. Somatosensory-evoked responses during carotid endarterectomy. Anesth Analg. 1982;61(10):879.
83. Morawetz RB, DeGiorlami U, Ojemann RG, Marcoux FW, Crowell RM. Cerebral blood flow determined by hydrogen clearance during middle cerebral artery occlusion in unanesthetized monkeys. Stroke. 1978;9(2):143.
84. Moresoli P, Habib B, Reynier P, Secrest MH, Eisenberg MJ, Filion KB. Carotid stenting versus endarterectomy for asymptomatic carotid artery stenosis: a systematic review and meta-analysis. Stroke. 2017;48:2150–7.
85. Moritz S, Kasprzak P, Arlt M, Taeger K, Metz C. Accuracy of cerebral monitoring in detecting cerebral ischemia during carotid endarterectomy. A comparison of transcranial Doppler sonography, near-infrared spectroscopy, stump pressure, and somatosensory evoked potentials. Anesthesiology. 2007;107(4):563.
86. Moura LMVR, Shafi MM, Ng M, Pati S, Cash SS, Cole AJ, et al. Spectrogram screening of adult EEGs is sensitive and efficient. Neurology. 2014;83(1):56–64.
87. Myers RR, Stockard JJ, Saidman LJ. Monitoring of cerebral perfusion during anesthesia by time-compressed Fourier analysis of the electroencephalogram. Stroke. 1977;8(3):331.
88. Neuloh G, Schramm J. Monitoring of motor-evoked potentials compared with somatosensory evoked potentials and microvascular Doppler ultrasonography in cerebral aneurysm surgery. J Neurosurg. 2004;100(3):389.
89. Nogueira RG, Jadhav AP, Haussen DC, Bonafe A, Budzik RF, Bhuva P, et al. Thrombectomy 6 to 24 hours after stroke with a mismatch between deficit and infarct. N Engl J Med. 2018;378(1):11–21.
90. North American Symptomatic Carotid Endarterectomy Trial Collaborators. Beneficial effect of carotid endarterectomy in symptomatic patients with high-grade carotid stenosis. Ann Intern Med. 1991;115(6 Suppl. 2):34.
91. Nwachuku EL, Balzer JR, Yabes JG, Habeych ME, Crammond DJ, Thirumala PD. Diagnostic value of somatosensory evoked potential changes during carotid endarterectomy: a systematic review and meta-analysis. JAMA Neurol. 2015;72:73–80.
92. Paiva T, Campos J, Baeta E. EEG monitoring during endovascular embolization of cerebral arteriovenous malformations. Electroencephalogr Clin Neurophysiol. 1995;95(1):3.
93. Palatinsky E, DiScenna A, McDonald H, Whittingham T, Selman W. SSEP and BAEP monitoring of temporary clip application and induced hypotension during cerebrovascular surgery. In: Intraoperative monitoring techniques in neurosurgery. McGraw-Hill; 1994. p. 61–71.
94. Pandey P, Kansara A, Thirumala P, Tamkus AA, Xavier AR. Neurophysiological monitoring with brainstem evoked potentials can be a valuable tool for patients undergoing vertebrobasilar stenting and angioplasty-initial experience. J Clin Neurophysiol. 2013;30(1):55–8.
95. Park D, Kim BH, Lee SE, Jeong E, Cho K, Park JK, et al. Usefulness of intraoperative neurophysiological monitoring during the clipping of unruptured intracranial aneurysm: diagnostic efficacy and detailed protocol. Front Surg. 2021;8:631053.
96. Paulsen RD, Steinberg GK, Norbash AM, López JR, Marks M. Embolization of rolandic cortex arteriovenous malformations. Neurosurgery. 1999;44(3):479.
97. Pedrini L, Tarantini S, Cirelli MR. Intraoperative assessment of cerebral ischaemia during carotid surgery. Int Angiol. 1998;17:10.
98. Pennekamp CWA, Bots ML, Kappelle LJ, Moll FL, de Borst GJ. The value of near-infrared spectroscopy measured cerebral oximetry during carotid endarterectomy in perioperative stroke prevention. A review. Eur J Vasc Endovasc Surg. 2009;38:539–45.

99. Perez-Borja C, Meyer JS. Electroencephalographic monitoring during reconstructive surgery of the neck vessels. Electroencephalogr Clin Neurophysiol. 1965;18(2):162.
100. Phillips JLH, Chalouhi N, Jabbour P, Starke RM, Bovenzi CD, Rosenwasser RH, et al. Somatosensory evoked potential changes in neuroendovascular procedures: incidence and association with clinical outcome in 873 patients. Neurosurgery. 2014;75(5):560–6.
101. Pokras R, Dyken ML. Dramatic changes in the performance of endarterectomy for diseases of the extracranial arteries of the head. Stroke. 1988;19(10):1289–90.
102. Quiñones-Hinojosa A, Alam M, Lyon R, Yingling CD, Lawton MT. Transcranial motor-evoked potentials during basilar artery aneurysm surgery: technique application for 30 consecutive patients. Neurosurgery. 2004;54(4):16.
103. Rampil IJ, Holzer JA, Quest DO, Rosenbaum SH, Correll JW. Prognostic value of computerized EEG analysis during carotid endarterectomy. Anesth Analg. 1983;62(2):186.
104. Redekop G, Ferguson G. Correlation of contralateral stenosis and intraoperative electroencephalogram changes with risk of stroke during carotid endarterectomy. Neurosurgery. 1992;34(2):191.
105. Reynolds MR, Derdeyn CP, Grubb RL, Powers WJ, Zipfel GJ. Extracranial-intracranial bypass for ischemic cerebrovascular disease: what have we learned from the Carotid Occlusion Surgery Study? Neurosurg Focus. 2014;36(1):E9.
106. Rigamonti A, Scandroglio M, Minicucci F. A clinical evaluation of near-infrared cerebral oximetry in the awake patient to monitor cerebral perfusion during carotid endarterectomy. J Clin Anesth. 2003;17(6):426.
107. Ritzenthaler T, Cho TH, Luis D, Berthezene Y, Nighoghossian N. Usefulness of near-infrared spectroscopy in thrombectomy monitoring. J Clin Monit Comput. 2015;29(5):585–9.
108. Ritzenthaler T, Cho TH, Mechtouff L, Ong E, Turjman F, Robinson P, et al. Cerebral near-infrared spectroscopy a potential approach for thrombectomy monitoring. Stroke. 2017;48(12):3390–2.
109. Rowed DW, Houlden DA, Burkholder LM, Taylor AB. Comparison of monitoring techniques for intraoperative cerebral ischemia. Can J Neurol Sci. 2004;31(3):347.
110. Sahaya K, Pandey AS, Thompson BG, Bush BR, Minecan DN. Intraoperative monitoring for intracranial aneurysms: the Michigan experience. J Clin Neurophysiol. 2014;31:563–7.
111. Sasaki T, Kodama N, Matsumoto M, Suzuki K, Konno Y, Sakuma J, et al. Blood flow disturbance in perforating arteries attributable to aneurysm surgery. J Neurosurg. 2007;107(1):60–7.
112. Saver JL, Goyal M, Bonafe A, Diener H-C, Levy EI, Pereira VM, et al. Stent-retriever thrombectomy after intravenous t-PA vs. t-PA alone in stroke. N Engl J Med. 2015;372(24):2285–95.
113. Schramm J, Koht A, Schmidt G. Surgical and electrophysiological observations during clipping of 134 aneurysms with evoked potential monitoring. Neurosurgery. 1990;26(1):61.
114. Schweiger H, Kamp HD, Dinkel M. Somatosensory-evoked potentials during carotid artery surgery: experience in 400 operations. Surgery. 1991;109:602.
115. Shaaban-Ali M, Momeni M, Denault A. Clinical and technical limitations of cerebral and somatic near-infrared spectroscopy as an oxygenation monitor. J Cardiothorac Vasc Anesth, WB Saunders. 2021;35:763–79.
116. Sharbrough F, Messick J, Sundt TM. Correlation of continuous electroencephalograms with cerebral blood flow measurements during carotid endarterectomy. Stroke. 1973;4(4):674.
117. Shaw DA, Venables GS, Cartlidge NEF, Bates D, Dickinson PH. Carotid endarterectomy in patients with transient cerebral ischaemia. J Neurol Sci. 1984;64(1):45–53.
118. Shiban E, Wunderlich S, Kreiser K, Lehmberg J, Hemmer B, Prothmann S, et al. Predictive value of transcranial evoked potentials during mechanical endovascular therapy for acute ischaemic stroke: a feasibility study. J Neurol Neurosurg Psychiatry. 2016;87(6):598–603.
119. Simon MV, Chiappa KH, Kilbride RD, Rordorf GA, Cambria RP, Ogilvy CS, et al. Predictors of clamp-induced electroencephalographic changes during carotid endarterectomies. J Clin Neurophysiol. 2012;29(5):462–7.
120. Sloan MA. Prevention of ischemic neurologic injury with intraoperative monitoring of selected cardiovascular and cerebrovascular procedures: roles of electroencephalography,

somatosensory evoked potentials, transcranial Doppler, and near-infrared spectroscopy. Neurol Clin. 2006;24(4):631.

121. Steiger HJ, Schäffler L, Boll J, Liechti S. Results of microsurgical carotid endarterectomy – a prospective study with transcranial Doppler and EEG monitoring, and elective shunting. Acta Neurochir. 1989;100(1–2):31–8.
122. Sundt TM. The ischemic tolerance of neural tissue and the need for monitoring and selective shunting during carotid endarterectomy. Stroke. 1983;14(1):93.
123. Sundt TM, Sharbrough FW, Anderson RE, Michenfelder JD. Cerebral blood flow measurements and electroencephalograms during carotid endarterectomy. J Neurosurg. 1974;41(3):310.
124. Sundt TM, Sharbrough F, Piepgras DG. Correlation of cerebral blood flow and electroencephalographic changes during carotid endarterectomy with results of surgery and hemodynamics of cerebral ischemia. Mayo Clin Proc. 1981;56:533.
125. Symon L. The relationship between CBF, evoked potentials and the clinical features in cerebral ischaemia. Proc 23rd Scand Neurol Congr Acta Neurol Scand. 1980;62:175.
126. Symon L, Crockard HA, Dorsch NWC, Branston NM, Juhasz J. Local cerebral blood flow and vascular reactivity in a chronic stable stroke in baboons. Stroke. 1975;6(5):482.
127. Takamura Y, Motoyama Y, Takatani T, Takeshima Y, Matsuda R, Tamura K, et al. Motor evoked potential monitoring can evaluate ischemic tolerance to carotid artery occlusion during surgery. J Clin Monit Comput. 2021;35(5):1055–62.
128. Tanabe J, Ishikawa T, Moroi J. Safe time duration for temporary middle cerebral artery occlusion in aneurysm surgery based on motor-evoked potential monitoring. Surg Neurol Int. 2017;8(1):79.
129. Thiagarajan K, Cheng HL, Huang JE, Natarajan P, Crammond DJ, Balzer JR, et al. Is two really better than one? Examining the superiority of dual modality neurophysiological monitoring during carotid endarterectomy: a meta-analysis. World Neurosurg. 2015;84(6):1941–1949.e1.
130. Thirumala PD, Thiagarajan K, Gedela S, Crammond DJ, Balzer JR. Diagnostic accuracy of EEG changes during carotid endarterectomy in predicting perioperative strokes. J Clin Neurosci, Churchill Livingstone. 2016;25:1–9.
131. Thirumala PD, Udesh R, Muralidharan A, Thiagarajan K, Crammond DJ, Chang YF, et al. Diagnostic value of somatosensory-evoked potential monitoring during cerebral aneurysm clipping: a systematic review. World Neurosurg. 2016;89:672–80.
132. Tiberio G, Floriani M, Giulini SM. Monitoring of somatosensory evoked potentials during carotid endarterectomy: relationship with different haemodynamic parameters and clinical outcome. Eur J Vasc Surg. 1991;5(6):647.
133. Trojaborg W, Boysen G. Relation between EEG, regional cerebral blood flow and internal carotid artery pressure during carotid endarterectomy. Electroencephalogr Clin Neurophysiol. 1973;34(1):61–9.
134. Udesh R, Natarajan P, Thiagarajan K, Wechsler LR, Crammond DJ, Balzer JR, et al. Transcranial doppler monitoring in carotid endarterectomy: a systematic review and meta-analysis. J Ultrasound Med. 2017;36(3):621–30.
135. Wahr J, Tremper KK, Samra S, Delpy DT. Near-infrared spectroscopy: theory and applications. J Cardiothorac Vasc Anesth. 1996;10(3):406.
136. Wassmann H, Fischdick G, Jain KK. Cerebral protection during carotid endarterectomy–EEG monitoring as a guide to the use of intraluminal shunts. Acta Neurochir. 1984;71(1–2):99.
137. Whittemore AD. Carotid endarterectomy and alternative approach. Arch Surg. 1980;115(8):940.
138. Wilent WB, Belyakina O, Korsgaard E, Tjoumakaris SI, Gooch MR, Jabbour P, et al. Intraoperative vascular complications during 2278 cerebral endovascular procedures with multimodality IONM: relationship between signal change, complication, intervention and postoperative outcome. J Neurointerv Surg. 2021;13(4):378–82.
139. Wöber C, Zeitlhofer J, Asenbaum S. Monitoring of median nerve somatosensory evoked potentials in carotid surgery. J Clin Neurophysiol. 1998;15(5):429.

140. Yu Y, Zhang K, Zhang L, Zong H, Meng L, Han R. Cerebral near-infrared spectroscopy (NIRS) for perioperative monitoring of brain oxygenation in children and adults. Cochrane Database Syst Rev. 2018;1(1):CD010947.
141. Zampella E, Morawetz RB, McDowell HA. The importance of cerebral ischemia during carotid endarterectomy. Neurosurgery. 1991;29(5):727.
142. Zhu F, Chui J, Herrick I, Martin J. Intraoperative evoked potential monitoring for detecting cerebral injury during adult aneurysm clipping surgery: a systematic review and meta-analysis of diagnostic test accuracy. BMJ Open. 2019;9:e022810.

Chapter 29
Intraoperative Neurophysiologic Monitoring for Thoracic and Thoracoabdominal Aortic Procedures

Felix W. Chang and Jaime R. López

Abbreviations

ACP	Antegrade cerebral perfusion
AH	Abductor hallucis
ASA	Anterior spinal artery
BCR	Bulbocavernosus reflex
CMAP	Compound muscle action potential
CPB	Cardiopulmonary bypass
CSF	Cerebrospinal fluid
CT	Computed tomography
DHCA	Deep hypothermic circulatory arrest
ECI	Electrocerebral inactivity
EMG	Electromyography
EP	Evoked potential
HCA	Hypothermic circulatory arrest
IONM	Intraoperative neurophysiologic monitoring
mA	Milliamps
MAP	Mean arterial pressure
MEP	Motor evoked potential

F. W. Chang (✉)
Department of Neurology and Neurological Sciences, Stanford University, Stanford, CA, USA
e-mail: felixchang@stanford.edu

J. R. López
Department of Neurology and Neurological Sciences, Stanford University, Stanford, CA, USA

Department of Neurosurgery (Courtesy), Stanford University, Stanford, CA, USA

S. M. Verst et al. (eds.), *Intraoperative Monitoring*,
https://doi.org/10.1007/978-3-030-95730-8_29

MRA	Magnetic resonance angiography
NPV	Negative predictive value
PPV	Positive predictive value
PSA	Posterior spinal artery
RCP	Retrograde cerebral perfusion
SACP	Selective antegrade cerebral perfusion
SCBF	Spinal cord blood flow
SCI	Spinal cord injury
SNAP	Sensory nerve action potential
SSEP	Somatosensory evoked potential
TA	Tibialis anterior
TAAA	Thoracoabdominal aortic aneurysm
TcMEP	Transcranial motor evoked potential
TEVAR	Thoracic endovascular aortic repair

Introduction

Spinal cord ischemia and infarction has been a well-recognized and feared complication of thoracic aortic and thoracoabdominal aortic surgery since its earliest days. Development of spinal cord infarction can lead to paraparesis or paraplegia, a devastating neurologic injury. In 1951, Lam and Aram reported one of the first known thoracic aortic repairs. In their report, this initial patient developed marked lower extremity weakness and neurogenic bladder postoperatively, with partial recovery at discharge. Historical rates of paraparesis and paraplegia have been reported at 16% [99]. Surgeries of the thoracic or thoracoabdominal aorta carry a high risk of spinal cord ischemia as it is necessary to temporarily or permanently interrupt the intercostal or segmental arteries which supply the spinal cord. Following interruption of these arteries, the spinal cord will have increased reliance on the collateral network supplied by other blood vessels not arising from the aorta, such as the vertebral artery or the hypogastric vascular network. If this collateral network is not sufficient, then spinal cord ischemia will occur.

A variety of methods have been investigated and implemented over time that have lowered the rate of spinal cord injury. IONM, the use of intraoperative neurophysiologic testing to monitor the integrity of neural structures, has gained popularity since its introduction in the field. IONM techniques can accurately identify intraoperative spinal ischemia to help guide intraoperative and potentially postoperative management. The goals of this chapter are as follows:

1. Review the vascular anatomy of the spinal cord.
2. Describe the neurologic injury which can occur in procedures of the descending aorta.
3. Describe the neuroprotective measures that can be taken.
4. Review the evidence base for the various IONM modalities.
5. Illustrate the practical aspects of IONM with clinical cases.

Vascular Anatomy of the Spinal Cord

To understand and recognize intraoperative spinal cord ischemia, a detailed knowledge of the vascular anatomy of the spinal cord is required. There can be great variability in the exact vasculature between patients, which may explain why some patients are more susceptible to injury than others.

The overall blood supply of the spinal cord can be described as a collateral network with many different inputs. The anterior two thirds of the spinal cord is usually supplied mainly by the anterior spinal artery (ASA), which runs longitudinally along the anterior surface of the spinal cord. The posterior third of the spinal cord is usually supplied by two posterior spinal arteries (PSAs), which run longitudinally along the posterior surface of the spinal cord and parallel to each other. The ASA and PSA give rise to penetrating sulcal arteries which feed the interior portions of the cord.

Along the thoracic and lumbar regions, the spinal cord receives blood flow from segmental arteries. These arise in pairs from the descending aorta. In the thoracic region, these segmental arteries are known as posterior intercostal arteries. Above T3, multiple segmental arteries may arise from the aortic arch or costocervical trunk as the superior intercostal artery. Below T3, each pair usually supplies a single spinal segment, and there are typically nine of these pairs. In the lumbar region, the segmental arteries are known as lumbar segmental arteries, with usually four pairs [86]. There are extensive communications between the segmental arteries at each level. At some levels, the segmental arteries will give off branches, anterior and posterior radiculomedullary arteries (or radicular arteries), which supply the spinal cord (see Fig. 29.1).

At the cervical level, the ASA usually arises at the foramen magnum and is formed from branches descending from the vertebral arteries. The ASA extends to the conus medullaris distally [86]. Anterior radiculomedullary arteries derived from the segmental arteries provide additional blood flow to the ASA as it travels caudally. Although named and often drawn as a single continuous artery, the ASA may be better thought of as a series of anastomotic vascular loops derived from Y-shaped feeding arteries. Between these larger arteries, many connections exist, creating a continuous network of vascular arcades [48]. See Fig. 29.2.

The PSAs originate at the level of the foramen magnum and are usually supplied by branches from the vertebral or posterior inferior cerebellar arteries. As the PSA descends, it is reinforced by blood supply from the posterior radiculomedullary arteries, which arise from the segmental arteries at each level [86]. Similar to the ASA, the PSAs can be discontinuous and can potentially cross from one side to the other at different levels. The PSA can be thought of as a ladder-like longitudinal network [48]. Transverse and oblique branches from the ASA and PSA form anastomoses between the arteries, forming the pial plexus. The pial plexus does not provide much collateral flow between the ASA and PSA, especially in the thoracolumbar regions. Compared to the ASA, the PSA has lower vascular resistance, as the PSA has more connections between large vessels. Higher resistance, among

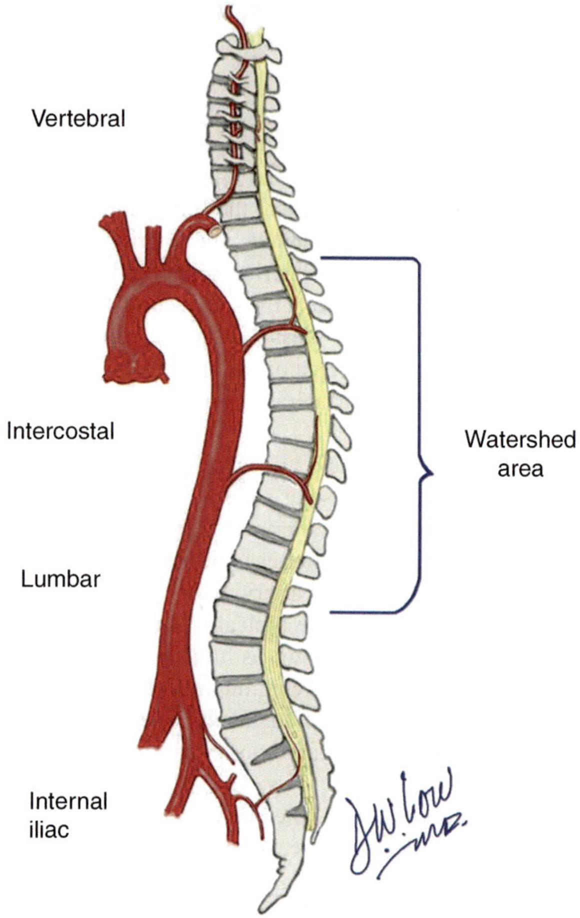

Fig. 29.1 Radiculomedullary (radicular) arteries are given off branches of the intercostal and lumbar segmental arteries every few spinal levels. These arteries reinforce the spinal cord blood flow at these levels. Watershed zones exist between radicular artery segments. The lower thoracic cord is more prone to ischemia as there is less collateral flow present and may be mainly dependent on the artery of Adamkiewicz (arteria radicularis magna). (Reprinted with permission from Cheung AT, López JR. Spinal Cord Ischemia Monitoring and Protection. Evidence-Based Pract Perioper Card Anesth Surg. 2021;323–43. Copyright 2021 Springer Nature Switzerland AG)

other reasons, means the ASA is relatively more susceptible to ischemia than the PSA [48]. Porcine studies have shown that there is a high dependence on epidural arcades to provide immediate backup flow during aortic occlusion [56]. As the blood supply of the spinal cord is a collateral network, it is logical to assume that increasing perfusion pressure by increasing mean arterial pressure and/or decreasing cerebrospinal fluid pressure can augment blood flow and reverse ischemia.

As the ASA is often discontinuous, areas between two feeding arteries can be susceptible to ischemia. Watershed levels have been observed at T1, T5, and T8–T9 [17, 40, 41]. The largest thoracolumbar anterior radiculomedullary artery is the artery of Adamkiewicz or arteria radicularis magna. This arises between T8 and L2 in 75% of patients but can also range from T5 to L4 [12, 16, 49, 60]. The artery of Adamkiewicz is important, as there is minimal collateral blood supply to the cord in the region the artery of Adamkiewicz supplies. There are typically no other anterior radiculomedullary feeders that arise below the level of the artery of Adamkiewicz

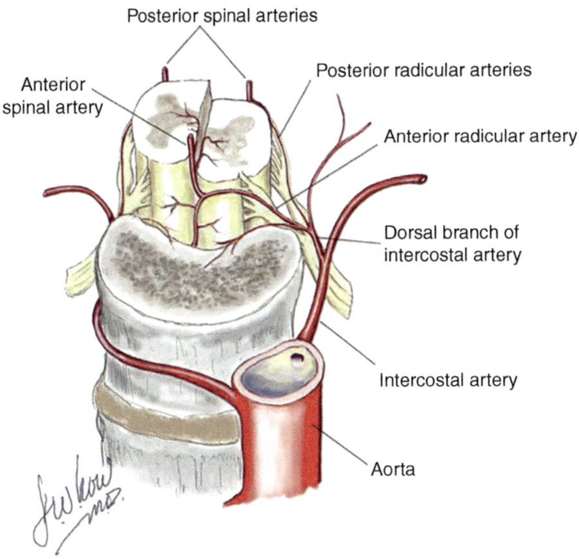

Fig. 29.2 A transverse section of the spinal cord shows the typical blood supply at a given spinal level. A pair of segmental (intercostal or lumbar) arteries is given off from the descending aorta. These give rise to the anterior and posterior radiculomedullary (radicular) arteries, which reinforce blood supply to the anterior spinal artery and posterior spinal arteries. (Reprinted with permission from Cheung AT, López JR. Spinal Cord Ischemia Monitoring and Protection. Evidence-Based Pract Perioper Card Anesth Surg. 2021;323–43. Copyright 2021 Springer Nature Switzerland AG)

[86]. The levels at which radiculomedullary arteries arise vary between patients. Embryologically, initially these occur at regular intervals at every thoracolumbar spinal level. As development continues however, these regress at irregular segments, explaining the variability between patients [113]. The vascular anatomy of the spinal cord is of importance in thoracic aortic and thoracoabdominal procedures, as they involve periods of clamping of the descending aorta and can involve sacrifice of the intercostal arteries.

Overview of Spinal Cord Ischemia and Stroke in Procedures of the Descending Aorta

Incidence

In Svensson et al. [99], a retrospective study of 1509 patients and 1679 thoracoabdominal aortic aneurysm (TAAA) repairs between 1960 and 1991 at a single center and one of the largest single studies on outcomes in TAAA, the overall incidence of paraplegia or paraparesis was 16% (234 of 1509 patients). The incidence of stroke was 3% (39 of 1509 patients). In a more contemporary study, by Coselli et al. [20], the rate of paraplegia/paraparesis was lower, likely the result of many improvements in surgical techniques over time. The authors looked at 2286 TAAA repairs at a single institution between 1986 and 2007 and found an incidence of 6.3% of spinal cord injury (SCI), and 1.7% of stroke.

Thoracic endovascular aortic repair (TEVAR) was first approved in the USA in 2005 following the GORE TAG trial [72]. It was initially thought that TEVAR may have been associated with a lower risk of spinal cord ischemia. Compared to open repair, the aorta is not cross-clamped during TEVAR, which avoids any reperfusion syndrome and causes less physiological disturbances. In the original GORE TAG trial, which enrolled patients with isolated descending thoracic aortic aneurysms, 3% (4 of 142) of patients developed paraplegia, and 4% (5 of 152) stroke [72]. In Buth et al. [13], paraplegia or paraparesis was seen in 2.5% (15 of 606) of patients, and stroke was observed in 3.1% (19 of 606) of patients. A prospective comparison of surgical and endovascular repair was performed by Greenberg et al. [42]. The authors evaluated 724 patients and found no statistically significant difference in the incidence of SCI between the open and endovascular repair (7.5% vs 4.3%, $p = 0.08$). Similar rates of injury were also noted between the two techniques across different extent repairs. Unfortunately, the stroke incidence was not reported. Although not certain, the lower incidence of SCI in earlier studies was likely due to populations with less extensive aneurysms being enrolled. In subsequent studies rates appeared similar in TEVAR. Ullery et al. [105] reported 2.8% (12 of 425) of patients with SCI, Scali et al. [88] reported an incidence of 9.2% (68 of 741), and Dias et al. [26] reported an incidence of SCI of 31%.

Risk Factors

In Svensson et al. [99], several risk factors for SCI were identified in open TAAA repair, which included total aortic clamp time, the extent of aortic repair, presence of aortic rupture, age, history of renal dysfunction, and concurrent presence of a proximal aortic aneurysm. Crawford extent II patients (proximal descending aorta to below the renal arteries), which made up 29% of patients (442 of 1509), had the highest incidence of SCI, at 31.5%, and additionally had a stroke rate of 5%. Figure 29.3 illustrates the Crawford classification system for aneurysms. Compared to extent I aneurysms (proximal descending aorta to the upper abdominal aorta), extent II aneurysms had an odds ratio of 1.73 for injury. The odds ratio for spinal cord injury compared to extent I aneurysms was 0.33 in extent III (distal descending aorta to the abdominal aorta) and 0.18 in extent IV (abdominal aorta). To summarize, the risk of SCI in descending order is extent II, extent I, extent III, and extent IV, which corresponds to increases in the involvement of the thoracic aorta. Each additional minute of aortic clamp time was associated with an odds ratio of 1.02 for paraplegia/paraparesis. In Coselli et al. [20], extent II repairs again showed the highest incidence of SCI at 6.3%, compared to 3.3% in extent I, 2.6% in extent III, and 1.4% in extent IV.

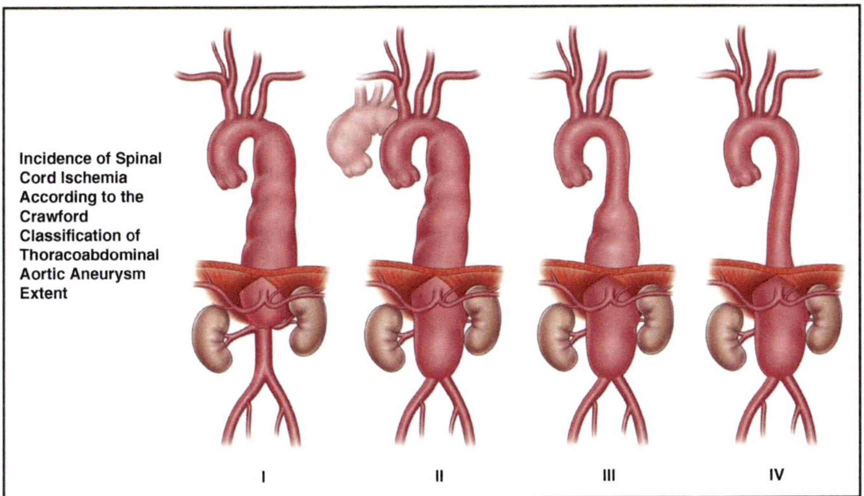

	I	II	III	IV
Endovascular Repair	10%	19%	5%	3%
Open Surgical REpair	14%	22%	10%	2%

Fig. 29.3 The rates of spinal cord ischemia from Greenberg et al. [42] in endovascular and open surgical repair of TAAA are shown according to their Crawford class. (Reprinted with permission from Cheung AT, López JR. Spinal Cord Ischemia Monitoring and Protection. Evidence-Based Pract Perioper Card Anesth Surg. 2021;323–43. Copyright 2021 Springer Nature Switzerland AG)

The degree of repair in TEVAR was similarly found to be one of the main risk factors for developing SCI in Greenberg et al. [42], who compared endovascular and open surgical repair of TAAA. In extent II repair, where the highest rate of SCI occurred, the rate of SCI was 19% in endovascular repair and 22% in open repair. In TEVAR as well, multiple studies confirmed extent of repair/length of aortic graft as the main risk factor for spinal cord ischemia [9, 26, 88]. Some of the other risk factors that have also been identified include age, history of renal insufficiency, and duration of procedure [13, 88].

Timeframe

SCI following TAAA repair can be seen in an immediate or delayed fashion. Most studies define immediate as occurring less than one day postoperatively. Delayed injury can occur after 1 day, or even several weeks later. In Greenberg et al. [42], which compared open and endovascular repair, most SCI tended to be delayed (more than 1 day postoperatively), 71% in the open repair group and 87% in the endovascular group. A similar trend was observed in Ullery et al. [105] where 83% of spinal cord injuries were delayed. Etz et al. [33] also observed in a series of 858 TAAA repairs that of the total of 20 patients (2.3%) who developed paraplegia, 3 of

20 occurred intraoperatively, 10 of 20 occurred with 48 hours of surgery despite intact somatosensory evoked potentials (SSEPs) at the end of surgery, and 7 of 20 occurred later. Estrera et al. [30] retrospectively analyzed factors that predicted delayed neurologic deficit in TAAA repair in 854 patients. The overall neurologic deficit rate was 6.9%, and the rate of delayed deficit was 2.7%. They found that preoperative renal dysfunction, acute dissection, and extent II repair were significant predictors of a delayed deficit. Additionally, the authors found that using adjuncts such as distal aortic perfusion and CSF drainage was associated with an increased risk of delayed ischemia ($p < .03$). They suggested this was because patients that previously developed immediate neurologic deficit instead developed delayed deficits due to the intraoperative protective effects of these adjunctive measures.

Protective Measures Against Cerebral and Spinal Cord Ischemia

There are a variety of methods in use to decrease the risk of ischemia of the brain and spinal cord. In the following section, we will review the most common of these methodologies. Understanding the principles of these techniques and their intersection with IONM facilitates more accurate monitoring and modifications in the procedure in response to IONM changes. The techniques discussed vary in use at different institutions, and there may be a preference for a particular technique at each institution. A discussion of how these techniques compare to each other is beyond the scope of this chapter.

Hypothermia

Hypothermia to 27 °C was first described by Lewis and Taufic [66] in 1953. Deep hypothermia was first described in cardiothoracic surgery in 1975 by Griepp et al. [44] who described cooling to 14 °C in aortic arch replacement. The introduction of hypothermia facilitated the development of increasingly complex surgeries. Procedures involving the aorta may necessitate temporarily stopping perfusion to the brain and/or spine. Neural tissues are highly metabolically active and sensitive to ischemia. Hypothermia mainly reduces injury by greatly reducing the global cerebral metabolic rate for glucose and oxygen, reducing the metabolism by 5–7% for every 1 °C decrease in temperature [29]. The reduction in cerebral or spinal metabolism allows for temporary interruption of perfusion while decreasing risk of ischemic injury.

Deep hypothermic circulatory arrest (DHCA) involves circulatory arrest and deep hypothermia, which is defined as 14.1–20 °C [104]. Hypothermia is achieved prior to circulatory arrest. Some of the advantages of this include a bloodless surgical field and no need to clamp the proximal aorta [61]. Disadvantages include hypothermic tissue damage, long cardiopulmonary bypass (CPB) times, coagulopathy, and possible neurocognitive effects [106, 111, 112]. DHCA time is limited to around 45 minutes. Gega et al. [39] showed that patients undergoing aortic arch surgery with DHCA lasting >40 minutes had a stroke rate of 13.1% compared to 3.3% in cases <40 minutes.

From an IONM perspective, it is likely that there will be no monitorable EEG, SSEPs, or transcranial motor evoked potentials (TcMEPs) during DHCA, as the low temperature, once reached, will usually obliterate these signals. Additionally, in any procedure with circulatory arrest, defibrillation may be needed prior to closure. Disconnecting the amplifier from the patient's body prior to any defibrillation is advised to avoid any potential damage to equipment.

Moderate hypothermic circulatory arrest (MHCA) is similar to DHCA, except with a targeted temperature of 20.1 °C–28 °C [102]. MHCA was introduced in an attempt to address some of these disadvantages of DHCA. MHCA is typically combined with cold perfusion to the brain, initially with retrograde cerebral perfusion (RCP) but now more commonly antegrade cerebral perfusion (ACP) (to be discussed further in the next section). The rationale for MHCA is that by providing cold blood to the brain, the benefit of greatly reduced cerebral metabolism is maintained, while some of the systemic disadvantages can be mitigated [5]. This technique has gained popularity since its introduction. Some disadvantages of MHCA+ACP are related to the presence of increased catheters compared to DHCA. There is a potential for catheter-induced trauma to the neck vessels, aortic dissection, air embolism, and embolism of atherosclerotic plaques [114]. DHCA tends to be necessary in thoracic aortic and thoracoabdominal aortic repair when cross-clamping of the proximal aorta is not feasible due to excessive plaque or fragility of the vessel in that area [111, 112].

Perfusion Strategies

There are a variety of perfusion strategies in use to avoid injury to neural structures, as well as other organs. These strategies can sometimes be used together and in conjunction with varying degrees of hypothermia. Understanding these strategies can help in determining which structures may be at higher risk for ischemia.

Cardiopulmonary Bypass (CPB)

Cardiopulmonary bypass is a technique that, as the name suggests, bypasses the heart and lungs, allowing for surgery to take place on cardiovascular structures, such as the aorta. The CPB circuit involves several components. Blood is removed from the body through venous cannulation and suction from the surgical field where it goes to a reservoir. Roller and/or centrifugal pumps at multiple points help propel the blood through the circuit. Along the circuit are filters, heat exchangers, and oxygenators. The blood is then brought back to the body through arterial cannulation sites [87]. In TAAA surgery, common sites of venous cannulation include the right atrium and left femoral vein. Arterial cannulation sites can include the left femoral artery, proximal aorta, and visceral vessels [62]. Exact sites of cannulation will vary between surgeries and surgeons. Complications of CPB include bleeding, air embolism, arterial dissection, systemic inflammation, platelet dysfunction, plaque embolization, and clotting [87].

Left Heart Bypass (LHB)

Left heart bypass is an alternative bypass technique to CPB. The pulmonary vein or left atrium is cannulated, blood is pumped out of the body in a system with a heat exchanger, and a distal site is cannulated. In TAAA, the left femoral artery is a frequently chosen cannulation site. Retrograde flow allows perfusion of the distal aorta and right leg. Unlike CPB, no oxygenation occurs outside the body during LHB as the blood is removed from the body after passing through the lungs. This means that single lung physiology must be sufficient for oxygenation for LHB to be possible. LHB can also reduce left ventricular strain (which is increased during surgery due to proximal aortic clamping) and allows more immediate control of hemodynamics [1, 90].

Retrograde Cerebral Perfusion (RCP)

Retrograde cerebral perfusion involves a perfusion catheter being placed in the superior vena cava, and cold, oxygenated blood being perfused to the brain in a retrograde fashion [4]. RCP theoretically may help in removing embolic material, as the flow is retrograde. It also is simpler to employ compared to antegrade cerebral perfusion. However, a porcine study by Ehrlich et al. [28] showed that there was negligible cerebral capillary flow during RCP and that some of the advantage seen from RCP may be facilitated by more efficient cooling.

Antegrade Cerebral Perfusion (ACP)

Antegrade cerebral perfusion or selective antegrade cerebral perfusion (SACP) involves perfusing the brain by placing perfusion catheters into the aortic branches supplying the brain. Blood flows in an antegrade fashion (physiologically) in this technique. This can be done either unilaterally or bilaterally. Common cannulation sites include the right axillary, innominate, common carotid artery, and/or the left common carotid artery [4]. If unilateral perfusion is utilized, the patient must have sufficient collateral cerebral blood flow, or the contralateral hemisphere will become ischemic. ACP is often combined with MHCA, with cold, oxygenated blood being directly perfused to the brain [6]. Excessive flow can cause cerebral edema [4]. The use of catheters in the vessels brings with it the risks of embolization and dissection.

Pharmacologic

There are many medications which have been studied for neuroprotection. There is at most weak evidence for their benefit. These agents include corticosteroids, inhaled anesthetics, propofol, lidocaine, magnesium, thiopental, mannitol, and others. The proposed mechanism of neuroprotection includes reducing excitotoxicity, reducing cerebral edema, reducing inflammation, stabilizing the electrochemical membrane, and reducing calcium influx [73].

Lumbar Drain

Spinal cord perfusion pressure is related to mean arterial pressure (MAP) and cerebrospinal fluid (CSF) pressure. Increasing MAP can increase the perfusion pressure and decreasing the CSF pressure does the same. The MAP can be controlled through a variety of pharmacologic and other methods. A lumbar drain, a catheter inserted into the CSF space, can drain CSF and decrease pressure, thereby increasing perfusion pressure. The use of lumbar drains in TAAA has been the subject of several meta-analyses. The earliest, by Cinà et al. [19], analyzed 14 studies, including 3 randomized control trials, and found 1396 patients in which a lumbar drain was used. The pooled odds ratio of all studies for paraplegia was 0.3. In a Cochrane review by Khan et al. [59], a pooled odds ratio of 0.48 was found, with the conclusion that there was limited data for the use of CSF drainage and that more studies were needed. Khan et al. [116] found that the relative risk of spinal cord injury was 0.44 when CSF drainage was used. A subgroup analysis found that there was no benefit for late spinal cord injury. Some of the possible complications of a lumbar drain include over-drainage resulting in subdural hematoma, spinal epidural hematoma, meningitis, and low CSF pressure headache necessitating epidural blood patch.

Reimplantation of Intercostal and Other Segmental Arteries

From an anatomic perspective, reimplantation of intercostal arteries and/or other segmental arteries makes sense. Major branches of the aorta like the celiac, superior mesenteric, inferior mesenteric, and renal arteries are regularly anastomosed to the graft to prevent ischemia of visceral organs. However, unlike the visceral organs, the spinal cord is supplied by a series of many smaller arteries arising from the aorta. Attaching all of these small vessels to the graft might substantially increase operative and ischemic time exposing the patient to higher rates of morbidity and mortality. In one of the first reported TAAA repairs, Lam and Aram [63] determined that the intercostal arteries at the level of the aneurysm were minimally functional, as pressure on the aneurysm sac following clamping did not result in a decrease of the sac size, and no reimplantation was performed. Since then, a number of different strategies for reimplantation have been explored. There is no clear consensus on the extent of reimplantation of intercostal and lumbar arteries that is preferred, and practice varies between surgeons. Strategies include limited reimplanting, reimplanting based on evoked potential changes, regular reimplanting of a subset of vessels, and reimplanting based on preoperative radiologic imaging [31, 32, 85]. It should be noted that in TEVAR, the intercostal arteries will be excluded in areas of graft coverage, as there is no way to reimplant them endovascularly.

In a retrospective series of 343 patients undergoing surgical TAAA repair by Safi et al. [85], the effect of intercostal reimplantation at levels from T7 to T12 was studied. The authors found that when T11 and T12 intercostal arteries were reimplanted or already occluded, patients had a lower rate of neurologic deficits ($p < .006$ for occlusion and $p < .03$ for reimplantation). Additionally, in patients where T11 and T12 were ligated, the rate of neurologic deficit was much higher, at 50%, compared to 12.9% in the reimplanted group. Reimplantation of T9 or T10 intercostal arteries was associated with a reduction in late neurologic deficits ($p = .05$) but did not modify early or overall neurologic deficits. Similarly, in Svensson et al. [100], a series of 99 patients, the authors reported that in patients who had one or more arteries at T11, T12, or L1 oversewn, the rate of neurologic deficit was 48% vs 27% in patients who had these vessels reattached or already occluded ($p = .05$). Oversewing all T11–L1 arteries was associated with a deficit in 63% vs 25% in patients where T11–L1 arteries were reattached ($p = 0.01$). Reattachment of all vessels from T7 to L4 did not show statistical significance in neurologic deficit.

Ross et al. [84] looked at segmental artery reimplantation in 132 patients undergoing TAAA repair with reimplantation of T8–L2 segmental arteries. The patients undergoing reimplantation were a consecutive cohort, compared to surgeries performed prior to the adoption of reimplantation at the authors' institution. They found that postoperative paraplegia was lower in the reimplantation group, with 0 of 41 patients in the reimplantation group developing paraplegia, compared to 8 of 91 (8.8%) in the non-reimplantation group ($p = .05$). They also noted that the average cross-clamp time was not significantly different between the two groups (30.3 vs 31.0 minutes in the reimplantation group).

Additional studies have been performed that have attempted to identify important intercostal arteries, such as the artery of Adamkiewicz, for reimplantation preoperatively. Williams et al. [110] performed spinal angiography preoperatively on 131 patients with extent I or extent II aneurysms undergoing surgical repair. They identified the artery of Adamkiewicz in 43% of patients and subsequently reimplanted it in those patients. Patients who did not have it identified had reimplantation of a set of intercostals with the level based on the surgeon's judgment. In the patients who had this artery identified, it was noted that 0 of 45 patients with degenerative aneurysms had spinal cord dysfunction, compared to 9 of 55 patients (16%) who did not have the artery of Adamkiewicz identified ($p = 0.01$). When comparing the whole population, there was no difference as this included patient with aortic dissection. In this study, they observed that in degenerative aneurysms, more intercostals were found to be occluded, and there was a robust paravertebral collateral network compared to patients with dissection, where they found almost always open intercostals. Therefore, in degenerative aneurysms a single pair of open intercostals may have much greater relative importance on spinal cord perfusion than in dissection. Mell et al. [74] looked at using magnetic resonance angiography (MRA) for identification of the artery of Adamkiewicz, the major intercostal source of this artery, and the anterior spinal artery. They were able to identify the intercostal artery supplying the artery of Adamkiewicz in 23 of 27 patients (85%). No patients developed paraplegia. The study was not able to make a conclusion on outcome given its small size. Reimplanted intercostal arteries appear to be patent over time. David et al. [24] reported that nine of ten patients demonstrated patency of reimplanted segmental arteries on 24-month follow-up computed tomography (CT) scans.

In a study that analyzed the impact of intercostal artery reimplantation on paralysis risk in TAAA repair by Acher et al. [2], the authors evaluated 655 patients and found that intercostal artery reimplantation reduced the rate of paralysis from 4.83% to 0.88%. They also determined that intercostal blood flow accounts for 20% of the risk of paraplegia, while the remaining risk was related to factors affecting collateral blood flow and metabolism (as determined by calculating the effect on risk of MAP, cardiac function, CSF drainage, and other neuroprotective measures).

More recently, some have questioned the practice of reimplantation of intercostal arteries. Wynn et al. [109] analyzed 805 patients undergoing thoracic aortic and TAAA repair. In this cohort, patients from 2005 to 2013 underwent intercostal reimplantation from T7 to L2, while patients from 1989 to 2005 did not. They found no statistically significant difference in SCI in groups with and without intercostal reimplantation (5.1% vs 8.8%, $p = 0.152$). A subgroup analysis of extent II patients also did not find a significant difference. A power calculation confirmed the study was appropriately powered to detect a difference. They concluded that the current neuroprotective measures were sufficient to prevent spinal cord ischemia associated with intercostal artery sacrifice.

Etz et al. [32] also felt that routine reimplantation of intercostal vessels was unnecessary. The authors conducted a study on 100 patients with the use of transcranial MEP (TcMEP) and SSEP monitoring where serial segmental arteries were sacrificed. TcMEPs were recorded from the tibialis anterior and abductor pollicis, stimulation was supramaximal, and a 50% amplitude decrement was considered critical. SSEPs were stimulated from the bilateral posterior tibial nerves. The authors sacrificed an average of 8 segmental artery pairs overall, with an average of 4.5 pairs sacrificed in the T7–L1 region, where the artery of Adamkiewicz usually arises from. They had two cases of postoperative paraplegia. One of these patients had intraoperative dissection with prolonged lower body ischemia with SSEP/MEP loss, and the other developed paraplegia following a postoperative respiratory arrest. Three patients had reversible MEP/SSEP changes, relieved by lightening anesthesia or raising MAP. The authors suggested one reason for their good outcomes may have been that they sacrificed segmental arteries prior to opening the aneurysm sac, limiting backbleeding and reducing steal. Backbleeding refers to the retrograde flow out of the spinal cord into the hypotensive aorta that can occur after the aneurysm is opened. This causes a steal phenomenon, reducing spinal cord perfusion.

Some surgeons prefer to guide intercostal artery reimplantation based on MEP/SSEP changes, as these might identify critical segments intraoperatively [31]. The use of evoked potentials will be discussed further in the subsequent section on the monitoring of TAAA repair.

Relationship of Regional Spinal Cord Blood Flow and Evoked Potentials

In the previous chapter on the monitoring of cerebrovascular disorders, we discussed that the relationship between SSEP, electroencephalography (EEG), and regional cerebral blood flow has been well described. Having a good understanding of the relationship between regional blood flow and electrophysiologic studies can lead to more precise correlation of changes in signals being related to ischemia. For spinal cord ischemia, the relationship is not well established; there have been a few similar studies in animals but not to the same extent as for cerebral blood flow.

There have been a few studies which have evaluated regional spinal cord blood flow in porcine, rabbit, and sheep models. In Haldenwang et al. [45], motor evoked potentials (MEPs) and regional spinal cord blood flow (SCBF) were measured in pigs undergoing a frozen elephant trunk surgery (a hybrid procedure with open aortic arch replacement and thoracic endovascular stenting of the proximal descending aorta). Half the pigs were randomized to have their thoracic segmental arteries from T4 to T13 clipped. Spinal cord blood flow was measured by tracking fluorescent microspheres, MEP stimulation was performed with epidural electrodes, and the pigs were cooled to 28 °C.

Thoracic SCBF was not significantly changed at baseline versus during selective cerebral perfusion, and there was no significant difference seen between the clipped and non-clipped groups. The clipped group did have significantly less hyperperfusion after CPB ended compared to the non-clipped group. Lumbar SCBF declined greatly in clipped and non-clipped groups during selective cerebral perfusion, with no difference between the two groups. In the group with segmental artery clipping, lumbar SCBF declined from 7.79 ml/min/100 g at baseline to 1.15 ml/min/100 g and 1.26 ml/min/100 g at 60 and 90 minutes, respectively. In the non-clipped group, the change was from 9.09 ml/min/100 g at baseline to 2.71 ml/min/100 g and 1.20 ml/min/100 g at 60 and 90 minutes, respectively. All groups saw a significant increase in SCBF above baseline following the end of CPB. MEP amplitudes were lower in clipped vs non-clipped groups in the vastus medialis and tibialis anterior muscles at all time points after baseline. MEPs were roughly 50% below baseline amplitude. External oblique MEPs showed a small difference between groups at certain time points. All animals showed evidence of spinal cord necrosis to varying degrees on histology. In the lumbar spinal cord, significantly more necrosis was seen in clipped group vs non-clipped group (Kleinman score of 6 vs 2.5). A Kleinman score of 6 corresponds to central necrosis involving the posterior and anterior horns and parts of white matter. A score of 2 represents necrosis of one posterior horn, and a score of 3 represents necrosis of both posterior horns.

Although we cannot establish an exact relationship between SCBF and MEP amplitude from this study, we do see that an approximately 50% amplitude reduction compared to smaller amplitude reductions of approximately 20% or less was associated with significantly more histologic necrosis. Additionally, SCBF of around 1.15–1.26 ml/min/100 gram was associated with a 50% amplitude reduction in this model. Although the non-clipped group reached similar trough levels of lumbar SCBF, MEP amplitude changes and histologic necrosis were significantly different from the clipped group. This may indicate that there may be other factors beyond the measurable regional SCBF that cause these changes.

In a rabbit model, Fan et al. [35] looked at SCBF measured by the hydrogen electrode technique and spinal cord evoked potentials (peripheral sensory stimulation with recordings at the spinal cord). Ischemia was induced at the T2 level of the aorta using a balloon. In the thoracic segment, regional SCBF was 34.28 ml/min/100 g in the ischemic group vs 55.28 in the control group. The latency of the N1 peak was 0.45 ms in the ischemic group vs 0.15 ms in the control group. The amplitude was reduced to 2.39 μV in the ischemic group from 4.18 μV in the control group. This corresponds to a roughly 45% decrease in amplitude. In the lumbar segment, regional SCBF was 99.99 ml/min/100 g in the control group and 53.2 in the ischemic group. N1 latency was 0.14 in the control and 0.34 in the ischemic group. N1 amplitude was 6.43 μV vs 2.95 μV in the control and ischemic groups. This represents a 55% decrease in amplitude. This study is difficult to generalize as it is in rabbits, and uses spinal cord evoked potentials, but we do see that a 50% amplitude reduction in the sensory evoked potential was associated with ischemia. This similarly showed that the lumbar segment appeared more sensitive to ischemia.

Also in rabbits, Murakami et al. [79] studied the relationship of TcMEPs and spinal cord ischemia induced by balloon occlusion of the infrarenal aorta. TcMEPs were observed to rapidly disappear following occlusion of the aorta. After reperfusion, the amplitude of the TcMEPs was found to be inversely proportional to the length of ischemia. Rabbits with longer ischemic times had lower post-recovery TcMEP amplitudes. Rabbits with post-recovery amplitudes of <75% of baseline were found to have significantly more neurologic deficits than those with higher recovery levels. Additionally, the recovery amplitude as a percentage of baseline correlated linearly with the number of remaining neurons in the spinal cord.

The relationship of SSEPs and SCBF was looked at closely in Kaplan et al. [55] using a sheep model with measurement of SCBF with radiolabeled microspheres and ischemia induced with aortic cross-clamping 1 cm distal to the origin of the left subclavian artery. Seven of 11 sheep had SSEP changes in this study following cross-clamping of the aorta. In this study, a 50% amplitude reduction in the cortical SSEP was noted at 4.8 minutes after cross-clamping, with disappearance of the cortical SSEP occurring at 7.8 minutes. The cortical SSEP reappeared 16 minutes after cross-clamping. Regional SCBF ranged from 41.2 to 62.8 ml/min/100 g in the cervical, thoracic, and lumbar segments at baseline. Following cross-clamping, the regional SCBF dropped to 0.5 to 5.7 ml/min/100 g in the thoracic and lumbar segments and was in a similar range at the point of the initial evoked potential change, and after 30 minutes of clamp time. After unclamping, hyperemia was noted. In the group without evoked potential changes, thoracic and lumbar SCBF was similar to the group with changes immediately following aortic clamping. After 30 minutes of clamping however, thoracic and lumbar SCBF was significantly higher in the group without SSEP change. Cervical SCBF was much higher in the group without SSEP changes immediately following clamping compared to the group with SSEP changes (105 vs 50 ml/min/100 g). This suggests that the ability to increase cervical flow may be involved in reducing injury, though not in a way that is reflected on regional SCBF measurements.

One major limitation of this study is that the sheep were not placed on bypass, and loss of EPs may have been due to limb ischemia. In support of this is the fact that the peripheral sensory evoked potential (stimulation was at the posterior tibial nerve and recorded at the hip) disappeared in at least three of the sheep and was the first EP to reappear after unclamping as spinal cord ischemia should not affect peripheral nerve function. Correlation of SCBF and SSEP amplitude was not possible with the data in this study.

Laschinger et al. [64] also showed changes in SSEP amplitude despite unchanged spinal cord blood flow in a study of dogs. They found that when distal aortic perfusion pressures were lowered from 70 mmHg to 40 mmHg, the amplitude of the SSEPs decreased from 6.48 mV to 5.00 mV ($p < 0.05$). Spinal cord blood flow was not significantly changed from baseline at any region with this change in perfusion pressure. After the distal aortic pressure was lowered below 40 mmHg, there was loss of SSEPs, which reappeared after the pressure was raised to 70 mmHg. Spinal cord blood flow below 40 mmHg was not reported.

Osenbach et al. [80] looked at SSEP and MEP amplitude in a rabbit model of spinal cord ischemia. Ischemia was produced with balloon occlusion of the infrarenal aorta. Ischemia was induced for 30, 60, and 90 minutes. MEPs were obtained with epidural stimulation electrodes with recording of D-waves at the spinal cord. SSEPs were recorded epidurally with stimulation at the distal cord. Regional SCBF was measured using radiolabeled microspheres. Regional SCBF was recorded at the conus, lumbar enlargement, upper lumbar cord, and thoracic cord. Thoracic regional SCBF was unchanged with occlusion. Upper lumbar regional SCBF declined from 21.3–36.8 to 14.1–20.3 ml/100 g/min following occlusion. At the lumbar enlargement, regional SCBF declined from 24.7–39.4 to 2.7–4.7 ml/100 g/min, with hyperemia occurring after reperfusion. At the conus, regional SCBF declined to nearly 0 following occlusion, with mild hyperemia after reperfusion. SCBF was not significantly different at differing occlusion times. MEP and SSEP amplitude were measured at baseline, and after recovery post-ischemia. Both MEP and SSEP post-recovery amplitude successively decreased with longer ischemic times. At 30, 60, and 90 minutes of ischemic time, SSEP post-recovery amplitude was 81.5%, 71.4%, and 39.9%. MEP post-recovery amplitude was 58.2%, 35.5%, and 27.1%.

This study has several limitations that do not allow further generalization. In contrast to other studies where occlusion occurred more rostrally, the aorta was occluded at the level of the infrarenal aorta, which might explain why thoracic regional SCBF was not significantly affected by occlusion in this study. D-waves were measured for MEPs, which have different characteristics compared to myogenic MEPs. MEP amplitude was reported as post-recovery amplitude, which is less useful than knowing the maximal decrement in amplitude or amplitude during the ischemic period. There are additional studies that analyze regional SCBF and evoked potentials but in the context of compressive lesions and trauma, which likely reflects a different injury mechanism than pure ischemia.

TcMEPs have also been shown to correlate with histopathologic outcome following ischemia. Lips et al. [67] ligated segmental arteries in pigs as a model of spinal cord ischemia. One group of animals was exposed to ischemia for 10 minutes, with TcMEPs reduced to >75% below baseline amplitude. This group had normal motor function and no evidence of infarction 72 hours after the experiment. In another group, reduced TcMEP signals were seen for >60 minutes, resulting in paraplegia and massive spinal cord infarct. In two animals with TcMEP loss for 40 minutes, there was normal function and moderate infarction seen at 72 hours.

In total, these studies reflect that both SSEPs and TcMEPs/MEPs demonstrate decrements in amplitude in response to ischemia. There is no data that yet shows an exact relationship between evoked potential amplitude and regional SCBF. The existing studies vary greatly in methodology used to elicit the evoked potentials. There exists a lag between onset of ischemia and change in evoked potentials. The exact regional SCBF at which ischemia transforms into infarct is unclear. Even with unchanged levels of measured regional SCBF following aortic occlusion, histologic evidence of spinal cord necrosis can be present. Nevertheless, in many of these studies, changes in SSEPs and TcMEPs were reversible, indicating they can be used to identify impending injury, though the exact threshold before reversible injury progresses to permanent is not established in contrast to the cerebrovascular literature.

Monitoring of Thoracic and Thoracoabdominal Aortic Repair

Monitoring open or endovascular repair of the descending thoracic aortic is an involved process and can require the use of many IONM modalities. In this section we will review these modalities and their evidence base.

EEG

As covered in the previous chapter on monitoring cerebrovascular disorders, EEG is a sensitive and specific modality for detecting cerebral ischemia with a well-established response to changes in regional cerebral blood flow. The rates of stroke can range from 1.7% to 3% and are in a similar range to stroke rates from CEA (Taylor et al. 1991; Svensson et al. 1993) [20, 99, 102]. Studies focusing specifically on EEG for the detection of cerebral ischemia in TAAA were not found, but there were some studies that mentioned the use of EEG as a part of multimodality monitoring. Much of the literature applying to EEG monitoring for cerebrovascular disorders would also be relevant for TAAA monitoring for cerebral ischemia and can be reviewed in detail in Chap. 28. Stroke occurring during TAAA repair would likely be embolic or due to ischemia. As TAAA repair requires manipulation of the aorta, potentially CPB and the introduction of catheters to various vessels, there is a risk of emboli forming. The diseased aorta itself could also be the source of emboli. In SACP, if a unilateral perfusion strategy is chosen, EEG changes of hemispheric ischemia can indicate inadequacy of the patient's cerebrovascular collateral system.

In a series of 71 patients undergoing hemiarch replacement with moderate HCA and SACP by Keenan et al. [57], the authors observed several findings. Prior to circulatory arrest, 66% of patients showed a continuous EEG, some with periodic complexes and the remainder in burst suppression. Following circulatory arrest, abrupt loss of activity on EEG was seen in 45% of patients, which resolved when unilateral SACP restored flow, except for two patients (6.2%). One patient had loss of left-sided activity, which resolved when they were converted to bilateral SACP. The other patient had global loss of activity and was placed back on CPB for additional cooling before reinitiation of circulatory arrest.

In surgeries in which DHCA is performed, EEG can be used to guide the targeted temperature. Electrocerebral inactivity or ECI (formerly used terminology includes isoelectric, flat, or electrocerebral silence) of the EEG indicates sufficient cooling. The purpose of DHCA is to reduce the cerebral metabolic rate for neuroprotection during circulatory arrest. Michenfelder and Milde [77] showed in dogs cooled to 7 °C that ECI was initially seen at 12 °C. The cerebral metabolism measured at 13 °C and 7 °C was the same and reflected only the direct effect of the temperature on metabolism. In a similar study in dogs by Mezrow et al. [76], the EEG was felt to have achieved ECI at 8 and 13 °C, though qEEG power showed remaining activity at 13 °C compared to 8 (6% of baseline power vs 1%). Cerebral oxygen metabolism was 8% of baseline at 8 °C and 19% of baseline at 13 °C. From these animal studies, we can conclude that ECI correlates with the minimal amount of cerebral metabolism possible and that there is no further benefit to going below the temperature at which ECI is seen.

Although earlier studies showed that low temperatures were necessary to obtain ECI, later studies showed that the temperature required in humans to achieve ECI was variable. Stecker et al. [97] looked at EEG findings during cooling in 109 patients. Nasopharyngeal temperature, which was thought to best approximate brain temperature, was tracked. During cooling, the first notable EEG change to occur is the appearance of unilateral or bilateral periodic complexes at 29.6 °C ± 3 °C, which appeared in 60% of patients. Burst suppression appeared at temperatures 24.4 °C ± 3 °C, and ECI occurred at 17.8 °C ± 4 °C with a range of 12.5 °C to 27.2 °C. Given the variability required to achieve ECI in patients, EEG can be useful in guiding temperature management and avoiding unnecessarily low temperatures. Similar findings were seen in Coselli et al. [21], where the nasopharyngeal temperature required for ECI varied between 10.1 °C and 24.1 °C.

In another study by James et al. [54], it was found that cooling to 12.7 °C achieved ECI in 95% of patients. 7% of patients achieved ECI when cooled to 18 °C. Patient-specific factors were analyzed to see if any were predictive of the temperature or cooling time necessary to achieve ECI. No factors with good predictive value were found, reinforcing the need for EEG to determine this endpoint.

SSEP

Prior to the development of TcMEPs, SSEPs were the sole modality available for spinal cord monitoring. One of the first uses of SSEPs in thoracic aortic repair was reported by Cunningham et al. [23] in 1982 where in a series of seven patients, they reported six SSEP changes reversed by surgical maneuvers, no patients had spinal cord injury, and one died intraoperatively from myocardial infarction. Schepens et al. [89] evaluated a series of 43 patients undergoing TAAA repair with SSEP monitoring. They noted a false negative rate of 5%; 28% of patients had transient SSEP decrease with no subsequent clinical deficit, 30% of patients had loss of SSEPs with some recovery, resulting in one patient with postoperative paraplegia, and one patient had persistent loss of SSEP and developed postoperative paraplegia. When SSEP changes occurred in this study, interventions made included increasing mean arterial pressure, increasing distal aortic perfusion, and reimplantation of intercostal arteries. There are many additional reports on the use of SSEP monitoring [38, 114].

SSEPs subsequently also began being reported as a method of identifying important intercostal arteries. Griepp et al. [43] reported sequentially clamping intercostal arteries and sacrificing them if there was no SSEP change after 8–10 minutes of occlusion. Paraplegia was greatly reduced compared to surgeries performed prior to SSEP use (2% vs 8%, $p < .008$). SSEP changes were reversible in 3 of 95 patients with perfusion improving interventions. Pillai et al. [82] also reported using SSEP guided intercostal reimplantation in a series of 131 patients. Fifty-two patients had SSEP guidance, while the remainder had routine intercostal reimplantation without SSEP guidance. Patients without SSEPs had their surgeries between 1999 and 2005 while patients with SSEPs occurred between 2005 and 2010. Of the patients with SSEPs, 73.1% had SSEP changes. If SSEP changes did not resolve with measures to increase perfusion, then intercostal reimplantation was performed, which occurred in 28.8% of patients. There was significantly less reimplantation in the SSEP guided group (28.8% vs 59.5%). Immediate paraplegia was not significantly different and occurred in 1.9% of the SSEP group and 2.5% of the non-SSEP group.

A larger review of SSEP use and predicting outcome was conducted by Achouh et al. [3]. A series of 444 patients were reviewed who underwent thoracic aorta and TAAA repair with SSEP monitoring. They found that the sensitivity of SSEPs for immediate neurologic deficit was 62.5% and specificity was 81.2% with an NPV of 99.2%. The overall rate of immediate deficit was 1.8%, the rate of delayed neurologic deficit was 3.2%, and SSEP changes occurred in 19.6% of patients, with 25%

of those being persistent SSEP changes. Patients with delayed deficit did not have any SSEP changes. The authors report the sensitivity analysis was limited as cases with reversible SSEP changes due to interventions are classified as false positives which can decrease sensitivity. This is a general problem with assessing sensitivity accurately in the IONM literature. The false negative rate can be more useful, though not reported in this study. Crawford et al. [22] reported with SSEP monitoring a false negative rate for immediate deficits of 13% in 198 patients. As SSEPs only measure dorsal column function in the spinal cord, it is not surprising that it can result in "false negative" monitoring for motor deficits. It is critical to understand what a test is assessing. In the case of SSEPs, they are evaluating posterior column sensory function, not motor function. Thus, if there are no SSEP changes and the patient develops postoperative isolated motor deficits, then this is not a "false negative." Instead, it is a true negative because sensory function was not altered. Thus, spinal cord injury confined only to the anterior cord and sparing the dorsal columns would have no effect on the SSEPs.

Overall, the literature shows that SSEPs have a reasonable negative predictive value even when used to predict motor function, but cases of postoperative motor deficits do occur. The false positive rate is somewhat high, as limb ischemia can also cause SSEP changes, though more complex technical setups can help differentiate between peripheral and spinal cord ischemia.

Non-limb SSEPs

Given the issue of potential limb ischemia confounding the interpretation of SSEPs, non-limb SSEPs present one potential solution to this problem. Pelvic sites and thoracic dermatomes are potential targets. In our institution, our protocol for monitoring thoracic aortic and thoracoabdominal aortic aneurysm repair includes pudendal and perianal nerve SSEPs. These sites have higher amplitudes compared to dermatomal SSEPs and are not in the surgical field. We have reported the use of these non-limb SSEPs in TAAA, but it has not otherwise been studied [65]. The disadvantages of these modalities include that these are more technically difficult to elicit, are small in amplitude, and are adversely affected by anesthetics which can make it difficult to obtain reliable signals for monitoring. The expected latency of the P1 peak is around 37 ms [81]. As these potentials are not expected to change during limb ischemia, their presence can make distinguishing spinal ischemia from limb ischemia simpler.

TcMEP

After the introduction of TcMEPs in the late 1990s, the technique quickly gained popularity for monitoring, as it reflected the integrity of the corticospinal pathway, and was not a surrogate marker for paralysis as SSEPs were. TcMEPs did not

displace SSEPs however; instead they were frequently combined as multimodality monitoring. Most studies on TcMEP use in TAAA also include SSEP monitoring.

The use of TcMEPs in monitoring TAAA surgery began in the late 1990s. Meylaerts et al. [75] reported one of the first series in which the performance of TcMEPs was compared with SSEPs in 38 patients. Eighteen of 38 patients showed decrements in TcMEP amplitude with SSEP changes concurrently noted in 5 of these 18 patients. SSEP changes lagged behind TcMEP changes. Thirteen of these TcMEP changes followed aortic cross-clamping. The change in amplitude ranged from complete loss to a 50% reduction. TcMEP changes occurred between 3 and 30 minutes after what was determined to be the provoking event. TcMEP changes were reversed in all patients, and no patients developed paraplegia. Recovery time for the TcMEP ranged from 1 to 45 minutes after corrective action was taken. In 11 patients, segmental artery implantation caused return of signals, and in the remaining 7 patients, the corrective action was increasing distal aortic perfusion or systemic blood pressure. TcMEP use was reported by many authors in the following years, with studies showing that TcMEPs predicted neurologic deficit well and resulted in change in operative management [50–52, 70, 98, 107].

There have been several studies on the predictive performance of multimodality monitoring. Shine et al. [92] studied 60 patients undergoing TAAA surgical repair with TcMEP, SSEP, and H reflex monitoring. TcMEPs had a sensitivity of 88% and specificity of 65% for spinal ischemia. The negative predictive value of no changes after 20 minutes of aortic cross-clamping was 96%. Keyhani et al. [58] evaluated SSEPs and TcMEPs in a series of 233 patients undergoing surgical TAAA repair. The NPV of no SSEP/TcMEP changes was >98% for immediate neurologic deficit. They did not find any variables associated with a delayed deficit. Irreversible changes were highly associated with immediate deficit, with an odds ratio of 21.9 for SSEP changes, and 60.8 for TcMEP changes. In this study, MEPs had a higher false positive rate than SSEPs. Sensitivity of persistent TcMEP and SSEP changes for immediate deficit was 62.5% and 37.5%.

Ter Wolbeek et al. [103] observed a high accuracy of SSEP/TcMEP monitoring in their series of 97 patients undergoing endovascular or surgical repair of TAAA. They found a sensitivity of 93% and specificity of 96% for neurologic deficits. Liu et al. [68] found a sensitivity and specificity for MEP/SSEP changes of 100% and 92.2% for paraplegia. Six patients had persistent signal changes, which resulted in one case of transient paraplegia and one case of permanent paraplegia. Patients with no change in SSEP or TcMEPs or reversible changes had no neurologic deficits.

A meta-analysis of SSEPs and MEPs in open TAAA repair was conducted by Fok et al. [37]. They identified 15 studies with 1720 patients, of which 1297 had TcMEP monitoring. There was a single prospective trial, with the remainder of trials conducted retrospectively. The warning criteria used were an amplitude reduction of 50% in six studies, 75% in five studies, and total loss in one study. 69.6% of patients had normal TcMEPs throughout the case. When TcMEP amplitude dropped, recovery was seen in 83.1% of patients. In patients with persistently reduced TcMEP amplitude, 92% of these patients developed permanent neurologic deficits. Five studies also used SSEPs, in 322 of the total patients. SSEP changes were seen concurrently with MEP changes 26% of the time (though only two studies reported on this). 0.9% of patients developed permanent neurologic deficit despite normal TcMEPs, though these were all cases of delayed onset deficit, which TcMEPs would not necessarily be expected to predict.

Tanaka et al. [101] also reported a meta-analysis of TcMEP monitoring in TAAA surgical repair. Sixteen studies with 1368 patients were found for analysis with an overall paraplegia rate of 3.9%. Warning criteria ranged from loss to a 50% amplitude reduction in TcMEP. The pooled sensitivity of TcMEP changes was 89.2% and the pooled specificity was 99.3%. A subgroup analysis showed that total TcMEP loss as a warning criterion had a sensitivity of 75% and a specificity of 99%. Sensitivities and specificities for a 75% amplitude reduction were 67% and 96% and for a 50% amplitude reduction 55% and 93%. From this, the authors concluded that total MEP loss was a better warning criterion to use.

Overall, TcMEPs add additional sensitivity compared to SSEPs. False negatives with TcMEP monitoring are rare. The combination of both results in a high negative predictive value. TcMEPs also respond quickly to ischemia and allow corrective intraoperative actions to be taken.

Segmental Artery Reimplantation

Many centers have reported using TcMEPs to guide the reimplantation or ligation of segmental arteries. Etz et al. [32] used MEP/SSEP guided segmental artery sacrifice in a series of 100 patients, with 2 patients developing postoperative neurologic deficit. They sacrificed an average of eight segmental artery pairs in each patient and reported no changes in the EPs. Hamaishi et al. [46] reported infusing cold blood into the aneurysm and tracking TcMEP changes in 14 patients. They found that in six of eight cases, TcMEP amplitude decreased and intercostal reimplantation was performed. The amplitude of the TcMEP recovered in four of six patients after reimplantation. One of the two patients with persistent TcMEP loss developed paraplegia postoperatively, while the other patient died of multi-organ failure prior to postoperative neurologic assessment. In the group of patients without TcMEP changes, all intercostals were ligated and no patients developed paraplegia. Estrera et al. [31] reported performing intercostal reimplantation only if TcMEPs or SSEPs changed in a series of 105 open repairs. They noted TcMEP loss in 50% of cases; one patient had persistent TcMEP changes and developed neurologic deficit postoperatively, while the other patients with TcMEP loss had no neurologic deficits develop.

Delayed Onset Spinal Cord Ischemia

Although intraoperative TcMEPs are good for assessing immediate neurologic deficits, they have not been found to be particularly predictive of delayed ischemia occurring in the postoperative setting. A few centers have reported using TcMEPs in the postoperative setting for additional monitoring. Usually, TcMEPs are not well tolerated by awake patients; however, following thoracic aortic and TAAA repair, patients are often still intubated and sedated, making this potentially feasible and necessary, as the clinical neurological exam may be hard to obtain accurately. Jafarzadeh et al. [53] reported performing TcMEPs postoperatively every hour until patients were weaned off of sedation and the ventilator. They reported that this helped with management of blood pressure and CSF drainage but had not collected enough patients yet to perform any statistical analysis.

See et al. [91] reported the use of intraoperative TcMEP monitoring to help guide BP management in the postoperative period. Between 2005 and 2010, patients were monitored until the end of aortic cross-clamping. Between 2010 and 2014, monitoring was extended to beyond the end of aortic cross-clamping. During this period of the surgery, the lowest systolic blood pressure at which no TcMEP changes were seen was used to estimate the safe range of blood pressure that could be used in the postoperative setting. The authors found that patients who received this "extended MEP monitoring" had an estimated means odd ratio of 0.15 for delayed spinal cord ischemia ($p < 0.01$). TcMEP changes seen in this period consisted of smaller amplitudes of the lower extremity TcMEPs in response to changes in blood pressure. The exact degree of amplitude change in this period was not reported. The authors suggested that TcMEP monitoring in the postoperative setting may be of use as well.

Paradoxical Increase in Amplitude

It has been observed that TcMEPs can sometimes paradoxically increase in amplitude following spinal cord injury [115]. The likely mechanism of this is injury to a subset of upper motor neurons leading to decreased inhibition and enhancement of the myogenic MEP response. If the injury progressed so that all the upper motor neuron axons responsible for generating a given muscle signal are injured, then a TcMEP would not be expected. If there is a focal increase in amplitude of TcMEPs without a change in stimulation parameters or anesthetic values, then there should be increased suspicion for this type of paradoxical response.

Hypothermia

Hypothermia in moderate and deep hypothermic circulatory arrest can have a significant effect on evoked potential monitoring. In many cases, deep hypothermia results in no monitorable evoked potentials during the critical period of cross-clamping. Shinzawa et al. [94] reported how TcMEPs changed with temperature during deep hypothermia in 15 patients. During the cooling phase, 12 of 15 patients had loss of the hand TcMEP before a nasopharyngeal temperature of 16 °C. The remaining patients had loss of the hand TcMEP once circulatory arrest began. Leg TcMEPs disappeared before 16 °C in 10 of 15 patients, with the remainder disappearing after circulatory arrest. The MEP latencies increased linearly as temperature decreased. In the hand, the latency increased from 21.5 to 46.4 ms at 21 °C. The leg increased from 42.3 to 77.0 ms at 22 °C. MEP amplitude recovered to around 50% at 25 °C during rewarming; however, it subsequently decreased in amplitude during the rest of rewarming. In general, the hand recovered before the leg, with half of patients recovering the hand potential below 20 °C. There was greater variability of the temperature at which the leg recovered, with five patients recovering between 21 and 30 °C, two below that, and eight above that. The hand also recovered faster, within 20 minutes in two thirds of the patients. Latency improved linearly during rewarming. Figures 29.4 and 29.5 show an example of typical SSEP and TcMEP changes due to deep hypothermia.

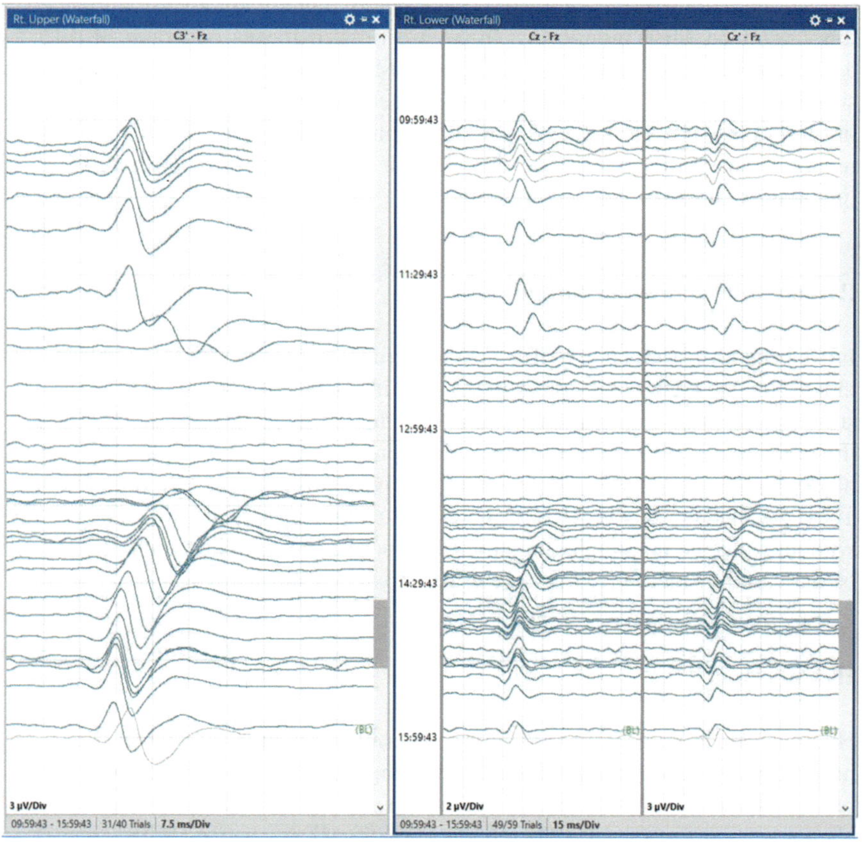

Fig. 29.4 The right median nerve and posterior tibial nerve SSEPs are shown during deep hypothermia to 20 °C and subsequent rewarming. The SSEPs are shown in chronological order, with earlier traces occurring at the top. EEG electrocerebral inactivity was seen at 21.9 °C. The right leg SSEP disappeared around 24 °C and reappeared at 25.9 °C

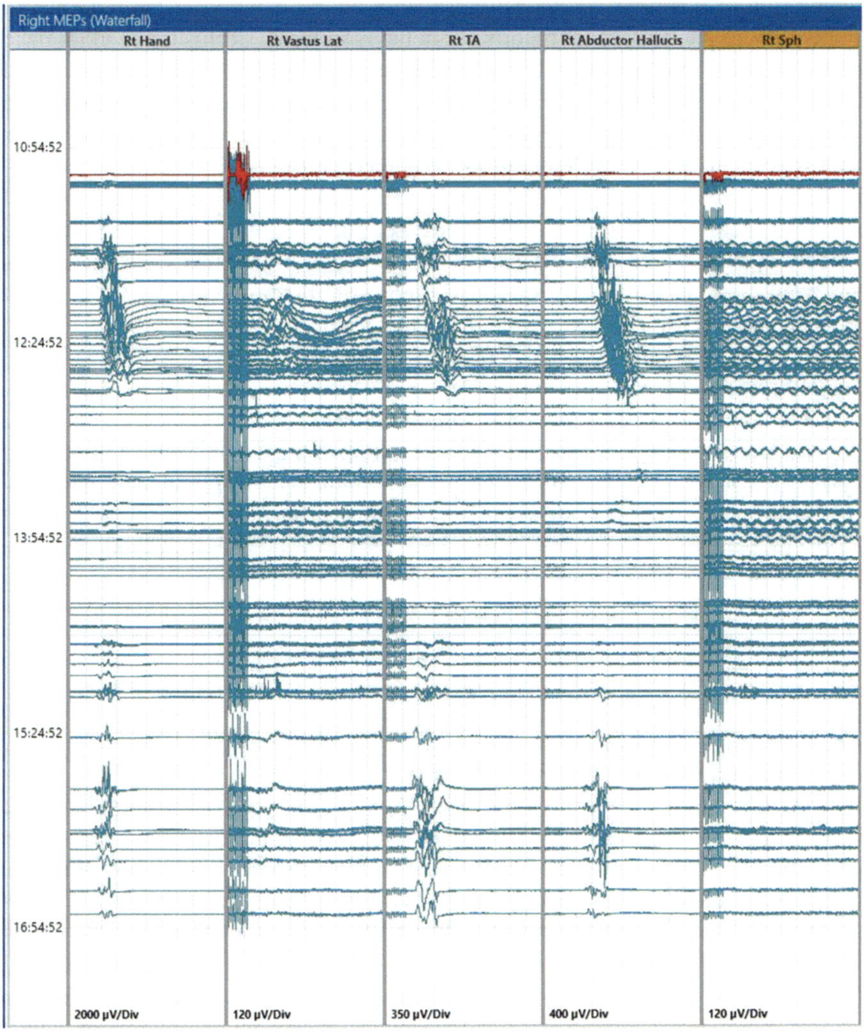

Fig. 29.5 Right-sided TcMEPs (from the right hand, vastus lateralis, tibialis anterior, abductor hallucis, and anal sphincter) during deep hypothermia to 20 °C and subsequent rewarming are shown

Bulbocavernosus Reflex (BCR)

The bulbocavernosus reflex is the reflex contraction of the external anal sphincter following penile or clitoral stimulation. This reflex arc is mediated by the sacral cord and sacral afferent/efferents, specifically of the S2–S4 region. This reflex can also be elicited and recorded with electrophysiologic techniques and has been used intraoperatively, most frequently in sacral surgeries [25, 96]. Intraoperative monitoring of this reflex provides information on the function of the sacral cord. Though there are no specific reports about the monitoring of this reflex in thoracic aortic and/or thoracoabdominal aortic aneurysm repair, it is part of our institutional monitoring protocol for these cases. From a technical standpoint, it requires no additional electrode setup if electrodes are already placed for pudendal nerve SSEPs and external anal sphincter monitoring. From a monitoring perspective, it has several advantages. It can be run frequently and without movement unlike the anal sphincter TcMEP, and it is not averaged; therefore a signal can be elicited more quickly than pudendal and perianal SSEPs. However, it is sensitive to anesthetics and neuromuscular blockade [96]. The warning criteria for interpreting BCR are not well established. Morota [78] found that when using postoperative urinary complications as the outcome in spinal cord lipomas, the positive predictive value (PPV) and NPV of a >75% reduction in amplitude of the response were 100% and 97.9%, respectively. A 50–75% reduction in amplitude had a PPV of 53.8% and NPV of 98.5%. A less than 50% reduction in amplitude had a PPV of 25.8% and NPV of 100%. In a study by Cha et al. [14] of pediatric patients undergoing cord untethering, BCR loss was used as a warning criteria. The authors found that BCR loss had a PPV of 44.4% at discharge and NPV of 87.7% for postoperative voiding dysfunction. At our institution, our practice is to use BCR loss as warning criteria.

Near-Infrared Spectroscopy (NIRS)

NIRS, also referred to as cerebral oximetry, relies on near-infrared light to determine regional oxygen saturation in tissues. The use of NIRS for cerebral ischemia in aortic procedures does not differ much from the procedures used for cerebrovascular disorders. A more detailed description of the technique and review of its use in cerebrovascular disorders can be found in the preceding chapter.

There are some recent reports of using NIRS for paraspinal oximetry to assess spinal cord ischemia [69]. Boezeman et al. [10] reported measuring the regional hemoglobin oxygen saturation in 15 patients undergoing open TAAA repair. The reference optode was placed at T3 and the active optode at T12, calculating a T12/T3 ratio. All patients also underwent TcMEP monitoring. They found that in patients who had a >50% decrease in area under the curve of the TcMEP, the T12/T3 ratio was lower ($p < 0.037$). Currently, this technique is still under investigation.

Monitoring of TEVAR

The general principles of monitoring the endovascular repair of thoracic and thoracoabdominal aortic aneurysms are similar to monitoring surgical repair. One of the main differences is that segmental arteries will be excluded during placement of the endograft and reimplantation of the segmental arteries is not possible.

There is less extensive experience of TcMEP and SSEP use in TEVAR but with overall similar results. Weigang et al. [108] looked at 21 patients undergoing TEVAR with TcMEP and SSEP monitoring. They found that deployment of the endograft resulted in transient loss of the TcMEP and SSEP in 14% of patients, with TcMEP changes occurring first. All changes were reversed by increasing blood pressure and draining CSF and these patients developed no complications. One patient with normal EPs developed delayed paraparesis 3 weeks after the procedure. Banga et al. [8] monitored SSEPs/TcMEPs in a series of 49 patients. 63% of patients had TcMEP/SSEP changes. Of these patients, 39% had their EPs return to baseline after interventions (increasing MAP and CSF drainage), one patient had persistent TcMEP loss and developed postoperative neurologic deficits, and the remainder of the patients had improvement of their EPs after lower extremity perfusion was restored. When persistent SSEP/TcMEP loss occurred, the authors would leave the procedure incomplete and allow continued flow into the aneurysm sac. Maier et al. [71] reported in a patient with SSEP/TcMEP loss after placement of the endograft, the procedure was stopped and subsequently completed 4 months later with the patient developing no neurologic deficits.

Bafort et al. [7] reported a single case where, with SSEP monitoring, test occlusion of the aneurysm was performed in a high-risk patient for 15 minutes prior to endograft deployment. There were no changes in the SSEPs and the patient developed no complications.

Differentiating Spinal Ischemia from Peripheral (Limb) Ischemia

Differentiation of spinal cord ischemia from peripheral ischemia is a critical skill in monitoring procedures of the thoracic aorta. Peripheral ischemia, or limb ischemia, is a common occurrence in thoracic aortic and thoracoabdominal aortic repair both with and without assisted circulation techniques. Often, the lower body below the distal aortic clamp is perfused by a perfusion catheter cannulating the common femoral artery through retro- and anterograde flow. If perfusion pressure is too low, then limb ischemia can develop. Additionally, the contralateral leg from the perfusion catheter may develop ischemia more easily, as it receives less blood than the ipsilateral leg. During the period of no perfusion during distal aortic anastomosis, limb ischemia may develop as well. Limb ischemia, although not ideal, can be tolerated for part of the surgery. From the orthopedic literature, where surgery is often performed with tourniquets, it is thought <2 hours of tourniquet time is tolerated. With times <2 hours, although muscle atrophy and electrophysiologic changes can be detected at short-term follow-up, the long-term outcomes are the same [36]. It is unlikely that the duration of limb ischemia in thoracic aortic repair will exceed 2 hours.

Similar to spinal ischemia, limb ischemia can cause a decrement or obliteration of the SSEPs and TcMEPs. The pattern of changes and preservation of certain signals can be relied on for differentiation. It has been reported in the literature that in cases of limb ischemia or peripheral nerve compression, sensory nerve action potentials (SNAPs) change prior to compound muscle action potentials (CMAPs). Chowet et al. [18] serially measured median nerve SNAPs and CMAPs in 12 healthy subjects, without a history of neurologic symptoms or neurologic disorders, who had their wrists placed in a hyperextended position. All 12 subjects developed significant decrement in the amplitude of their SNAPs, sufficient to qualify as conduction block (>80% reduction of baseline), and 2 of 12 volunteers had a significant decrement in their CMAP. In a similar study by Hofmeijer et al. [47], median nerve SNAPs and CMAPs were recorded in five healthy subjects who had arm ischemia induced by a blood pressure cuff. Median nerve SNAPs were observed to disappear at 30 minutes in all subjects, and CMAPs at 35 minutes in all subjects. Additional excitability studies were also performed during this study. Their conclusion was that sensory axons were more vulnerable to ischemia than motor axons. This may be mediated by sensory axons possessing a larger persistent sodium current than motor axons, and therefore being more dependent on the sodium-potassium pump to maintain their ion gradients. At our institution we have also observed that in cases of intraoperative peripheral nerve ischemia and compression, SSEP changes preceded MEP changes [15].

Therefore, in cases of limb ischemia, we would expect the cortical SSEP to manifest a change preceding any MEP changes. The expected change would be a reduction in amplitude and possible disappearance, as well as progressive prolongation in latency. This prolongation in latency is not seen in many other scenarios. The common other scenario the shift in latency can be seen is in hypothermia. The SSEP change can precede the MEP change by at least several minutes. If a SSEP change is noted, it is important to increase the frequency that TcMEPs are being checked. When MEP changes occur, they tend to initially manifest in more distal leg muscles, such as the abductor hallucis (AH), before changes are evident in proximal muscles, as the distal leg is likely more ischemic. The proximal leg may be spared, which is a reason why sampling proximal leg muscles (such as the vastus lateralis or rectus femoris) can be useful. Additionally, if the perfusion catheter is placed on the left leg, then the right leg may develop changes first.

In spinal ischemia, MEP changes often precede SSEP changes. Dong et al. [27] observed that when SSEP and MEP changes occurred together, the SSEP changes appeared 3–12 minutes after TcMEP changes. Weigang et al. [108] similarly observed that MEP changes occurred prior to SSEP changes. Meylaerts et al. [75] noted a delay of 2–34 minutes. This is probably because the anterior cord, where the corticospinal tracts and anterior horn cells are located, is more dependent on the intercostal arteries than the posterior cord, where the dorsal columns are located. Thus, ischemia may occur in the anterior cord first. However, it is important to remember that spinal cord vasculature has high variability between individuals, and this expected pattern may not always occur. Additionally, in the spinal cord, the dorsal columns are only comprised of white matter tracts, as their synapses occur above the level of cervico-medullary junction. Compared to gray matter, such as the anterior horn cells, white matter is more resistant to ischemic injury [34].

To increase our ability to rapidly identify limb ischemia, it is our practice to place pulse oximetry probes on both legs when monitoring these procedures. Pulse oximetry changes have been shown to precede SSEP changes by an average of 3 minutes in limb ischemia caused by retraction on the iliac artery in anterior lumbar surgery [11]. If pulse oximetry shows intact oxygenation when an IONM change occurs, then the observed evoked potential (EP) changes are more likely to be a case of spinal cord ischemia. If the pulse oximetry has a low reading, then it is less helpful, as spinal cord and limb ischemia could be simultaneously present. Even though simultaneous spinal cord and limb ischemia is less likely to occur, careful interpretation of all the EPs is necessary to determine the cause of the change. In surgery performed without assisted circulation techniques, limb ischemia is more frequent. Following the loss of limb EPs due to peripheral ischemia, we can only rely on the non-limb EPs to determine the integrity of the cord.

Non-limb EPs are also important in differentiating peripheral from spinal ischemia. The modalities we use to monitor these include the BCR, perianal SSEP, pudendal SSEP, and anal sphincter MEP. These signals are all mediated by sacral roots to the spinal cord. Unfortunately, these EPs are not always reliably obtained in each patient. If present at baseline, then their persistence supports intact spinal cord function and provides evidence against the presence of critical levels of spinal cord ischemia. Therefore, if these EPs remain present and unchanged while leg TcMEP/SSEP changes are occurring, then this can be interpreted as being consistent and suggestive of limb ischemia. As some of these techniques are not frequently used outside of monitoring this type of surgery, it is important to maintain a good familiarity with them, as they can be essential in differentiating spinal and limb ischemia. Using a combination of these patterns and signs can make differentiating spinal cord ischemia and limb ischemia clearer.

Definition of Critical Changes

Criteria for critical changes can vary depending on the interpretation of the literature. If generalized effects such as anesthesia, temperature, or technical factors have already been ruled out, we defined the following as critical changes: new focal slowing on the EEG; 50% or more reduction in the amplitude of the cortical SSEP; an increase of 1 ms or more of the central conduction time of the SSEP; 50% reduction in MEP amplitude; and loss of the BCR.

Possible Interventions in Response to Critical Changes

In most scenarios, after IONM changes occur, the surgical or procedural management of the case is altered. Below we list some of the strategies that can be used upon encountering changes.

Open Surgical Repair

(a) Increase mean arterial pressure, if no contraindication.
(b) Drain CSF from lumbar drain, if no contraindication.
(c) Reimplant intercostal/lumbar arteries.
(d) Transfuse blood.
(e) Increase distal aortic perfusion.
(f) Ligate backbleeding intercostal vessels if present.
(g) Selectively perfuse intercostal arteries.
(h) Convert from unilateral SACP to bilateral SACP if cerebral ischemia is suspected.

TEVAR

(a) Increase mean arterial pressure, if no contraindication.
(b) Drain CSF from lumbar drain, if no contraindication.

Stimulating and Recording Techniques

There are a variety of stimulation and recording protocols that exist for obtaining evoked potentials. A full discussion of different parameters is beyond the scope of this chapter; however, we will present the parameters used at our institution, which we have found produce consistent and reproducible EPs. The stimulation and recording techniques used for EEG, median nerve SSEPs, posterior tibial nerve SSEPs, and TcMEPs can be found in same section in Chap. 28, the preceding chapter on the monitoring of cerebrovascular disorders. For thoracic aortic and TAAA repair, we have more extensive coverage of lower limb TcMEPs compared to cerebrovascular disorders. Typically, the bilateral hand (first dorsal interosseous muscle linked to the abductor pollicis brevis), vastus lateralis, tibialis anterior, extensor hallucis longus, abductor hallucis, and external anal sphincter are sampled. Bilateral median or ulnar nerve SSEPs, posterior tibial nerve SSEPs, and eight-channel EEG are performed.

Pudendal Nerve SSEPs

For pudendal nerve SSEPs, placement of the stimulating electrodes will differ between male and female patients. In male patients, we place standard surface stimulation electrodes on the dorsal surface of the penis. The cathode is placed proximally, closer to the body. The anode is placed several centimeters distal to the

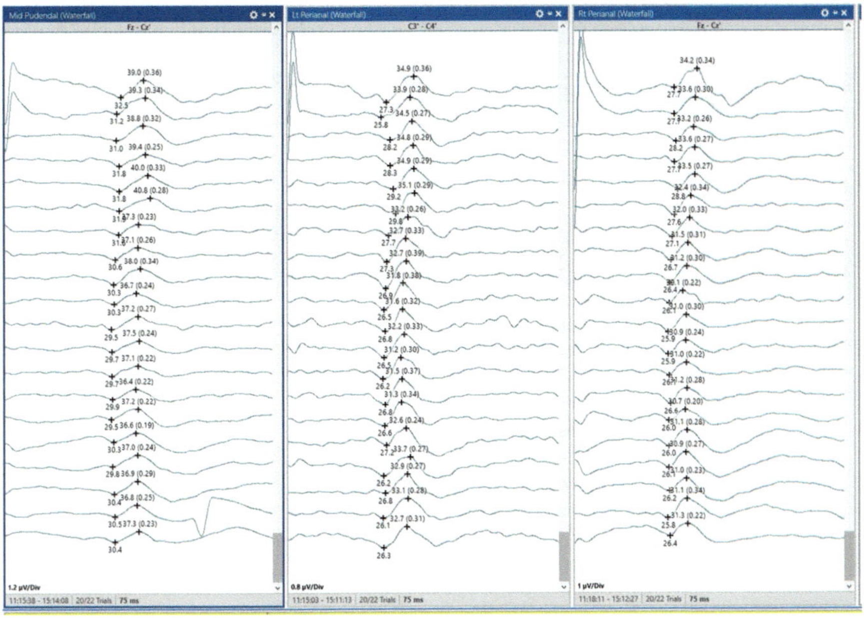

Fig. 29.6 An example of pudendal and perianal SSEPs is shown. The box on the left shows the pudendal nerve SSEP in a male patient. The two boxes on the right show left and right perianal SSEPs. The latency of the N and P components is labelled in ms on each trace, with the amplitude in μV shown in parentheses

cathode. For female patients, we place two sets of surface electrodes, one on the left and one on the right. The cathode is placed immediately lateral of the clitoris on each side. The anode is placed a few centimeters below the cathode, between the labia majora and minora on each side. Recording electrodes for the cortical and subcortical responses are the same as for limb SSEPs. The stimulation current ranges from 20 to 50 milliamps (mA) typically. The stimulation frequency ranges from 2 to 4 Hz. Filters are set at 30 Hz to 3 kHz. The number of required averages ranges from 200 to 300. Figure 29.6 shows an example of pudendal SSEPs.

Perianal Nerve SSEPs

For perianal nerve SSEPs, two sets of standard surface stimulation electrodes are placed, one on each side of the anus. The anodes are placed at the 3 and 9 o'clock position from the anus when looking at the patient from a lithotomy position. The cathodes are placed several centimeters laterally from the anodes. Recording electrodes for the scalp and subcortical potentials is the same as for limb SSEPs. The stimulation current ranges from 20 to 50 mA typically. The stimulation frequency ranges from 2 to 4 Hz. Filters are set at 30 Hz to 3 kHz. The number of required averages ranges from 200 to 300. Figure 29.6 shows an example of perianal SSEPs.

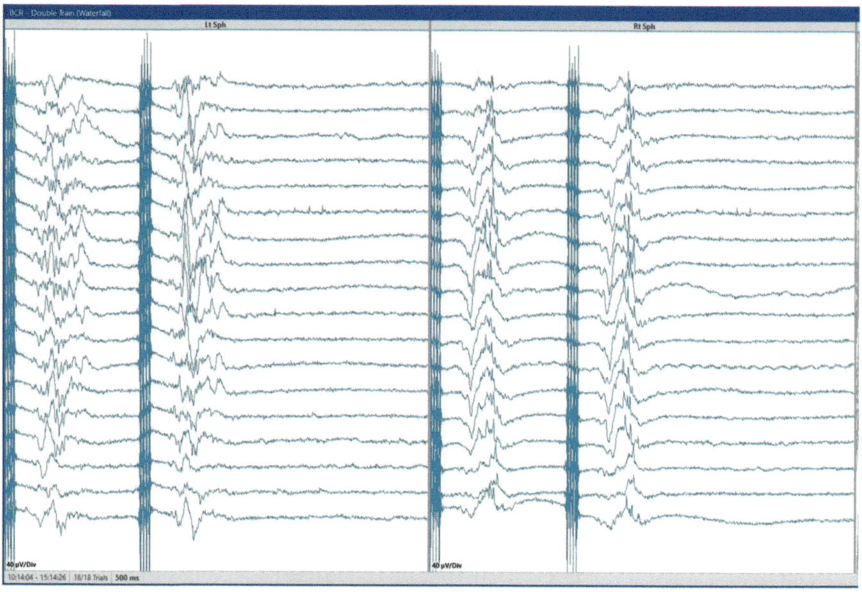

Fig. 29.7 An example of the BCR waveform obtained from double train stimulation is shown here. Recordings are from the "left" and "right" anal sphincter

BCR

The electrophysiological BCR involves stimulating the pudendal nerve and recording at the external anal sphincter. As monitoring TAAA repair at our institution already involves placement of pudendal nerve and anal sphincter electrodes, monitoring the BCR requires no additional electrode placement. For the external anal sphincter, two pairs of subdermal needle electrodes are placed on each side of the anus and secured with tape.

For stimulation, a double-train multipulse stimulus is used; we have found this results in an elicitable reflex in a higher proportion of patients, consistent with the literature [83, 93, 95]. The stimulus current is typically between 20 and 60 mA. The first and second trains consist of pulses of 4, with an interstimulus interval of 3 ms, a pulse width of 500 µs, and an inter-train interval of 150 ms. Recording is done with a time base of 50 ms/division, and a default sensitivity of 50 µV/division. Filters are set at 30 Hz and 3 kHz. Recording is made from both pairs of anal sphincter electrodes. In the case of female patients, where there are two pairs of stimulating electrodes, both are separately used for stimulation. An example of the BCR can be seen in Fig. 29.7.

Common Pitfalls

Open repair of thoracic aortic and thoracoabdominal aortic aneurysms is often procedure with high blood loss compared to other procedures monitored in IONM. Care should be taken to shield all reusable equipment and cables appropriately from blood, which will make case breakdown faster. Defibrillation is sometimes needed in these cases. It is important to make sure the defibrillation current is not directed into the amplifier, such as by disconnecting the amplifier cable during defibrillation, as this may damage equipment.

Conclusion

The use of IONM in thoracic aortic and thoracoabdominal aortic aneurysm surgery has evolved and grown greatly since its inception. Monitoring of these procedures requires a detailed knowledge of the anatomy and physiology of spinal cord ischemia, clinical neurophysiology, the various surgical approaches, and the many available neuroprotective adjunctive measures. Fortunately, the overall rate of paraplegia has decreased since thoracic aortic and TAAA repair was first introduced. The exact contribution of IONM to this improvement is unclear, as many neuroprotective adjunctive measures were concurrently introduced. Nevertheless, a large evidence base has shown the usefulness of IONM techniques in thoracic aortic and TAAA surgery. IONM has been shown to have a strong negative predictive value for immediate spinal cord injury. However, the literature remains limited by the lack of prospective controlled trials, which ethically are currently difficult to justify. Delayed paraplegia remains a persistent problem, and whether neurophysiologic monitoring has a role in detecting this remains to be explored.

Case Examples

Case Example 1

A 58-year-old man presented with chest pain. His imaging (Fig. 29.8a) showed a distal arch and extent I descending thoracic aortic aneurysm. The case, an open repair, was performed at normothermia with CPB. The first change in this case was noted in the left arm (Fig. 29.8b). The proximal aortic clamp was placed distal to the left carotid artery, and the left subclavian artery had an additional clamp placed at its takeoff from the aorta. The left common femoral artery was cannulated. The distal clamp was placed above the T10 intercostal arteries. Around 20 minutes following this, a >50% decrease in amplitude of the left arm SSEP was seen. The hand

MEP amplitude was unchanged. Approximately 15 minutes after this, the anastomosis to the left subclavian artery was completed and perfusion restored. The SSEP quickly returned to baseline following this. The EEG remained at baseline during the period of SSEP changes. This change was thought to be limb ischemia due to clamping of the subclavian artery. This follows the general pattern of SSEP changes preceding MEP changes in limb ischemia. It is likely if the ischemia continued for longer, the hand MEP would also be lost.

Around the same time as the left arm SSEP change, a change in the right leg SSEP was noted, followed by the left leg. This quickly progressed to loss of both leg SSEPs (Fig. 29.8c). Distal aortic perfusion was increased several times with little improvement seen. Eight minutes after the right leg SSEP change, the right leg TcMEPs were noted to be lost (Fig. 29.8d). The left leg TcMEPs remained intact at the tibialis anterior (TA) and showed a decreasing amplitude in the left AH. The TA and anal sphincters show an increase in amplitude around this time due to an increase in stimulation voltage. The BCR and perianal SSEPs remained unchanged during this period (Fig. 29.8e,f).

It was felt that these changes represent limb ischemia for several reasons. The SSEP change occurred before the MEP change. The SSEP changes occurred in the right leg before left leg, which would be expected as the perfusion catheter was in the left common femoral artery. The TcMEP changes occurred in distal leg muscles before proximal muscles in the left leg. Additionally, the anal sphincter TcMEPs, BCR response, and perianal SSEPs representing distal cord function remained present and unchanged from baseline.

Fig. 29.8 (**a**) A 3D reconstruction of the aneurysm from the CT angiogram is shown. (**b**) The left median nerve SSEP is shown, with traces appearing in chronological order. The earlier traces appear at the top. Timing of the clamping of the left subclavian artery is shown by the solid arrow. The hollow arrow shows the timing of unclamping of the left subclavian artery. (**c**) The bilateral posterior tibial nerve SSEPs are shown chronologically, with earlier traces appearing at the top. Decrement in amplitude and subsequent loss of the right posterior tibial SSEP can be seen at around 12:51 (solid arrow). The left posterior tibial nerve SSEP shows the same trend beginning around 13:05 (hollow arrow). (**d**) The bilateral TcMEPs are shown in chronological order, with earlier traces appearing at the top. At 12:59 (solid arrow), loss of the right vastus lateralis, tibialis anterior, and abductor hallucis and decreased amplitude of the left abductor hallucis are seen. (**e**) The BCR response is shown, with recordings from the left and right anal sphincters. The black arrow indicates when distal aortic perfusion was stopped for the distal anastomosis. The BCR is lost shortly after this. (**f**) Perianal SSEPs are shown. The pudendal is not shown as it was unreliable at baseline. Attenuation of the perianal SSEP can be seen, which corresponded with the timing in change of the BCR. (**g**) Following the pause in distal aortic perfusion, there was an increase in EMG activity in the anal sphincter. At baseline there was no EMG activity. After several minutes this EMG activity quieted down, and it was noted the BCR response was lost. (**h**) Bilateral TcMEPs are shown chronologically following Figure 29.8d in time. Re-emergence of the signals from the legs can be seen once CPB was weaned off (solid arrow). (**i**) The bilateral posterior tibial nerve SSEPs are shown again. The left posterior tibial nerve SSEP returns following CPB being weaned off (black arrow). The right posterior tibial nerve SSEP also returns but in a more delayed fashion (hollow arrow). (**j**) The BCR was more delayed in returning than the other signals. Return was not seen until the end of the case

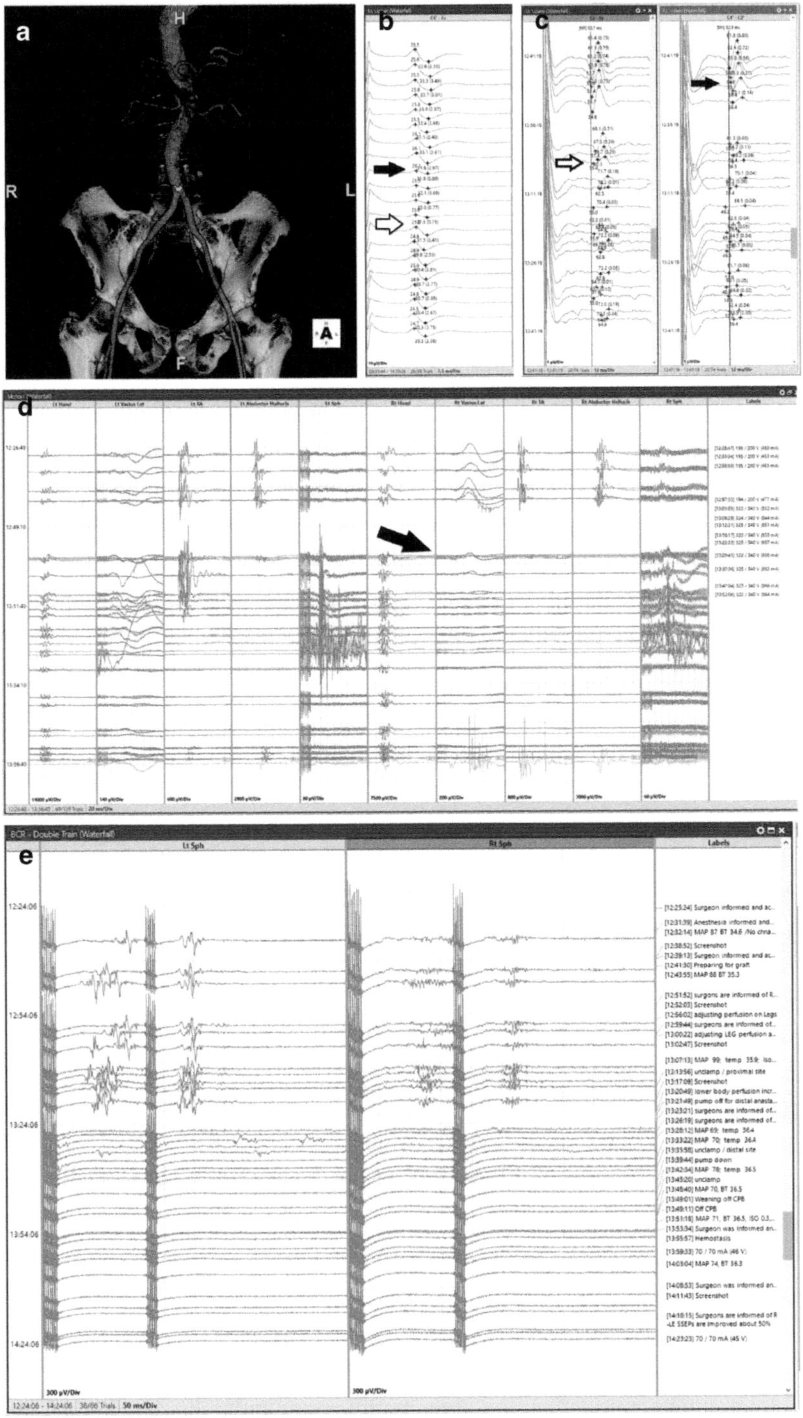
a
H
R
L
F
b
c
d
e
BCR - Double Train (Waterfall)
Lt Sph
Rt Sph
Labels
12:24:06
12:54:06
13:24:06
13:54:06
14:24:06
300 μV/Div
300 μV/Div
12:24:06 - 14:24:06 | 36/86 Trials | 50 ms/Div

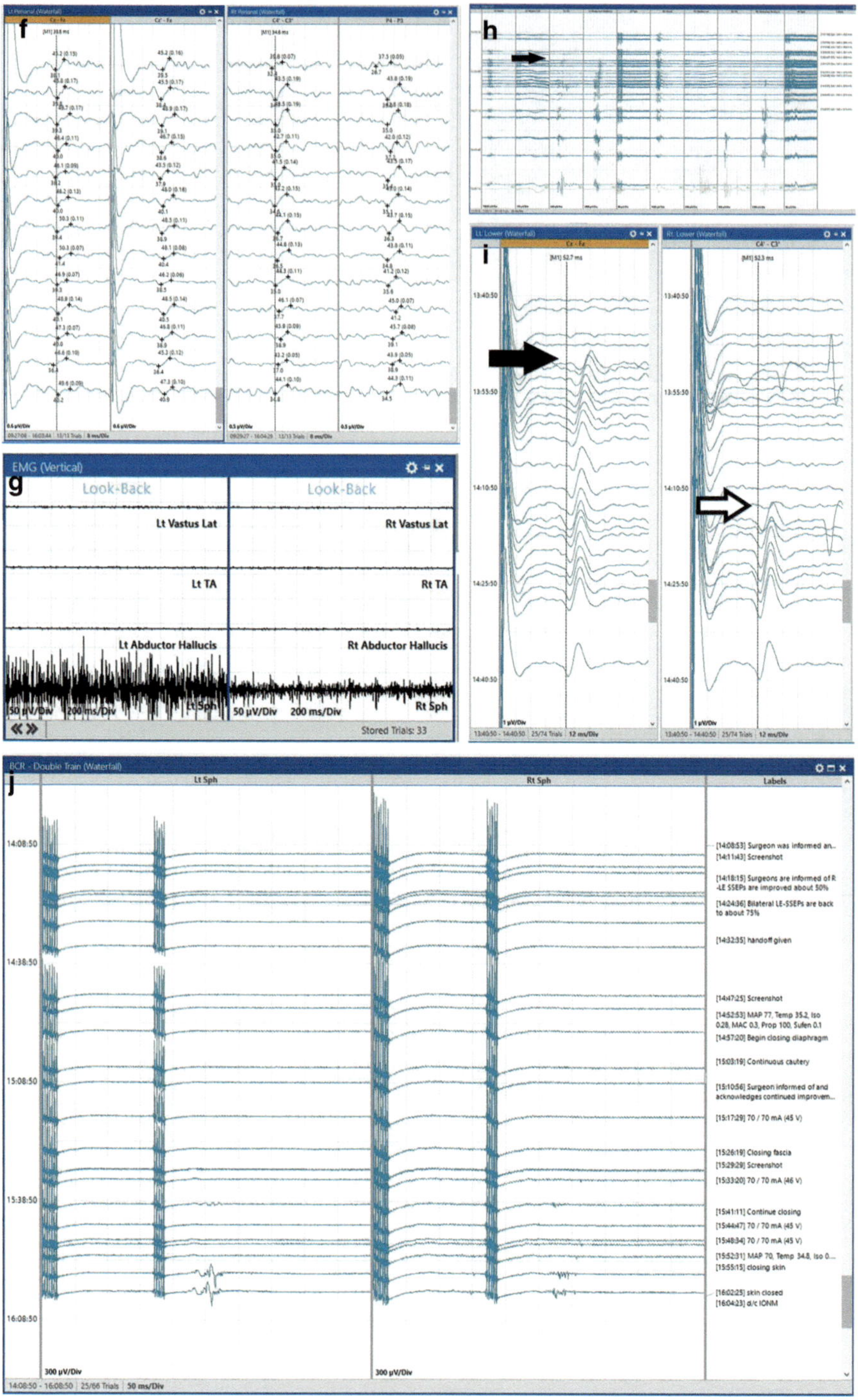

Fig. 29.8 (continued)

When distal aortic perfusion was stopped for the distal anastomosis, additional changes occur. The free-running electromyography (EMG) shows active large amplitude spontaneous activity from the anal sphincter (Fig. 29.8g), which had not been present at baseline. After several minutes this anal sphincter EMG stops. Following this, the BCR is no longer seen (Fig. 29.8e) and the anal sphincter TcMEP is also lost (Fig. 29.8d). The perianal SSEPs were reduced in amplitude as well. The changes were now felt to reflect spinal ischemia. Once the distal anastomosis was completed and perfusion restored, an improvement in the signals began to be seen. The left leg SSEP and TcMEPs return first followed later by the R leg TcMEPs and SSEPs (Fig. 29.8h,i). The sphincter TcMEP also reappears. The BCR does not reappear until the end of the case (Fig. 29.8j). The amplitude of the TcMEP responses appeared similar to the baseline amplitude, though the stimulation voltage was higher than at baseline. The patient awoke with an intact neurological exam.

This case illustrates that by relying on modalities mediated by the distal cord (BCR, perianal SSEPs), it can be possible to distinguish spinal cord ischemia from limb ischemia even when limb ischemia has already resulted in the loss of leg EPs. Another takeaway from this case is that arm ischemia can also occur during these cases if the distal arch is involved. The neuromonitoring alerts in this case resulted in an increase of the distal aortic perfusion and MAP to reduce limb and spinal ischemia. Being able to differentiate the initial change in the leg EPs as limb ischemia rather than spinal ischemia was useful in determining that intercostal reimplantation was not needed in this case. Spinal ischemia only occurred once perfusion to the segment of aorta distal to the graft (below the T10 intercostal level) was not perfused. This suggests that the critical segmental arteries for spinal cord perfusion in this patient lie outside of the aneurysm and below the graft level.

Case Example 2

A 74-year-old woman with a past medical history of an extent II TAAA was initially scheduled for nonemergency surgical repair; however, 1 week prior to her scheduled surgery, she presented with flank pain and was found to have a ruptured aneurysm. Her neurological exam was intact at baseline. Imaging showed an 8.4x4.6 cm aneurysm with active extravasation at the T10–T11 level. Surgery was conducted with mild hypothermia, CPB, and SACP (with unilateral perfusion of the left common carotid artery).

Following aortic cross-clamping, loss of the bilateral leg TcMEPs is seen in the next trace (Fig. 29.9a). Bilateral leg SSEP loss is seen 33 minutes after the TcMEP changes (Fig. 29.9b). It was felt that this change represented spinal cord ischemia, as the MEP changes occurred before SSEP changes. Additionally, the proximal leg TcMEPs were affected at the same time as the distal leg TcMEPs. There were no reliable BCR or pudendal or perianal SSEPs to provide further evidence of spinal or limb ischemia. The surgeon was alerted and the decision was made to place a graft at the T11 intercostals (Fig. 29.9c). Following the connection of this graft to a

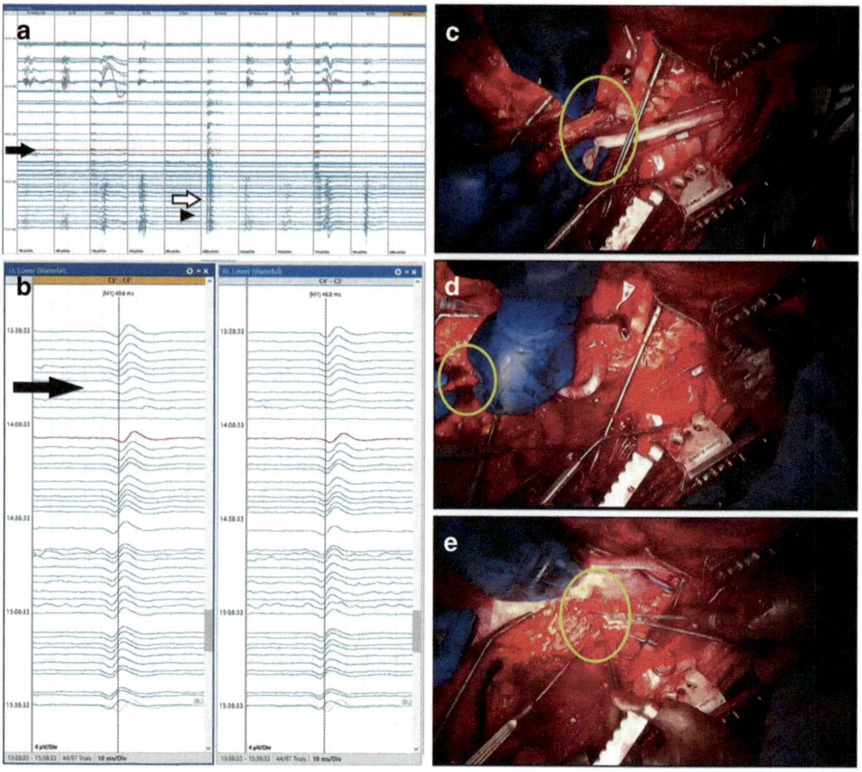

Fig. 29.9 (**a**) The bilateral TcMEPs are shown chronologically. No left-hand channel is present, as it was sterilely prepped. The first red trace is just prior to the initiation of CPB and aortic cross-clamping. Loss of the bilateral leg signals is seen in the following traces. The solid arrow marks the start of perfusion of the intercostal graft. The leg TcMEPs begin to return after some delay. The hollow arrow shows interruption of perfusion to the intercostal graft so that it can be anastomosed to the main graft. The solid arrowhead shows when the intercostal graft begins to be perfused again after being attached to the main graft. (**b**) The bilateral posterior tibial nerve SSEPs are shown chronologically. Decrement and then loss of the bilateral leg SSEPs is shown by the solid arrow. The red trace marks the first trace following the start of perfusion to the intercostal graft. SSEP changes were delayed by approximately 30 minutes following MEP loss. (**c**) The yellow circle shows a graft being attached to a pair of T11 intercostals in an end-to-side fashion. (**d**) The yellow circle shows the perfusion catheter being inserted into the intercostal graft. (**e**) The yellow circle shows the intercostal graft (which has been trimmed) being attached to the main graft

perfusion catheter (Fig. 29.9d), the leg SSEPs immediately return to their baseline amplitude (Fig. 29.9b). The TcMEPs return ~10–15 minutes after this catheter is placed. A mild reduction is seen in the leg TcMEP amplitudes when the perfusion catheter is removed so that the intercostal graft can be anastomosed to the main aortic graft (Fig. 29.9e). This improves once perfusion is again restored. At the conclusion of the case, the EPs appeared to be at baseline values.

No immediate postoperative exam was able to be performed on the patient due to sedation. Late on post-op day 1, the patient was noted to have left leg paresis. Later in the day, this evolved to bilateral leg plegia. The MAP was maintained with a goal of greater than 85. Over the course of the next week, the patient had some improvement in strength and was discharged with approximately 2/5 strength in the legs. Despite the improvement of the TcMEP and SSEPs following T11 intercostal reimplantation, the patient developed what appeared to be delayed spinal cord ischemia. Delayed ischemia remains difficult to prevent in these patients, and we do not know if the intraoperative interventions prevented a more devastating neurologic outcome.

Case Example 3

A 57-year-old woman with a history of FBN1 gene mutation, causing type A aortic dissection status post-repair, presents with growth of an infrarenal abdominal aortic aneurysm to beyond 5 cm. A surgical repair is planned with CPB. Approximately 25 minutes after aortic cross-clamping, loss of the right leg SSEP is seen (Fig. 29.10a). The bilateral iliacs were clamped as the distal clamp site in this case. The left common femoral artery was cannulated. The right leg TcMEPs were found to be absent approximately 7 minutes after the SSEP change (Fig. 29.10b). The left extensor hallucis longus appears flat in a few traces, but this is an artifact due to amplifier saturation. The distal right leg muscles were affected more than the proximal. The right vastus lateralis TcMEP remained present though attenuated. Pulse oximetry showed the right toe saturation as lower than the left. The change of SSEPs before TcMEPs, pulse oximetry, and distal leg muscles affected first supported limb ischemia in the right leg. As both iliacs were clamped in this case, there was no route for retrograde perfusion of the right leg. Once the anastomosis was finished and the bilateral iliac arteries unclamped, the right leg EPs quickly returned to baseline.

Case Example 4

A 69-year-old woman with a chronic aortic dissection and extent III TAAA (Fig. 29.11a) presents for planned surgical repair. Following aortic cross-clamping and the opening of the aneurysm sac, loss of the bilateral leg TcMEPs is seen (Fig. 29.11b). Some improvement is seen with an increase in the MAP. Following

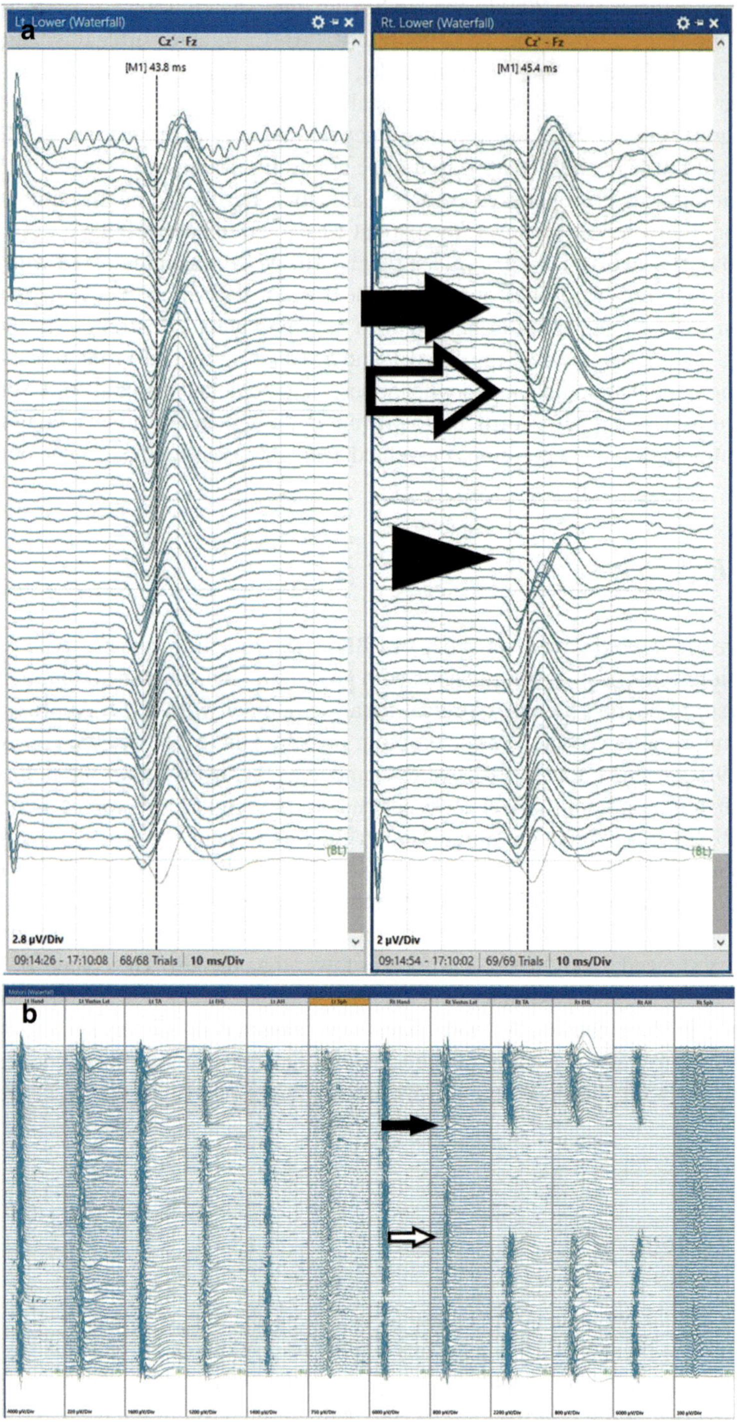
Lt. Lower (Waterfall)
Cz' - Fz
[M1] 43.8 ms
2.8 µV/Div
09:14:26 - 17:10:08
68/68 Trials
10 ms/Div
Rt. Lower (Waterfall)
Cz' - Fz
[M1] 45.4 ms
2 µV/Div
09:14:54 - 17:10:02
69/69 Trials
10 ms/Div
a
b

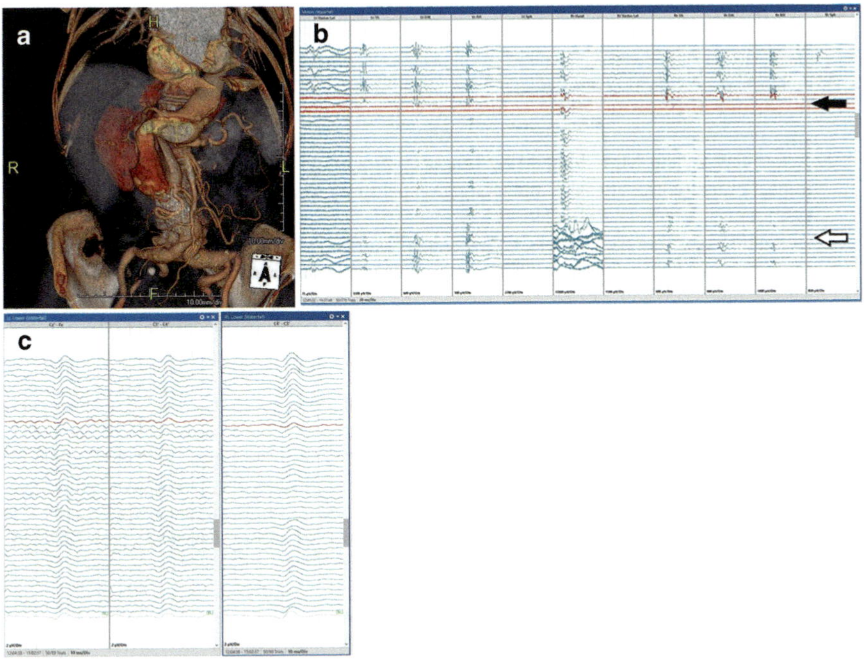

Fig. 29.11 (**a**) A 3D reconstruction from the CT angiogram demonstrating the extent III aneurysm is shown. (**b**) Bilateral TcMEPs are shown chronologically. Loss of leg TcMEPs is seen following opening of the aneurysm sac (solid arrow). Some improvement is seen with an increase in the MAP. The signals greatly improve after backbleeding lumbar arteries are ligated (hollow arrow). (**c**) Bilateral posterior tibial nerve SSEPs are shown chronologically. The right leg SSEP is affected more than the left. The SSEP change was delayed compared to the TcMEP change. The amplitude of the right leg SSEP improved after ligation of the backbleeding vessels as well

the TcMEP changes, right>left leg SSEP amplitude reductions were also seen (Fig. 29.11c). This was felt to represent spinal cord ischemia as the TcMEP changes preceded the SSEP changes and equally involved the proximal and distal leg. The BCR, anal sphincter TcMEP, pudendal SSEP, and perianal SSEP were not reliably obtained in this case and could not be used as additional evidence. The surgeon noted profuse backbleeding from some of the lumbar segmental arteries and ligated these. Following this, the EPs improved back to baseline, supporting that this was spinal cord ischemia. Backbleeding can result in a steal phenomenon which decreases spinal cord perfusion.

Fig. 29.10 (**a**) Bilateral posterior tibial nerve SSEPs are shown chronologically. The solid arrow shows when the proximal aortic clamp and bilateral iliac arteries were clamped distally. The left common femoral artery was perfused off the CPB circuit. Approximately 25 minutes later, the right leg SSEP changes, as indicated by the hollow arrow. Following the completion of distal anastomosis and perfusion of the graft, the SSEP returns (solid arrowhead). (**b**) Bilateral TcMEPs are shown chronologically. The solid arrow shows reduction in amplitude of the right leg TcMEPs. Perfusion of the main graft is followed by return of the right leg TcMEPs (hollow arrow)

References

1. Acher CW, Wynn M. Thoracic and Thoracoabdominal aneurysms: open surgical treatment. In: Sidawy A, Perler B, editors. Rutherford's vascular surgery and endovascular therapy. 9th ed. Amsterdam: Elsevier; 2019. p. 987–1007.
2. Acher CW, Wynn MM, Mell MW, Tefera G, Hoch JR. A quantitative assessment of the impact of intercostal artery reimplantation on paralysis risk in thoracoabdominal aortic aneurysm repair. Ann Surg. 2008;248(4):529–38.
3. Achouh PE, Estrera AL, Miller CC, Azizzadeh A, Irani A, Wegryn TL, et al. Role of somatosensory evoked potentials in predicting outcome during Thoracoabdominal aortic repair. Ann Thorac Surg. 2007;84(3):782–8.
4. Alnajar A, Aleong EF, Azhar MZ, Azarrafiy R, Lamelas J. Review of cerebral perfusion strategies for aortic surgery with application for minimally invasive approaches. J Card Surg. 2020;35(12):3539–44.
5. Anttila V, Kiviluoma K, Pokela M, Rimpiläinen J, Mäkiranta M, Jäntti V, et al. Cold retrograde cerebral perfusion improves cerebral protection during moderate hypothermic circulatory arrest: a long-term study in a porcine model. J Thorac Cardiovasc Surg. 1999;118(5):938–45.
6. Bachet J, Guilmet D, Goudot B, Dreyfus GD, Delentdecker P, Brodaty D, et al. Antegrade cerebral perfusion with cold blood: a 13-year experience. Ann Thorac Surg. 1999;67(6):1874–8.
7. Bafort C, Astarci P, Goffette P, El Khoury G, Guerit J-M, de Tourtchaninoff M, et al. Predicting spinal cord ischemia before endovascular Thoracoabdominal aneurysm repair: monitoring somatosensory evoked potentials. J Endovasc Ther. 2002;9(3):289–94.
8. Banga PV, Oderich GS, De Souza LR, Hofer J, Cazares Gonzalez ML, Pulido JN, et al. Neuromonitoring, cerebrospinal fluid drainage, and selective use of iliofemoral conduits to minimize risk of spinal cord injury during complex endovascular aortic repair. J Endovasc Ther. 2016;23(1):139–49.
9. Bisdas T, Panuccio G, Sugimoto M, Torsello G, Austermann M. Risk factors for spinal cord ischemia after endovascular repair of thoracoabdominal aortic aneurysms. J Vasc Surg. 2015;61(6):1408–16.
10. Boezeman RPE, Van Dongen EP, Morshuis WJ, Sonker U, Boezeman EHJF, Waanders FGJ, et al. Spinal near-infrared spectroscopy measurements during and after thoracoabdominal aortic aneurysm repair: a pilot study. Ann Thorac Surg. 2015;99(4):1267–74.
11. Brau SA, Spoonamore MJ, Snyder L, Gilbert C, Rhonda G, Williams LA, et al. Nerve monitoring changes related to iliac artery compression during anterior lumbar spine surgery. Spine J. 2003;3(5):351–5.
12. Brockstein B, Johns L, Gewertz BL. Blood supply to the spinal cord: anatomic and physiologic correlations. Ann Vasc Surg. 1994;8(4):394–9.
13. Buth J, Harris PL, Hobo R, van Eps R, Cuypers P, Duijm L, et al. Neurologic complications associated with endovascular repair of thoracic aortic pathology: incidence and risk factors. A study from the European Collaborators on Stent/Graft Techniques for Aortic Aneurysm Repair (EUROSTAR) Registry. J Vasc Surg. 2007;46(6):1103.
14. Cha S, Wang KC, Park K, Shin HI, Lee JY, Chong S, et al. Predictive value of intraoperative bulbocavernosus reflex during untethering surgery for post-operative voiding function. Clin Neurophysiol. 2018;129(12):2594–601.
15. Chang FW, Nguyen V, Le S, Lee L, Cho SC, López JR. Outcomes and patient characteristics of intraoperative peripheral somatosensory evoked potentials (SSEP) changes. American Clinical Neurophysiology Society Annual Meeting; 2021 Feb 10–14.
16. Charles YP, Barbe B, Beaujeux R, Boujan F, Steib JP. Relevance of the anatomical location of the Adamkiewicz artery in spine surgery. Surg Radiol Anat. 2011;33(1):3–9.
17. Cheshire WP, Santos CC, Massey EW, Howard JF. Spinal cord infarction: etiology and outcome. Neurology. 1996;47(2):321–30.

18. Chowet AL, Lopez JR, Brock-Utne JG, Jaffe RA. Wrist hyperextension leads to median nerve conduction block: implications for intra-arterial catheter placement. Anesthesiology. 2004;100(2):287–91.
19. Cinà CS, Abouzahr L, Arena GO, Laganà A, Devereaux PJ, Farrokhyar F. Cerebrospinal fluid drainage to prevent paraplegia during thoracic and thoracoabdominal aortic aneurysm surgery: a systematic review and meta-analysis. J Vasc Surg. 2004;40(1):36–44.
20. Coselli JS, Bozinovski J, LeMaire SA. Open surgical repair of 2286 Thoracoabdominal aortic aneurysms. Ann Thorac Surg. 2007;83(2):S862.
21. Coselli JS, Crawford ES, Beall AC, Mizrahi EM, Hess KR, Patel VM. Determination of brain temperatures for safe circulatory arrest during cardiovascular operation. Ann Thorac Surg. 1988;45(6):638–42.
22. Crawford ES, Mizrahi EM, Hess KR, Coselli JS, Safi HJ, Patel VM. The impact of distal aortic perfusion and somatosensory evoked potential monitoring on prevention of paraplegia after aortic aneurysm operation. J Thorac Cardiovasc Surg. 1988;95(3):357–67.
23. Cunningham JN, Laschinger JC, Merkin HA, Nathan IM, Colvin S, Ransohoff J, et al. Measurement of spinal cord ischemia during operations upon the thoracic aorta. Initial clinical experience. Ann Surg. 1982;196(3):285–96.
24. David N, Roux N, Douvrin F, Clavier E, Bessou JP, Plissonnier D. Aortic aneurysm surgery: long-term patency of the reimplanted intercostal arteries. Ann Vasc Surg. 2012;26(6):839–44.
25. Deletis V, Vodusek DB. Intraoperative recording of the bulbocavernosus reflex. Neurosurgery. 1997;40(1):88–93.
26. Dias NV, Sonesson B, Kristmundsson T, Holm H, Resch T. Short-term outcome of spinal cord ischemia after endovascular repair of thoracoabdominal aortic aneurysms. Eur J Vasc Endovasc Surg. 2015;49(4):403–9.
27. Dong CCJ, MacDonald DB, Janusz MT. Intraoperative spinal cord monitoring during descending thoracic and thoracoabdominal aneurysm surgery. Ann Thorac Surg. 2002;74:S1873.
28. Ehrlich MP, Hagl C, McCullough JN, Zhang N, Shiang H, Bodian C, et al. Retrograde cerebral perfusion provides negligible flow through brain capillaries in the pig. J Thorac Cardiovasc Surg. 2001;122(2):331–8.
29. Erecinska M, Thoresen M, Silver IA. Effects of hypothermia on energy metabolism in mammalian central nervous system. J Cereb Blood Flow Metab. 2003;23:513–30.
30. Estrera AL, Miller CC, Huynh TT, Azizzadeh A, Porat EE, Vinnerkvist A, et al. Preoperative and operative predictors of delayed neurologic deficit following repair of thoracoabdominal aortic aneurysm. J Thorac Cardiovasc Surg. 2003;126(5):1288–94.
31. Estrera AL, Sheinbaum R, Miller CC, Harrison R, Safi HJ. Neuromonitor-guided repair of thoracoabdominal aortic aneurysms. J Thorac Cardiovasc Surg. 2010;140(6 SUPPL):S131.
32. Etz CD, Halstead JC, Spielvogel D, Shahani R, Lazala R, Homann TM, et al. Thoracic and Thoracoabdominal aneurysm repair: is reimplantation of spinal cord arteries a waste of time? Ann Thorac Surg. 2006;82(5):1670–7.
33. Etz CD, Luehr M, Kari FA, Bodian CA, Smego D, Plestis KA, et al. Paraplegia after extensive thoracic and thoracoabdominal aortic aneurysm repair: does critical spinal cord ischemia occur postoperatively? J Thorac Cardiovasc Surg. 2008;135(2):324–30.
34. Falcao ALE, Reutens DC, Markus R, Koga M, Read SJ, Tochon-Danguy H, et al. The resistance to ischemia of white and gray matter after stroke. Ann Neurol. 2004;56(5):695–701.
35. Fan T, Wang CC, Wang FM, Cheng F, Qiao H, Liu SL, et al. Experimental study of the protection of ischemic preconditioning to spinal cord ischemia. Surg Neurol. 1999;52(3):299–305.
36. Fitzgibbons PG, Di Giovanni C, Hares S, Akelman E. Safe tourniquet use: a review of the evidence. J Am Acad Orthop Surg. 2012;20:310–9.
37. Fok M, Jafarzadeh F, Sancho E, Abello D, Rimmer L, Howard C, et al. Is there any benefit of neuromonitoring during descending and thoracoabdominal aortic aneurysm repair? Innov Technol Tech Cardiothorac Vasc Surg. 2015;10(5):342–8.

38. Galla JD, Ergin MA, Lansman SL, McCullough JN, Nguyen HK, Spielvogel D, et al. Use of somatosensory evoked potentials for thoracic and thoracoabdominal aortic resections. Ann Thorac Surg. 1999;67:1947–52.
39. Gega A, Rizzo JA, Johnson MH, Tranquilli M, Farkas EA, Elefteriades JA. Straight deep hypothermic arrest: experience in 394 patients supports its effectiveness as a sole means of brain preservation. Ann Thorac Surg. 2007;84(3):759–67.
40. Gharagozloo F, Larson J, Dausmann MJ, Neville RF, Gomes MN. Spinal cord protection during surgical procedures on the descending thoracic and thoracoabdominal aorta: review of current techniques. Chest. 1996;109(3):799–809.
41. Gillilan LA. Veins of the spinal cord: anatomic details; suggested clinical applications. Neurology. 1970;20(9):860–8.
42. Greenberg RK, Lu Q, Roselli EE, Svensson LG, Moon MC, Hernandez AV, et al. Contemporary analysis of descending thoracic and thoracoabdominal aneurysm repair a comparison of endovascular and open techniques. Circulation. 2008;118(8):808–17.
43. Griepp RB, Ergin MA, Galla JD, Lansman S, Khan N, Quintana C, et al. Looking for the artery of Adamkiewicz: a quest to minimize paraplegia after operations for aneurysms of the descending thoracic and thoracoabdominal aorta. J Thorac Cardiovasc Surg. 1996;112(5):1202–15.
44. Griepp RB, Stinson EB, Hollingsworth JF, Buehler D. Prosthetic replacement of the aortic arch. J Thorac Cardiovasc Surg. 1975;70(6):1051–63.
45. Haldenwang PL, Prochnow N, Baumann A, Buchwald D, Häuser L, Schlömicher M, et al. Spinal cord ischemia after selective cerebral perfusion in a porcine "frozen elephant trunk" simulation model. Ann Thorac Surg. 2015;99(5):1624–31.
46. Hamaishi M, Orihashi K, Takahashi S, Isaka M, Okada K, Sueda T. Transcranial motor-evoked potentials following intra-aortic cold blood infusion facilitates detection of critical supplying artery of spinal cord. Eur J Cardio-thoracic Surg. 2008;33(4):695–9.
47. Hofmeijer J, Franssen H, van Schelven LJ, van Putten MJAM. Why are sensory axons more vulnerable for ischemia than motor axons? PLoS One. 2013;8(6):e67113.
48. Hong MK-Y, Hong MK-H, Pan W-R, Wallace D, Ashton MW, Taylor GI. The angiosome territories of the spinal cord: exploring the issue of preoperative spinal angiography: laboratory investigation. J Neurosurg Spine. 2008;8(4):352–64.
49. Hyodoh H, Shirase R, Akiba H, Tamakawa M, Hyodoh K, Yama N, et al. Double-subtraction maximum intensity projection MR angiography for detecting the artery of Adamkiewicz and differentiating it from the drainage vein. J Magn Reson Imaging. 2007;26(2):359–65.
50. Jacobs MJ, Mess W, Mochtar B, Nijenhuis RJ, Statius Van Eps RG, Schurink GWH. The value of motor evoked potentials in reducing paraplegia during thoracoabdominal aneurysm repair. J Vasc Surg. 2006;43(2):239–46.
51. Jacobs MJHM, Meylaerts SA, De Haan P, Mol BAD, Kalkman CJ. Assessment of spinal cord ischemia by means of evoked potential monitoring during thoracoabdominal aortic surgery. Semin Vasc Surg. 2000;13(4):299–307.
52. Jacobs MJHM, Meylaerts SA, De Haan P, De Mol BA, Kalkman CJ, Cherry J, et al. Strategies to prevent neurologic deficit based on motor-evoked potentials in type I and II thoracoabdominal aortic aneurysm repair. J Vasc Surg. 1999;29(1):48–59.
53. Jafarzadeh F, Bashir M, Yan T, Harrington D, Field ML, Kuduvalli M, et al. Setting up and utilizing a service for measuring perioperative transcranial motor evoked potentials during thoracoabdominal aortic surgery and thoracic endovascular repair. Interact Cardiovasc Thorac Surg. 2014;18(6):748–56.
54. James ML, Andersen ND, Swaminathan M, Phillips-Bute B, Hanna JM, Smigla GR, et al. Predictors of electrocerebral inactivity with deep hypothermia. J Thorac Cardiovasc Surg. 2014;147(3):1002–7.
55. Kaplan BJ, Friedman WA, Gravenstein N, Richards R, Davis RF. Effects of aortic occlusion on regional spinal cord blood flow and somatosensory evoked potentials in sheep. Neurosurgery. 1987;21(5):668–75.

56. Kari FA, Wittmann K, Saravi B, Puttfarcken L, Krause S, Förster K, et al. Immediate spinal cord collateral blood flow during thoracic aortic procedures: the role of epidural arcades. Semin Thorac Cardiovasc Surg. 2016;28(2):378–87.
57. Keenan JE, Wang H, Ganapathi AM, Englum BR, Kale E, Mathew JP, et al. Electroencephalography during Hemiarch replacement with moderate hypothermic circulatory arrest. Ann Thorac Surg. 2016;101(2):631.
58. Keyhani K, Miller CC, Estrera AL, Wegryn T, Sheinbaum R, Safi HJ. Analysis of motor and somatosensory evoked potentials during thoracic and thoracoabdominal aortic aneurysm repair. J Vasc Surg. 2009;49(1):36–41.
59. Khan SN, Stansby G, Group CV. Cerebrospinal fluid drainage for thoracic and thoracoabdominal aortic aneurysm surgery. Cochrane Database Syst Rev. 2012;(10):CD003635.
60. Koshino T, Murakami G, Morishita K, Mawatari T, Abe T, Svensson L. Does the Adamkiewicz artery originate from the larger segmental arteries? J Thorac Cardiovasc Surg. 1999;117(5):898–905.
61. Kouchoukos NT, Masetti P, Rokkas CK, Murphy SF. Hypothermic cardiopulmonary bypass and circulatory arrest for operations on the descending thoracic and thoracoabdominal aorta. Ann Thorac Surg. 2002;74(5):S1885–7.
62. Kouchoukos NT, Wareing TH, Izumoto H, Klausing W, Abboud N. Elective hypothermic cardiopulmonary bypass and circulatory arrest for spinal cord protection during operations on the thoracoabdominal aorta. J Thorac Cardiovasc Surg. 1990;99(4):659–64.
63. Lam CR, Aram HH. Resection of the descending thoracic aorta for aneurysm; a report of the use of a homograft in a case and an experimental study. Ann Surg. 1951;134(4):743–52.
64. Laschinger JC, Cunningham JN, Baumann FG, Isom OW, Spencer FC. Monitoring of somatosensory evoked potentials during surgical procedures on the thoracoabdominal aorta: II. Use of somatosensory evoked potentials to assess adequacy of distal aortic bypass and perfusion after thoracic aortic cross-clamping. J Thorac Cardiovasc Surg. 1987;94(2):266–70.
65. Lee L, Lee J, Jones E, Cho SC, Nguyen V, Le S, et al. Novel intraoperative neurophysiologic monitoring (IONM) techniques during thoracic endovascular aortic repair (TEVAR) to rapidly assess central spinal cord versus peripheral limb ischemia. Neurology. 2016;86(16):4.192.
66. Lewis FJ, Taufic M. Closure of atrial septal defects with the aid of hypothermia; experimental accomplishments and the report of one successful case. Surgery. 1953;33(1):52–9.
67. Lips J, De Haan P, De Jager SW, Vanicky I, Jacobs MJ, Kalkman CJ. The role of transcranial motor evoked potentials in predicting neurologic and histopathologic outcome after experimental spinal cord ischemia. Anesthesiology. 2002;97(1):183–91.
68. Liu LY, Callahan B, Peterss S, Dumfarth J, Tranquilli M, Ziganshin BA, et al. Neuromonitoring using motor and somatosensory evoked potentials in aortic surgery. J Card Surg. 2016;31(6):383–9.
69. Luehr M, Mohr FW, Etz CD. Indirect Neuromonitoring of the spinal cord by near-infrared spectroscopy of the Paraspinous thoracic and lumbar muscles in aortic surgery. Thorac Cardiovasc Surg. 2015;64(4):333–5.
70. MacDonald DB, Janusz M. An approach to intraoperative neurophysiologic monitoring of thoracoabdominal aneurysm surgery. J Clin Neurophysiol. 2002;19(1):43–54.
71. Maier S, Shcherbakova M, Beyersdorf F, Benk C, Kari FA, Siepe M, et al. Benefits and risks of prophylactic cerebrospinal fluid catheter and evoked potential monitoring in symptomatic spinal cord ischemia low-risk thoracic endovascular aortic repair. Thorac Cardiovasc Surg. 2019;67(5):379–84.
72. Makaroun MS, Dillavou ED, Kee ST, Sicard G, Chaikof E, Bavaria J, et al. Endovascular treatment of thoracic aortic aneurysms: results of the phase II multicenter trial of the GORE TAG thoracic endoprosthesis. J Vasc Surg. 2005;41(1):1–9.
73. Manetta F, Mullan CW, Catalano MA. Neuroprotective strategies in repair and replacement of the aortic arch. Int J Angiol. 2018;27(2):98.

74. Mell MW, Wynn MM, Reeder SB, Tefera G, Hoch JR, Acher CW. A new intercostal artery management strategy for Thoracoabdominal aortic aneurysm repair. J Surg Res. 2009;154(1):99–104.
75. Meylaerts SA, Jacobs MJ, van Iterson V, De Haan P, Kalkman CJ, Van Iterson V, et al. Comparison of transcranial motor evoked potentials and somatosensory evoked potentials during thoracoabdominal aortic aneurysm repair. No title. Ann Surg. 1999;230(6):742.
76. Mezrow CK, Midulla PS, Sadeghi AM, Gandsas A, Wang W, Dapunt OE, et al. Evaluation of cerebral metabolism and quantitative electroencephalography after hypothermic circulatory, arrest and low-flow cardiopulmonary bypass at different temperatures. J Thorac Cardiovasc Surg. 1994;107(4):1006–19.
77. Michenfelder JD, Milde JH. The effect of profound levels of hypothermia (below 14°C) on canine cerebral metabolism. J Cereb Blood Flow Metab. 1992;12(5):877–80.
78. Morota N. Intraoperative neurophysiological monitoring of the bulbocavernosus reflex during surgery for conus spinal lipoma: what are the warning criteria? J Neurosurg Pediatr. 2019;23(5):639–47.
79. Murakami H, Tsukube T, Kawanishi Y, Okita Y. Transcranial myogenic motor-evoked potentials after transient spinal cord ischemia predicts neurologic outcome in rabbits. J Vasc Surg. 2004;39(1):207–13.
80. Osenbach RK, Hitchon PW, Mouw L, Yamada T. Effects of spinal cord ischemia on evoked potential recovery and postischemic regional spinal cord blood flow. J Spinal Disord Tech. 1993;6(2):146–54.
81. Pelliccioni G, Piloni V, Sabbatini D, Fioravanti P, Scarpino O. Sex differences in pudendal somatosensory evoked potentials. Tech Coloproctol. 2014;18(6):565–9.
82. Pillai JB, Pellet Y, Panagopoulos G, Sadek MA, Abjigitova D, Weiss D, et al. Somatosensory-evoked potential-guided intercostal artery reimplantation in thoracoabdominal aortic aneurysm surgery. Innov Technol Tech Cardiothorac Vasc Surg. 2013;8(4):302–6.
83. Rodi Z, Vodušek DB. Intraoperative monitoring of the bulbocavernosus reflex: the method and its problems. Clin Neurophysiol. 2001;112(5):879–83.
84. Ross SD, Kron IL, Parrino PE, Shockey KS, Kern JA, Tribble CG, et al. Preservation of intercostal arteries during thoracoabdominal aortic aneurysm surgery: a retrospective study. J Thorac Cardiovasc Surg. 1999;118(1):17–24.
85. Safi HJ, Miller CC, Carr C, Iliopoulos DC, Dorsay DA, Baldwin JC, et al. Importance of intercostal artery reattachment during thoracoabdominal aortic aneurysm repair. J Vasc Surg. 1998;27(1):58–68.
86. Santillan A, Nacarino V, Greenberg E, Riina HA, Gobin YP, Patsalides A. Vascular anatomy of the spinal cord. J Neurointerv Surg. 2012;4(1):67–74.
87. Sarkar M, Prabhu V. Basics of cardiopulmonary bypass. Indian J Anaesth. 2017;61(9):760.
88. Scali ST, Wang SK, Feezor RJ, Huber TS, Martin TD, Klodell CT, et al. Preoperative prediction of spinal cord ischemia after thoracic endovascular aortic repair. J Vasc Surg. 2014;60:1481–1490.e1.
89. Schepens MAAM, Boezeman EHJF, Hamerlijnck RPHM, ter Beek H, Vermeulen FEE. Somatosensory evoked potentials during exclusion and reperfusion of critical aortic segments in Thoracoabdominal aortic aneurysm surgery. J Card Surg. 1994;9(6):692–702.
90. Schepens MAAM, Defauw JJAM, Hamerlijnck RPHM, Vermeulen FEE. Use of left heart bypass in the surgical repair of Thoracoabdominal aortic aneurysms. Ann Vasc Surg. 1995;9(4):327–38.
91. See RB, Awosika OO, Cambria RP, Conrad MF, Lancaster RT, Patel VI, et al. Extended motor evoked potentials monitoring helps prevent delayed paraplegia after aortic surgery. Ann Neurol. 2016;79(4):636–45.
92. Shine TSJ, Harrison BA, De Ruyter ML, Crook JE, Heckman M, Daube JR, et al. Motor and somatosensory evoked potentials: their role in predicting spinal cord ischemia in patients undergoing thoracoabdominal aortic aneurysm repair with regional lumbar epidural cooling. Anesthesiology. 2008;108(4):580–7.

93. Shinjo T, Hayashi H, Takatani T, Boku E, Nakase H, Kawaguchi M. Intraoperative feasibility of bulbocavernosus reflex monitoring during untethering surgery in infants and children. J Clin Monit Comput. 2019;33(1):155–63.
94. Shinzawa M, Minatoya K, Ohnishi Y, Yoshitani K, Irie T, Ogino H. Changes of motor evoked potentials during descending thoracic and thoracoabdominal aortic surgery with deep hypothermic circulatory arrest. J Anesth. 2012;26(2):160–7.
95. Skinner S, Chiri CA, Wroblewski J, Transfeldt EE. Enhancement of the bulbocavernosus reflex during intraoperative neurophysiological monitoring through the use of double train stimulation: a pilot study. J Clin Monit Comput. 2007;21(1):31–40.
96. Skinner SA, Vodušek DB. Intraoperative recording of the Bulbocavernosus reflex. J Clin Neurophysiol. 2014;31(4):313–22.
97. Stecker MM, Cheung AT, Pochettino A, Kent GP, Patterson T, Weiss SJ, et al. Deep hypothermic circulatory arrest: I. Effects of cooling on electroencephalogram and evoked potentials. Ann Thorac Surg. 2001;71(1):14–21.
98. Sueda T, Okada K, Watari M, Orihashi K, Shikata H, Matsuura Y. Evaluation of motor- and sensory-evoked potentials for spinal cord monitoring during thoracoabdominal aortic aneurysm surgery. Jpn J Thorac Cardiovasc Surg. 2000;48(1):60–5.
99. Svensson LG, Crawford ES, Hess KR, Coselli JS, Safi HJ. Experience with 1509 patients undergoing thoracoabdominal aortic operations. J Vasc Surg. 1993;17(2):357–70.
100. Svensson LG, Hess KR, Coselli JS, Safi HJ. Influence of segmental arteries, extent, and atriofemoral bypass on postoperative paraplegia after thoracoabdominal aortic operations. J Vasc Surg. 1994;20(2):255–62.
101. Tanaka Y, Kawaguchi M, Noguchi Y, Yoshitani K, Kawamata M, Masui K, et al. Systematic review of motor evoked potentials monitoring during thoracic and thoracoabdominal aortic aneurysm open repair surgery: a diagnostic meta-analysis. J Anesth Springer. 2016;30:1037–50.
102. Taylor DW, Whisnant JP. Beneficial effect of carotid endarterectomy in symptomatic patients with high-grade carotid stenosis. Ann Intern Med. 1991;115(6 SUPPL. 2):34.
103. Ter Wolbeek C, Hartert M, Conzelmann LO, Peivandi AA, Czerny M, Gottardi R, et al. Value and pitfalls of neurophysiological monitoring in thoracic and thoracoabdominal aortic replacement and endovascular repair. Thorac Cardiovasc Surg. 2010;58(5):260–4.
104. Tian DH, Yan TD. Consensus on hypothermia in aortic arch surgery. Hear Lung Circ. 2014;23(1):e47–8.
105. Ullery BW, Cheung AT, Fairman RM, Jackson BM, Woo EY, Bavaria J, et al. Risk factors, outcomes, and clinical manifestations of spinal cord ischemia following thoracic endovascular aortic repair. J Vasc Surg. 2011;54(3):677–84.
106. Uysal S, Lin HM, Fischer GW, Di Luozzo G, Reich DL. Selective cerebral perfusion for thoracic aortic surgery: association with neurocognitive outcome. J Thorac Cardiovasc Surg. 2012;143(5):1205–12.
107. Van Dongen EP, Schepens MA, Morshuis WJ, Ter Beek HT, Aarts LP, De Boer A, et al. Thoracic and thoracoabdominal aortic aneurysm repair: use of evoked potential monitoring in 118 patients. J Vasc Surg. 2001;34(6):1035–40.
108. Weigang E, Hartert M, Siegenthaler MP, Pitzer-Hartert K, Luehr M, Sircar R, et al. Neurophysiological monitoring during thoracoabdominal aortic endovascular stent graft implantation. Eur J Cardiothorac Surg. 2006;29:392–6.
109. Wynn M, Acher C, Marks E, Acher CW. The effect of intercostal artery reimplantation on spinal cord injury in thoracoabdominal aortic aneurysm surgery. J Vasc Surg. 2016;64:289–96.
110. Williams GM, Roseborough GS, Webb TH, Perler BA, Krosnick T, Safi HJ, et al. Preoperative selective intercostal angiography in patients undergoing thoracoabdominal aneurysm repair. J Vasc Surg. 2004;39(2):314–21.
111. Yoo JS, Kim JB, Joo Y, Lee WY, Jung SH, Choo SJ, et al. Deep hypothermic circulatory arrest versus non-deep hypothermic beating heart strategy in descending thoracic or thoracoabdominal aortic surgery. Eur J Cardio-thoracic Surg. 2014;46(4):678–84.

112. Yoo JS, Kim JB, Jung S-H, Choo SJ, Chung CH, Lee JW. Surgical repair of descending thoracic and thoracoabdominal aortic aneurysm involving the distal arch: open proximal anastomosis under deep hypothermia versus arch clamping technique. J Thorac Cardiovasc Surg. 2014;148(5):2101–7.
113. Zawiliński J, Litwin JA, Nowogrodzka-Zagórska M, Gorczyca J, Miodoński AJ. Vascular system of the human spinal cord in the prenatal period: a dye injection and corrosion casting study. Ann Anat. 2001;183(4):331–40.
114. Ziganshin BA, Elefteriades JA. Deep hypothermic circulatory arrest. Ann Cardiothorac Surg. 2013;2(3):303.
115. Zileli M, Schramm J. Motor versus somatosensory evoked potential changes after acute experimental spinal cord injury in rats. Acta Neurochir. 1991;108(3–4):140–7.
116. Khan NR, Smalley Z, Nesvick CL, Lee SL, Michael LM. The use of lumbar drains in preventing Spinal cord injury following thoracoabdominal aortic aneurysm repair: An updated systematic review and meta-analysis. Vol. 25, Journal of Neurosurgery: Spine. J Neurosurg Spine; 2016. p. 383–93.
117. Guérit JM, Verhelst R, Rubay J, Khoury G, Matta A, Dion R. Multilevel somatosensory evoked potentials (SEPs) for spinal cord monitoring in descending thoracic and thoracoabdominal aortic surgery. Eur J Cardio-thoracic Surg. 1996;10(2):93–104.

Part VII
Pheripheral Nerve Surgery

Chapter 30
Peripheral Nerve: Neurophysiology as a Tool to Optimize Topographic Accuracy and Surgical Planning

Maria Rufina Barros

Abbreviations

BPI	Brachial plexus injury
CMAPs	Compound muscle action potentials
EDX	Electrodiagnostic exam
EMG	Electromyography
fEMG	Free-running electromyography
HFF	High-frequency filter
IONM	Intraoperative neurophysiological monitoring
LFF	Low-frequency filter
MEPs	Motor-evoked potentials
MRI	Magnetic resonance imaging
MU	Motor unit
NAP	Nerve action potential
NEE	Needle electrode examination
PN	Peripheral nerve
SEPs	Sensory-evoked potentials
SNAPs	Sensory nerve action potentials
Tc-MEP	Transcranial motor-evoked potential
tEMG	Trigger electromyography

M. R. Barros (✉)
Department of Intraoperative Monitoring, Neurological Institute of Espirito Santo, Vitória, ES, Brazil

Department of Neurophysiology, Vitoria Apart Hospital (VAH), Vitória, ES, Brazil
e-mail: mariabarros@vah.com.br

S. M. Verst et al. (eds.), *Intraoperative Monitoring*,
https://doi.org/10.1007/978-3-030-95730-8_30

Introduction

Traffic accidents are considered a public health problem. They are ranked among the first causes of violent deaths worldwide, particularly in developing countries. Every minute in Brazil, one person dies or is seriously injured as a result of motorcycle accident [1]. By affecting mostly the young and economically active population, this high rate of motorcycle accidents generates a great social and economic impact, overloading the public health and the social security systems [11]. Every year, thousands of youths lose their lives or are removed from the employment market permanently at an early age.

Hence, we deliberately focus on the management of traumatic brachial plexus injuries (BPIs), given the high incidence in our country, the huge complexity, and the technical divergences involved in this issue.

In BPI, the clinical history and physical examination, added to preoperative electrodiagnostic examination (EDX), provide the most important tools to define the diagnosis, prognosis, and surgical planning [33].

The correct management of BPI, even in polytrauma referral centers, demands the engagement of the whole team. It is necessary to be aware of the main aspects inherent to this kind of injury [29] and the anatomical complexity involved (Fig. 30.1): (1) accuracy in the topographic diagnosis, as the outcome depends on this; (2) attention to the possibility of multiple nerve injuries in more than one topography and with different levels of severity; (3) choosing the ideal time window

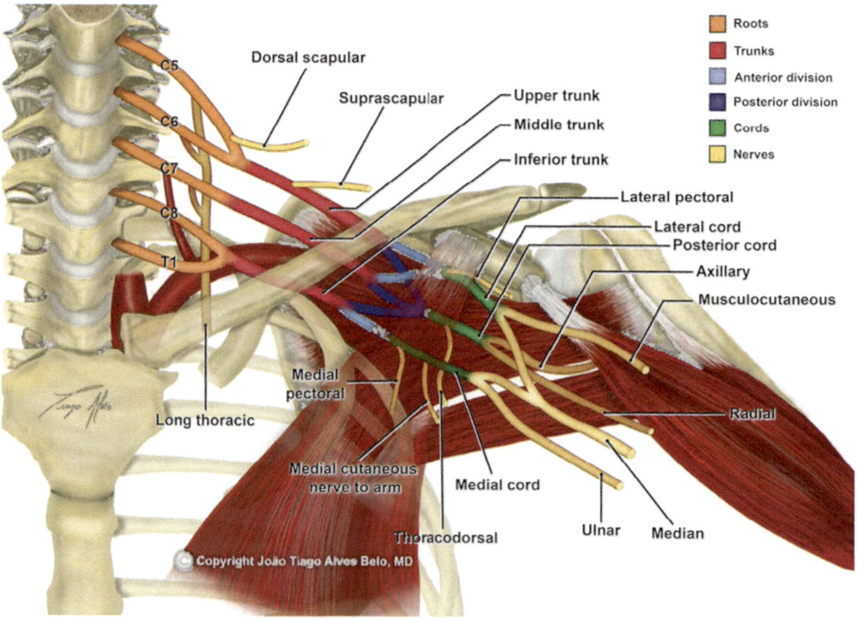

Fig. 30.1 Anatomical complexity of the brachial plexus

for the intervention; (4) planning the most suitable surgical approach [31], whether neurolysis, grafting, transfers, or a combination of all of them for the same patient.

All diagnostic tests performed preoperatively, whether EDX [7], the computed tomographic myelography (CTM), and magnetic resonance imaging (MRI), carry their percentage of failure to define precisely the topography and severity of the injury and, consequently, to estimate the prognosis [28]. Particularly, concerning nerve root avulsion, the intraoperative neurophysiology can move forward in relation to preoperative diagnostic studies.

The majority of BPI are closed injuries, secondary to traction and stretching [17]. The surgical approach to this kind of injury usually occurs around 6 months after the trauma. We highlight the fact that, this time window, allows the reinnervation process of subclinical lesions in the possible donor nerves. Thus, even if not clinically evident, this donor may have suffered a considerable axonal loss, and may not qualify as the ideal donor (author's personal observation).

The nerve action potential (NAP) development technique cannot be overlooked. Since Kline and Happel's pioneer work in the 1960s and until present day, the NAP is the most widely used modality in peripheral nerve monitoring [21, 22]. Rarely, there will be a peripheral nerve surgical approach where it is not performed. We aim to highlight the importance of mastering, executing, and applying it properly.

In our country, despite the alarming rates of motorcycle accidents, few neurophysiologists are involved with peripheral nerve monitoring. Our goal, besides encouraging and introducing colleagues to the NAP's proper execution, is to demonstrate that EDX and intraoperative neurophysiologic monitoring (IONM) are tools that can effectively modify the surgical planning. Consequently, they directly impact the outcome of traumatic, tumoral, or compressive peripheral nerve surgical approaches.

Last but not least, IONM should be considered as a complement to preoperative assessments of clinical evaluation, imaging, and EDX. To better explain our reasoning and protocol, one should make a parallel with epilepsy surgery, in which intraoperative EEG is a continuity of the preoperative EEG assessment.

NAP: Past, Present, and Future

Despite all the propaedeutics and preoperative planning, the final decision about the ideal surgical management relies on the NAP, if it is detectable or not. Considering that NAP is the main neurophysiological test performed in practically all surgical approaches to the peripheral nerve, it is fundamental that we first discuss its concept, technique, and applicability.

Most peripheral nerve injuries result from blunt trauma and maintain some degree of continuity. A positive NAP means that a satisfactory reinnervation process is underway and that enough axons are conducting distal to the lesion [21]. This response expresses the functionality of approximately 4000–5000 myelinated axons with a diameter greater than or equal to 5 microns [19, 33].

The diversity in caliber and myelination of these fibers will be reflected in the characteristics of the recorded responses, which can have low amplitude, prolonged latency, and slow conduction velocity. However, when dealing with damaged nerves, it is not the individual analysis of these parameters that matters. The proper interpretation of the functional status of those fibers will base surgeon's decision making as follows: (1) A positive NAP usually implies in performing only neurolysis and/or split repair. (2) A negative NAP involves a more complex approach by employing grafts or transpositions.

A neural fascicle may exhibit an intact appearance on its external surface and be internally disrupted. Hence, a decision based on visual inspection alone can be completely wrong. We suggest as further reading the outstanding texts of Susan E. Mackinnon [26], who was responsible for spreading the term "VI-degree lesion" (Fig. 30.2). Indeed, there can be coexistence of grade I (preserved) to grade V (transected) fascicles in the same neural segment. Mackinnon and Dellon modified Sunderland's classification [40] to include the mixed lesion pattern (grade VI), which more closely matches to clinical practice.

Some neuromas in continuity, despite their bad appearance, have positive NAPs and histological organization compatible with axonal maturation. Conversely, other nerves, apparently preserved and without a neuromatous appearance, do not conduct across and distally to the lesion. These nerves, if biopsied, exhibit a more compromised fascicular architecture, incompatible with a satisfactory regeneration process [19]. For this reason, surgeons and neurophysiologists should not be impressed by the appearance but rather perform NAP on absolutely all lesions in continuity (Fig. 30.3).

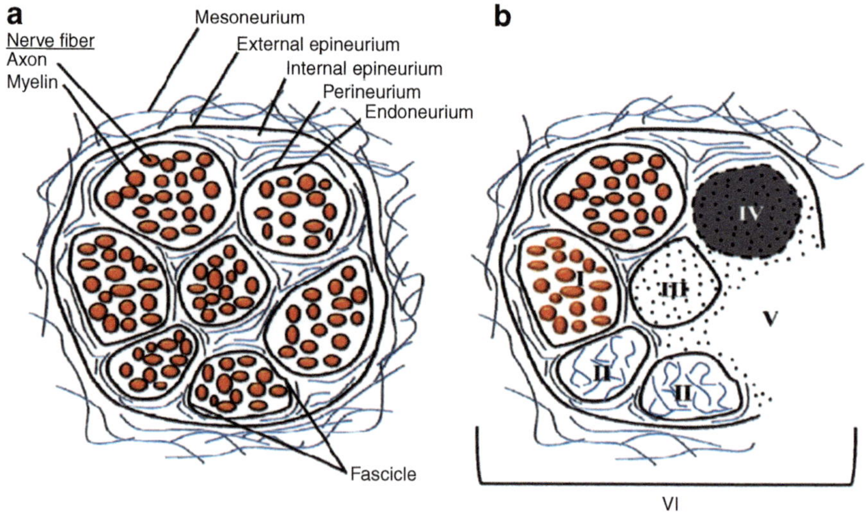

Fig. 30.2 Sunderland grade VI injury. (**a**) Normal nerve. (**b**) Classification of nerve injury. (Courtesy of the Thieme, with permission)

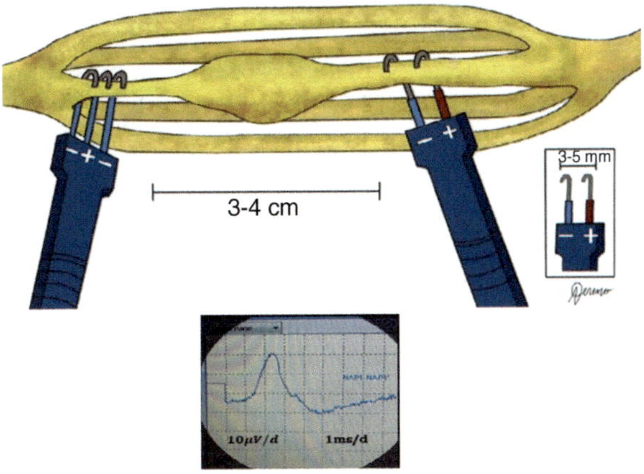

Fig. 30.3 NAP recording on a neuromatous segment. Illustration to highlight the optimal distance between the two probes with the correct positioning of the bipolar probe: cathode proximally oriented and the ideal distance between the probe tips

Ideal "Time Window" for NAP Recording

In acute continuity injuries, NAP is useful to identify conduction block in the damaged nerve segment. But, during this period, one cannot distinguish between neuropraxia, axonotmesis, and/or neurotmesis. The time window for performing NAP must be tailored considering the mechanism and particular pattern of the damage [19, 38]:

(a) *8 weeks to 4 months* – in focal or known partial lesions, like injuries at the site of bone fractures or secondary to gunshot wounds
(b) *16 weeks to 6 months or longer* – in closed stretch injuries such as BPI, since these tend to be more diffuse and multiple
(c) *Any time after diagnosis* – on tumoral lesions or entrapments.

In this context, the NAP recording bridges the gap that is left by the EDX ambulatory tests. Especially in more proximal lesions, the presence of NAP around the 6th and 8th weeks allows the identification of a regenerative process that would rather take months to be detected by conventional EDX.

Following an axonotmesis, once the communication between the axon and the cell body has been disrupted, a complex sequence of events along the distal axonal stump begins: mobilization of various pro-inflammatory and phagocytic factors that culminate with the disintegration of the motor plate [10]. For a satisfactory functional recovery, an axonal regeneration rate of 1 mm/d or 1 inch/month is required [37]. In proximal lesions like traumatic BPI, despite all the conditions for satisfactory reinnervation being favorable, it takes months for the axonal sprouting cone to cover the distance to the terminal innervated muscle. This time-lapse is usually incompatible with a satisfactory reinnervation process [26].

NAP Instrumentation and Equipment Setup Step by Step

Over the last decades, there has been an impressive development of the hardware and software of IONM systems. Currently, most devices provide the necessary setup for NAP studies. Regardless of all technological upgrades, the NAP registration is always a challenge for beginners. For this reason, we strongly recommend, as a complementary reading, the pioneers' description of the NAP technique [19, 20, 22, 33, 41].

For NAP registration, if a tourniquet is being used at the extremity, it must be deflated approximately 20 minutes before the recordings due to the ischemia effects. Also, the administration of any local anesthetic should be avoided, since its action can result in conduction block.

Electrodes for Stimulus and Recording

The NAP is a response "time-locked" with the stimulus. A huge stimulus artifact and a neurobiological signal indistinguishable from noise can be registered on the screen if unproper probes are being used. A tripolar probe should be used for stimulation and a bipolar one for recording (Fig. 30.4). The tips of both should be J- or hook-shaped, to softly support the nerve during recordings. This allows the nerve being tested to be moved away from the adjacent tissues and fluids, reducing spread and shunting [22]. Additionally, for achieving a high-quality recording, it is recommended to use larger-caliber electrodes to record from larger nerves, and thinner and more delicate electrodes to record from the smaller ones [20] (Fig. 30.5).

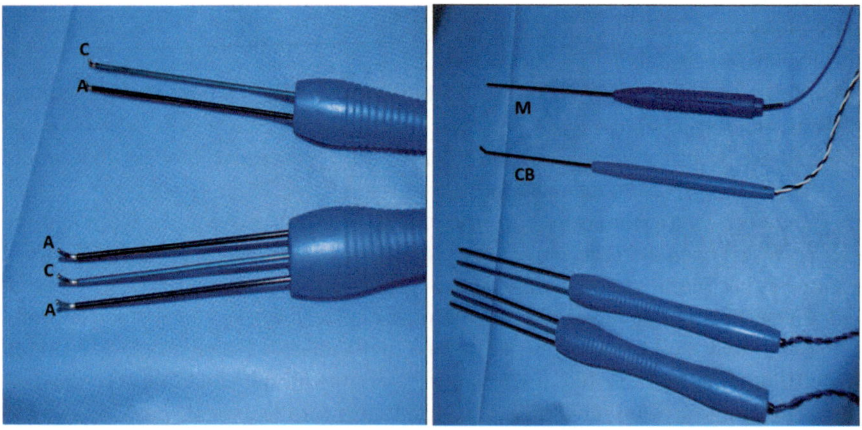

Fig. 30.4 Probes configuration with J- or hook-shaped tips for NAP stimulation and recording: (A) anode, (C) cathode; (CB) concentric bipolar probe to choose fascicles, (M) monopolar probe not suitable for peripheral nerve IONM

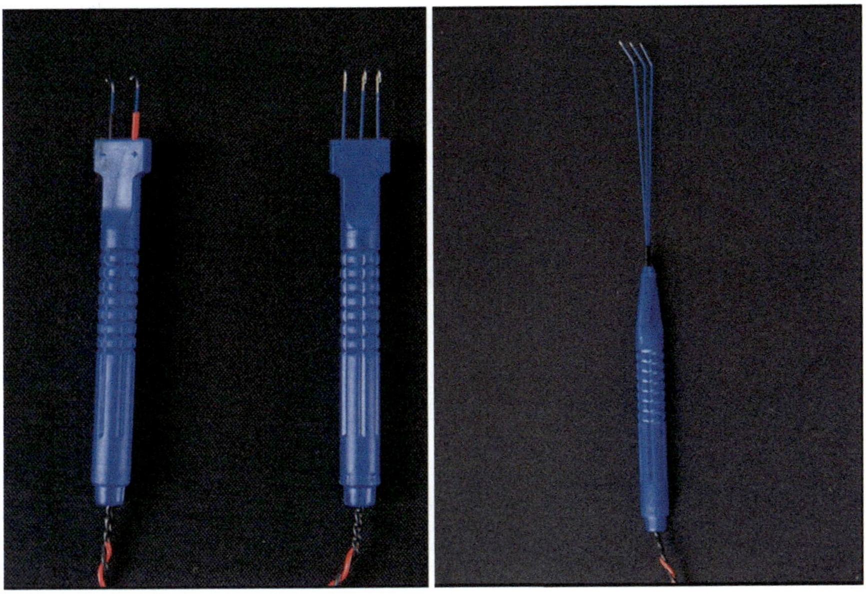

Fig. 30.5 Thinner and more delicate probes for smaller nerves

The whole team should be aware of the following concepts and to correctly choose and use the supplies involved:

(a) *Tripolar probes for stimulation* – The tripolar probe arrangement consists of a centrally positioned cathode between two externally interconnected anodes. This stimulus configuration generates two current paths, thus creating a potential difference between the internal active pole and the two external anodes. It delivers a more focal stimulation, reducing the longitudinal spread and the probability of contaminating CMAP recordings. In this stimulation paradigm, if a lower current intensity reaches the muscle, the stimulus artifact will be reduced (Figs. 30.3 and 30.4).
(b) *Bipolar probe for registration* – For NAP registration, the cathode pole must be positioned proximally to avoid anodal block (Fig. 30.3).
(c) *Ideal spacing between the probes' tips and proportionality of the distance between stimulus and register* – There are technical reasons for keeping a proportional spacing between the tips of both the stimulus and recording probes (Fig. 30.3).

  C.1 *Regarding the stimulus,* there is an inverse relationship between the separation of the probe tips and the intensity of the stimulus required to depolarize the nerve: distances smaller than 3 mm are not only insufficient to stimulate the nerve, but also require a higher stimulus intensity, and higher stimulus intensity results in larger stimulus artifact [33]. For effective stimulation in large neural tissue structures, such as the sciatic nerve or brachial plexus elements, the separation between the probe tips must be greater than *3 mm or 5 mm,* but this can be as much as *7 mm* [20].

C.2 *Regarding recording,* in the bipolar configuration, one tip will be more active capture pole, while the other will be the less active pole. But if the two recording tips are too close to each other, the NAP will have its amplitude drastically reduced or may not be recorded at all, since it originates from damaged nerves with impaired responses. Moreover, the nerve is composed by axons of varying diameters and fibers in different stages of remyelination, which implies in different depolarization thresholds. There may be an increased temporal dispersion due to the differences in conduction velocities among the fibers; consequently, the impulses will arrive at the recording pole at different times. Therefore, a bipolar probe with very short spacing between the tips may not register the entire response, losing the slowest components.

C.3 *The distance between stimulus and recording* is also very important (Fig. 30.3). Before starting the NAP study, the nerve should be exposed to a length of 3–4 cm, which is the minimal distance that must be maintained between the two probes. If too close to each other, the after-slope of stimulus artifact will contaminate the NAP response, even if tripolar probe is used [33].

Filter: Are You Aware of the NAP's Frequency Range?

The answer to this question determines the band-pass filters. A NAP response lies at a frequency range of 1000 Hz [41]. Taking a look to the Fourier's transformation model is essential to better understand how to eliminate frequencies above and below this range but preserve the NAP frequency signal.

The Fourier's transformation model converts waveform data presented in time domain, into frequency domain [2] and enables to choose the best band-pass filter. The electrical response generated by NAP is a very small signal and must be amplified. Yet, by this amplification process, more noise is incorporated into the signal and must be cut out to allow a clearer definition. The band-pass filters need to be properly chosen in order to eliminate noise without overfiltering the signal [19, 20, 33].

- *High-Frequency Filter (HF)*: Equal or greater than **2500 Hz.** If the High Filter is lower or equal to **1000 Hz**, it will impair NAP amplitude, leading to a lower response, because it is within the NAP's frequency range. Therefore, do not forget that the High Filter influences the amplitude and morphology of the response.
- *Low-Frequency Filter (LFF):* Around **10 Hz or 5 Hz**, although sometimes **2 or 1 Hz** may be necessary. This is the filter that we will change first when the stimulus artifact is contaminating the response to the point of interfering with its correct analysis. By changing the LFF, it is possible to switch the stimulus artifact recorded on the screen to an opposite direction, and thereby move it away from

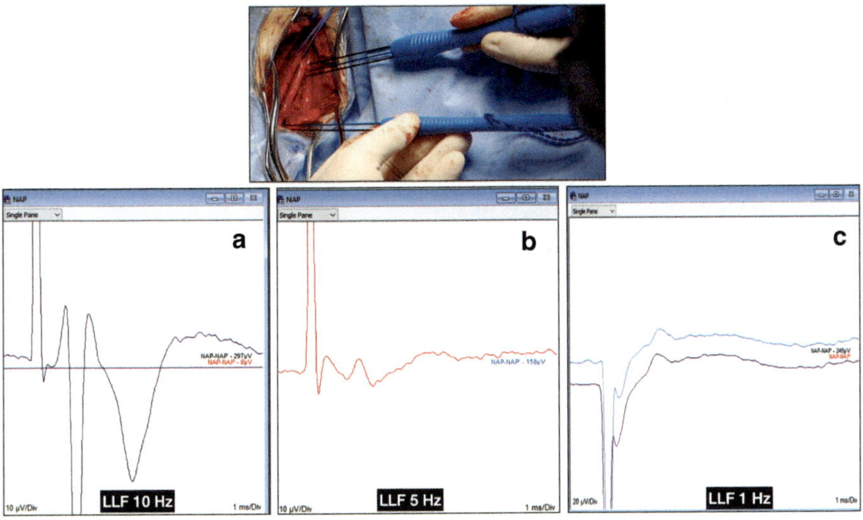

Fig. 30.6 In this case, a huge stimulus artifact initially hindered the NAP recording (**a**). The surgeon held on the probes in place, while the neurophysiologist quickly searched for the best filter setting. The first option was to adjust the low-frequency filter (**b**, **c**) in order to split the stimulus artifact in the opposite direction, enabling to observe the onset of the NAP

the onset of the NAP response [39]. To illustrate this scenario, see the sequence of filter settings made for a NAP record with a huge stimulus artifact (Fig. 30.6).

- Only after a high-quality recording has been acquired, the stimulation should proceed by the inching technique to properly assess the entire nerve segment (Fig. 30.7). Of note, both HFF and LFF can interfere with NAP morphology. Hence, proper adjustments must be made at each new recording, since the operating room environment's noise level changes may occur.
- *Notch Filter:* If the notch filter is already built into the equipment, it is recommended to keep it off. Similar to somatosensory-evoked potentials (SSEPs), if the notch filter is turned on, an artifact very similar to the biological signal may be generated. This is called the "ringing effect."

Gain and Sweep Setup

The NAP amplitude is directly proportional to the size of the stimulated nerve and the number of depolarized fibers. A sciatic nerve NAP has proportionally larger amplitude than a suprascapular nerve NAP. But in general, it does not exceed 200 μV approximately. Therefore, a gain of 20–50 μV per division is sufficient. Regarding the sweep setting, Crum and Strommen have proposed a simple and rational guide: presuming a conduction velocity of *50 m/s*, the ideal time base can be matched using the calculation of *1 ms per 5-cm distance*. A time base of 0.5–2.0 ms by division is suitable, but should be increased for longer distances [4].

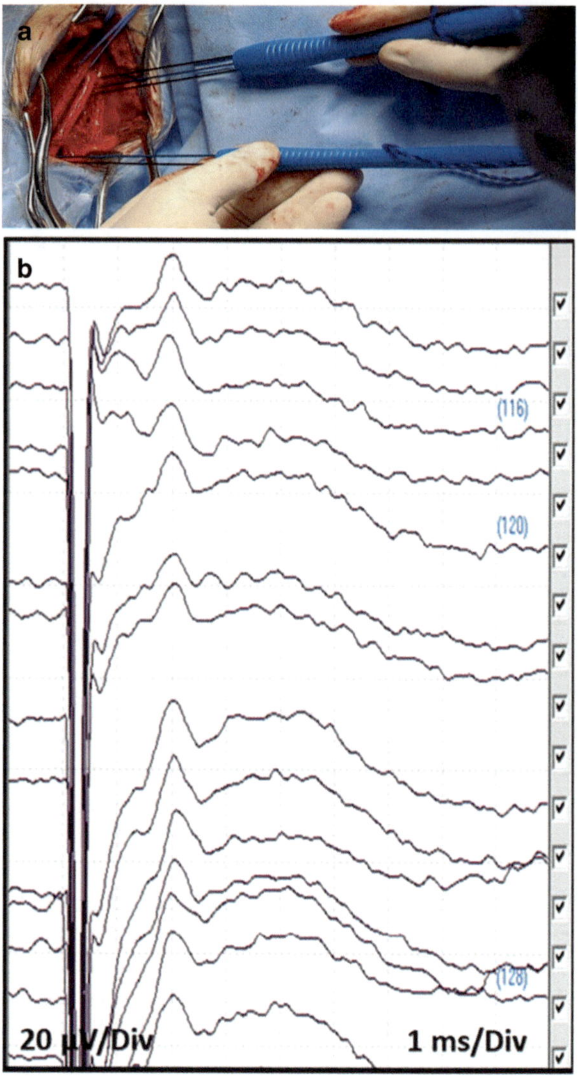

Fig. 30.7 (**a**) NAP with the inching technique in order to assess the whole nerve segment. (**b**) Recording after setting the low-frequency filter to 1 Hz and switching the stimulus artifact downward

Stimulus Setup: Duration, Intensity, and Frequency

The NAP stimulation threshold, like other electrically evoked responses, is resultant from the interaction between pulse duration and current intensity in the applied stimulus. If the duration is too short, one must increase the intensity to reach the threshold.

A. *Stimulus Duration:* Since the stimulus artifact will be more pronounced with larger pulse duration, it is recommended to start with the shortest possible pulse duration, around *0.05–0.1 ms* with adjustments in intensity and, if necessary, to increase the pulse duration additionally. A better understanding about rheobase and chronaxie concepts allows for greater accuracy in stimulus configuration and improves efficiency in threshold determination. Since it is beyond the scope of this chapter, we suggest as complementary reading [32]. The chronaxie concept is applied to express the relative excitabilities of different fibers correlating with the pulse duration: – *large and medium size fibers* short pulse 0.1–0.2 ms; – *smaller myelinated fibers* 0.3 ms; – *unmyelinated fibers* 0.5 ms [5]. Veale et al. [43] studied human ulnar nerves, and correlated pulse duration with the preferentially depolarized fiber and concluded that short-pulse duration was sufficient to depolarize motor fibers, which is the main goal of the NAP, while a large-pulse duration would be necessary to depolarize sensory fibers [43]. Remember that when dealing with damaged nerves, fibers in regeneration process with higher thresholds will always be present.

B. *Stimulus Intensity:* In neurophysiological practice, the stimulus intensity should always be supramaximal, in order to elicit the highest response amplitude and this concept also applies to the NAP. But the higher the stimulus intensity, the greater the stimulus artifact and the probability to elicit volume-conducted responses from distal muscles [30]. Different pulse and intensity adjustments may be necessary depending on the change in functional status caused by the injury. Considering the pulse duration of **0.05–0.2 ms**, the average intensity of **3–15 V or 1–5 mA** would be sufficient in most cases to achieve the stimulation threshold. In some circumstances, a higher intensity of up to **50 V or 20 mA** is required [4, 22]. The presence of fibrosis and extensive scar tissue surrounding the nerve change tissue conductance and the relationship between rheobase and chronaxie.

C. *Stimulus Frequency:* Being a direct recording of the nerve, the NAP stimulus frequency should be kept low, always around **2.1 Hz** or less. This is crucial to avoid heat injury that may happen when the charge delivered directly to the nerve is high (review Chap. 4). In this way, keeping a low stimulus frequency compensates for the short pulse duration, which is primarily chosen because of the motor fiber threshold and the high stimulus intensities required in cases with a lot of scar fibrosis.

D. *Grounding:* the stimulus artifact after slope (up- or down-slope) can be the greatest obstacle to successful NAP recording. For more than 10 years now, we have been using a larger surface electrode, positioned as close as possible to the stimulated nerve segment, that is, for stimulation and recording at the brachial plexus (BP), it can be placed at the scapular region, while for the lumbosacral plexus, at the thigh (Fig. 30.8). This electrode must be connected to the common ground position of the respective recording channels.

Summarizing Always start the NAP recording with the shortest pulse duration possible but sufficient to achieve the motor fiber thresholds. Increasing the pulse duration will be necessary only when the intensity increment is not sufficient to override the rheobase value. In these cases, keep the stimulus frequency low as compensation.

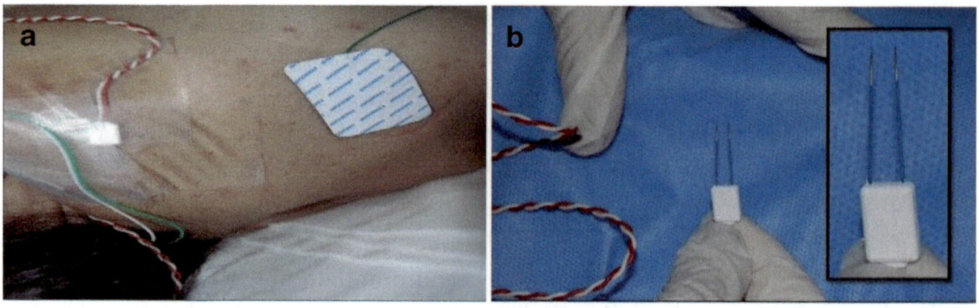

Fig. 30.8 (**a**) Large surface ground to NAP recordings. (**b**) Insulated needles to tEMG/CMAP and MEP recordings

IONM in Peripheral Nerve Surgery Beyond the NAP

In the last decades, the progress in IONM has been immense. The neurophysiologists have moved from the laboratories, where electrical safety and grounding are more adequate, to the operating rooms, where they must deal with a huge noise load contaminating the electrically evoked neurobiological signal.

This partnership between neurophysiologists and surgeons has become mutually rewarding: the formers have broadened their view regarding surgical demands, which has enabled more streamlined monitoring protocols. Accordingly, the surgeons have acquired multimodal functional assessment performed routinely. Therefore, it enhanced accuracy in surgical reasoning, beyond the outpatient EDX had previously achieved, especially regarding blunt and proximal injuries.

In the author's opinion, performing multiple IONM modalities, including somatosensory-evoked potentials (SSEPs), motor-evoked potentials (MEPs), free run EMG, and trigger EMG, allows a more precise identification regarding the nerve segment that should be stimulated in priority. Multimodal IONM provides additional information to analyze difficult situations as follows: (1) When there is no response by the donor stimulation, is this donor appropriate? Was double crushing previously excluded by EDX? (2) Identification of unexpected viability ("good NAP"), pointing to preganglionic lesions.

Electrodiagnostic Studies: Preoperative Protocol

In this section, we discuss the neurophysiological modalities from a comprehensive patients´ management perspective. Along the last decade, we developed a protocol in which pre- and intraoperative neurophysiologies are interconnected and mutually complementary. The patient is evaluated in our clinical neurophysiology laboratory, as the first step. The intraoperative protocol, including the sequence of testing, is decided jointly with the surgical team, based on the preoperative clinical evaluation and EDX. Teamwork enhances the pinpoint of information from perioperative EDX that can most probably benefit the decision making during the approach.

At our institution, the experience inside the operating room has influenced the ambulatory EDX assessment protocols and vice versa. Therefore, we are currently performing the EDX with focus on surgical planning. It aims to provide the surgeon with a more detailed report about the injury's topography and which sensory-motor domains are more affected. We believe that a target-guided EDX makes IONM easier and more dynamic.

It is not the scope of this chapter to discuss concepts and techniques of perioperative EDX but rather to help the neurophysiologist to set a proper IONM protocol. Anatomical references, myotome chart, and patterns of injury can be found in Chaps. 3 and 11.

EDX Special Considerations

Some limitations must be considered especially in closed and proximal traumatic injuries:

4.1.1 *Impossibility of assessment of the proximal sites,* which are inaccessible to the conduction study.

4.1.2 *The ideal time window between injury and EDX*: (A) Decline in amplitude of the sensory nerve action potentials (SNAPs) is seen from day 5 on, with the maximum drop estimated at 10–11 days after injury. (B) Compound muscle action potentials (CMAPs) drop from day 3 with a nadir around day 7. (C) Denervation signs on needle examination are detected around the third or fourth week, 21 days post injury on average [7].

4.1.3 *EDX parameters are limited in proximal lesions, leading to impossibility of establishing the prognosis and, consequently, the management strategy.* As previously mentioned, under ideal conditions, the regeneration rate can reach 1 mm/d [21], which implies in a long period of time until the sprouting cone reaches the target muscle in distal extremity. During this period, EDX does not add information on nerve viability. Yet, about 18–24 months after injury, there is an important neuromuscular degeneration and the presence of fibromatous scars, hindering the outcome [27]. Therefore, during this gap, NAP is mandatory to properly check on nerve fibers viability.

Despite all these limitations, EDX is fundamental for decision making, providing relevant information regarding topography, severity, multiplicity of lesions, double crush injuries, and donor selection, among others. For this reason, we strongly recommend well-done EDX studies, in order to ensure correct topographical diagnosis and reasoning. The neurophysiologist in charge of the IONM should initially analyze the EDX technical quality, since incomplete EDX compromises the identification of the injured sensory and motor domains.

Traumatic BPI is usually a closed injury difficult to diagnose, offering a challenging scenario. Perioperative EDX is time-consuming, because it implies in the inclusion of unusual sensory and motor nerves and muscles. It should be individualized for each patient, according to clinical deficits and enclosing a comprehensive assessment of the most probable lesion topographies. We follow the algorithm proposed by Ferrante and Wilbourn [6–9], starting with the evaluation of each BP's sensory and motor domain (Figs. 30.9 and 30.10). It is imperative to be familiar with its complex anatomical organization and topographical landmarks to identify the proximal level of the injury, pre- or postganglionic, primary branches, trunks, divisions, cords, and terminal branches (Fig. 30.1). The electrophysiological pattern of the injury depends on the combined analysis of SNAPs, CMAPs, and the needle electrode examination (NEE). They are equally important and necessary, as each one of them adds complementary information.

The axonal loss pattern is predominant in BPI, although the demyelinating pattern can occur in less severe cases. Although it is beyond the scope of this chapter to go deeper into the physiopathology of these lesions, some neurophysiological aspects are relevant for diagnosis: (1) The SNAPs and CMAPs amplitudes are the parameters that have the best correlation with the severity of axonal loss, because they reflect the number of axons that remain conducting. (2) The latency and conduction velocity reflect only the depolarization threshold of the fast conducting fiber contingent and may remain normal even in situations with severe axonal loss [7].

Normative values are determined by each laboratory based mainly on the patient's age and height. In general, and ruling out comorbidities, the best comparison score is with the patient himself or herself through the evaluation of the contralateral extremity. Amplitude lower than 50% in relation to the contralateral side should be valorized.

Performing Perioperative EDX

Sensory Nerve Conduction

Like other authors [7, 27, 35], we suggest starting and including a wider selection of sensory nerves in the evaluation (Fig. 30.9). The SNAPs must be recorded from lateral antebrachial cutaneous, superficial radial, median (thumb – D1, index – D2, middle finger – D3), ulnar (little finger – D5), and medial antebrachial cutaneous nerves.

The SNAPs may stay unchanged in preganglionic lesions, since the cell body of sensory fibers is located in the preserved ganglion. Conversely, low-amplitude SNAP, abolished CMAP, and denervation potentials in NEE can also be seen in the preganglionic pattern of injury. To avoid misinterpretation, the amplitudes should be compared with the contralateral side and valued only if smaller than 50%. The SNAPs should not be used as indicators of improvement in postoperative tests,

Box 1
The SNAP domains of the trunk and cord elements

Upper trunk
- LABC (100%)
- Med-D1 (100%)
- Radial (60%)
- Med-D2 (20%)
- Med-D3 (10%)

Middle trunk
- Med-D2 (80%)
- Med-D3 (70%)
- Radial (40%)

Lower trunk
- Uln-D5 (100%)
- MABC (100%)
- Med-D3 (20%)

Lateral cord
- LABC (100%)
- Med-D1 (100%)
- Med-D2 (100%)
- Med-D3 (80%)

Posterior cord
- Radial (100%)

Medial cord
- Uln-D5 (100%)
- MABC (100%)
- Med-D3 (20%)

Abbreviations: LABC, lateral antebrachial cutaneous NCS; MAB, medial antebrachial cutaneous NCS; Med-D1, medial NCS recording from first digit; Med-D2, median NCS recording from second digit; Med-D3, median NCS recording from third digit; S-Radial, superficial radial NCS; Ula-D5, ulnar NCS recording from fifth dogot.

Fig. 30.9 Ferrante [7]: The SNAP domains of the trunk and cord elements. (Courtesy of the Elsevier, with Permission)

because these responses hardly return to normal value even with satisfactory reinnervation.

According to Ferrante, EDX should start with sensory nerve conduction studies, since the sensory fiber pathways of each domain are well established and known. The great vulnerability of the sensory nerves to axonal loss makes them cornerstones in locating the lesion topography.

Motor Nerve Conduction

We suggest selecting nerves and muscles according to the motor domain [7], evaluating in priority: spinal accessory (trapezius), axillary (deltoid), musculocutaneous (biceps), radial (extensor indicis, extensor digititorum communi), median (abductor pollicis brevis, flexor carpi radialis), ulnar (abductor digiti minini, flexor carpi ulnaris) (Fig. 30.10).

Since the CMAPs amplitude is the parameter that best correlates with the severity of the injury until satisfactory reinnervation occurs, we emphasize the importance of comparison with the contralateral limb.

Box 2
The CMAP domains of the trunk and cord elements

Upper Trunk
- Musc-biceps
- Ax-deltoid
- Radial-EDC

Middle Trunk
- Radial-EDC

Lower Trunk
- Median-APB
- Ulnar-ADM
- Ulnar-FDI
- Radial-EIP
- Radial-EDC

Lateral cord
- Musc-biceps

Posterior cord
- Ax-deltoid
- Radial-EDC
- Radial-EIP

Medial cord
- Median-APB
- Ulnar-ADM
- Ulnar-FDI

Abbreviations: Ax-deltoid, axillary NCS, recording deltoid;Median-APB, median NCS, recording abductor policis brevis;Musc-biceps, musculocutaneous NCS, recording biceps; Radial-EDC, radial NCS, recording extensor digitorum communis; Radial-EIP. radial NCS, recording extensor indicis proprius; Ulnar-ADM, ulnar NCS, recording abductor digiti minimi; Ulnar-FDi, ulnar NCS, recording first dorsal interosseous.

Fig. 30.10 Ferrante [7]: The CMAP domains of the trunk and cord elements. (Courtesy of the Elsevier, with Permission)

For a numerical reference, we suggest using the formula [27]:

$$U - A / U \times 100 = \%\text{of axon loss}$$

U = CMAP amplitude of contralateral side
A = CMAP amplitude of injured side

The score of severity is based on the estimated percentage (%) of axonal loss: the abolition or nondetection of CMAP indicates the absence of viable axons at the moment of the EDX; **>75%** = severe axonal loss and **50–75%** = moderate axonal loss.

Usually, closed lesions do not undergo surgery immediately, but are followed up for a period of 6–8 months. Sequential EDX can identify an escalation in CMAP amplitude, which is compatible with progressive reinnervation. Yet, waiting longer than 18–24 months for surgical repair is incompatible with nerve viability for grafting, as previously discussed. In this scenario, it is necessary to use other neurophysiological tools, now in the intraoperative context (see NAP section).

Needle Electrode Examination

In muscles of proximal topography, in which no CMAP can be obtained, the NEE is of great value [35]. Within 15–21 days after the trauma, the needling of these muscles already registers signs of active denervation with fibrillation potentials and positive sharp waves, which allows defining proximally the injury extension.

Although there is a straight proportion between the number of denervated muscle fibers and the number of fibrillation potentials recorded in the muscle, in the spectrum of BPI, even mild or moderate lesions can show expressive fibrillation potentials, especially in the more distal muscles because of the high innervation rate in these muscles [7].

NEE identifies mild-to-moderate axonal lesions, in cases of normal sensory or motor nerve conduction studies. Analysis of the motor unit action potentials (MUAPs) morphology is a relevant step in the EDX. Following the acute phase, when denervation may have ceased, NEE evaluates the progression of reinnervation by recording nascent MUAPs, related to collateral sprouting or to proximo-distal axonal growth.

The MUAPs will change their morphology parallel to the time elapsed [35]: in an earlier phase of reinnervation, the NEE will register unstable polyphasic and low-amplitude MUAPs. In a later phase, these MUAPs will have larger amplitudes and longer durations with high recruitment frequencies (neurogenic pattern). Of note, during this period, the CMAP neuroconduction studies may exhibit normal amplitude and thereby underestimate the severity of axonal loss. Therefore, at this stage of MUAPs remodeling, only the NEE by identifying a reduced recruitment and a rarefied interferential pattern can estimate the injury severity (Fig. 30.11b).

Case Example 30.1
In the sequence of Figs. 30.11 and 30.12a, b, we show the case of a patient referred to our institution to perform a BP surgical repair due to a severe upper trunk injury (Sunderland V). In the first EDX, performed in another institution, it was diagnosed only an injury restricted to the upper trunk, with normal middle and lower trunks. Based on this initial diagnosis, the surgical plan was to perform an Accessory-Suprascapular and Ulnar-Musculocutaneous Anastomosis.

In our Institution, as part of our IONM protocol, we performed a preoperative EDX focusing on the ideal surgical planning and assessment of possible donors, in order to eliminate partial lesions not identified in routine exams.

To our surprise, we detected a severe injury of the ulnar nerve branch to the Flexor Carpi Ulnaris (Fig. 30.11), due to a previously traumatic elbow lesion specifically impairing this branch and sparing the distal ulnar branches (the only ones evaluated in the first EDX).

As the Flexor Carpi Ulnaris Branch is the donor for Oberlain 1, the surgical planning was changed to Oberlain 2, in which the donor is the median nerve fascicle to the Pronator Teres muscle coaptated to the musculocutaneous.

In Fig. 30.12a, b we highlight how tEMG is a useful tool in the correct identification and selection of fascicles. It allows the surgeon, in real time, to accurately map the fascicle that has been chosen.

Many surgical approaches to the BP occur on average 4–6 months after the traumatic event. So, in this phase the NEE is more important than the nerve conduction study. Considering that, following the trauma acute phase, the NEE may show a very rarefied interferential pattern with few motor units being recruited, identifying subclinical injuries. This injury pattern detected by the NEE is compatible with significant axonal loss, regardless of preserved CMAPs amplitudes. In this case example, we show this scenario and justify the rationale for our protocol, connecting preoperative EDX with IONM, which has been positively impacting our outcomes in surgical approaches to BPI.

This case pinpoints the importance of the interaction between EDX and IONM, as extremely useful tools in peripheral nerves surgical approaches.

In author's opinion, the amplitude recovery of MUAPs during the reinnervation phase requires careful attention while selecting the donor nerve during the EDX. If it is erroneously assumed that a normal CMAP means an unaffected domain and no comprehensive NEE is performed, a reinnervated territory will not be identified. This misinterpretation can be more frequently seen in late performed EDX, with reinnervation in progress. Therefore, the damage of potential donors could be overlooked, if they were chosen based solely on CMAP amplitude values. For better understanding of this concept, we show Case Example 30.1, in which a previously selected donor was rejected after performing a new EDX at our institution, in

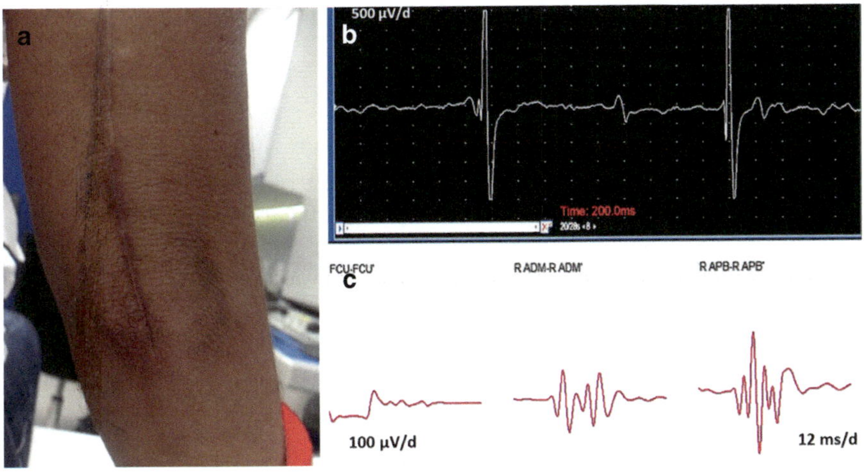

Fig. 30.11 (**a**) Elbow trauma had occurred previously to BPI: ulnar nerve branch to the flexor carpi ulnaris was adhered to the fibrous scar. (**b**) NEE examination of the flexor carpi ulnaris muscle: rarefied interferential pattern. (**c**) Myogenic cortical MEP as a complementary tool for injury identification and corroboration with EDX findings. This donor was discarded and replaced by another one. See next figure

accordance to our surgical planning protocol. All possible donors should be evaluated with NEE [36], in order to accurately estimate their degree of axonal loss.

To accurately evaluate the distribution of fibrillation potentials in the acute phase and the subsequent analysis of MUAPs morphology changes in the chronic phase, the findings should be interpreted jointly with SNAPs and CMAPs neuroconduction studies. Two opposite scenarios point to severe lesion: (A) recording of abundant fibrillation potentials and low-amplitude CMAPs; (B) recording of preserved SNAPS and CMAPs, but with large amplitude and high frequency MUAPs in NEE. The muscles selection must be made according to their respective motor domains aiming to maintain a close topographic correlation with their respective nerve origin and pathway along the BP elements. Muscles belonging to the same domain present similar patterns of involvement, except in the occurrence of multiple injuries.

Muscles innervated by branches originating from multiple segments of the BP must be included in the NEE [7]. Sequential needling of the most proximal to the most distal is essential for delimiting the most proximal injury level. Additionally, for muscles innervated by BP proximal nerves, in which CMAP studies can be unfeasible, the NEE gains relevance [35] in topography identification.

Therefore, for the EDX-NEE, we suggest assessing in priority:

- **Anterior Primary Ramus (APR)**
  - *C5–C6–C7 → Long Thoracic Nerve → Serratus Anterior*
  - *C5 → Dorsal Scapular Nerve → rhomboideus major*

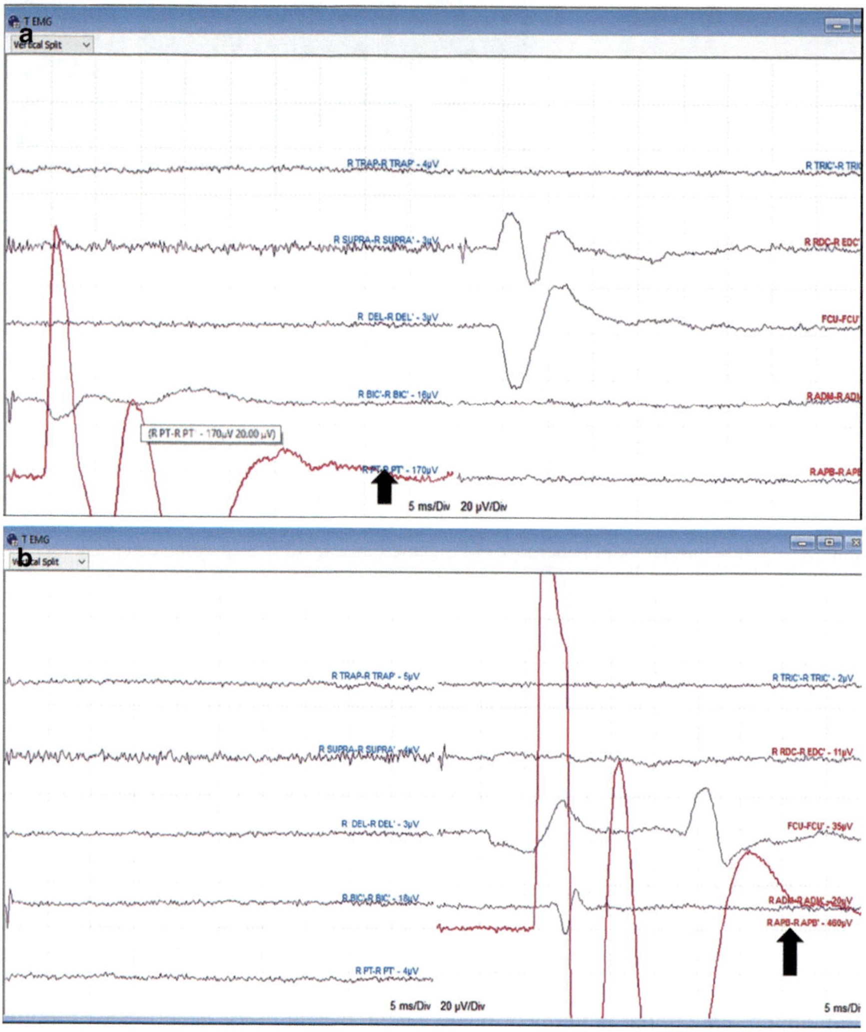

Figs. 30.12 (**a**, **b**) Continuation of the previous figure, the surgical strategy changed to Oberlain 2, taking the median nerve as the donor. The black arrows show how tEMG is a useful tool for the surgeon to identify and choose the most suitable donor fascicle: the ideal is the pronator teres fascicle (**a**) and not the abductor pollicis brevis (**b**) in order not to impair hand movements

1. **Trunks**
   - Superior trunk → *Suprascapular nerve* → *Infraspinatus/Supraspinatus*
2. **Cords**
   - Lateral cord → *Musculocutaneous nerve* → *Biceps brachi*
   - Posterior cord → *Axillary nerve* → *Deltoid*
   - Medial cord → *Ulnar nerve* → *First dorsal interossei*

3. **Terminal Branches**

   - Median nerve → *Abductor pollicis brevis*
   - Radial nerve → *Extensor digitorum communis*
   - Ulnar nerve → *First dorsal interosseous*
   - Musculocutaneous nerve → *Biceps brachi*
   - Axillary nerve → *Deltoid*

Intraoperative Protocol

Free Run and Trigger Electromyography

Free Run Electromyography

Continuous free-running electromyography (fEMG) enables recording of electrical activity from skeletal muscles innervated by nerves or roots potentially at risk. Thus, the main goal of fEMG is monitoring the occurrence of spontaneous discharges, and identifying them as pathological or not, to properly alert the surgeon [13].

The pattern of discharges recorded by fEMG may differ in morphology, activation behavior, and firing frequency. Tonic and phasic discharges should be recognized and properly interpreted [18]:

- *Tonic Discharge:* This is also called neurotonic discharge and includes repetitive episodes of activity from grouped motor units. It can occur in short bursts lasting several milliseconds, or prolonged trains lasting ≤1 min with a frequency around 50–200 Hz. It may occur if the nerve is dangerously manipulated, submitted to compression, contusion, stretching, or cutting.
- *Phasic Discharge*: This is also called "burst," is a short discharge, and maintains relative synchronicity. These bursts arise from direct mechanical contact between the nerve and the surgical instruments, with brief and immediate activation of some motor units [16].

A deep review about the predictive value of neurotonic discharges in different surgical contexts has been covered in Chaps. 21 and 26. Thus, this section focusses on particularities regarding peripheral nerve IONM.

Neurotonic discharges may occur with equal magnitude and frequency in circumstances that do not pose risk of nerve injury [12, 14] such as sudden metabolic changes altering the membrane excitability, heat propagation from electrocautery, "light" anesthesia, or irrigation with cold saline solution. Of note, fEMG cannot be monitored during the cautery use and the parameters may require reevaluation after its prolonged use. It is paramount that the neurophysiologist be aware of the surgical maneuvers step by step, to properly contextualize these discharges as an alert or not, thus avoiding false warnings.

Differently from ischemia and traction conditions, a sharp nerve section may be silent or show only an isolated burst. Furthermore, the disconnected nerve's distal stump can still be activated by mechanical irritation and electrical stimulation, leading to a misinterpretation regarding the nerve continuity and maintenance of nerve conduction.

Last but not the least, previously damaged nerves are less prone to present neurotonic discharges when compared to healthy ones; thus, fEMG may skip further intraoperative injuries.

Trigger Electromyography

Trigger electromyography (tEMG) is performed by applying an electrical stimulus to a motor nerve, root, or BP elements and recording the CMAP from the corresponding myotomes. The tEMG is used for neural structures identification, allowing the surgeon to (1) identify variations either anatomical, or secondary to injury; (2) attest if a nerve is sensory or motor; (3) assess safe distance between the nerve and surgical devices.

Adequation of the stimulation protocol may be necessary if, besides the traumatic injury, there is a pre-existing pathology like a long-standing compression of the nerve, trunk, or root. Under these circumstances the stimulation threshold may be two to three folds higher [15].

Specifically in peripheral nerve surgeries that involve nerve transfer, tEMG is an indispensable tool. It enables a correct identification of appropriate fascicles from the donor nerve, which will be coaptated to the damaged motor nerve [29]. It is fundamental to isolate target fascicles, for example, those who innervate the forearm muscles aiming to avoid the ones responsible for hand movements. Thus, you can accurately identify and properly select the ulnar nerve fascicles to the flexor ulnaris carpi muscle (Oberlain1) or the median nerve fascicles to the pronator teres muscle (Oberlain 2) (Fig. 30.12a, b).

Although tEMG can be applied with either bipolar or monopolar probes, the goal should be the maximum selectivity with minimum spread of the response. Hence, the monopolar technique with the cathode over the stimulated nerve and a distant anode leads to unreliable results (Fig. 30.13). Bipolar stimulation, by enabling a more focused response and lower spread, should be chosen preferentially in peripheral nerve surgery approaches. Therefore, we emphasize not to use a monopolar probe due to the spread magnitude that interferes with the other channels (Fig. 30.13).

Stimulus Setup

I- Bipolar Probe

I.a- The stimulation in the surgical field to identify neural structures and assess functional viability should be carried out with the bipolar probe with J- or hook-shaped tips. It softly supports the nerve during recordings to keep it away from the fluids and thus minimizes the spread (Fig. 30.4).

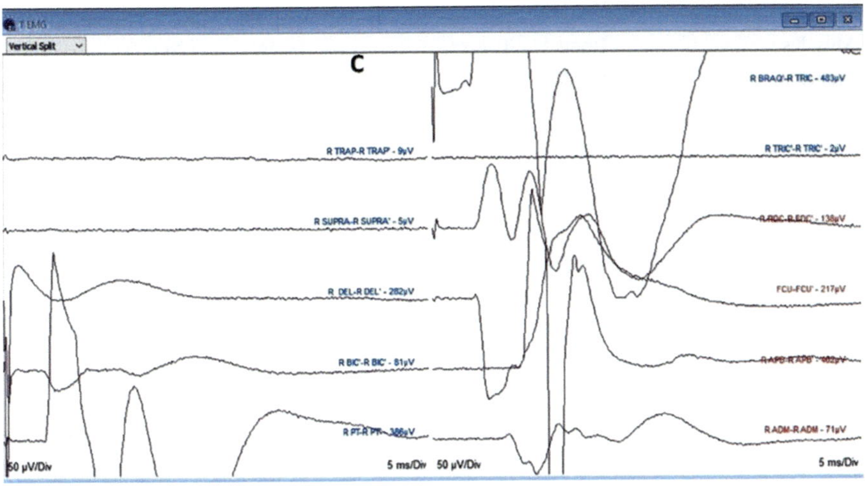

Fig. 30.13 Probe monopolar due to the magnitude of the spread is not suitable for identifying and choosing fascicles

I.b- A donor nerve stimulation should be performed with a concentric bipolar probe to identify and select fascicles (Fig. 30.4). It enables the mapping and following of the fascicles' somatotopy in different regions of the nerve: ventral, dorsal, or lateral (Fig. 30.12a, b).

II- Intensity, Duration, and Frequency

Please go back to NAP section to review specific considerations regarding each of these parameters:

- *Pulse duration* – **0.1–0.2 ms** – *target to large- and medium-sized fibers*
- *Intensity* – **1–15 V or 0.5–5 mA or higher**
- *Frequency* – **2.1 Hz or higher**

III- Recording Setup

III.a- Muscles Selection: It may change according to injury topography and surgical approach. Usually, they are the same and assessed in preoperative EDX and intraoperative MEP (see section "Needle Electrode Examination" and Table 30.1).

III.b- Recordings: Recordings are made with subdermal needles in bipolar montage, with active and reference electrodes inserted close to the muscle motor point (see Chap. 3). For deeper muscles, insulated needles of a suitable size must be chosen (Fig. 30.8). It enhances selectivity, since the tip picks up only the closest motor unit potentials. Hence, there is no "contaminated" response from neighbor muscles.

III.c- Sweep and Gain: The sweep length should be set based on the most relevant data to be analyzed. Ideally, different windows should be used for fEMG and tEMG [16]:

Table 30.1 Protocol for Tc-MEP recording

Muscles	Roots	Trunks	Cords	Nerves
Trapezius[a]	C3–C4			Accessory
Infraspinatus	C5–C6	Upper	*	Suprascapular
Deltoid	C4–C5	Upper	Posterior	Axillary
Brachioradialis	C5–C6	Upper	Posterior	Radial
Biceps brachii	C5–C6	Upper	Lateral	Musculocutaneous
Pronator teres[b]	C6–C7	Upper, middle	Lateral	Median
Extensor digitorum	C7–C8	Upper, middle, lower	Posterior	Radial
Flexor carpi ulnaris[c]	C8–T1	Lower	Medial	Ulnar
Extensor indicis	C7–C8	Lower	Posterior	Radial
Abductor pollicis brevis	C8–T1	Lower	Medial	Median
Abductor digiti minimi	C8-T1	Lower	Medial	Ulnar

Adapted from Ferrante [7]
(*) Trunk level
[a]Frequent donor
[b]Oberlain 2 donor
[c]Oberlain 1 donor

- *Long Sweep (2–10 s):* Although it provides enough time for discharges the pattern and duration to be recorded, it compresses the MUPs morphology too much, and hinders the artifacts recognition.
- *Short Sweep (30–200 ms):* It enables a clear distinction between artifacts and potentials morphology. However, very short time-window may limit analysis (like discharge duration).

It may be necessary to interchange between different sweeps for analysis optimization.

The sweep choice always depends on both the particularities of the monitored case and the protocol used.

(a) **fEMG**: Gain 50–300 μV; Sweep 50–200 ms/division: both parameter settings should enable proper recording and analysis of amplitude and frequency.
(b) **tEMG:** 20–200 μV; Sweep 5–20 ms/division: parameters are adjusted to improve analysis of latency and morphology of electrically evoked response.

- **Filters:** Low-frequency filter (LFF) 10–30 Hz; high-frequency filter (HFF) 2–10 kHz.

Somatosensory-Evoked Potential

The SSEP methodology and basic concepts have already been detailed in Chap. 8.

The somatosensory-evoked potential (SSEP) is extremely helpful during surgical explorations of traumatic BPI. The anatomical appearance of BP during surgery can be very misleading, as nerve roots may be in pseudo-continuity. For this reason, performing SSEPs is helpful in testing if the anatomically preserved nerve roots or trunks present functional continuity [23]. The surgical approach greatly differs in pre- and postganglionic lesions: only stumps in functional continuity, that are centrally connected to the spinal cord, are amenable to grafting. SSEP aims to identify pre- or postganglionic injury pattern.

The traumatic BPI is a challenging scenario with multiple injuries, frequently with varying levels of severity. There may even be a double damage to the same structure in different topography distribution. We strongly suggest performing SSEPs prior to NAP, because it is imperative to determine if and which sensory roots are avulsed.

A normal NAP can be generated by sensory fibers distal to the dorsal root ganglion, despite the complete root avulsion and central disconnection with the medulla. Based on the presence or absence of cortical SSEPS response, we will be able to better interpret the NAP [19].

Stimulation

The stimulation can be done directly at roots C5, C6, C7, C8, T1 using a bipolar probe. The radial, median, and ulnar nerves can also be stimulated. Direct nerve root or brachial plexus trunk stimulation requires a slightly different protocol than that used for mixed nerves: square wave pulses at **0.5–5 mA**; pulse duration **0.1–0.3 ms**; frequency **3.17 Hz** [30].

Recording

The recording may be as follows: (1) *subcortical at the Erb point (N9)* or cervical *Csp* (N13); (2) cortical contralateral C3′–Cz or C4′–Cz or C3′–C4′ (N20–25), keeping in mind that these latencies may be slightly prolonged. It is possible to record the SSEPs directly from the nerve root or trunk by using a bipolar probe when the stimulus is made distally on the nerve. The recording setup is **sweep 5 ms/division, gain of 2–5 μV/division.**

Band-Pass Filters

Low Filter 30 Hz; High Filter 3000 Hz. It may be necessary to change to unusual band-pass filters like keeping the **LFF in 30–50 Hz** and change the HFF to **750–500 Hz** during direct nerve recording and stimulation.

When the stimulation is carried out by the surgeon, the number of averages is limited. Nevertheless, it is possible to record reproducible responses. In cases with multiple root avulsions, no subcortical or cortical SSEP potentials can be recorded, even using multiple stimulation sites.

Motor-Evoked Potential

Transcranial motor-evoked potential (Tc-MEP) is a neurophysiological modality that is still seldomly applied to peripheral nerves monitoring. Many authors do not consider it a reliable tool when it comes to IONM of roots, plexuses, and peripheral nerves because of supposed limitations; most of them are described in detail by Nair [30]: (1) Tc-MEP activates a small subset of descending motor axons and anterior horn cells, evoking responses in muscles supplied by multiple roots. (2) Intramuscular recording with needle electrodes provides a very limited sample, which is restricted to the electrode reading area. (3) Recordings performed distally to the lesioned site. (4) All myotomes of each root are not evaluated. (5) Great intertrial variability.

Regarding level of recommendation, MEP corresponds to class III, type C as long as it is performed by skilled personnel and considering its limitations and confounding factors [25]. For peripheral nerves approaches, it is classified as type U due to insufficient data. Nevertheless, we routinely perform Tc-MEP in all BPI surgical explorations, since, as neurophysiologists, we are familiar with its application and interpretation. Based on our 10 years-experience, we pinpoint the following features:

1. The amplitude and polyphasia of the recorded potentials are clearly different in myotomes innervated by the injured structures compared to myotomes with intact innervation (Figs. 30.14, 30.15, 30.16, and 30.17). In combined lesions of C5 and C6 or C8 and T1, although the double motor domain is common, it is possible to identify reduced or absent responses. Yet, by partial diffuse BPI or in

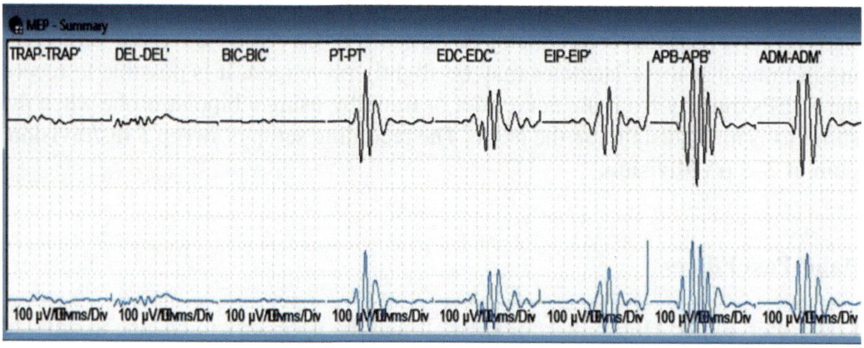

Fig. 30.14 Tc-MEP using total intravenous anesthesia (TIVA) with strict anesthetic level control through spectral EEG. In this case, one can easily identify the injury by the responses of the trapezius, deltoid, and biceps, respectively, C3–C4–C5–C6 roots. The injury involved the spinal root of the accessory nerve, a frequent donor, which was ruled out for anastomosis purposes

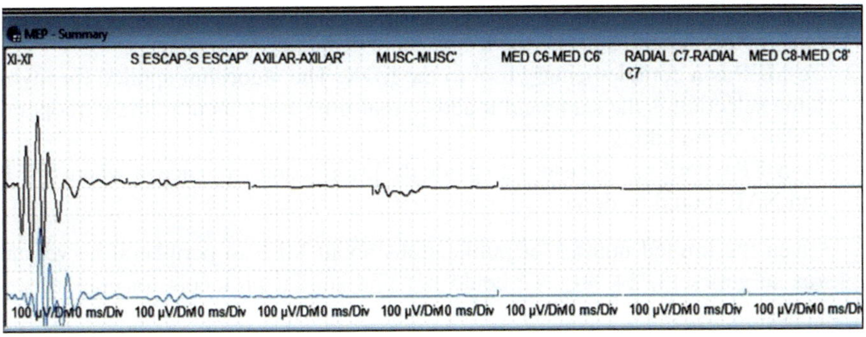

Fig. 30.15 Total avulsion pattern (C5–T1), already diagnosed in the preoperative exams. MEP response recorded only in the accessory (trapezius). Suprascapular (infraspinatus), musculocutaneous (biceps brachi), median C6–C7 (pronator teres), radial C7 (extensor digitorum communis), median C8 (abductor pollicis brevis)

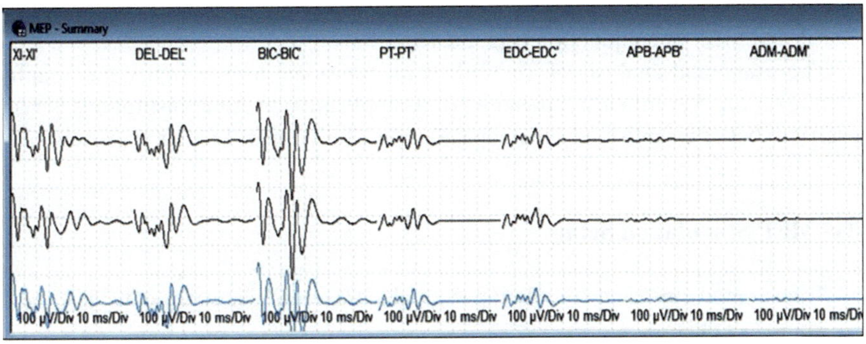

Fig. 30.16 Diffuse involvement pattern: postganglionic at C5–C6–C7 (partial motor impairment, as shown by MEP), preganglionic at C8–T1, as confirmed by NAP, MEP, and PESS

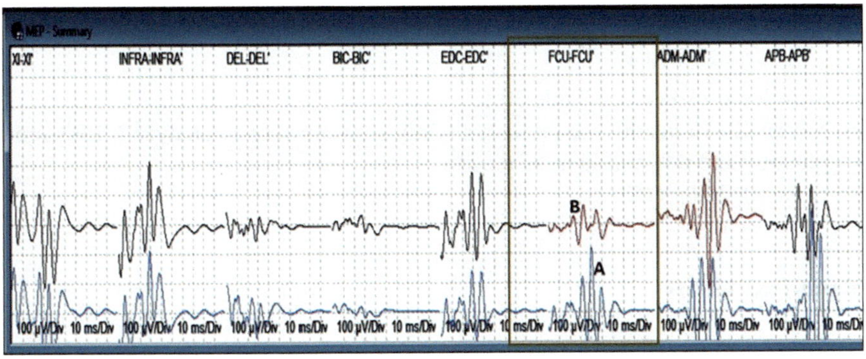

Fig. 30.17 Sharp wound restricted to the upper trunk of the brachial plexus (deltoid and biceps brachi), distal to the suprascapular nerve (infraspinatus muscle with preserved MEP). Anastomosis with coaptation of the flexor carpi ulnaris to the musculocutaneous was carried out. (A) preharvesting (B) postharvesting of the flexor carpi ulnaris fascicle. Note the reduction in the response of the flexor carpi ulnaris without change in the response of the abductor digiti minimi

isolated C7 lesions, the overlapping of more than one nerve root for each muscle renders the identification of the lesion more difficult.
2. Tc-MEP is a complementary tool to the EDX. The algorithm applied for myotome selection is the same and it adds a real-time assessment to the intraoperative decision making.
3. Tc-MEP recordings are useful to guide the priority and sequence of where SSEP and NAP should be done.

Given the limited number of publications about MEP in peripheral nerve and plexus surgeries [3, 24, 44], we could not find similar protocols for comparison purposes.

The motor domain chart is outlined in Table 30.1. We aim to replicate, by similarity, Ferrante's concept that muscles belonging to the same domain [7] show similar patterns of injury: MEP's response of smaller amplitudes and fewer phases, in general, are recorded in the myotomes of the lesioned motor domains. It is important to emphasize that the pre- or postganglionic injury pattern is not diagnosed based solely on Tc-MEP analysis. For this purpose, it is necessary to analyze NAP, SSEP, and MEP in conjunction (Fig. 30.16).

The usage and analysis of Tc-MEP is an additional tool to injury topography identification. Nevertheless, spreading of its application by other institutions is necessary to better establish its accuracy and replicability in BPI repair approaches.

Tc- MEP Stimulation Setup

- Transcranial electrical stimulation through corkscrew electrodes at C3/C4
- Train:7–9 pulses
- Duration: 75 us ms
- Intensity: 200–500 V

Tc-MEP Recording Setup

- *Muscles of choice*, see Table 30.1.
- *Sweep* 12–15 ms/div, we prefer a slightly slower sweep to analyze MEP's morphology and polyphasia more clearly.
- *Gain* 50–200 μV/div.

Band-Pass Filters

Low filter 10–100 Hz; high filter 2000–2500 Hz.

The Multiplicity of Injuries and the Donor Nerve Assessment

In polytrauma, multilevel compromise of the BP is frequently observed as previously mentioned in the EDX preoperative section. In addition to proximal injury at the nerve roots and BP elements, overlapping injuries can also occur in more distal topographies, even without clinical manifestation. Nerve injuries may be found at bone fracture sites or secondary to vascular injury [34, 42].

We consider this particularity in the surgical management of BPI quite important, because if the potential donor nerves are damaged and not diagnosed, the entire surgical outcome can be compromised.

In a targeted way, we highlight the following nerves:

1. Accessory nerve may show significant damage, especially in the prefixed plexus, compromising its role as a good donor for anastomosis purposes (Fig. 30.14).
2. Suprascapular nerve is prone to damage in case of local impact injuries and in shoulder dislocations.
3. Axillary nerve can be damaged in humerus fractures or vascular trauma involving the axillary artery.
4. Radial nerve may be involved in humerus and radius fractures.
5. Ulnar nerve can be injured in elbow fractures or after a long hospitalization with improper bed positioning (Fig. 30.11).
6. Compression secondary to compartment syndromes may involve all terminal branches of radial, median, and ulnar nerves, most frequently in lesions of the infraclavicular portion of the brachial plexus.

Therefore, we fully agree with Schreiber et al. [36] when he stated that the health and integrity of the donor nerve and the corresponding muscle should be routinely assessed by EDX. It is a fundamental tool capable of predicting the outcome of a nerve transfer surgery.

Anesthesia

This subject has already been extensively discussed in other chapters (review Chap. 5). In our Institution, we prioritize total venous anesthesia with propofol and opioid, and we carefully monitor anesthetic level through spectral EEG. Since we perform Tc-MEP in practically all cases, we do not use any type of neuromuscular blocker, even when the NAP recording is challenging.

Final Statements

We emphasize that the our multimodal IONM protocol is feasible in other peripheral nerves approaches like form entrapment and tumoral lesions.

In our experience, the application of dermatomeric SSEPs and NAP elicited by transcranial electrical stimulation has limited use in IONM. Accordingly, these responses are hard to acquire and they are usually contaminated by huge artifacts, rendering their analysis difficult. We are working to improve their application in our protocol to enhance reliability.

Conclusion

In this chapter, we revisited and highlighted essential technical aspects to set proper protocols for stimulation and recording techniques during peripheral nerves approaches. Detailing their particularities and challenges may encourage other institutions and colleagues to take part in these surgeries. Adding MEP in the protocol can potentially improve outcome and is a helpful tool in many ways. Since the neurophysiological modalities are complementary to each other, the combined analysis of data facilitates and streamlines their interpretation. Multimodality provides greater accuracy in the identification of the lesion topography and enhances the decision making.

Last but not least, EDX should be considered a fundamental part of the management of this patients and should not be overlooked.

References

1. dos Anjos KC. Implicações sociais e econômicas nos pacientes vítimas de acidentes com motocicleta internados no IOT-HCFMUSP [Internet] [Mestrado em Ortopedia e Traumatologia]. São Paulo: Universidade de São Paulo; 2012 [cited 2021 Jun 4]. Available from: http://www.teses.usp.br/teses/disponiveis/5/5140/tde-09012013-170224/.
2. Bracewell RN. The Fourier transform and its applications. 3rd ed. Boston: McGraw Hill; 2000.
3. Burkholder LM. Neurogenic motor evoked potentials: role in brachial plexus surgery. J Neurosurg. 2003;98:4.
4. Crum BA, Strommen JA, Stucky SC. Peripheral nerve stimulation and monitoring during operative procedures. Muscle Nerve. 2007;35(2):159–70.
5. Deandres J. Peripheral nerve stimulation in the practice of brachial plexus anesthesia: a review. Reg Anesth Pain Med. 2001;26(5):478–83.
6. Ferrante MA. Brachial plexopathies: classification, causes, and consequences. Muscle Nerve. 2004;30(5):547–68.
7. Ferrante MA. Electrodiagnostic assessment of the brachial plexus. Neurol Clin. 2012;30(2):551–80.
8. Ferrante MA, Wilbourn AJ. The utility of various sensory nerve conduction responses in assessing brachial plexopathies. Muscle Nerve. 1995;18(8):879–89.

9. Ferrante MA, Wilbourn AJ. Electrodiagnostic approach to the patient with suspected brachial plexopathy. Neurol Clin. 2002;20(2):423–50.
10. Geuna S, Raimondo S, Ronchi G, Di Scipio F, Tos P, Czaja K, et al. Chapter 3: Histology of the peripheral nerve and changes occurring during nerve regeneration. In: International review of neurobiology [Internet]. Elsevier; 2009 [cited 2021 Jun 6]. p. 27–46. Available from: https://linkinghub.elsevier.com/retrieve/pii/S0074774209870037
11. Greve JMD, Resende MR, da Silva HB, Andreuccetti G, Bernini CO, Leyton V. Factors related to motorcycle accidents with victims: an epidemiological survey. Med Express [Internet]. 2018 [cited 2021 Jun 4];5. Available from: http://www.medicalexpress.net.br/details/328/factors-related-to-motorcycle-accidents-with-victims%2D%2Dan-epidemiological-survey
12. Harper CM. Intraoperative cranial nerve monitoring. Muscle Nerve. 2004;29(3):339–51.
13. Harper CM, Daube JR. Facial nerve electromyography and other cranial nerve monitoring. J Clin Neurophysiol [Internet]. 1998;15(3). Available from: https://journals.lww.com/clinicalneurophys/Fulltext/1998/05000/Facial_Nerve_Electromyography_and_Other_Cranial.4.aspx.
14. Holland NR. Intraoperative electromyography. J Clin Neurophysiol. 2002;19(5):10.
15. Holland NR, Lukaczyk TA, Riley LHI, Kostuik JP. Higher electrical stimulus intensities are required to activate chronically compressed nerve roots: implications for intraoperative electromyographic pedicle screw testing. Spine [Internet]. 1998;23(2). Available from: https://journals.lww.com/spinejournal/Fulltext/1998/01150/Higher_Electrical_Stimulus_Intensities_Are.14.aspx.
16. Kartush JM, Rice KS, Minahan RE, Balzer GK, Yingling CD, Seubert CN. Best practices in facial nerve monitoring. Laryngoscope [Internet]. 2021 [cited 2021 Aug 20];131(S4). Available from: https://onlinelibrary.wiley.com/doi/10.1002/lary.29459.
17. Kim DH, Cho Y-J, Tiel RL, Kline DG. Outcomes of surgery in 1019 brachial plexus lesions treated at Louisiana State University Health Sciences Center. J Neurosurg. 2003;98(5):1005–16.
18. Kim S-M, Kim SH, Seo D-W, Lee K-W. Intraoperative neurophysiologic monitoring: basic principles and recent update. J Korean Med Sci. 2013;28(9):1261.
19. Kline DG. Nerve action potential recordings. In: Kline and Hudson's nerve injuries [Internet]. Elsevier; 2008 [cited 2021 Jun 8]. p. 75–85. Available from: https://linkinghub.elsevier.com/retrieve/pii/B978072169537250013X.
20. Kline DG. Management of nerve injuries (with emphasis on Nerve Action Potential (NAP) recordings). In: Sindou M, editor. Practical handbook of neurosurgery [Internet]. Vienna: Springer Vienna; 2009 [cited 2021 Jun 18]. p. 1588–609. Available from: http://link.springer.com/10.1007/978-3-211-84820-3_94.
21. Kline DG, Hackett ER, May PR. Evaluation of nerve injuries by evoked potentials and electromyography. J Neurosurg. 1969;31(2):128–36.
22. Kline DG, Happel LT. A quarter century's experience with intraoperative nerve action potential recording. Can J Neurol Sci. 1993;20(1):3–10.
23. Landi A, Copeland S, Parry C, Jones S. The role of somatosensory evoked potentials and nerve conduction studies in the surgical management of brachial plexus injuries. J. Bone Joint Surg Br Vol. 1980;62-B(4):492–6.
24. MacDonald DB, Stigsby B, Al Homoud I, Abalkhail T, Mokeem A. Utility of motor evoked potentials for intraoperative nerve root monitoring. J Clin Neurophysiol. 2012;29(2):118–25.
25. Macdonald DB, Skinner S, Shils J, Yingling C, American Society of Neurophysiological Monitoring. Intraoperative motor evoked potential monitoring – a position statement by the American Society of Neurophysiological Monitoring. Clin Neurophysiol. 2013;124(12):2291–316. https://doi.org/10.1016/j.clinph.2013.07.025. Epub 2013 Sep 18. PMID: 24055297.
26. Mackinnon SE. Nerve surgery. New York: Thieme Publishers; 2015. p. 1–40.
27. Mansukhani K. Electrodiagnosis in traumatic brachial plexus injury. Ann Indian Acad Neurol. 2013;16(1):19.

28. Mazal AT, Faramarzalian A, Samet JD, Gill K, Cheng J, Chhabra A. MR neurography of the brachial plexus in adult and pediatric age groups: evolution, recent advances, and future directions. Expert Rev Med Devices. 2020;17(2):111–22.
29. Moran SL, Steinmann SP, Shin AY. Adult brachial plexus injuries: mechanism, patterns of injury, and physical diagnosis. Hand Clin. 2005;21(1):13–24.
30. Nair DG. Intraoperative mapping of roots, plexuses, and nerves. J Clin Neurophysiol. 2013;30(6):613–9.
31. Noland SS, Bishop AT, Spinner RJ, Shin AY. Adult traumatic brachial plexus injuries. J Am Acad Orthop Surg. 2019;27(19):705–16.
32. Ranck JB. Which elements are excited in electrical stimulation of mammalian central nervous system: a review. Brain Res. 1975;98(3):417–40.
33. Robert EG, Happel LT, Kline DG. Intraoperative nerve action potential recordings. Neurosurgery. 2009 ;65(suppl_4):A97–104.
34. Rubin DI. Diseases of the plexus. Continuum Lifelong Learn Neurology. 2008;14:156–79.
35. Rubin DI. Brachial and lumbosacral plexopathies: a review. Clin Neurophysiol Pract. 2020;5:173–93.
36. Schreiber JJ, Feinberg JH, Byun DJ, Lee SK, Wolfe SW. Preoperative donor nerve electromyography as a predictor of nerve transfer outcomes. J Hand Surg Am. 2014;39(1):42–9.
37. Seddon HJ, Medawar PB, Smith H. Rate of regeneration of peripheral nerves in man. J Physiol. 1943;102(2):191–215.
38. Shin AY, Spinner RJ, Steinmann SP, Bishop AT. Adult Traumatic Brachial Plexus Injuries. J Am Acad Orthop Surg. 2005;13(6):15.
39. Simon MV. Intraoperative neurophysiology: a comprehensive guide to monitoring and mapping. New York: Demos Medical Publishing; 2019.
40. Sunderland S. A classification of peripheral nerve injuries producing loss of function. Brain. 1951;74:491–516.
41. Tiel RL, Happel LT, Kline DG. Nerve action potential recording method and equipment. Neurosurgery. 1996;39(1):103–9.
42. Tsao BE, Wilbourn AJ. The medial brachial fascial compartment syndrome following axillary arteriography. Neurology. 2003;61(8):1037–41.
43. Veale JL, Mark RF, Rees S. Differential sensitivity of motor and sensory fibres in human ulnar nerve. J Neurol Neurosurg Psychiatry. 1973;36(1):75–86.
44. Wiertel-Krawczuk A, Huber J. Standard neurophysiological studies and motor evoked potentials in evaluation of traumatic brachial plexus injuries – a brief review of the literature. Neurol Neurochir Pol. 2018;52(5):549–54.

Part VIII
Head and Neck Surgery

Chapter 31
Monitoring in Facial, Neck, and Ear Surgeries

Karina Maria Alécio de Oliveira, Estela Lladó-Carbó, Ricardo José Rodriguez Ferreira, Marcus Vinícius Magno Gonçalves, and Marina Azzi Quintanilha

Abbreviations

BLR	Blink reflex
CB-MEP	Corticobulbar motor-evoked potential
CVNM	Continuous intraoperative stimulation of the vagus nerve
ECA	External carotid artery
EEG	Electroencephalography
EMG	Electromyography
EMG-fr	Electromyography free run
EMG-st	Trigged electromyography

K. M. A. de Oliveira (✉)
Department of Neurology and Neurophysiology, Clinica Stela de Monitoramento Clínico e Cirúrgico em Neurologia, Brasília, DF, Brazil

E. Lladó-Carbó
Clinical Neurophysiology Department, Neurotoc - Intraoperative Neuromonitoring company-(Spain), HM Catalunya Hospital, Barcelona, Spain

R. J. R. Ferreira
AACD - Disabled Child Care Association, São Paulo, SP, Brazil

Dr Ricardo Ferreira Clinic, São Paulo, SP, Brazil

Spine Surgery Department at Orthopedics and Trauma Institute of Clinical Hospital of the University of São Paulo Medical School, São Paulo, SP, Brazil

M. V. M. Gonçalves
Neurologist and Neurophysiologist, Neurology at the University of the Region of Joinville (UNIVILLE), Joinville, Brazil

M. A. Quintanilha
Cervical and Head Surgery Department, CICAP, Centro Clínico Sudoeste, Brasília, DF, Brazil
e-mail: adm@institutoazzi.com.br

S. M. Verst et al. (eds.), *Intraoperative Monitoring*,
https://doi.org/10.1007/978-3-030-95730-8_31

ETE	Orotracheal tube electrode
FN	Facial nerve
GN	Glossopharyngeal nerve
HNE	Head, neck and ear approaches
ICA	Internal carotid artery
IONM	Intraoperative neurophysiology monitoring
IONMm	Multimodal intraoperative neurophysiology monitoring
IONMu	Unimodal intraoperative neurophysiology monitoring
LAR	Laryngeal adductor reflex
LCCA	Left common carotid artery
MEP	Motor-evoked potentials
RCCA	Right common carotid artery
RLN	Recurrent laryngeal nerve
SLN	Superior laryngeal nerve
SSEP	Somatosensory-evoked potential
TOF	Train of four
VNS	Vagus nerve stimulation

Introduction

Intraoperative neurophysiologic monitoring (IONM) during head, neck, and ear (HNE) approaches aims to perform a functional topographic diagnosis and monitor the functionality of the neural structures in real time during the surgery. It prevents imminent nerve damage and predicts postoperative nerve function [1]. Although the incidence of palsy is low in experienced hands, when permanent, it impairs patient's quality of life and triggers litigation for malpractice [2]. IONM, if properly performed and documented, offers some protection in a litigious environment [2].

Ideally, HNE IONM is composed of several and simultaneous or interspersed modalities of neurophysiological studies including free run (EMG-fr) and stimulated (EMG-st) electromyography, laryngeal adductor reflex (LAR), somatosensory-evoked potentials (SSEP), motor-evoked potential (MEP), electroencephalography (EEG), and train of four techniques (TOF).

Mapping associated with EMG-fr are the most used methods, generally performed by technicians. Yet, technical difficulties, like those related to artifacts, may lead to false-positive and false-negative alarms, compromising the outcome [1]. Despite of that, the incorporation of mapping has promoted better surgical results. IONM differs from the conventional neural approach in HNE surgeries, reported in most papers (since most papers deal only with nerves mapping instead of IONM). Mapping is a localizer test, performed intermittently by the surgeon aiming to identify neural structures. Monitoring is a more complex neurophysiological technique, composed of different tests, covering sensory and motor pathways, done continuously and almost independently from the surgeon. It is performed by a skilled neurophysiologist. Monitoring includes mapping, but mapping is not at all the same as monitoring. For more about this issue, refer to Chap. 2.

There are various pathologies addressed in HNE surgery, like thyroid, parathyroids, parotids, submandibular glands neoplasms, thyroid goiters, thyroglossal cyst, lymphadenopathies, jugular glomus, carotid diseases, skin tumors, anterior cervical arthropathy, carotid endarterectomy, cholesteatoma dissections, otitis media and treatment for deafness by cochlear electrode implantation, and treatment of epilepsy by means of *vagus* nerve stimulator implant [3]. This chapter focus on IONM for their approach.

Anatomy, Function, and Damage Consequences

For a better understanding of IONM techniques in HNE surgeries, the main anatomical structures involved will be presented below.

- Nerves: Facial, cochlear vestibular, glossopharyngeal, *vagus* and its branches (recurrent laryngeal and upper laryngeal nerves), accessory, hypoglossal, and phrenic, involving motor, sensory, and autonomic pathways. Phrenic nerve is of concern, since it originates from the cervical roots C3, C4, and C5, and has a cervical trajectory before reaching the diaphragm.
- Vessels: Common carotid arteries, internal and external carotids, external jugular vein, and lymph chains at different cervical levels.
- Medium and inner ear: There is an intimate relationship of these structures with the facial nerve in internal meatus and its emergence through the skull.

Facial Nerve (VII)

The facial nerve (FN) originates in the facial (motor) nerve nucleus in the pons at the brainstem, emerges from the lateral surface of brainstem at the pontine-medullary junction, goes toward the internal acoustic meatus, and passes through the FN canal in the petrous portion of the temporal bone (Fig. 31.1).

Among its different segments, stands out the FN trunk localized behind the posterior wall of the internal auditory canal. At the facial canal, in petrous part of temporal bone, where the small sensory and large motor roots fuse and enlarge at the geniculate ganglion, the FN gives off the grater petrosal nerve, which carries preganglionic parasympathetic fibers to the lacrimal gland, for the pterygopalatine ganglion and taste fibers. Two more branches emerge along the bony canal, the nerve to stapedius, the chorda tympanum, and preganglionic parasympathetic fibers.

The extracranial portion of the FN runs just anterior to the external ear. The first extracranial branch is the posterior auricular nerve, providing motor innervation to some muscles around the ear. Some branches innervate the posterior belly of the digastric muscle and the stylohyoid muscle. The main trunk (motor root) continues into the parotid gland (The parotid gland is innervated by the glossopharyngeal nerve.). Within the parotid gland, the FN first divides in two branches (zygomatic temporal and cervical facial branches) and finally gives off five branches: temporal, zygomatic, buccal, marginal mandibular branch, and cervical branch (Fig. 31.2).

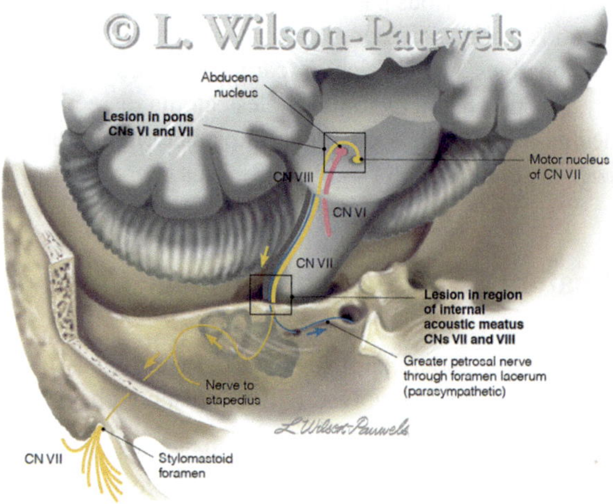

Fig. 31.1 Intracranial FN trajectory. (With permission from Wilson-Pauwels, L., Akesson EJ, Stewart, PA, Spacey, SD. Cranial Nerves in Healthy and Disease, second Edition, 2002)

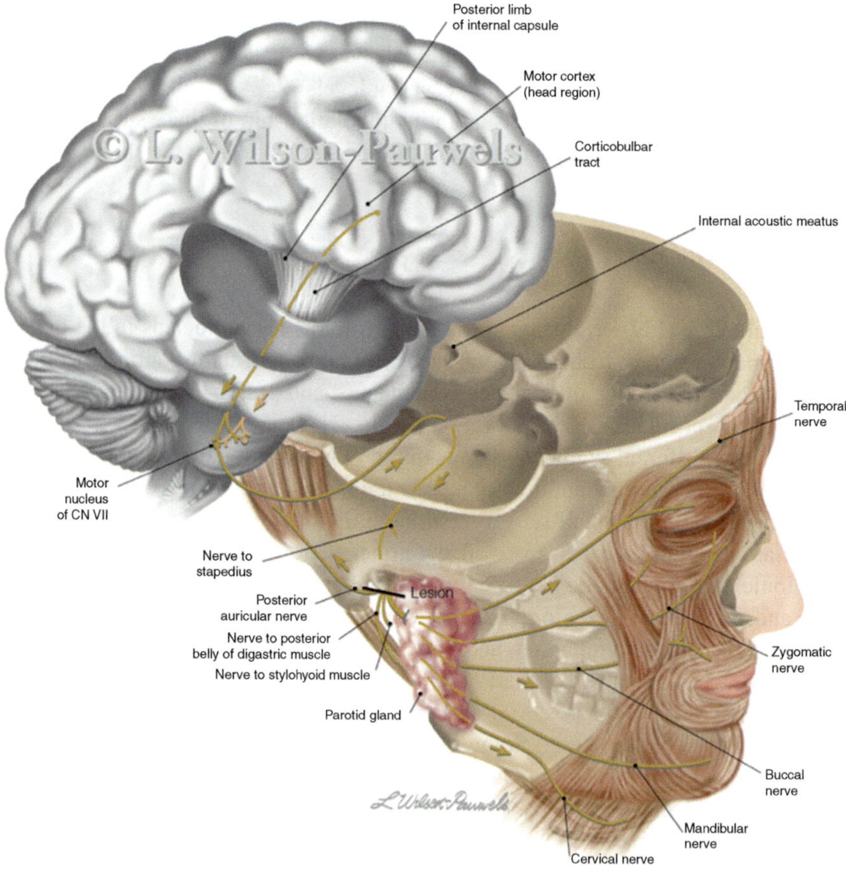

Fig. 31.2 Extracranial FN trajectory. (With permission from Wilson-Pauwels, L., Akesson EJ, Stewart, PA, Spacey, SD. Cranial Nerves in Healthy and Disease, second Edition, 2002)

These branches are responsible for the motor supply to the facial muscles. Damage or injury may result in facial palsy, including partial or total loss of facial mimic, abundant tearing, salivation, and loss of taste and hearing.

Anatomists have tried to build a classification to unify different patterns observed during FN dissection. Yet, due to its plexiform arrangement with several ramifications of the terminal branches, favoring difficulties during the parotid gland surgery, many different classifications have been proposed.

Vestibulocochlear Nerve (VIII)

The vestibulocochlear nerve originates in the pontine bulb groove of the brainstem, penetrates the temporal bone through the internal acoustic meatus, crossing the meatus along with the FN and intermediate nerve. It has two branches, the vestibular and the cochlear branches, both closely related. The vestibular part innervates the vestibular system, and the cochlear part innervates the cochlea.

Glossopharyngeal Nerve (IX)

The glossopharyngeal nerve (GN) has altogether 4 nuclei located in the medulla oblongata: ambiguous, inferior salivary, spinal of the trigeminal nerve, and solitary nucleus.

The GN originates in the bulb, in the posterior lateral groove in the form of root filaments that together form the nerve trunk, and follows out of the skull through the jugular foramen (Fig. 31.3). At this level, it expands into two ganglia, upper and lower, and moves toward the internal and external carotid stems, makes an anterior lower loop. The GN has 6 branches: (1) the tympanic nerve offers fibers to the parotid gland, carrying parasympathetic fibers, and eventually becomes the lesser petrosal nerve, exiting the skull via the foramen oval and synapsing in the otic ganglion, (2) branch to the stylopharyngeal muscle, (3) branch to carotid sinus, which communicates with the *vagus* nerve to carry signals from the baroreceptors in the carotid sinus and chemoreceptors in the carotid body (helping in blood pressure, blood oxygen, and CO2 level regulation), (4) pharyngeal branches, which join with the pharyngeal branches of the va*gus* nerve and sympathetic nerves form the pharyngeal plexus and innervate the muscles of the pharynx, (5) tonsillar branches, which provides sensory innervation to the palatine tonsil, and (6) lingual branches, which supply the vallate papillae, mucous membrane, and follicular glands of the posterior tongue.

The glossopharyngeal nerve is a mixed nerve, with sensory and motor functions, responsible for the sensitivity of the anterior 2/3 of the tongue, pharynx, and auditory tube, and for the motor mars of larynx muscles. The paralysis of the glossopharyngeal nerve is associated with alterations of the phonator apparatus characterized by paralysis of the vocal cords and severe pain in the palatine tonsils, soft palate, lateral and posterior part of the pharynx, and base of the tongue.

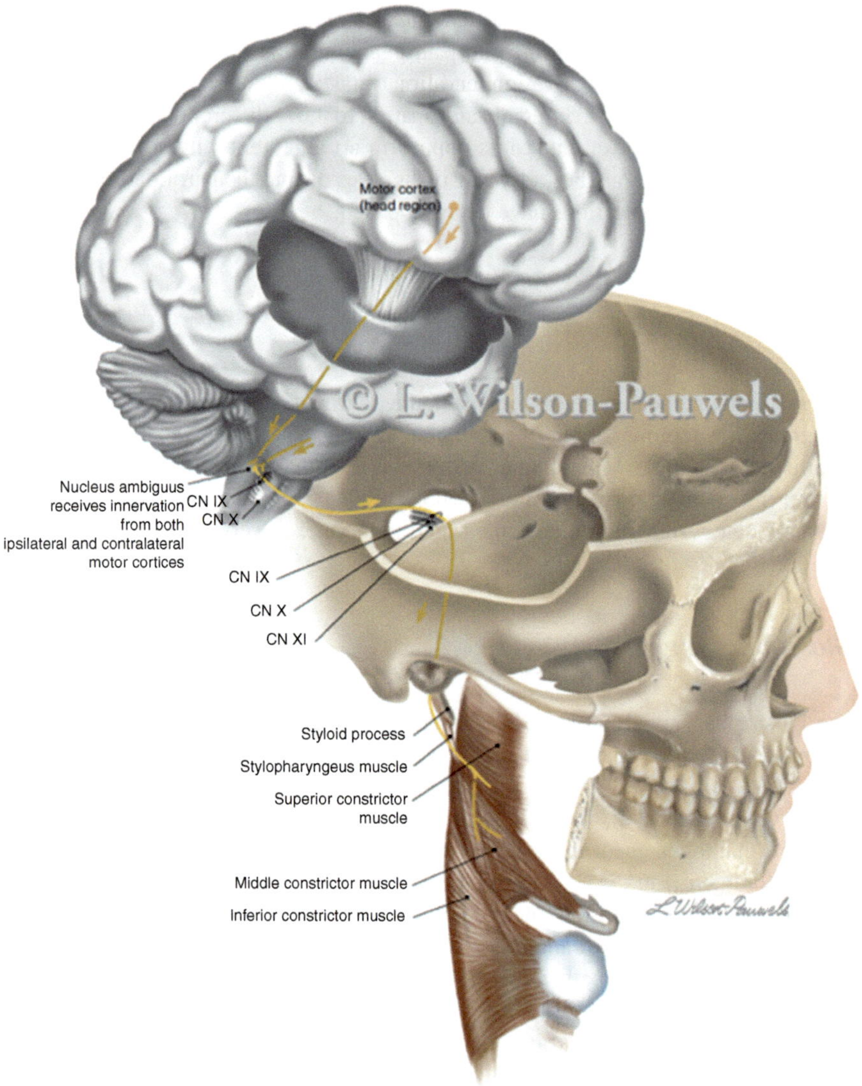

Fig. 31.3 Glossopharyngeal nerve trajectory. (With permission from Wilson-Pauwels, L., Akesson EJ, Stewart, PA, Spacey, SD. Cranial Nerves in Healthy and Disease, second Edition, 2002)

Vagus Nerve (X)

The origin of the vagus nerve occurs in the middle third of the posterolateral groove of the bulb, dorsal to inferior olive, and exits from the skull by the jugular foramen. It has two ganglia, the superior, also called the jugular, and the inferior. The vagus descends through the neck in the carotid sheath, laterally to the internal and common carotid arteries and medially to the internal jugular vein, reaches the thoracic

Each monitored anatomical structure poses graphical tracings with morphology, amplitude, and latency specific to its physiology. Small differences in the assembly of templates for stimulation and stimulus acquisition may occur depending on the normative values used by each laboratory and neurophysiologist. The initial graphics are obtained immediately after the anesthesia and will be used as baselines throughout the procedure. The on-going monitoring allows for immediate identification of any alteration of function and allows the surgeon to quickly react to avoid any further stretch or injury.

Stimulated and Spontaneous EMG

EMG is largely used in multimodal IONM protocols. Detailed information on the technique is available in Chap. 11. The inadvertent use of neuromuscular blockers should be ruled out before starting by performing TOF.

EMG-fr

EMG-fr is used in the study of peripheral nerves at rest.

Paired subdermal needles or surface electrodes or hook-wires are necessary to record motor activity. Among the surface electrodes stands out the orotracheal-cannula electrode (ETE), which is used in surgeries in which the study of the vocal cords is necessary (Fig. 31.5) [6]. There are also orotracheal cannulas with built-in wire electrodes, which pose a higher risk of causing perforating lesions in orotracheal path structures [7].

A-trains present the highest correlation with neuronal injury [8] (Fig. 31.6a). Detailed analysis of EMG-waveform characteristics can provide more accurate warning criteria than solely continuous acoustic EMG through loudspeakers.

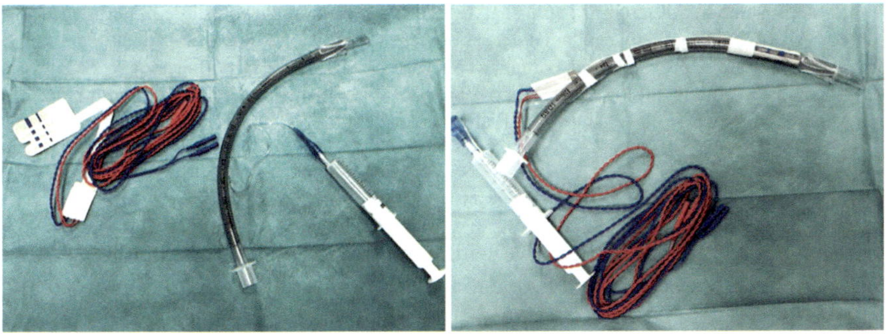

Fig. 31.5 ETE. Laryngeal electrode is usually designed to easily fit any ET tube, with stripes for easy placement. Commonly, they show optimal impedance

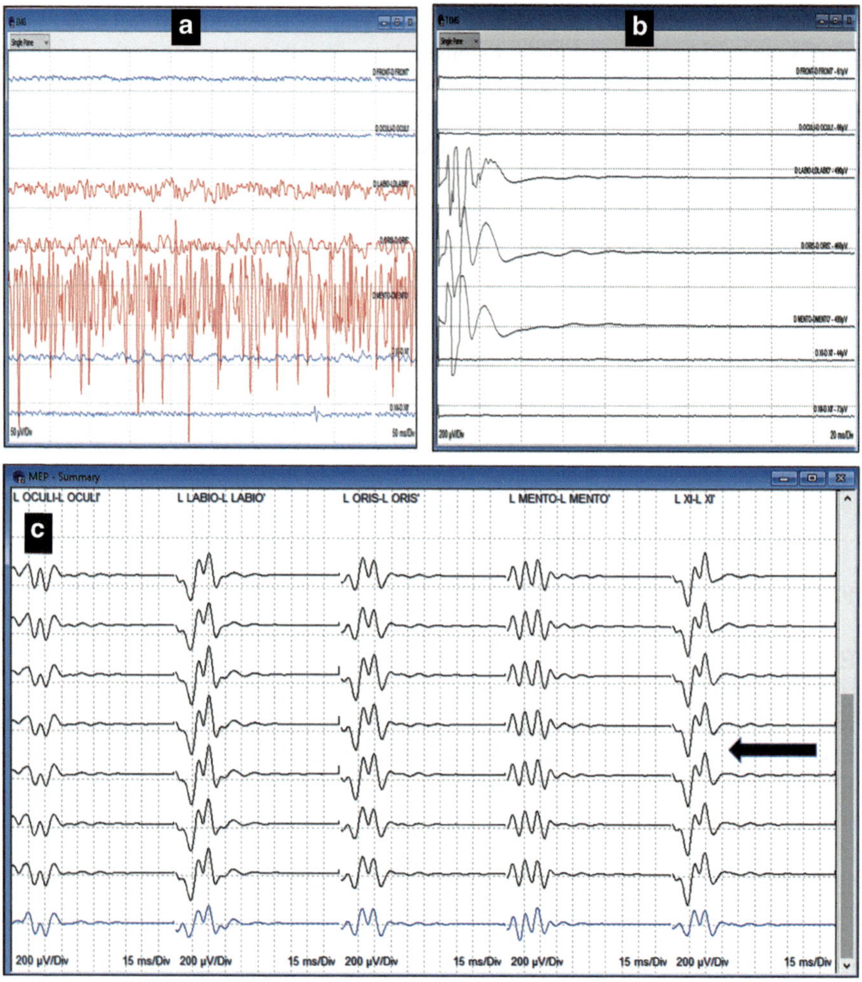

Fig. 31.6 (**a**) Free-run EMG showing discharges on *mentalis* during surgical access in a parotid tumor approach. (**b**) Although it is unusual to record such a finding, the surgeon performed triggered EMG to map for displaced facial nerves branches. Positive findings confirmed the proximity to *mentalis* fascicle, preventing its damage. This case illustrates the importance of recording several branches of the facial nerve due to possibility of its branches´ displacement, with respect to any standard pattern. (**c**) Unchanged MEP after the discharged (occurrence signalized the arrow)

EMG-st

Mapping aims to identify the nerve within the surgical field. Stimulation is done to ensure the integrity of structures due to the risk of punctual injury during tissue dissection, traction, and hemostasis. Initial potentials from the recurrent, superior laryngeal, vagus end others nerves should be obtained before manipulation for further comparison during the approach.

Either a monopolar or a bipolar nerve stimulator (either with double tips or concentric tip) may be used for mapping purposes. Monopolar probes provide more sensitivity, while bipolar enhances specificity. The stimulation protocol is composed by short duration single pulses of 50–60 μs up to 200 μs at 3.1 Hz. Usually, the final charge is a matter of pulse duration versus intensity, meaning that the shorter the pulse, higher the intensity, resulting in even final charges. Thus, current intensities up to 5 mA may be used with pulses of 50–60μS, while 2 mA is recommended for larger pulses [9]. Normally, short durations and low intensities of 1–2 mA is enough to produce replicable responses in a healthy nerve. In case of fibrous or infiltrating tissue or elements that dissipate the current (blood, saline, etc.), upper charges should be used to safely locate neural structures.

The stimulation results in a compound muscle action potential (CMAP) from each recorded muscle. Nerve stimulation is usually not limited to one point on nerve. It is necessary to explore its path to identify possible focal lesion sites (inching technique). Mapping of the nerves takes place during several surgical stages (e.g.: pre-, trans-, and post-lobe excision) to confirm integrity and reduce false negatives. Functional assessment is limited, since the nerve can still maintain unchanged CMAP distally to the damaged point. Hence, integrity assessment relies fully on the most proximal CMAP elicited.

During robotic or intraoral approaches, a 25 cm-length monopolar stimulator, with a straight tip of 200 mm, is used, due to the need to couple the electrode to the robot and the distance traveled by the stimulator to the access of the target nerve. Recordings are made with an ETE.

The clip-type nerve stimulator may be used for the *vagus* nerve. However, its use is related to neuronal suffering due to prolonged stimulation or direct nerve compression.

For EMG-st, the identification of motor response of the stimulated nerve is the crucial element of the study (Figs. 31.6b and 31.7). Outcome prediction is related to final to baseline CMAP amplitude. Accordingly, reduction greater than 50% from baseline predicts new deficits, which will be even worse in case of loss of the motor response, considering the same stimuli points and in the absence of changes in the anesthetic patterns. Major criterion for loss of function is the final absence of nerve response.

SSEP and MEP

They aim to evaluate cortical perfusion in surgeries in proximity to carotid plexus irrigation, since they pose risk of stroke. MEP for corticospinal tract aims to evaluate internal carotid as well as middle and anterior cerebral arteries perfusion territories.

MEP stimulation and SSEP records are performed through corkscrew electrodes placed on the scalp according to the 10–20 EEG system. Usually, we perform bilateral median or ulnar nerves SSEP, using Fz-C3´/C4'and MEP stimulating at C3/

Fig. 31.7 Triggered EMG results during parotid, showing unexpected positive facial nerve temporal branch

C4-Cz and Cz-Cz + 6 cm and recording on limb muscles (contralateral hand and foot). Further details in Chaps. 8 and 9, respectively.

For SSEP, the increase in latency greater than 10% and the reduction of amplitude greater than 50% are considered as predictive factors of neuronal injury. For MEP, amplitude deterioration of 50–70% inspires care, being higher than 80% compatible with injury.

Corticobulbar Motor-Evoked Potentials (CB-MEP)

The CB-MEP aims to monitor the motor pathway from the motor cortex to the muscles innervated by the motor cranial nerves. For more details and pitfalls, refer to Chap. 21. During HNE surgeries, electrical stimulation is applied over C3/Cz or C4/Cz for eliciting responses from the targeted muscles (percutaneously recorded with 76 μm diameter hook-wire or subdermal electrodes passing through 27-gauge needles, guided by electromyogram (EMG) feedback) [10].

CB-MEP is a reliable monitoring test of the functional integrity of motor cranial nerves (masseter, facial, glossopharyngeal, vagus, accessory, and hypoglossal). There is no additional cost, since it is recorded in the same channels used for EMG-fr.

Laryngeal Adductor Reflex (LAR)

The LAR is applicable to all surgeries where vagal nerve integrity may be compromised [11]. It represents a novel method for intraoperatively assessing the vagus nerve reflex arc, composed by a sensorial afferent component (through superior laryngeal nerve) and a motor efferent response (through recurrent laryngeal nerve). The LAR or glottic closure reflex has the function of protecting the aspiration of objects. Thus, the motor efferent activates the tiroarytenoid and cricoarytenoid lateral muscles, adducting the vocal cords. For further details on LAR, please refer to Chap. 12.

There are two expected responses after stimulation, a bilateral R1 and a contralateral R2. Usually, R1 is the measured response during IONM for HNE surgeries. R1 has an average latency of 22 + −3 ms, and mean amplitude of 300 + -180uV (Fig. 31.8a and b).

To obtain its components, it is recommended to stimulate with biphasic pulse with width from 500 to 1500 ms and intensity up to 15 mA. Bandwidth should be set between 20 to 1000 Hz with a curve duration equal to 100 ms. Its scan should be between 10 to 15 ms-division and amplitude with sensitivity of 100 mV-division. There is a special designed ETE composed of six channels, from which two poles are used for stimulation and four poles for recording.

The intraoperative loss of LAR response has been considered as a major criterion of neuronal injury, while transient disappearance with recovery may not correlate with new deficits [12]. It requires TIVA and no use of neuromuscular pharmacological blockers.

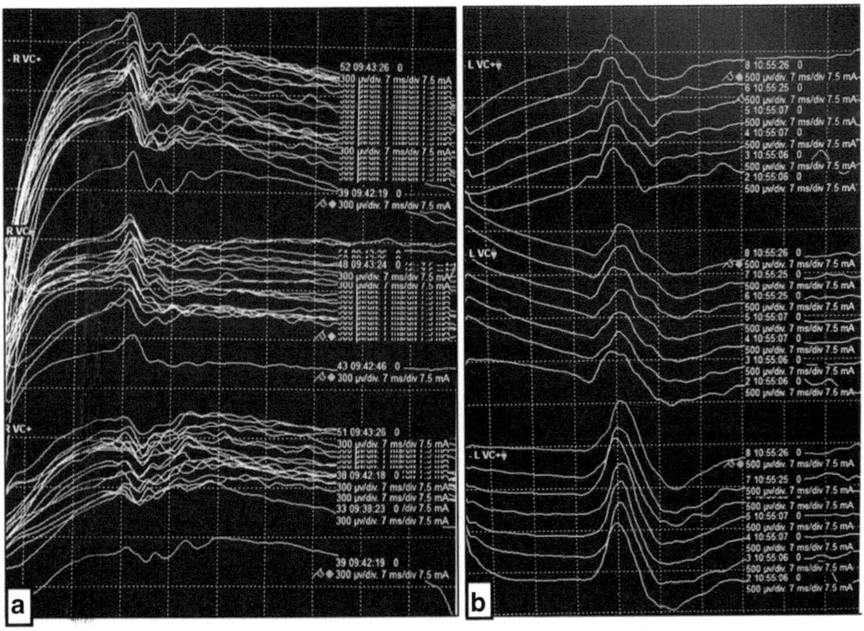

Fig. 31.8 (**a**) Right (300uV/ div and 7 ms/ div) and (**b**) Left LAR (500uV/ div and 7 ms/ div). Traces of LAR in a 63-year-old-woman who underwent total thyroidectomy (right thyroid carcinoma). Bilateral stable LAR recordings throughout the approach, showing that the reflex can be successfully recorded during TIVA. Patient presented no new deficit

EEG

EEG recordings at Fz-C3'and/or Fz-C4' and FZ-Cz aims to evaluate the level of anesthesia, cerebral epileptogenic activity, and cerebral perfusion during the procedure. The asymmetrical slowing of the waves is considered an alert signal for reduced cortical perfusion. The changes may be reversible depending on the severity of the impairment and reactional maneuvers performed by the surgeon. Usually, transient intraoperative deterioration with partial or total recovery may determine transient or no new deficits. In the presence of unreversed neurophysiological changes, permanent deficits might occur.

Additionally, EEG is a useful tool in anesthesia depth assessment. Presence of theta low voltage waves with a compressed spectral array (CSA) between 10 and 14 Hz is correlated with a deep sedation level, according to our experience. Changes in EEG, such as burst-suppression pattern (deep anesthetic level) or alpha/beta rhythms (superficial anesthetic level), are considered out-of-normality range and informed to the anesthesiologist team. EEG activity correlates with proper anesthesia depth and enables optimal IONM.

Further details on this subject can be found in Chap. 10.

Facial Nerve Monitoring in Parotid Surgery

Facial nerve injury remains the most feared complication of parotid gland surgery. The incidence of permanent facial paresis after parotidectomy may be as high as 9% (permanent facial nerve weakness), while the incidence of transient facial nerve weakness may range from 14% to 64% [13]. Risk factors impact the outcome, like previous parotid surgery, malignant tumor, more extensive surgery for larger tumors (located in the deep lobe), total parotidectomy, and previous inflammatory conditions.

Is there Evidence to Perform Facial Nerve Monitoring during Parotid Surgeries?

The use of intraoperative facial nerve monitoring during parotid gland surgery among Otolaryngologist-Head and Neck Surgeons continues to be a matter of debate. In a systematic review (mostly using passive continuous facial nerve monitoring or EMG-fr combined with EMG-st), the incidence of immediate and permanent postoperative weakness following parotidectomy was significantly lower in the monitored group (23.4% immediate, 5.7% permanent) versus the unmonitored group (38.4% immediate, 13.6% permanent). However, there was no significant difference when only prospective data was analyzed [14].

An important limitation of those studies is that it was not described how many intraoperative alerts resulted in surgeon's maneuvers to protect the facial nerve. Indeed, the protective reaction is usually ignored in the reports, since it prevents damage to the nerve, being classified as "false positive." *Yet, it is a true positive alert* resulting in effective preventive reaction. Thus, continuous multimodal IONM diminishes the risk of facial nerve injury to less than 2% and improves the surgical excision and/or debulking of previously inoperable tumors [15].

IONM Protocol

The goals of intraoperative facial monitoring in parotid surgery include the following:

Intermittent facial nerve mapping (EMG-st) + active continuous facial nerve monitoring (through EMG-fr and CB-MEP).

1. Subdermal paired needle electrodes are placed in the following muscles: frontalis (temporal branch), orbicularis oculi (zygomatic branch), nasalis and orbicularis oris (buccal branch), mentalis (marginal mandibular branch), and platysma (cervical branch).
2. Early identification of the facial nerve trunk as it exits the stylomastoid foramen, since it can be displaced posteriorly when the tumor is located close to the nerve's exit, or superiorly or inferiorly if distal to the main trunk.
3. Intraoperative identification of the distal branches of the facial nerve (intermittent facial nerve mapping) during surgical dissection and quantify the innervating contribution of each branch to the target muscle.
4. Warning the surgeon of unexpected facial nerve anatomy.
5. Warning the surgeon of significant changes in facial CMAP amplitude (recorded after using the mapping technique) and CB-MEP .
6. Reduce mechanical trauma to the nerve, if necessary.
7. Evaluation and prognosis of nerve function at the end of the surgery.

Our multimodal IONM protocols in parotid surgeries include EEG (to maintain a deep level of anesthesia), TOF (absence of muscle relaxant), EMG-fr, (continuous anomalous discharge monitoring), EMG-st (intermittent facial nerve mapping, and CB-MEP (active continuous facial nerve monitoring). In some considered high-risk cases, we tend to perform preoperative mapping (if muscle relaxant has already been washed away).

EMG-fr

It is a continuous but passive form of monitoring based on EMG signals following nerve injury or irritation [16]. During the procedure, the neurophysiologist analyzes any neurotonic discharges, communicating the changes to the surgeon for immediate recovery maneuvers.

EMG-st

Mapping aims to identify the trajectory and to evaluate the functional status, by using a handheld probe. Baselines identify latency and amplitude values at the beginning, which will be compared to CMAP during and at the end of the surgery. For nerve identification, the stimulus intensity should be adjusted to the threshold level at which a CMAP response is elicited. That will allow the surgeon to check the facial's nerve functionality at different stages of the surgery and will provide an objective comparison of the facial nerve functional status at different time points of the procedure.

Monopolar stimulation probe is the most common used, unless there is the necessity to identify some very specific branches and to avoid the spread of current; then, the use of concentric bipolar stimulation probes is recommended. Note that the surgeons feel very comfortable with the presence of sound-guided stimulation feedback, so it may be important to set up the audio EMG settings. In tumors involving specific branches of the facial nerve, monitoring should focus on the correspondent muscles [17] (Fig. 31.7). Figure 31.9 shows a selective CMAP response in the *nasalis* muscle, after mapping a nerve branch in a tumor involving the buccal branch of the facial nerve. In such a case, amplitude changes in *nasalis* should be

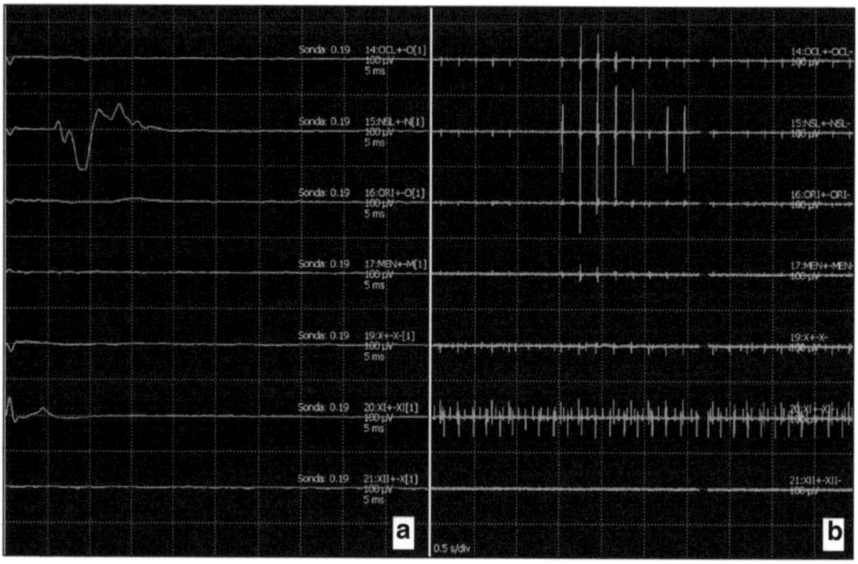

Fig. 31.9 (**a**) EMG-st: CMAP response recorded selectively on the *nasalis* muscle after monopolar stimulation (0.19 mA) of a nerve branch across a parotid tumor. (**b**) EMG-fr recordings from VII, X, XI, and XII lower cranial nerves. Notice neurotonic discharges mostly in the *nasalis* muscle due to manipulation of its innervation branch during tumor dissection

continuously compared with the amplitude of additional monitored muscles outside the field of dissection (*oculi* or *mentalis*).

Active Continuous Facial Nerve Monitoring (Neuromonitoring)

This method was described by Ulkatan et al. [18]. The neurophysiologic principles are similar to the clip electrode method for the vagus nerve [19]. Ulkatan methodology is based on the placement of 1) a needle stimulating electrode behind the ear toward the stylomastoid foramen, to act as a cathode and (2) a surface stick pad electrode over the mastoid process as an anode. CMAP recordings are done with two subdermal needle electrodes inserted in the muscles above mentioned. This method suffers no interference from the monopolar coagulator and requires a specific training from both the surgeon and the neurophysiologist. Teamwork communication is mandatory.

Once CMAP baselines are stablished, they will be compared with other CMAPs elicited at short intervals during the surgery. It is recommended to alert the surgeon when the CMAP's amplitude drop is significant in one or more branches of the facial nerve.

Preoperative Facial Nerve mapping's

Goal is to give the surgeon a topographical perspective of the facial nerve in distorted anatomy by marking the path of its branches on the skin surface [20]. It should be done at threshold intensity so that the branches are selectively stimulated, which is observed by the muscle twitching. It is an additional test in case of CB-MEP, resulting in extracranial nerve activation.

CB-MEP

The role of CB-MEP in parotid approaches is still to be determined. It may interfere with the surgeon's performance due to the temporal muscle twitch that is noticed during the electrical stimulation. Yet, the technique adds valuable information on the integrity of several cranial nerves and can be applied through a well-coordinated teamwork between the surgeon and the neurophysiologist. It enables a continuous facial nerve monitoring.

Recommendations The use of multimodal IONM during parotid surgeries is the most recommended protocol to monitor neural integrity. The combination of the above-mentioned tests is a promising new methodology in which the functional status of the facial nerve is always assessed (Fig. 31.10). Additionally, a fluent communication between surgical and neurophysiologic monitoring teams increases effectiveness of the procedure.

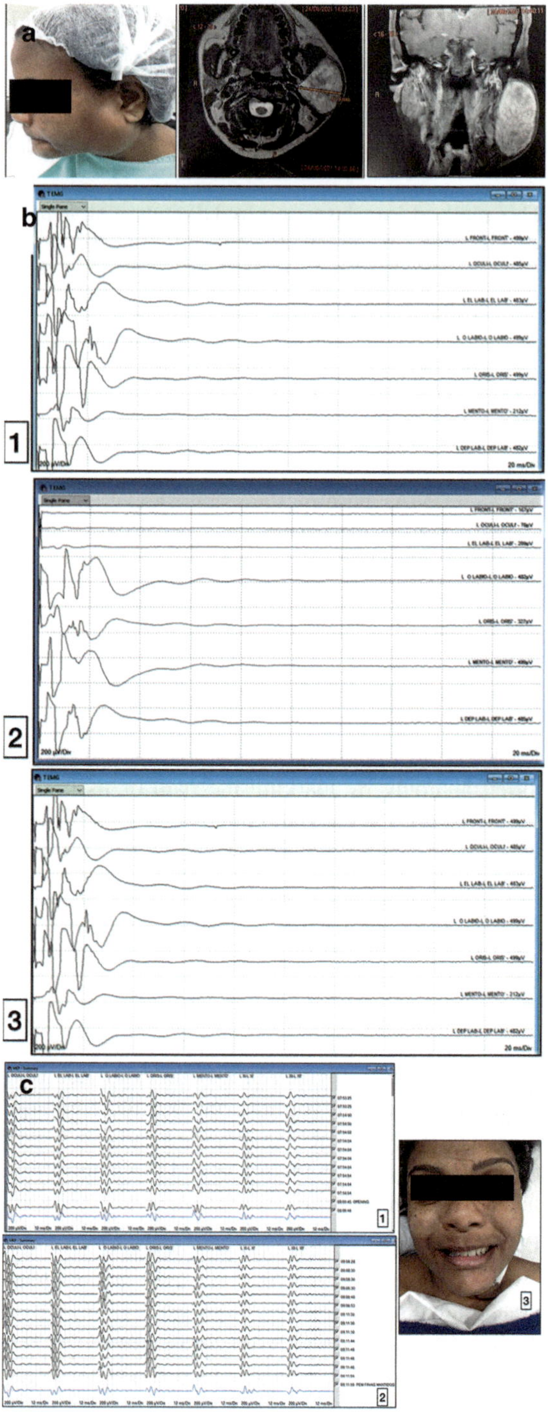

Fig. 31.10 (**a–c**) Female, 40 years old, tumoral lesion in the left parotid gland: pleomorphic adenoma. Neurophysiological protocol: Bilateral median PESS C3'-C4'. Spectral EEG. CB-MEP C3/C4-Cz: T05, ISI 2.5, I 230–250 mV, Dur 75 µs. Free EMG: 50 µV/Div, 50 ms/Div. tEMG: Int 0.2–5.0 mA, dur 0.1–0.2 ms, 2.79 Hz. Selected muscles: frontalis, orbicular oculi, orbicular oris (lips), orbicular oris, upper lip elevator, mentalis, lower lips depressor. (**a**) Preoperative clinical aspect and MRI, showing a measurement of 7.6 X 5.8 X 4.2 cm tumor. (**b**) 1 & 3: Initial and final mapping at the Facial nerve trunk threshold of 0.3 mA; 2: Mapping during resection: selective buccal and mandibular branches. (**c**) 1 & 2: MEP recordings from beginning until the end of surgery, showing stable and unchanged potentials. 3: immediate clinical status after wake-up from anesthesia, showing no facial nerve deficit facial nerve deficit

The Use of Multimodal IONM during Thyroid Surgeries

> *"I am convinced that the best management of recurrent laryngeal nerve injuries is of a preventative character"* Frank Lahey 1938, Boston.
>
> *"It is the author's inflexible rule to never resect the second lobe of the thyroid gland in the bilateral procedure until the integrity of the RLN on the first side has been proven."* Victor Riddell 1970, St. George's Hospital London.

Thyroid surgeries have seen a boom in recent years due to improvement in diagnosis of small papillary tumors (<1 cm) with ultrasound. Although a more conservative management has been tried, thyroidectomy rates have grown in countries with high incidence of papillary tumors.

Among the possible complications related to thyroid surgery, damage to the recurrent laryngeal nerve (RLN) is one of the most common. The signs and symptoms of the nerve injury vary from transient paresis with hoarseness and disturbances of the voice, to permanent damage including the need for tracheostomy in rare cases. Hence, monitoring systems are necessary in an attempt to avoid RLN lesion, improve the safety of the surgical procedure, and maintain patient's quality of life.

The larynx is innervated by two branches of the vagus nerve: the SLN that carries afferent sensory input from the supraglottic and glottic larynx, and the RLN, which is related to sensory nerve supply of the infraglottic region and provides motor innervation to laryngeal muscles (except for the cricothyroid muscle, which is innervated by the SLN).

In the surgical field, the RLN is located either by the palpation and or by identification of the inferior thyroid artery. Then, gentle dissection is performed caudally to the artery in the plane of the tracheoesophageal groove. Palpation might not be reliable, especially in cases of previous surgeries, anatomic variation, the presence of large multinodular goiter, or inflammatory adenopathies.

EMG-fr and EMG-st

Intraoperative mapping of the RLN started in Europe and was first described by Flisberg and Lindholm (1960). Since then, different RLN recording techniques have been reported. We name some:

1. *Laryngeal palpation after RLN stimulation* to observe muscle twitch.
2. *Direct into vocal cord:* A) hook wires inserted via direct vision using an endoscopic technique (done by the neurophysiologist or anesthesiologist); B) direct but blind subdermal needles insertion through the cricothyroid membrane (applied by the surgeon himself or herself within the surgical field). Although easy to perform, the needle placement is blind, which can cause hematoma of the vocal cords, misplacement, or cuff perforation. We recommend option B execution only if it is not possible to perform option A or 3.

3. ETE: Endotracheal tube that consists of a low-pressure cuffed silicone elastomer endotracheal tube with either integrated bilateral paired stainless-steel wire electrodes or with a laryngeal electrode with stripes that fit any ET tube (Fig. 31.5).

Options 1 and 2 record the CMAP resulting from the vocal cord adduction elicited by RLN stimulation with a hand-held probe and register spontaneous firing through EMG-fr channels. Table 31.1 compares the abovementioned recording techniques.

The fundamental IONM technique during thyroid approaches is vagus nerve branches stimulation. In selected cases, it can be performed transcutaneously using superficial electrodes, aiming to set a baseline CMAP to check on RLN integrity (before the beginning of the surgery) and to verify the correct placement of the recording electrodes. It is mostly performed during surgery using different handheld probes for intermittent mapping. Its obvious limitation is the risk of nerve injury in between 2 stimulations. Additionally, lesion proximal to the site of stimulation will go undetected, since Wallerian degeneration will take around 7 days to occur.

Thus, the functional assessment of RLN is limited to the moment of stimulation and is fully dependent that it is performed proximally to the damaged site.

Intermittent nerve stimulation is performed with a monopolar hand-held stimulating probe with a subdermal sternal reference. Single stimulus of 0.1 ms duration, with maximum intensity 2 mA and a repetition rate of 4 Hz, is applied. Loss of signal is defined as a CMAP amplitude below 100 μV with an absent posterior cricoarytenoid muscular twitch response on laryngeal palpation during vagal and RLN stimulation (following Catherine F.Sinclair's et al. criteria).

Table 31.1 Comparison between different RLN IONM techniques

	Cricothyroid membrane	Hook wires in vocal cord	ETE
CMAP amplitude	1.5–3.0 mV High	1.6–1.8 mV High	300–400 uV Low
Impedances	Low	Low	High
Muscle relaxant	No	No	No
Validity	100%	100%	70%
Laterality specific	Yes	Yes	No
Respiratory rate influence	No	No	Yes
Inconvenient	Invasive Needles into the operating field Cuff punction	Invasive Slow execution Costs Laryngoscopy	Noninvasive Artifact Difficult intubation False + Signal loss
Level of difficulty	Low	High	Moderate/high
Assistance	Surgeon	Surgeon, neurophysiologist, anesthesiologist	Anesthesiologist, Neurophysiologist

Continuous Intraoperative Stimulation of the Vagus Nerve

To reduce the gap between intermittent stimulation and to map the entire RLN continuously, continuous intraoperative stimulation of the vagus nerve (CVNM) proximal to the exit point of the RLN has been introduced [21]. It relies on exposure of the RLN and/or vagus nerves for placement of electrodes, being an invasive technique. Mapping is carried out by positioning an electrode directly on the course of the vagus nerve proximally to the RLN origin. The EMG signal is recorded from the ETE and reproduced both visually and acoustically, and analysis includes amplitude and latency. The optimal stimulation intensity is 1 mA (fibers A and B), which hinders any side effects related to recruitment of the C vagal fibers. The negative pulse is rectangular, with 0.1–0.2 ms duration, and a frequency of 1 Hz.

The electrodes used for CVNM of the RLN differ by geometry and design. They can present (a) open (b) closed, and (c) half-closed conformation. Open design may require that the electrode simply leans on the surface of the nerve (partial dissection) or that it surrounds (360° dissection) the RLN. Regarding the stimulation mode, electrodes differ in monopolar, bipolar, and tripolar [22].

Yet, many reports show evidence that CVNM may cause serious patient harm. In a prospective, noncontrolled trial of CVNM in a cohort of 20 nonrandomly selected patients undergoing thyroid and parathyroid surgery, David J Terris et al. reported hemodynamic instability and reversible vagal neuropraxia in 2/9 patients (the trial was aborted at patient n° 9) [23]. The stimulation clamp became dislodged 11 times in 5 cases and was replaced in 7 of those instances. Although it may.

Occasionally provide meaningful information, the risk-benefit ratio does not favor widespread adoption.

LAR

Sinclair et al. have recently described a novel methodology for assessing laryngeal and vagus nerve integrity based on the recording of the LAR, which relies on the placement of ETEs for stimulating and recording laryngeal responses (11). The technique monitors the entire vagal reflex arc, including sensory, motor, and brainstem pathways. LAR seems to be a viable method of monitoring RLN and vagus nerve integrity during surgery.

Technical attention should be taken to avoid rotation of the endotracheal tube, which may result in loss of response of the reflex components, thus determining the presence of false positives.

The LAR is elicited by electrical stimulation of the contralateral vocal cord to the operative field using the right or left ETEs (e.g., for a left thyroid goiter surgery, we stimulate the right vocal cord and record on the left vocal cord). The contralateral R1 (cR1) and R2 (cR2) responses are defined as the short- (R1) and long-latency (R2) responses, elicited in the contralateral vocal fold muscles relative to the stimulating side (Fig. 31.11).

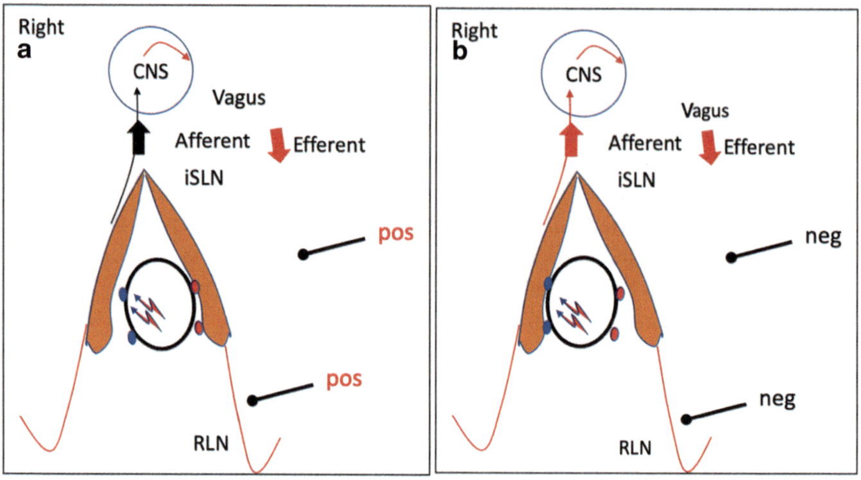

Fig. 31.11 **LAR:** ETE displacement during surgery at the left side. *Courtesey of Dr Xavier Guirao, Head of Unit of Endocrine and Head & Neck Surgery.* (**a**) **LAR with right side displacement:** Right ETE displacement leading to Left-LAR negative: no afferent stimulus (through ipsilateral SLN). Left RLN and vagus nerve mapping, positive (pos). Surgical field visualization: Laryngeal twitch present after any stimulation point. (**b**) **LAR with left side displacement:** Left side ETE displacement: no afferent input (through ipsilateral SLN). Left RLN and vagus nerve mapping: negative (neg). Right-LAR negative due to no afferent stimulus from the left vocal cord. Surgical field visualization: Laryngeal twitch positive at any stimulation point

Catherine F.Sinclair et al. included 134 nerves-at-risk in a prospective trial with continuous LAR monitoring during neck endocrine surgeries. Significantly more postoperative vocal cord paralysis ($P < 0.001$) was seen among patients with an amplitude decrement (opening-to-closing) >60% or with absolute closing amplitude <100 μV [24]. The LAR-continuous-IONM was highly sensitive to RLN stretch or compression. Three different derivations were constructed for recording each LAR elicited: (1) electrode 1 versus electrode 2 (being both from the same side of the endotracheal tube); (2) electrode 1 versus reference electrode (placed at the sternum); and (3) electrode 2 versus reference electrode at the sternum.

We strongly recommend the use of a noninvasive RLN IONM. We use the following alarm and prognostic criteria, based on Sinclair et al.:

1. If amplitude response decreases >50% compared to baseline amplitude, impending nerve injury is possible, and the surgeon should be warned, and the tissue released.
2. If the amplitude decreases >60% of baseline and does not recover with tissue relaxation, postoperative nerve and vocal fold dysfunction are likely.

IONM Protocol for HNE Approaches

Prior to the Entrance of the Patient into the Operating Room (Being the Patient Still Awake)

The surgeon makes a percutaneous laryngeal ultrasound, which is a well-tolerated noninvasive exam, in order to (1) visualize in real time the vocal cord movements (abduction-adduction maneuvers) and (2) locate vagus nerve in the neurovascular bundle (helps with a better and faster macroscopic intraoperative location, prior to the mapping)

Preparation for an Effective ETE Recording and Stimulation

After induction of general anesthesia with TIVA and using a short-acting muscle relaxant (succinylcholine) only for intubation purposes, the patient is intubated either with an ETE or with an adhesive laryngeal electrode that fits the size of the tube. Once tube's position has been checked (impedances) and readjusted, if necessary, baseline LAR is performed from both sides, and amplitude and latency values are recorded. Only after those circumstances, the tube can be fixed. Tracheal secretions may hinder LAR recordings, since it compromises electrode impedance and originates artifacts. It is recommended to aspirate secretions and stablish new baselines prior to the beginning of the surgery. In patients with many secretions, and if there are not contraindications, atropine may be indicated (which reduces secretions in the mouth and respiratory passages and relieves the constriction and spasm in respiratory passages).

Multimodal Protocol

1. TOF technique (4 out of 4 twitches are recommended before taking LAR baselines)
2. EEG (stable sedative status)
3. EMG-fr of the vocal cords (recorded through the endotracheal tube electrodes)
4. Intermittent mapping of the SLN (*), RLN, and vagus nerve, adding marginal mandibular branch of the facial nerve (*mentalis* muscle), phrenic nerve (G1: electrode 5 cm above xiphoid process; G2: ipsilateral to the stimulation side 16 cm infero-lateral from G1 over the chest margin) and accessory nerve (trapezius or sternocleidomastoid muscles) in total thyroidectomy surgeries with cervical lymph node excision.

5. LAR recording from right and left vocal cords.

*(*)The superior laryngeal nerve gives off the external branch of the superior laryngeal nerve (EBSLN), which runs medial to the superior pole vessels to innervate the cricothyroid muscle. This motor nerve (*i.e., *Amelita Galli-Curci nerve) increases tension of the vocal cords, allowing for high notes. Injury to the nerve leads to a weak, low voice that fatigues easily and lacks projection. Patients may also have problems with aspiration.*

Both intermittent stimulation and LAR technique are applied during the following critical stages of the surgery: (1) dissection of prethyroidal muscles (F1); (2) superior lobe dissection (F2); (3) midlobe dissection (F3); (4) inferior lobe dissection (F4); (5) pretracheal fascia dissection (F5); (6) Berry's ligament (suspensory ligament of the thyroid gland) dissection (F6); and (7) lobectomy (F7). In this way, amplitude and latency values are pointed after intermittent stimulation as follows:

- Step 1. SLN (S1). Signal beginning F2 stage.
- Step 2. SLN (S2). Signal at the end of F2 stage.
- Step 3. Vagus nerve (V1). Signal beginning F3.
- Step 4. RLN (R1). Signal beginning F3.
- Step 5. RLN (R2). Signal at the end of F7.
- Step 6. Vagus nerve (V2). Signal at the end of F7.

In many thyroid surgeries, transient decreases in LAR amplitude without concomitant increases in reflex latency may occur during surgical maneuvers that put traction on the RLN mostly during midlobe dissection stage (F3) and Berry's ligament dissection (F6). Releasing the tissue as well as changing surgery's approach into the inferior lobe dissection resulted in the recovery of LAR amplitude (Fig. 31.12). Most probably, no change in LAR predicts good outcome (Fig. 31.13).

During all stages of the procedure, intermittent mapping and LAR technique are frequently applied and surgeon should be informed if any significant changes are observed, so recovery measures can be taken in order to prevent nerve injury.

Role of CB-MEP

In addition to the above protocol, the main author and editors add the CB-MEP as another IONM modality:

1. The muscles for CB-MEP recording are the same ones already used in EMG.
2. The terminal branches of the facial nerve are the most prone to damage. Therefore, a sudden CB-MEP drop in only one branch with unchanged response in the others is a relevant information.
3. Interaction with the surgeon regarding muscle twitch is managed similarly to other surgical procedures.

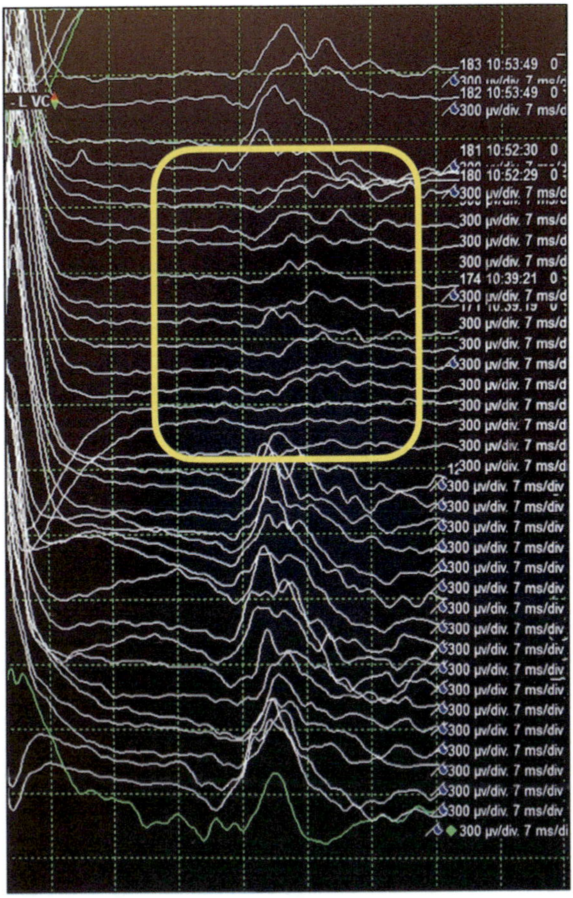

Fig. 31.12 Consecutive traces of the left LAR in a 56-year-old woman who underwent total thyroidectomy (left thyroid carcinoma), showing reversible changes from baseline. The change correlated with surgical maneuvers that put stretch and compression directly on the left RLN during midpole dissection phase (F3). LAR recovered to baseline value after 3 minutes by simply relaxing the tissue and irrigating with warm saline. No new immediate deficits were observed

Recommendation The use of multimodal IONM during neck surgeries is the most recommended protocol to monitor neural integrity of the SLN, RLN, and vagus nerve. Combination of different neurophysiological tests is promising to promote continuous vagus nerve monitoring. Yet, it requires expertise from the neurophysiologist and anesthesiologist's team in combination with the surgeon's familiarity with the techniques.

The Use of Multimodal IONM in Mastoid and Cochlear Implant Surgeries

Iatrogenic injury to the facial nerve (FN) is one of the most devastating complications of mastoid surgery. Some authors have found the incidence of FN injury in primary otologic procedures to be as high as 1% and 4% [25]. During revision

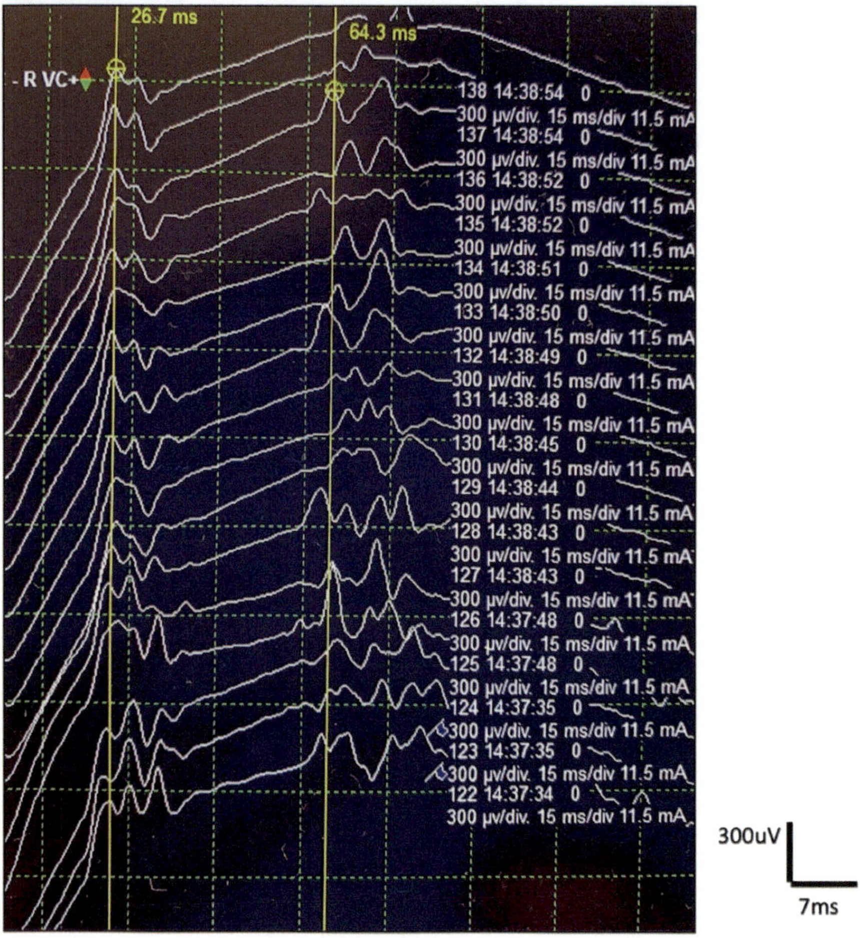

Fig. 31.13 Traces of right LAR in a 54-year-old woman who underwent total thyroidectomy (thyroid goiter).The surgery started on the right side, with a reproducible and stable Right LAR: R1 (26.7 ms) and R2 (64.4 ms) with similar amplitude values in both components. No changes were recorded during the procedure with perfect correlation with normal postoperative neurological status

procedure, it was reported to be more than double when compared to primary operations at 4% to 10% and 0.6% to 3.7%, respectively [26].

Despite technological advances, such as the introduction of the operating microscope and delicate surgical drill, and the availability of preoperating imaging, the overall risk of iatrogenic FN paralysis remains considerably high [27]. In an epidemiological study, 82% of otologic FN injuries were caused by mastoid surgery [28]. In a retrospective study of 5 years, Ryu et al. demonstrated 43% (6 cases) of iatrogenic FN injuries had occurred in tympanic segment, 28.5% (4 cases) of injuries in second genu combined with tympanic segment, and 28.5% (4 cases) of injuries in mastoid segment [27].

Indexed bibliography in mastoid and cochlear implant surgeries describes mainly EMG-st of FN, which corresponds to unimodal or incomplete intraoperative neurophysiological monitoring (IONMu) [29]. The same applies to the surgeries with robotic cochlear implantation [30].

Multimodal intraoperative neurophysiological monitoring (IONMm), by means of its two stages of mapping and monitoring, should yield precise information to the surgeon about the functioning of FN. The neurophysiological feedback lets surgeons correlate their actions over a given surgical time, based on the IONMm findings, allowing them to interrupt maneuvers, retreat, and, with this, prevent neurological lesions. This type of information is supplied to the surgical team throughout all stages of the procedure.

IONMm include FN CB-MEP, EMG-fr, and EMG-st and blink reflex (BLR) to assess FN functional integrity. EMG-st technique is used solely to map the FN proximity. It determines, through the depolarization threshold found, the distance of the monopolar stimulator in relation to the FN and offers feedback on if this distance can be considered safe. However, we emphasize that EMG-st is not a monitoring technique, but rather only a mapping tool. It does not allow the monitoring of ongoing lesions related to stretching, thermal, or traction events. EMG-fr may show spontaneous discharges elicited by mechanical or deleterious maneuvers although the direct effect on outcome may not be linear (more details in Chap. 21). CB-MEP assesses the entire cranial nerve motor pathway, including branches that are not directly visualized by the surgeon. Thus, we highlight that unimodal IONM (IONMu) is incomplete to diagnose most of the lesions that could occur, being essential to monitor the FN with all the tests above mentioned.

Neurophysiologists are properly skilled to offer beyond an IONMu, which most probably ends to enhance good outcome. Hence, we suggest that IONMm be conducted in all mastoid surgeries, including mastoidectomies and cochlear implant surgery. FN CB-MEP should be routinely used to reduce the risk of reversible and irreversible neural damages. During an implant surgery, FN CB-MEP it is generally performed until the implant is placed. Yet, Yellin et al., 2016 reported safe use of CB-MEP in patients with cochlear implants [31].

Thus, we suggest the adoption of fundamental steps during mastoidectomies and cochlear implant surgeries to perform CB-MEP [32]:

1. Muscles recordings should include muscles innervated by several FN branches namely: temporal (frontalis), zygomatic (orbicular oculi), buccal (orbicular oris), and marginal mandibular (mentalis). CB-MEP is performed **during the entire surgery including the drilling phase for access to the cochlea**. We use montage C3 (+) versus Cz (−) for left hemispheric stimulation and C4 (+) versus Cz (−) for right hemispheric stimulation [33]. Verst et al. [34] advocated montage C5 (+) versus Cz (−) for left hemispheric stimulation and C6 (+) versus Cz (−) for right hemispheric stimulation, because this corresponds better to the anatomy of M1 for the corticobulbar pathways. Our experience shows that deterioration

of the responses can occur during the drilling by thermal nerve injury. In practice, the surgeon reacts: stopping the drilling and waiting 1 to 3 minutes for us to continuously evaluate the FN CB-MEP. CB-MEP amplitude reduction greater than 50% may be associated with irreversible damage of the FN. This criterion is usually useful in acoustic neuroma surgery [35]. We suggest the same criterion to mastoid and implant cochlear surgeries.
2. After the access, the surgeon uses a monopolar stimulator probe to map and locate the FN. EMG-st applies pulses lasting 0.1 ms or 100 us, since with this pulse duration, 1 mA implies 1 mm distance to the nerve. It was estimated through animal study that a stimulation of 3.0 mA is safe to prevent FN damage during middle ear surgery [36].
3. The BLR technique may elicit R1 component during brainstem IONM and TIVA [37]. The protocol demands multipulse stimulation, with an interstimulus interval of 2 ms, an intensity of 20–40 mA, and a train repetition rate of 0.4 Hz over the supraorbital nerve [33]. BLR might be considered a new tool for IONMm in mastoid and implant cochlear surgeries.

Recommendations Multimodal IONM is highly recommended to monitor neural integrity, but unfortunately, they are not yet widely used during mastoidectomies and cochlear implants. We use of IONMm in all mastoid surgeries that require IONM, except in patients with previous cochlear implant.

Vagus Nerve Stimulation

Unilateral vagus nerve pacemaker implantation is used to manage refractory epilepsy. Our protocol aims to assess cerebral perfusion and cranial nerves´ function.

- EMG-fr and EMG-st with subdermal needles insert into the soft palate (IX) and tongue (XII) and ETE (X).
- LAR.
- SSEP of median nerves.
- MEP with recordings in both hands (brevis thumb adductor).
- CB-MEP for cranial nerves.
- TOF.
- EEG for anesthetic level and cerebral perfusion assessments.

Glomus Carotideo

It is a complex approach that poses risk mainly to cerebral perfusion and nearby cranial nerves (Fig. 31.14).

Our protocol includes the following:

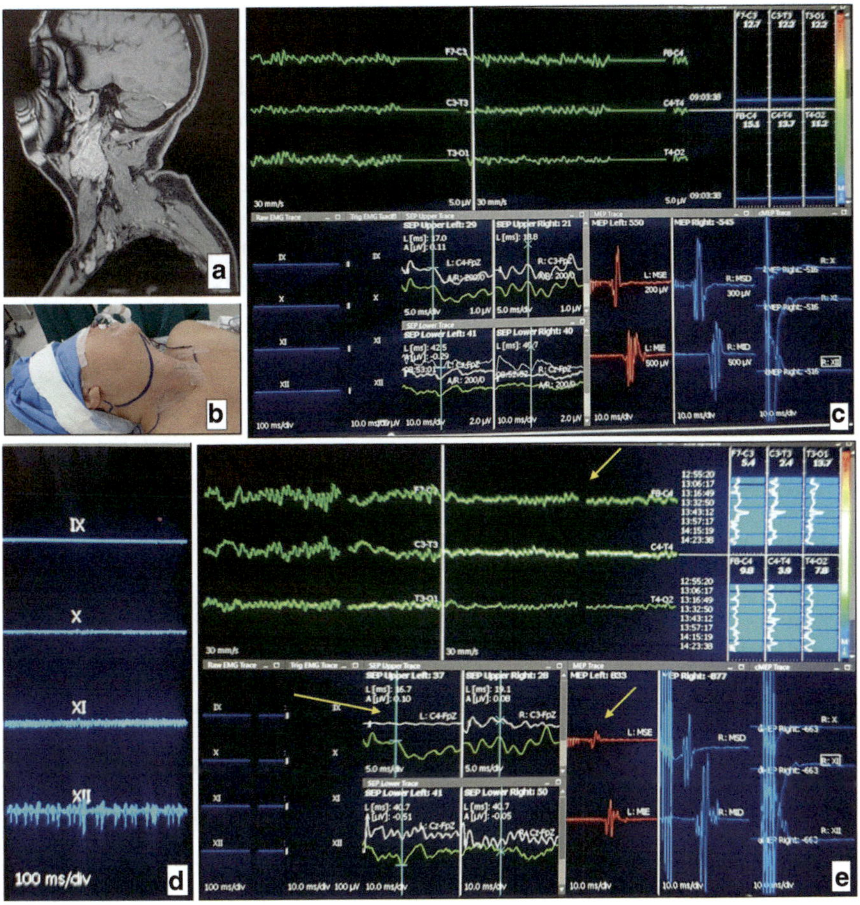

Fig. 31.14 Man, 55 year old, with a solid hard mass in the right neck. (**a**) MRI showing a right carotid paraganglioma (**b**) patient positioning (**c**) IONMm protocol included EMG-fr, EMG-st, and CB-MEP of IX, X, XI, and XII cranial nerves, MEP of both hands and feet, bilateral median and tibial nerves SSEP, EEG. (**d**) Tumor dissection led to A-trains recorded in EMG-fr of the XII (**e**) During caudal tumor manipulation: deterioration and loss of N20 of left upper limb, followed by drop in left upper limb MEP and EEG amplitude drop on right hemisphere (signed with yellow arrows). Surgery was stopped until full recovery of the neurophysiological responses. Patient presented no new neurological deficit

- EMG-fr and EMG-st with subdermal needles insert into the soft palate (IX), ETE (X), trapezius (XI) and tongue (XII).
- LAR.
- SSEP of median and tibial nerves.
- MEP with recordings in both hands and feet (brevis thumb adductor and abductor haluccis brevis).
- CB-MEP for cranial nerves.
- TOF.
- EEG for anesthetic level and cerebral perfusion assessments.

Conclusion

HNE surgeries pose risk to peripheral nervous system and cerebrovascular perfusion. Multimodal IONM enhances the identification of adverse events and contributes to better outcome.

In this chapter, we highlighted the importance of active continuous cranial nerve monitoring during several approaches. Particularly, we recommend the addition of LAR and CB-MEP in the IONM protocols to improve normative data development among different centers and to enhance patient's safety during HNE surgeries.

References

1. Stankovic P, Wittlinger J, Georgiew R, Dominas N, Hoch S, Wilhelm T. Kontinuierliches intraoperatives Neuromonitoring (cIONM) in der Kopf-Hals-Chirurgie – eine Übersicht [Continuous intraoperative neuromonitoring (cIONM) in head and neck surgery-a review. German version]. HNO. 2020;68(11):801–9. German. https://doi.org/10.1007/s00106-020-00823-2. PMID: 32157335; PMCID: PMC7591407.
2. Schneider R, Machens A, Lorenz K, Dralle H. Intraoperative nerve monitoring in thyroid surgery-shifting current paradigms. Gland Surg. 2020;9(Suppl 2):S120–8. https://doi.org/10.21037/gs.2019.11.04. PMID: 32175252; PMCID: PMC7044089.3.
3. González HFJ, Yengo-Kahn A, Englot DJ. Vagus Nerve Stimulation for the Treatment of Epilepsy. Neurosurg Clin N Am. 2019;30(2):219–30. https://doi.org/10.1016/j.nec.2018.12.005. PMID: 30898273; PMCID: PMC6432928.
4. Werner JA. Historischer Abriss zur Nomenklatur der Halslymphknoten als Grundlage für die Klassifikation der Neck-dissection [Historical outline on the nomenclature of neck lymph nodes as a basis of neck dissection classification]. Laryngorhinootologie. 2001;80(7):400–9. German. https://doi.org/10.1055/s-2001-15711. PMID: 11488152.5.
5. Li Y, Liu K, Ke Y, Zeng Y, Chen M, Li W, Liu W, Hua X, Li Z, Zhong Y, Xie C, Yu H. Risk Factors Analysis of Pathologically Confirmed Cervical Lymph Nodes Metastasis in Oral Squamous Cell Carcinoma Patients with Clinically Negative Cervical Lymph Node: Results from a Cancer Center of Central China. J Cancer. 2019;10(13):3062–9. https://doi.org/10.7150/jca.30502. PMID: 31281484; PMCID: PMC6590044.
6. Dralle H, Sekulla C, Lorenz K, Brauckhoff M, Machens A. German IONM Study Group. Intraoperative monitoring of the recurrent laryngeal nerve in thyroid surgery. World J Surg. 2008;32(7):1358–66. https://doi.org/10.1007/s00268-008-9483-2.
7. Alerta de Tecnovigilância-SISTEC 2190 -Richards – KIT Canula para estimulação recorrente com sonda estimuladora NIM Response – Potencial de Evento Adverso Grave ao dobrar excessivamente a cânula. Área: GGMON. Número: 2190. Ano: 2017.
8. Romstöck J, Strauss C, Fahlbusch R. Continuous electromyography monitoring of motor cranial nerves during cerebellopontine angle surgery. J Neurosurg. 2000;93(4):586–93. https://doi.org/10.3171/jns.2000.93.4.0586. PMID: 11014536.
9. Wojtczak B, Sutkowski K, Krzysztof Kaliszewski K, Głód M, Marcin BM. Experience with intraoperative neuromonitoring of the recurrent laryngeal nerve improves surgical skills and outcomes of non-monitored thyroidectomy. Langenbeck's Arch Surg. 2017;402(4):709–17. https://doi.org/10.1007/s00423-016-1449-5.
10. Deletis V, Fernández-Conejero I, Ulkatan S, Rogic M, Lladó-Carbó E, Hiltzik D. Methodology for intra-operative recording of the corticobulbar motor evoked potentials from cricothyroid muscles. Clin Neurophysiol. 2011;122(9):1883–9.

11. Sinclair CF, Maria TJ, Tapia OR, Ulkatan S, Deletis V. A novel methodology for assessing laryngeal and vagus nerve integrity in patients under general anesthesia. Clin Neurophysiol. 2017;128(7):1399–405. https://doi.org/10.1016/j.clinph.2017.03.002. ISSN 1388-2457.
12. Cirocchi R, Arezzo A, D'Andrea V, Abraha I, Popivanov GI, Avenia N, Gerardi C, Henry BM, Randolph J, Barczyñski M. Intraoperative neuromonitoring versus visual nerve identification for prevention of recurrent laryngeal nerve injury in adults undergoing thyroid surgery. Cochrane Database Syst Rev. 2019;1(1):CD012483. https://doi.org/10.1002/14651858.CD012483.pub2. PMID: 30659577; PMCID: PMC6353246.
13. Jin H, Kim BY et al. Incidence of postoperative facial weakness in parotid tumor surgery: a tumor subsite analysis of 794 parotidectomies. BMC Surg. 2019;19(1):199.
14. Chiesa-Estomba CM, Larruscain-Sarasola E, et al. Facial nerve monitoring during parotid gland surgery: a systematic review and meta-analysis. Eur Arch Otorhinolaryngol. 2021; 278 (4):933–43.
15. Ulkatan S, Waner M, et al. New methodology for facial nerve monitoring in extracranial surgeries of vascular malformations. Clin Neurophysiol. 2014;125 (4):849–55.
16. Romstöck J, Strauss C, et al. Continuous electromyography monitoring of motor cranial nerves during cerebellopontine angle surgery. J Neurosurg. 2009; 93(4): 586–93.
17. Fan CJ, Cosetti MK, Levitin GM, Ulkatan S. Intermittent and continuous monitoring of the facial nerve: from the ear to the neck. Current Otorhinolaryngology Reports. Nerve monitoring in head and neck surgeries C.Sinclair. 2021;
18. Ulkatan S, Waner M, et al. New methodology for facial nerve monitoring in extracranial surgeries of vascular malformations. Clin Neurophysiol. 2014;125 (4):849–55.
19. Kandil E, Mohsin K, et al. Continuous vagal monitoring value in prevention of vocal cord paralysis following thyroid surgery. Laryngoscope. 2018;128(10):2429–32.
20. Bly RA, Holdefer RN, et al. Preoperative facial nerve mapping and guide pediatric facial vascular anomaly resection. JAMA Otolaryngol Head Neck Surg. 2018;144(5):418–26.
21. Lamadé U, et al. A new system for continuous recurrent laryngeal nerve monitoring. Minimally Invasive Therapy & Allied Technologies. 6.
22. Kim HY, et al. Technical instructions for continuous intraoperative neural monitoring in thyroid surgery. J Endocr Surg. 2018;18(1):61–78.
23. Terris DJ, Chaung K, Duke WS. Continuous vagal nerve monitoring is dangerous and should not routinely be done during thyroid surgery. World J Surg. 2015;39(10):2471–6.
24. Sinclair CF, Téllez MJ, Ulkatan S. Noninvasive, tube-based, continuous vagal nerve monitoring using the laryngeal adductor reflex: feasibility study of 134 nerves at risk. Head Neck. 2018;40(11):2498–506.
25. Harner SG, Daube JR, Ebersold MJ. Electrophysiologic monitoring of facial nerve during temporal bone surgery. Laryngoscope. 1986;96:65–9.
26. Wilson L, Lin E, Lalwani A. Cost-effectiveness of intraoperative facial nerve monitoring in middle ear or mastoid surgery. Laryngoscope. 2003;113:1736–45.
27. Ryu NG, Kim J. How to avoid facial nerve injury in Mastoidectomy? J Audiol Otol. 2016;20(2):68–72.
28. Hohman MH, Bhama PK, Hadlock TA. Epidemiology of iatrogenic facial 1 nerve injury: a decade of experience. Laryngoscope. 2014;124:260–5.
29. Casano K, Giangrosso G, Mankekar G, Sevy A, Mehta R, Arriaga M. Additional benefits of facial nerve monitoring during Otologic surgery. Otolaryngol Head Neck Surg. 2020;163(3):572–6.
30. Ansó J, Dür C, Gavaghan K, Rohrbach H, Gerber N, Williamson T, Calvo EM, Balmer TW, Precht C, Ferrario D, Dettmer MS, Rösler KM, Caversaccio MD, Bell B, Weber S. A Neuromonitoring approach to facial nerve preservation during image-guided robotic Cochlear implantation. Otol Neurotol. 2016;37(1):89–98.
31. Yellin JL, Wiggins CR, Franco AJ, Sankar WN. Safe transcranial electric stimulation motor evoked potential monitoring during posterior spinal fusion in two patients with cochlear implants. J Clin Monit Comput. 2016;30(4):503–6.

32. Fernández-Conejero I, Deletis V. Transcranial electrical stimulation and monitoring. J Neurosurg. 2014;120:291–2.
33. Deletis V, Fernández-Conejero I. Intraoperative monitoring and mapping of the functional integrity of the brainstem. J Clin Neurol. 2016;12(3):262–73.
34. Verst SM, Sucena AC, Maldaun MV, Aguiar PH. Effectiveness of C5 or C6-Cz assembly in predicting immediate post operative facial nerve deficit. Acta Neurochir. 2013;155:1863–9.
35. Amano M, Kohno M, Nagata O, Taniguchi M, Sora S, Sato H. Intraoperative continuous monitoring of evoked facial nerve electromyograms in acoustic neuroma surgery. Acta Neurochir. 2011;153(5):1059–67; discussion 1067.
36. Park E, Kim H, Han HM, Choi IH, Jung HH, Im GJ. The optimal and safe intensity for facial nerve stimulation during intraoperative neuromonitoring in middle ear surgery. PLoS One. 2019;14(8):e0221748.
37. Deletis V, Urriza J, Ulkatan S, Fernandez-Conejero I, Lesser J, Misita D. The feasibility of recording blink reflexes under general anesthesia. Muscle Nerve. 2009;39:642–6.

Part IX
Epilepsy Surgery

Chapter 32
Intraoperative Monitoring in Epilepsy Surgery

Vera Cristina Terra, Marcelo Volpon, and Hélio Rubens Machado

Abbreviations

CSF	Cerebrospinal fluid
CT	Computed tomography
ECoG	Electrocorticography
EEG	Electroencephalography
HFO	High-frequency oscillation
IEEG	Intracranial electroencephalography
iMRI	Intraoperative magnetic resonance imaging
MRI	Magnetic resonance image
SEEG	Stereo-electroencephalography
US	Ultrasonography
VEEG	Video-electroencephalography monitoring

V. C. Terra (✉)
Centro de atendimento Integral das Epilepsias, Nossa Senhora das Graças Hospital, Rua Alcides Munhoz, Curitiba – PR, Brazil
e-mail: vera.terra@epicentrocuritiba.com.br

M. Volpon
Center for Epilepsy Surgery & Department of Surgery and Anatomy, Ribeirão Preto Medical School of the University of São Paulo, Ribeirão Preto, SP, Brazil

H. R. Machado
Center for Epilepsy Surgery, Department of Surgery and Anatomy, Ribeirao Preto Medical School, University of Sao Paulo, Ribeirao Preto, Sao Paulo, Brazil
e-mail: hrmachad@fmrp.usp.br

S. M. Verst et al. (eds.), *Intraoperative Monitoring*,
https://doi.org/10.1007/978-3-030-95730-8_32

Introduction

Epilepsy is a quite common disease, with an incidence of around 50 per 100,000 patients per year. It has a bimodal distribution with two peaks: in infants, especially within the first few years of life and in people over the age of 50 years [65, 66, 87]. It is estimated that around 100 children for each 10,000 live births will develop recurrent seizures in the first year of life, and the general prevalence of pediatric epilepsy is around 0.2% [65, 66, 87]. Surgery is an effective treatment for pharmacological refractory epilepsy, and resective surgery remains the main type of procedure, although a trend to move away from large, open, surgical procedures, to minimally invasive, neuromodulatory, disconnective, or ablative resection has been noted over time [21]. Overall, the goal of epilepsy surgery is to achieve satisfactory seizure control; nevertheless, partial seizure reduction is already sufficient to produce significant behavioral and cognitive improvement, particularly when considering children [77].

In most epilepsy surgery centers, each individual patient case is discussed in a case conference that review all obtained data and a final decision is made. One of the data presented is the video-electroencephalography (VEEG) used noninvasively to identify epileptogenic zone and, together with magnetic resonance image (MRI) and neuropsychological evaluation, guide epilepsy surgery. However, sensitivity of VEEG can be low due to interference from the dura, skull, and scalp, needing the positioning of electrodes near the current source, in other words, in the surface of the brain [108]. This technique is called electrocorticography (ECoG). Electrophysiological monitoring can be performed acutely in the operation room or chronically, for longer periods, in the ward [108]. Recently, the concept of epileptogenic network has emerged, recognizing that multiple brain connections may be responsible for seizures generation and reinforcing the importance of intracranial electroencephalographic recording (IEEG) [101].

Adjuncts to Surgery

Several neurosurgical adjuncts are available that, along with ECoG, allow for precise tailoring of surgical resection of lesion with unclear margins and/or near eloquent areas, including neuronavigation, neuroendoscopy, intraoperative ultrasonography (US), intraoperative magnetic resonance imaging (iMRI), and robot-assisted surgery [21]. Although they might not be widely available in all epilepsy surgery centers, mostly due to their high cost and logistic issues, the current medical literature has several clinical studies confirming their usefulness [21, 84]. Wurm et al. [106] had already proved the value of neuronavigation in epilepsy surgery by linking individual anatomical, pathological, and functional data in a series of 223 cases [106]. Our team, likewise, has performed a systematic literature review and concluded that, although well-designed research studies evaluating the role of neuronavigation are required, neuronavigation tends to help produce higher rates of seizure control, a reduced need for reoperations, and lower rates of complications or postoperative neurological deficits [84]. In addition, Roessler et al. reported on their large series of 415 epilepsy patients treated with resective surgery, with the aid of neuronavigation and iMRI, 49 patients (11.8%) went on to have surgery extension, which resulted in an Engel class I outcome in 72.7% [72]. The greatest likelihood of an Engel Class I outcome was found in patients with cavernoma, hippocampal sclerosis, and low-grade epilepsy associated tumors, and their rates of postoperative neurological deficits were also lower.

Neuronavigation

Neuronavigation systems supply intraoperative orientation, localization, and guidance with a high level of accuracy and precision [23]. Basically, they use a reference device, which may be attached to the patient's head (for electromagnetic systems) or to the head holder, using a specific bracket. Then, several anatomical landmarks within the patient's face and head are registered, and neuronavigation softwares will merge previous radiological scans with these acquired three-dimensional points. The surgeon is then able to check the location of any given structures and lesions, as well as to follow the progress of surgical dissections (Fig. 32.1). Relative drawbacks of neuronavigation include brain shift after the egress of cerebrospinal fluid and/or parenchyma, and the inability to have real-time images [23]. Concurrent use and fusion of intraoperative US scans has come up to overcome this [75].

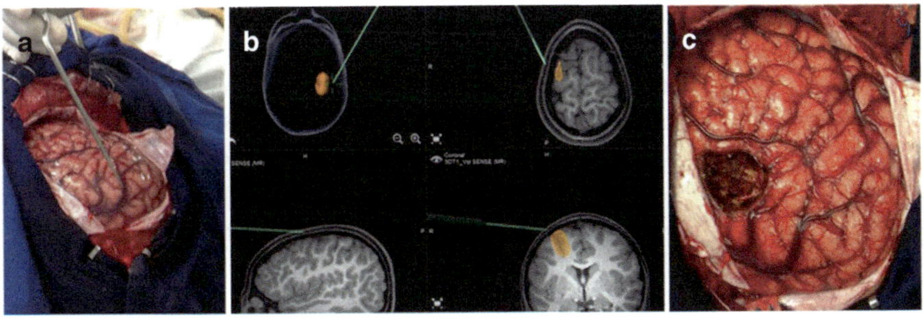

Fig. 32.1 Case of a 6-year-old boy operated for a front-rolandic focal cortical dysplasia type IIA with the use of neuronavigation and ECoG. (**a**): Intraoperative location of the lesion, with the neuronavigation scans seen in (**b, c**): Photograph after complete removal of the lesion. Patient is seizure-free with no deficits on follow-up

Intraoperative Ultrasonography

Intraoperative ultrasonography is also known to improve the intraoperative detection of epileptogenic lesions and the extent of resection of the epileptogenic zone [56]. US correlates well with presurgical imaging, with a resolution comparable to MRI, and allows for more tailored resections by facilitating the delineation of the dysplastic tissue [1]. Some US advanced tools, such as elastography (quantitative assessment of elasticity values), even permit intraoperative real-time tissue mapping by differentiating normal and pathological epileptogenic tissues [56].

Intraoperative MRI (iMRI)

Similarly, iMRI provides real-time and high-quality intraoperative images and is a valuable tool in a neurosurgeon's armamentarium [74]. It has been shown to be a great contribution in a variety of pathologies and patient populations, helping surgeons to achieve their surgical goals of maximal resection while minimizing morbidity and reducing operative time [50]. iMRI mitigates the brain shift phenomenon; other benefits include clear-cut evaluation of the extent of resection, prompt identification of surgical complications, and better postoperative outcomes [21, 33]. It has few limitations, such as cost, logistic, and safety concerns, which are gradually being overcome.

ECoG

The use of intraoperative ECoG varies within centers and depends on the underlying seizure etiology, neurophysiologist, and neurosurgeon experience [108]. It is based on the concept that epilepsy is a disease that involves both nonseizing and seizing activity and once the stability is broken, and a seizure starts, a large network is recruited. ECoG may be a method to study these networks even if seizures are not recorded [110]. ECoG was first realized in 1935 by Föster and Altembürger and then in 1936 by Gibbs, Lennox, and Gibbs (cited in [52]). However, the systematic use of ECoG in epilepsy surgery was achieved by Walker et al. [99] (cited in [52]) and Penfield and Flanigin [70].

ECoG recordings are done intraoperatively through the craniotomy and should be done prior to, during, and following resection with a combination of subdural and depth electrodes. Subdural electrodes can be slipped under the dura beyond the craniotomy to cover unexposed areas [42]. Typically, intraoperative neurophysiological monitoring is used mainly to outline the tissue that gives rises to epileptiform activity (the epileptogenic zone) and enable wider cortical resections that might lead to better seizure control; map out cortical function and thus make surgical dissection safer; and predict the chances of success after surgery based on persistent or afresh spikes [25]. However, it also may be indicated to a better evaluation of interictal activity distribution at the time of implantation of subdural/depth electrodes for chronic extraoperative intracranial EEG studies.

ECoG allows investigation of the cortical convexity and can be particularly helpful in the identification of the irritative and seizure onset zones and their relationship with functionally eloquent cortex [110]. ECoG should not be a fishing expedition [42], and, in this scenario, resection must be delineated carefully considering the epileptogenic focus, provided by the combination of preoperative MRI, VEEG, and neuropsychological evaluation and their relation to functionally eloquent cortex [110]. So ECoG should be indicated in all patients in which a proper noninvasive lateralization and regionalization of the epileptogenic zone has been possible, but the limits of resection should be established more precisely during surgery [86]. The diagnostic techniques should enable us to understand the interplay among diseased tissue, the epileptogenic network, and the healthy brain. The absence of a structural lesions on MRI may be a challenge, since the triad described above is broken and may have repercussions on long-term seizure control [53].

In lesional epilepsy surgery, the resection extension is generally the key prognostic impacting seizure outcome and, in many situations, the epileptogenic zone exceeds the lesion itself. In these cases, ECoG may be a reliable method to delimit brain resections. Roessler et al. [72] observed that almost 30% of patients with long-term epilepsy-associated tumors had an intraoperative need for additional resection, although the surgeon had the impression that the lesion had been totally resected. However, other authors evaluating the patterns of spread in patients with porencephaly, Lennox-Gastaut syndrome, and West syndrome observed that the use of ECoG could result in more focal resections, reducing the risk of neurological deficits [71].

In 2016, Jayakar et al. published a consensus based expert recommendation on the utility of intracranial EEG recording. In this consensus, the authors evaluated recommendations to chronic subdural and deep EEG recording, but many aspects discussed there may be considered when evaluating the indications of ECoG (Table 32.1). As in chronic evaluation, ECoG is a complement of noninvasive

Table 32.1 Recommendations for ECoG use in epilepsy surgery

When consider?	Is there a reasonable hypothesis to justify ECoG? There are limitations of the scalp and functional imaging data Information obtained during ECoG will change the resection plan
Modality	Intraoperative recording Electrodes placed under direct visualization (subdural or depth electrodes
Limitations	Almost only interictal activity Limited registration time Effect of anesthesia on EEG and functional mapping Cost
Risk / morbidity	Minimal risks of bleeding related to electrode insertion Small incremental risk related to length of anesthesia

Modified from [42]

evaluation providing more precise information on the localization of the presumed epileptogenic zone. In this way, ECoG is unwarranted when it is not expected to change the surgical plain. The major advantages of ECoG are avoiding the discomfort, risks, and costs of chronic intracranial electrodes, with no need for a second surgical procedure that includes implantation of electrodes, extraoperative intracranial VEEG recording, and electrodes removal with or without neurosurgery [42]. The authors also pointed out the main limitation: the time of recording is restricted and generally lasts 20–60 minutes, rarely ictal events are recorded, and resection is based only on interictal epileptiform activity. Also, depth electrodes positioning is less accurate (without stereotactic guidance) and, for practical reasons, less electrodes are used, although larger areas may be sampled sequentially. Although ECoG realization involves a high cost due to the electrodes it carries virtually no risk/morbidity other than the small incremental risk related to prolongation of anesthesia and is considered a noninvasive intracranial EEG recording modality [42].

Electrodes and Registration Techniques

ECoG may be done with electrodes positioned in subdural position (strips, grids, or a spider-like device) or depth in the brain. The choice of electrode type depends on the individual neurosurgeon's / neurophysiologist preference, anatomic considerations accessibility, and costs [78, 108] and is tailored for each patient. The neurophysiologist must keep in mind that subdural electrode coverage is limited and did not contemplate deep sources [31]. Although there is no minimum number of contacts for a ECoG register, the number of contacts and their positioning are closely related to registered area: the greater the number of contacts used, the greater the area studied. Considering this, use of strips or the spider-like device allows an easier repositioning of electrodes during registration with studies of different areas with different combinations obtained sequentially, allowing a better delimitation of the epileptogenic zone, as if a puzzle is being assembled [31, 42].

For practical reasons, ECoG generally uses fewer electrodes compared to that used in chronic extraoperative VEEG recording (subdural or depth) and all IEEG electrodes share some common recording features: they have a high spatial resolution and give precise information. However, they have a spatial limitation, with only a small portion of the brain tissue being sampled by each contact. This is an estimated sphere of 5 mm area beyond its boundaries. As Jayakar et al. [42] said, IEEG is "blind" if the electrodes are placed in insufficient number or distant from the focus, reinforcing the importance of a clear hypothesis before surgery.

For ECoG the most used electrodes are made of nickel-chromium or platinum-iridium, compounds nonmagnetic compatibly with intraoperative MRI [42]. The main electrodes options are described below and illustrated in Fig. 32.2.

1. *Silicone plastic strips or grids*: Electrodes are coated with silicone plastic. Typically, the diameter of each contact is 5 mm and the distance between con-

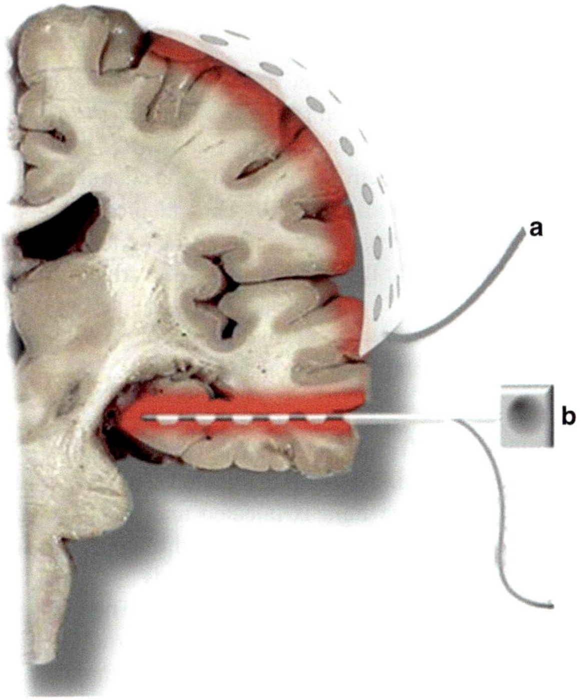

Fig. 32.2 Types of invasive monitoring in epilepsy. (**a**): subdural cortical electrodes. (**b**): depth electrodes (SEEG)

tacts is 10 mm. Their main advantage is enabling optimal contiguous coverage, mapping exploration, and sampling of the cerebral cortex [62], making them particularly useful for superficial lesions and the determination of its anatomic and functional relationships. The main disadvantages of the subdural method are related to the inability to record and assess deep structures such as the insular cortex, orbitofrontal cortex, cingulate gyrus, and depths of sulci, among others. The number of contacts is variable and may be between 4 and 64 [24, 37, 42]. They are put directly in contact with the cortex.

2. *Spider like device*: This is a kind of electrode system that uses a collection of individual somewhat rigid wire electrodes that is placed over exposed surface of the cortex. These electrodes are secured in a metal frame that is attached to the skull or to the surgical table with a clamp [108]. The tip of the electrodes is covered with a conductive material that touches the cortex. Electrodes can be positioned individually in the brain surface, with spacing between contacts adjusted according to the are to be studied. This kind of electrode cannot be used for interhemispheric or basal foci [42].
3. *Depth electrodes*: These are needle-shaped electrodes used more frequently to chronic register of mesial temporal structures or deep lesions [42, 108]. For ECoG, electrodes are usually inserted under direct visual or neuronavigational system guidance and a hybrid register may be obtained combining subdural and depth electrodes [42, 108].

Subdural Evaluation

Traditionally, ever since the first works of Penfield and Jasper in 1939 [69], invasive eletrophysiological monitoring has been performed with the use of subdural electrodes, which are put in direct contact with the cortical surface to be explored. The use of subdural electrodes is usually considered in the following conditions: lack of lateralization or localization of the epileptogenic zone, discordant information on noninvasive studies, the presence of the epileptogenicity near eloquent cortex, and the need to define the relationship of the area to be resected to a lesion present on MRI [22]. Their implantation must take into consideration some patient features such as site of disease, age, and results of preoperative testing. They might also be used for electrical stimulation and thus better define motor and language areas, for instance.

Implantation Technique of Strips and Grids
After dural opening, recording electrodes are gently placed in contact with the brain and isotone saline fluid is injected underneath contacts to facilitate the register. Strips can be slipped under the dura through a burr-hole or below the borders of a craniotomy, if necessary. The larger grids most often require a large craniotomy, to be placed under direct visualization [42]. The most used skin incisions are as follows: question-mark shaped, starting at the root of the zygoma and extending superiorly; barn door shaped, which facilitates implantations involving multiple lobes, starting anteriorly at the line of hair insertion, and following paramedian posteriorly over the lambdoid suture; and the classic bicoronal or ¾ bicoronal incision, which provides wide exposure of the frontal lobes, by which allows for more posterior approaches. Other incisions can be used, depending on the surgery to be performed.

Subsequent craniotomies and durotomies should be wide, allowing for a complete intraoperative electrographic study and exposing the more relevant anatomical references (Fig. 32.3). Care should be taken in children who may have a thickened cranial bone layer due to the use of antiseizure medication and trauma; in addition, their venous sinuses and other superficial vascular structures may be dislocated, due to the cerebral atrophy present in many of these patients, so attention must be taken when slipping and positioning the electrodes. Once the strips have been positioned as desired, electrodes are connected to EEG device for registering brain activity.

If chronic IEEG register is necessary, the proximal leads of the electrodes should be tunneled obliquely through the scalp with a trocar, taking care to not change the strip/grid position. Then electrodes are fixed with a nylon or silk purse-string suture placed around each exiting lead, to inhibit or prevent cerebrospinal fluid (CSF) leakage and to anchor the lead to prevent migration. Each strip is carefully identified, and the location annotated. Intraoperative test recordings are performed to confirm proper electrode functioning [37]. The dura, bone, and skin are then closed as usual, with particular care with the former to prevent CSF leaks, and postimplant radiological images (computer tomography – CT and/or MRI) are obtained to certify electrode positioning.

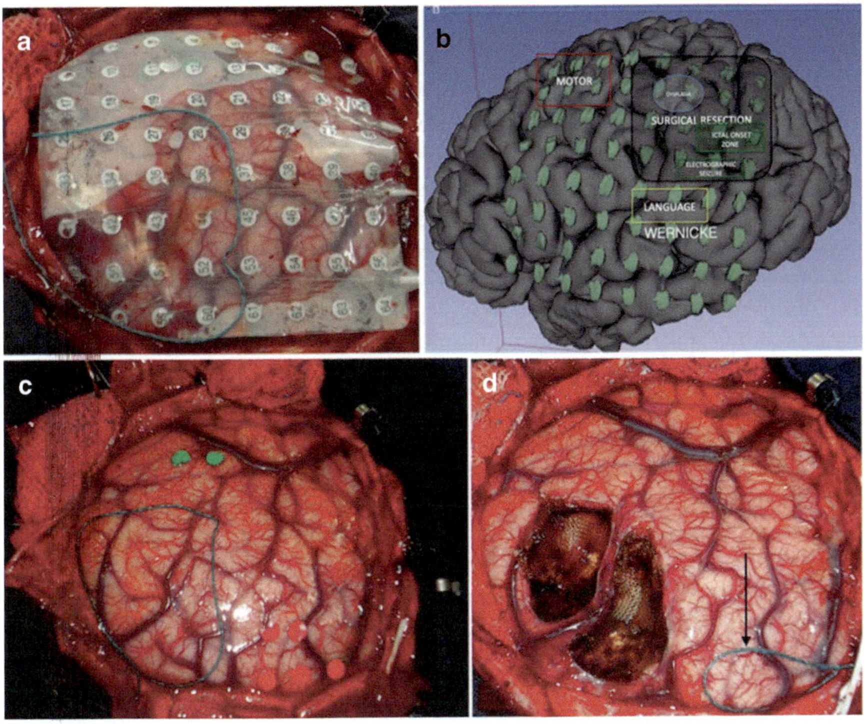

Fig. 32.3 A 10-year-old boy with seizures since 14 months of age. (**a**): Position of subdural grids. (**b**): Cortical map after MRI reconstruction with the proposed surgical strategy avoiding language and motor areas. (**c**) and (**d**): Pre- and postresection intraoperative photographs, respectively. Pathology: Cortical dysplasia type II B. Patient has rare seizures (Engel II) in a 5-year follow-up

Stereo-Electroencephalography Technique (SEEG)

SEEG has been developed by the French neurosurgeon Jean Talairach and his colleague neurologist Jean Bancaud in the 1960s [4]. Its methodological principles remain similar to the ones originally described, which are based on anatomical and electroclinical correlations with the main aim to conceptualize the three-dimensional spatial–temporal organization of the epileptic discharge within the brain [15]. In order to get proper SEEG recordings, the formulation of preimplantation hypotheses is the single most important element in the process of planning the placement of electrodes. If the preimplantation hypotheses are incorrect, the placement of the depth electrodes will be inadequate and the interpretation of the SEEG recordings will not give access to the definition of the epileptogenic zone [2].

SEEG is the method of choice for analyzing the spatiotemporal dynamics of the epileptogenic network [2]. It has the advantages of allowing extensive and precise deep brain recordings and stimulations (to localize seizure onset zone) with minimal associated morbidity [34]. Although the indications of SEEG are constantly expanding, classical clinical scenarios for depth exploration include MRI-negative cases, discordance between noninvasive electroclinical and imaging modalities, multiple epileptogenic lesions amenable to resection, and overlapping with eloquent cortex [2]. SEEG should also be considered in the following situations: deep-seated or difficult-to-cover location of the suspected epileptogenic zone; failure of a previous subdural invasive study to clearly outline the exact location of the seizure onset zone; need for extensive, bihemispheric explorations; and when the preoperative evaluation is suggestive of extended network involvement [15]. It is a discussion if acute implantation of depth electrodes can disrupt neuronal activity, generating spikes that do not represent epileptogenic zone and so its use in acute recordings should be evaluated with caution [42, 108].

Surgical Technique

Depth electrodes implantation for chronic registers follows standard stereotaxic techniques (Fig. 32.4). After a concise implantation plan has been designed, the stereotactic frame is positioned in the operating room, and then the patient is taken to the CT or MRI, where scans are obtained with the frame in situ. Then, pre-, and postframing scans are fused, using appropriate softwares (usually, stereotactic systems come with their own software), which also give the precise coordinates for

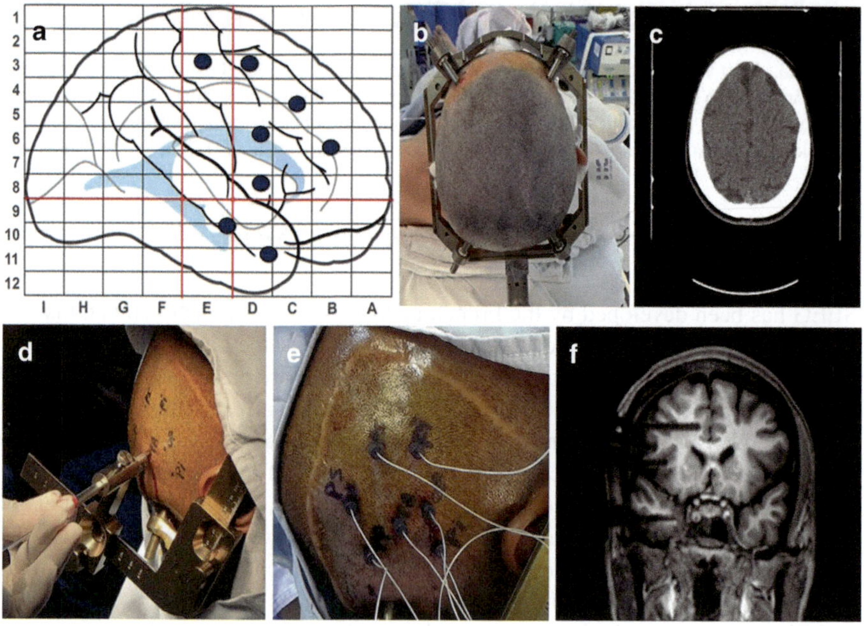

Fig. 32.4 Implantation of SEEG. (**a**): Preoperative planning. (**b**): Positioning of the stereotactic frame. (**c**): CT scan with the frame positioned. (**d**): Burr-hole insertion of the depth electrodes. (**e**): After insertion, electrodes are fixed with correspondent bolts. (**f**): Postoperative T1-weighted MR image showing the position of the electrodes

insertion. Desired targets are reached using commercially available depth electrodes in various lengths and number of contacts, depending on the specific brain region to be explored. The electrodes are implanted through 2.5-mm-diameter drill holes, using an orthogonal or oblique orientation [34]. As for superficial electrodes, post-operative scans are merged with previous ones to provide precise location of each electrode. A detailed vascular presurgical evaluation, including angiographic studies (angio-CT or angio-MRI), is fundamental to avoid hemorrhagic complications, which, along with infection and other minor problems, are reportedly quite infrequent, occurring in less than 1.3% of cases [61].

EEG Analysis: Interictal and Ictal Classical Pattern

After electrodes (subdural, spider, or depth) are positioned, for acquisition a reference lead and a ground lead are necessary. Personally, we use intraoperatively, dura mater in two distant points (one reference and the other ground leads). For ground lead is also possible that the electrode be positioned in an extracranial position. ECoG may be analyzed with a common reference or in a bipolar montage (the first option is the most used). Then electrodes are connected to a digital EEG monitoring system and signals were filtered (low filter of 0.03 and a variable high filter), with a 60 Hz filter and sensitivity adjusted from 50 mV to 200 mV [78]. High filter may be opened to register high oscillation frequencies (HFO – ripples and fast ripples):80–490 Hz. The possibility of registration of these frequencies is related to equipment capacity, and they will be discussed later [24]. The general principle is that the higher the signal (desired waveform) and the lower the noise/interference, the more accurate, reliable, and interpretable the recording will be [47].

The duration of ECoG monitoring is variable, and some authors consider five minutes enough [108] but ideally it should last 20 to 60 minutes [42]. In fact, register is considered satisfactory if epileptic activity is observed and the epileptogenic zone could be delimited [78]. EEG recording should be carried out by a certified clinical neurophysiologist, and electrographic signals are usually identified through visual observation. The rate, location, and time of onset of the observed spikes and/or electrographic seizures are analyzed before any cortical procedure is done. After a period of ECoG registration, methods of stimulation may be used to induce epileptogenic activity, either interictal or ictal. These methods include pharmacological activation (that will be discussed below) or direct cortical stimulation of the brain, using a handheld bipolar electrode or register electrodes themselves. In this situation, ECoG should be recorded from adjacent electrode contacts to determine the threshold for eliciting after-discharges [108].

When analyzing EEG obtained during ECoG, as in any EEG register, background is firstly evaluated. Background evaluation can provide valuable information concerning the brain functioning and the waveform pattern varies with the different locations of electrodes, pre-existing lesions, preoperative medications, and anesthetic drugs [14]. If awakening register is obtained, posterior alpha rhythm and rolandic mu rhythm may be observed at the same topography as that observed in scalp recordings [29]. If patient is under general anesthesia, the amount of anesthesia given will modulate EEG pattern, which can vary from a continuous and mixed activity, with fast and slow rhythms to a burst-suppression pattern, and in this situation, the ECoG record will be inconclusive. The neurophysiologist must be careful not to confuse sharp activity of bursts with real epileptiform activity. For a good register, anesthetics should be suspended at least 10 minutes before acquisition beginning [29]. Background activity may also be dominantly composed of diffuse and continuous fast rhythm, differentiated of epileptiform activity, since this one is usually more localized and suffer variations with time. Fig. 32.5 demonstrates examples of electrographic patterns observed during ECoG recordings.

One major problem of ECoG register may be the artifacts, and they need to be corrected or discarded when analyzing EEG sign at the beginning of the register. They can be divided into artificial or physiological. The most common artificial artifact is powerline noise (50 or 60 Hz) that is usually induced to the acquisition system and may present as high-frequency harmonic signs. Instrumentation and electrodes artifacts are also common, and this later one may be due to electrodes positioned near the scalp or cranial nerve foramen or defective electrodes. Defective electrodes positioned as common reference may render the entire register ineligible if not corrected. Physiological artifacts may be related to natural pulsation of the brain tissue driven by respiration, cerebral-spinal fluid pulsation, and hearth rhythm (blood flow and pulsation in vessels), muscle artifacts (especially in awake surgery), and eye movements [64].

Considering epileptiform activity, first interictal discharges are highlighted. The morphology of spikes is remarkably similar when comparing cortex and scalp registers, besides the large difference in amplitude that must be compensated for sensibility changes. The presence of multifocal spikes usually signals widespread pathology and may correlate with a worst seizure control outcome. Interictal epileptiform discharges are classified according to the patterns described by Palmini et al. [67] and summarized by San-Juan et al. [78]. More than one pattern may be observed in the same patient:

- Sporadic spikes, spikes occurring at an irregular time interval with a focal or multifocal distribution.
- Rhythmic continuous spikes occurring at regular time intervals for at least 10 seconds, with frequency of 1 Hz.
- Bursts of spikes with at least one second duration with a frequency of 10 Hz or greater.
- Recruiting discharges, rhythmic spike activity characterized by increased amplitude and decreased frequency (electrocorticographic seizures).

The pattern of rhythmic continuous spikes discharges is usually more restricted than the more diffuse interictal spiking and may be related to epileptic onset zone, being a marker of the perilesional electrographic abnormalities [67]. This activity may be represented for the following patterns:

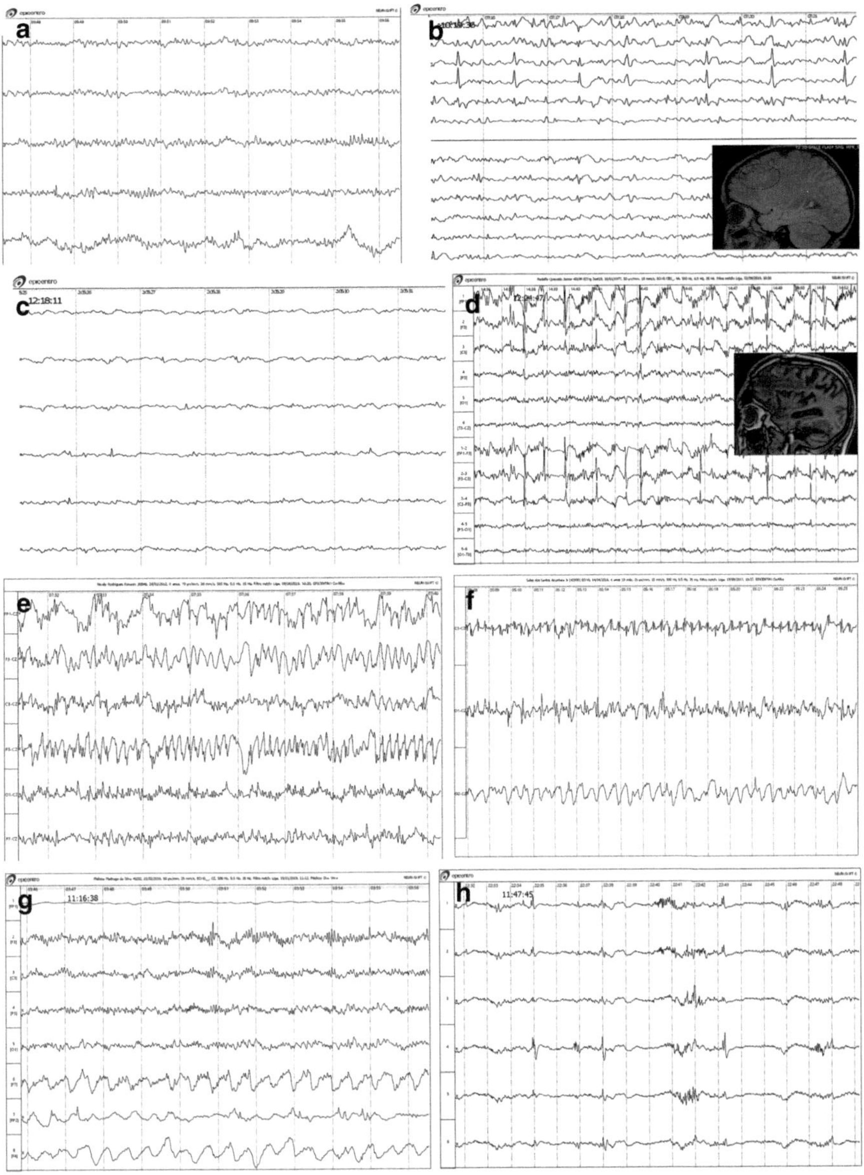

Fig. 32.5 Examples of ECoG patterns. (**a**): Normal continuous background activity; (**b**): Pacient with frontal cortical dysplasia with frequent interictal spikes; (**c**): Postresection of the same patient as in (**a**); (**d**): Rhythmic continuous spikes in a patient with a posttraumatic destructive frontal lesion. (**e and f**): ictal pattern in a patient with tuberous sclerosis (**e**) and hemimegalencephaly (**f**); (**g**): Pulse artifact mimiking a focal slowing; (**h**): HFO in a patient with normal MRI and temporal lobe epilepsy

- Repetitive electrographic seizures (recruiting prolonged trains of rhythmic activity): in this pattern, isolated spikes progressively increase in frequency and rhythmicity until approximately 12 to 16 Hz, for several seconds, and is followed by focal slowing or attenuation of the recording.
- Repetitive bursting discharges: bursts or trains of spikes at 10 Hz or faster with variable duration (usually 5 to 10 seconds) that disappear abruptly.
- Continuous or quasicontinuous rhythmic spikes: prolonged trains of rhythmic spikes or sharp waves at 1–8 Hz, for more than 10 seconds.

Resection of these patterns is correlated with a better surgical outcome. However, the resection of isolated spikes or newly developed spikes (observed only after resection) has controversial benefit for surgical outcome.

Although interictal activity is usually identified in ECoG, the same cannot be said of ictal patterns. As already mentioned, the ictal pattern is easily obtained in chronic recordings; however, it is not frequent to record seizures in acute ECoG. When present, the most common electrographic pattern is low-voltage fast activity; sharp activity at ≤13 Hz; low-frequency high-amplitude periodic spikes; burst of high-amplitude polyspikes; spike-and-wave activity; and delta brush [26] and these patterns are readily identified. If no spontaneous seizures are seen, some authors recommend its induction, and this will be discussed later in this chapter.

Other electrographic abnormalities observed in ECoG are high-frequency oscillation (HFO) patterns, a transient oscillatory pattern occurring synchronously, with short duration and that stand out from the background activity. This activity may be obscured by background noise of ECoG recordings and may not be observed if equipment does not have a noise attenuation system [24, 110]. Filter parameters should be set to band-pass of 80–240 Hz for ripple range and 250–500 Hz for fast ripples and occur at the slope of epileptiform spike. They should be differentiated from physiological HFO that usually occurs in functionally eloquent areas (paracentral, hippocampus, and occipital cortex) and have a longer duration. Also, physiological HFO seems to be intermixed with an oscillatory background activity, whereas HFO observed in a flat background is more suspicious to reflect epileptic activity [28]. The higher the frequency of HFO, the more localized and specific for the epileptogenic focus it appears to be. Visual HFO analyses is time consuming and should be differentiated from artifacts.

HFOs were originally discovered with the use of depth and microelectrodes and since then have been considered a biomarker of epileptogenicity. HFO may be found in all types of pathologies and may be evoked to direct brain electrical stimulation near and far away epileptic zone onset [90, 93].

When analyzing ripples and fast ripple patterns, different results were described in literature. Fast ripples usually occur more focally than ripples and spikes, and they are probably generated by local pathological connections of neuronal clusters [91]. It is important to clarify that even fast ripples may be more widespread and be observed in areas far away from the epileptogenic zone. In this way, it is important to realize serial registers, with the first one been done just after brain exposure. Then a resection is programed and should be restricted to the lesion or the area first supposed to be involved with seizures generation. After this first resection, a new ECoG register is done, and the resection may be increased based on this new register. The removal of the first target region may lead to the disappearance of the HFO pattern. If epileptogenicity is still observed, resection should be extended and a new ECoG register done. This sequence may be repeated as often as necessary, including recordings after final resections. The discovery of persistent fast ripples on these repeated measurements could indicate that more cortical tissue should be removed [28, 60, 92–94, 110]. In this way, to assure the highest chance of surgical success, ECoG should be repeated throughout surgery, as it is the only way to ensure complete resection of epileptogenic areas [24, 27, 95].

Talking about ripples and spikes, the affirmation above is not so clear. Ripples occur more frequently than fast ripples and are found over larger areas. Some authors have demonstrated that the presence of residual ripples and isolated spikes does not predict recurrence of seizures [28, 91, 93, 110], while other authors suggested presurgical ripples also appear to be related with epileptogenic region [40, 105]; Worrell and Gotman, 2011]. Ripples have been implicated in learning and memory consolidation, and it seems that ripples associated with spikes or seizures are probably epileptogenic [31, 92, 93, 96].

Eloquent Areas Stimulation and Surgery in Awake Patients

Testing function during surgery requires direct cortical/ subcortical stimulation of the eloquent area, which often require active patient participation [39]. ECoG register and direct stimulation may be obtained in awake patients and is an alternative when the epilepsy focus is adjacent to eloquent cortex. Awake surgery for epilepsy has certain advantages, such as intraoperatively mapping, allowing identification of eloquent areas, ECoG record without influence of anesthesia, maximizing the yield. However, some disadvantages are also present and are related to the limited intraoperative time and dependence of patient cooperation. Awake surgery is not feasible in all patients, especially in younger age and patients with intellectual disabilities and/ or psychiatric problems [42, 54, 97] and although it can be performed in persons younger than 15 years, it is essential that patient is suitable to cooperate [47]. As this procedure is potentially challenging for patients, it is essential that the procedure is useful for epilepsy surgery [54].

To realize awake surgery, usually, patient is under general anesthesia with a laryngeal mask during skin and skull opening, dura is soaked with local anesthetics, and the patient is then awakened. Intraoperative brain mapping and monitoring is performed and, at the end of the surgery, patient is again put under general anesthesia [32, 42, 54]. It is essential that patients do not have pain or seizures during this phase of surgery and patients should be trained with the environment of the operative room and the protocol test that is going to be used during surgery [47, 97]. For more details on anesthesia and pain management of the awake patient, refer to Chap. 9.

Direct cortical and subcortical stimulation may be done with a handheld probe (Fig. 32.6) or subdural grids/strips, usually consisting of a bipolar stimulation. To ensure that electrical activation has not spread beyond the electrode tips, the amplitude

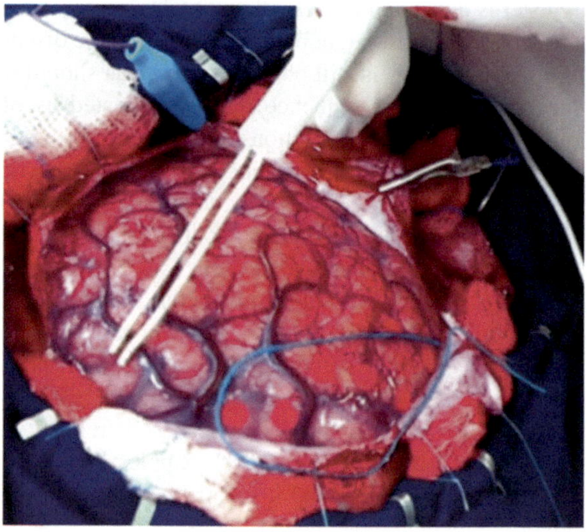

Fig. 32.6 Brain stimulation during ECoG. Handheld probe is stimulation hand motor area and epileptogenic cortex is delimited with the blue line. Red dots represent the areas with the greatest epileptogenicity

of the stimulation should not induce after-discharges [39, 108]. Usually, a biphasic current with an initial intensity of 1.5 to 2 mA is applied to cortex [32]. Intensity of stimulation is increased until a clear response is obtained, and a double check should be done with response reproduction [47]. Stimulation should be stopped if a functional response is obtained; a sustained after-discharges is evoked, if stimulation induces seizures or if the maximal intensity current is applied and no response is obtained [7, 8]. Throughout the process, an extensive map should be made with the points studied in the cortical surface, considering which areas should be resected and which ones represent functional eloquent areas and should be maintained.

In stimulation of motor cortex and the corticospinal tract, it is easy to see the response by looking for muscle twitches and stimulation can be done in asleep or awake patients [19, 97]. Even while eloquent cortex is preserved, interrupted connections with subcortical regions may lead to postsurgical functional deficits. Thus, motor cortex or white matter region should be stimulated during resection to minimize the risk of motor deficits [39].

Language stimulations require a more complex protocol or even spontaneous talk and can only be done in awake patients [49, 97]. Intraoperative language mapping during awake surgery is the gold-standard method for surgery if language area is implicated in the epileptogenic zone and direct electrical stimulation enables to identify cortical and subcortical language areas and pathways [19]. Cortex not associated with language hits is stimulated with increased intensity to a maximum of 10 to 12 mA before being deemed potentially nonessential [32]. Awake surgery is indicated in patients with lesions in the dominant opercular region, inferior part of the precentral gyrus, posterior half of the temporal lobe, and supramarginal and angular gyri of the parietal lobe [47]. Patients with impairment of language functions considering understanding, reading, and object naming are not suitable for awake surgery [47]. Awake surgery in patients with temporal lobe epilepsy should be done only if eloquent language area is suspected to be involved in seizure onset zone.

Other functions that can be stimulated are visual, cognitive (such as visuospatial functions, calculation), and memory [76, 97]. The use of neuropsychological tests during awake brain stimulation is not comparable to a standard neuropsychological assessment, and the main paradigms used are described in Table 32.2. Chapter 19 details language protocols tailored to patient individual characteristics.

Table 32.2 Main paradigms used to stimulate functional cortical areas during epilepsy surgery. Modified from [76]

Function	Test
Language	Active language task (patient naming visually presented words) and rest task (patient silent) Category: Fluency Naming: Color, days of week, months of year, tools, animals and unique persons, object picture, verb, famous people, action picture Counting forward or backward Language comprehension by matching sentence to pictures Questions like "what is your name?" "tell me where you are?" Reading sentences Recognition of pictures with a distraction task Repetition Semantic associations Sentence construction Verb generation Word and sentence comprehension Writing sentences
Motor/sensory	Continuous movements (flexion–extension of arm and fingers) Finger tapping Sensory motor profile awake scale (different sensory and motor tasks, e.g., blink eyes, lift knee, sensory awareness of fingers) Simple repetitive movements of the contralateral upper limb Voluntary rhythmic movements (alternating touching between tip of the thumb with the other fingers)
Memory	World span (repeating 3 words immediately)
Visuospatial	Line bisection Line matching (angle) Modified picture-naming test Presentation of 2 objects diagonally on screen divided in 4 quadrants Target cancelation
Calculation	Single digit addition, subtraction or multiplication
Emotions	Describing mental states based on eye region of human faces (Reading the mind in the eyes test) Emotional recognition task Labeling of facial emotion expressions
Executive functions	Go/no-go test Stroop test
Music	Musical tasks (comparing melodies, identifying if a melody was a waltz or march, reading a short excerpt) Reading (without singing) an excerpt of a score Singing words of a familiar song

Neurosurgical Aspects

Epilepsy surgery is the most effective treatment for select patients with drug-resistant epilepsy. In the recent years, there is an increase in the practice of extra-temporal resections, particularly in the context of surgery for nonlesional epilepsy, probably related to the development of new and better diagnostic techniques and neuroimaging modalities [44]. In this way, IEEG recording are increasingly needed, and with more experience, better results are expected. The approach should be individualized to each patient and lobe of suspicion of epilepsy onset zone, and some specific surgical techniques and EEG findings will be discussed.

Temporal Lobe Surgery and ECoG

Temporal lobe epilepsy is the most common form of refractory epilepsy in adults, and in about one-third of the patients, seizures are related to hippocampus sclerosis (HS). The surgical treatment of temporal epilepsy must be tailored individually. In adults, more than 70% of patients have mesial temporal sclerosis, in contrast with children, in whom only 40% have mesial temporal sclerosis, whereas 40% have focal cortical dysplasia and 20% tumors [36]. Less than 25% of these patients remain seizure-free only on medication for more than one year, and surgery is the best nonpharmacological treatment [63]. The occurrence of dual neocortical and mesial pathology is not infrequent, requiring an elaborated presurgical strategy that must encompass surrounding dysplastic tissue.

Traditionally, the technique for temporal lobe surgery is the antero-mesial lobectomy: starting with a 4.5–5 cm lateral neocortical resection, the temporal horn of the ipsilateral ventricle is entered, and up to 2.5–3 cm of the hippocampal head along with the amygdala is removed. Some patients do not need resection of the mesial structures and in others, a wider lateral resection toward the occipital lobe is required (Fig. 32.7); these decisions are made with the guidance of intraoperative neurophysiological data.

In patients with temporal lobe epilepsy related to mesial temporal sclerosis, the realization of ECoG is controversial and studies did not clearly answer this question [89]. Nowadays, standard resection is usually the rule and recent studies have demonstrated excellent surgical prognosis with this type of resection in up to 75–80% of patients [45]. Considering this, some authors concluded that ECoG is not necessary for anterior medial temporal lobectomy secondary to HS to tailor resection [78, 108, 110]. With this evidence, the presence of residual spikes after standard temporal lobectomy can be observed in up to 62% of patients and considering that ECoG register electrical activity from a very confined region, this may lead to false localization of interictal/ictal onset zone and then its resection may not make sense [68, 81, 100]. However, other authors suggested that resection of isolated spikes in lateral neocortical temporal lobe even in HS patients has a prognostic value, with an

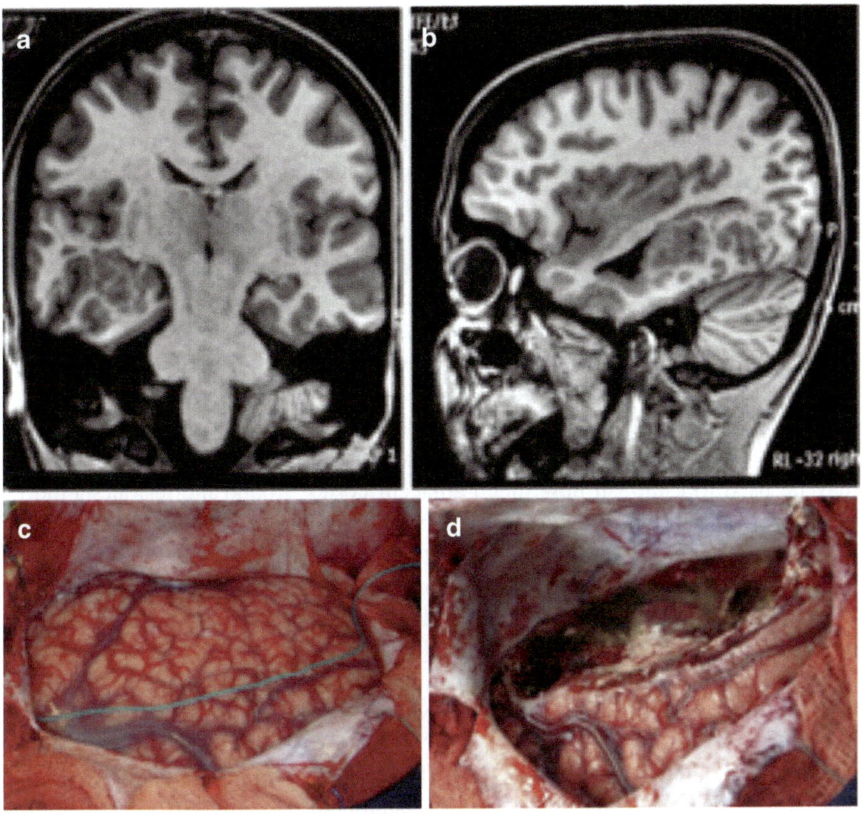

Fig. 32.7 Tailored left temporal lobectomy. Case of an 11-year-old child with a 4-year history of complex partial seizures, 4–5 per day. (**a** and **b**): Respectively, coronal and sagittal T1-weighted MRI scans showing a large right temporal cortical malformation. ECoG confirmed epileptogenesis beyond the lateral limits of the temporal lobe, toward and posterior to the preoccipital notch. (**c**): Planned excision according to ECoG and radiological findings. (**d**): Postresection photograph showing the resection cavity

increase in the number of patient's being seizure-free in long-term follow-up [55, 57, 98, 103]. Groups that perform selective amygdalohippocampectomy demonstrated that patients with mesial basal interictal discharges restricted to the temporal lobe have better surgical results [12]. In patients with neocortical lesions associated with mesial temporal sclerosis, ECoG can contribute to an individualized resection, allowing the identification of areas with active interictal activity and areas without electrographic changes and it seems that in patients without HS, resection of interictal spikes is related to better postsurgical outcome [108]. In this way, in patients with structural lesions such as tumors, postinfectious lesions, vascular malformations, ischemic or inflammatory lesions, traumatic encephalomalacia, and malformations of cortical development (that includes focal cortical dysplasia, polymicrogyria, nodular heterotopia, hamartomas, etc.), tailored resections are associated with improved outcomes, and usually, the resection limits can be set by interictal / ictal electrographic abnormalities activity registered during surgery by ECoG [59, 63, 108].

In patients with negative MRI findings, acute intraoperative ECoG can be used, and surgery undertaken when interictal spikes are restricted to temporal lobe. In patients in whom acute ECoG demonstrates extratemporal spikes, chronic monitoring of the mesial structures or anterior temporal tip with subdural or depth electrodes might lead to a more precise definition of the epileptogenic zone. Therefore, intraoperative ECoG may be useful in identifying a subset of patients with MRI negative temporal lobe epilepsy who could benefit from surgery directly without the need for chronic electrocorticography [53].

Burkholder et al. [9] showed that presence of unilateral interictal epileptiform discharges in scalp EEG and complete resection of intraoperative ECoG spikes were the two variables correlated with good postoperatively seizure outcome in patients with normal MRI and in patients with brain lesions. Intraoperative ECoG may be used to establish how much adjacent cortex around the lesion should be removed, contributing to determine complete resection of adjacent irritative zone [78, 108]. Tripathi et al. [88] showed that about 90% of patients with postsurgical good outcome (Engel I and II) showed an improvement in postresection spikes in ECoG register [78, 88]. In these patients, HFO, when present, has been proposed to be a biomarker of the epileptogenic zone [109].

Considering patients with malformations of cortical development, especially patients with focal cortical dysplasia, more widespread area of lesion than that recognized by MRI may be present and ECoG increases the chance of resection of potentially epileptogenic cortex [82, 83, 108]. An ECoG signature of this condition consists of prolonged trains of rhythmic epileptogenic activity [67].

Another electrographic pattern that may be observed in temporal lobe epilepsy ECoG is interictal regional delta slowing. Tao et al. [85] have shown that this pattern was highly correlated with neocortical seizure onset zones, mostly that located in the anterior and basal temporal regions. Mesial onset seizures typically propagated into lateral cortex where interictal regional delta slowing originates, suggesting that this pattern may be associated with an epileptic network [85].

Extratemporal Surgery and ECoG

In patients with extratemporal epilepsy, the delimitation of ictal onset zone is even more difficult than in patients with temporal lobe epilepsy. In adults, most epileptic foci are on the temporal lobe; in children, however, extratemporal epilepsy is more frequent, and up to 20% of surgical procedures for drug-resistant epilepsy involve exclusively resection of brain areas outside the temporal lobe [11, 17]. According to recent studies, seizure freedom is less likely to be achieved in such cases, but careful patient selection and presurgical workup, alongside a meticulous surgical technique, can surely improve outcome of extratemporal resections [3]. For all these reasons, intraoperative monitoring and electrocortical mapping have a paramount importance in this context, and we have used it very frequently, in around 80% of our cases of cortical dysplasia [86], to help tailor resections, contributing to define the extent of the irritative zone in relation to lesions [18].

In nonlesional extratemporal resections, ECoG may have more limited value and chronic intracranial recordings may provide more accurate information on the delimitation of the resection [48]. In this way, some authors suggested that ECoG is valuable in determining the extent of resection only in the presence of a structural lesion and the association with neuronavigation may improve lesion resection efficacy and then surgical outcome [13]. If the lesion was not been completely removed, seizures may continue despite the removal of the epileptogenic zone [6, 30, 48].

For extratemporal surgery, the importance of a thorough preoperative work-up and a proper careful surgical indication is of utmost importance. Obviously, lesionectomies should be considered in the presence of a circumscribed single epileptogenic lesions (Fig. 32.8); nevertheless, as is the case of epilepsy associated with tumors, electrophysiological monitoring should still be undertaken to make sure all epileptogenic tissues are removed (including surrounding focal cortical dysplasia, such as type IIIB). Potential candidates for frontal surgical procedures usually present with epilepsy clinically manifested by tonic/clonic seizures (reflecting involvement of Brodmann area 6 or 4), hypermotor seizures, or disperceptive seizures [43], whereas focal seizures with unilateral temporo-parieto-occipital (TPO) onset or generalized seizures with asymmetrical clinical or electroencephalographic features are clinically seen in posterior quantic disconnection patients [17]. Anyway, in patients submitted to lesionectomies, serial ECoG should determine the need to extend the initial resection, particularly in patients with dysplastic lesions [38, 79].

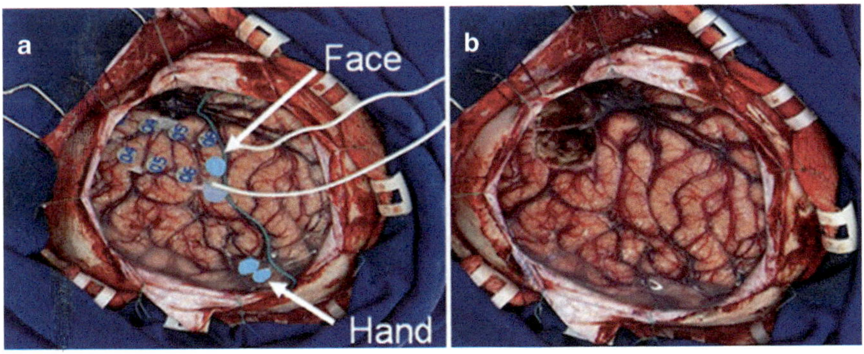

Fig. 32.8 Lesionectomy of an inferior frontal gyrus focal cortical dysplasia. (**a**): Cortical strips are placed over the dysplastic lesion, for delineation of its posterior margins, as well as the face and hand motor areas are localized with electrocortical stimulation. (**b**): After resection. Patient is currently seizure-free

As mentioned above, disconnective procedures are presently preferable to traditional lobectomies, because they reduce complications related to extensive resections, such as massive blood loss, hydrocephalus, and longer operating times, while achieving equivalent seizure outcomes [46]. Extratemporal surgical techniques can be broadly divided into lesionectomy, frontal lobectomy or disconnection, posterior quadrant disconnection, and hemispheric procedures (hemispherectomy and hemispherotomy).

Disconnective Procedures

All disconnective procedures start with the recognition of the central lobe, which consists of the precentral (motor) and postcentral (sensitive) gyri on the lateral surface, which must be respected and preserved. The central lobe is located over the sylvian fissure and lies slightly obliquely until it reaches the midline. The paracentral lobule in the medial surface is limited posteriorly by the ascending marginal ramus of the cingulate sulcus. For more details on gyri and sulci anatomy, refer to Chap. 4.

For frontal disconnections, surgery begins with a cortical supraorbital incision, is performed along the anterior skull base, just above the most lateral aspect of the sphenoid wing, which is followed transversally until the midline is reached. The disconnection continues to the frontal convexity, parallel to the precentral sulcus. At this point, the lateral ventricle is entered, guiding the whole lateral disconnection. The incision then meets the interhemispheric fissure, and the falx is followed for medial cortical dissection. Finally, a transverse corpus callosotomy from within the ventricle is performed.

Temporal-parietal-occipital disconnections (Fig. 32.9) begin with an intraparietal disconnection, which is performed with a standard microsurgical cortical incision orthogonally just posterior to the postcentral gyrus. The white matter along the whole length of the incision is deepened to reach the tissue along the falx, and the disconnection is done up to the pia along the falx to reach the sagittal sinus superiorly and the level of the corpus callosum inferiorly. The incision that has reached the corpus callosum and opened the ventricle is curved posteriorly in an intraventricular parasagittal plane, and all fibers entering the posterior corpus callosum are interrupted. This would interrupt all the parieto-occipital commissural fibers as they reach the corpus callosum. Then, for temporal disconnection, another cortical incision is made over the superior temporal gyrus (T1), heading toward the temporal horn of the lateral ventricle, where the amygdala is identified and is then resected along with the uncus. Completion of the hippocampectomy is performed last. In some patients, the epileptogenic zone is contained within the limits of the parieto-occipital region, and the temporal steps described above might be skipped (parieto-occipital disconnection).

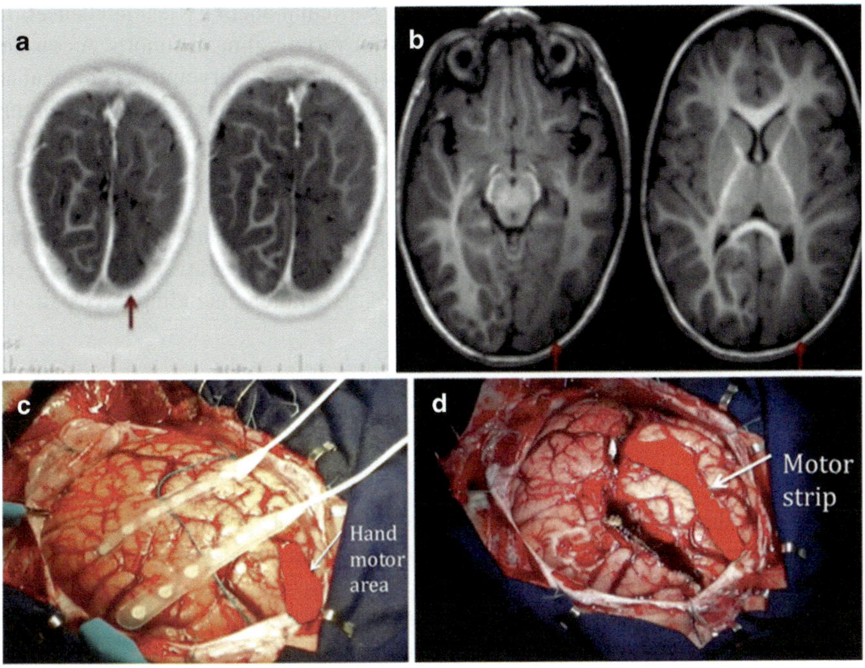

Fig. 32.9 Temporal-parietal-occipital disconnection. (**a** and **b**): MRI scans of a 6-year-old girl showing a large posterior quadrant cortical malformation. (**c**): Intraoperative ECoG and delineation of the hand motor area as depicted; the blue string shows the location of the cortical incision. (**d**): Photograph after disconnection, with preservation of the motor strip

ECoG in Pediatric Population

As in adult patients, ECoG is often performed before resection, and typically before subdural or depth electrode placement in children undergoing intraoperative monitoring. Preresection ECoG provides insight into the location of the seizure onset zone (SOZ) in most children considering interictal spikes and the presence of electrographic seizures. These findings are highly concordant with the SOZ and can guide resection and obviate the need for further chronic invasive testing [35, 51]. Also, resection of HFOs in children is associated with a better postsurgical outcome [28, 105].

The Pediatric Epilepsy Surgery Task Force of the International League Against Epilepsy (ILAE) Commissions of Pediatrics and Diagnostics undertook the task of formulating recommendations for diagnostic evaluation in localizing the epileptogenic region or critical cortex and to guide clinical care in children [41]. These recommendations strive to achieve an optimal balance between extreme overutilization and underutilization of ancillary tests. Neither the position of doing all diagnostic tests possible nor insisting on one particular ancillary test lends itself to scientific scrutiny or meets the complex needs of various clinical cohorts. A consensus was reached among the experts that early surgical intervention is critical in infants with severe epilepsy to prevent developmental arrest/ regression [16]. In this way, especially in children with tumors and malformation lesions ECoG is always indicated [86].

In children, mapping of eloquent areas must be evaluated carefully. Most services consider mapping motor areas intraoperatively and language mapping in chronic records. However, Lohkamp et al. [51] observed that awake brain surgery was psychologically well tolerated by 48 out of 50 children, including three patients under the age of 10.

Anesthesia

Anesthesia should not prevent the evaluation of EEG background and the recording of electrographic abnormalities, and in this way, correct doses and concentration of anesthetic agents must be known. They have an impact on neuronal transmission and synapses and can either produce a dose-dependent depression or overexcitability activity of the brain [20]. These effects may be unpredictable, and if not tailored for each patient may occasionally render the study unhelpful [42]. Beta activity initially increases with most anesthetic agents, followed by diffusely slow theta and delta activity. Sufentanil, Fentanyl, Alfentanil, Propofol, Methohexital and Thiopental enhance epileptiform activity, in a dose-dependent manner. Other drugs, such as halothane, barbiturates, benzodiazepines, isoflurane, and sevoflurane, decrease this activity [54]. Deep anesthesia may mask the generation of spontaneous abnormal spikes or HFO, often leading to a pattern of burst-suppression and should be avoided [108].

Considering each drug individually, opioids (Fentanyl, Remifentanil, Sufentanil, and Alfentanil) produce a smaller effect on EEG when compared with intravenous or inhalational anesthetics, and because of their excellent analgesic properties, they are an important component of balanced general anesthesia. Inhalation agents (such as nitrous oxide, enflurane, isoflurane, and sevoflurane) are in general accepted to be used during ECoG studies for mapping epileptiform and epileptogenic foci. Also dexmedetomidine does not hinder interpretation of EEG and causes no new epileptiform activity: it is safe to be used during ECoG and functional mapping. However, Etomidate and Ketamine can decrease the after-discharge threshold, and it should be avoided during direct electrical cortical stimulation [13, 47].

Neuromuscular-blocking agents is fundamental to the anesthetic procedure and its use during epilepsy surgery is beneficial for EEG acquisition. However, they must be avoided for motor mapping, since they decrease the muscle tone, causing muscle paralysis and then preventing or decreasing motor response [47].

In summary, before ECoG, both intravenous and inhaled drugs are weaned down or stopped, and low-dose opioid infusion or dexmedetomidine may be continued. Muscle relaxants may be needed to prevent movements. In this way, patients submitted to epilepsy surgery with ECoG, and eloquent cortex mapping procedure, need a superficial anesthesia and it is important to warn patient preoperatively about the risk of awareness during surgery [13]. Table 32.3 summarizes the effects of main sedative and anesthetic drugs [14, 20].

In some cases, epilepsy surgery needs eloquent cortex mapping, and, in this situation, patient should be awaked during surgery. Considering that, a guideline for

Table 32.3 Effect of drugs in ECoG pattern and brain mapping

Drug	Effects on EEG	Brain mapping
Midazolam	Increases theta and delta slowing with superimposed fast activity Decreases alpha activity	Do not use before functional mapping
Pentobarbital	Increases fast frequencies at low doses Depressant effect to burst suppression at higher doses Significantly suppresses EEG activities	Do not use before functional mapping
Thiopental	Activation of spikes with *bolus*	
Propofol	Low dose: Mild activation of fast frequency High dose: Burst suppression	May be used in low doses to activate interictal spikes
Fentanyl Remifentanil Sufentanil Alfentanil*	Smaller effect on EEG Low dose: Loss of beta waves and a slowing of alpha waves High dose: Diffuse theta and delta waves	May induce interictal spikes and lower seizure threshold *Avoid during cortical stimulation. May be used in bolus to potentiate seizures
Nitrous oxide Sevoflurane Isoflurane Enflurane	Increase beta and gamma range Slow theta and delta oscillation High doses: Burst suppression pattern	Combination of nitrous oxide and isoflurane has a less suppressive EEG effect May be used for mapping epileptiform and epileptic foci
Etomidate	Low dose: Is proepileptic High dose: Burst suppression pattern	Increases the functional mapping threshold
Ketamine	Produces fast oscillations on the high beta and low gamma frequencies Nonspecific activation of IEA especially in limbic structures	Decreases seizure threshold
Dexmedetomidine	Low dose: Minimal effect on background IEA, slow delta oscillations High dose: Increase amplitude of delta oscillations	Causes no new spike foci or seizure activity

IEA interictal epileptiform activity
* Activation most effective and specific when compared with remifentanil and fentanil [13]

awake craniotomy for brain mapping has been proposed [14, 24, 47, 108]. For more details on anesthesia and patient's management during awake craniotomy, refer to Chap. 9.

Other factors that should be considered in anesthesia during ECoG and brain mapping is temperature, hypoxemia, and blood pressure. Decrease of these parameters progressively slows EEG pattern, and extreme drops may induce a burst suppression pattern or even an isoelectric register [5, [109]. Carbon dioxide concentration may lead to delta slowing, followed by burst suppression and isoelectric pattern with hypocapnia as well as hypercapnia [47].

Pharmacological Activation

The basic principle of pharmacological activation is to selectively increase the cortical excitability, particularly of the irritative zones to produce an increase in interictal epileptiform activity. A successful activation is usually quoted as either an increase in the frequency of spiking, an increase in the spike distribution, or both. However, there are doubts about how well the induced area matches with the epileptogenic zone, making this activation controversial among authors. Some suggested that activation may be nonspecific, does not carry any localization values, and may lead to localization confusion and failed surgery [14], and thus, pharmacologic activation of epileptiform discharges should never be preferred to spontaneous alterations occurring in the pre-excision ECoG and it would seem reasonable to consider its use if pre-excision ECoG has no discharges [10]. The use of postexcision ECoG in general is sufficiently dubious, and the practice of pharmacologic activation during this recording cannot be recommended [10]. In this way, from a clinical point of view, it is important to realize that events remote from the epileptogenic lesion, whether these are spikes or HFOs, spontaneous or evoked, always should be considered carefully in relation to anatomy and etiology of the epilepsy [95].

Disagreeing with what was suggested above, some authors indicated that anesthetic agents are safe to be used as pharmacological activation method. Thus, Remifentanil (300 μg/kg bolus) and Propofol (50–175 mg) may facilitate localization of the epileptogenic zone, while minimizing resection of nonepileptogenic eloquent brain tissue [102]. Other authors suggested that Alfentanil (20–100 μg/kg) should be the better opioid for intraoperative activation of the ECoG in neurosurgical patients undergoing resection of a temporal lobe epileptic focus, and neither alfentanil nor remifentanil activated epileptiform activity in nonepileptic brain tissue [58]. Also, Methohexital (25–100 mg) is considered safe and reliable for activating epileptogenic foci during acute ECoG recordings [107]. Other drugs that may be used are Enflurane, Sevoflurane and Fentanyl. However, Sato et al. [80] demonstrated that nitrous oxide (50–70%) significantly decreased spikes during ECoG, with great interference in ECoG results and should be turned off before EEG register begins.

Conclusion

Intraoperative ECoG has been used by epilepsy surgeons for over six decades and after a period of skepticism, ECoG seems to be back in the focus of interest for intraoperative guidance of resecting epileptogenic tissue. In epilepsy surgery, to obtain the best seizure control outcome, one of the most important factors is the complete resection of the lesion and the principle that justifies the use of ECoG in epilepsy surgery is its capacity to delineate the irritative zone and the ictal zone; together these zones form the epileptogenic zone, which is the area in the cerebral cortex capable of generating epileptogenic seizures [73, 78, 108]. San-Juan [78] demonstrated three groups of postresection ECoG: (1) without residual epileptiform activity, (2) with residual epileptiform activity, and (3) de novo postresection epileptiform activity. Seizure-free at mean follow-up of 19.2 months in relation to the postresection ECoG patterns was as follows: 38/58 (65%) without residual epileptiform activity, 11/29 (40%) with residual epileptiform activity, and 6/17 (35%) de novo postresection epileptiform activity and the Kaplan-Meier curves with the dichotomous variable seizure-free versus nonseizure-free groups showed a significant tendency in the survival curves for seizure-free when no residual epileptiform activity is observed in postresective ECoG. When removing brain tissue, neurosurgeons aim to retain brain function to the maximal extent possible, since neurons and networks around and inside a lesion may still contribute usefully to a function [39]. In this way, ECoG seems to be one of the best methods to combine the minimum of tissue removed and the maximum of epileptogenic tissue resected to achieve seizure postoperative control.

References

1. Akeret K, Bellut D, Huppertz HJ, Ramantani G, König K, Serra C, Regli L, Krayenbühl N. Ultrasonographic features of focal cortical dysplasia and their relevance for epilepsy surgery. Neurosurg Focus. 2018;45(3):E5.
2. Alomar S, Jones J, Maldonado A, Gonzalez-Martinez J. The stereo-electroencephalography methodology. Neurosurg Clin N Am. 2016;27(1):83–95.
3. Ansari SF, Maher CO, Tubbs RS, et al. Surgery for extratemporal non-lesional epilepsy in children: a meta-analysis. Childs Nerv Syst. 2010;26:945–51.
4. Bancaud J, Talairach J, Waltregny P, et al. Stimulation of focal cortical epilepsies in topographic diagnosis. (Clinical EEG and SEEG study). Rev Neurol (Paris). 1968;119(3):320–5. (in French).
5. Banoub M, Tetzlaff JE, Schubert A. Pharmacologic and physiologic influences affecting sensory evoked potentials: implications for perioperative monitoring. Anesthesiology. 2003;99(3):716–37. https://doi.org/10.1097/00000542-200309000-00029.
6. Blume W, Girvin J, Kaufman J. Childhood brain tumors presenting as chronic uncontrolled focal seizure disorder. Ann Neurol. 1982;12:538–41.
7. Borggraefe I, Catarino CB, Rémi J, Vollmar C, Peraud A, Winkler PA, Noachtar S. Lateralization of cortical negative motor areas. Clin Neurophysiol. 2016;127(10):3314–21. https://doi.org/10.1016/j.clinph.2016.08.001.

8. Brainer-Lima PT, Brainer-Lima AM, Brandt CT, Carneiro GS, Azevedo HC. Mapeamento da área motora durante a cirurgia de tumor intracraniano: fatores que podem modificar a intensidade da estimulação [Intraoperative mapping of motor areas during brain tumor surgery: electrical stimulation patterns]. Arq Neuropsiquiatr. 2005;63(1):55–60. Portuguese. https://doi.org/10.1590/s0004-282x2005000100011.
9. Burkholder DB, Sulc V, Hoffman EM, Cascino GD, Britton JW, So EL, Marsh WR, Meyer FB, Van Gompel JJ, Giannini C, Wass CT, Watson RE Jr, Worrell GA. Interictal scalp electroencephalography and intraoperative electrocorticography in magnetic resonance imaging-negative temporal lobe epilepsy surgery. JAMA Neurol. 2014;71(6):702–9. https://doi.org/10.1001/jamaneurol.2014.585.
10. Cascino GD. Pharmacological activation. Electroencephalogr Clin Neurophysiol Suppl. 1998;48:70–6.
11. Centeno RS, Yacubian EM, Sakamoto AC, et al. Pre-surgical evaluation and surgical treatment in children with extratemporal epilepsy. Childs Nerv Syst. 2006;22:945–59.
12. Chen X, Sure U, Haag A, Knake S, Fritsch B, Muller HH, Becker R, Oertel WH, Bertalanffy H, Hamer HM, Rosenow F. Predictive value of electrocorticography in epilepsy patients with unilateral hippocampal sclerosis undergoing selective amygdalohippocampectomy. Neurosurg Rev. 2009;29(2):108–13.
13. Cho DY, Lee WY, Lee HC, Chen CC, Tso M. Application of neuronavigator coupled with an operative microscope and electrocorticography in epilepsy surgery. Surg Neurol. 2005;64(5):411–7. https://doi.org/10.1016/j.surneu.2005.02.023; discussion 417-8.
14. Chui J, Manninen P, Valiante T, Venkatraghavan L. The anesthetic considerations of intraoperative electrocorticography during epilepsy surgery. Anesth Analg. 2013;117(2):479–86. https://doi.org/10.1213/ANE.0b013e318297390c.
15. Cossu M, Cardinale F, Castana L, Nobili L, Sartori I, Lo RG. Stereo-EEG in children. Childs Nerv Syst. 2006;22(8):766–78. https://doi.org/10.1007/s00381-006-0127-2.
16. Cross JH, Jayakar P, Nordli D, Delalande O, Duchowny M, Wieser HG, Guerrini R. Mathern GW; international league against epilepsy, subcommission for Paediatric epilepsy surgery; commissions of neurosurgery and Paediatrics. Proposed criteria for referral and evaluation of children for epilepsy surgery: recommendations of the subcommission for pediatric epilepsy surgery. Epilepsia. 2006;47(6):952–9. https://doi.org/10.1111/j.1528-1167.2006.00569.x.
17. D'Argenzio L, Colonnelli MC, Harrison S, et al. Seizure outcome after extratemporal epilepsy surgery in childhood. Dev Med Child Neurol. 2012;54:995–1000.
18. Dash GK, Rathore C, Jeyaraj MK, Wattamwar P, Sarma SP, Radhakrishnan K. Predictors of seizure outcome following resective surgery for drug-resistant epilepsy associated with focal gliosis. J Neurosurg. 2018;1:1–9. https://doi.org/10.3171/2018.3.JNS172949; Epub ahead of print.
19. De Witte E, Satoer D, Robert E, Colle H, Verheyen S, Visch-Brink E, Mariën P. The Dutch linguistic intraoperative protocol: a valid linguistic approach to awake brain surgery. Brain Lang. 2015;140:35–48. https://doi.org/10.1016/j.bandl.2014.10.011.
20. Dineen J, Simon MV, Nozari A. Intraoperative neurophysiology – a comprehensive guide to monitoring and mapping. 2nd Edition. 2019:59–80.
21. Dorfer C, Rydenhag B, Baltuch G, Buch V, Blount J, Bollo R, Gerrard J, Nilsson D, Roessler K, Rutka J, Sharan A, Spencer D, Cukiert A. How technology is driving the landscape of epilepsy surgery. Epilepsia. 2020;61(5):841–55. https://doi.org/10.1111/epi.16489.
22. Dubeau F, McLachlan RS. Invasive electrographic recording techniques in temporal lobe epilepsy. Can J Neurol Sci. 2000;27(Suppl 1):S29–34, discussion S50–S52.
23. Enchev Y. Neuronavigation: geneology, reality, and prospects. Neurosurg Focus. 2009;27(3):E11.
24. Fedele T, Ramantani G, Burnos S, Hilfiker P, Curio G, Grunwald T, Krayenbühl N, Sarnthein J. Prediction of seizure outcome improved by fast ripples detected in low-noise intraoperative corticogram. Clin Neurophysiol. 2017;128(7):1220–6. https://doi.org/10.1016/j.clinph.2017.03.038.

25. Fernández IS, Loddenkemper T. Electrocorticography for seizure foci mapping in epilepsy surgery. J Clin Neurophysiol. 2013;30(6):554–70.
26. Ferrari-Marinho T, Perucca P, Dubeau F, Gotman J. Intracranial EEG seizure onset-patterns correlate with high-frequency oscillations in patients with drug-resistant epilepsy. Epilepsy Res. 2016;127:200–6. https://doi.org/10.1016/j.eplepsyres.2016.09.009.
27. Feyissa AM, Worrell GA, Tatum WO, Mahato D, Brinkmann BH, Rosenfeld SS, ReFaey K, Bechtle PS, Quinones-Hinojosa A. High-frequency oscillations in awake patients undergoing brain tumor-related epilepsy surgery. Neurology. 2018;90(13):e1119–25. https://doi.org/10.1212/WNL.0000000000005216.
28. Frauscher B, Bartolomei F, Kobayashi K, Cimbalnik J, Van't Klooster MA, Rampp S, Otsubo H, Höller Y, Wu JY, Asano E, Engel J Jr, Kahane P, Jacobs J, Gotman J. High-frequency oscillations: the state of clinical research. Epilepsia. 2017;58(8):1316–29. https://doi.org/10.1111/epi.13829.
29. Frauscher B, von Ellenrieder N, Zelmann R, Doležalová I, Minotti L, Olivier A, Hall J, Hoffmann D, Nguyen DK, Kahane P, Dubeau F, Gotman J. Atlas of the normal intracranial electroencephalogram: neurophysiological awake activity in different cortical areas. Brain. 2018;141(4):1130–44. https://doi.org/10.1093/brain/awy035.
30. Fried I, Kim J, Spencer D. Limbic and neocortical gliomas associated with intractable seizures: a distinct clinico-pathological group. J Neurosurg. 1994;34:815–23.
31. Fujiwara H, Leach JL, Greiner HM, Holland-Bouley KD, Rose DF, Arthur T, Mangano FT. Resection of ictal high frequency oscillations is associated with favorable surgical outcome in pediatric drug resistant epilepsy secondary to tuberous sclerosis complex. Epilepsy Res. 2016;126:90–7. https://doi.org/10.1016/j.eplepsyres.2016.07.005.
32. Gamble AJ, Schaffer SG, Nardi DJ, Chalif DJ, Katz J, Dehdashti AR. Awake craniotomy in arteriovenous malformation surgery; the usefulness of cortical and subcortical mapping of language function in selected patients. World Neurosurg. 2015; https://doi.org/10.1016/j.wneu.2015.06.059.
33. Giordano M, Samii A, Lawson McLean AC, Bertalanffy H, Fahlbusch R, Samii M, Di Rocco C. Intraoperative magnetic resonance imaging in pediatric neurosurgery: safety and utility. J Neurosurg Pediatr. 2017;19(1):77–84.
34. Gonzalez-Martinez J, Bulacio J, Alexopoulos A, et al. Stereoelectroencephalography in the "difficult to localize" refractory focal epilepsy: early experience from a north American epilepsy center. Epilepsia. 2013;54(2):323–30.
35. Greiner HM, Horn PS, Tenney JR, Arya R, Jain SV, Holland KD, Leach JL, Miles L, Rose DF, Fujiwara H, Mangano FT. Preresection intraoperative electrocorticography (ECoG) abnormalities predict seizure-onset zone and outcome in pediatric epilepsy surgery. Epilepsia. 2016;57(4):582–9. https://doi.org/10.1111/epi.13341.
36. Harkness W. Temporal lobe resections. Childs Nerv Syst. 2006;22(8):936–44.
37. Hitti FL, Buch VP, Kennedy BC, Vogel TW, Heuer GG, Goodman RR, Baltuch GH, Storm PB. Peg, strip, and grid implantation. In: Baltuch GH, Cukiert A, editors. Operative techniques in epilepsy surgery. New York: Thieme; 2020. p. 22–8.
38. Holmes M, Wilensky A, Ojemann G, et al. Hippocampal or neocortical lesion on magnetic resonance imaging do not necessarily indicate site of ictal onset in partial epilepsy. Ann Neurol. 1999;45:461–5.
39. Huberfeld G, Trébuchon A, Capelle L, Badier JM, Chen S, Lefaucheur JP, Gavaret M. Preoperative and intraoperative neurophysiological investigations for surgical resections in functional areas. Neurochirurgie. 2017;63(3):142–9. https://doi.org/10.1016/j.neuchi.2016.10.008.
40. Jacobs J, Zijlmans M, Zelmann R, et al. High-frequency electroencephalographic oscillations correlate with outcome of epilepsy surgery. Ann Neurol. 2010;67:209–20.
41. Jayakar P, Gaillard WD, Tripathi M, Libenson MH, Mathern GW. Cross JH; task force for Paediatric epilepsy surgery, Commission for Paediatrics, and the diagnostic Commission of the International League against Epilepsy. Diagnostic test utilization in evaluation for

resective epilepsy surgery in children. Epilepsia. 2014;55(4):507–18. https://doi.org/10.1111/epi.12544; Epub 2014 Feb 11.
42. Jayakar P, Gotman J, Harvey AS, Palmini A, Tassi L, Schomer D, Dubeau F, Bartolomei F, Yu A, Kršek P, Velis D, Kahane P. Diagnostic utility of invasive EEG for epilepsy surgery: indications, modalities, and techniques. Epilepsia. 2016;57(11):1735–47. https://doi.org/10.1111/epi.13515.
43. Jeha LE, Najm I, Bingaman W, Dinner D, Widdess-Walsh P, Lüders H. Surgical outcome and prognostic factors of frontal lobe epilepsy surgery. Brain. 2007;130(Pt 2):574–84.
44. Jehi L, Friedman D, Carlson C, Cascino G, Dewar S, Elger C, Engel J Jr, Knowlton R, Kuzniecky R, McIntosh A, O'Brien TJ, Spencer D, Sperling MR, Worrell G, Bingaman B, Gonzalez-Martinez J, Doyle W, French J. The evolution of epilepsy surgery between 1991 and 2011 in nine major epilepsy centers across the United States, Germany, and Australia. Epilepsia. 2015;56(10):1526–33. https://doi.org/10.1111/epi.13116.
45. Jeong SW, Lee SK, Hong KS, Kim KK, Chung CK, Kim H. Prognostic factors for the surgery for mesial temporal lobe epilepsy: longitudinal analysis. Epilepsia. 2005;46(8):1273–9.
46. Kawai K. Epilepsy surgery: current status and ongoing challenges. Neurol Med Chir (Tokyo). 2015;55:357–66.
47. Kayama T, Guidelines committee of the Japan awake surgery conference. The guidelines for awake craniotomy guidelines committee of the Japan awake surgery conference. Neurol Med Chir (Tokyo). 2012;52(3):119–41. https://doi.org/10.2176/nmc.52.119.
48. Keene DL, Whiting S, Ventureyra EC. Electrocorticography. Epileptic Disord. 2000;2(1):57–63.
49. Kovac S, Scott C, Rugg-Gunn F, Miserocchi A, Vollmar C, Rodionov R, McEvoy A, Diehl B. Unusual cortical stimulation findings: connectivity between primary motor and supplementary motor areas. Epilepsy Behav. 2010;19(4):639–42. https://doi.org/10.1016/j.yebeh.2010.09.006.
50. Levivier M, Wikler D, Massager N, Legros B, Van Bogaert P, Brotchi J. IRM opératoire et chirurgie de l'épilepsie (Intraoperative MRI and epilepsy surgery). Neurochirurgie. 2008;54(3):448–52. French.
51. Lohkamp LN, Mottolese C, Szathmari A, Huguet L, Beuriat PA, Christofori I, Desmurget M, Di Rocco F. Awake brain surgery in children-review of the literature and state-of-the-art. Childs Nerv Syst. 2019;35(11):2071–7. https://doi.org/10.1007/s00381-019-04279-w; Epub 2019 Aug 3.
52. Longo PW, Pupo PP, Lemmi O, Pazzanese O, Mattos Pimenta A. A eletrocorticografia como meio de orientação na terapêutica cirúrgica da epilepsia. Arq. Neuro-Psiquiatr. 10(3). São Paulo July/Sept. 1952.
53. Luther N, Rubens E, Sethi N, Kandula P, Labar DR, Harden C, Perrine K, Christos PJ, Iorgulescu JB, Lancman G, Schaul NS, Kolesnik DV, Nouri S, Dawson A, Tsiouris AJ, Schwartz TH. The value of intraoperative electrocorticography in surgical decision making for temporal lobe epilepsy with normal MRI. Epilepsia. 2011;52(5):941–8. https://doi.org/10.1111/j.1528-1167.2011.03061.x.
54. Maesawa S, Nakatsubo D, Fujii M, Iijima K, Kato S, Ishizaki T, Shibata M, Wakabayashi T. Application of awake surgery for epilepsy in clinical practice. Neurol Med Chir (Tokyo). 2018;58(10):442–52. https://doi.org/10.2176/nmc.oa.2018-0122.
55. Mathern GW. Epilepsy surgery patients with cortical dysplasia: present and future therapeutic challenges. Neurology. 2009;72(3):206–7.
56. Mathon B, Amelot A, Carpentier A, Clemenceau S. Intraoperative real-time guidance using ShearWave Elastography for epilepsy surgery. Seizure. 2019;71:24–7.
57. McBride MC, Binnie CD, Janota I, Polkey CE. Predictive value of intraoperative electrocorticograms in resective epilepsy surgery. Ann Neurol. 1991;30:526–32.
58. McGuire G, El-Beheiry H, Manninen P, Lozano A, Wennberg R. Activation of electrocorticographic activity with remifentanil and alfentanil during neurosurgical excision of epileptogenic focus. Br J Anaesth. 2003;91(5):651–5. https://doi.org/10.1093/bja/aeg241.

59. Morino M, Ishibashi K, Hara M. Surgical treatment of tempo- ral lobe epilepsy associated with subcortical ectopic gray matter under the guidance of intraoperative electrocorticography. Seizure. 2004;13(7):470–4.
60. Mouthaan BE, Van't Klooster MA, Keizer D, Hebbink GJ, FSS L, Ferrier CH, Van Putten MJAM, Zijlmans M, Huiskamp GJM. Single pulse electrical stimulation to identify epileptogenic cortex: clinical information obtained from early evoked responses. Clin Neurophysiol. 2016;127(2):1088–98. https://doi.org/10.1016/j.clinph.2015.07.031.
61. Mullin JP, Shriver M, Alomar S, Najm I, Bulacio J, Chauvel P, Gonzalez-Martinez J. Is SEEG safe? A systematic review and meta-analysis of stereo-electroencephalography-related complications. Epilepsia. 2016;57(3):386–401.
62. Najm IM, Bingaman WE, Luders HO. The use of subdural grids in the management of focal malformations due to abnormal cortical development. Neurosurg Clin N Am. 2002;13(1):87–92.
63. Nayak CS, Bandyopadhyay S. Mesial Temporal Lobe Epilepsy. In: StatPearls [Internet]. Treasure Island (FL): StatPearls Publishing; 2020.
64. Nejedly P, Kremen V, Sladky V, Cimbalnik J, Klimes P, Plesinger F, Mivalt F, Travnicek V, Viscor I, Pail M, Halamek J, Brinkmann BH, Brazdil M, Jurak P, Worrell G. Multicenter intracranial EEG dataset for classification of graphoelements and artifactual signals. Sci Data. 2020;7(1):179. https://doi.org/10.1038/s41597-020-0532-5.
65. Obeid M, Wyllie E, Rahi AC, Mikati MA. Approach to pediatric epilepsy surgery: state of the art, part I: general principles and presurgical workup. Eur J Paediatr Neurol. 2009;13(2):102–14.
66. Obeid M, Wyllie E, Rahi AC, Mikati MA. Approach to pediatric epilepsy surgery: state of the art, part II: approach to specific epilepsy syndromes and etiologies. Eur J Paediatr Neurol. 2009;13(2):115–27.
67. Palmini A, Gambardella A, Andermann F, Dubeau F, da Costa JC, Olivier A, Tampieri D, Gloor P, Quesney F, Andermann E, et al. Intrinsic epileptogenicity of human dysplastic cortex as suggested by corticography and surgical results. Ann Neurol. 1995;37(4):476–87. https://doi.org/10.1002/ana.410370410.
68. Panov F, Li Y, Chang EF, Knowlton R, Cornes SB. Epilepsy with temporal encephalocele: characteristics of electrocorticography and surgical outcome. Epilepsia. 2016;57(2):e33–8. https://doi.org/10.1111/epi.13271.
69. Penfield W. The epilepsies: with a note on radical therapy. N Engl J Med. 1939;221:209–18.
70. Penfield W, Flanigin H. Surgical therapy of temporal lobe seizures. Arch Neurol A Psychiat. 1950;64:491–500.
71. Rassi-Neto A, Ferraz FP, Campos CR, Braga FM. Patients with epileptic seizures and cerebral lesions who underwent lesionectomy restricted to or associated with the adjacent irritative area. Epilepsia. 1999;40(7):856–64.
72. Roessler K, Hofmann A, Sommer B, Grummich P, Coras R, Kasper BS, Hamer HM, Blumcke I, Stefan H, Nimsky C, Buchfelder M. Resective surgery for medically refractory epilepsy using intraoperative MRI and functional neuronavigation: the Erlangen experience of 415 patients. Neurosurg Focus. 2016;40(3):E15. https://doi.org/10.3171/2015.12.FOCUS15554.
73. Roessler K, Heynold E, Buchfelder M, Stefan H, Hamer HM. Current value of intraoperative electrocorticography (iopECoG). Epilepsy Behav. 2019;91:20–4. https://doi.org/10.1016/j.yebeh.2018.06.053.
74. Rogers CM, Jones PS, Weinberg JS. Intraoperative MRI for brain tumors. J Neuro-Oncol. 2021;151(3):479–90.
75. Roth J, Biyani N, Beni-Adani L, Constantini S. Real-time neuronavigation with high-quality 3D ultrasound SonoWand in pediatric neurosurgery. Pediatr Neurosurg. 2007;43(3):185–91.
76. Ruis C. Monitoring cognition during awake brain surgery in adults: a systematic review. J Clin Exp Neuropsychol. 2018;40(10):1081–104. https://doi.org/10.1080/13803395.2018.1469602.

77. Ryvlin P, Cross JH, Rheims S. Epilepsy surgery in children and adults. Lancet Neurol. 2014;13(11):1114–26. https://doi.org/10.1016/S1474-4422(14)70156-5.
78. San-Juan Y, Alonso-Vanegas MA, Trenado C, Hernández-Segura N, Espinoza-López DA, González-Pérez B, Cobos-Alfaro E, Zúñiga-Gazcón H. Fernández-González de Aragón MDC, Hernandez-Ruiz a. Electrocorticographic patterns in epilepsy surgery and long-term outcome. J Clin Neurophysiol. 2017;34(6):520–6. https://doi.org/10.1097/WNP.0000000000000407.
79. Santos MV, Machado HR. Extratemporal disconnective procedures for the treatment of epilepsy in children. Epilepsia. 2017;58(Suppl 1):28–34.
80. Sato Y, Sato K, Shamoto H, Kato M, Yoshimoto T. Effect of nitrous oxide on spike activity during epilepsy surgery. Acta Neurochir. 2001;143(12):1213–5. https://doi.org/10.1007/s007010100016; discussion 1215-6.
81. Schwartz TH, Bazil CW, Walczak TS, Chan S, Pedley TA, Goodman RR. The predictive value of intraoperative electrocorticography in resections for limbic epilepsy associated with mesial temporal sclerosis. Neurosurgery. 1997;40:302–9.
82. Sisodiya SM, Fauser S, Cross JH, Thom M. Focal cortical dysplasia type II: biological features and clinical perspectives. Lancet Neurol. 2009;8(9):830–43. https://doi.org/10.1016/S1474-4422(09)70201-7.
83. Sisodiya SM, Fauser S, Cross JH, Thom M. Focal cortical dysplasia type II: biological features and clinical perspectives. Lancet Neurol. 2009;8(9):830–43. https://doi.org/10.1016/S1474-4422(09)70201-7.
84. Sonvenso DK, Itikawa EN, Santos MV, Santos LA, Trevisan AC, Bianchin MM, Pitella FA, Kato M, Carlotti CG Jr, Busatto GF, Velasco TR, Santos AC, Leite JP, Sakamoto AC, Machado HR, Nunes AA, Wichert-Ana L. Systematic review of the efficacy in seizure control and safety of neuronavigation in epilepsy surgery: the need for well-designed prospective studies. Seizure. 2015;31:99–107.
85. Tao JX, Chen XJ, Baldwin M, Yung I, Rose S, Frim D, Hawes-Ebersole S, Ebersole JS. Interictal regional delta slowing is an EEG marker of epileptic network in temporal lobe epilepsy. Epilepsia. 2011;52(3):467–76. https://doi.org/10.1111/j.1528-1167.2010.02918.x. Epub 2011 Jan 4.
86. Terra VC, Thomé U, Rosset SS, Funayama SS, dos Santos AC, dos Santos MV, Sakamoto AC, Machado HR. Surgery for focal cortical dysplasia in children using intraoperative mapping. Childs Nerv Syst. 2014;30(11):1839–51. https://doi.org/10.1007/s00381-014-2459-7; Epub 2014 Oct 9.
87. Thijs RD, Surges R, O'Brien TJ, Sander JW. Epilepsy in adults. Lancet. 2019;393(10172):689–701. https://doi.org/10.1016/S0140-6736(18)32596-0.
88. Tripathi M, Garg A, Gaikwad S, Bal CS, Chitra S, Prasad K, Dash HH, Sharma BS, Chandra PS. Intra-operative electrocorticography in lesional epilepsy. Epilepsy Res. 2010;89(1):133–41. https://doi.org/10.1016/j.eplepsyres.2009.12.007.
89. Vale FL, Vivas AC, Manwaring J, Schoenberg MR, Benbadis SR. Temporal lobe epilepsy and cavernous malformations: surgical strategies and long-term outcomes. Acta Neurochir. 2015;157(11):1887–95. https://doi.org/10.1007/s00701-015-2592-4; discussion 1895.
90. van Klink NE, Van Klooster MA, Zelmann R, et al. High frequency oscillations in intra-operative electrocorticography before and after epilepsy surgery. Clin Neurophysiol. 2014;125:2212–9.
91. Van't Klooster MA, Leijten FS, Huiskamp G, Ronner HE, Baayen JC, Van Rijen PC, Eijkemans MJ, Braun KP, Zijlmans M, HFO study group. High frequency oscillations in the intra-operative ECoG to guide epilepsy surgery ("The HFO Trial"): study protocol for a randomized controlled trial. Trials. 2015;16:422. https://doi.org/10.1186/s13063-015-0932-6.
92. Van't Klooster MA, Van Klink NE, Leijten FS, Zelmann R, Gebbink TA, Gosselaar PH, Braun KP, Huiskamp GJ, Zijlmans M. Residual fast ripples in the intraoperative corticogram predict epilepsy surgery outcome. Neurology. 2015;85(2):120–8. https://doi.org/10.1212/WNL.0000000000001727.
93. Van't Klooster MA, Van Klink NE, Leijten FS, Zelmann R, Gebbink TA, Gosselaar PH, Braun KP, Huiskamp GJ, Zijlmans M. Residual fast ripples in the intraoperative corticogram predict epilepsy surgery outcome. Neurology. 2015;85(2):120–8. https://doi.org/10.1212/WNL.0000000000001727.

94. Van't Klooster MA, NEC VK, Van Blooijs D, Ferrier CH, KPJ B, FSS L, GJM H, Zijlmans M. Evoked versus spontaneous high frequency oscillations in the chronic electrocorticogram in focal epilepsy. Clin Neurophysiol. 2017;128(5):858–66. https://doi.org/10.1016/j.clinph.2017.01.017.
95. Van't Klooster MA, Van Klink NEC, Zweiphenning WJEM, Leijten FSS, Zelmann R, Ferrier CH, Van Rijen PC, Otte WM, Braun KPJ, Huiskamp GJM, Zijlmans M. Tailoring epilepsy surgery with fast ripples in the intraoperative electrocorticogram. Ann Neurol. 2017;81(5):664–76. https://doi.org/10.1002/ana.24928.
96. Vaz AP, Inati SK, Brunel N, Zaghloul KA. Coupled ripple oscillations between the medial temporal lobe and neocortex retrieve human memory. Science. 2019;363(6430):975–8. https://doi.org/10.1126/science.aau8956.
97. Vigren P, Eriksson M, Duffau H, Wretman A, Lindehammar H, Milos P, Richter J, Karlsson T, Gauffin H. Experiences of awake surgery in non-tumoural epilepsy in eloquent localizations. Clin Neurol Neurosurg. 2020;199:106251. https://doi.org/10.1016/j.clineuro.2020.106251.
98. Vossler DG, Kraemer DL, Haltiner AM, Rostad SW, Kjos BO, Davis BJ, Morgan JD, Caylor LM. Intracranial EEG in temporal lobe epilepsy: location of seizure onset relates to degree of hippocampal pathology. Epilepsia. 2004;45(5):497–503.
99. Walker AE, Marshall C, Beresford E. Electrocorticographic characteristics of the cerebrum in posttraumatic epilepsy. In: Epilepsy, vol. 26. A. Res. Nerv. A. Ment. Dis., Williams and Wilkins Co.; 1947. p. 502–15.
100. Wang MY, Wang J, Zhou J, Guan YG, Zhai F, Liu CQ, Xu FF, Han YX, Yan ZF, Luan GM. Identification of the epileptogenic zone of temporal lobe epilepsy from stereo-electroencephalography signals: a phase transfer entropy and graph theory approach. Neuroimage Clin. 2017;16:184–95.
101. Wang Y, Sinha N, Schroeder GM, Ramaraju S, McEvoy AW, Miserocchi A, de Tisi J, Chowdhury FA, Diehl B, Duncan JS, Taylor PN. Interictal intracranial electroencephalography for predicting surgical success: the importance of space and time. Epilepsia. 2020;61(7):1417–26. https://doi.org/10.1111/epi.16580.
102. Wass CT, Grady RE, Fessler AJ, Cascino GD, Lozada L, Bechtle PS, Marsh WR, Sharbrough FW, Schroeder DR. The effects of remifentanil on epileptiform discharges during intraoperative electrocorticography in patients undergoing epilepsy surgery. Epilepsia. 2001;42(10):1340–4. https://doi.org/10.1046/j.1528-1157.2001.05901.x.
103. Wennberg R, Quesney F, Olivier A, Dubeau F. Mesial temporal versus lateral temporal interictal epileptiform activity: comparison of chronic and acute intracranial recordings. Electroencephalogr Clin Neurophysiol. 1997;102:486–94.
104. Worrell G, Gotman J. High-frequency oscillations and other electrophysiological biomarkers of epilepsy: clinical studies. Biomark Med. 2011;5:557–66.
105. Wu JY, Sankar R, Lerner JT, Matsumoto JH, Vinters HV, Mathern GW. Removing interictal fast ripples on electrocorticography linked with seizure freedom in children. Neurology. 2010;75:1686–94.
106. Wurm G, Ringler H, Knogler F, Schnizer M. Evaluation of neuronavigation in lesional and non-lesional epilepsy surgery. Comput Aided Surg. 2003;8(4):204–14.
107. Wyler AR, Richey ET, Atkinson RA, Hermann BP. Methohexital activation of epileptogenic foci during acute electrocorticography. Epilepsia. 1987;28(5):490–4. https://doi.org/10.1111/j.1528-1157.1987.tb03677.x.
108. Yang T, Hakimian S, Schwartz TH. Intraoperative ElectroCorticoGraphy (ECog): indications, techniques, and utility in epilepsy surgery. Epileptic Disord. 2014;16(3):271–9. https://doi.org/10.1684/epd.2014.0675.
109. Yang J, Skaggs DL, Chan P, Shah SA, Vitale MG, Neiss G, Andras LM. Raising mean arterial pressure alone restores 20% of intraoperative neuromonitoring losses. Spine. 2017; https://doi.org/10.1097/BRS.0000000000002461.
110. Zijlmans M, Zweiphenning W, van Klink N. Changing concepts in presurgical assessment for epilepsy surgery. Nat Rev Neurol. 2019;15(10):594–606. https://doi.org/10.1038/s41582-019-0224-y.

Part X
Movement Disorders Surgery

Chapter 33
Neurophysiological Guidance for Movement Disorder Surgery

Denise Spinola Pinheiro and Erich Fonoff

Abbreviations

CSPTC	Cortico-striatal-pallidal-thalamic-cortical
CT	Computed tomography
cZI	Caudal zona incerta
DBS	Deep brain stimulation
DTI	Diffusion tensor imaging
Gd	Gadolinium contrast media
GPe	External segment of the globus pallidus
GPi	Internal segment of the globus pallidus
IONM	Intraoperative neurophysiological monitoring
LFP	Local field potential
MER	Microelectrode recording
MR	Magnetic resonance
PD	Parkinson's disease
SNr	Substance nigra pars reticulata
STN	Subthalamic nucleus
SW	Susceptibility weighted
Vc	Caudal ventral sensory nucleus
Vim	Ventral intermediate nucleus

D. S. Pinheiro (✉)
Department of Neurology, Universidade Federal de São Paulo, São Paulo, SP, Brazil
e-mail: denise.pinheiro@unifesp.br

E. Fonoff
Department of Neurology, University of São Paulo, São Paulo, SP, Brazil
e-mail: fonoffet@usp.br

S. M. Verst et al. (eds.), *Intraoperative Monitoring*,
https://doi.org/10.1007/978-3-030-95730-8_33

Voa	Ventral oral anterior
Vop	Ventral oral posterior
ZI	Zona incerta

Background

The use of intraoperative neurophysiological monitoring (IONM) during surgical procedures has developed extensively in the past decade and has become an important adjunctive technique, adding more safety to surgical approaches. In stereotactic surgery, the outcome results are intimately related to the target definition and adverse effect prevention. In functional neurosurgery, more specifically in stereotactic-guided procedures directed to deep-seated targets in the brain, as in movement disorder surgery, IONM aims to prevent potential nervous tissue damage and add elements to the decision-making of final target localization. Deep brain stimulation (DBS) is currently the most applied therapeutic technique for movement disorders, alleviating symptoms in conditions such as Parkinson's disease (PD), essential tremor and tremor syndromes, and different types of dystonia. The targets of implants vary according to the experience of centers, diagnosis, and predominant symptoms. The most performed targets are in the subthalamic area, as the subthalamic nucleus (STN) itself, rostral or caudal zona incerta or the posterior subthalamic area, internal segment of the globus pallidus (GPi), and thalamus as the nucleus ventral intermediate nucleus (Vim), nucleus ventral oral anterior or posterior, or the centromedian/parafascicular nuclear complex [17].

Neural Circuitry of Movement Disorders

Although the pathophysiology of movement disorders is not completely understood, successful therapeutic interventions are currently performed in targets previously used for focal ablation such as the thalamus and the GPi. However, the growing anatomo-physiological knowledge of the cortico-striatal-pallidal-thalamic-cortical (CSPTC) circuit provides additional targets like the subthalamic nucleus, and currently gives insights for the development of new targets and understanding of adverse effects of interventions. The important development of new therapeutic targets in functional neurosurgery depends on the comprehension of the intricate circuitry and its reactions to neuromodulation or neuroablation.

There are at least five parallel circuits that connect the basal ganglia, thalamus, and cortex and are related to oculomotor, limbic, prefrontal, and motor functions. These circuits originate in different areas of the frontal lobe and pass through the basal ganglia and thalamus before returning to the cortical region of origin [3]. The motor circuit is directly involved in the pathophysiology of PD and has been studied extensively in an animal model using (1-methyl-4-phenyl-1,2,3,6-tetrahydropyridine (MPTP) [11, 35, 39]. This dysfunctional circuit originates in the precentral area and passes through the striatum (caudate and putamen), serving as an input structure to the basal ganglia, while the GPi and substance nigra pars reticulata (SNr) are used as output structures. This information is organized anatomically through a direct monosynaptic pathway and an indirect multisynaptic pathway. In the direct pathway, the information is transmitted directly from the putamen to the output structures. In the indirect pathway, the information passes through the GPi and STN before reaching the output pathway. There is a reciprocal regulation between the two pathways, as the direct pathway is related to movement initiation, while the indirect pathway seems to suppress it.

In PD, the reduction of dopamine in the substantia nigra pars compacta accentuates the activity of the indirect pathway, leading to GPi and SNr hyperactivity. This inhibits thalamocortical activation, reduces frontal activity, and it is responsible for classic motor symptoms of the disease such as tremor, rigidity, bradykinesia, gait disturbances, and postural changes [33]. Experimental studies in MPTP monkeys lead to the inclusion of the STN as an important nucleus in this circuitry and the pathological hyperactivity in Parkinson-like changes in the circuit. Based on that, deep brain stimulation of the STN was proposed and tested in patients. Different from GPi and Vim, targets derived from empirical data, the STN, as therapeutic target for PD, was entirely created in the laboratory and currently is one of the most used targets in movement disorder surgery. IONM played a paramount role in the translational application of the experiential findings, because it confirmed the hyperactivity of neurons in the STN initially found in MPTP models. From the very beginning, STN stimulation was proposed for bilateral approach as a new modulatory therapy avoiding lesions.

In dystonia, this dysfunctional mechanism of the circuit is not well understood, as no alterations of neurotransmitters or specific components have been evidenced, and electrophysiological studies suggest dysfunction in the communication pattern between structures of the circuit [38]. In general, dystonic movements occur when inhibition fails to reach network loops that are not directly related to the motor task intended. In normal conditions, surrounding inhibitory information is normally required to select appropriate commands for each motor task. Impulses originating from the motor cortex go through the basal ganglia circuits that act as a filter to enroll specific neuronal networks, while inhibiting unwanted surrounding circuits outside the core motor behavior engram. In dystonia, this mechanism is lost giving rise to cocontractions agonist-antagonist muscles associated with impaired sensory-motor integration disclosing the occurrence of dystonic symptoms. Rather than the narrow involvement of cerebral cortex and the basal ganglia, multiple levels of integration of sensory-motor information including the thalamus and cerebellar circuits and spinal circuitry as well.

The pathophysiology of essential tremor involves GABAergic dysfunction of the cerebellar dentate nucleus and brain stem connecting nuclei, possibly caused by sluggish neurodegeneration in these regions with loss of Purkinje cells, leading to tremulous activity within the cerebello-thalamo-cortical circuit. Apparently, the degeneration of both Purkinje cells and neighboring GABAergic neurons (basket cells) increases their connections, resulting in rewiring and reorganization of neuronal connections within the cerebellum. Slow circuit reorganization alters network parameters such as the strength and directionality of interregional coupling, producing changes in oscillating patterns of cerebellothalamic loops that worsens tremor and induces mild ataxia with time.

Surgery

Successful movement disorder surgery requires precise placement of the electrode within the target nucleus. This is achieved using stereotactic techniques based on a combination of preoperative and perioperative imaging, electrophysiological mapping with microelectrode recording (MER), stimulation, and intraoperative clinical evaluation of the implanted electrode.

Stereotactic-guided procedures can be performed using different stereotactic frames depending on the availability. However, almost all frames used currently worldwide are isocentric and support either stereo-CT scan or stereo-MRI. Nowadays, stereotactic planning is performed with assistance of computer software capable of fusing different image modalities and incorporating them into the stereotactic space, also referred as the Talairach space. Once the patient's image is acquired with the frame on, every cubic millimeter within the brain receives stereotactic coordinates. The isocentric method simplifies the simulation of multiple trajectories, allowing the chosen trajectory plan to be performed accurately by having the target coordinates and given antero-posterior and latero-lateral angles. Different image modalities can be used in the deep brain implants procedures. However, stereo-CT fused into preoperative MRI or stereo-MRI is the most employed one. In addition to target definition, MRIs can show anatomical landmarks and structures that should be avoided in the trajectory planning, adding safety to the procedure. The T1 gadolinium MRI sequence can be merged into the stereo-CT to show of the convexity and opercular sulci, the lateral and third ventricles, and brainstem borders and blood vessels. In addition, SW images show small vessels, especially veins deep seated within the gray and white matter. Different T2-weighted MR sequences are also employed to clearly show the limits between gray and white matter, and iron deposits with various intraparenchymal nuclei and white matter tracts that can also be used to refine the target definition [40]. Iron deposits appear hypointense (dark) regions in the upper midbrain marking the position of the subthalamic nucleus (STN), the red nucleus, substantia nigra, mammillary bodies, segments of globus pallidum and white matter tracts as the internal capsule, anterior commissure, mammillothalamic tract, fornix, and others (Figs. 33.1 and 33.2).

On top of image-guided anatomical target definition, a microdrive conducts 1–5 microelectrodes, depending on the microrecording technique to refine the targeting.

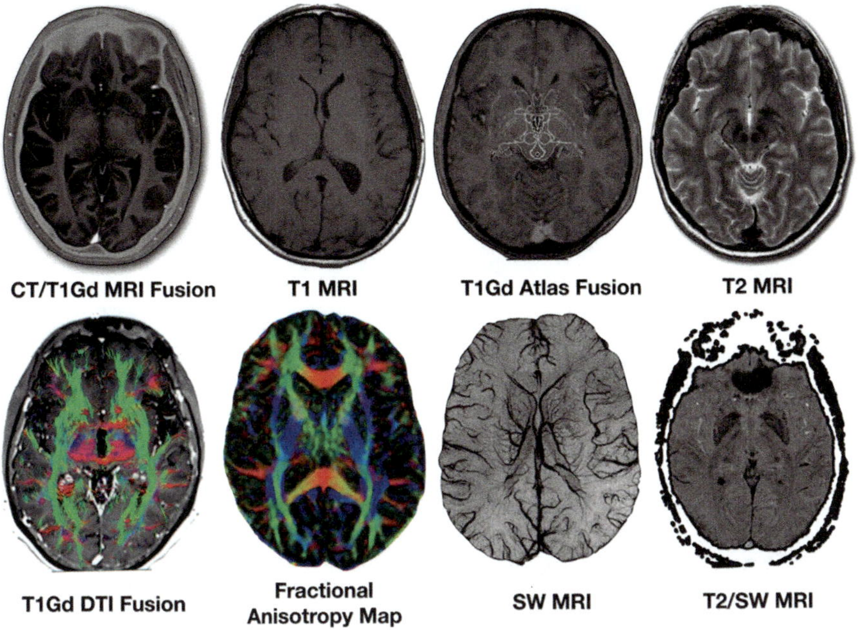

Fig. 33.1 Typical image modalities used for functional stereotactic procedures. Each image sequence is employed for a purpose to show either the target itself or structures that should be avoided during trajectory planning

Microelectrodes are mounted into the microdrive parallel channels that conduct to the center of the target separated by 2 mm center-to-center distance covering the region. In our practice, 3 microelectrodes are used routinely in subthalamic nucleus implants allowing the mapping of the trajectory, which gives a 3D idea of the nucleus based on the type of neuronal activity. The patient is usually kept under sedatives for most of the procedure time length, but he or she can be awakened during the micro-recording mapping followed by intraoperative neurological examination.

Deep brain stimulation has provided the possibility of treatment of bilateral movement disorders, such as PD, essential tremor, and generalized dystonia. Most of the patients benefit from bilateral procedures as it is preferentially performed in the same approach routinely throughout the world. Our group has been dedicated to the development of simultaneous bilateral procedures, which required changes in the stereotactic frame providing the possibility of performing bilateral and simultaneous microrecording [18]. Besides the open field for research in neurophysiology, bilateral simultaneous procedures have recognizably shortened the procedure time and increased accuracy, avoiding misplacing of DBS leads due to brain shifting. This stereotactic system allows independent coordinates in the same frame for each hemisphere (Fig. 33.3) [4–6, 23].

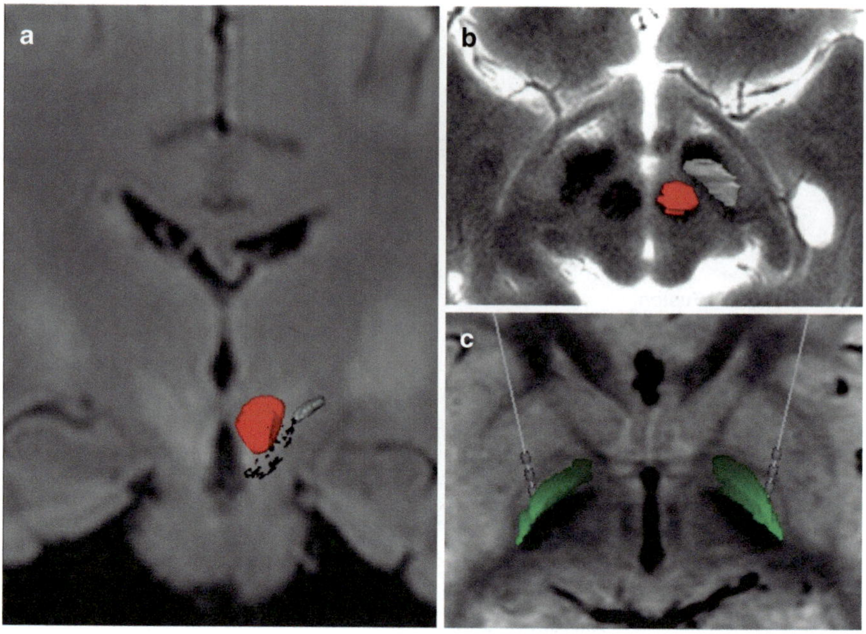

Fig. 33.2 (**a**) Coronal section of a T1 MRI showing 3D reconstruction of the red nucleus (red), the subthalamic nucleus (gray), and the island of cells of the substantia nigra (black). (**b**) Axial section of a T2 MRI showing iron deposit (dark) on the right corresponding to the red nucleus (red), the subthalamic nucleus (gray) on the left. (**c**) Axial perspective view of a T2 MRI showing the region of the globus palladium and 3D reconstruction of the GPi (green) and 3D simulation of a deep brain stimulation electrode and a typical trajectory. Images given by Eduardo Alho and Rodrigo Paul from São Paulo-Würzburg Electronic Atlas of the Human Brain

Microelectrode Recording

The main goal of a neurophysiological evaluation is to confirm the electrode's location within the target, because better surgical results depend on accurate placement of the electrode in the target nucleus [29]. Several neurophysiological methods can be used, such as impedance measurements, macroelectrode recording, semi-microelectrode recording, and evoked potentials, but the most frequently used are MER and local field potential (LFP).

MER involves recording extracellular action potentials from the cells near the electrode using a system attached to the stereotactic frame called a microdrive, which is used to advance or retract the MER electrode [8, 9] (Fig. 33.4). Depending on the proposed trajectory, the MER usually starts 10–20 mm above the estimated target, moves gradually, and may exceed the target by a few millimeters. One to three trajectories are often performed. The recording of a single trajectory is used to confirm the electrode's location, while the use of multiple trajectories aims to access

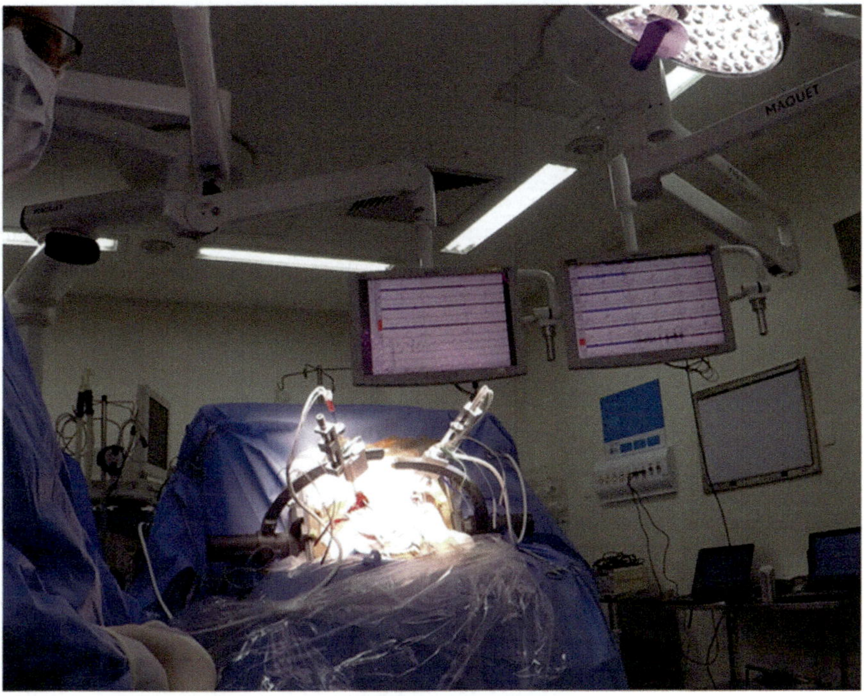

Fig. 33.3 Simultaneous bilateral procedure performed during a bilateral STN DBS implant in a Parkinson's disease patient. Image shows two stereotactic isocentric arches mounted with one microdrive each recording from 3 channels from each side (left and right) (Bramsys/Micromar System, São Paulo, Brazil). Microrecording of subthalamic neuronal activity in two different screening fed by two dedicated amplifiers

a larger area of the target, obtain a detailed physiological mapping of the nucleus, and define the borders.

The physiological characteristics of neuronal activity, with emphasis on cell firing frequency and changes in baseline activity, are analyzed. The recording of more distant cells cannot be differentiated from baseline noise. The pattern of neuronal firing in the target nuclei is characteristic and differs from the firing pattern of nearby structures, which delimits the borders of these nuclei. Cellular firing is also assessed at the frequency of the tremor and in response to sensory stimulation and/or active and passive limb movements.

Two firing patterns are found: a burst pattern, which is defined as a period in which a significantly high number of firings occur compared to that in a quieter period, and an oscillation pattern, which is defined as a pattern of neuronal activity in which discharges occur periodically and may be regular or irregular [27]. The signals are visualized on the equipment's display, transmitted through a speaker, and interpreted by an experienced neurophysiologist.

Fig. 33.4 Microdrive system

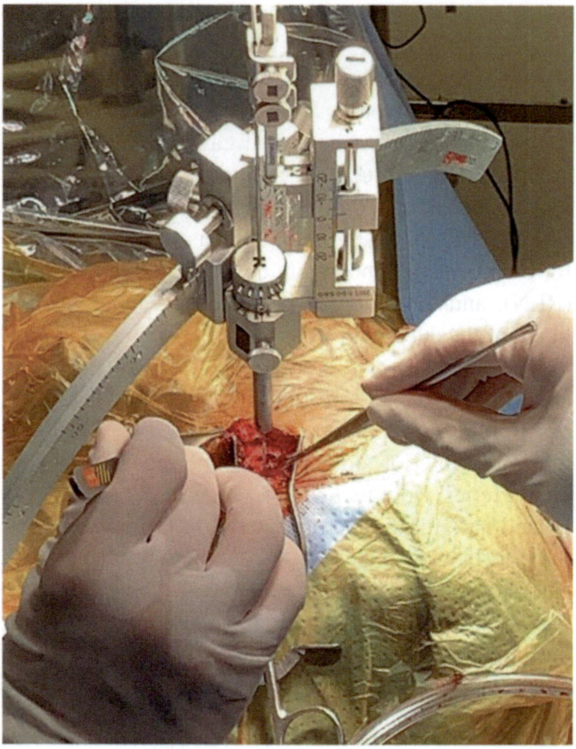

This system allows the simultaneous or sequential record of five different trajectories spaced 2 mm apart. Commercially available MER electrodes have a conically shaped tip with a maximum length that is significantly shorter than the diameter of the smallest cells and impedance of 0.3–1 MΩ at 1 KHz, which allows the capture of the extracellular action potential of nearby cells. The electrodes also have a proximal macroelectrode contact, usually 1.5–3 mm above the recording tip used for LFP capture and intraoperative electrical stimulation testing.

Despite the significant evolution in imaging method quality, MER is essential, and several centers use some form of intraoperative electrophysiological evaluation [1]. MER aims to confirm electrode placement within the target nucleus and, most importantly, define the sensorimotor part, the region where increased neuronal activity occurs in response to activation maneuvers that corresponds to the region where the best clinical response is achieved with the electrode implantation.

After the electrophysiological evaluation, electrical stimulation is performed using the tip of the MER electrode and/or the stimulation halo positioned a few millimeters above. The objective is to evaluate the therapeutic efficacy by mimicking the efficacy of the definitive lead before its placement. Electrical stimulation is also used to estimate the proximity of neighboring structures by evaluating the side effects.

After the desired trajectory is defined, the DBS electrode is located and the macrostimulation performed using the contacts of the electrode itself. It is made with an external stimulator that resembles chronic therapeutic stimulation. This is usually performed using bipolar stimulation between adjacent electrode contacts. This step assesses the stimulation intensity (voltage or current) required to achieve clinical efficacy and side effects. The goal is to achieve the greatest suppression of motor symptoms associated with the least presence of side effects. The difference between these two thresholds, clinical efficacy, and side effects is called therapeutic window.

The unfavorable aspects of MER are described in the literature and include increased surgical time, hemorrhage, and pneumocephalus, which can lead to brain shift with reduced accuracy of stereotactic localization [16, 21, 28]. Despite its safety, a correlation has been described between the risk of intracranial hemorrhage and the number of trajectories performed and is estimated to be 3% for MER-related bleeding and 0.6% for the occurrence of permanent deficits [12].

Subthalamic Nucleus

The STN is a small biconvex lens-shaped structure located ventral to the thalamus with a maximum rostrocaudal extent of 13.2 mm and mediolateral extent of 8–9 mm [7, 22]. Its neighboring structures are the anterolateral corticospinal/corticobulbar tract, dorsoposterior medial lemniscus, anteroventral nerve III fibers, and posteromedial red nucleus. The dorsal border is formed by the zona incerta (ZI) and Forel's field, while the ventral border is formed by the substantia nigra pars reticulata (SNr).

The STN is functionally divided into motor, limbic, and associative regions. The limbic region is positioned in the anteromedial region of the nucleus. The sensory-motor region, the ideal target of the DBS electrode, is in the dorsal posterolateral region of the nucleus and confirmed by the presence of movement-evoked neural response [2, 24].

During the typical microrecording trajectory, the first structure recorded is the thalamus, which shows variable neuronal activities. However, most trajectories pass through the ventrolateral nuclei of the thalamus, reticular nucleus, ventral oral anterior (Voa), and ventral oral posterior (Vop) and show irregular low-frequency cell firing with intermittent high-frequency bursts depending on the nucleus recorded.

Baseline activity is reduced in the ZI and Forel's field, because they are rich in white matter bundles and sparse high-voltage firing is observed.

The proximity of the electrode to the STN is preceded by a sudden increase in baseline activity. Entry into the nucleus is characterized by intense cellular activity with multiple neuronal firings at a frequency of 37 ± 17 Hz. The cells of the STN exhibit two types of firing patterns: a population of cells that fire to a clustered burst-like trend more characteristic of the dorsal region of the nucleus, and another population of cells that exhibit intense tonic activity with irregular firing more characteristic of the deep regions of the nucleus. In about 10% of patients with parkinsonian tremor, it is possible to visualize the firing of a population of burst-like cells in the tremor frequency [10].

The sensorimotor region of the STN, located in the dorsolateral region of the nucleus, is defined as the region in which increased neuronal activity occurs in response to passive or active maneuvers of the contralateral face, shoulder, arm, wrist, leg, and foot regions [36]. The best clinical response to stimulation was observed when the electrode is positioned in this region. Somatotopy exists with the motor cortex, in which the cells related to the arm are more lateral and those related to the leg are more medial. Neurons located in the ventral and medial regions of the STN are connected to the associative and limbic cortical regions.

At the ventral border of the STN, a decrease in cell activity occurs. Upon exiting the STN, the microelectrode passes through a narrow silent 1- to 2-mm region before entering the SNr. The SNr is differentiated from the STN by its lower cellular density; therefore, it is more easily isolated with its high-amplitude regular firing, and frequency of approximately 50–70 Hz [37] (Fig. 33.5).

The intense neuronal activity of the STN contrasts with the low frequency or nearly silent activity of neighboring structures, such as the lateral internal capsule and the dorsal ZI and Forel's field. Based on the MER findings, localization within the nucleus is possible. The absence of cellular recordings in the thalamus suggests a more anterior and/or lateral trajectory. If cellular spiking in the thalamus is present but the STN recording is short, the trajectory may be more posterior or medial. Absence of the SNr suggests a more lateral trajectory.

The neurophysiologist should be aware that a more medial trajectory may record cell firing from the red nucleus, which has a similar electrophysiological recording to that of the STN. The presence of a typical ventral and medial STN recording that is incompatible with imaging, a lack of clinical improvement, and the presence of

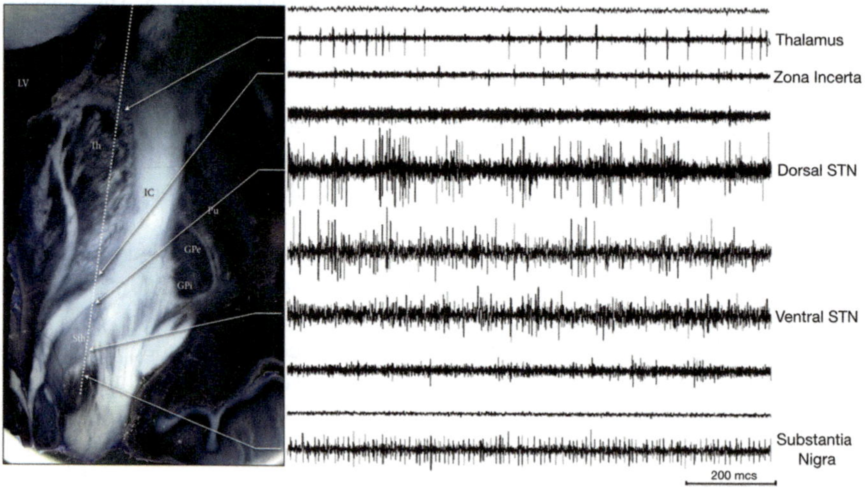

Fig. 33.5 Microelectrode mapping showing recording segments (on the right) obtained from sequential sites in the depth of thalamus-subthalamic region following a routine trajectory (white inclined dotted line) from the thalamus down to the substantia nigra. Coronal section of human brain histologic preparation dyed with galocianine. Images given by Helmut Heinsen from São Paulo-Würzburg Electronic Atlas of the Human Brain [23]

autonomic side effects with a sensation of heat, sweating, and oculomotor alteration suggests a red nucleus recording [31].

An optimal trajectory presents an extension of at least 4 mm associated with kinesthetic activity in the dorsolateral region of the STN and defined dorsal and ventral borders recognizing cellular firing patterns from the anterior thalamus, ZI, and SNr.

After recording, intraoperative high-frequency stimulation is administered in the proximal portion of the MER. When the trajectory is optimal, improvement is noted in parkinsonian motor symptoms such as rigidity, bradykinesia, and tremor. Stimulation also plays a key role in the assessment of side effects because of the large number of structures around the nucleus. When the electrode is too lateral (e.g., close to the internal capsule), stimulation can cause dysarthria and tonic contraction of the contralateral muscles, especially those of the face and hand. Spread of the current to the posteromedial lemniscus region produces persistent contralateral upper- and lower-limb paresthesia that must be differentiated from the transient paresthesia induced by the increased current that lasts around 10 seconds. A sensation of nausea suggests a more medial trajectory, whereas ipsilateral monocular deviation of the eye and pupillary changes indicate the activation of oculomotor fibers. More anterior stimulation induces a uni- or bilateral sensation of heat, sweating, or mydriasis [34].

After implantation of the DBS lead, the macrostimulation test is repeated with a definitive lead with the same objectives of assessing clinical benefits and the occurrence of side effects. Often, the introduction of the DBS electrode reduces the patient's signs and symptoms before the start of the test stimulation. This is caused by the microlesion effect and probably related to mechanical disruption of the tissue due to the positioning of the electrode, a benefit similar to that seen in pallidotomy or thalamotomy.

The clinical benefit of intraoperative stimulation is evident in PD, because the patient stops the medication 6–12 hours before surgery. The appearance of dyskinesias during stimulation is indicative of a good antikinetic effect with chronic stimulation and good lead placement; consequently, a good result is achieved. This usually occurs in patients who present dyskinesia in response to levodopa and are usually contralateral to stimulation, but it can be ipsilateral or global [31].

The appearance of side effects from the stimulation of neighboring structures with low thresholds may limit the therapeutic efficacy of DBS lead. A more lateral trajectory demonstrates orofacial and appendicular contractions in addition to contraversive eye movement. A more medial trajectory may be evidenced by reduced clinical efficacy with no obvious side effects, only eye deviation caused by stimulation of oculomotor nerve fibers. Stimulation of the ventral STN or SNr may occasionally produce effects such as hypomania, anxiety, and pseudobulbar responses [30].

Optimal placement of the DBS electrode suppresses motor symptoms at low stimulation intensity and exhibits side effects at high stimulation intensity, allowing a good therapeutic window for the treatment of PD.

Internal Segment of the Globus Pallidus

The GPi is the target of DBS in PD and dystonia. The globus pallidus is a part of the lenticular nucleus. The external segment of the globus pallidus (GPe) forms the lateral and dorsal border of the GPi, the internal capsule forms the posteromedial border, and the optic tract forms the ventral border. The putamen is separated from the GPe by the external medullary lamina, and the GPe is separated from the GPi by the internal medullary lamina. Another lamina separates the external from the internal segment of the GPi. Each of these laminas is surrounded by cells called border cells that have a characteristic presentation in the MER and are important in the anatomical differentiation of the structures described above.

For PD and dystonia, the trajectory is directed to the motor region of the nucleus in the ventral and posterior regions of the GPi. In PD, this target is preferred when patients present with signs of cognitive changes. Typically, this trajectory passes through the striatum and the GPe before reaching the GPi. Usually, the recording begins 15–20 mm above the target in the putamen with the presence of spontaneous sparse activity at a frequency of 1–10 Hz. Between the putamen and the GPe lies in the first laminar layer, identified by the decrease in electrical activity associated with the presence of border cells. These cells exhibit a typical regular high amplitude firing with a frequency of 34 ± 19 Hz [22, 25, 26]. Entry into the GPe is marked by increased baseline activity associated with two types of cells. The Pausers cells have an irregular moderate- to high-amplitude firing with a frequency of 20–60 Hz and some periods of an asynchronous pause of hundreds of milliseconds. Burster cells are generally smaller than pauser cells and are identified by short high-frequency bursts. It is important to differentiate the burster cells from the X-cells that represent cell death caused by mechanical trauma, which are time-related and have high-frequency decreasing amplitude. The GPe exit is marked by a reduction in baseline activity, followed by border cells.

In PD, GPi entry is marked by increased baseline activity with a high density of neurons and two predominant classes of cells: tremor cells that fire at the patient's tremor and tonic regular high-frequency-firing cells (60–100 Hz) with few pauses compared to GPe. The GPi is subdivided into external and internal segments, both of which show similar cellular recording patterns; however, the GPIe shows lower cellularity. In the motor region of the nucleus, similar to what occurs in the STN, many cells respond to active and passive contralateral movements of the face and limbs. The motor region of the GPi is somatotopically organized with the representation of the dorsomedial leg and the ventrolateral arm [38].

In dystonia, the frequencies of Gpe and Gpi cells are similar, and differentiation is caused by reduced cell activity on the laminae and the detection of border cells.

At the bottom of the GPi, there was a decrease in baseline activity associated with the border cells followed by the optic tract. Photic stimulation delivered with the dark room evoked modulation of the baseline signal and cellular response at the frequency of stimulation (Fig. 33.6).

A typical GPi trajectory is 5–7 mm in length. More anterior trajectories pass through the optic tract, while more posterior trajectories are directed toward the

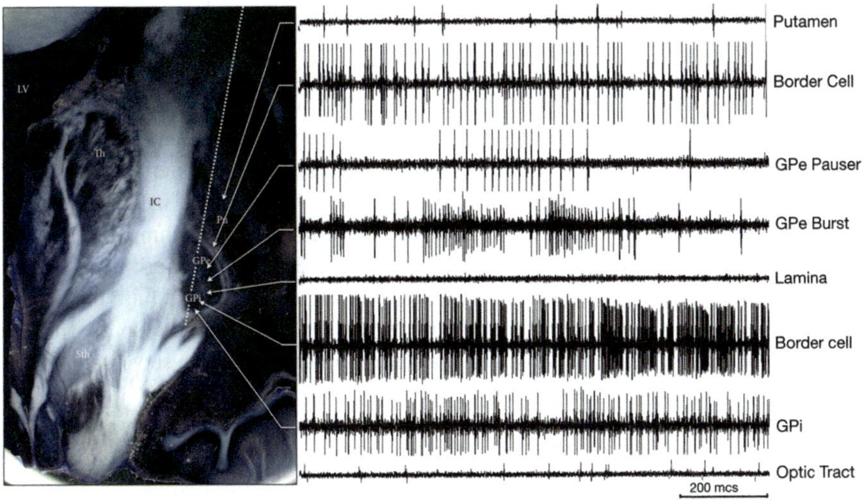

Fig. 33.6 Microelectrode mapping showing recording segments (on the right) obtained from sequential sites in the depth of striato-pallidal region following a routine trajectory (white inclined dotted line) from the putamen down to the GPi. Coronal section of human brain histologic preparation dyed with galocianine. Images given by Helmut Heinsen from São Paulo-Würzburg Electronic Atlas of the Human Brain [23]

internal capsule. Stimulation near the optic tract produces phosphenes, and stimulation near the internal capsule produces dysarthria and contralateral tonic contractions of the face and limbs. If stimulation with MER indicates a safe distance from the internal capsule and the optic tract, the DBS electrode is implanted.

Macrostimulation is performed to determine the thresholds for clinical and side effects. When motor symptoms are evident at low intensities, the electrode should be readjusted laterally and anteriorly. Side effects related to the optic tract are less frequent because of the safe distance from the optic tract, and usually, the most distal electrode is not stimulated.

Ventral Intermediate Nucleus

The Vim is a target for surgical treatment of tremor. The electrode is guided to the ventrolateral region of the thalamus, which is the motor area of the nucleus.

There is a well-defined physiological correlation between the motor and sensory nuclei of the thalamus, despite receiving afferents from distinct regions. The Vim receives afferents from the cerebellum, while the caudal ventral sensory nucleus (Vc) receives afferents from the spinothalamic and medial lemniscus. Understanding spatial and somatotopic organization is crucial, because electrode placement is guided to the homuncular region of the patient's tremor. The somatotopic organization of the Vim resembles onion shells in which activity related to the lower limbs is more external and usually found in the upper, lateral, and lower regions of the nucleus, and the face corresponds to the innermost area of the nucleus.

The MER usually begins at 15 mm above the target. In the dorsal region of the thalamus, neuronal activity tends to be sparse with low- and low-amplitude bursts. As the electrode reaches the more caudal regions, the voluntary activity is replaced by cells that passively fire for joint motion. The pathway may traverse the Voa and Vop nuclei, where tonic activity is found by contralateral active voluntary movement of the upper and lower extremities. Entry into Vim is accompanied by an increase in neuronal activity, and two types of cells are encountered: tremor cells and kinesthetic cells. The tremor cells have a rhythmic firing pattern with the tremor frequency, which can be synchronized with the electromyographic recording of the patient's tremor. Kinesthetic cells, typical of the Vim thalamus, are sensitive to muscle spindle activation and respond to movement [19].

Posterior to the Vim lies the Vc or sensory thalamus. Electrode entry into the Vc is marked by a shift of the baseline signal with the appearance of high-amplitude cells that are highly sensitive to light touch. With more anterior displacement within the Vc, neurons become more responsive to proprioception, as evidenced by joint capsule activation. Neurons at the Vim/Vc border exhibit a response to pressure from the arm and leg muscles. The Vc is used to guide the trajectory to the Vim, which is usually 2–3 mm anterior to it.

Once the boundary is identified, the kinesthetic evaluation is initiated to identify a mediolateral somatotopic correlation, since the somatotopy of the Vc and Vim nuclei are almost identical. If the purpose of the surgery is to control an upper-extremity tremor, the cells related to passive movement of the upper limb must be identified.

The DBS electrode is implanted in the region containing neurons with kinesthetic receptive fields at 2–4 mm anterior to the border of the sensory relay nucleus [22]. Often, insertion of the DBS electrode suppresses tremor. A shallow trajectory results in few contacts within the nucleus and lower electrode efficacy.

Evaluation of the side effects caused by stimulation is essential, and it is mandatory to obtain tremor suppression in the absence of sustained paresthesia. Very lateral trajectories activate corticobulbar and corticospinal fibers that cause contralateral tonic muscle contraction. Persistent paresthesia at low stimulation intensities indicates proximity to the Vc. High-intensity stimulation that does not suppress the tremor or induce paresthesia suggests an anterior trajectory. The presence of dysarthria suggests a medial trajectory.

Subthalamic Region and Fields of Forel

Although microrecording only provides data from neuronal activity recorded from the vicinity of the cell bodies, it is logical that this will only be useful in targets found in nuclear regions or with the gray matter. Targets located within the white matter consisting of connecting fibers usually do not benefit from MER. However, there are techniques that can be employed, recording from neighboring nuclei from a known

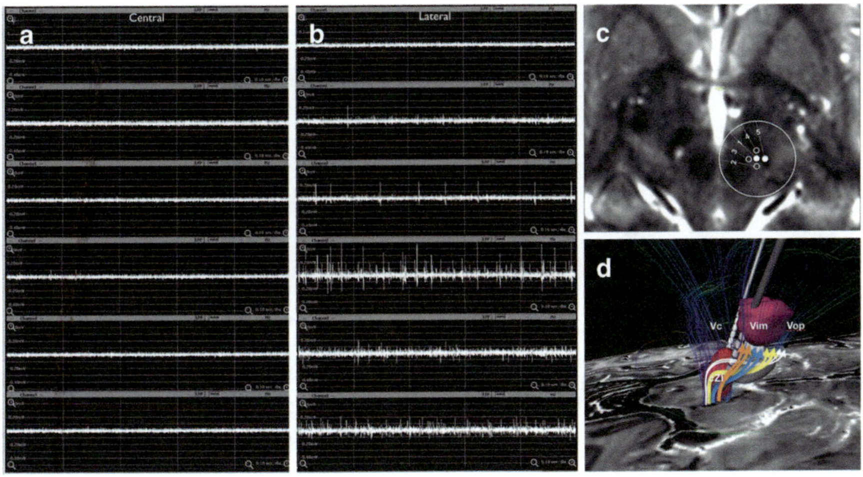

Fig. 33.7 (**a**, **b**) Center and lateral parallel MER tracks showing mostly physiological silence, what corroborates a region of fibers with roughly no cells, while in the neighboring channel which consisted by zona incerta followed by the subthalamic nucleus typical activity was recorded from the roof of the nucleus after (dorsal STN). (**c**) Illustrative image showing the axial T2 MRI with the target placed in the caudal zona incerta (cZI) with a scaled representation of the microdrive showing center and lateral channels being used. Electrode tip was placed in the center channel to treat tremor in the caudal zona incerta (cZI) coming from a trajectory from the Thalamus (Vim) [15, 20] (**d**) Lateral view of a 3D reconstruction of the subthalamic region including red nucleus (red), the subthalamic nucleus (gray) and the thalamic Vim (purple) showing a final location of the DBS lead implanted in the Vim in the same trajectory of posterior subthalamic area. Vc; ventrocaudal nucleus of thalamus, Vim; ventralis intermedius nucleus of thalamus, Vop; ventralis oralis posterior nucleus of thalamus, cZI; Caudal Zona incerta. White, yellow, orange and blue curved arrows illustrate the cerebellar input fiber into the thalamus. Images given by Erich Fonoff and Eduardo Alho from São Paulo-Würzburg Electronic Atlas of the Human Brain

distance from the target itself. This is the case for the targets in the Fields of Forel and other targets in the subthalamic region. Figure 33.7 shows the target placed in the caudal zona incerta (central channel of the microdrive); the corresponding microrecording remains mostly silent, which corroborates a region of fibers with small number of neurons, while in the neighboring channel, which consisted by zona incerta followed by the subthalamic nucleus typical, activity was recorded from the roof of the nucleus after (dorsal STN). Electrode was placed in the center channel.

Local Field Potential

Depth recordings in functional neurosurgery reveal that a change occurs in the rhythmic neuronal oscillatory activity in the structures that compose the CSPTC. These activities can be detected as LFP in the MER electrode or recorded directly from the DBS electrode [14].

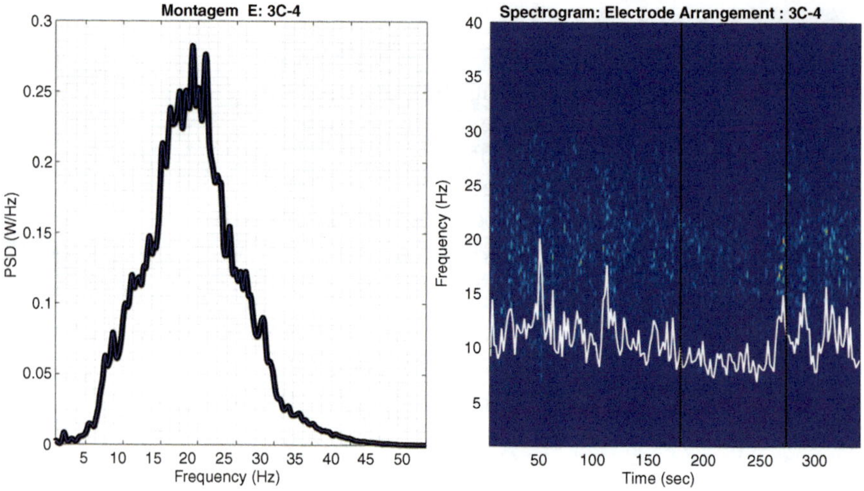

Fig. 33.8 Power spectral density (PSD) and spectrogram related to subthalamic nucleus local field potential in a Parkinson's disease surgery. In the spectrogram it is highlighted (by black bars) the patient moving hand where there is an amplitude suppression. Signal analysis developed by Jean Faber

The LFP represents the sum of extracellular potentials from multiple neurons and generates oscillatory brain activities that are divided into different frequency-based bands. The number of neurons recorded depends on the area of the recording electrode and the density of the cells around the electrode. Activity peaks at the beta frequency (13–30 Hz) are identified in the basal ganglia and motor cortex of PD patients and correlated with rigidity and bradykinesia (Fig. 33.8) [32].

In the model proposed by Brown [13], beta activity impairs motor function via an antikinetic effect and, on the other hand, oscillations in gamma frequency have been called prokinetic rhythms. In STN, the presence of beta activity is most evident in the dorsolateral sensory-motor area of the nucleus, which is the most effective region for DBS electrode implantation. In patients treated with L-dopa or those without PD, beta activity was not identified.

LFP has been used as a biomarker for target confirmation. Since these cells represent an aggregate of neurons, they are more resistant to physiological fluctuations and more easily compared by physicians and institutions, allowing standardization of the data analysis and interpretation. The LFP is a neurophysiological modality used in closed-loop therapy.

The use of DBS electrode contacts with better beta activity improves the efficacy of surgery treatment, because it interrupts these pathological oscillations and improves bradykinesia.

Conclusion

Electrophysiologic mapping is essential in movement disorder surgeries. The accurate definition of the borders and the identification of the sensory-motor region are fundamental for a better placement of the electrode in the target nucleus and consequent clinical improvement. The recent use of LFP improved the understanding of the functional patterns of the basal ganglia and their connections with the cortex, optimizing the use of DBS through closed-loop therapy.

Acknowledgments I am thankful for the knowledgeable inputs from Professor Helmut Heinsen, Dr. Eduardo Alho, Rodrigo Paul, and Jean Faber.

References

1. Abosch A, Timmermann L, Bartley S, et al. An international survey of deep brain stimulation procedural steps. Stereotact Funct Neurosurg. 2013;91:1–11. https://doi.org/10.1159/000343207.
2. Alexander GE, Crutcher MD, DeLong MR. Basal ganglia-thalamocortical circuits: parallel substrates for motor, oculomotor, "prefrontal" and "limbic" functions. Prog Brain Res. 1990;85:119–46.
3. Alexander GE, DeLong MR, Strick PL. Parallel organization of functionally segregated circuits linking basal ganglia and cortex. Annu Rev Neurosci. 1986;9:357–81. https://doi.org/10.1146/annurev.ne.09.030186.002041.
4. Alho EJL, Alho ATDL, Grinberg L, et al. High thickness histological sections as alternative to study the three-dimensional microscopic human sub-cortical neuroanatomy. Brain Struct Funct. 2018;223:1121–32. https://doi.org/10.1007/s00429-017-1548-2.
5. Alho EJL, Alho ATDL, Horn A, et al. The ansa subthalamica: a neglected fiber tract. Mov Disord. 2020;35:75–80. https://doi.org/10.1002/mds.27901.
6. Alho EJL, Fonoff ET, Di Lorenzo Alho AT, et al. Use of computational fluid dynamics for 3D fiber tract visualization on human high-thickness histological slices: histological mesh tractography. Brain Struct Funct. 2021;226:323–33. https://doi.org/10.1007/s00429-020-02187-3.
7. Bejjani BP, Dormont D, Pidoux B, et al. Bilateral subthalamic stimulation for Parkinson's disease by using three-dimensional stereotactic magnetic resonance imaging and electrophysiological guidance. J Neurosurg. 2000;92:615–25. https://doi.org/10.3171/jns.2000.92.4.0615.
8. Benabid AL, Koudsié A, Benazzouz A, et al. Deep brain stimulation of the corpus luysi (subthalamic nucleus) and other targets in Parkinson's disease. Extension to new indications such as dystonia and epilepsy. J Neurol. 2001;248:37–47. https://doi.org/10.1007/PL00007825.
9. Benabid AL, Krack PP, Benazzouz A, et al. Deep brain stimulation of the subthalamic nucleus for Parkinson's disease: methodologic aspects and clinical criteria. Neurology. 2000;55:S40–4.
10. Benazzouz A, Breit S, Koudsie A, et al. Intraoperative microrecordings of the subthalamic nucleus in Parkinson's disease. Mov Disord. 2002;17(Suppl 3):S145–9. https://doi.org/10.1002/mds.10156.
11. Bergman H, Wichmann T, Karmon B, DeLong MR. The primate subthalamic nucleus. II. Neuronal activity in the MPTP model of parkinsonism. J Neurophysiol. 1994;72:507–20. https://doi.org/10.1152/jn.1994.72.2.507.

12. Binder DK, Rau GM, Starr PA. Risk factors for hemorrhage during microelectrode-guided deep brain stimulator implantation for movement disorders. Neurosurgery. 2005;56:722–32; discussion 722–732. https://doi.org/10.1227/01.neu.0000156473.57196.7e.
13. Brown P. Bad oscillations in Parkinson's disease. J Neural Transm Suppl. 2006:27–30. https://doi.org/10.1007/978-3-211-45295-0_6.
14. Brown P, Williams D. Basal ganglia local field potential activity: character and functional significance in the human. Clin Neurophysiol. 2005;116:2510–9. https://doi.org/10.1016/j.clinph.2005.05.009.
15. Contreras Lopez WO, Azevedo AR, Cury RG, et al. Caudal zona incerta/VOP radiofrequency lesioning guided by combined stereotactic MRI and microelectrode recording for posttraumatic midbrain resting-kinetic tremor. World Neurosurg. 2016;86:316–20. https://doi.org/10.1016/j.wneu.2015.09.031.
16. Deep-Brain Stimulation for Parkinson's Disease Study Group, Obeso JA, Olanow CW, et al. Deep-brain stimulation of the subthalamic nucleus or the pars interna of the globus pallidus in Parkinson's disease. N Engl J Med. 2001;345:956–63. https://doi.org/10.1056/NEJMoa000827.
17. Florence G, Sameshima K, Fonoff ET, Hamani C. Deep brain stimulation: more complex than the inhibition of cells and excitation of fibers. Neuroscientist. 2016;22:332–45. https://doi.org/10.1177/1073858415591964.
18. Fonoff ET, Azevedo A, Angelos JSD, et al. Simultaneous bilateral stereotactic procedure for deep brain stimulation implants: a significant step for reducing operation time. J Neurosurg. 2016;125:85–9. https://doi.org/10.3171/2015.7.JNS151026.
19. Garonzik IM, Hua SE, Ohara S, Lenz FA. Intraoperative microelectrode and semi-microelectrode recording during the physiological localization of the thalamic nucleus ventral intermediate. Mov Disord. 2002;17(Suppl 3):S135–44. https://doi.org/10.1002/mds.10155.
20. Ghilardi MGDS, Ibarra M, Alho EJL, et al. Double-target DBS for essential tremor: 8-contact lead for cZI and Vim aligned in the same trajectory. Neurology. 2018;90:476–8. https://doi.org/10.1212/WNL.0000000000005076.
21. Gorgulho A, De Salles AAF, Frighetto L, Behnke E. Incidence of hemorrhage associated with electrophysiological studies performed using macroelectrodes and microelectrodes in functional neurosurgery. J Neurosurg. 2005;102:888–96. https://doi.org/10.3171/jns.2005.102.5.0888.
22. Gross RE, Krack P, Rodriguez-Oroz MC, et al. Electrophysiological mapping for the implantation of deep brain stimulators for Parkinson's disease and tremor. Mov Disord. 2006;21(Suppl 14):S259–83. https://doi.org/10.1002/mds.20960.
23. Hamani C, Florence G, Heinsen H, et al. Subthalamic nucleus deep brain stimulation: basic concepts and novel perspectives. eNeuro. 2017;4:ENEURO.0140-17.2017. https://doi.org/10.1523/ENEURO.0140-17.2017.
24. Hamani C, Saint-Cyr JA, Fraser J, et al. The subthalamic nucleus in the context of movement disorders. Brain. 2004;127:4–20. https://doi.org/10.1093/brain/awh029.
25. Hutchison WD, Allan RJ, Opitz H, et al. Neurophysiological identification of the subthalamic nucleus in surgery for Parkinson's disease. Ann Neurol. 1998;44:622–8. https://doi.org/10.1002/ana.410440407.
26. Hutchison WD, Lozano AM, Davis KD, et al. Differential neuronal activity in segments of globus pallidus in Parkinson's disease patients. Neuroreport. 1994;5:1533–7. https://doi.org/10.1097/00001756-199407000-00031.
27. Kaneoke Y, Vitek JL. Burst and oscillation as disparate neuronal properties. J Neurosci Methods. 1996;68:211–23. https://doi.org/10.1016/0165-0270(96)00081-7.
28. Khan MF, Mewes K, Gross RE, Škrinjar O. Assessment of brain shift related to deep brain stimulation surgery. Stereotact Funct Neurosurg. 2008;86:44–53. https://doi.org/10.1159/000108588.

29. Kinfe TM, Vesper J. The impact of multichannel microelectrode recording (MER) in deep brain stimulation of the basal ganglia. Acta Neurochir Suppl. 2013;117:27–33. https://doi.org/10.1007/978-3-7091-1482-7_5.
30. Koeglsperger T, Palleis C, Hell F, et al. Deep brain stimulation programming for movement disorders: current concepts and evidence-based strategies. Front Neurol. 2019. https://doi.org/10.3389/fneur.2019.00410.
31. Krack P, Fraix V, Mendes A, et al. Postoperative management of subthalamic nucleus stimulation for Parkinson's disease. Mov Disord. 2002;17(Suppl 3):S188–97. https://doi.org/10.1002/mds.10163.
32. Kühn AA, Tsui A, Aziz T, et al. Pathological synchronisation in the subthalamic nucleus of patients with Parkinson's disease relates to both bradykinesia and rigidity. Exp Neurol. 2009;215:380–7. https://doi.org/10.1016/j.expneurol.2008.11.008.
33. Obeso JA, Rodriguez-Oroz MC, Rodriguez M, et al. Pathophysiology of levodopa-induced dyskinesias in Parkinson's disease: problems with the current model. Ann Neurol. 2000;47:S22–32; discussion S32–34.
34. Pollak P, Krack P, Fraix V, et al. Intraoperative micro- and macrostimulation of the subthalamic nucleus in Parkinson's disease. Mov Disord. 2002;17:S155–61. https://doi.org/10.1002/mds.10158.
35. Rezai AR, Machado AG, Deogaonkar M, et al. Surgery for movement disorders. Neurosurgery. 2008;62:SHC809–39. https://doi.org/10.1227/01.neu.0000316285.52865.53.
36. Rodriguez-Oroz MC, Rodriguez M, Guridi J, et al. The subthalamic nucleus in Parkinson's disease: somatotopic organization and physiological characteristics. Brain. 2001;124:1777–90. https://doi.org/10.1093/brain/124.9.1777.
37. Sterio D, Zonenshayn M, Mogilner AY, et al. Neurophysiological refinement of subthalamic nucleus targeting. Neurosurgery. 2002;50:58–69. https://doi.org/10.1097/00006123-200201000-00012.
38. Vitek JL. Pathophysiology of dystonia: a neuronal model. Mov Disord. 2002;17(Suppl 3):S49–62. https://doi.org/10.1002/mds.10142.
39. Wichmann T, Bergman H, DeLong MR. The primate subthalamic nucleus. III. Changes in motor behavior and neuronal activity in the internal pallidum induced by subthalamic inactivation in the MPTP model of parkinsonism. J Neurophysiol. 1994;72:521–30. https://doi.org/10.1152/jn.1994.72.2.521.
40. Zrinzo L, Foltynie T, Limousin P, Hariz M. Image-guided and image-verified deep brain stimulation. Mov Disord. 2013;28:254–4. https://doi.org/10.1002/mds.25302.

Part XI
Special Topics

Chapter 34
IOM in Pelvic Floor: Gynecological and Urological Surgeries

Ricardo José Rodriguez Ferreira, Emília Caram Bordini, Guillermo Martín-Palomeque, Lidia Cabañes-Martinez, and Nucelio Luiz De Barros Moreira Lemos

Abbreviations

ANS	Autonomic nervous system
BCR	Bulbocavernous reflex
EAS	External anal sphincter
EMG	Electromyography
EMG-fr	Electromyography free-run
EMG-tg	Electromyography triggered
IAS	Internal anal sphincter
ICP	Intracavernous pressure
IONM	Intraoperative neurophysiological monitoring
IVP	Intravesical pressure

R. J. R. Ferreira (✉) · E. C. Bordini
AACD - Disabled Child Care Association, São Paulo, SP, Brazil

Dr Ricardo Ferreira Clinic, São Paulo, SP, Brazil

Spine Surgery Department at Orthopedics and Trauma Institute of Clinical Hospital of the University of São Paulo Medical School, São Paulo, SP, Brazil

G. Martín-Palomeque · L. Cabañes-Martinez
Clinical Neurophysiology, Hospital Ramón y Cajal, Madrid, Spain

N. L. D. B. M. Lemos
Gynecology Department, University of Toronto, Toronto, ON, Canada

S. M. Verst et al. (eds.), *Intraoperative Monitoring*,
https://doi.org/10.1007/978-3-030-95730-8_34

N	Nerve
SNS	Somatic nervous system
SSEP	Somatosensory-evoked potential
TcMEP	Transcranial motor-evoked potential
TIVA	Total intravenous anesthesia

Introduction

Since the early 1900s, radical hysterectomy for cervical cancer is advocated in order to increase survival rates [21]. However, it is associated with increased functional morbidity, like high rates of urinary retention, constipation, and sexual dysfunction [9, 34].

Radical laparoscopic resection of deeply infiltrating endometriosis has been related to similar sequelae since the 1990s. Although wide resection has promoted symptomatic relief for patients, it has been frequently related to autonomic nerves injury [28, 32], urinary symptoms, and rectal and sexual dysfunction [2, 5, 8, 11].

This scenario applies to urological surgeries, especially those related to prostate neoplasms, since wide and radical resections are related to high prevalence of urinary incontinence and erectile dysfunction. Currently, neural preservation has been considered a goal during these approaches.

In this context, intraoperative neurophysiology monitoring (IONM) emerged as an important adjuvant to map and monitor the main pelvic neural structures of somatic and autonomic nervous systems (ANS). Concerning the somatic nervous system, the main structure of interest is the *pudendal nerve*. In the case of the ANS, although the methods are continuously improving, there are still limitations and accuracy.

This chapter focuses on IONM during gynecological and urological pelvic floor surgeries.

Pelvic Floor Anatomy and Physiology

The pelvic floor is composed of muscles, ligaments, and fascia that act as a support for the bladder, reproductive organs, and rectum. This function is performed through ligaments, fascia, and muscles (Eickmeyer 2017). The pelvic floor muscles receive innervation through somatic, visceral, and central pathways.

The main somatic nerve of the pelvic floor is the pudendal nerve.

The main autonomic fibers are the hypogastric plexuses (sympathetic) and the pelvic splanchnic nerves (parasympathetic).

Thus, *the anorectal, urinary, and sexual functions are under mixed control, that is, autonomic and somatic.*

The *levator ani* muscle is the largest and strongest muscle of the pelvic floor and is innervated by the sacral nerve roots (S2–S5) (Fig. 34.1a–c). The striated urethral

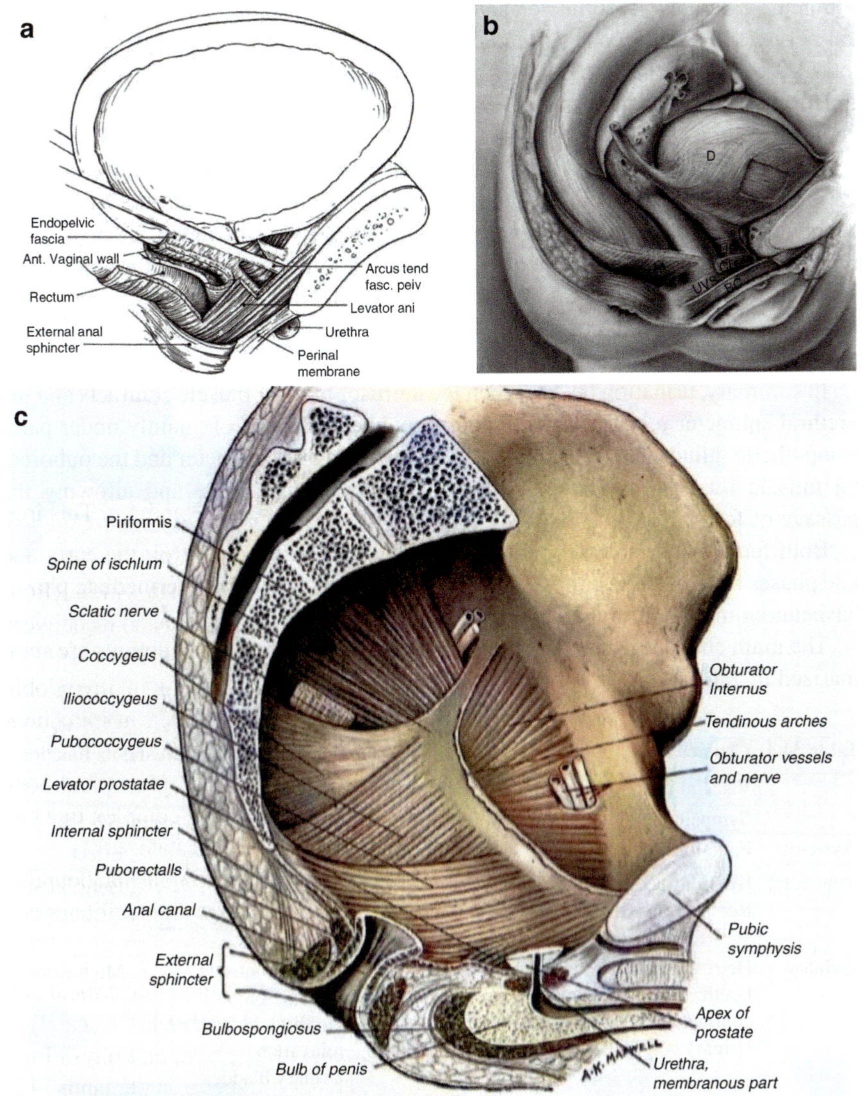

Fig. 34.1 Pelvic floor. (**a**) Lateral view of the components of the urethral support system. Note how the levator ani muscles support the rectum, vagina, and urethrovesical neck. Also note how the endopelvic fascia beside the urethra attaches to the levator ani muscle; contraction of the levator muscle leads to elevation of the urethrovesical neck. Puborectalis muscle is removed for clarity. (With permission from Ashton-Miller and DeLancey [1]). (**b**) Lateral view of urethral and pelvic floor muscular anatomy. BC denotes bulbocavernosus, CU compressor urethrae, D detrusor, LA levator ani, US urethral sphincter, UVS urethrovaginal sphincter. Puborectalis muscle is removed for clarity. (With permission from Ashton-Miller and DeLancey [1]). (**c**) Pelvic aspect of left levator ani and coccygeus. The superior gluteal vessels and nerve have been cut close to the upper border of piriformis, the anal canal has been divided below the anorectal flexure, and the greater part of the prostate has been removed. The constituent parts of the levator ani are shown. (Adapted from de Groat and Yoshimura [4], with permission)

sphincter, external anal sphincter, and perineal muscles are innervated by the pudendal nerve (somatic nervous system (SNS) [3]. The motor points of the pelvic floor muscles we use in our protocol are shown in Chap. 3 – (Pictures 3.49 and 3.50). The function of the pelvic floor muscles is to support the pelvic organs with coordination between contraction and relaxation.

The pelvic floor provides active support through a constant state of muscle contraction and passive support from the surrounding connective tissue and fascia. With an increase of the intra-abdominal pressure, the pelvic floor muscles reflexively contract with upward movement, closing the vagina and the urethral and anal sphincters. This action is important for maintaining continence. Pelvic floor relaxation, on the other hand, occurs only briefly and intermittently during normal urination and defecation processes (Eickmeyer 2017).

In summary, urination occurs when the detrusor bladder muscle contracts and the urethral sphincter relaxes, through autonomic nervous control, mainly under parasympathetic influences. Defecation occurs when the anal sphincter and the puborectal muscle relax simultaneously, opening the rectoanal angle and allowing the passage of feces.

Both female and male sexual responses are under mixed control: the early and late phases have somatic control by the pudendal nerve, and the intermediate phases have autonomic control, mainly by the parasympathetic.

The main characteristics of the innervation of the ANS and its functions are summarized in Table 34.1.

Table 34.1 Characteristics of the innervation of the autonomic nervous system and its functions

	Visceral innervation – functional effects			
	Sympathetic – thoracolumbar		Parasympathetic – sacral S2–SS	
Systems	Function	Effect	Function	Effect
Anorectal	IAS contraction Rectal relaxation/filling	Fecal continence	IAS relaxation Rectal mobility/emptying	Defecation
Urinary	Detrusor muscle relaxation Urethral–bladder neck contraction Urinary continence	Urinary continence	Detrusor muscle contraction Urethral–bladder neck relaxation Urinary bladder emptying	Micturition
Sexual	Bulbospongiosus muscle contraction	Ejaculation	Cavernous corpus filling secretion	Penile erection Lubrification

IAS internal anal sphincter

Pelvic Floor Surgeries and Neural Structures at Risk

Due to the complex anatomy that involves pelvic floor surgeries, the main structures at risk from a neurological point of view must be highlighted, as well as their division (somatic or autonomic). This differentiation is particularly important to guide the neurophysiological protocol to be adopted in each surgical procedure.

In summary, in pelvic floor surgeries, the neurological structures at risk are listed below; they are also show in Fig. 34.1a–c.

- Central pathways: somatic.
- Conus medullaris and cauda equina: somatic and autonomic.
- Sacral roots S1–S5: somatic and autonomic.
- Pudendal nerve (sensory branches: dorsal nerve of penis and clitoris; motor branches: perineal nerve and inferior rectus nerve): somatic.
- Hypogastric plexus (sympathetic fibers): autonomic.
- Splanchnic plexus (parasympathetic fibers): autonomic.
- Pelvic plexus, rectal plexus, bladder plexus, prostate plexus (mixed sympathetic and parasympathetic fibers): autonomic.

Of the structures mentioned, the pudendal nerve and its branches have less exposure in these surgeries, since its anatomical position, below the *levator ani* muscle, confers relative protection (Fig. 34.1a). The splanchnic and pelvic plexuses, as well as their branches to the bowel, bladder, and prostate, are the most vulnerable in open, laparoscopic, and robotic approaches (Fig. 34.2).

Intraoperative Pelvic Floor Neurophysiology

Neurophysiological evaluation in pelvic floor surgeries should be divided into tests for somatic nervous system or for ANS. They are summarized in Table 34.2.

Neurophysiological Tests: Somatic Nervous System

The main neurophysiological tests for evaluation of the SNS in pelvic floor surgeries are transcranial motor-evoked potentials (TcMEPs), somatosensory-evoked potentials (SSEPs), bulbocavernous reflex (BCR), free run and triggered electromyography (EMG).

Figure 34.3 shows a multimodal IOM for evaluation of the somatic nervous system with all the tests mentioned above.

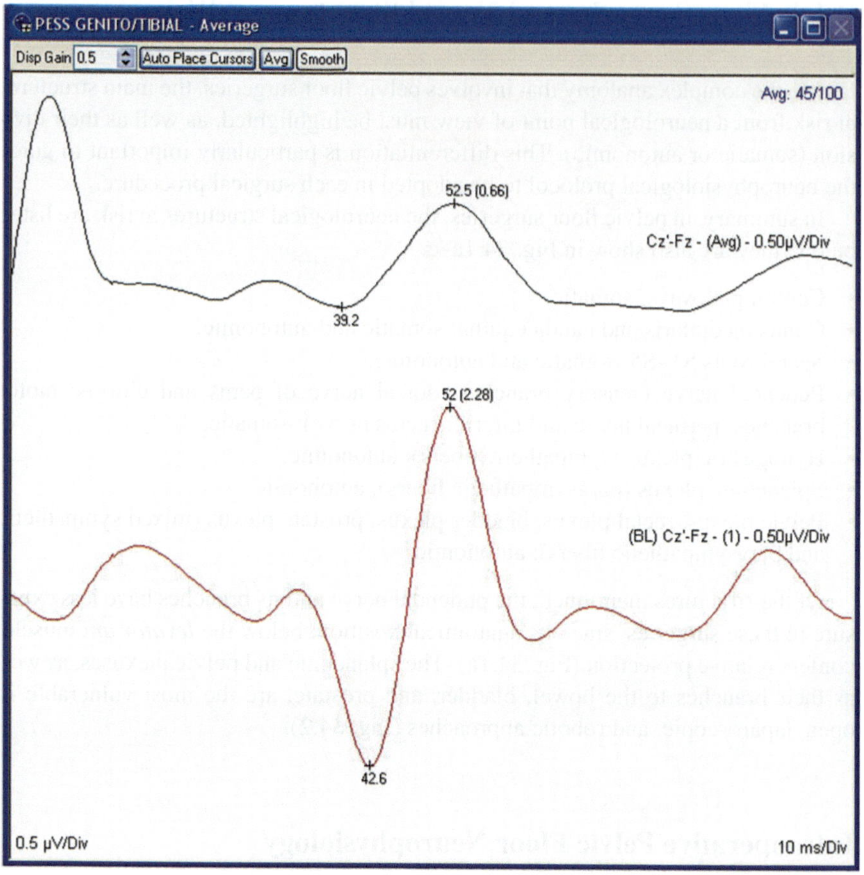

Fig. 34.2 Pudendal and tibial SSEP. SSEP recording Cz′/Fz. Upper trace: SSEP genitocortical – stimulation at dorsal nerve of the clitoris. Bottom trace: SSEP tibial nerve – stimulation at the ankle

Table 34.2 IOM tests during pelvic surgeries (Multimodal protocol)

INTRAOPERATIVE NEUROPHYSIOLOGICAL TESTS – MULTIMODAL PROTOCOL	
SOMATIC NERVOUS SYSTEM	**AUTONOMIC NERVOUS SYSTEM**
TcMEP	IVP – INTRA VESICAL PRESSURE
SSEP	ICP – INTRA CAVERNOUS PRESSURE
BCR – SOMATIC / SOMATIC	BCR – AUTONOMIC/SOMATIC
EMG – FREE RUN / TRIGGERED	IAS – EMG INTERNAL ANAL SPHINCTER

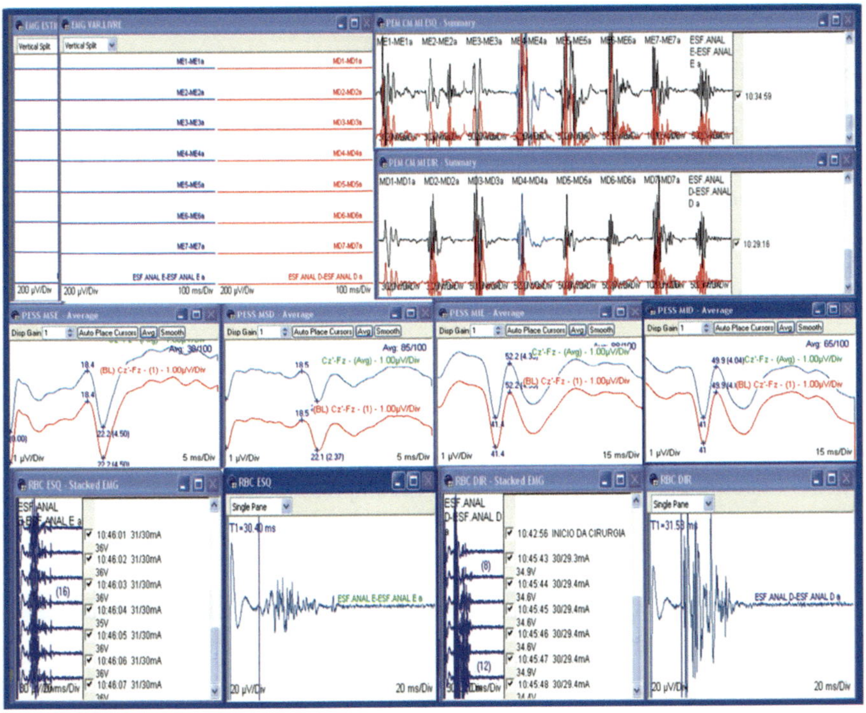

Fig. 34.3 Multimodal IOM of the SNS. Upper responses: EMG (free run and triggered); TcMEP. Middle responses: SSEP (ulnar and tibial nerves). Lower responses: BCR (Somatic-Somatic, responses of external anal sphincter)

TcMEP

TcMEP should *always* be performed in these surgeries, as it can continuously monitor the motor pathway, including motor roots, plexuses, and nerves at risk.

The myotomes suggested in our protocol, with their respective innervation, are as follows: *Cremaster/Labia Majora* (genitofemoral nerve (n)), *Adductor magnus* (obturator n.), *Iliopsoas* (femoral n.), *Quadriceps femoris* (femoral n.), *Tibialis anterior* (deep fibular n.), *Fibularis longus* (superficial fibular n.), *Gastrocnemius* (tibial n.), *Abductor hallucis* (medial plantar n.), external anal sphincter (EAS) (pudendal n.), *Transversalis perineum superficialis* (pudendal n.). Refer to Chap. 3 for anatomical atlas.

Electrodes should also be placed on the upper limbs as sentinels. We usually use the m. abductor digiti minimi (ulnar n.).

Whenever TcMEP is performed, the surgeon must be notified in order to remove the instruments (laparoscopic surgeries) or the robot blades (robotic surgeries).

The technique for TcMEP stimulation was described in Chap. 9.

SSEP

SSEP should be performed routinely, because it can continuously monitor the sensory function of peripheral nerves, roots, dorsal spine, and cerebral cortex.

We use SSEP of the tibial, ulnar, and pudendal nerves. Recording channels for pudendal nerve SSEPs are the same as the tibial n. (Cz′/Fz) (Fig. 34.2).

For technical details of SSEP, see Chap. 8.

BCR (Somatic-Somatic)

BCR is specifically important, because it can provide sensory and motor data about the pudendal nerve, one of the main neural structures involved in these procedures.

Additionally, initial BCR may diagnose the pre-existence of asymmetries or lack of responses. Final recordings document the maintenance, worsening, or improvement of neurological status after surgical decompression – Fig. 34.4.

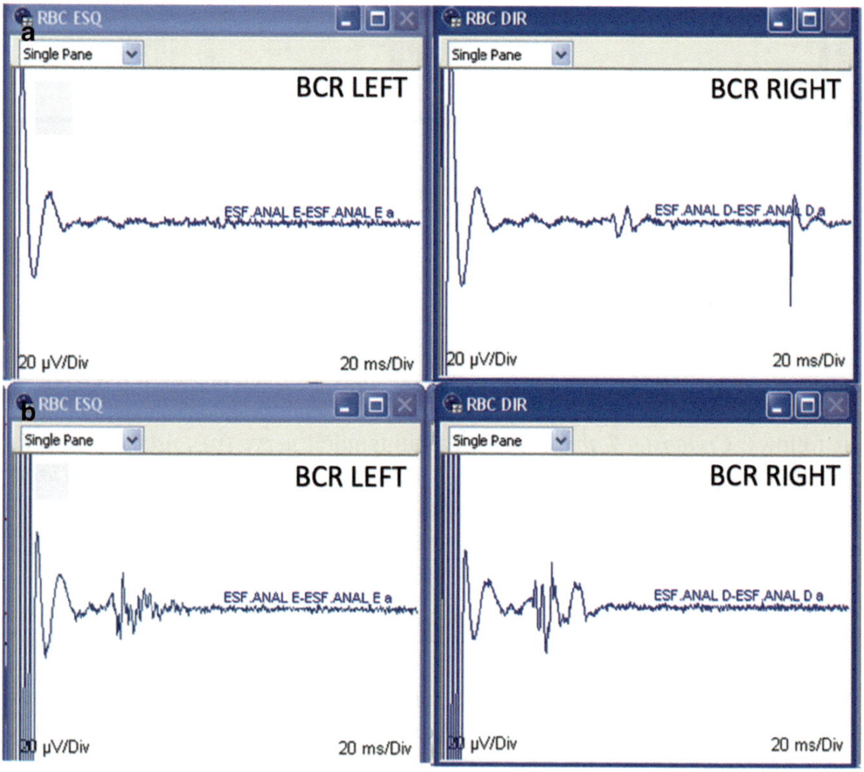

Fig. 34.4 External anal sphincter BCR. (**a**) Pre-decompression: absent responses. (**b**) After decompression: BCR was present, translating improvement of neurophysiological responses

BCR: Stimulation

The stimulation of the dorsal n. of the clitoris or dorsal n. of the penis is performed with the use of a pair electrodes, using needles for women (one at each side of the clitoris) and surface electrodes for men as shown in Fig. 34.5.

The stimulus is usually performed using a single pulse or train-of-four (inter-stimulus interval of 2 ms); duration of 500 μs; intensity of 40–60 mA.

Due to the anatomical proximity of the left and right branches of the dorsal n. of the clitoris, it may be difficult to individualize the stimulation. Nevertheless, in our protocol, the side differentiation is made by the recording responses: left or right perineum and external anal sphincter.

BCR: Recording

BCR is recorded with electrodes placed in the right and left EAS and superficial transverse muscles of the perineum [*Cabañes and Martín-Palomeque – unpublished data*]. The double-recording technique is important to evaluate two branches of the pudendal nerve: inferior rectal n. and perineal n.– Fig. 34.6. Thus, it enables the

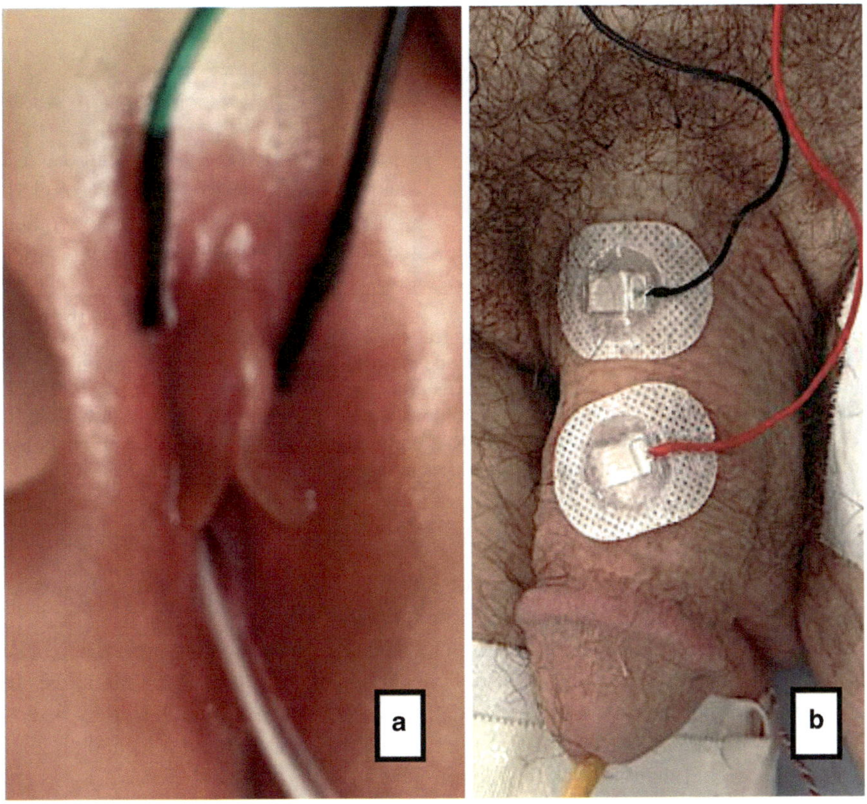

Fig. 34.5 Electrode's placement BCR for stimulation. (**a**) Dorsal nerve of the clitoris. (**b**) Dorsal nerve of the penis

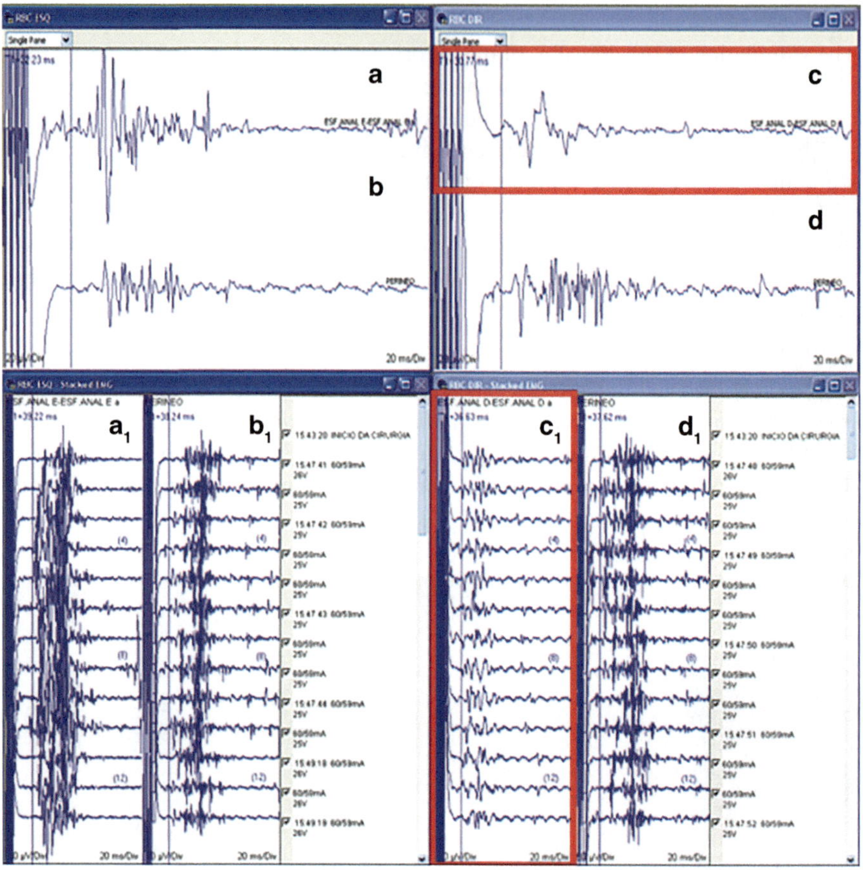

Fig. 34.6 BCR responses – double recording technique. The figure shows BCR responses of the external anal sphincter (upper traces **a** and **c**), and perineal (bottom traces **b** and **d**), distinguishing the pudendal nerve into its branches: inferior rectal nerve and perineal nerve. **a** and **b**: Left BCR single responses; **c** and **d**: Right BCR single responses. **a1** and **b1**: Left BCR waterfalls responses; **c1** and **d1**: Right BCR waterfalls responses. **Red rectangle**: reduced amplitude and asymmetrical responses in the right external anal sphincter branch, validating the diagnosis of exclusive involvement of this branch

DIAGNOSIS of selective impairment of one of the branches. This is especially important in patients with pudendal nerve entrapment.

The positioning of the EAS needle electrodes is of particular importance. The insertion and fixation must be carefully checked, since it is one of the main tests in this surgical approach. It is recommended to selectively record each side by inserting a pair of needles on the left (analog clock position at 1 h and 5 h) and another pair on the right (analog clock position at 7 h and 11 h) – Fig. 34.7.

BCR parameters to be evaluated are latency, amplitude, and duration. Normal latency values range between 30 and 40 ms. Amplitude and duration should be compared side by side, mainly to consider the symmetry of the response – Fig. 34.8.

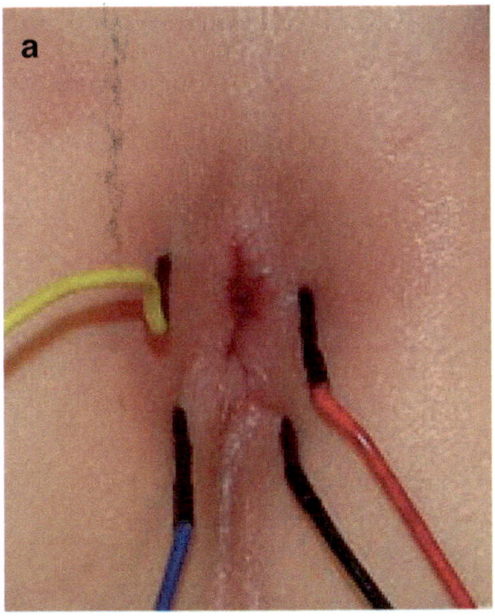

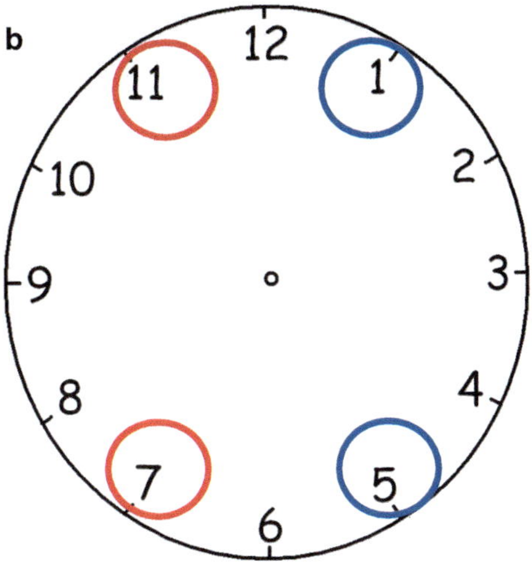

Fig. 34.7 Placement of electrodes – external anal sphincter. (**a**) Needle electrodes placed in external anal sphincter following the analog clock positioning. (**b**) Analog clock for comparison showing right (red circles: 11 h and 7 h) and left (blue circles: 1 h and 5 h) positions

Free-Run EMG

Free-run EMG is used for continuous monitoring, since it provides real-time information of roots and nerves. The assessment includes the same myotomes as the TcMEP.

Free-run EMG may show neurotonic discharges during direct or indirect manipulation (traction), which should be reported to the surgical team. These events must be evaluated by more frequently performed TcMEP.

EMG Triggered

EMG triggered remains in these surgeries as an important tool for mapping the somatic neural structures of the intraoperative field; in laparoscopic surgeries, this test can be considered *essential*, since visualization is more difficult in this approach, making the mapping fundamental for the correct identification of the structures. The myotomes are the same as above mentioned.

Stimulation may be done with a monopolar or bipolar stimulator probe – our preference is for the bipolar stimulator. Due to the characteristics of the procedure, the stimulator must be longer than usual: usually, a 40-cm long stimulating probe should be used. This length enables the mapping during any type of the surgical approach (open, laparoscopic, and robotic).

Usually, the differentiation of the S2 and S3/S4 roots is of particular importance. This distinction can be made based on the responses obtained, as shown in Fig. 34.9:

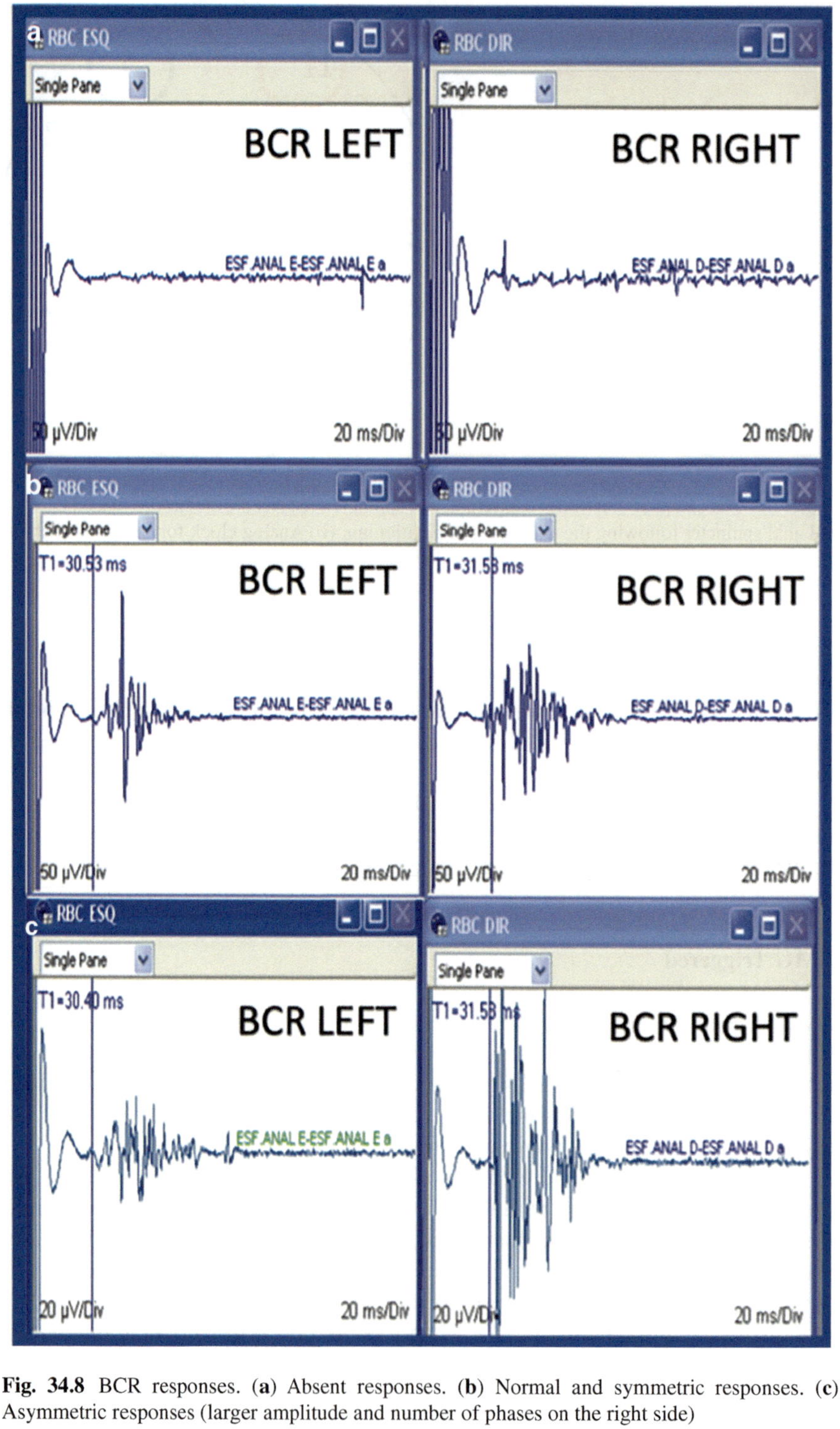

Fig. 34.8 BCR responses. (**a**) Absent responses. (**b**) Normal and symmetric responses. (**c**) Asymmetric responses (larger amplitude and number of phases on the right side)

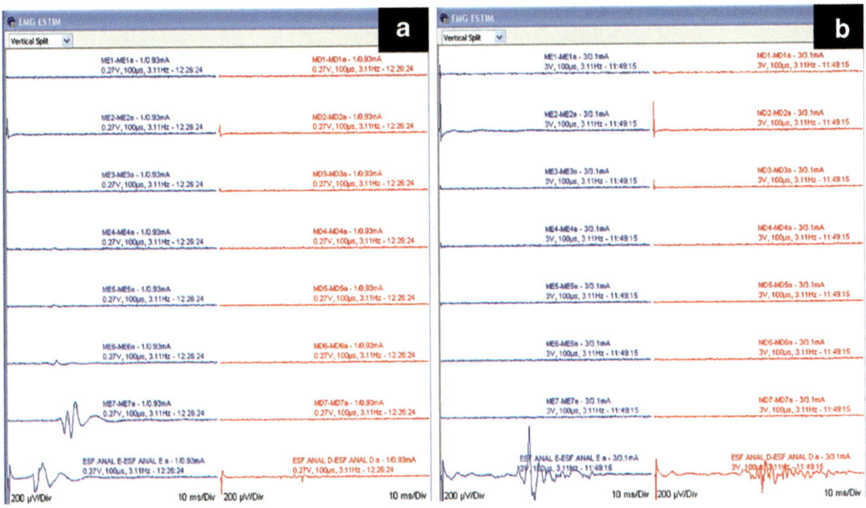

Fig. 34.9 EMG-triggered responses. (**a**) S2 responses: abductor hallux and external anal sphincter; (**b**) S3/S4 responses: responses present only in the external anal sphincter. Blue: left; Red: right. *Myotomes: 1 – Cremaster/Labia Majora. 2 – Iliopsoas. 3 – Quadriceps femoris. 4 – Tibialis anterior. 5 – Fibularis longus. 6 – Gastrocnemius. 7 – Abductor hallux. 8 – External anal sphincter*

- S3/S4 roots: responses present *only* in the anal sphincter.
- S2 root: responses present in abductor hallux (with or without response in anal sphincter).

Neurophysiological Tests: Autonomic Nervous System

Stimulation of the fibers of the ANS results in more variable responses of longer latencies than that elicited for SNS. Additionally, there is no recording of muscle contraction, but rather of the changes of intravesical/intracavernous pressure. Thus, conventional IOM techniques are not suitable for this purpose.

When parasympathetic nervous system stimulation is performed, the effects observed will be (a) increased intravesical pressure, due to contraction of the detrusor bladder muscle; (b) increased intracavernous pressure, due to relaxation of the smooth muscles and filling of the corpus cavernosum.

These pressure changes can be registered with a pressure transducer, and their main limitation is that they are not continuously monitored, that is, *they can only be mapped*. Mapping is an intermittent act that depends on surgeon's participation, while monitoring can be continuously performed by the neurophysiologist, enabling the identification of risky events in time to start a recovery maneuver.

In terms of anesthesia, although some studies suggest the possibility of using inhaled agents, in our practice, we use only TIVA, because it is related to more stable and reproducible responses.

Intravesical Pressure (IVP)

A three-way Foley catheter system is used, connected to a pressure transducer attached to a properly calibrated cystomanometer. This equipment measures and records the pressure variations after intraoperative parasympathetic stimulation and the consequent contraction of the detrusor muscle.

The preparation for the test should be done by emptying the urinary bladder and then filling it with 300–400 ml of saline solution. This step is important, because complete bladder filling allows a more sensitive recording of the small variations in detrusor muscle contraction, avoiding false negatives.

The stimulation is performed in the parasympathetic plexus, with a bipolar stimulator probe with a minimum length of 40 cm, as previously mentioned (section "EMG Triggered"). The stimulation protocol is continuous stimulation for 30 s, with a frequency of 30 Hz, duration of 0.2 ms or 200 μs, and intensity of 10–20 mA.

The test is considered positive; that is, there is direct stimulation of the parasympathetic neural pathways, demonstrating their integrity, when the threshold of 4 cm of H_2O is reached within 20 s – Fig. 34.10. If after 30 s of stimulation, there is no change in pressure, or changes that do not reach 4 cm of H_2O, the stimulation is considered negative. In the latter case (negative test), there are three possible

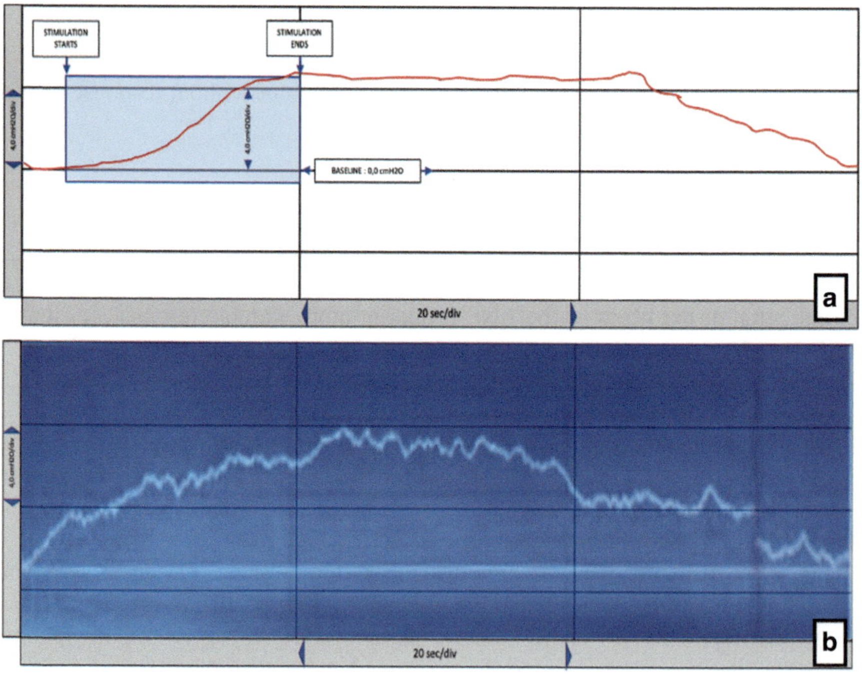

Fig. 34.10 Intravesical and intracavernous pressure. (**a**) Scheme of a positive mapping: increase in the pressure over 4 cm of H_2O in less than 20 s. (**b**) Real case of IVP changes during a neurovascular bundle mapping in a prostatectomy surgery

interpretations: (1) there was no precise localization of the parasympathetic neural structures, (2) there is a lesion in this neural pathway, or (3) inadequate setting/preparation for the test (false negative).

To avoid false results, complete bladder filling prior to testing, and accurate stimulation protocol should be applied.

Intracavernous Pressure (ICP)

A system consisting of a catheter, pressure transducer, and a 19G–23G butterfly needle is used. In our protocol, we use the 19-gauge (19G) butterfly needle.

The system is prepared by completely filling the catheter ports (transducer and butterfly) with saline solution. The butterfly needle is inserted into one of the corpora cavernosa and attached to suitable equipment for the analysis of pressure variations. Since the two corpus cavernosum are interconnected, there is no distinction between right and left. To check if the system is working, the penis must be manually compressed while monitoring changes in the recorded pressures. The stimulation may be carried out after testing the system.

The stimulation and the protocol for response analysis are done in the same way as described in the section "Intravesical Pressure (IVP)" – Fig. 34.10.

Bulbocavernosus Reflex (BCR) [Autonomic-Somatic]

BCR is usually performed through the somatic fibers, as mentioned above. However, it can also evaluate the sympathetic nervous system, with the stimulation of the internal urethral sphincter. This way, the afferent pathways are the fibers of the sympathetic nervous system, and the efference is somatic, via the pudendal nerve.

The stimulation is performed with urethral catheter electrode built in a Foley catheter and the recording is the external anal sphincter.

The main difference between the two BCR responses (Somatic-Somatic vs. Autonomic-Somatic) is the *latency*. In the Autonomic-Somatic BCR, the latency is longer, around 60–65 ms. The major limitation of this technique is the possibility that intraurethral stimulation may spread to the dorsal nerve of the clitoris or the dorsal nerve of the penis, with consequent recording of double responses.

EMG: Internal Anal Sphincter (IAS)

EMG of the internal anal sphincter is one of the methods used to check anal function. The IAS is situated between the rectal canal and the external anal sphincter (EAS) and is innervated exclusively by the autonomic nervous system, through parasympathetic and sympathetic fibers. For this reason, the control of the IAS is totally involuntary. Under physiological conditions, it remains constantly contracted (sympathetic tone) and presents relaxation (parasympathetic) only with the stimulus of the arrival of the fecal bolus. Thus, parasympathetic stimulation should show up in the EMG recordings as an interruption of the contraction (relaxation).

A dual assessment protocol with the same stimulus is possible by performing stimulation of the parasympathetic nerves and recording through the IAS-EMG channel and the cystomanometry [17, 19].

However, in our protocol, we did not use the IAS-EMG test, due to the possibility of false result by interference of EAS contraction. It is a confounding factor even with the use of teflon or coaxial EMG needles placed transanally under endosonographic guidance.

Protocol: IOM in Gynecological Surgeries

The main surgeries involving the gynecological pelvic floor are endometriosis, gynecological or lumbosacral plexus tumors, radical hysterectomy in cervical cancer, pudendal nerve entrapment, neuromodulation catheter implantation, or analgesic infusion catheter. These surgeries may be open, laparoscopic, or robotic.

IOM in these surgeries is performed using the following tests: (1) TcMEP, (2) SSEP, (3) EMG (free run and triggered), (4) BCR (Somatic-Somatic and Autonomic-Somatic).

A practical approach with a step-by-step protocol for the neurophysiologist is given below.

In these surgeries, we do not routinely perform mapping, through direct stimulation of the hypogastric plexus (sympathetic nervous system). As a monitoring test of the autonomic nervous system, the BCR Autonomic-Somatic can be used in this surgery.

Step-by-Step Setting Protocol: Gynecological Surgery

A. *Preoperative*

- Anesthesia: Prepare the patient as mentioned in the previous chapters. Use preferentially TIVA and perform bite-block protection after intubation.
- Urethral catheterization (Foley catheter) must be done *before* the insertion of the electrodes in the clitoris, perineum, and anal sphincter region. This prevents accidental displacement of the electrodes. In addition, the placement of the electrodes in this region should preferably be done under sterile conditions, after appropriate degerming, by a trained neurophysiologist, especially in cases where there is associated uterine manipulation.

- *Positioning of the electrodes for recording.*
  The electrodes should be placed on the myotomes as described above (section "TcMEP"). The placement of the EAS electrodes should be done carefully as mentioned in section "BCR (Somatic-Somatic)".
  Electrodes should also be placed on the upper limbs as sentinel.
- *Positioning electrodes for stimulation:*
  Lower limbs: electrodes for tibial nerves SSEP.
  Upper limbs: electrodes for ulnar nerves SSEP (sentinel).
  Clitoris: electrodes on the dorsal nerve of the clitoris for BCR and SSEP of the pudendal nerve (Fig. 34.5).
- *Anode electrode positioning* (for the intraoperative stimulation phase by the surgeon when using a monopolar stimulator probe): surface electrode on the portion of the *Quadratus lumborum*, ipsilateral to the surgical approach.
- *Positioning of the corkscrew electrodes on the scalp:* Electrodes are placed according to 10–20 EEG guidelines for TcMEP and SSEP.

IOM Sequence After Baselines of Tc-MEP, SSEP, BCR, EMG

B. *Intraoperative*

- *Mapping* of neural structures with a monopolar or bipolar stimulating probe, held by the surgeon (triggered EMG).
- *Monitoring:*
- perform Tc-MEP, SSEP, and BCR intermittently.
- EMG free run: In these surgeries, transient genitofemoral and/or obturator nerve retraction may be required. The free run EMG may demonstrate neurotonic discharges during direct or indirect manipulation (traction). They should be reported to the team, and if they are frequent or long lasting, TcMEP should be performed more frequently, which could identify reduced amplitude in the responses of the labia majora/ adductor muscles compared to baselines.

The abovementioned tests cited should be done intermittently in order to continuously monitor the structures at risk. In pudendal entrapment surgeries, control with TcMEP and BCR should be done immediately after release. In patients under general anesthesia, the phenomenon of BCR accommodation does not occur. Thus, a BCR amplitude deterioration or loss of response should be immediately communicated to the surgical team, as they are usually a true positive event. It may lead to interruption of the surgery.

Protocol: IOM in Urologic Surgeries

Among the pelvic floor urological surgeries, the most important is the *prostatectomy*. In this section, we discuss open, laparoscopic, and robotic prostatectomy approaches, which pose risks to both the somatic and autonomic nervous systems. Thus, multimodal IOM should *always* be performed. Yet, from a neurological point of view, one of the main objectives in this surgery is to preserve the autonomic functions – erection and urination. In this context, the correct *mapping* of the ANS stands out as one of the main concerns. It is noteworthy that there is not yet an adequate technique to maintain continuous *monitoring* of the ANS.

IOM uses the following tests: (1) TcMEP, (2) SSEP, (3) EMG (free run and triggered), (4) BCR (Somatic-Somatic and Autonomic-Somatic), (5) IVP – intravesical pressure (cystomanometry), (6) ICP – intracavernous pressure, (7) IAS-EMG (we do not use it in our practice – as mentioned before). Technical details have been mentioned in previous sections of this chapter.

The main particularity in prostate surgeries is the mapping of the neurovascular bundle in the periphery of the prostate [6, 16]; this will be issued below with a specific stimulation protocol. Of note, the anatomy of the neurovascular bundle presents large anatomical variations.

Stimulation Protocol (Martín-Palomeque [26] *– Ramon y Cajal Protocol)*

The responses to these stimuli can be analyzed in the ICP and IVP tests.

The stimulus protocol is as previously mentioned (continuous stimuli for 30 s, with a frequency of 30 Hz, duration of 0.2 ms, and intensity of 10–20 mA), using a bipolar stimulation probe of 40 cm. The stimulation sites for adequate mapping are performed considering the prostate as a sphere, subdivided into base, middle, and apex, right and left – Fig. 34.11a.

As shown in Fig. 34.11b, stimulation is executed following an analog clock scheme. Epidemiologically, the highest concentration of fibers in the neurovascular bundle is found at the base of the prostate, in its rectal portion [6]. The approach performed in surgeries for prostatectomy as well as the anatomical position of the prostate and the periprostatic neurovascular bundle are shown in Fig. 34.12.

Stimulation sites:

(a) Base of prostate, right side
(b) Right neurovascular bundle
(c) Right prostatic apex
(d) Base of the prostate, left side
(e) Left neurovascular bundle
(f) Left prostatic apex

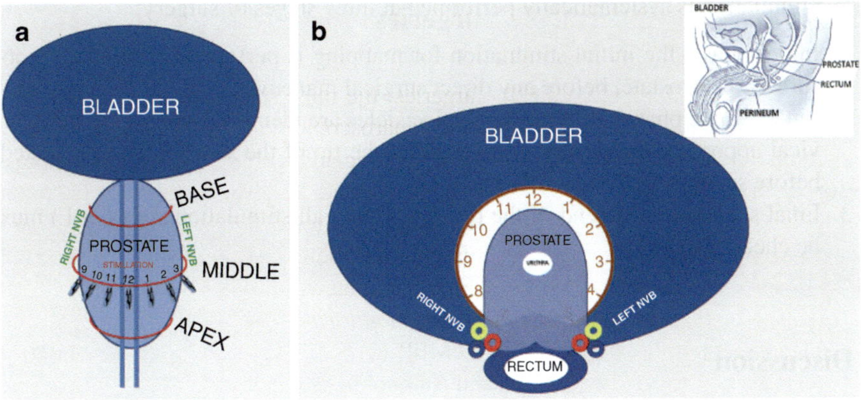

Fig. 34.11 Prostate neurovascular bundle mapping scheme. (**a**) Coronal view of the prostate with stimulation sites. (**b**) Axial view of the prostate with the neurovascular bundle and comparison with the analog clock for stimulation. NVB neurovascular bundle

Fig. 34.12 Anatomical schematic of the prostate: surgical access routes (red arrows) and their relationships with the neurovascular bundle, fascia, and rectum. (Reprinted with permission from Stolzenburg et al. [35])

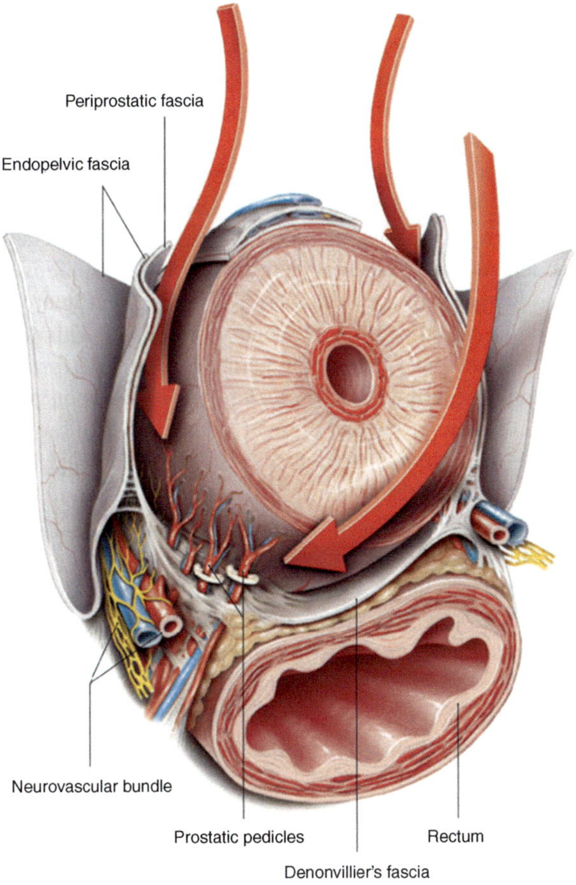

Stimulation is systematically performed at three stages of surgery:

1. Initial phase: the initial stimulation for mapping is performed soon after exposure of the prostate, before any direct surgical maneuver.
2. Intermediate phase: once the seminal vesicles are identified and after a transcervical approach, the plexuses surrounding the tip of the vesicles are stimulated, before sectioning the vascular pedicles.
3. Final stage: after the end of the prostatectomy, all stimulation sites (A–F) must be checked again.

Discussion

IOM in Gynecological Pelvic Floor Surgeries

Surgeries to treat cervical cancer, total hysterectomy, radical resection of deeply infiltrated endometriosis, and pudendal nerve entrapment may damage somatic and autonomic nervous systems, negatively affecting bladder, rectal, and sexual functions (vaginal lubrication and edema) [2, 5, 8, 11, 23, 24]. The neural structures that may be damaged are the pelvic sympathetic and parasympathetic neural pathways – superior hypogastric plexus, hypogastric nerves, pelvic splanchnic nerves, and inferior (pelvic) hypogastric plexus.

Japanese gynecologists were the first to describe a technique for cervical cancer surgery with nerve sparing in the 1960s [10] and years later, this concept was introduced in Europe by other groups [13, 14, 29, 37]. They created the so-called LANN (Laparoscopic Neuronavigation) technique, which is based on the use of neural tissue mapping in the intraoperative field, direct neurostimulation, and identification and dissection of intrapelvic nerves [30, 31]. This technique should be recognized as a precursor of the current neural mapping performed with triggered EMG. In the original described LANN technique, sacral roots were stimulated with a bipolar laparoscopic probe and clinical visualization of motor responses (such as leg, foot, finger, and gluteus movements) was necessary [23, 31].

Currently, preservation of function, reduction of morbidity, and quality of life are pursued goals. In this sense, the LANN technique associated with a multimodal IOM promotes a safe and accurate identification of the sacral roots. This avoids an imprecise and unreliable analysis based solely on clinical patient movements. Hence, the responses recorded after triggered EMG do not always correspond to the clinically detectable movements, which highlights that the neurophysiological method is more sensitive. Multimodal IOM includes continuous free run EMG, which is an ongoing technique that can detect depolarizations arising from neural manipulation or traction, without the need of stimulation. It enlarges the assessment of the integrity of the sacral roots and pudendal nerve by allowing their monitoring through Tc-MEP, SSEP, and BCR testing. If any of these responses change, the surgeon can be alerted and may lead to possible changes in the surgical approach strategy.

IOM in Pelvic Floor Surgeries: Urologic

Prostate cancer is the most frequently diagnosed type of cancer among men, frequently leading to radical prostatectomy, with a 10-year survival rate approaching 90% [27]. The occurrence of urinary incontinence and erectile dysfunction remains a significant problem [18, 20, 27]. Koehler et al. [20] report that the percentage of postoperative erectile dysfunction ranges from 12% to 83%, depending on the surgical technique used, patient age, clinical factors (intercurrent diseases such as diabetes), presurgical erectile function, and other social factors. Such complications cause great impact on the quality of life, since survival rates are excellent.

In a pioneering collaboration between surgeons and pathologists, it was Walsh and Donker (1982) who identified the anatomical course of the neurovascular bundles that supposedly contain the cavernous nerves. Later, Walsh et al. [39], Walsh and Schlegel [38] extrapolated these findings to describe a surgical technique that attempted to respect these nerve structures in radical prostatectomy procedures. Sexual potency could be fully preserved in 74–83% of his patients using his technique (depending on the type and extent of surgery).

Following this context, Lue et al. [25] demonstrated that the cavernous nerves could be stimulated electrically, causing erection. Yet, the mapping was not accurate, that is, the stimulation resulted in electrical spread; therefore, it was not possible to precisely locate the course of the nerve fibers. Later, to facilitate the proposed stimulation technique, a device was developed to simultaneously stimulate the cavernous nerves and measure penile tumescence, with a ring connected to a pressure transducer – the so-called CaverMap. At an early stage, results looked positive: in the case series by Walsh et al. [40], stimulation with the CaverMap demonstrated a sensitivity of 87.8% and specificity of 54% in localizing the neurovascular bundle. In this series, 71–78% of patients maintained sexual potency at the 12-month postoperative follow-up.

However, despite these apparently positive initial results, Holzbeierlein et al. [15] concluded that CaverMap did not provide adequate mapping of the cavernous nerves. They reported that positive responses did not necessarily correlate with the precise anatomical location of the cavernous nerves, since (a) they could be observed by stimulating at sites remote to the nerves and (b) changes in penile tumescence occurred as a consequence of anesthesia, medications, surgical manipulation, and other factors.

Rehman et al. [33] and Terada et al. [36] described methods using pressure changes in the corpora cavernosa after autonomic nerve fiber stimulation. The authors concluded that ICP through stimulation of the NVB is a simple, reproducible, and reliable method of assessing cavernous nerve preservation. In Terada's [36] case series, it was possible to map the cavernous nerves positively in 91% of patients.

More recent studies, such as the review conducted by Matthew in 2005, which evaluated data from papers published from 1996 to 2004, indicated that rates of erectile dysfunction after radical prostatectomy could range from 25% to 75%. He pointed out that approximately 60% of those patients reported emotional distress related to sexual dysfunction.

In the series by Martín-Palomeque et al. [26], 91.6% of the evaluated patients showed positive responses after stimulation: positivity as a change in ICP at 4 cm H_2O. Thus, also in this study, ICP was shown to be effective as a mapping technique.

Given these data, the need for a more precise neurological evaluation during prostatectomy surgeries arises.

Limitations

All the techniques mentioned for evaluating the ANS still have limitations. Specifically, they are mapping techniques that may localize nerve structures, but do not monitor them continuously. The preoperative status of the patients regarding age, erectile dysfunction, urinary incontinence, and the presence of comorbidities such as diabetes and polyneuropathy, and the extent of the prostate tumor may negatively impact the outcome.

An additional limitation is the anatomical variability of the neural structures. The authors Espinosa-Medina et al. [7] even arouse questions on the attributed functions and anatomical location of the sympathetic and parasympathetic nervous system, which have been considered sedimented in the literature, since the works of Gaskell [12] and Langley [22].

The results of Martín-Palomeque et al. [26], although considered preliminary, robustly (about 91%) demonstrated the possibility of mapping and localizing neurovascular bundle.

Conclusion

In pelvic floor surgeries, there is a complex and intricate nervous system accompanying the pelvic viscera, with sympathetic and parasympathetic plexuses and nerves, along with the somatic nervous system.

Nerve lesions can cause neurological dysfunction and lead to serious functional impairment of activities of daily living, including urinary and fecal incontinence, and sexual impairment (male and female).

IOM protocols are quite similar to those used in other medical specialties. However, there are fundamental particularities (especially concerning BCR), and the association with specific methods, such as cystomanometry, intracavernous pressure, and assessment of the internal anal sphincter.

In gynecological pelvic floor surgeries, the hypogastric (sympathetic) plexus is one the most important structures at risk. Yet, there is as no safe and reliable technique for its mapping. Luckily, it is usually easily detectable in macroanotomy.

Multimodal IOM can reliably evaluate the somatic nervous system, by mapping with triggered EMG and monitoring through EMG-fr, TcMEP, SSEP, and BCR, hence improving its preservation.

Urological pelvic floor surgeries (prostatectomy) are still a great challenge for neurophysiology, since the autonomic nervous system depends on the mapping of the neurovascular bundle. Some of the described techniques present satisfactory results regarding mapping. Yet, the impossibility of performing continuous monitoring of the structures at risk may negatively impact the outcome. For this reason, the use of multimodal IOM, with continuous monitoring of the pudendal nerve (BCR, free run EMG, SSEP, and TcMEP), is mandatory during prostatectomy surgeries, since this nerve participates in the first and last stages of erection.

For these reasons, New studies are needed to improve the existing techniques and develop a method to continuously monitor the autonomic nervous system.

References

1. Ashton-Miller JA, DeLancey JO. Functional anatomy of the female pelvic floor. Ann N Y Acad Sci. 2007;1101:266–96. https://doi.org/10.1196/annals.1389.034. Epub 2007 Apr 7. PMID: 17416924.
2. Ballester M, Chereau E, Dubernard G, Coutant C, Bazot M, Daraï E. Urinary dysfunction after colorectal resection for endometriosis: results of a prospective randomized trial comparing laparoscopy to open surgery. Am J Obstet Gynecol. 2011;204(4):303–6. https://doi.org/10.1016/j.ajog.2010.11.011.
3. Corton MM. Anatomy of pelvic floor dysfunction. Obstet Gynecol Clin N Am. 2009;36:401–19.
4. de Groat WC, Yoshimura N. Anatomy and physiology of the lower urinary tract. Handb Clin Neurol. 2015;130:61–108. https://doi.org/10.1016/B978-0-444-63247-0.00005-5. PMID: 26003239.
5. Dubernard G, Piketty M, Rouzier R, Houry S, Bazot M, Darai E. Quality of life after laparoscopic colorectal resection for endometriosis. Hum Reprod. 2006;21(5):1243–7.
6. Eichelberg C, Erbersdobler A, Michl U, Schlomm T, Salomon G, Graefen M, Huland H. Nerve distribution along the prostatic capsule. Eur Urol. 2007;51(1):105–10; discussion 110-1. https://doi.org/10.1016/j.eururo.2006.05.038. Epub 2006 Jun 12. PMID:16814455.
7. Espinosa-Medina I, Saha O, Boismoreau F, Chettouh Z, Rossi F, Richardson WD, Brunet JF. The sacral autonomic outflow is sympathetic. Science. 2016;354(6314):893–7. https://doi.org/10.1126/science.aah5454. PMID: 27856909; PMCID: PMC6326350.
8. Fanfani F, Fagotti A, Gagliardi ML, Ruffo G, Ceccaroni M, Scambia G, et al. Discoid or segmental rectosigmoid resection for deep infiltrating endometriosis: a case-control study. Fertil Steril. 2010;94:444–9.
9. Fishman IJ, Shabsigh R, Kaplan AL. Lower urinary tract dysfunction after radical hysterectomy for carcinoma of cervix. Urology. 1986;28(6):462–8.
10. Fujiwara T. Surgery for cervical cancer (in Japanese). Tokyo: Igakutoshyosyuppan; 1984.
11. Gabriel B, Nassif J, Trompoukis P, Lima AM, Barata S, Lang-Avérous G, Wattiez A. Prevalence and outcome of urinary retention after laparoscopic surgery for severe endometriosis--does histology provide answers? Int Urogynecol J. 2012;23(1):111–6. https://doi.org/10.1007/s00192-011-1492-2.
12. Gaskell WH. On the structure, distribution and function of the nerves which innervate the visceral and vascular systems. J Physiol. 1886;7:1–80.

13. Höckel M, Konerding MA, Heussel CP. Liposuction-assisted nerve-sparing extended radical hysterectomy: oncologic rationale, surgical anatomy, and feasibility study. Am J Obstet Gynecol. 1998;178(5):971–6.
14. Höckel M, Horn LC, Hentschel B, Höckel S, Naumann G. Total mesometrial resection: high resolution nerve-sparing radical hysterectomy based on developmentally defined surgical anatomy. Int J Gynecol Cancer. 2003;13(6):791–803.
15. Holzbeierlein J, Peterson M, Smith JAJR. Variability of results of cavernous nerve stimulation during radical prostatectomy. J Urol. 2001;165:108–10.
16. Kaiho Y, Nakagawa H, Saito H, Ito A, Ishidoya S, Saito S, Arai Y. Nerves at the ventral prostatic capsule contribute to erectile function: initial electrophysiological assessment in humans. Eur Urol. 2009 Jan;55(1):148–54. https://doi.org/10.1016/j.eururo.2008.09.022. Epub 2008 Sep 24. PMID: 18835086.
17. Kauff DW, Bremm RP, Lang H, Kneist W. Laparoscopic pelvic neuromonitoring permits superior nerve-sparing technical and electrophysiological aspects of the open and laparoscopic approach. Biomed Eng/Biomed Tech. 2014;59:356–9. https://doi.org/10.1515/bmt-2014-4151.
18. Kirschner-Hermanns R, Jakse G. Quality of life following radical prostatectomy. Crit Rev Oncol Hematol. 2002;43:141–51.
19. Kneist W, Kauff DW, Lang H. Laparoscopic neuromapping in pelvic surgery: scopes of application. Surg Innov. 2014;21(2):213–20. https://doi.org/10.1177/1553350613496907. Epub 2013 Jul 25. PMID: 23892318.
20. Koehler N, Holze S, Gansera L, et al. Erectile dysfunction after radical prostatectomy: the impact of nerve-sparing status and surgical approach. Int J Impot Res. 2012;24:155–60.
21. Kraima AC, Derks M, Smit NN, van de Velde CJ, Kenter GG, DeRuiter MC. Careful dissection of the distal ureter is highly important in nerve-sparing radical pelvic surgery: a 3D reconstruction and immunohistochemical characterization of the vesical plexus. Int J Gynecol Cancer. 2016;26(5):959–66. https://doi.org/10.1097/IGC.0000000000000709.
22. Langley JN. The autonomic nervous system: part I. Cambridge: W. Heffer; 1921.
23. Lemos N, Souza C, Marques RM, Kamergorodsky G, Schor E, Girão MJ. Laparoscopic anatomy of the autonomic nerves of the pelvis and the concept of nerve-sparing surgery by direct visualization of autonomic nerve bundles. Fertil Steril. 2015. pii:S0015-0282(15)01649-0. https://doi.org/10.1016/j.fertnstert.2015.07.1138.
24. Lemos NLBM, Ribeiro R, Fernandes GL, Abrão MS, Moretti-Marques R. Nerve-sparing routes in radical pelvic surgery. In: Gomes-da-Silveira G, da Silveira G, Pessini S, editors. Minimally invasive gynecology. Cham: Springer; 2018. https://doi.org/10.1007/978-3-319-72592-5_6.
25. Lue TF, Gleason CA, Brock GB, Carroll PR, Tanagho EA. Intraoperative electrostimulation of the cavernous nerve: technique, results and limitations. J Urol. 1995;154(4):1426–8. https://doi.org/10.1016/s0022-5347(01)66882-4. PMID: 7658549.
26. Martín-Palomeque G, Cabañes-Martínez L, de Blas Beorlegui G, Moreno Galera MDM, López JR, Burgos FJ, Regidor Bailly-Baillière I. Novel mapping method for the intraoperative neurophysiologic monitoring of sexual function during prostate surgery. J Clin Neurophysiol. 2018;35(6):463–7. https://doi.org/10.1097/WNP.0000000000000506. PMID: 30320663.
27. Matthew AG, Goldman A, Trachtenberg J, et al. Sexual dysfunction after radical prostatectomy: prevalence, treatments, restricted use of treatments and distress. J Urol. 2005;174:2105–10.
28. Nezhat C, Nezhat F, Pennington E, Nezhat CH, Ambroze W. Laparoscopic disk excision and primary repair of the anterior rectal wall for the treatment of full-thickness bowel endometriosis. Surg Endosc. 1994;8:682–5.
29. Possover M, Stöber S, Plaul K, Schneider A. Identification and preservation of the motoric innervation of the bladder in radical hysterectomy type III. Gynecol Oncol. 2000;79(2):154–7.
30. Possover M, Rhiem K, Chiantera V. The "laparoscopic neuro- navigation" – LANN: from a functional cartography of the pelvic autonomous neurosystem to a new field of laparoscopic surgery. Min Invasive Ther Allied Technol. 2004;13:362–7.

31. Possover M, Chiantera V, Baekelandt J. Anatomy of the sacral roots and the pelvic splanchnic nerves in women using the LANN technique. Surg Laparosc Endosc Percutan Tech. 2007;17(6):508–10.
32. Redwine DB, Wright JT. Laparoscopic treatment of complete obliteration of the cul-de-sac associated with endometriosis: long-term follow-up of en bloc resection. Fertil Steril. 2001;76(2):358–65.
33. Rehman J, Christ GJ, Kaynan A, et al. Intraoperative electrical stimulation of cavernosal nerves with monitoring of intracorporeal pressure in patients undergoing nerve sparing radical prostatectomy. BJU Int. 1999;84:305–10.
34. Seski JC, Diokno AC. Bladder dysfunction after radical abdominal hysterectomy. Am J Obstet Gynecol. 1977;128(6):643–51.
35. Stolzenburg J-U, McNeill A, Liatsikos EN. Nerve-sparing endoscopic extraperitoneal radical prostatectomy. BJU Int. 2008;101:909–28. https://doi.org/10.1111/j.1464-410X.2008.07544.x.
36. Terada N, Arai Y, Kurokawa K, et al. Intraoperative electrical stimulation of cavernous nerves with monitoring of intracorporeal pressure to confirm nerve sparing during radical prostatectomy: early clinical results. Int J Urol. 2003;10:251–6.
37. Trimbos JB, Maas CP, Deruiter MC, Peters AA, Kenter GG. A nerve-sparing radical hysterectomy: guidelines and feasibility in Western patients. Int J Gynecol Cancer. 2001;11(3):180–6.
38. Walsh PC, Schlegel PN. Radical pelvic surgery with preservation of sexual function. Ann Surg. 1988;208(4):391–400. https://doi.org/10.1097/00000658-198810000-00001. PMID: 3178328; PMCID: PMC1493736.
39. Walsh PC, Lepor H, Eggleston JC. Radical prostatectomy with preservation of sexual function: anatomical and pathological considerations. Prostate. 1983;4(5):473–85. https://doi.org/10.1002/pros.2990040506. PMID: 6889192.
40. Walsh PC, et al. Efficacy of first-generation Cavermap to verify location and function of cavernous nerves during radical prostatectomy: a multi-institutional evaluation by experienced surgeons. Urology. 2001;57:491–4.

Index

A

Accessory nerve, 752
Adauri Bueno de Camargo, MD, 18–19
Adverse effects of IOM
  biting and movement, 102
  bleeding and bruising, 104
  cardiac arrhythmias, 104
  infections, 104
  seizures and after discharges, 103
Alfredo Torres Castellon, MD, PhD, 22
Alpha-agonists, 466
American Clinical Neurophysiology Society (ACNS), 439
American Society for Neurophysiologic Monitoring (ASNM), 166
Anesthesia, 358, 560
Anesthesia Positioning Care, 468
Anomia, 361
Antegrade cerebral perfusion (ACP), 670
Anterior interbody fusion (ALIF), 505–509
Anterior Primary Ramus (APR), 729
Anterior spinal artery (ASA), 663, 664
Arcuate fasciculus (AF), 310–312, 374
Autonomic nervous system (ANS)
  BCR, 853
  EMG-IAS, 853, 854
  ICP, 852, 853
  intravesical pressure, 852, 853
  parasympathetic nervous system, 851
Awake craniotomy
  anesthetic technique, 289–291, 294
  brain mapping, 338
    central nervous system structural basis, 341
    chronaxie and rheobase, 341, 342
    direct cortical motor evoked potential (MEP), 336
    effectiveness, 338
    high frequency, 339, 340, 342, 343
    hodotopy, 335
    language tests, 337
    low frequency, 338–340, 343
    monopolar *vs.* bipolar probe, 344, 345
    stimulation parameters, 338
    tablet fixation, 336
    triggering language and cognitive tasks, 345, 347, 348
    true positives and negative results, 343
  complications, 295–297
  definition, 287
  DES, 350, 351
  description, 328
  electrical protocol, 328
  glioblastoma and extend of resection, 329, 330
  language, brain, mapping, 328
  low-grade glioma surgery, 329
  maximal safe resection, 330
  patient selection and preparation, 288, 289, 331, 332
  pharmacological effects, 294–296
  preoperative imaging, 332, 334
  risks, 348–350
  safe resection, 330
  task and mapping triggering, 345–346
  teamwork, 288
  technical nuances, 334, 335

S. M. Verst et al. (eds.), *Intraoperative Monitoring*,
https://doi.org/10.1007/978-3-030-95730-8

B
Benzodiazepines, 115
Biological electrical artefacts, 108
Bispectral analysis (BIS), 118, 119
Bispectral index (BIS), 464, 465
Bite injury, 103
Blink reflex (BR)
anesthetic considerations, 239
clinical assessment, 240–242
hypnotic drugs, 238
practical application, 242, 243
R1 and R2 response, 238
recording parameters, 239
stimulation parameters, 239
Boston Naming Test, 360
Brachial plexus injuries (BPIs), 712, 713
Brainstem auditory evoked potentials (BAEPs)
anesthesia, 138
auditory pathway anatomy, 132
auditory pathway fibers, 132
children, 138
definition, 129
dendritic processes, 132
drilling and cerebellar retraction, 138
efficacy, 139
equipment, 131, 132
limitations, 139
qualifications, 130, 131
repetitive auditory stimulation, 130
stimulation and recording technique, 133–135
uses, 130
warning criteria, 135–137
waveforms, 133
Brain surface
brain mapping techniques, 265
brain ranges, 253
cerebral functions, 263
cortex, 253
cortical functional maps, 264, 265
cytoarchitecture, 259–261
diencephalon and the telencephalon, 253
DWI, 265
encephalon, 253
fMRI, 264
FT, 265
infratentorial compartment, 253
intrinsic connectivity, 261–263
minimal common brain, 265
multi-modal parcellation, 266, 267
PET, 264
residual WHO grade II glioma, 266
sulcal pattern, 254–259
Brazilian Society of Clinical Neurophysiology (SBNC), 42
Broca's aphasia, 304
Broca's theory, 302
Bulbocavernosus reflex (BCR), 556, 557, 685–687, 845–850, 853

C
Calculation complexity, 368
Capacitor and filters, 95
Cardiopulmonary bypass (CPB), 669, 670
Carlo Domênico Marrone, MD, 24–26
Carotid endarterectomy, 220, 221
Carotid endarterectomy (CEA), 613
CaverMap, 859
CENEPSI Bioengineering Laboratory, 13, 14
Central conduction time (CCT), 614
Cerebral aneurysm surgery, 628–630
Cerebral blood flow (CBF), 113
and arterial pressure, 114
and cerebral metabolic rate ($CRMO_2$), 113, 114
inhaled halogenated anesthetics, 114–116
Cerebral blood volume, 112–113
Cerebral oxygen metabolic rate ($CMRO_2$), 113
Cerebrovascular disorders
cerebral aneurysm surgery, 628–630
cerebral AVMs, 630
critical changes, 635, 636
definition, 612
EC-IC bypass surgery, 631
high-grade carotid artery stenosis
anesthesia, 618
continuous EEG monitoring, 616, 617
critical intraoperative EEG changes, 619
history, 615
ischemia, 618
MEPs monitoring, 623, 624
NIRS, 626, 627
quantitative EEG, 619–621
SSEP monitoring, 621–623
surgical and endovascular procedures, 615, 616
transcranial doppler, 624–626
INR, 631–635
patient history, 640–651
recordings, 637–639
regional cerebral blood flow, 613–615
stimulation, 637, 638
Cervical spinal surgery
anterior approach

advantage, 516
disadvantage, 516
intraoperative, 519–521
preoperative, 516–519
classification, 514
C5 palsy, 532, 533
decompression and screw placement, 514
endoscopic approach, 523, 524
IONM, 515
clinical evidence, 530–532
D-wave, 525–527
electromyography, 528–530
mMEP, 524, 525
SSEPs, 526–528
pathologies, 515
posterior approach
advantage, 521
disadvantage, 521
intraoperative, 522, 523
preoperative, 521, 522
posterior compression, 514
white cord syndrome/spinal cord reperfusion injury, 533, 534
Charges (Q), 91
Classic language model, 302–304
Clinic-anatomical correlation method, 302
Cochlear implant surgery, 771, 773, 774
Color Naming, 369
Compound motor action potential (CMAP), 551, 553
Compound motor unit action potential (CMUAP), 389
Compound muscle action potentials (CMAP), 58, 59
Conduction aphasia, 302, 303
Conductivity of material, 91
Connectionism theory, 263
Contemporary language model, 304–306
Continuous direct cortical motor evoked potential (DC MEP), 279
Continuous intraoperative stimulation of the vagus nerve (CVNM), 767
Contraindications to IOM
electronic implants, 105–106
pacemakers, 105
Conus medullaris, 570, 571
Cortical mapping, 278
Corticobulbar Motor-Evoked Potentials (CB-MEP), 237, 407–409, 758
"compound" CMUAP, 413
evaluation and prognostic scores, 412, 413
limitations, 411, 414, 415
recording parameters, 410, 412
stimulus parameters, 410
C5 palsy, 532, 533
C5 syndrome, 514
Cytoarchitecture, 259–261

D

Deep brain stimulation (DBS), 819, 821
Deep hypothermic circulatory arrest (DHCA), 668
Delayed onset spinal cord ischemia, 682, 683
Dexmedetomidine, 119
Diffuse intrinsic brainstem gliomas, 422
Diffusion tensor imaging (DTI), 306, 307
Diffusion-weighted imaging (DWI), 265
Direct cortical stimulation (DCS), 10
Direct electrical stimulation (DES), 302, 358
Dual task, 364–365
Dural manipulation, 334
D-wave collision technique, 599
D-wave inter-spinous ligament technique (DWILT), 526, 527

E

Education level (EL), 359
Electrical artifacts, 106–107
Electrical charges, 91–92
Electrocardiogram (EKG), 208
Electric current (i), 90–92
Electric displacement, 94
Electrocorticography (ECoG), 10
Electroencephalogram (EEG)
anesthetic agents, 118
anesthetic drugs, 120
artifacts, 207–209
bilateral and generalized attenuation, 219
bispectral analysis (BIS), 118, 119
burst suppression, 218, 219
cardiac surgery, 221
carotid endarterectomy, 220, 221
definition, 118
display velocity, 206, 207
electrode types, 205
epileptiform activity/seizures, 120, 217
filter settings, 206
generalized slowing, 218
graphics, 209–215
inhaled anesthetics, 120
interhemispheric asymmetry, 220
IOM documentation, 221, 222
neurophysiological electrocerebral activity evaluation, 203

Electroencephalogram (EEG) (*cont.*)
in operating room, 215–217
pathology, 204
recording, 204–205
seizure, 120
sensitivity, 207
TIVA, 118, 119
unexpected awakening, 217
Electromyography (EMG)
bipolar stimulation, 233
definition, 226
equipment setup and screen display, 234
free run EMG (fEMG), 226, 229–231, 234, 235
hook wires, 228
low-frequency filter, 234
monopolar stimulation, 232, 233
muscle recording, 228
protocol, 228, 229
subdermal needle electrodes, 227
surface electrodes, 227
triggered stimulus (tEMG), 226, 231, 232
Electronic implants, 105–106
Emotion and Behavior Task, 373
Energy, 93
Epilepsy surgery
adjuncts
clinical studies, 782, 783
ECoG, 784–786
iMRI, 784
intraoperative ultrasonography, 784
neuronavigation, 783
anesthesia, 804–806
electrodes and registration technics
depth electrodes, 787
IEEG, 786
SEEG, 789, 790
silicone plastic strips/grids, 786
skin incisions, 788
spider like device, 787
subdural evaluation, 788
subdural position, 786
surgical technique, 790, 791
eloquent areas stimulation, 795–797
incidence, 782
interictal and ictal classical pattern, 791–796
neurosurgical aspects
disconnective procedures, 802
extratemporal surgery and ECoG, 800–802
pediatric population, 803, 804
temporal lobe epilepsy, 798–800
Epileptiform activity, 120
Essential tremor, 819
Evidence-based medicine (EBM), 46
Extracranial-intracranial (EC-IC) bypass, 631

F

Facial nerve (FN), 747–749
Faraday's 2nd law, 62
Federal Board of Biomedicine (Conselho Federal de Biomedicina - CFBM), 44
Fiber dissection, 306
Fiber tractography (FT), 265
Foundation for Teaching and Research in Health Sciences of the Federal District (FEPECS), 26
Fourier's transformation model, 718
Fourth ventricle's floor mapping
afferent and efferent nuclei, 424
anatomy, 421, 422
brainstem cavernoma, 422
brainstem lesions resection, 424
continuous dynamic mapping, 426, 427
corticobulbar bundles, 425
corticobulbar tracts and cranial nerve trajectories, 428
cranial nerve motor nuclei, 425
dorsal safe entry zones, 424
exophytic brainstem gliomas, 422
facial colliculus, 423
first line treatment, 422
grey matter nuclei and white matter tracts, 423
image guidance, 421
LAR significant change (LAR-SC), 428
lateral lemniscus, 425
medial lemniscus, 425
narrow infrafacial triangle, 424
neurophysiological mapping techniques, 422
neurophysiological mapping tools, 426, 427
neurophysiological methods, 422
"peripheral" response, 427
pilocytic astrocytoma, 428
safe entry zones, 424
suprafacial triangle, 424
Francisco José Carchedi Luccas, MD, 14–16, 18
Freehand technique, 480
Free run electromyography (frEMG), 389, 575, 731, 732

anatomical and functional preservation, 401, 402
A-train, 402–406
B-bursts, 402
B-spikes, 402
intermedius nerve, 406, 407
neurotonic train, 402
trains B and C, 402
Free-running spontaneous EMG (fEMG), 548–550
Frontal aslant tract (FAT), 312, 313, 375

G
GABAergic dysfunction, 819
Gary Gronich, MD, 12–14
General anesthesia, 116–117
Geschwind area (GA), 377
Globus pallidus (GPe), 828, 829
Glomus Carotideo, 774, 775
Glossopharyngeal nerve (GN), 749
Glossopharyngeal neuralgia, 433
Grading of Recommendations Assessment, Development and Evaluation (GRADE) method, 47
Grounding, 95–99
Ground loop currents, 98
Gynecological surgeries, 858
intraoperative, 855
preoperative, 854, 855

H
Hagen-Poiseuille relation, 112
Head, neck and ear (HNE) approaches
accessory nerve, 752
anatomical structures, 747
arterial vascular system-common carotid, external and internal, 753, 754
facial nerve, 747–749
facial nerve injury
CB-MEP, 763
CMAPs, 763
EMG-fr, 761
EMG-st, 762, 763
evidence, 760, 761
incidence, 760
preoperative facial nerve mapping, 763
protocol, 761
Glomus Carotideo, 774, 775
glossopharyngeal nerve, 749
hypoglossal nerve, 753
incidence, 746
lymphatic vases, 754
mapping, 746
mastoid and cochlear implant surgeries, 771, 773, 774
neurophysiological techniques
anesthesia, 754
CB-MEP, 758
EEG, 760
EMG-fr, 755, 756
EMG-st, 756, 757
LAR, 758, 759
SSEP and MEP, 757, 758
thyroid surgeries
CB-MEP, 770
CVNM, 767
EMG-fr and EMG-st, 765, 766
HM Catalunya Hospital, Barcelona, 769–772
LAR, 767, 768
RLN, 765
vagus nerve, 750–752
vagus nerve stimulation, 774
vestibulocochlear nerve, 749
Hematimetric control, 467, 468
Hemifacial spasm (HFS), 433
Hemodynamic control, 467
Hickok-Poeppel model, 305
High-frequency filter (HF), 718
High-grade carotid artery stenosis
anesthesia, 618
continuous EEG monitoring, 616, 617
critical intraoperative EEG changes, 619
history, 615
ischemia, 618
MEPs monitoring, 623, 624
NIRS, 626, 627
quantitative EEG, 619–621
SSEP monitoring, 621–623
surgical and endovascular procedures, 615, 616
transcranial Doppler, 624–626
Hodotopy, 304, 335
Hoffmann reflex, 558, 559
Human connectome project, 266, 267
Hypoglossal nerve, 753
Hypothermia, 668, 669, 683

I
Impedance, 94
Inferior fronto-occiptal fasciculus (IFOF), 314, 316–318, 375

Inferior longitudinal fasciculus (ILF), 318, 319, 376
Inhalational agents, 295–296
Inhaled halogenated anesthetics, 114–116
Intensity x Pulse Duration x Stimulator Electrode Diameter, 92
Internal anal sphincter (IAS), 853, 854
International Society of Intraoperative Neurophysiology (ISIN), 7
Interventional neuroradiologic (INR) procedures, 631–635
Intracavernous pressure (ICP), 852, 853
Intracranial pressure (ICP), 112
Intramedullary spinal cord tumors (IMSCT)
  dorsal column mapping techniques
    antegrade recording of spinal SEPs, 596, 597
    Gracilis SEP phase reversal technique, 598, 599
    PT NAPs, 594–596
  D-wave monitoring, 591–595
  free electromyography monitoring, 594
  interpretation, 603–605
  MEPs, 590, 591
  modalities, 589, 590
  motor pathways mapping techniques
    direct stimulation, 600, 601
    double-train stimulation technique, 601, 602
    D-wave collision technique, 599
  neurophysiological monitoring protocol, 603
  pathologies, 588, 589
  SEPs, 590
Intraoperative neurophysiologic monitoring (IONM), 547
  in Brazil
    academic training, 29
    evidence and level of recommendation, 46–48
    evidence-based practice (EBP), 46
    evolution of equipment, 30, 32
    goals of, 40
    initial steps, 40
    law 3.268/1957, 42
    mapping *vs.* monitoring, 43
    medical assistants/technicians role, 44–45
    medical legal and ethics aspects, 41, 42
    medical professionals qualification, 42, 43
    monitoring operators, 53
    of late 1980s and early 1990s, 10–13
    pioneering neurophysiologists, 12, 14, 15, 17–20, 22–28
    planning steps, 40
    quality of evidence, 47
    reliability, 51, 52
    remote IONM, 50, 51
    remote/on-site neurophysiologist, 49
    requirements, 40
    SNBC, 32–35
    strength of recommendation, 47
    technicians in neurophysiology, 28
    training, 43, 44
    training challenges, 29, 30
  cerebrovascular disorders (*see* Cerebrovascular disorders)
  cervical spinal surgery
    clinical evidence, 530–532
    D-wave, 525–527
    electromyography, 528–530
    mMEP, 524, 525
    SSEPs, 526–528
  clinical papers, 3
  description, 3
  ISIN Rio 2015, 9, 10
  in Latin America
    international mentors and societies, 6, 7
    origin, 5, 6
    Special Interest Group (SIG), 7, 8
  LIFS
    ALIF, 505–509
    LLIF, 497–504
  SDR, 569, 570 (*see* Selective dorsal rhizotomy (SDR))
  timeline, 4, 5
Intraoperative optimization, 359
Intravenous agents, 296–297
Intravesical pressure (IVP), 852, 853
Intrinsic connectivity, 261–263
Invasive electrodes, 90
Item response theory (IRT), 360

J

JAMA study, 330
José Alberto Nunes Sobrinho, MD, 26

K

Ketamine, 466
Kirchhoff's laws, 93
Klinger's technique, 306, 307

L

L4 and L5 roots sectioning, 582
Language assessment, 333
Language comprehension, 304
Language network
  arcuate fasciculus, 310–312
  connectivity patterns, 307
  frontal aslant tract, 312, 313
  ILF, 318, 319
  inferior fronto-occiptal fasciculus, 314, 316–318
  MdLF, 314, 315
  superior longitudinal fasciculus, 308–310
  U fibers, 307, 308
  uncinate fasciculus, 320
Laryngeal adductor reflex (LAR), 244–248, 759, 767, 768
Lateral lumbar transpsoas interbody fusion (LLIF), 497–504
Left heart bypass (LHB), 670
Left inferior frontal area, 377
Lidocaine, 465
Lipomeningocele, 543
Local field potential (LEP), 831, 832
Loss of motor potentials, 108
Lower limb somatosensory-evoked potentials (SSEPs), 555, 556
Low-frequency filter (LFF), 718
Lumbar interbody fusion surgeries (LIFS)
  complications, 496
  IONM
    ALIF, 505–509
    LLIF, 497–504
Lumbar vertebra, 476
Luxury perfusion, 114

M

Magnesium sulfate, 466
Marek-Marsel Mesulam, 263
Maria Lúcia Furtado de Mendonça, MD, 22–24
Maria Rufina Barros, MD, 26–28
Masseteric reflex, 243–244
Mastoid surgery, 771, 773, 774
Math test, 359
Mechanical thrombectomy, 634
Memory tasks, 367
  verbal, 367
  visual, 368
  working memory, 368
Microelectrode recording (MER), 822–825
Microvascular decompression (MVD)
  BAEPs, 437–440
  classifications, 431
  common indications, 431
  complications, 433–435
  electromyography, 440, 442–444
  FMEP monitoring, 446–448
  incidence of, 431
  intraoperative monitoring, 435–437
  lateral spread response, 444–446
  outcomes
    glossopharyngeal neuralgia, 433
    hemifacial spasm (HFS), 433
    trigeminal neuralgia, 432
  surgical techniques, 432
  symptoms, 431
Middle longitudinal fasciculus (MdLF), 314, 315
Middle-posterior temporal lobe, 377–378
MLF, 376
Moderate hypothermic circulatory arrest (MHCA), 669
Motor evoked potentials (MEP), 554, 555
  anatomy and physiology of motor system, 182
  applications and safety, 198, 199
  D-wave, 184, 185, 525–527
  electrical stimulation, 184
  electrode placement, 186–191
  interpretation and alarm criteria, 196, 197
  I-wave, 184
  muscle MEP (mMEP), 185, 186, 524, 525
  neurophysiological registration, 184
  recording, 195
  stimulus parameters, 193, 194
  Sylvian fissure, 182
Motor function monitoring, 271–272
Motor nerve conduction, 726, 727
Motor recovery prediction, 279–281
Motor unit action potentials (MUAPs), 727
Movement *(t)*, 91
Movement disorders
  globus pallidus (GPe), 828, 829
  LFP, 831, 832
  MER, 822–825
  neural circuitry, 818–820
  STN, 825–827
  subthalamic region and fields of forel, 830, 831
  surgery, 820–823
  ventral intermediate nucleus, 829, 830

Muscle motor point
CMAP, 58, 59
definition, 57
gluteus minimus, 80
M. abductor hallucis, 79
M. abductor pollicis brevis, 75
M. abdutor digiti minimi, 75
M. adductor brevis, 77
M. adductor longus, 77
M. Biceps brachii, 71
M. bíceps femoris–long head, 81
M. bíceps femoris–short head, 82
M. brachiorradialis, 72
M. Bulboespongiosus, 85
M. Crycothyroid, 67
M. Deltoid, 70
M. diaphragm, 75
M. extensor carpi radialis, 72
M. extensor digitorum, 72
M. extensor hallucis longus, 78
M. extensor indicis, 74
M. external anal sphincter, 87
M. external urethral sphincter, 86
M. flexor carpi radialis, 73
M. flexor carpi ulnaris, 74
M. frontalis, 64
M. gastrocnemius, 79
M. Genioglossus, 67
M. gluteus maximus, 80
M. gluteus medius, 80
M. iliacus, 77
M. infraspinatus, 70
M. intercostalis, 76
M. internal anal sphincter, 86
M. Ischiocavernosus, 84
M. Levator labii superioris alaeque nasi, 65
M. masseter, 68
M. Mentalis, 66
M. obliquus abdominis, 76
M. occipitalis, 64
M. Orbicularis oculi, 65
M. orbicularis oris, 66
M. perineal transversus, 83
M. Platysma, 66
M. pronator teres, 73
M. Rectus abdominais, 76
M. rectus femoris, 78
M. Semimembranosus, 81
M. semitendinosus, 81
M. Sternocleidomastoid, 69
M. supraespinatus, 70
M. Temporalis, 68
M. tensor fasciae latae, 82
M. tibialis anterior, 78
M. trapezius, 69
M. triceps brachii, 71
morphology and amplitude of motor potentials, 62, 63
muscle-potentials generators, 58, 59
obese patients, 62
peripheral CMAP AND mMEP, 63
practical manuals, 58
recording electrodes, 59, 60, 62
Muscle recordings, 472
Myelomeningocele, 542

N

Near-infrared spectroscopy (NIRS), 626, 627
Needle electrode examination (NEE), 727–731
Nerve action potential (NAP)
caliber and myelination, 714
development, 713
filters, 718–720
gain and sweep setup, 719
stimulation and recording, 715–718
stimulus duration, intensity and frequency, 720–722
time window, 715
VI-degree lesion, 714
Neuromuscular blockers, 467
Neuronavigation systems, 783
Neurophysiological signal modalities, 90
Neurophysiological tools, 277–279
Newtonian fluids, 112
Non-biological electrical artefacts, 107–108
Non-equipotential grounds, 97
Notch filter, 719
Number counting, 360

O

Object naming (ON), 359–362
Ohm's law, 92, 93
Ohy-Maldaun Fast Track Cognitive Test (OMFTCT), 333
Opioid anesthetics, 116
Optic radiation (OR), 376

P

Pacemakers, 105–106
Parkinson’s disease (PD), 819
Pelvic floor
anatomy and physiology, 840, 842
autonomic nervous system

BCR, 853
EMG-IAS, 853, 854
ICP, 852, 853
intravesical pressure, 852, 853
parasympathetic nervous system, 851
gynecological surgeries, 858
intraoperative, 855
preoperative, 854, 855
limitations, 860
neurological structures at risk, 841, 843
somatic nervous system, 844
BCR, 845–850
EMG – triggered, 851
EMG triggered, 849, 851
free-run EMG, 849
SSEP, 846
TcMEP, 845
survival rates, 840
urologic surgeries, 856–860
Peripheral nerves
anesthesia, 739
BPI, 712, 713
electrodiagnostic studies
clinical evaluation, 722
limitations, 723–726
motor nerve conduction, 726, 727
NEE, 727–731
sensory nerve conduction, 724, 725
intraoperative protocols
fEMG, 731, 732
MEP, 734, 736–738
SSEP, 734, 735
trigger electromyography, 732–734
IONM, 722
multiplicity of injuries and donor nerve assesment, 738, 739
NAP
caliber and myelination, 714
development, 713
filters, 718–720
gain and sweep setup, 719
stimulation and recording, 715–718
stimulus duration, intensity and frequency, 720–722
time window, 715
VI-degree lesion, 714
Phasic discharge, 731
Phonation and articulation, 302
Posterior spinal arteries (PSA), 663
Posterior tibial (PT), 590
Posterior tibial nerve action potentials (PT NAPs), 594–596
Power spectral density (PSD), 832
Preoperative language assessment, 359
Preoperative magnetoencephalography, 332
Preserving language, 302
Propofol, 116, 119
Prostate cancer, 859
Pudendal nerve somatosensory-evoked Potential (pSSEP), 556

R
Read the Mind in Eyes Task (RMET), 373
Recording myotomes, 575
Recurrent laryngeal nerve (RLN), 765
Regional cerebral blood flow (rCBF), 613–615
Resistance, 92, 93
Retrograde cerebral perfusion (RCP), 670
Root excitability, 581

S
Safety paradigms
electric stimulation, 99
excitotoxicity and electrochemical damage, 100, 101
leakage current or equipment malfunction, 100
preventive measures, 102
thermal injury and burns, 101, 102
2021-2022 SBNC directory´s recommendations, 48
Seizure onset zone (SOZ), 803
Selective dorsal rhizotomy (SDR)
conventional laminotomy technique, 572
historical evolutionary aspects, 569, 570
IONM
anesthesia, 573
EMG artifacts, 582, 583
equipment set up, 573
flowchart, 582, 583
free electromyography, 575
L4 and L5 roots sectioning, 582
recording and stimulator probes and anodal/cathodal stimulation, 574
recording myotomes, 575
recording of threshold, 581
root excitability, 581
tetanic stimulation, 577–580
tetanic stimulations, 581
threshold stimulation, 575–577
minimally invasive approach, 570, 571
muscle tonus and spasticity, 566–568
patients selection, 568, 569
Semantics, 365–366

Sensory function monitoring, 273
Sensory nerve conduction, 724, 725
Short-term visual and verbal memory, 359
Silvia Mazzali-Verst, MD, PhD, 20–22
Skull base surgery
bulbar IX and X nerves, 388
CoMEP, 389, 407–409
"Compound" CMUAP, 413
evaluation and prognostic scores, 412, 413
limitations, 411, 414, 415
recording parameters, 410, 412
stimulus parameters, 410
correct needling, 389–392
free run electromyography (frEMG), 389
anatomical and functional preservation, 401, 402
A-train, 402–406
B-bursts, 402
B-spikes, 402
intermedius nerve, 406, 407
neurotonic train, 402
trains B and C, 402
multifactorial data, 388
neurophysiological tests, 388
prognostic parameters, 388
trigger electromyography (tEMG), 389
bipolar stimulation, 394–396
continuous facial mapping, 401
mapping application, 392–394
monopolar cathodal stimulation, 394–397
threshold and amplitude analyzing, 397, 398
unusual responses to stimulation, 398–401
voltage/current system, 397
SLF, *see* Superior longitudinal fasciculus
Society of Clinical Neurophysiology (SBNC), 32–35
Somatic nervous system (SNS), 844
BCR, 845–850
EMG triggered, 849, 851
free-run EMG, 849
SSEP, 846
TcMEP, 845
Somatosensory evoked potentials (SSEPs), 526–528
anatomy, 169
anesthetic agents and muscle relaxants, 175, 176
averager, 168
blood pressure and temperature, 176
blood supply, 169, 170
channels, 167
efficacy, 176
electrodes, 167
filter settings, 168
limitations, 177
professional and technical monitoring, 166
stimulation and recording technique, 170, 173, 174
time-base, 168
uses, 166
warning criteria, 175
waveforms, 170–173
Spectral edge frequency (SEF), 210
Spinal cord blood flow (SCBF), 674–676
Spinal cord ischemia (SCI) and stroke
ACP, 670
BCR, 685–687
CPB, 669, 670
critical changes, 689, 690
differentiation, 687–689
EEG, 677–679
hypothermia, 668, 669
intercostal and segmental arteries, 671–674
LHB, 670
lumbar drain, 671
paraplegia, 667
pharmacologic, 671
RCP, 670
regional spinal cord blood flow and evoked potentials, 674–677
risk factors, 666, 667
SSEPs, 679, 680
stimulation and recording protocols, 690–693
TcMEPs, 680–684
TEVAR, 666
Spinal cord reperfusion injury, 533, 534
Spinal cord retethering, 545–547
Spinal deformity surgery
anatomical structures, 461
anesthesia, 464
alpha-agonists, 466
Anesthesia Positioning Care, 468
BIS, 464, 465
hematimetric control, 467, 468
hemodynamic control, 467
ketamine, 466
lidocaine, 465
magnesium sulfate, 466
neuromuscular blockers, 467
thermal control, 468
TIVA, 464

decision-making algorithm, 482–486
development, 461
evidence level, 486–488
factors, 460
history, 462, 463
improvement, 461
intraoperative
pedicle instrumentation, 475–482
protocol, 471–475
multimodal IONM, 463
neuromuscular scoliosis, 463
osteotomized segments, 461
planes, 460
preoperative, 469–472
Spoken language, 302
Spontaneous speech production, 303
Stereo-electroencephalography technique (SEEG), 789, 790
Stroop task, 366
Subcortical mapping, 274–276
Subthalamic nucleus (STN), 819, 825–827
Subthalamic region and fields of forel, 830, 831
Succinylcholine, 116
Superior longitudinal fasciculus (SLF), 308–310, 375
Superior temporal artery–middle cerebral artery (STA-MCA) bypass, 631
Sylvian fissure, 305
Synthetic opioids, 119

T

Tabes dorsalis, 569
Temporal lobe epilepsy, 798–800
Tests combinations *versus* brain area, 378
Tethered cord syndrome (TCS)
anatomy, 540
anesthesia, 560
BCR, 556, 557
definition, 540
diagnosis, 541
electromyography
fEMG, 548–550
tEMG, 550, 551, 553
Hoffmann reflex, 558, 559
IONM, 547
lower limb SSEPs, 555, 556
motor evoked potential, 554, 555
multimodal protocols, 547, 548
neurosurgeon
clinical evaluation, 542
closed spinal dysraphism, 545
occult spinal dysraphism, 545
open spinal dysraphism, 544, 545
prenatal evaluation, 542, 543
spinal cord retethering, 545–547
surgical treatment, fetal stage, 543, 544
pSSEP, 556
Thoracic aortic and thoracoabdominal aortic aneurysms
historical rates, 662
patient history, 693, 694, 697–699, 701
SCI and stroke
ACP, 670
BCR, 685–687
CPB, 669, 670
critical changes, 689, 690
differentiation, 687–689
EEG, 677–679
hypothermia, 668, 669
intercostal and segmental arteries, 671–674
LHB, 670
lumbar drain, 671
paraplegia, 667
pharmacologic, 671
RCP, 670
regional spinal cord blood flow and evoked potentials, 674–677
risk factors, 666, 667
SSEPs, 679, 680
stimulation and recording protocols, 690–693
TcMEPs, 680–684
TEVAR, 666
vascular anatomy, 663–665
Thoracic endovascular aortic repair (TEVAR), 666
Thoracic vertebra, 476
Thyroid surgeries
CB-MEP, 770
CVNM, 767
EMG-fr and EMG-st, 765, 766
HM Catalunya Hospital, Barcelona, 769–772
LAR, 767, 768
RLN, 765
TongardR Healthnology, 517
Tonic discharge, 731
Total intravenous anesthesia (TIVA), 118, 119, 464
Transcranial motor-evoked potential (Tc-MEP), 736
Transpedicular neurophysiologic navigation, 480–482

Trigeminal Neuralgia, 432
Triggered EMG, 550, 551, 553

U
Uncinate fasciculus (UF), 320, 375
Upper motor neurons (UNM), 182
Urologic surgeries, 856–860

V
Vagus nerve, 750–752
Vagus nerve stimulation (VNS), 752, 774
Ventral intermediate nucleus, 829, 830
Verbal naming (VN), 363, 364
Verst-Maldaun-Language Assessment (VMLA), 333
  VMLA-ON, 360
Vestibulocochlear nerve, 749
Visual evoked potential (VEP)
  anesthesia and systemic factors, 159, 160
  definition, 144
  flash-light stimulation, 144
  intraoperative techniques
    asleep techniques, 146, 148–150
    bipolar and monopolar stimulation, 155, 158
    bipolar stimulation parameters, 154
    clinical evaluation and tractography images analysis, 159
    direct electrical stimulation (DES), 155, 156
    double picture naming task (DPNT), 157
    dual stimulation technique, 154
    interpretation and warning signs, 151–153
    monopolar electrode, 154
    registration, 150, 151
    subcortical-cortical evoked potentials, 154
    tractography, 159
    VMLA-semantic, stroop test, 156
  tumor resection, 144
  visual pathways, 145–148
Visual tasks
  line bisection test, 371
  target cancellation task, 371
  visual field and reading, 369, 370
  visuospatial function, 371
Visual word form area (VWFA), 376

W
Wernicke-Geschwind language model, 303, 304
White cord syndrome, 533, 534
Working memory (WM), 368
Writing & drawing, 372
Writing dysfunction vs. site, 372

GPSR Compliance

The European Union's (EU) General Product Safety Regulation (GPSR) is a set of rules that requires consumer products to be safe and our obligations to ensure this.

If you have any concerns about our products, you can contact us on ProductSafety@springernature.com

In case Publisher is established outside the EU, the EU authorized representative is:

Springer Nature Customer Service Center GmbH
Europaplatz 3
69115 Heidelberg, Germany

Batch number: 10732057

Printed by Printforce, the Netherlands